History of Medicine
for
the first and second year medical student

William J. Keller, Ph.D.

Printed in the United States of America.
Printed on recycled, acid-free paper.

First printing, December 2019.
Second printing, September 2020.
Third printing, January 2021.

Library of Congress Control Number: 2019917402.

ISBN 978-1-7340308-0-8 (paperback).
ISBN 978-1-7340308-1-5 (hardcover).

Publisher's Cataloging-in-Publication Data.

Names: Keller, William J., 1954- author.
Title: History of medicine : for the first and second year medical student / William J. Keller, PhD.
Description: Johns Island, SC : William J. Keller, 2019. | Includes bibliographical references and index.
Identifiers: LCCN 2019917402 (print) | ISBN 978-1-7340308-0-8 (paperback) | ISBN 978-1-7340308-1-5 (hardcover)
Subjects: LCSH: Medicine--History. | Medicine, Ancient. | Medical sciences. | Medicine--Study and teaching. | BISAC: MEDICAL / History. | MEDICAL / Education & Training.
Classification: LCC R131 .K45 2019 (print) | LCC R131 (ebook) | DDC 610.9--dc23.

Website: historyofmedicinebook.com.
The author request all comments and inquires be emailed to:
    historyofmedicinebook@gmail.com.

Table of Contents

Preface

The purpose of this book is to provide medical students and others interested in the history of medicine, a well referenced, readable resource, which succinctly describes the evolution of medical knowledge from 3500 BC to present day. This book offers an opportunity to systematically follow in chronological order, major discoveries, major events, influential people, and institutions most responsible for moving medical knowledge forward or impeding its forward progress. The book is organized into 10 conventional disciplines, typically studied by medical students during their first two years of medical school; histology, anatomy, physiology, biochemistry, behavioral sciences, neurosciences, microbiology, immunology, pharmacology, and pathology. Given scientific and medical knowledge is dynamic and changes with time, this book offers an opportunity to understand the evolution of how and why we have come to our present state of scientific and medical knowledge. Additionally, this book dispels common myths and corrects much misinformation which has become a part of the general public's and many medical students' knowledge about the history of medicine.

Much effort has been committed to ensuring the accuracy of information contained in this book. I am solely responsible for the accuracy of all information. I used primary sources whenever available, located and read original articles of historical significance, had many articles translated from their original languages into English, and relied heavily upon electronic information available from scholarly sources, accessed from around the world by way of computer based electronic media. Considerable time and efforts were made to discover the true history, rather than rely upon secondary sources or others' synthesis of information. Many books currently available in the market, on the history of medicine, rely heavily upon secondary and tertiary sources. This book relies almost exclusively on original, primary sources and offers over 2,700 primary reference sources. The process of investigation, synthesis, and preparation of this manuscript was completed over a 15 year period, with much attention placed upon ensuring the highest of quality and scholarly standards.

As a medical student and future physician your time is in high demand. Select a chapter or chapters that are of the most interest to you. Begin there. Chapters have been written to stand alone. It is not necessary to read the entire book from beginning to end. Initially read the sections which hold the most interest for you. I image you will return frequently, using this book as a reference, to more fully understand the history of the materials you are learning in your medical school courses. When you have a brief moment of free time, randomly read a few paragraphs or pages. You might be surprised how much information you will retain over the course of a busy semester.

As a medical student, take this opportunity to think about how and why our medical knowledge is what it is today. Be open to new ideas. Be willing to challenge medical dogma. Be open to and willing to change your thinking in the presence of new information. Acknowledge facts change. Be willing to propose new, thoughtful, and innovative alternatives to existing knowledge and practices. Do not blindly accept or uncritically embrace medical dogma. Be willing to think independently and for yourself. Be willing to lead rather than follow. These are exciting times in medicine. I encourage you to embrace all of its experiences and opportunities. Do consider making a difference, now as a medical student and throughout your professional medical career, as a practicing physician. Knowing the history of medicine will make you a more knowledgeable physician and will allow you to more fully appreciate the efforts of those whom have come before you and those whom will come after you, as the history of medicine continues to be written.

WJK

Acknowledgments

A brief note of appreciation. Thank you to all of the medical and graduate students whom I have had the sincere pleasure to teach and learn from over the past 40 years. Thank you to all of the academic librarians around the world, whom have worked with me to locate original sources, translate documents, and contributed so much to ensuring the quality and accuracy of information contained in this volume. A special note of appreciation is due Prof. Jacalyn Duffin of Queen's University. She offered kind, thoughtful, encouragement to pursue my interest in the history of medicine when I was a young Assistant Professor of Medical Neurosciences, many, many, many years ago. Finally, thank you to my many professors and faculty colleagues, whom have encouraged and supported independent thought in academia and have braved the oftentimes unpleasant consequences of challenging scientific and medical dogma. Thank you all.

WJK

Chapter 1

Medical Histology

Definition.

Histology is "…the science concerned with the minute structure of cells, tissues, and organs in relation to their functions…" (1997)[1]. The term is derived from the Greek "histos" meaning tissue and "logos" meaning the study of a subject. The National Institutes of Health defines histology simply as "…the study of the structure, composition, and function of tissues…" (2010)[2]. As a medical student you might simply define histology as the microanatomy course you take during first semester medical school and which is designed to complement your gross anatomy course. Studying histology and gross anatomy provide you with the opportunity to examine, explore, and understand the same part of the body from two very different perspectives.

Introduction.

Independent of the definition(s) you choose, histology is a core, foundation course in the medical education of every medical student today and provides the basic knowledge necessary to begin to understand normal and abnormal biological tissues. For the moment, accepting Steadman's definition above (1997)[1], you will need at least three crucial elements to satisfy the definition: a collection of cells forming a tissue, tools necessary to study the collection of cells, and a matrix of knowledge in which to relate tissue structure to function.

This chapter explores the historical development of medical histology from its earliest beginnings in the ancient civilizations of Mesopotamia, Egypt, and Greece to its current state today, as practiced by modern Western medicine. Emphasis is placed upon the development of medical histology as a professional and scientific based discipline. Particular attention is devoted to developing an understanding of the fluid conceptual matrixes used across time and the factors which most influenced change. Influential people whom have shaped the discipline throughout history are briefly presented, along with milestone discoveries, which have led us to our current knowledge base, and the way we understand and practice medical histology today. The material is presented within a contextual matrix of other commonly recognized world events, whenever it makes sense, in order to provide a more global perspective from which to understand the people, events, and contributions. The chapter is organized chronologically for quick reference and consistency with other chapters.

History.

Histology has a relative short recorded history, spanning less than 400 years.

Early Records, 3500 BC - 500 BC.

There is very little recorded evidence of systematic or scientific study of micro-anatomical tissues, during this early period. Early records do reveal an interest and study of biological structures, with primary focus placed upon simply identifying regional internal and external gross anatomical structures. Casual observations are being made between the similarities and differences of human and animals gross anatomical structures and tissues. There is no evidence at this time, observations are being made at the cellular level.

Perhaps recently discovered Tablets, from the ancient civilization of Mesopotamia, now being translated by academics JoAnn Scurlock (1953-) and Burton Andersen (1932-), will yield information of the ancient civilizations' understanding of histology, in the same way the Tablets have revealed the Ancient's understanding of gross anatomy (2005)[3].

Evidence does suggest the Ancients are aware of magnification, perhaps viewing objects through droplets of water. It is not unreasonable to believe someone might have viewed human tissue through such a simple form of magnification, giving mankind its first glimpse of the structural foundation of life. Histology will have to wait until the early-1000s, for regular use of magnifying glasses in the Middle East and the mid-1600s for the regular use of magnifying glasses and early light microscopes in Western Europe, to systematically exam tissues, at the cellular level.

Antiquity, 500 BC - 500 AD.

The primary unit of scientific study during Antiquity is gross anatomical structure and not the micro-anatomical unit.

There is very little written evidence today any systematic or scientific observations of biological tissues at the micro-anatomical level occurs during Antiquity. Evidence does exist, indicating people did have knowledge of magnification and did use burning glasses for practical daily life. It is reasonable to believe someone did indeed inspect biological tissues under a magnifying glass, only to fail to record their observations, thereby losing the observations to time and history.

The written historical record reveals systematic study and substantial advances in gross anatomy flourish during this period. Dissection of humans are permitted and span from the opening of the first medical school by the Greek natural philosopher Alcmaeon of Croton circa 600 BC to the fall of the Roman Empire circa 475 AD. Significant contributions to the knowledge of gross anatomy are made by the Greeks e.g. Hippocrates, Aristotle, Herophilus, and Galen; however, none are known to have contributed to the study of micro-anatomy or worked consistently with the aid of magnification.

Antiquity is characterized by investigations and comparisons of gross anatomical structures. Systematic investigations of tissues, using magnification techniques, will not appear until 1021 AD. Even then examination by magnification is limited to gross tissues and the cellular world of tissues remains unknown.

Middle Ages (Medieval Times), 500 AD - 1400 AD.

There is very little evidence any systematic, micro-anatomical observations of biological tissues occurs in Western Europe during the Middle Ages. This is not surprising given the geo-political, social, and economic events occurring in Western Europe. Little emphasis and few resources are devoted to scientific discovery. This is a time for physical survival and daily existence, rather than pursuit of new intellectual knowledge. Much time and energy is devoted to war between neighboring countries. Intellectual investigation, philosophical reflection, and academic scholarship are displaced by simple, rote translation and rerecording of medical knowledge identified, developed, and carefully recorded by the Ancient civilizations.

Thousands of clay tablets and papyri, written in original languages e.g. Greek, are translated and recorded into Latin, the official and approved language of the newly organized Christian based religions of Western Europe. The great majority of these translations are funded by the Christian and Catholic Churches. Scientific and medical knowledge is frequently reinterpreted during translation to better fit within the matrix of organized religions' belief systems. Organized religions having the greatest influence at this time are Christianity, Catholicism, Judaism, and Islam. All organized religions contribute to modifying medical knowledge during translations to better fit with the teachings of their particular religious beliefs.

Medical knowledge has been in the past, is today, and will be in the future modified and oftentimes determined by external factors, which have nothing to do with scientific objectivity. Often funding sources determine what will be investigated, how it will be investigated, and what will constitute acceptable findings. Can you think of any other factors or influences which have affected the scientific and medical knowledge base from which we draw today, whenever we practice modern professional science or modern professional medicine? External factors influencing science and medicine today are similar in many ways to the external factors influencing science and medicine thousands of years ago. As medical students and future practicing physicians, it is important to be aware of these influences and how they have shaped and continue to shape the professional knowledge base.

OK… back to the Middle Ages and histology.

Relatively isolated from the events in Western Europe, in modern-day Iraq, significant advances are being made in optics, magnification, and a new methodological approach to studying the natural world. These advances and their application open a new window from which to study the natural world, including the human body. New tools and original thought provide the necessary means to advance scientific knowledge exponentially. As new discoveries are made, old knowledge and associated dogma begin to be reexamined by the scientific communities. New discoveries and new interpretation of old knowledge meet with much resistance from faith based organized religions.

Ibn al-Haytham (965 AD-1035 AD) Iraqi Muslim scientist, makes several substantial contributions, which prove to effect the course of science and histology for the next thousand years (1021AD/2007)[4]. Two contributions are most notable within our context here.

First, Ibn al-Haytham (translated into Latin as Alhazeni) is responsible for writing and compiling "The Book of Optics", circa 1021 AD. "The Book of Optics" is a seven volume collection of observations, experiments, results, and synthesis of information, following a process which will later be termed the scientific method. Volumes I, II, and III are devoted to the theory of vision, physiology of the eye, anatomy of the eye, and perception. Volumes IV, V, VI, and VII are devoted to traditional physical optics. This landmark collection of old and new knowledge remains a landmark in the advancement and collection of knowledge in the fields of optics and physics today. "The Book of Optics" provides the first written evidence of systematic investigations of magnification. The original text is written in Arabic, as "Kitab al Manazir" and is translated into Latin as "De Aspectibus", during the late-1100s and early-1200s by the Spanish. Subsequently, the Book is translated into Italian, as "Prospettiva" during the 1300s. All seven volumes are first published in type set print, in Germany, during the late-1500s (1572)[5]. Recent English translations of "The Book of Optics" are offered by Mark Smith (1021AD/2001,2006,2008,2010)[6,7,8,9].

Second, Ibn al-Haytham introduces a method of scientific thought and systematic investigation we collectively term today, the scientific method. The method follows a systematic hypothetico-deductive process and utilizes systematic, repeatable experiments as the preferred method, whenever investigating the natural world, including the human body. This epistemological approach stands in marked contrast to the authoritative, dogmatic approaches of organized religion which dominate Western Europe at this time.

The Middle Ages produce very few specific contributions to histology from Western Europe, hold the translations of the ancient civilizations' medical and scientific knowledge base into Latin. However, in the Middle East, exceptional contributions by Ibn al-Haytham, in areas of magnification and introduction of the scientific method, lay the foundation upon which histology will build, as a scientific based discipline, into present day modern histology.

Early Modern, 1400 AD - 1800 AD.

The Early Modern Period witness the early beginnings of modern histology with its roots anchored firmly in the mid-1600s. The Renaissance of Western Europe is well underway and a return to original discoveries and investigations into the natural sciences.

Robert Hooke (1635-1703), a non-physician, is one of the first modern historical figures associated with laying the foundation upon which the field of histology, as a science based discipline will build. An English microscopist, he coins the term "cell". His landmark publication "Micrographia: Or some physiological descriptions of minute bodies made by magnifying glasses, with observations and inquires there upon" provides one of the first publications which systematically evaluates microstructures, using magnification as its primary tool for observation (1665)[10]. "Micrographia" offers the medical community and public at large, the first publication which demonstrates the power of examining objects, biological and static, under the magnifying lens. His drawings of cork, plant cells, eye of a fly, louse, gnat, edge of a razor, point of a needle, and just about anything else you can think of impressively demonstrates the power of this tool for investigating and understanding biology in a new way.

Robert Hooke's application of magnification to the study of microstructure and microorganisms is unlike anything previously reported. He applies an existing technology in a new way and opens a new door, which allows us to view the living world in ways never considered before.

Marcello Malpighi (1628-1694) Italian anatomist, capitalizes upon recent improvements in the microscope and is credited with the first microscopic description of human tissues; describing microscopic structure of the renal glomeruli, pulmonary alveoli, capillaries, taste buds, blood, liver, brain, and skin (1661,1666,1666,1666)[11,12,13,14]. He is first to see red blood cells under a microscope and attributes the color of blood to these cells (1666)[15]. Marcello Malpighi's microscopic observations and descriptions stand in contrast with those of Robert Hooke. Marcello Malpighi describes tissues of internal organs, while Robert Hook focuses instead on plants, insects, and non-biological objects. Marcello Malpighi makes additional notable contributions in the area of embryology, using the microscope as the primary tool in describing the developmental growth of the chick embryo, inside the egg (1673)[16].

Antonie van Leeuwenhoek (1632-1721) Dutch textile inspector is recognized by most as making considerable contributions to the foundation of histology and microbiology through his refinement in the microscope and high quality lenses. He is credited with being the first to observe and report single cell organisms, which he terms animalcules (modern-day microorganisms). He is credited with the first microscopic observations of muscle fibers, spermatozoa, bacteria, and the flow of blood through capillaries.

His major contributions are in the refinement of the microscope, as a tool for systematic study of tissues. Van Leeuwenhoek develops a simple and rapid glass technique which permits the rapid production of lenses capable of magnification on the order of 300x. Seven of van Leeuwenhoek microscopes are known to exist today and are housed in the Utrecht University Museum, Netherlands and Deutsches Museum in Munich (1981)[17].

Antonie van Leeuwenhoek is not a physician or scientist by education or training, rather a Dutch textile inspector and owner of a very successful drapery business in Amsterdam. His interest in developing magnifying lenses stems not from an interest in science or medicine, rather from a need to better inspect cloth. Through an intermediary, Dutch physician Regnerus de Graaf (1641-1673), Antonie van Leeuwenhoek submits his microscopic observations to the Royal Society of London for the Improvement of Natural Knowledge (England's Academy of Science) (1673)[18].

Van Leeuwenhoek's microscopic observations are first met with enthusiasm from the Society in 1673. However, enthusiasm quickly sours when he submits his microscopic observations of single celled organisms, in a letter to the Society dated October 1676 (1677)[19]. The submissions so disturb the Society's dogma on life itself and given single cell organisms are entirely unknown at the time, the Society challenges van Leeuwenhoek's submission, questions his credibility, and dispatches a review committee to observe van Leeuwenhoek to determine if indeed his observations and mind are sound. The Society in 1680 determines he and his observations are indeed sound and begin the process of reevaluating the scientific basis of life itself. Given the new information, the Church soon begins to reevaluate its long held position on spontaneous generation.

While van Leeuwenhoek contributes to the foundation of histology and science with his lenses used in the microscope, progress might have been more rapid had he disclosed his technique for producing the lenses. Records report he is fearful of others stealing his technique and believes he never receives his rightful recognition, by the scientific and medical communities. He keeps his secrets of how he makes his lenses and they are lost to the scientific and medical communities with his death. No one can reproduce the lenses or untangle the production technique for over three centuries. During the 1950s, Clair Stong, an amateur scientist and Westinghouse electrical engineer, unravels the secrets and replicates the lens production techniques used by Antonie van Leeuwenhoek. The secret lies in fusing thin glass threads rather than polishing. Utilizing the glass thread fusing technique to create a lens, Clair Stong successfully creates several lenses, and successfully produces working van Leeuwenhoek design microscopes (1952)[20].

Van Leeuwenhoek never publishes his works, however his original papers and correspondences to the Royal Society have recently been examined by Brian Ford (1939-) independent research biologist (1981)[21]. Van Leeuwenhoek's papers and letters have remained relatively undisturbed in the Society's vaults for over three centuries. As the papers are translated, more information is becoming available as to van Leeuwenhoek's contributions in the area of magnification, the application of magnification to the study of biological tissues, the impact both professional and cultural whenever scientific dogma is challenged, and realities of potentially justified reservations in sharing knowledge with the scientific and medical communities.

Marie Francois Xavier Bichat (1771-1802) French histologist is credited with the first systematic investigation of tissues, using tissues as the primary unit of study. He is one of the many fathers of histology. Marie Bichat introduces the term "tissue" into the scientific literature, from the French word "tissue", meaning woven materials. Bichat relies upon systematic, detailed dissections of tissues as his primary source of information and seldom uses the microscope. Using only hand lenses he identifies 21 tissues e.g. glandular, fibrous, mucus. He offers his belief the body is made of different tissues and these tissues can be isolated, studied, and affected by disease processes.

The approach of studying tissues, rather than the entire organism, sets Bichat apart from others around him. He encourages doctors to perform frequent autopsies, in order to better understand the relationship between disease and changes in tissues. Marie Bichat offers the scientific and medical communities the first substantive publications in the field of histology, "Traite des membranes en general et de diverses membranes en particulier" (1800)[22] and "Anatomie Generale" (1801)[23].

In brief summary, the Early Modern period witness the laying of the early foundations for modern histology. Robert Hook offers the first observations of cells under the microscope and his seminal publication "Micrographia". Marcello Malpighi offers his first reports of the microscopic observations of the renal glomeruli, pulmonary alveoli, capillaries, brain, and other internal human organ tissues. He offers the first microscopic description of sequential embryotic growth and development. Antonie van Leeuwenhoek improves the lenses used in microscopy and creates the technology to image objects and single cell organisms at 300x magnification. He reports his observations of the existence of single cell organisms and forces professional science and medicine to reevaluate dogma, which has remained in place for the past 1,500 years. Marie Bichat proposes the systematic investigation of biological tissues, using tissues as the primary unit of study, and offers the first substantive publications in the new scientific based discipline that will later be termed Histology.

The foundation for histology is now in place. Conceptually, investigators are beginning to think about microscopic organisms, the cell matrix structures of biological tissues, and how body tissues change with pathologies. The developing discipline now has the necessary technology to move the discipline forward and to systematically study the body at a new level of analysis, the cell.

Middle Modern, 1800 AD - 1900 AD.

The Middle Modern period of the 1800s witness an explosion of new knowledge and advances in the field of histology. Significant advances are being made in magnification, offering considerable improvements in the microscope. Fixation and staining techniques are introduced and refined. New and improved microtomes provide the necessarily thin tissue samples for study with the light microscope, opening a new and yet unexplored world to scientific discovery and investigation.

Many, but not all scientists of the period, are skeptical of the microscope, holding it in contempt and thinking it to be detrimental to the progress of biology. Microscopic anatomy is viewed by several respected scientists as "…pure fancy…", "…star gazing…", and "…celestial anatomy…" (1984)[24].

The new discipline is named "Histology" by German anatomist August Mayer (1787-1868) (1819)[25]. The term is derived from the Greek words "histo" meaning woven material and "logos" meaning study. Histology soon becomes an accepted scientific discipline, quickly produces new scientific knowledge, and necessitates a complete re-evaluation of scientific, medical, and religious dogma.

Thomas Hodgkin (1798-1866) British pathologist and Joseph Lister (1786-1869) London wine merchant, amateur microscopic enthusiast, and father of his more famous son Joseph Lister (1827-1912) (of antiseptic theory fame), offer a landmark paper, applying microscopic technology to observe and then report erythrocytes have no nuclei (1827)[26]. In the same paper, Thomas Hodgkin and Joseph Lister report their observations of striations in skeletal (striated) muscles (1827)[26]. Their report of no nuclei in mature RBCs presents information at great odds with current dogma and observations made over the previous two hundred years. The scientific community simply rejects their findings and attributes their inability to find a nucleus, in the mature red blood cell (RBC), as the result of limits in microscopic resolution. Only later and with much resistance will Thomas Hodgkin and Joseph Lister's findings be accepted by the scientific and medical communities.

Joseph Lister (the father) solves a major problem restricting the resolution of microscopic imaging. The problem is light bends at different angles, depending upon where light hit a lens, thereby distorting and blurring the viewed image (spherical aberration). Similarly wavelengths of different colors refract to differing degrees, resulting in halos of colors around different parts of a viewed image (chromatic aberration). Joseph Lister is first to describe and report a corrected optical system for the compound microscope, which successfully corrects for both spherical and chromatic aberrations (1830)[27]. Solving this problem, eliminates a major technological problem limiting microscopic observations for the previous two hundred years.

Johannes Evangelista Purkinje (1787-1869) Czech Republic anatomist, identifies several specialized, microscopic structural and functional components within tissues, including the sweat glands of the skin (1833)[28]; the inhibitory neuronal cell layer located in the cerebellar cortex, termed the Purkinje cell layer (1837)[29]; and the specialized cardiac muscle tissue which conducts electricity from the AV node to the ventricles of the heart, the Purkinje fibers (1839)[30]. Additionally, he introduces the term "protoplasm" into the scientific literature, for the substance found inside of cells (1839,1840)[31,32].

A brief side note about Purkinje; in 1823 he publishes his first observations on fingerprints. The paper describes and illustrates nine distinct fingerprint patterns which have become the basis of fingerprint classification system used today, 195 years after Joseph Purkinje first describes the basic fingerprint patterns (1823)[33].

Johannes Muller (1801-1858) German physiologist and comparative anatomist, contributes to histology in his advocacy of a specific epistemological approach. He advocates a systematic approach, utilizing close observation and pattern identification of biological tissues. This investigative approach stands in contrast to the empty theorizing and blind empiricism, employed by many of his colleagues. Johannes Muller's approach influences many of his students e.g. Jakob Henle, Rudolf Virchow, and Theodore Schwann. Perhaps you recognize these names and associate major contributions with each one.

Just as Johannes Muller influenced his students, your medical school professors are influencing you, contributing to how you think about medicine, and how you will practice medicine when you become a practicing physician. It is OK to let them know someday how much they influenced you. Sometimes it takes years before you realize it. Drop them a note or email and say thank you.

Perhaps you recognize a more concrete contribution made by Johannes Muller. He introduces the Mullerian duct. Remember from embryology, this structure develops into the Fallopian tubes in females and disappears in males (1830)[34].

Friedrich Gustav Jakob Henle (1809-1885) German anatomist, pathologist, and student prosector for Johannes Muller, makes multiple and substantial contributions to histology. Jakob Henle describes, details, and draws the renal loops, human epithelia, and lymphatic system. His book "General Anatomy", published in 1841 discusses general histology and presents a classification system of tissues still used today (1841)[35]. This 1,043 page book represents the first comprehensive treatment of histology. It offers a revision of Marie Bichat's 21 tissue classification system and places tissues into the four main tissues categories recognized today; epithelial, connective, muscular, and nervous (1841)[35].

While Henle is most often remembered by medical students for his renal Loops, he makes additional and significant contributions. For example, he is first to report and understand disease tissues are a modification of normal tissues. He co-founds a theory which states microorganisms are the causative factor producing disease (1840)[36]. Along with his student Robert Koch, they formulated the Henle-Koch postulates. The Henle-Koch postulates are still used today and establish four criteria to establish a causal relationship between a suspected microorganism and a specific disease. See the Pathology chapter of this book for a more complete discussion of the Henle-Koch postulates.

Rudolf Virchow (1821-1902) German pathologist, focuses his attention on the pathologies of cells. In particular he makes several notable contributions to the way the profession thinks about diseases of organs and tissues. He challenges the dogma of the day regarding the origin of disease and argues disease is the resultant consequence of disordered cells and cellular processes. He offers an early description of leukemia cells and is among the first to report a case of leukemia in the professional literature (1845)[37]. One year later, he challenges current dogma which states most diseases are caused by inflammation of veins (phlebitis) and proposes many of these disease conditions actually result from clots of blood inside of blood vessels (thrombosis) and portions of the thrombus can dislodge and move through blood vessels and lodge in smaller vessels (emboli) resulting in infarction of tissues (1846a,1846b)[38,39]. It is in these publications he first introduces the terms "thrombosis" and "emboli" into the professional medical literature (1846a,1846b)[38,39]. The terms are still used in medicine today, over 172 years since they are first introduced into the literature.

Rudolf Virchow plays an important role in moving histology forward, as a developing and maturing scientific discipline, by co-founding a new journal, devoted specifically to the advancement of the union between histology, pathology, physiology, and clinical medicine. The new journal, "Archi fur Pathologische Anatomie und Physiologie und fur Klinische Medizin" [Archives of Pathological Anatomy and Physiology, and of Clinical Medicine] offers its first issue in 1846. The journal quickly becomes one of the most prominent journals of the period. Rudolf Virchow takes over sole editorial duties for the journal, after his co-founder's death (Heinrich Reinhardt (1819-1852)) in 1852. The journal soon becomes known simply as "Virchow's Archives". The journal, now titled "Virchow's Archives: The European Journal of Pathology", continues publication today, now 172 years since its first issues, as a highly respected, peer reviewed, monthly medical journal, focusing upon all aspects of human pathology, especially at the cellular level.

Note: Rudolf Virchow originally founded the journal having become dissatisfied with editors of established journals rejecting his submissions for publication. Many new journals throughout the history of medicine are founded upon similar grounds.

Additional contributions to histology are made by Rudolf Virchow in his development and experimental investigations of the relatively new and revolutionary Cell theory, originally proposed by Polish embryologist and histologist Robert Remak (1815-1865). In brief, Robert Remak's theory states the origin of cells is the result of the division of pre-existing cells (1852)[40]. This revolutionary conceptualization directly challenges medical dogma and opens a new line of investigations. Rudolf Virchow openly plagiarizes much of Robert Remak's work on the origin of cells and attributes the originality of the work to himself (1860)[41]. So goes another example in the history of medicine of one professional claiming priority for discovery or creative new ideas of another. See the Pathology chapter of this book for details and a discussion of this issue, as it relates to Rudolf Virchow.

Theodor Schwann (1810-1882) German physiologist and student of Johannes Muller is most recognized by medical students today as the person responsible for identifying the myelin producing Schwann cells, which surround peripheral nervous system neurons (1839)[42]. Perhaps of greater importance and unknown to many medical students is he makes at least three, equally if not more significant contributions to histology.

First, he and Matthias Schleiden (1804-1881) revolutionize the field of biology when they present their Cell theory (1839,1847)[43,44]. Cell theory, in brief states the cell is the basic unit of structure for all living things; all living things are composed of cells; and all new cells are produced from pre-existing cells. Secondly, Schwann openly challenges the dogma of spontaneous generation and provides a series of microscopic observations in support of his position. Third, Schwann challenges his mentor Johannes Muller and breaks with scientific and religious dogma and the doctrine of Vitalism.

Vitalism, in brief states the functions of living organisms are the result of vital principles distinct from biochemical reactions; the processes of life are not explicable by laws of physics and chemistry alone; and that life is in some part self-determined. Schwann's challenge of this doctrine necessitates a reexamination of medical, scientific, and religious beliefs. Prior to Schwann's challenge, disease and illness are conceptualized within the matrix of an imbalance in the vital energies, whether these vital energies are defined as four humors (Hippocrates), four temperaments (Galen), qi and prana (Eastern religion), or the soul (Christian religion). Today, and consistent with Schwann's early conceptualizations, disease and illness are conceptualized within the matrix of physical and biochemical disturbances in otherwise healthy tissues.

Theodor Schwann devotes much of his life examining the functional relationships between microscopic structure, function, and the physical-chemical bases of life. Schwann coins the term "metabolism" to define the chemical changes which occur inside of cells. Albert von Kolliker (1817-1905) Swiss anatomist and physiologist writes of Schwann, in "A Manual of Human Microscopic Anatomy", "…if Bichat founded histology more theoretically by laying down and consistent working out a system, Schwann has, by his investigations established it on facts…" (1860, p.2)[45].

Trivia: Theodor Schwann's dissertation, "De necessitate æris atmosphærici ad evolutionem pulli in ovo incubato", written in partial fulfillment of the academic requirements for his doctorate degree, addresses breathing inside of a hen's egg and demonstrates air is necessary for the development of the embryo (1834)[46].

Robert Remak (1815-1865) Polish histologist, embryologist, and also a student of Johannes Muller, makes his major contributions to histology by publishing his revolutionary discovery, the origin of new cells is from the division of pre-existing cells (1852)[47]. His proposal of this new conceptualization as to the origin cells so challenges established medical and scientific dogma his work is simply rejected by the scientific and medical communities. It will be decades later before this revolutionary idea begins to receive acceptance from the established scientific and medical communities. Advancements in microscopy and the works by Theodor Schwann and others provide the scientific based evidence to support Robert Remak's proposed origin of cells and revolutionizes the long standing doctrine of spontaneous generation of cells, held by the scientific, medical, and religious communities.

Robert Remak is responsible for several firsts. He uses the relatively new microscopic technology to identify the location of neuronal cell bodies of peripheral motor nerves to be the spinal cord of the central nervous system (1838)[48]. He identifies and describes neurofibrils, the intra-cellular structure which provide the cytoskeletal structure to neurons (1838)[48]. He additionally identifies and describes the six layer cytoarchitectural structure of the cerebral cortex recognized today. Robert Remak, an oftentimes unrecognized name in medical history, is responsible for the classification of embryological tissues into the three categories we use today ectoderm, mesoderm, and endoderm (1850)[49].

Rudolph Albert von Kolliker (1817-1905) Swiss histologist, makes many contributions to the new and developing discipline of histology. He is first to describe in detail, smooth muscle and striated muscle, and recognize they are made up of different assemblies of nucleated cells (1849)[50]. He is first to describe the muscles of the arterial walls and recognize nerve fibers are continuous with their nerve cell bodies (1862-63)[51]. His microscopic observations of the nervous systems tissues, in combination with those of Robert Remak, lay the foundation for correctly understanding the central and peripheral nervous systems.

Perhaps his best known publication, the two volume set "A Manual of Human Histology" provides an up to date compellation of scientific studies, in an integrated format, and includes thoughtful discussions of the burgeoning field of microscopic anatomy (1853,1854)[52]. This two volume publication discusses the development of histology, where the field has been, where it is today in the mid-1800s, and where it should go in the future. The publication encourages students and practitioners to focus not on structure alone and to extend observations and thought to the study of normal and abnormal chemical processes of tissues.

The first half of the century makes much progress in laying the foundation of histology. The discipline places an emphasis on microscopic, scientific based descriptions of the structures of biological tissues. Technical developments contribute to the advancement of histology as a science and with increasing relevance to the practicing medical clinician. For example, the familiar 3x1 inch glass microscope slide is standardized in 1839 by the Microscopical Society of London and commercial glass cover slips first appear courtesy of Chance Brothers of Birmingham in 1840. These simple technological advancements provide histology new and sharper tools to investigate the microanatomy of biological tissues. The ability to view and systematically study the cell provides the scientific data in support of the newly proposed Cell theory. Technological advancements, often simple, coupled with thoughtful conceptualization and independent synthesis of the current knowledge base, as in this case, revolutionize medical and scientific dogma and help establish histology as a legitimate scientific discipline.

By mid-1800s, calls are made from the leaders in the field to move beyond description of structure and to investigate aggressively the chemical and metabolic property of living tissues.

The second half of the century responds to the calls from pioneer leaders in histology. Developments in technology offer the necessary equipment to study cells and tissues in much greater detail. The microscope, a primary tool of histology continues to improve while offering greater resolution powers and solutions to distorted imaging. Refinement of the microtome permits thinner slices of tissues, more suitable for the light microscope. Tissue fixation is introduced and innovative staining techniques improve significantly, allowing for sharing of stable tissue samples between multiple investigators and identification of cellular structures previously never seen. Histology, incorporates investigations into the chemical and metabolic properties of tissues and cells as part of the identified areas of investigation, for this relatively new discipline.

In order to fully appreciate the history of histology, one must appreciate not only the people who made significant contributions but also appreciate the tools of the discipline. Several and significant advances in histology, during the second half of the 1800s are directly related to the improvement in the tools used by the profession. These tools provide the necessary technology, which will help to challenge and revolutionize the medical and scientific dogma, held firmly for over a thousand years.

One such technological advance made during the second half the 1800s is the introduction of fixation. The chemical process by which fresh biological tissues are preserved from decay, insuring preservation for extended periods of time. This development eliminates the need to immediately examine biological tissues freshly harvested. Fixation additionally permits the same tissues sample to be shared between scientists. A few tissue samples fixed during the 1700s and many more from the 1800s survive today (1977)[53].

Formalin, introduced as a fixative, substantially improves the process of preserving biological tissues (1893,1893,1894)[54,55,56]. Formalin allows tissues to better retain their original biological form and extends the time a sample can be examined. Formalin remains a popular fixative today, over 125 years after it is first serendipitously discovered and introduced by German physician Ferdinand Blum (1865-1959), while studying the potential use of water diluted solutions of formaldehyde as a potential bactericide, for Bacillus antracis, B. typhi, Staphylococcus aureus, and Proteus species. (1893,1893,1894)[57,54,56].

Important developments in technology of histology include advancements in the precision cutting capabilities of the microtome. Early in the 1800s biological tissues are sliced thinly by hand with a razor, and sandwiched between slides for inspection under the light microscope. Unfortunately, the tissues decay relatively quickly and the hand razor technique fail to generate sufficiently thin slices to maximize the capabilities of the microscope of the period. An improved microtome begins to solve this problem (1839,1979)[58,59].

Early forms of the microtome, termed cutting machines, were available for slicing tissues as early as 1770. The first useful microtome was introduced by English optician, instrument and globe maker George Adams, Jr. (1750-1795) and improved 28 years later in 1798, by Scottish watchmaker Alexander Cummings (1733-1814) and professional mica slide-maker Robert Custance (1740-1799). However, it is not until Johannes Purkinje's medical student, Gabriel Valentin (1810-1883) introduces the Valentin knife, that true advances are made in the preparation of biological tissues suitable for the light microscope (1839)[58]. The Valentin knife is a double blade razor with a slice adjuster. According to French biologist Charles Chevalier, it proves to be one of the first truly useful tools, capable of reliably producing sufficiently uniform thin tissue sections, for use with the light microscope. Chevalier coins the term "microtome", from the Greek "mikro" meaning small and "tome" meaning slice (1839)[58].

The modern rotary microtome is introduced circa 1885 with major improvements to the instrument having been made by Horace Darwin (1851-1928), Charles Darwin's son. The rotary microtome contributes significantly to the advancement of histology, providing a much needed tool. Popularity of the rotary microtome contributes to the founding and financial success of the Cambridge Scientific Instrument Company, the scientific instrument company founded by Horace Darwin in 1891 to meet the increase demand for the new microtome. The Company manufactures highly prized microtomes well into the 1970s (sic).

Staining techniques also make significant advances and contributions to histology, during the last half of the 1800s. In that biological tissues have little inherent contrast, staining provides a technique to highlight not only the cell itself but structures and materials inside of the cell.

Several of the stains introduced during the 1800s are still being used today in varying forms. For example, German anatomist Heinrich Wilhelm von Waldeyer-Hartz (1836-1922) introduces his "hematoxylin stain" used in staining DNA and RNA (1863)[60]; Italian neuroscientist Camillo Golgi (1843-1926) introduces his "la reazione nera" black reaction, silver nitrate stain, allowing to view the entire microanatomy of neurons (1873)[61]; German chemist A. Wissowzky introduces his hematoxylin and eosin "H&E stain" (1876)[62]; German bacteriologists Franz Ziehl (1859-1926) and Friedrich Neelsen (1854-1898) introduce their "acid-fast stain" used to identify bacteria responsible for tuberculosis (1882,1883)[63,64]; Danish bacteriologist Christian Gram (1853-1938) introduces his stain for bacterial cell walls (Gram stain) (1884a,1884b)[65,66]; Italian L. Daddi introduces his "Sudan III stain" for lipids (1896)[67]; and German pathologist Karl Weigert (1845-1904) introduces his stain for visualizing elastin (Weigert stain) (1898)[68].

These new staining techniques make previously poorly visible tissues now visible, for segregation from other tissues and making components within tissues now visible for detail study. The contributions of stains and staining techniques cannot be overstated in their roles in contributing to the advancement of histology as a scientific discipline. Contributions of the 1800s to development of methods and technologies outweigh most all other contributions to histology during this period.

Trivia: Hematoxylin is derived from the extract of the heartwood of the Haematoxylum campechianum tree. The tree is native to Mexico and Central America. Its dyeing properties are well known in Central America, long before it is brought to Western Europe by Spanish explorers, soon after the "discovery" of the Americas. Hematoxylin is first used in Western Europe to dye fabrics and first used in microscopy during the 1840s (1958)[69].

Heinrich Wilhelm von Waldeyer-Hartz (1836-1922) German anatomist introduces the hematoxylin stain and uses this dye to make landmark observations which guide the direction of histology. Combining microscopic observation and his newly developed stain, he is able to study the intra-nuclear filaments of chromatin, which later will be recognized as essential elements involved in cell division. Heinrich Wilhelm von Waldeyer-Hartz introduces the term "chromosome" (colored bodies) into the scientific literature to describe these structures which absorb the new stain (1888)[70].

Building upon the works of Camillo Golgi and Santiago Ramon y Cajal, Heinrich Wilhelm Waldeyer-Hartz uses new stains to clearly visualize the primary structural components of the neuron e.g. cell body, dendrites, axons, as well as visualize the synapse between neurons. He is among the first to describe the neuron as a self- contained, discrete anatomical unit. His observations coupled with thoughtful analysis and synthesis of recent advances in histology result in the proposal of his revolutionary theory, termed the "Neuron doctrine" (1891)[71].

The Neuron doctrine, in brief simply states the neuron is the primary structural and functional unit of the nervous system and communication occurs between neurons across a small synaptic space. In the same year, Wilhelm Waldeyer-Hartz introduces the term "neuron", derived from the Greek meaning "wire", into the scientific and medical literature (1891)[71]. Wilhelm Waldeyer-Hartz provides histology a foundation upon which the field would quickly build over the next one hundred years.

Camillo Golgi (1843-1926) Italian physician and scientist is most remembered for his original contributions in developing silver impregnation methods "the black reaction", used primarily for the staining and study of neural tissues. His silver staining techniques reveal for the first time the entire neuron, including the cell body, axon, and dendritic processes. While most medical students will recognize him for his work in identifying the intracellular organelle the Golgi apparatus (1886)[72], he also discovers the sensory receptor in tendons (1880)[73], and is first to report the unique anatomy of the distal convoluted tubules of the kidney and attachment to the afferent arterials of the glomerulus (1889)[74].

Perhaps one of Camillo Golgi's most unrecognized contributions is his systematic study of malaria. He is responsible for detailing the life cycle of the plasmodium falciparum and relating the timing of fevers to the life cycle of the parasite (1892)[75].

Santiago Ramón y Cajal (1852-1934) Spanish histologist applies the metal staining techniques introduced by Golgi to the microscopic study of brain tissues and provides details on the structure and connectively of neural structures. As an exceptionally talented artist, Cajal makes exquisite detailed drawings of his observations of neural structures. Many are reproduced for educational purposes. You are likely to find an example of his drawings in your neuroscience textbook today.

Santiago Ramon y Cajal's detailed observations provide scientific evidence which requires reexamination of the medical dogma of the period. Prior to Santiago Ramon y Cajal's observations, medical and scientific dogma holds the central nervous system is comprised of a single continuous anatomical structure, composed of contiguous cells fused together, and forming a massive mesh (reticular) network. The network functions as a collective singular structure. This is the Reticular theory, proposed by German anatomist Joseph von Gerlach (1820-1896) and serves as the predominant anatomical model from which to understand the anatomy of the central nervous system, between 1871 and 1891 (1872)[76]. The Reticular anatomical model is replaced by Wilhelm Waldeyer-Hartz's newly proposed Neuron doctrine (1891)[77]. The Neuron doctrine holds the central nervous system is composed of discrete cells, which communicate with each other across synaptic junctions between cells.

Santiago Ramon y Cajal shares the 1906 Nobel Prize in Physiology or Medicine with Camillo Golgi. Santiago Ramon y Cajal is recognized for his interpretation of the histological evidence supporting the Neuron doctrine and Camillo Golgi's is recognized for his innovative staining techniques which make Cajal's observations possible (1906)[78]. Santiago Ramon y Cajal is an ardent proponent of the Neuron doctrine, while Camillo Golgi is an equally ardent proponent of the Reticular doctrine. The two men never persuade the other to change their respective positions, in regard to the organizational structure of the nervous system. Both men use the same tools, methods, and view essentially the same histological specimens. So goes a scientist's commitment to one's own theoretical matrix, whenever interpreting objective findings.

Trivia: Joseph von Gerlach, originator of the Reticular theory, is among the first to apply photomicrography to medical research. He publishes "Die photographie als hilsmittel microskopischer forschung" [Photography as a tool in microscopic science] and discusses the practical applications of microphotography to the study of medicine (1863)[79].

Investigators from Europe lead the rapid advances being made in the discipline of medical histology during the 1800s. Oftentimes lost in the many European contributions is a single American professor, Edmund Peaslee.

Edmund Peaslee (1814-1878) American Professor of Anatomy at Dartmouth College, Professor of Pathology and Physiology at the New York Medical College and Professor of Surgeries at the Medical School of Maine, offers the first systematic and comprehensive book in the English language on human histology (1857)[80]. The book provides an organized collection of histology knowledge to date and advocates histology move from simple observation and description of tissues to focus more on the associated physiology of tissue structure and relevance to disease processes.

Wilhelm His, Sr. (1831-1904) Swiss anatomy professor is usually not recognized by medical students and perhaps confused with his son Wilhelm His, Jr. (1863-1934) cardiologist who discovers the specialized tissues in the heart, which help synchronize its contractions (Bundle of His). Wilhelm His, Sr., however makes significant contributions in histology through his contributions in fixation, microtome development, recognizing axons have free endings, recognizing axonal growth during embryological development, recognizing the numerous neuritic outgrowths from the neuronal cell body, and introducing the term "dendrite", from the Greek meaning tree, into the scientific and medical literature, and finally his contribution of a brief 34 page book printed in 1865, "Die Haute und Hohlen des Korpers", in which he first introduces the term "endothelium" and offers observations of endothelial tissue (1865)[81].

Julius Cohnheim (1839-1884) German pathologist, one of Rudolf Virchow's students, and perhaps one of the most under recognized figures in medicine, is first to report his observation of movement of white blood cells from systemic vascular circulation into surrounding infected tissues (1868)[82]. Although diapedesis had been theorized two decades earlier by William Addison (1802-1881), limits in microscope resolution and histology techniques prohibited visualization of the process until Julius Cohnheim's report in 1868 (1868)[82].

Louis Antoine Ranvier (1835-1922) one of the most prominent histologists of the second half of the 1800s is responsible for first identifying the gaps between the myelin producing Schwann cells, in the peripheral nervous systems, the nodes of Ranvier (1878)[83]. He provides the necessary anatomical evidence to understand propagation of neuronal signals down myelinated peripheral nerves (salutatory conduction). His work is presented in several publications of the period, yet none so comprehensively than the two volume set prepared by himself, Ernst Heinrich Weber (1795-1878) (Weber Test fame - lateralizing hearing deficits), and Ernst Weber's younger brother, Wilhelm Eduard Weber (1804-1891), "Lecons sur histologie de systeme nervoeus" [Lessons on the histology of the nervous system] (1878)[83].

Theodor Hermann Meynert (1833-1892) German anatomist frequently contributes to a more complete understanding of the cytoarchitectural organization of the cerebral cortex and other brain structures. He is an influential professor of two of his most recognizable students Sigmund Freud and Carl Wernicke. Theodor Meynert devotes much of his professional life to establishing psychiatry as a science and studying the relationship between brain and mental processes. Much of the evidence appears in several publications and is summarized in his 1884 textbook titled "Psychiatrie: Klinik der Erkrankungen des Vorderhirns" [Psychiatry: Clinic on the Diseases of the Forebrain] (1884)[84]. Theodor Meynert is perhaps most remembered today by medical students for the Nucleus Basalis of Meynert, located in the brain's frontal lobes and whose degeneration is closely associated with dementia of the Alzheimer's type (1982)[85].

Salomon Stricker (1834-1898) Austrian histologist builds upon the works of William Addison and Julius Cohnheim and makes significant contributions in the study of leukocyte diapedesis, contractility of vascular walls, cell division, and the extracellular matrix. Among his many original contributions, perhaps his most important contribution is his ability to bring together large amounts of information and then make the information available to the scientific and medical communities at large. He edits several comprehensive histology textbooks and provides much needed English translations. Salomon Stricker edits "A Manual of Histology" and draws together some of the most influential histologists of the time. Each contributor offers a chapter in their respective areas of interests e.g. Salomon Stricker (general methods of investigation; general characteristics of the cell; development of the cell), Theodor Meynert (brain), J. Arnold (muscles), Frederick von Recklinghausen (lymphatic systems), Max Shultze (nervous system), Wilhelm Waldeyer-Hartz (auditory nerve and cochlea; ovaries), W. Muller (spleen), and Theodor Leber (blood vessels of the eye) to highlight only a few (1872)[86]. Each chapter is translated into English and provides a readable compilation of the state of histology knowledge of this period. "A Manual of Histology" is issued and translated under Salomon Striker's direction and supervision specifically for the medical student.

Soon Salomon Stricker offers another influential edited multivolume, the much more comprehensive "Manual of Human and Animal Histology" volume 1 (1870), volume 2 (1872), volume 3 (1873). This multivolume collection offers a detailed, integrated treatment of human and animal histology (English translations) (1870,1872,1873)[87]. Many of the same notable contributors to Stricker and Buck's smaller "Manual of Histology" provide chapters to this expanded work. This book is soon recognized as the most authoritative and comprehensive text in histology, since Kolliker's text a quarter century earlier. Today, over one hundred forty-eight years later, it is considered one of the landmark publications in the discipline of Histology.

Hans Christian Gram (1853-1938) Danish scientist develops the staining technique still used today, which differentiates bacteria into two large groups, Gram positive and Gram negative, based upon properties of the cell walls (1884)[88].

Charles Scott Sherrington (1857-1952) English histologist identifies and studies the segmental distribution of the anterior and posterior spinal nerve roots, is among the first to investigate and map the sensory dermatomes, and discovers muscle spindles are responsible for initiating the stretch reflex (1894,1898)[89,90]. He is first to recognize every posterior spinal nerve root receives input from a particular segment of skin with some overlap from adjacent dermatomes. Charles Sherrington postulates the law of reciprocal innervation, essential for normal movement and which states when contraction of a muscle is stimulated there is a simultaneous inhibition of its antagonist muscle. Charles Sherrington is credited with introducing the term "synapse" into the scientific literature, coming from synaptein the Greek for "syn" together and "haptein" to clasp. Charles Sherrington shares the 1932 Nobel Prize in Physiology or Medicine with Edgar Adrian (1889-1977) for "…their discoveries regarding the functions of the neuron…" (1932)[91].

In summary, in the first half of the 1800s histology witnesses many advances and histology establishes itself as a valuable scientific discipline. Hodgkin and Lister report no nucleus exists in erythrocytes. Purkinje details the inhibitory layer of cells in the cerebellar cortex and discovers the sweat gland. Muller advocates an epistemological approach to histology, which guides advances in the discipline for 100 years. Henle introduces his Loops, details the lymphatic systems, introduces classification of tissues into four categories epithelial, connective, muscular, neural, and postulates a relationship between microorganisms and diseased tissues. Schwann offers the Cell theory and rejects Vitalism. Remak introduces classification of tissues into ectoderm, mesoderm, endoderm and proposes cells are the result of the division of preexisting cells and not spontaneous generation. Virchow openly plagiarizes Remak and additionally describes the leukemia cell. Kolliker publishes the first textbook devoted to human histology, details skeletal and smooth muscle noting the different nucleated cell assemblies, describes muscles of arterial walls, and recognizes nerve fibers are continuous with their cell body.

The second half of the 1800s witness the introduction of numerous technological advances e.g. stains and staining procedures, formalin, improved microtomes, and microscope resolutions. Waldeyer introduces hematoxylin stain, identifies chromosomes, and proposes the Neuron doctrine. Golgi introduces his silver stain, identifies intracellular organelles, and details the life cycle of the parasite responsible for malaria. Cajal rejects the Reticular theory, embraces the Neuron doctrine, and meticulously draws the microscopic anatomy of neurons. Gram introduces his stain for bacteria cell walls. Ziehl and Neelsen introduce their acid-fast stain and identify bacteria responsible for tuberculosis. Blum develops formalin and offers a revolutionary process for fixation of biological tissues. Cohnheim observes vascular diapedesis. His, Sr. describes neuronal axon growth during embryonic development. Ranvier identifies his Nodes and explains salutatory conduction. Meynert correlates histological changes in cerebral tissues with psychiatric disorders. Stricker provides a compressive manual of histology for medical students. Sherrington maps the dermatomes. Overall, the 1800s are one hundred good and very productive years for medical histology.

Late Modern, 1900 AD - 2000 AD.

The first half of the 1900s reveals continued progress, characterized by improvements in the tools, techniques, and an increased application to medicine. The existence of stem cells are first postulated, frozen section techniques developed, staining procedures for neurons improved, new stains for amyloid and glycogen are introduced, histochemistry and immunohistochemistry are founded, and the first electron microscope is introduced.

Louis Wilson (1866-1942) American pathologist provides one of the first significant contributions to histology, at the beginning of the century. Working in the established labs of the new Mayo Clinics in Minnesota and a few make shift labs he builds in a barn on his own residential property, Louis Wilson modifies the frozen section procedure to allow immediate microscopic examination and rapid intraoperative diagnosis of tissues removed during surgery (1905)[92].

Thomas Cullen (1868-1953) Canadian gynecologist working at John Hopkins Hospital (Cullen sign fame) and Ludwig Pick (1866-1944) German pathologist from the City Hospital Friedrichshain-Berlin (East Berlin) (Niemann-Pick disease and phenochromocytoma fame), offer similar frozen section procedures ten years before Louis Wilson introduces his procedure in America (1895,1897)[93,94]. However, it is Louis Wilson's procedure which proves to be most useful and is accepted by the medical and surgical communities. Louis Wilson's procedure, with modifications is still being used at the Mayo Clinics today.

Franz Nissl (1860-1919) German histologist develops staining techniques for selectively visualizing neuronal cell bodies and RNA and details the staining technique in his landmark paper "Ueber eine neue Untersuchungsmethode des Centralorgans zur Feststellung der Localisation der Nervenzellen" [About a new method of investigation of the central organ to determine the localization of the nerve cells] (1894)[95]. Franz Nissl completes important and influential investigations into the correlations between psychiatric signs and symptoms with changes in brain glia cells, cerebral blood vessels, components of blood, and assorted brain tissues. He systematically investigates the relationships between changes in cerebral cortex and the clinical condition known as dementia (1896a,1896b,1899,1904)[96,97,98,99].

Perhaps, most medical students today will recognize him for his staining techniques, which allows him to identify numerous intracellular structures, including the protein producing rough endoplasmic reticulum (RER) of the neuron (Nissl substance) and extra nuclear ribosomes (Nissl granules) (1894a,1894b)[100,101]. Franz Nissl works with Alois Alzheimer for seven years, becomes good friends, publish several papers together, and a six volume landmark publication in the rapidly developing discipline of histology; "Histologische und histopathologische Arbeiten über die Grosshirnrinde" [Histological and histopathological studies on the cerebral cortex] (1908-1918)[102].

Trivia: Franz Nissl is the best man at Alois Alzheimer's wedding in 1894.

Aloysius (Alois) Alzheimer (1864-1915) German psychiatrist contributes significantly to advancing histology through his many microscopic investigations of brain tissues and their correlation with patient behavior. Alois Alzheimer is perhaps recognized most immediately for his published observations of patient AD (Auguste Deter). She is the 55 year old female psychiatric patient, who upon her death provides her brain for histological inspection by Alzheimer, Franz Nissl, and others working in the Munich laboratories of Emil Kraepelin (1856-1926). In his landmark 1908 publication, "Uber eine eigenartige Erkrankung der Hirnrinde" [About a peculiar disease of the cerebral cortex] Alzheimer uses Nissl's staining techniques to identify the plaques and tangles which will become the defining neurohistological characteristics of Alzheimer's disease for the next 100 plus years (1908)[103].

While most remembered for his contribution to identifying the neuropathological changes associated with Alzheimer's disease, Alois Alzheimer spends much more of his professional life investigating microscopic changes in brain tissues and associating the changes with other observed and reported behaviors of patients. Alzheimer studies and occasionally publishes detailed observations on brain- behavior relationships, including brain arterial sclerosis, syphilis, epilepsy, "Huntington disease", "Wilson disease", and several white matter diseases. In his later years, Alzheimer focuses heavily upon brain-behavior relationships associated with changes in glia cells rather than brain neurons.

Trivia: Alzheimer's doctoral thesis in 1887 investigates the wax producing glands in the ear (1888)[104].

Korbinian Brodmann (1868-1918) German anatomist offers his cytoarchitectural analysis and descriptions of the brain's cerebral cortex. He identifies forty-seven (47) distinct regions, based upon histological observations, using Franz Nissl's staining techniques. These areas, now termed Brodmann areas, are still used today, over 100 years after he first introduces his areas to the scientific and medical communities. Korbinian Brodmann publishes his first cortical histologically based maps in 1909 and argues the cerebral cortex of the human shares the same cortical organization as other mammals (1909)[105]. While many have subsequently proposed alternative cytoarchitectural mappings of the cerebral cortex, none have stood the test of time or have ever been as well accepted as Brodmann's. Over time Brodmann's areas have been associated with specific function; for example Area 4 for fine voluntary movement; Area 22 (Broca's area) for normal language production; Area 44 (Wernicke's area) for normal comprehension of spoken language, Area 17 for normal vision, and Areas 3, 1, 4 for normal tactile somato-sensation.

Advances in technology and innovative uses of old technologies contribute significantly to the advancement of every new discipline. So, too is the case with histology. Many, new, innovative, staining, histochemical, and immunohistochemical procedures are introduced during the late-1800s and early-1900s.

Hans Bennhold (1893-1976) German internist develops the first truly useful stain for amyloid, introducing the Congo red stain (1922)[106]. Five years later psychiatrist Paul Divry (1889-1967), biochemist Marcel Florkin (1900-1979), and pathologist Jean Firket (1890-1958) add their contribution, visualizing apple-green birefringence, when amyloid is stained with Congo red and exposed to polarized light (1927)[107].

Gyorgy Gomori (1904-1957) Hungarian histochemist and Hideo Takamatsu (1911-1979) Japanese histochemist, working independently in separate labs, first report the innovative and original procedures for demonstrating the presence of alkaline phosphatase in tissue sections (1939,1939)[108,109]. Histology is now able to supplement structural staining techniques and moves towards investigations of physiology and chemistry of tissues, in addition to simple structure. Enzyme histochemistry broadens the area of investigations and proves pivotal in the history and development of medical histology.

Albert Coons (1912-1978) American immunologist recognizes it is possible to tag an antibody with a colored label without loss of its antigen binding capacity (immunofluorescence) (1941)[110]. Albert Coons and Melvin Kaplan (unknown-) are first to apply the technique to identify antigen in tissue sections (1950)[111]. Ultimately, this inspired concept leads the way to the new and important diagnostic tool of immunocytochemistry.

Joseph McManus (1911-1980) Canadian histologist introduces "periodic acid Schiff" (PAS) staining for the purpose of staining glycogen in tissues (1948)[112]. The PAS stain is frequently used today to distinguish between different types of glycogen storage diseases. McManus pioneers the field of histochemistry during the 1940s and 1950s. He studies the kidney and coins the term "juxtaglomerular complex" (1942)[113]. McManus is a pioneer and ardent supporter of the combined MD/ PhD training program. In addition to his technical contributions to histology he writes a thoughtful book which examines the history of medicine from a philosophical perspective (1963)[114].

Much of the early-1900s are characterized by advances and application of staining and light microscopic techniques. Limits of both are quickly reached. In an effort to better visualize subcellular structure and associated tissue processes a new and alternative technology is required.

Ernst Ruska (1906-1988) and Max Knoll (1897-1968) together introduce the first electron microscope prototype in 1931. Ruska devotes the rest of his professional career to improving the electron microscope while his colleague Max Knoll moves into television technologies. From the perspective of medicine, it is Ruska's brother Helmut Ruska (1908-1973) who spearheads the application of the electron microscope to biological tissues and medical applications. He is the first scientist to study sub-microscopic structures of bacteria phages and viruses with an electron microscope. In the 1940s, he publishes numerous articles reporting his research, including "Die Bedeutung der Ubermikroskopie fur die Virusforschung" [The Significance of Electron Microscopy for Virus Research] (1939)[115]. Ernst Ruska is awarded the 1986 Nobel Prize in Physics or Medicine for "…fundamental work in electron optics, and for the design of the first electron microscope…" (1986)[116].

The second half of the 1900s reveals rapid advances in tools, techniques, and expands histology into new and exciting areas of investigation. Great advances are made in the microscopic technologies; improved application for staining continues; histochemistry and immunohistochemistry become a part of routine medical practices; adult neurogenesis is introduced; stem cells are identified and application to medicine are quickly recognized; innovative microscale biotechnologies are introduced; functional human cells are grown in 3-dimension ex vivo; tissue engineering is introduced and expands exponentially; regenerative medicine is founded; and digital computer based technologies revolutionize histology, including how histology is taught in medical schools.

Joseph Altman (1925-2016) American biologist and independent investigator at Massachusetts Institute of Technology (MIT) is among the first to recognize adult neurogenesis and report the adult brain can and does generate new functional connections between neurons within the central nervous system. He and his research group publish a series of papers during the mid-1960s demonstrating new growth of neuronal cells in the mature adult brain, by utilizing titrated thymidine autoradiology to label cells (1967)[117]. His original observations so challenge scientific dogma they are initially largely ignored by the scientific and medical communities.

Michael Kaplan (1952-) American research biologist builds upon the earlier work of Joseph Altman. Michael Kaplan in the 1970s and 1980s, combines titrated thymidine labeling and electron microscopy and confirms adult neurogenesis (1979,1985)[118,119]. Today, over five decades after Altman and Kaplan first introduced the idea and provided essential histological evidence, it is now reasonably well accepted, adult neurogenesis does occur in humans (1992,1998, 1999)[120,121,122].

Adult neurogenesis serves as a good example of how medical dogma changes with advancements in tools and techniques used within a field and the importance of thoughtful synthesis of information by scientists whom are not so easily dissuaded by dogma and the presses of colleagues.

Facts and truths you learn today in medical school may be untrue. No, your professors are not intentionally providing you with misinformation but rather the basic and clinical sciences are taught from the basis of current scientific and medical dogma. Learn to think and critically evaluate information for yourself. Don't rely upon others to do it for you.

OK…back to the history of histology.

Judah Folkman (1933-2008) American scientist, offers his seminal work in the area of angiogenesis, the process during which abnormal cell growth attracts new blood vessels to nourish and sustain growth. His initial original work into angiogenesis and recommended applications for innovative treatments for cancers are largely dismissed by the medical community (1971)[123]. After a decade of continued work, the scientific and medical communities slowly begin to accept Folkman's conceptualization and the possibility of anti-angiogenesis as a potential treatment for some cancers. Judah Folkman's angiogenesis model provides an important new conceptual matrix and results in the introduction and development of several new technologies. Today, angiogenesis inhibitors are common in the treatment of several specific cancers e.g. multiple myeloma and colon cancers.

The term "stem cell" is first introduced to the scientific community during the 1907 meeting of the Congress of the Hematological Society in Berlin by Russian histologist Alexander Maksinmov (1874-1928). He postulates the existence of stem cells, which he refers to as "polyblasts", within a matrix of hematopoiesis (1909)[124]. Not until the early-1960s are stem cells physically identified. Stem cells quickly become and continue to remain an area of much excitement and research. With applications of stem cell research apparent in medicine, religious, political, and societal pressures constrain advances in stem cell research throughout the second half of the 1900s and early-2000s.

Ernest McCulloch (1926-2011) Canadian cell biologist and James Till (1931-) Canadian biophysicist are first to report evidence of stem cells, as self-renewing cells in bone marrow (1963,1963)[125,126]. Their work provides the foundation from which research over the next 50 years will build.

Tissue engineering is first introduced during the early-1980s and provides significant and exciting advancements in histology. This relatively new field of tissue engineering defined by American biochemical engineer Robert Langer and transplant researcher Joseph Vacanti American as "…an interdisciplinary field that applies the principles of engineering and life sciences towards the development of biological substitutes that restore, maintain, or improve tissue function or a whole organ…", is arguably one of the most significant advances to impact histology during the late-1900s (1993)[127].

Robert Langer (1948-) American biochemical engineer is one of the first to introduce new biotechnologies which change the study of tissues forever. Robert Langer and Joseph Vacanti (1948-) are two of the most influential scientists in establishing and advancing tissue engineering. Their first landmark publication in "Science" introduces tissue engineering to a broad segment of the general scientific community (1993)[127]. The paper outlines a method for using resorbable polymer matrices as a vehicle for cell transplantation and growing human tissues. This seminal paper stimulates the imagination of others and stands as a landmark publication in a very young field. Foundational works by Langer, Vicanti, and others provide the necessary tools, techniques, creative imagination, and rigorous scientific thought, allowing tissue engineering to flourish as an active scientific and commercial venture for the balance of the 1900s.

Joseph Vacanti (1948-) American transplant researcher contributes significantly to the field of tissue engineering since its beginning. Robert Langer and Joseph Vacanti provide the first substantive article to the general scientific community, introducing the field and laying the foundation for research, for the next 25 years. Joseph Vacanti and Robert Langer provide a substantial proportion of the early work on growing human tissues in 3-dimentions. Their original approach in growing 3-dimentional human tissues remains the model still used today.

In brief, the approach of Robert Langer and Joseph Vacanti is to provide a "…scaffold made of an artificial, biodegradable polymer, seeding it with living cells and bathing the cells in growth factor. The cells can come from living tissue or stem cells. The cells multiply, filling up the scaffold, and growing into a three-dimensional tissue. Once implanted in the body, the cells recreate their proper tissue functions, blood vessels grow into the new tissue, the scaffold melts away, and lab-grown tissue becomes indistinguishable from its surroundings…" (2010)[128]. The technique has significant implications for future organ transplants and potentially eliminating the current problem of organ rejection by the recipient's immune system.

Before summarizing the history of medical histology during the 1900s, it makes sense to take a moment and examine the development of one particular technology, which has always been a primary tool in histology, the microscope. The 1900s witnesses many changes in the instrument. These changes contribute significantly to broadening the range of study available to histology as well as expanding the scientific knowledge base. Improvements in microscope technology are immediatcly incorporated into the clinical dimensions of medical histology and the microscope quickly become an indispensable tool in every practicing physician's medical office.

Do you remember the first time you looked through the eye piece of a microscope and the first microscopic image you viewed?

The modern traditional standard three objective lens light microscope, at the beginning of the 1900s has a 170x magnification and 0.9 micrometer resolution. Magnification and resolution continuously improves throughout the 1900s, resulting in 1200x magnification with 0.25 micrometer resolution by 1999. Magnification and resolution of early microscopes are restricted by visual light physics. With the development of improved imaging techniques during the 1900s, these early problems are minimized or eliminated. Introduction of florescent microscopy allows resolutions of approximately 10 nanometers and interference microscopy produces resolutions of 1 nanometer. For those of you who are light microscope purest, recently introduced Sarfus technology permits very impressive resolutions e.g. down to 0.3 nanometer with optical light microscopes.

The first electron microscopes is invented by German physicist Ernst Ruska and German electrical engineer Max Knoll, at the Berlin Technische Hochschule. The instrument offers magnification of 400x, with resolutions of approximately 0.2 micrometers (1932,1935)[129,130]. Initially, incapable of visualizing small intracellular organelles, the electron microscope advances to approximately 1,000,000x magnification capabilities, with 0.1 nanometer resolutions, by the end of 1999 (1999)[131]. Electron microscopes are first to visualize strains of DNA, initially coated with metals, in the 1960s and later more directly in the 1970s (1971)[132].

The first scanning tunneling microscope (STM) gives three-dimensional images of objects, down to the atomic level, is invented by German physicist Gerd Binnig (1947-) and Swiss physicist Heinrich Rohrer (1933-2013). Gerd Binnig submits the patent for the STM in 1980. At that time, he is advised not to release the STM information to the scientific community until the patent is finally approved and registered. Sound familiar? See earlier in this chapter, Antonie van Leeuwenhoek's reservations, during the late-1600s, regarding his disclosure of his innovative lens making techniques, which allowed viewing of single cell organisms for the very first time to a very disbelieving medical community. Binnig and Rohrer released their first STM publication in 1982 after securing a patent (1982)[133]. Gerd Binning and Heinrich Rohrer receive the 1986 Nobel Prize in Physics "…for their design of the scanning tunneling microscope…", six years after they filed for the original patent and only four years after they produced a working STM (1986)[134].

By the end of 1900s the scanning tunneling microscope (STM) is capable of magnification of 1,000,000,000x with 0.1 nanometer lateral and 0.01 nanometer depth resolution (1999)[135]. The scanning probe microscope can detect features as small as a single picometer (one thousandth of a nanometer), resolution of 1/20th of an individual atom.

The first digital microscopes are produced by Hirox Company Limited and the Keyence Corporation of Tokyo Japan in 1986. These scopes provide an attractive alternative to peering through the eye piece of a traditional microscope. The digital scope displays the image on a video screen, while simultaneously permitting the storage of the image on a computer disk. With a little additional software, three dimensional rotation of the sample tissue are made possible. As of 2010, you can purchase a digital microscope which plugs into your laptop computer's USB port, with magnification 200x, a built in digital camera, and 1.3 megapixel resolutions for under $100.00. Digital microscopy and virtual histology has become routine in teaching histology to medical students today.

So goes a much truncated presentation of the advances in microscope technologies and applications to histology during the 1900s. Certainly a difference from the 30x magnification, poor resolution, and absence of colors witnessed by Robert Hooke as he first described his observation of the cell, in his publication "Micrographia" (1665)[10], to the 1,000,000,000x STM available in 1999 (1999)[135].

In summary, in the second half of the 1900s, histology witnesses many advances. Wilson introduces the frozen section techniques. Nissl stains nucleic acids (RNA and DNA). Alzheimer reports the histological changes associated with early onset dementia. Brodmann details the cytoarchitecture of the cerebral cortex. Sherrington maps the dermatomes. Bemmjhold stains amyloid. McManus stains glycogen. Gormori and Takamatusu introduce enzyme histochemistry.

Coons introduces immunohistochemistry. Ruska and Knoll invent the electron microscope. Hirox and Keyence Corporations introduce digital microscopy. Altman introduces adult neurogenesis. Folkman introduces angiogenesis. McCulloch and Till demonstrate the existence of stem cells. Langer and Vacanti introduce tissue engineering and microscale biotechnologies.

Wow, what a century for histology.

Current Modern, 2000 AD - 2019 AD.

Currently, exciting new areas of rapid advancement are evident in the development of microscale biotechnologies for tissues, detailed imaging and chemical analyses of intracellular and intercellular processes of specific tissues, tissue engineering and associated manipulation of normal and abnormal tissues growth in vivo and ex vivo, and the computer based digital revolution opens new doors to the application of histology to the practice of clinical medicine.

One new and innovative technique, representative of the many emerging tools now available to the histologist is CLARITY (2013,2013,2013,2013)[136,137,138,139]. The procedure offers the histologist one more tool to better understand the structure, composition, and function of tissues.

Karl Deisseroth (1971-) Professor of Bioengineering, Psychiatry, and Behavioral Sciences at Stanford University and Kwanghum Chung (unknown-) Assistant Professor of Medical Engineering and Sciences introduce a new technology, which allows for making brain tissues transparent and labeling of specific proteins within tissues and permitting vivid visualization of cells and their relationship with other cells. They term the new technique CLARITY.

In brief, the CLARITY procedure is accomplished by placing a tissue in a transparent scaffolding matrix, then removing lipid components. What remains are proteins and nucleic acids. Contrast agents are introduced such as antibodies, DNA, or RNA labels, or fluorescent molecule tags, which bind to special target substances. Using specialized microscopy, a high resolution, three dimensional image can be observed. Equally exciting component of this new procedure is that it is possible to remove antibodies and reapply new ones, enabling the sample to be targeted with new antibodies targeting different proteins and generation of a new image. The procedure is now being used to image local neural circuits and trace specific neurotransmitter systems previously unseen. Preliminary studies reveal abnormal, ladder like connections appearing within and between neurons in a brain of an autistic child (2013)[136].

Medical education continues to rely upon histology as valued basic science and continues to be taught as a separate course in most USA medical school programs. While the emphasis has shifted from traditional microscopic study and traditional staining techniques to digital images, histology continues to provide the basis from which medical students can understand both normal and abnormal tissues functions.

Histology continues to play an important role today in the preparation of both research and clinical physicians. Tools have become sharper, techniques improved and new technologies introduced. The continued interdisciplinary approach to the investigation of tissues will secure histology's contributions to the medical sciences for the future.

References.

[1] Dirckx, J. (1997). Stedman's concise medical dictionary for the health professions. Third Edition. Baltimore: Williams and Wilkins.

[2] National Institutes of Health (2010) National Library of Medicine. Retrieved January 2010 from http://www.nlm.nih.gov/tsd/acquisitions/cdm/subjects49.html

[3] Scurlock, J. and Andersen, B. (2005). Diagnoses in Assyrian and Babylonian medicine: Ancient sources, translation, and modern medical analyses. Chicago: University of Illinois Press.

[4] Steffens, B. (2007). Ibn al Haytham - The first scientist. Profiles in Science. Greensboro, NC: Morgan Reynolds Publishing.

[5] Al-Haytham, I. (circa 1021,1572). Opticae Thesasaurus: Alhazeni Abris libri septem nunc primum edit. Basel: Friedrich Risner.

[6] Smith. A. (2001). Alhacen's theory of visual perception: A critical edition with English translation and commentary on the first three Books of Alhacen's De Aspectibus. Transactions of the American Philosophical Society, vol. 91, (4-5). Philadelphia: American Philosophical Society.

[7] Smith, A. (2006). Alhacen on the principles of reflection: A critical edition with English translation and commentary of Books 4 and 5 of Alhacen's De Aspectibus. Transactions of the American Philosophical Society, vol. 95 (2-3). Philadelphia: American Philosophical Society.

[8] Smith, A. (2008). Alhacen on image formation and distortion in mirrors: A critical edition with English translation and commentary of Book 6 of Alhacen's De Aspectibus. Transactions of the American Philosophical Society, vol. 98 (1-2). Philadelphia: American Philosophical Society.

[9] Smith, M. (2010). Alhacen on refraction: A critical edition with English translation and commentary of Book 7 of Alhacen's De Aspectibus. Transactions of the American Philosophical Society, vol. 100 (1-2). Philadelphia: American Philosophical Society.

[10] Hooke, R. (1665). Micrographia: Or some physiological descriptions of minute bodies made by magnifying glasses with observations and inquires there upon. London: Jo. Martyn and Allestry. Retrieved September 20, 2016 from https://ceb.nlm.nih.gov/proj/ttp/flash/hooke/hooke.html

[11] Malpighi, M. (1661). De pulmonibus. Philosophical Transactions of the Royal Society. London.

[12] Malpighi, M. (1666). De Lingua. In De viscerum structura excecitation anatomica. Bologna: Jacopo Monti.

[13] Malpighi, M. (1666). De Cerebro. In De viscerum structura excecitation anatomica.Bologna: Jacopo Monti.

[14] Malpighi, M. (1666). De Externo Tractus Organo. In De viscerum structura excecitation anatomica. Bologna: Jacopo Monti.

[15] Malpighi, M. (1666). Accedit dissertatio de polypo cordis. In De viscerum structura exercitation anatomica. Bologna, ex typographia Iacobi Montij. [English translation by J. Forrester (1995), Med. History, 39(4) Oct.:477-492. Cambridge University Press].

[16] Malpighi, M. (1673). Dissertatio epistolica de formation pulli in ovo. London: Philosophical Transactions of the Royal Society. London.

[17] Ford, B. (1981). Twenty years of Leenwenhoeck Specimens. Lab News, Sept p A4-A6 9/8/01, 13:53.

[18] Leeuwenhoek, A. (1673). A specimen of some observations made by a microscope, contrived by M. Leewenhoek in Holland, lately communicated by Dr. Regnerus de Graaf. Philos. Trans. R. Soc. London., 8:6037-6038.

[19] Leeuwenhoeck, A. (1677). Observations communicated to the publisher by Mr. Antony van Leeuwenhoeck, in Dutch letter of the 9th of October 1676: concerning little animals by him observed in rain-well-sea- and snow-water; as also in water wherein pepper had lain infused. Philos. Trans. R. Soc. London, 12:821-831.

[20] Stong, C. (1952). C. L. Stong Papers, 1952-1976. Smithsonian Institution, National Museum of American History: Archives Center Washington D.C. , Call number ACNMAH 0012.

[21] Ford, B. (1981). The van Leeuwenhoek Specimens, Notes and Records of the Royal Society, (1):37-59.

[22] Bichat, X. (1800). Traite des membranes en general et de diverses membanes en particulier. Paris: Ricahrd, Caille et Ravier.

[23] Bichat, X. (1801). Anatome Generale. Paris: Brosson and Gabon.

[24] Restak R. (1984). The Brain. New York: Bantam Books.

[25] Mayer, A. (1819). Uber Histologie and cine neue Eintheilung Gewebe de Menschilchen Kopers. [On histology and a new division of the tissues of the human body]. Bonn: Marcus.

[26] Hodgkin, T. and Lister, J. (1827). Notice of some microscopic observations of the blood and animal tissues. Philosophical magazine, 2:130-9.

[27] Lister, J. (1830). On the Improvement of Achromatic Compound Microscopes. Philosophical Transactions of the Royal Society, 120:187–200.

[28] Wendt, A. (1833). De epidermide humana. Dissertation supervised by J. Purkinje. University of Breslau.

[29] Ber. u. d. Versamml. Deutsch Naturf. U. Aerzte, 1837.

[30] Palicki, B. (1839). De musculari cordis structura. Dissertation supervised by J. Purkinje and G. Valentin. University of Breslau.

[31] Purkinje, J. (1839). Paper presented to the Silesian Society for National Culture, January 16, 1839. Introduces protoplasm.

[32] Purkinje, J. (1840a). Uebers. Arb. Verand. Schles. Ges. Vat. Kult., 16:81.

[33] Purkinje, J. (1823). Commentatio physiologico organi visus et en examine Systematis cutaneous. Breslau.

[34] Muller, J. (1830). Bildungsgeschichte der Genitalien.

[35] Henle, J. (1841). Allegemeine Anatomie: Lehre von den mischungs- und formbestandtheilen des menslichen körpers. Leipzig. Berlag von Leopold.

[36] Henle, J. (1840). Pathologische Untersuchungen. Berlin: Verlag von August Hirschwald.

[37] Virchow, R. (1845). Weisses Blut. Neue Notiz Geb Natur-u Heilk. 36:151-6.

[38] Virchow, R. (1846a). Die Verstopfung der lungenarterie und ihre folgen. Beitr. Exper. Path., 2:1.

[39] Virchow, R. (1846b). Thromboembolism. Beitr. Exper. Path., 2:227.

[40] Remak, R. (1852). Ueber extracellulare entstehung thierischer zellen und uber die vermehrung derselben durch theilung [About extracellular emergence of animal cells and the multiplication by division of the same]. Archiv fur Anatomie, Physiologie, und Wissenschaftliche Medicine, 47-57.

[41] Virchow, R. (1860). Cellular pathology as based upon physiological and pathological histology. London: John Churchill.

[42] Schwann, T and Schleyden, M. (1839). Microscopic investigations on the accordance in the structure and growth of plants and animals. Berlin. [English translation by the Sydenham Society, 1847. London.].

[43] Schwann, T. (1847) Microscopical Researches on the Similarity in the Structure and the Growth of Animals and Plants. Translated from the German (1839) by Henry Smith. London: Printed for the Sydenham Society; C and J Aslard, Printers.

[44] Schwann, T. (1839). Mikroskopische Untersuchungen über die Übereinstimmung in der Struktur und dem Wachstum der Thiere und Pflanzen. Berlin: Verlag der Sander'schen Buchhandlung, G.E. Reimer.

[45] Kolliker, A. (1860). A manual of human microscopic anatomy. [English translation by George Busk and Thomas Huxley for the Sydenham Society]. London.

[46] Schwann, T. (1834). De necessitate æris atmosphærici ad evolutionem pulli in ovo incubato. Doctoral dissertation. Berlin.

[47] Remak, R. (1852). Ueber extracelluläre Entstehung thierischer Zellen und über die Vermehrung derselben durch Theilung. Archiv für Anatomie, Physiologie und Wissenschaftliche Medicin., 47-57. Johannes Muller Editor, Berlin: Verlag von Weit et Comp. http://www.biodiversitylibrary.org/item/50176#290

[48] Remak, R. (1838). Observationes anatomicae et microscopicae de systematis nervosi structura. Doctoral dissertation. Berolini: Sumtibus et formis Reimerianis.

[49] Remak, R. (1850-1855). Untersuchungen über die Entwickelung der Wirbelthiere. 3 parts; Berlin: G. Reimer.

[50] Kolliker, A. (1849). Beitrage zur Kenntnis der glatten Muskeln. Zeitschr. Wiss. Zool., 1:48-87.

[51] Kolliker. A. (1862). Termination of nerves in muscles, as observed in the frog; and on the disposition of the nerves in the frog's heart. Proceedings of the Royal Society of London, 12:65-84.

[52] Kolliker, A. (1853,1854). A manual of human histology, vol. 1 and vol. 2. [Translated and edited by George Busk and Thomas Huxley for the Sydenham Society]. London: J. E. Adlard.

[53] Bracegirgle, B. (1977). The history of histology: A brief survey of sources. His. Sci., 15:77-101.

[54] Blum, F. (1893). Der formaldehyde als hartungsmittel. Z. Wiss. Mikrosc., 10:314.

[55] Gegner, C. (1893). Uber einige wirkungen des formaldehyds. Inaugrual dissertation zur erlangung der medizinischen doktorwurde vorgelegt der hohen medizinischen Fakultat der kgl. Bayer. Friedrich-Alexanders-Universitat zu Erlangen im Juli 1893. Erlangen: K.B. Hofbuchdruckerei von Aug. Vollrath.

[56] Blum, F. (1894). Notiz uber die Anwendung des Formaldehyds (Formol) als Hartungs-und Koneservierungsmittel. Anat. Anz., 9:229.

[57] Blum. F. (1893). Der formaldehyde als antisepticum. Munich Med. Wochenschur., 8 August: 601.

[58] Chevalire, C. (1839). Des microscopes et de leur usage. Paris.

[59] Bracegridle, B. (1979). A history of micro technique: the evolution of the microtome and the development of tissue preparation. London: Heinemann Educational Books.

[60] Waldeyer, W. (1863). Untersuchungen uber den Ursprung und den Verlauf des Axencylinders bei Wirbellosen und Wirbelthieren sowie uber dessen Endverhalten in der quesgestreiften. Muske faser Henle un Pfeufer, Zeits Nation Med., 20:193-256.

[61] Golgi, C. (1873). Sulla struttura della sostanza grigia del cervelo. Gazzetta Medica Italiana. Lombardia, 33:244-246.

[62] Wissowzky, N. (1876). Ueber das Eosin als reagenz auf Hamoglobin und die Bildung von Blutgefassen und Blutkorperchen bei Saugetier und Huhnerembryonen. Arch fur Mikroskopische Anatomie, December, (13)1:479-496.

[63] Ziehl, F. (1882). Zur farbung des tuberkelbacillum. Deutsche Medizinische Worchenschrift., 8:451-452.

[64] Neelsen, F. (1883). Ein casuistischer Beitrag zur Lehre von der tuberkulose. Zentralblatt fur Medizinische Wissenschaften, 28:497-501.

[65] Gram. C. (1884). Uber die isolierte Farbung der Schizomyceten in Schnitt und Trockenpraparaten. Forrtschritte der Medizin. 2 (6):185-189, March 15.

[66] Gram, C. (1884). Ueber die Farbung der Schizomyceten in Schnittenpraparaten, Congres periodique international des sciences medicales. 8th Session. Section de pathologies general et d'anatomie pathologique, 116-117. Copenhagen, Aug.:10-16.

[67] Daddi, L. (1896). Nouvelle method pour colorer la graisse dans les tissues. Archives Italiennes de Biologie., 26: 143-146. Original paper in Giornale d. R. Acc. Di medicina di Torino, No. 2. 1896.

[68] Weigert, C. (1898). A method for staining elastic fibers. Zbl. Allg. Path. Path. Anato., 9:289-292.

[69] Baker, J. (1958). Principals of biological microtechniques. London: Methuen., 172-174.

[70] Waldeyer, W. (1888). Uber karyokinese und ihre beziehungen zu den befruchtungsvorgagen. Archiv fur Mikroskopische Anatomie und Entwicklungsmechanik, 32:1-122.

[71] Waldeyer, W. (1891). Ueber einige neuere forschungen im gebiete der anatomie des centalnervensystems [About some new research in the field of anatomy of the central nervous system]. Deutsche medicinische Wochenschrift, Berlin. 17:1213-1218, 1244-1246, 1287-1289, 1331-1332, 1350-1356.

[72] Golgi, C. (1886). Studii sulla fina anatomia degli organi centrali del sistema nervoso. Milano.

[73] Golgi, C. (1880d). Sui nervi dei tendini dell'uomo e di altri vertebrati e di un nuovo organo nervosa terminale musculo-tendineo. Mem. Royal Academy of Sciences Tor., 32:359-385.

[74] Golgi, C. (1889). Annotazioni intomo all'istologia dei reni dell'uomo e di altri mammiferi e sull'istogenesi dei canaliculi oriniferi. Atti della Reale Accademia dei Lincei, Sez IV, Rendiconti, 5:334.

[75] Golgi, C. (1892). Action de la quinine sur les parasites malariques et sur les accès fébriles qu'ils determinant. H. Loescher.

[76] Gerlach, J. von. (1872). Ueber die Structur der grauen Substanz des menschlichen Grosshirns: Vorläufige Mittheilung' . Centrallblatt für die medicinischen Wissenschaften, 70:273-275.

[77] Waldeyer W. (1891). Ueber einigen neuere Forschungen im Gebiete die Anatomie des Centralnervensystems, Deutsche medicinische Wochenschrift. 70:1352-1356.

[78] Nobel Prize Foundation (1906). The Nobel Prize in Physiology or Medicine 1906. Royal Swedish Academy of Sciences. Stockholm. Retrieved June 2009 from www.nobelprize.org

[79] Von Gerlach, J. (1863). Die photographie als hulsmittel mikroskopischer forschung. Leipzig: Wilhelm Engelmann.

[80] Peaslee, R. (1857). Human histology in its relations to descriptive anatomy, physiology, and pathology. Philadelphia: Blanchard and Lea. Retrieved 8-19-2015 from address collections.nlm.nih.gov/catalog/nlm:nlmuid-61610050R-bk

[81] His, W. (1865). Die Häute und Höhlen des Körpers. Schweighauserische Universitäts-Buchdruckerei.

[82] Cohnheim J. (1868). Ueber entzuendung und eiterung. [On inflamation and suppuration]. Arch. Path. Anat. Physiol. Klin. Med., 40:1–79.

[83] Ranvier, L. and Weber, E. (1878). Lecons sur histologie du systeme nerveux. 2 volumes). [Lessons on the histology of the nervous system]. Paris: F. Savy.

[84] Meynert, T. (1884). Psychiatrie. Klinik der Erkrankungen des Vorderhirns [Clinic: On the diseases of the forebrain].

[85] Whitehouse, P., Price, D., Struble, R., Clark, A., Coyle, J., Delong, M. (1982). Alzheimer's disease and senile dementia: loss of neurons in the basalis forebrain. Science, 215:1237-1239.

[86] Stricker, S. (1872). A Manual of Histology [American translation by Henry Buck, 1872]. New York: William Wood and Company.

[87] Stricker, S. (1870,1872,1873). Handbuch der Lehre von den Geweben des Menschen und der Thiere. [Manual of human and comparative histology, vols 1,2,3.; English translation by Henry Power. London: The News Sydenham Society].

[88] Gram, H. (1884). Über die isolierte Färbung der Schizomyceten in Schnitt- und Trockenpräparaten. Fortschritte der Medizin., 2:185–9.

[89] Sherrington, C. (1894). On the anatomical constitution of nerves of skeletal muscles; and remarks on recurrent fibers in the ventral spinal nerve-root. J. Physiol., Oct 15; 17(3-4), 210.2-258.

[90] Sherrington, C. (1898). Experiments in examination of the peripheral distribution of the fibers of the posterior roots of some spinal nerves, Philosophical Transactions, B, 190:45-186.

[91] Nobel Prize Foundation (1932). The Nobel Prize in Physiology or Medicine 1932. Royal Swedish Academy of Sciences. Stockholm. Retrieved June 2009 from www.nobelprize.org

[92] Wilson, L. (1905). A method for the rapid preparation of fresh tissues for the microscope. J. Am. Med. Assoc., 45:1737.

[93] Cullen, T. (1895). A rapid method of making permanent specimens from frozen sections by the use of formalin. Johns Hopkins Hospital Bull., 6:67.

[94] Pick, L. (1897). A rapid method of preparing permanent sections for microscopical diagnosis. BMJ., 1:140-141.

[95] Nissl, F. (1894). Ueber eine neue Untersuchungsmethode des Centralorgans zur Feststellung der Localisation der Nervenzellen, [About a new method of investigation of the central organ to determine the localization of the nerve cells] Neurologisches Centralblatt, Leipzig, 13:507-508.

[96] Nissl, F. (1896a). Die bezienhungen der nervenzellsubstanzen zu den tatigen, ruhenden und eruedeten zellzustanden [The relationship of the nerve cel to the active substances, resting and tired cell states]. Allgemeine Zeitschrift fur Psychiatrie, 52:1147-1154.

[97] Nissl, F. (1896b). Mitteilungen zur pathologischen anatomie der dementia paralytica [Releases to pathological anatomy of paralytic dementia]. Archiv. fur Psychiatrie., 28:987-992.

[98] Nissl, F. (1899). Uber einige beziehungen zwischen nervenzellerkrankungen und gliosen erscheinungen bei verschiedenen psychosen [About some relaionships between nerve cell and glia disease symptoms in different psychoses]. Archiv. fur Psychiatrie un Nervenkrankheiten, Berlin. 32:656-676.

[99] Nissl, F. (1904). Zur histopathologie der paralytischen riendenerkrankung. In: Histologische und histopathologische arbeiten uber die grosshirnrinde mit besonderer berucksichtigung der pathologischen anatomie der geisteskrankheiten [For histopathology the paralytic cow disease. In: Histological and histopathological studies on the cerebral cortex with special emphasis on the pathological anatomy of mental illness]. Vol. 1. Jena: G. Fischer.

[100] Nissl, F. (1894a). Ueber eine neue untersuchungsmethode des centalorgans zur feststellung der localisation der nervenzellen [A new method of investigation of the central organ for determining the localization of the nerve cells]. Neurological Centrablatt, Leipzig, 13:507-508.

[101] Nissl, F. (1894b). Uber die sogenannten granula der nervenzellen [On the so-called granules of the nerve cells]. Neurologisches Centralblatt, Leipzig, 13:676-685; 781-789; 810-814.

[102] Nissl, F. and Alzheimer, A. (1908). Histologische und histopathologische arbeiten über die grosshirnrinde mit besonderer berucksichtingung der pathologischen anatomie der geisteskrankheiten. Jena: Verlag von Gustav Fischer.

[103] Alzheimer, A. (1908). Uber eine eigenartige Erkrankung der Hirnrinde [About a peculiar disease of the cerebral cortex], Allgemeine Zeitschrift fur Psychiatrie und Psychisch Gerichtliche Medizin, 64(1–2):146–148); [English translation by L. Jarvik and H. Greenson 1987, Alzheimer Dis Assoc Disord., 1(1):3–8.].

[104] Alzheimer, A. (1888). Uber die Ohren schmal drüsen [About the ears small glands (wax producing)] Doctoral dissertation. Würzburg: Druck und Verlag der Stahel'schen Univer. Buch and Kunsthandlung.

[105] Broadmann, K. (1909). Vergleichende Lokalisationslehre der Grosshirnrinde in ihren Principien, dargestellt auf grund des Zellenbaues. Leipzig, J. A. Barth Verlag. [English translation by Laurence J. Garey, Localisation in the Cerebral Cortex 1994 and 1999. London: Imperial College Press.].

[106] Bennhold, H., (1922), Eine specifische amyloidfärbung mit kongorot, Münchener Medizinische Wochenschrift, 44, 1537.

[107] Divry, P., Florkin, M., and Firket, J. (1927). Sur les proprietes otiques de l'amiloide. C. R. Soc. Biol., 97:1808-10.

[108] Gomoti, G. (1939). Microtechnical demonstration of phosphatase in tissue section. Proc. Soc. Exp. Biol. Med., 42:23-26.

[109] Takamatsu, H. (1939) Histologische und biochcmische studien ueber die phosphatase und deren verteilung in verschiedenen organwn und geweben. Trans. Soc. Path. Jap., 29:492-498.

[110] Coons, A., Creech, H., and Jones, R. (1941). Immunological properties of an antibody containing a fluorescent group. Proc. Exp. Biol. Med., 47:200-202.

[111] Coon, A. and Kaplan, M. (1950). J. Exp. Med., Jan. 1, 91(1):1-13.

[112] McManus, J. (1948). Histological and histochemical uses of periodic acid. Stain Technol., 23:99-108.

[113] McManus, J. (1942). The juxtaglomerular complex. The Lancet, 240(6214):394-396.

[114] McMannus, J. (1963). Fundamental ideas of medicine: A brief history of medicine. Springfield: Charles C. Thomas.

[115] Ruska, H., Borries, B., and Ruska, E. (1939). Die Bedeutung der Übermikroskopie für die Virusforschung [The significance of electron microscopy for virus research]. Archiv für die gesamte Virusforschung, 1:155-169.

[116] Nobel Prize Foundation (1986). The Nobel Prize in Physics 1986. Royal Swedish Academy of Sciences. Stockholm. Retrieved June 2009 from www.nobelprize.org

[117] Altman, J. and Das, G. (1967). Postnatal neurogenesis in the guinea pig. Nature. June 10, 214:1098-1101.

[118] Kaplan, M. (1979). Cell Proliferation in the Adult Mammalian Brain. PhD. Dissertation, May 1979. Boston University.

[119] Kaplan, M. (1985). Formation of neurons in young and senescent animals: An electron microscopic and morphological Analysis; Hope for a new neurology. New York Academy of Sciences, 57:173-192.

[120] Reynolds, B. and Weiss, S. (1992). Generation of neurons and astrocytes from isolated cells of the adult mammalian central nervous system. Science, 255(5052):1707-10.

[121] Eriksson P., Perfilieva E., Björk-Eriksson T., Alborn, A., Nordborg, C., Peterson, D., and Gage, F. (1998). Neurogenesis in the adult human hippocampus. Nat. Med., 4 (11):1313-7.

[122] Gould, E., Reeves, A., Graziano, M., and Gross, C. (1999). Neurogenesis in the neocortex of adult primates. Science, 286 (5439): 548–52.

[123] Folkman J. (1971). Tumor angiogenesis: therapeutic implications. New England Journal of Medicine, 285:1182-1186.

[124] Maximov, A. (1909). Der lymphozyt als gemeinsame stammzelle der verschiedenen blutelemente in der embryonalen entwicklung und im postfetalwn leben der sanfetiere [The lymphocyte as a stem cell common to the different blood elements in embryonic development and during the post fetal life of mammanls]. Folia Haematologica. 8:125-134.

[125] Becker, A., McCulloch, E., and Till, J. (1963). Cytological demonstration of the clonal nature of spleen colonies derived from transplanted mouse marrow cells. Nature, 197:452–454.

[126] Siminovitch, L., McCulloch, E., and Till, J. (1963). The distribution of colony-forming cells among spleen colonies. Journal of Cellular and Comparative Physiology, 62:327–336.

[127] Langer, R. and Vacanti, J. (1993). Tissue engineering. Science, 260 (5110):920 -926.

[128] Vacanti, J. (2010). Faculty profile. Massachusetts General Hospital. Retrieved January 2010 from http://www.massgeneral.org/research/researchlab.aspx?id=1129

[129] Knoll, M and Ruska, E. (1932). The electron microscope. Z. Physics, (78):318-339.

[130] Ruska, E. (1935). The electron microscope as ultra microscope. Research and Progress. (January) 1:18-19.

[131] Bozzola, J. and Russell, L. (1999). Electron microscopy: principles and techniques for biologists. Boston: Jones and Barlett.

[132] Griffith, J., Huberman, J., and Kornberg, A. (1971). Electron microscopy of DNA polymerase bound to DNA. J. Mol. Biol., 55:209-214.

[133] Binnig G., Rohrer, H., Gerber, C., and Weibel, E. (1982). Surface Studies by Scanning Tunneling Microscopy. Physical Review Letters, 49:57-60.

[134] The Nobel Prize Foundation (1986). Nobel Prize in Physics 1986. Royal Swedish Academy of Sciences. Stockholm. Retrieved June 2009 from www.nobelprize.org

[135] Bai, C. (1999). Scanning tunneling microscopy and its applications. 2nd edition, New York: Springer Verlag.

[136] Deisseroth, K. (2013). See through brain. Nature video. Retrieved 8-25-2016 from https://www.youtube.com/watch?v=c-NMfp13Uug&feature=youtu.be

[137] Underwood, E. (2013). Tissue imaging methods makes everything clear. Science. 340 (6129):131-132.

[138] Geaghan-Breiner, C. (2013). CLARITY Brain Imaging. Stanford University.

[139] Shen, H. (2013). See through brains clarify connections. Nature, April 10, 496(74444):151. doi:10.1038/496151a

Chapter 2

Medical Anatomy

Definition.

Anatomy is the science of morphology or structure of an organism. The word anatomy is derived from the Greek "anatome", which when translated into English means dissection, from "ana" apart + "tome" a cutting. Human anatomy is more restrictive in definition, restricting itself to describing the form and structure of the human body and its various parts (1997)[1].

Introduction.

The study of human anatomy has long been a part of the education of medical students. The importance of anatomy in medical education and the importance placed upon it by practicing physicians have fluctuated considerably throughout time. The scientific study of human anatomy and its application to the practice of medicine has always been influenced by religious beliefs, politics, geographic location, and medical dogma,

This chapter explores the historical development of medical anatomy from its earliest beginnings in the ancient civilizations of Mesopotamia, Egypt, and Greece to its current state today, in modern Western medicine. Emphasis is placed upon the development of medical anatomy as a professional and scientific based discipline. Particular attention is devoted to developing an understanding of the fluid conceptual matrixes used across time and the factors which most influenced change. Influential people whom have shaped the discipline throughout history are briefly presented, along with milestone discoveries, which have led us to our current knowledge base, and the way we understand and practice medical anatomy today. The material is presented within a contextual matrix of other commonly recognized world events, whenever it makes sense, in order to provide a more global perspective from which to understand the people, events, and contributions.

This chapter is written for you, the medical student, in an effort to broaden your knowledge base of anatomy. The intent is to go beyond information you will memorize during medical school and provide an opportunity for you to begin to appreciate where the discipline began, where it is today, and where you might take it in the future, while developing an additional appreciation of the people and events who have gone before you. The chapter is organized chronologically for quick reference and consistency with other chapters.

None of what follows will likely be on your USMLE Step I or Step II. This material will simply make you a more informed physician and professional, open your eyes to how truths in science and medicine change, and emphasize the need to be skeptical of professional dogma of the times.

History.

Early Records, 3500 BC - 500 BC.

Historical records allow us to trace the beginnings of the systematic study of medical human anatomy back to the earliest recorded histories of the ancient civilizations of the Sumerians circa 3500 BC, ancient Egyptians circa 3200 BC, Babylonians circa 2000 BC, ancient Greeks circa 1100 BC, and ancient Romans 750 BC.

Each ancient civilization make their own unique contributions to the scientific study of medical human anatomy. It makes little sense, based upon current scientific evidence, to argue who makes the first or the most significant contributions. In combination, the ancient civilizations all contribute to laying the foundation for the scientific study of the human body for medical purposes. Many scholars identify the earliest recorded beginnings to the appearance of formal written language.

One of the earliest written languages, revealing evidence of the study of anatomy for medical purposes, is the written language of ancient Sumeria, located in Mesopotamia (present day southern Iraq), circa 3500 BC. This early written language is termed cuneiform, denoting the wedge shape impression made by the pointed reed stylus used to mark clay tablets. Writings from these tablets reveal an ordered civilization, one engaged in much commerce, and which necessitated the development of a record keeping system. This written language system provides a nonperishable method with which to record and detail anatomical observations of the human body.

There is growing evidence, based upon the recent translation of clay tablets, written in the Mesopotamian written language of cuneiform, revealing centuries of accumulated and recorded medical knowledge. These tablets are revealing detailed observations, diagnostic criteria, recommended treatments, and associated prognoses of numerous medical conditions.

Recently, thousands of additional tablets have been discovered and are now being translated by scholars JoAnn Scurlock (1953-) and Burton Andersen (1932-) (2005)[2]. To date, there is no direct report human autopsies were ever performed in ancient Sumeria. However, the tablets do reveal hundreds of detailed anatomical reports of internal human organs and structures, both normal and diseased, which could not have been observed, detailed, and correlated with normal function, without opening the body. Overall, these tablets are now beginning to reveal a rather sophisticated collection of medical knowledge, including human anatomy.

These tablets are additionally revealing the Mesopotamian approach to knowledge. The Mesopotamians applied primarily and almost exclusively an empirical approach. The fundamental basis of the empirical approach to knowledge is that knowledge can best be derived from experience and evidence. Emphasis is placed upon information obtained from one's own sensory perception of the world, as revealed through seeing, hearing, tasting, smelling, and touching. From their empirically derived knowledge base they apply inductive reasoning, moving from a set of specific observation to generalized conclusions. The empirical-inductive approach characterizes the epistemological approach of ancient Mesopotamia and the approach that characterizes most advances in anatomical knowledge for the next 5,000 years.

The empirical-inductive approach stands in contrast to the rational-deductive process approach popularized by Greek philosophers and mathematicians during Antiquity, circa 500 BC-500 AD. The Greek emphasize careful intellectual reasoning to generate general rules of nature, which are then tested using deductive reasoning to evaluate the truth of the general rule. The rational-deductive approach minimizes experience in favor of careful intellectual reasoning, maintaining the position if well-reasoned premises are true, then the conclusions derived from the premises must then be true. Deductive reasoning is applied to the intellectually derived premises to evaluate the truth of the premises and provides a method of establishing new knowledge, moving from the general to the specific.

Both epistemological approaches have strengths and weaknesses. The fundamental differences in these two approaches are striking and provide a useful contextual matrix to better understand the methods used to acquire new knowledge throughout history. The approach preferred by the ancient civilizations of Mesopotamia, preferred throughout most all history, and most frequently applied to the discovery of new anatomical knowledge, is the empirical-inductive approach and method.

The Scurlock and Andersen tablets are providing much information regarding the scope and depth of anatomical knowledge of ancient Mesopotamia and favored epistemological approach applied in the discovery of new anatomical knowledge. As the ongoing translations of Scurlock and Andersen continue, the extent and depth of anatomical knowledge of the ancient civilizations of Mesopotamia will become more clear.

Before moving on to the ancient Egyptians contribution to human anatomy, recognition of the additional contributions of the Mesopotamian civilization is in order. To better understand this ancient civilization's contribution to anatomy it is of value to understand a few of their many other contributions.

The Mesopotamians develop an original and uniform numbering system, which is applied to the study of natural events, anatomy, and accounting. Have you ever wondered why there are 60 seconds in a minute, 60 minutes in an hour, 24 hours in a day, and 360 degrees in a circle? It is the result of the sexagenimal number system (base 60) created and developed by the Mesopotamians, circa 2000 BC. The system works well for measuring time, angles, geographic coordinates, and permits easy calculations of fractions, especially important in commerce. The sexgensimal number system predates the much more familiar decimal system (base 10) of the Egyptians, first recorded circa 2000 BC.

Which of the two systems do you believe most rapidly calculates ratios naturally occurring in human anatomy? Hint: See Leonardo da Vinci in his discussion of proportions in regard to drawing the human form, presented later in this chapter.

Ancient Egyptian civilization parallels the recorded development of Mesopotamia. Records suggest there was much sharing of knowledge and goods between the two civilizations. The Egyptians had no problem opening the body and removing parts for burial. Based upon available historical evidence, including several papyri dated to the time period, the ancient Egyptians maintained an excellent knowledge of human anatomy. While religious beliefs and cultural practices prohibited medical dissections owing to the strongly held belief the whole body must be preserved in order to reunite with the spirit after death, knowledge of human anatomy was considerable.

Egyptians make significant contributions to the field of comparative anatomy. Much of the knowledge of human anatomy popularly attributed to the ancient Egyptians, upon further scholarly inspection, reflects knowledge most likely acquired from lands outside of Egypt and simply incorporated into their knowledge base. The most obvious and likely source is the many writings of ancient Mesopotamia. Much of the human anatomical knowledge of Egypt is recognized as information simply recopied from much earlier records and subsequently integrated into Egyptian writings. This is not an unusual practice and is evident throughout the history of science and medicine.

Imhotep, circa 2900 BC credited founder of Egyptian medicine and architect of the Step Pyramid is responsible for recording most of the written record of anatomical knowledge we reference today, from ancient Egypt. He has been identified as the author of numerous papyrus scrolls, including three of the most notable papyri, the Edwin Smith, Georg Ebers, and Kahun. Each papyrus is named for the person who discovered or purchased the papyrus in modern times and not for the person(s) who authored the papyrus or the person(s) who translated them. Acknowledging theses three papyri are recopied several times throughout history, the papyri still provide a useful insights into the knowledge of anatomy of the ancient Egyptians, between 3200 BC and 500 BC.

Papyrus is a thick paper-like material produced from the insides of the papyrus plant which grows in the wetlands of the Egyptian Nile Delta. Papyrus is first produced circa 3000 BC and serves as a reasonable and portable writing surface. Papyrus provides an alternative to clay tablets and animal skin parchments. Papyrus is used in Egypt until early-1100 AD, at which time it is replaced almost completely by paper. Paper is invented in China circa 200 AD. Paper slowly makes its way to Egypt and Western Europe, through the Islamic world and where it rapidly replaces clay tablets, papyrus, and parchment, as the preferred writing surface.

Trivia: The word paper is derived from the Ancient Egyptian word "papyrus".

Edwin Smith papyrus (circa 1500 BC) is purchased in 1862 by American antiquities collector and dealer Edwin Smith (1822-1906). The Papyrus is first translated during modern times by Egyptologist James Breasted (1865-1935) (1930)[3]. The Papyrus is found in the ancient Egyptian city of Thebes (present day Luxor, Egypt). The Edwin Smith papyrus scroll is approximately 500 lines of text, written on both sides of the papyrus. The Papyrus is approximately15 feet in length. It contains 48 surgical cases, grouped according to anatomical lesion and associated signs and symptoms. The Papyrus describes internal and external human anatomy in detail, including brain, heart, liver, spleen, bladder, kidneys, and vessels. Remember, while the Edwin Smith papyrus is dated circa 1500 BC it reflects anatomical knowledge detailed in writing as early as 3000 BC. The original Edwin Smith's papyrus is housed at the New York Academy of Medicine, Rare Book Room, in New York City. A complete English translation can be found online (2009)[4].

Ebers papyrus (circa 1550 BC) is purchased in 1873 by German Egyptologist Georg Ebers (1837-1898) and first translated, during modern times by Heinrich Joachim (1890)[5] into German and later into English by Bendix Ebbell (1937)[6]. The papyrus is found in the ancient Egyptian city of Thebes (present day Luxor, Egypt). The Ebers papyrus is approximately 2,289 lines, written on

110 pages, stretching over 65 feet in length. This papyrus is much more complete than the Edwin Smith papyrus and describes anatomical systems, including the heart and the vessels of the systemic blood supply. The Ebers papyrus (circa 1550 BC)[7] is currently housed in the University of Leipzig Library, Special Collections, Leipzig, Germany. A complete English translation can be found online (2018)[8].

Kahun papyrus (circa 1800 BC) is found by English Egyptologist Flinders Petrie (1853-1942), during his first excavation (1888-1890) of the workers' village (Kahun), of the pyramid Senusret II, located in the middle Egyptian oasis region of Faiyum, Egypt. The Kahun papyrus is first translated into English by F. Griffith and published as "The Petrie Papyri: Hieratic Papyri from Kahun and Gurob" (1898)[9]. The Kahun papyrus describes several topics, including literature, veterinary medicine, mathematics, laws regarding wills, and the sale of slaves. Plates V (p31) and VI of the Papyrus are of most interest here, in regard to anatomy. The plates provide a detailed description of the anatomy associated with patient complaints and offers prescribed treatments, on topics of fertility, pregnancy, contraception, and gynecological disease. The Papyrus itself is dated circa 1800 BC. However, the Papyrus contains cumulative medical knowledge, especially in regard to female health issues, dating to early ancient Egypt, circa 3000 BC. The Kahun papyrus is currently housed at University College of London. A scanned copy of the papyrus can be viewed online (2009)[10].

In summary, the Early Records of anatomy (3500 BC-500 BC) reveal a reasonable understanding of internal human anatomy, as early as the ancient civilizations of Mesopotamia and Egypt. Dissections of animals are common with evidence suggesting human dissections likely occurred, based upon the detail descriptions recently revealed in tablets and papyri from the period. The sexagesimal and decimal numbering systems provides a uniform number based measurement system and is applied to the measurement of animals and the human body. Papyri replace clay tablets for recording anatomical knowledge. The Smith, Ebers, and Kahun papyri report anatomical knowledge from the ancient civilizations, circa 3500 BC-1550 BC. Written records reveal a working knowledge of human anatomy, with practical applications, and based on social and religious belief systems. While much information is available on human anatomy during this period, there is no written record of organized, systematic study of anatomy as a scientific discipline during this period.

Antiquity, 500 BC - 500 AD.

Antiquity witnesses the development and continuing interest in studying the anatomy of the human body. Anatomy is associated with function. Clinical signs and symptoms continue to be associated with damaged anatomy. Dissections become an important procedure and contribute significantly to the advancement of medical knowledge. Instruction in anatomy is introduced into the formal education and training of future physicians. The human body begins to be understood and conceptualized within the matrix of functional human anatomy. New conceptual matrixes are offered to explain normal and abnormal functions. Information is systematically collected, recorded, and organized. World centers for scholarship are established and anatomy is studied systematically. Many fundamentals of anatomy established during Antiquity continue to be taught in medical schools today. Antiquity is an exciting time for anatomy.

Medical historians often begin the discussion of Antiquity with the introduction of Hippocrates, circa 429 BC on the island of Cos. However, approximately 100 years before Hippocrates, another influential figure, Alcmaeon of Croton establishes the first medical school in Croton. Croton, a scholastic city is located on the coast of southern Italy (sole of the boot) and approximately 1,200 miles west-northwest of the island of Cos. Croton is heavily populated by the Greeks and is part of series of Greek settlements along the Gulf of Taranto (gulf between the heel and sole of the boot of Italy). We begin our discussion in Croton.

Alcmaeon of Croton (557 BC-491 BC) ancient Greek philosopher/scientist, is one of the most important contributors of anatomical knowledge of the period. He pioneers anatomical dissection and makes several celebrated contributions based upon his dissections. He clearly establishes the anatomical connections between the eye and the brain, via the optic nerves. He observes, when the optic nerve is cut the animal cannot see. His original and only known written work, "On Nature", is perhaps the first written record in Greek medicine. Only pieces of the original document remain. Most information regarding Alcmaeon is based upon the writings of subsequent scholars e.g. Galen, circa 150 AD (1896,1952,2008)[11,12,13].

Alcmaeon of Croton applies a rational approach to collecting knowledge and making anatomical observations. He assigns function to all anatomical structures he observes. He proposes the brain to be the structure responsible for conscious sensation, thought, and memory. He further speculates on such topics as sleep, wakefulness, and postulates sleep occurs when the cerebral blood vessels are filled and wakefulness occurs when they are emptied. He is first to propose the Doctrine of humors model, within which to conceptualize and understand body function and disease. Within the Doctrine of humors conceptual matrix, he describes a need for balance between humors to maintain good physical health. Alcmaeon's contribution to first proposing the Doctrine of humors model is acknowledged by subsequent Greeks scholars Aristotle and Galan. The writings of Aristotle and Galan therefore are in conflict with the popular belief which incorrectly assigns the proposal of the Doctrine of humors to Hippocrates.

So goes the questionable practice of assigning credit for contributions in science and medicine based upon popular lore rather than primary sources.

Hippocrates (460 BC-370 BC) is born on the Greek Island of Cos. This island is located in the Aegean Sea, between Greece and Turkey, approximately 4 km off the coast of Turkey. (For us Americans who break out in a cold sweat whenever measurements are expressed in the metric system units, 4 km is approximately 2.5 miles). The island is approximately 40 km long (approximately 25 miles) and 4 km wide. During Hellenistic Greece, the period between the death of Alexander the Great in 323 BC and the annexation of the classical Greek homelands by Rome in 146 BC, the island of Cos serves as a navy outpost and a favorite resort for education and higher learning. Hippocrates, a reluctant, itinerant clinician makes no substantial contributions to the advancement of anatomy. His name is referenced when referring to a collection of medical treatises and books, assembled circa 300 BC, reflecting the collective recorded medical knowledge of Greek medicine to that point in time.

The Hippocratic Collection is comprised of approximately seventy books and about sixty treaties representing a collection of fundamental Greek medicine. The collection is collected and assembled in the Great Library of Alexandria circa 300 BC. The Collection is multi-authored and can be loosely organized into ten general areas of medicine; anatomy, physiology, general pathology, diagnosis, prognosis, surgery, gynecology and obstetrics, mental illness, and ethics. Digitized copies of the first printed editions of the Hippocratic Collection are housed in the Bibiotheque Inter-Universitiarire de Medicine of Paris (1525-1595,2009)[14]. The anatomy collection reveals an absence of systematic, gross anatomical knowledge. The anatomy collection focuses upon detail description of the heart with little attention to other anatomical systems. Nerves are described as hollow tubes.

Aristotle (384 BC-322 BC) philosopher/scientist, born in the ancient Kingdom of Macedonia, located in the northeastern region of the Greek peninsula and residing most of his life in Athens, relies heavily upon dissection, as a primary tool and an essential source of new knowledge. He focuses on comparative anatomy, although there is evidence he does dissect many human bodies. Influenced by his teacher, the Greek philosopher Plato (428 BC-348 BC), Aristotle believes only the soul is sacred and not the body. The body is simply a physical structure to house the soul. Aristotle has no problem or issues with dissecting the human body. His approach is strictly empirical. That is, knowledge is best acquired through experiences and experiments. This approach stands in in contrast to the rational approach, embraced later by Greek mathematicians e.g. Archimedes and Euclid, which states knowledge is best acquired through reason and intuitions, independent of experience or experiments.

Aristotle is credited with being first to identify the structural differences between arteries and veins. He and his contemporaries contribute significantly to the understanding and offer detailed descriptions of organ systems. Aristotle advocates the position, all body parts have function and function can be observed through the use of experiments. This fundamental mindset for acquiring new knowledge provides the early foundation for the practice still encouraged in medical students today, over 2,000 years later. Every medical student learns early in their education the value of associating anatomical structure with physiology and clinical function.

Alexander the Great (355 BC-323 BC), the ancient king of Macedonia (located in the northeast peninsula of Greek) and general who invades Egypt at 22 years of age, is important in anatomy not for his contribution as a scientist or medical practitioner, but rather for establishing a new city in Egypt, Alexandria. The new City of Alexandria is located on the western end of the Nile delta and soon becomes the center and repository for all Western world knowledge. The City maintains a commitment to new learning and knowledge for more than a thousand years. In the new City, the Alexandrian Library is founded and assembles a great collection of Hellenistic literature and scientific knowledge. (Hellenistic period spans the period from the end of the wars of Alexander the Great circa 323 BC to the annexation of Greece by the Roman Republic circa 146 BC). Intellectuals and anatomists are summoned from all parts of the western world, including Greece and Rome, to contribute to the assembly and depository of world knowledge.

The Alexandrian Library houses several hundred thousand papyrus scrolls and tablets, detailing ancient and new world knowledge, in such diverse areas of mathematics, astronomy, physics, natural sciences, and anatomy. The Library serves not only as a repository of knowledge but as an active center in establishing new knowledge. The Library often provides stipends for international scholars and their families and provides the resources for diverse and numerous active research programs. The scholastic productivity within the Library places high demand for papyrus. Little if any papyrus is exported from the Nile delta during the most productive days of Alexandria. Consequently, the world searches for an alternative, resulting in the development of parchment, as a principal writing surface elsewhere in the world.

In reference to anatomy, the City and Libraries of Alexandria are committed to the protection of old knowledge and the search for new knowledge. In the search for new knowledge the City permits dissections of criminals, alive or dead. The City thrives as a world center of scholarship, knowledge, and learning. It is at Alexandria the subjects we regard as Basic Sciences today are differentiated into separate areas of investigation and study; for example the structure of the body (anatomy) is separated from the function of the body (physiology) for the purposes of scholarly investigations.

Archimedes (287 BC-212 BC) the mathematician responsible for the law of equilibrium of fluids, the study of equilibrium of mechanical forces (statics), and the physics which explains the principles of the lever, "…Give me a lever and I will move the world...", is one of several notable non-physicians residing in Alexandria during its early days.

Euclid (325 BC-265 BC) the mathematician responsible for proving the Pythagorean Theorem ($a^2 + b^2 = c^2$) and founding Euclidean geometry is one of the notable non-physician residents of the City, during its early days and contributes to the excitement of learning and education which becomes so much a part of Alexandria.

Archimedes and Euclid rely upon rationalism and deductive reasoning, as their primary method of discovery of new knowledge. This method stands in contrast to the methods of empiricism and inductive reasoning, which had been the gold standard for anatomical investigation in Alexandria. It is reasonable to believe the methods of rationalism and deductive reasoning utilized by Archimedes and Euclid may have been applied to the study of human anatomy. The two epistemological approaches stand in contrast to one another, while exemplifying the openness to new ways of discovering new knowledge evidenced in the City and Libraries of Alexandria.

Herophilus (335 BC-280 BC) born in Chalcedon (present day Turkey) is a notable Greek figure in the history of human anatomy. He provides one of the first documented, large series of human dissections. Herophilus is credited with completing over 600 human dissections, most upon condemned criminals. He compiles one of the first standardized registries of anatomical terms. While in residence in Alexandria, he performs frequent dissections of the human body and contributes substantially to the knowledge of human anatomy. His works greatly complement the existing anatomical knowledge based primarily upon comparative anatomy. His detailed dissections result in many early anatomical descriptions of the eye, retina, lymphatic system, brain, arachnoid mater, cerebral venous sinuses and confluence, cerebral ventricles, tendons, nerves, liver, and uterus. He reports arteries to be six times thicker than veins; details sections of the small intestines; and coins the term duodenum. Herophilus holds strongly to Greek dogma, emphasizing the role and function of the balance of humors model to explain normal and impaired physical health.

Trivia: The term duodenum is derived from the Greek word "duodka" meaning twelve finger-widths in length.

Erasistratus (304 BC-250 BC) another influential Alexandrian and pupil of Herophilus contributes his detailed descriptions of the nervous systems and details the differences between sensory and motor nerves. He believes, however, as did many of this period, nerves are hollow and conduct nervous spirits. He details the cerebrum and cerebellum and contributes significantly to the anatomical and physiological study of the respiratory and digestive systems, systematically studying and assigning function. He also describes the epiglottis and its function during swallowing. Erasistratus details the anatomy of the heart and offers the term tricuspid valve to describe the valve between the right atrium and right ventricle. Unlike Herophilus, he rejects current dogma of the humors doctrine. Erasistratus embraces instead the doctrine of atomic structure. In brief, the doctrine of atomic structure maintains the human body requires inspired air "pneuma" to fill the arteries and activate the structural atoms of the body via the "pneuma" filled nerves. More on this in the Physiology chapter.

The great Greek city of scholarship Alexandria, Egypt (sic) begins its decline soon after the City's invasion by Julius Cesar in 47 BC. The City and the Alexandrian Library, the world's depository of ancient knowledge and center for new learning is burned. The Library quickly falls into decay. The Library is intentionally and totally destroyed in 391 AD, during frenzied riots instigated by fanatical Christians and under orders of the Roman Empire to destroy all non-Christian temples. So goes the complex interactions observed throughout the history of medicine and science, between academic, scholastic, social, financial, political, and religious influences.

Aulus Celsus (14 AD-37 AD), Roman encyclopedist of the period and not to be confused with Celsius (1701-1744) the Swedish astronomer who reintroduced the centigrade standard in the thermometer, is an advocate of the dissection of human cadaver. Records reveal Celsus is also not a physician by training or avocation but a scholar from a wealthy family of means. He provides an extensive encyclopedia account of the history of medicine. His encyclopedia, "De Medicina" [On Medicine] outlines the history of medicine and provides description of most organ systems in the body (circa 30 AD)[15]. It is recognized as the best surviving treaties of Alexandrian medicine known today. Celsus' "De Medicina" survives for thousands of years and is the first medical writing to be printed in moveable type (Florence, circa 1478 AD). English translated sections are available online from the Loeb Library (2009)[16].

"De Medicina" is organized into eight chapters. Each chapter addresses topics of diet and exercise; causes of disease with diagnosis and prognosis; treatments of disease, including the common cold; anatomical description of disease; pharmacology, including opiates, laxatives, and diuretics; diseases of the skin; classical operations e.g. lithotomy and the removal of cataracts; and finally treatments of dislocations and fractures. These eight chapters are one part of a much larger encyclopedia set which details agriculture, military science, jurisprudence, philosophy, and oratory. Chapter four of "De Medicina" is devoted to anatomy and disease of specific parts of anatomy. "De Medicina" is required reading of medical students throughout the world for over one and a half centuries.

Today, Aulus Celsus is best remembered for the description of four cardinal signs and symptoms of inflammation; rubor, tumor, calor, and dolor [redness, swelling, heat, and pain]. Sound familiar? Yes, today in medical school you are taught some of the same information taught to medical students over 2,000 years ago.

Trivia: Aulus Celsus' encyclopedia, "De Medicina" is the first known text to translate Greek medical terms into Latin (circa 30 AD)[15].

Galen of Pergamum (129 AD-200 AD) philosopher and physician is arguably the most prolific and influential medical writer of all time. His writing influence medical thought and teachings for over 1500 years. He is born in one of the great cultural centers of the times, the Greek city of Pergamum, into a family of wealth and means. He lives most of his life in Rome were he writes prolifically on the subject of anatomy and surgery. Records reveal he employed 20 or more scribes at any one time, committing his dictation to the written record.

As physician to the gladiators, he has numerous opportunities to observe living human anatomy. He writes extensively on the subjects of bones, joints, muscles, and trauma. A confident, dogmatic, teleological position best characterizes his writing. His positions are always clear. Every structure has a function and he knows the function. Anyone who disagrees with him simply fails to appreciate the truth. His dogma and authoritarianism remains the fountain from which most educated persons will blindly drink for over a century. Galen's treatises on anatomy, based largely upon animal anatomy, becomes the major authoritative resource for human anatomy and medicine for the next 1500 years.

Specific contributions to anatomy attributed to Galen are detailed descriptions of the spinal cord; renal-urinary systems; neuromuscular systems; the laryngeal nerves; identification of seven pairs of cranial nerves; and proclaiming the body contains two separate blood systems, one for the scarlet blood of the arteries and one for the purple blood of the veins. Galan proposes arterial blood is the end product of venous blood passing through the muscular cardiac septum from the right cardiac ventricle into the left cardiac ventricle. Venus blood is produced by the liver. Galen encourages human dissection. However, yielding to external influences e.g. organized religions, most all of the anatomical dissections performed by Galen and his contemporaries are conducted on animals. Finding from the animal dissections are generalized to the human anatomy. Errors are made, yet few challenge the authoritative writings of Galen for more than a century.

Galen conducts his studies and publishes his writings on anatomy during the time of the Christian dominated Roman Empire. This period, approximately 150 years after the destruction of the City and Libraries of Alexandria, yields to the tremendously influential pressures of the newly founded Christian Church. The Christian belief system prohibits or at least discourages the dissection of human bodies. So goes another example in the history of medicine and science of external influences and pressures restricting the pursuit of new knowledge.

Human dissection is rare during the period of the Roman Empire. The last large series of human dissections is completed by Herophilus and Erasistratus of Alexandria, 350 years before Galen. No new large series of human dissections appear for another 1000 years. Mondino de'Luzzi's manuscript "Anathomia Mondini" offers the first major series of human dissections since Alexandria (1316)[17]. This manuscript is subsequently printed and serves as the first textbook based heavily upon human dissections.

Trivia: Over twenty revised manuscript copies of "Anathomia Mondini" circulate throughout Western Europe, before the manuscript is first printed in 1478. The development of the printing press, in Western Europe around the mid-1400s provides the new technology necessary to replace the traditional handwritten manuscript method of book production.

In summary, Antiquity (500 BC- 500 AD) witnesses the founding of the first medical school by Alcmaeon of Croton and establishes the systematic study of structure and function of the human body, utilizing systematic human dissections. Alcmaeon advocates the investigation and study of functional anatomy, associating function with every anatomical structure. The doctrine of balanced humors is introduced first by Alcmaeon, at the medical school located at Croton, Italy. Hippocrates, an itinerate, reluctant clinician makes no significant contributions to anatomy. The multi authored treaties reflecting fundamental Greek knowledge of medicine and sciences, termed the Hippocratic Collection, is collected and placed in the Great Library of Alexandria, located in Egypt. The Collection contains detailed anatomical descriptions of the human heart, and addresses diverse yet integrated topics of physiology, general pathology, diagnosis, prognosis, surgery, obstetrics, gynecology, mental illness, and ethics. Aristotle describes structural differences between arteries and veins, details major organ systems, and advocates the use of human dissection to be essential for the understanding of functional human anatomy. He, like Alcmaeon before him, advocates association of every anatomical structure with a specific function. The City and Libraries of Alexandria are established and serve as centers of knowledge and new learning. Herophilus provides the first known record of a larger series of human dissections, describes the gross anatomy of the brain, and coins the term duodenum. Erasistratus describes the valves of the heart and the different functions of sensory and motor peripheral nerves. The Great Library of Alexandria is intentionally destroyed by invading military forces led by Julius Caesar. The Library and its contents are destroyed for political and religious purposes. Aulus Celsus summaries anatomical and medical knowledge to date in encyclopedia form, describes the anatomy and function of most major organ systems, and introduces the four signs and symptoms of inflammation to medicine; rubor, tumor, calor, and dolar. Galen establishes the authoritative foundation of human anatomy, based primarily upon the dissection of animals, which will serve as anatomical dogma for the next 1,500 years.

Antiquity is characterized by much effort by ruling powers, hold the destruction of the Libraries of Alexandria, to preserve the accumulated medical knowledge of the Greeks and early civilizations. The search for new knowledge is encouraged and supported. Centers of learning and investigation are established. Centers for the training of future physicians are established in Croton, Italy, the Greek settlement of Cnidus, located on the Datca peninsula (Turkey), and on the Greek island of Cos. Advances are being made in anatomy. Organized religion e.g. Christianity, appears during mid-Antiquity and greatly slows the progress in understanding the functional anatomy of the human body. Political and social unrest further slow progress. The City and Library of Alexandria are destroyed. Other cities of learning and devoted to the discovery of new knowledge within the Greek and Roman empires wane academically and culturally. The Antonine Plague (165 AD-180 AD) (smallpox) and the Plague of Cyprian (250 AD-270 AD) (smallpox) move through Europe and a large proportion of the population is lost to the infections. Attention is redirected from epistemological pursuits to physical survival. Faith-based organized religion displaces science.

Middle Ages (Medieval Times), 500 AD - 1400 AD.

Anatomy witnesses few advances during the Middle Ages.

The Middle Ages defines the historical period between the fall of the Western Roman Empire circa 475 AD and the fall of the Eastern Roman (Byzantine) Empire and its capital city Constantinople (present day Istanbul, Turkey) circa 1450 AD. Few advances are made in anatomy or scientific knowledge in general, during this 1000 year period of European history. Newly founded organized religions, both Christian and Islam, influence tremendously the directions and methods applied in anatomy and other natural sciences. Scholarship moves from the ancient centers of learning to Christian monasteries scattered throughout Europe. Human dissection which yielded much new information during Antiquity is now prohibited by both the Christian Church, founded circa 30 AD and Islam, founded circa 610 AD.

Scholarship during the Middle Ages in Europe is restricted largely to compilation and translation of Greek records of knowledge into to Latin. Latin is the preferred language of learning throughout Europe and the official language of the Christian Church. With each translation of original text the influences of organized religion and biases soon begin to appear in the Latin translations. Errors in content and reinterpretations of information to better fit into religious belief systems prove common. In addition to the modification of knowledge during the translation process, many of the original ancient records are destroyed as the result of numerous religion sanctioned military campaigns, common during the period.

Political, economic, cultural, and religious influences suppress scientific thought and creative imagination. Religious, faith based beliefs replace scientific explanations. The Church becomes central to understanding anatomy and the natural sciences. The Church offers authoritative and dogmatic explanations of nature which cannot be explained by science of the day. For example, science is unable to provide an explanation for infectious diseases which are common in Europe and which have eliminated a substantial proportion of the population. The Church however, provides a dogmatic and easily understandable explanation widely accepted by the masses. Illness is simply a punishment from God for one's transgressions. Treatment for illness is prayer and penitence. True then and true today, in the absence of a plausible scientific explanation for a natural event almost any alternative will be entertained and oftentimes accepted in order to calm the uneasiness produced by the unknown.

Scientific advances in the scientific study of anatomy come to a halt in Europe. An outcast Christian sect known as the Nestorians, travel east carrying with them many original Greek manuscripts, including those of Aristotle and Galen. The Nestorians remain devoted to scholarship and learning and survive the religious turmoil of the regions for nearly a century. They establish a center of learning in southern Persia (present day Iraq) circa 800 AD and translate many of the original Greek records, especially Galen into Arabic. During the next 500 years the most extensive understanding of medicine and all significant advances in medicine and associated fields come from Persia and the Arabic Empire.

Abu Ibn al-Razi (865 AD-925 AD) notable Persian (present day Iran) scholar is one of several non-Western European polymaths making significant contributions during this period. Al-Razi believes medicine has nothing to do with religion and religion has no place in science. Al-Razi holds, medicine should be studied and subjected to critical analysis and not blindly accepted based upon faith. His treaties on medicine are thoughtful, well organized and follow what many would consider common scientific practices of today. He carefully describes every step of his experiments so others can reproduce them and offer support or rejection of his conclusions. He believes strongly in the organization and systematic categorization of information. Al-Razi is credited with being first to classify the natural world into the now familiar categories of animal, vegetable, and mineral.

Al-Razi makes several contributions to medicine, including a massive multi-volume encyclopedia like notebook titled "Kitab-al-Hawi fi al-tibb" [The Comprehensive Book on Medicine], which organizes medical treatments of disease anatomically, from the head down (circa 925 AD)[18]. He is credited with establishing a system for classifying skin rashes, providing the necessary observational criteria for differentiating smallpox from measles, and being first to write specifically on childhood disease. His most important contribution to anatomy lies in his advocacy of careful, systematic observation of the human body, coupled with thoughtful organization of the observations, followed by the dissemination of the observations to the professional community.

Greek medical knowledge returns to Europe circa 1075 AD with the arrival of Constantine the African (1020 AD-1087 AD) to the southern Italian city of Salerno. Constantine the African arrives from North Africa and is an established Greek and Islamic medical text translator. He is invited to Salerno by the local Archbishop. The purpose of the invitation is to have Constantine the African translate the original Greek writings of Aristotle, Hippocrates, and Galen, which have been translated from Greek into Arabic by the Nestorians, from Arabic into the language of the Church, Latin. Latin is the language of Western European scholars and most preferred by the Church.

Among the many scholarly translations completed by Constantine and of historical importance is the translation from Arabic into Latin of "Kitab Kamil as-Sina'a at-Tibbiyya" [The Complete Book of the Medical Arts] written by Persian physician Ali ibn Abbass al-Majusi (980 AD)[19]. This book contains a comprehensive treatment of Arabic medicine until 1000 AD. This text includes numerous topics such as the anatomy of the brain, nervous systems, and capillary systems.

Ibn al-Nafis (1213 AD-1288 AD) an Arabian physician and notable scholar during this period is an early proponent of human dissection and postmortem autopsy. He is credited with being the first to correctly describe both the pulmonary and coronary circulations. His careful observations, thoughtful analyses bolstered by human dissections disproves the dogma of Galan, as it pertains to the circulation of blood and which has been in place for 1400 years.

Ibn al-Nafis reports in his 1242 AD manuscript, titled "Sharh Tashrih al-Qanun Ibn Sina" [Commentary on Anatomy in Avicenna's Canon], "…blood in the right ventricle of the heart must reach the left ventricle by way of the lungs alone and not through a passage connecting the ventricle, as Galen maintained…" (1242)[20]. This relatively recently discovered manuscript by Muhyo Al-Deen Altawi (1924)[21] raises the question of whom is first to report and correctly describe the anatomy of the cardio-pulmonary circulation system; Ibu al Nifis (1242)[21], Michael Sevetus (1553)[22], Realdo Colombo (1559)[23], or as popularly taught to many medical students today, William Harvey (1628)[24].

Renewed interests in anatomy and other natural sciences return to Europe. Italy especially plays an important and influential role. Anatomy, as a scientific discipline, slowly begins its return as a respected field of study in southern and Western Europe. Contributions to the advancement of new knowledge reappear in Europe.

The Scuola Medica Salernitana [Medical School of Salerno] the first medical school of Medieval Europe, bases most of its teachings upon "The Complete Book of the Medical Arts" [Kitab Kamil as-Sina'a at-Tibbiyya] as translated by Constantine. Salerno soon becomes a city of scholarship and recognized site of medical learning. The School becomes legendary for its openness to new ideas, integration of multiple cultures Italian, Greek, Arab, Christian, Jewish, and Muslim, and an unprecedented openness to admit women students and faculty. The School holds true to the ancient Greek position of the doctrine of balanced humors, teaching an imbalance in the humors blood, phlegm, black bile and yellow bile are the central causes of illness. The School openly and passionately rejects the Church's position illness is the consequence of sin. The treatment for illness therefore is restoring the balance of the humors and not prayer and penance.

Frequent dissections of animals are conducted at Salerno and dissections are integrated into the medical school curriculum. Evidence of human dissections is less clear. One can only assume human dissection may have been conducted, given the recorded history of the School's openness to new ideas, renewed interests in the search for scientific knowledge, and relative freedom from the modifying influences of organized religions.

In northern Italy, in the city of Bologna, another influential medical school is founded circa 1200 AD, the Medical Faculty at the University of Bologna. Here too human dissection is permitted for the first time since the Christian dominated Roman Empire prohibited human dissection approximately 1,200 years earlier.

Mondino de'Luzzi (1275 AD-1326 AD) born in the northern Italian city of Bologna, a Professor of Medicine at the University of Bologna, reintroduces the Alexandrian School to anatomy. Mondino de'Luzzi advocates the use of human dissection as a primary source of anatomical knowledge and anatomy remains central to the training of every medical student. His manuscript "Anathomia Mondini" [Mondino's Anatomy] provides the text which will result in the first textbook of anatomy, based upon human dissections (1316)[25]. This textbook becomes the gold standard for medical students and medical education for the next 250 years. "Mondino's Anatomy" is only displaced by Andrea Vesalius's "Fabrica" (1543)[26].

Mondino de'Luzzi's original manuscript of "Anathomia Mondini" and subsequent textbook contains no illustrations. The text includes both Latin and Arabic terms. Thirty years later, Italian physician and engineer Guido de Vigenvano (1285-1345 AD) provides illustrations to the text, in "Anathomia Designata per Figures" (1345)[27]. This publication consist of 24 plates. Eighteen of the Plates have been lost to time. Plates XI-XVI are devoted to the spinal cord, brain, meninges and trepanning have survived (1926)[28].

Imagine just for a moment trying to learn human anatomy by standing over a cadaver, while your professor reads to you in Latin excerpts from Galen's treatises on anatomy, which are based upon dog anatomy, and for additional clarity, reads excerpts from Mondino de'Luzzi's textbook, based on human dissection but without any illustrations. Aghhh….

Trivia: The term "cadaver" originates form the Latin word "cadere" meaning "to fall dead". The term is introduced into the medical literature circa 1350 AD.

Many consider Mondino de'Luzzi to be one of the many fathers of Modern Anatomy.

The contributions of non-Western European scholars to the advancement of scientific and medical knowledge appear to be greatly underrepresented in the English medical and scientific literature. Today, with the availability of rapid access and translation capabilities, the specific contributions to the life sciences of these non-Western European scholars perhaps will become more evident soon.

In summary, the Middle Ages (500 AD-1400 AD) witness the influences of the organized religions of Christianity and Islam upon the direction and methods applied in the study of anatomy. Established empirical based scientific explanations of anatomy and other natural sciences are replaced by faith based religious dogma. Scholarship in Europe is limited to the compilation and translation of Greek knowledge into the language of the Church. An outcast Christian sect, the Nestorians, carry many original manuscripts of Aristotle and Galen east, into Persia (Iran) and out of war prone western and southern Europe. Centers of learning are established in Persia. Aba al-Razi advocates separation of science from religion and offers a method of scientific investigation still followed today. Constantine the African returns to southern Italy from North Africa and translates "The Complete Book of Medical Arts", from Arabic into Latin. The Medical School of Salerno is re-established and offers a progressive and open approach to the study of anatomy. The School admits women and thrives upon contributions from diverse cultural influences from outside of Italy. The School rejects religious dogma and returns to an empirical approach in the study of anatomy and medicine. Ibn al-Nafis describes cardio-pulmonary circulation and disproves Galen dogma on this topic. De'Luzzi reintroduces the Alexandria School approach to acquiring new knowledge and offers the first textbook based upon human dissection.

As the Middle Ages come to a close, the bubonic plague returns to Europe wiping out approximately one third of the entire population of Europe. Science and medicine fail to explain the concept of contagious disease. Many return to the solace and comfort offered by organized religion. Religion offers dogmatic explanations to questions science and medicine simply cannot answer. The general populous returns to organized religion and embraces Christian and Catholic dogma. Simply stated, the Church argues disease is the resultant consequence of committed mortal sins. Prayer and penance are the remedies. So goes the Middle Ages.

Early Modern, 1400 AD - 1800 AD.

The scientific study of anatomy flourishes during the Early Modern period. Anatomy reestablishes itself as a science based discipline. The human form is examined from scientific, biometric, and artistic perspectives. Anatomists and artists work cooperatively, often using human dissection to understand the human body. Major body organ and muscle systems are identified and detailed.

Western Europe transitions from the epistemological darkness of the Middle Ages into and through a cultural movement defined by the rebirth of scholarly learning, drawing heavily upon the classical sources, and implementation of significant education reform. You recognize this period as the European Renaissance. This period is characterized by intellectual revitalization. Renaissance scholars rely upon a humanistic method of learning and acquiring scientific knowledge. The humanistic approach is a method for acquiring new knowledge, based upon the premise new knowledge is best acquired through the recovery, interpretation, and assimilation of the knowledge and values of the ancient Greeks and Romans. Human anatomical structures and their associated function are now conceptualized within a matrix of mechanistic systems. Vitalism is replaced by laws of physics. Science, medicine, and the arts intermingled freely. Anatomy, as a scientific based discipline thrives.

Leonardo da Vinci (1452-1519) an Italian, from the vineyards and olive groves of Tuscany and arguably one of the greatest artistic painters of all times, is an anatomist. Perhaps you recognize him as the individual responsible for his drawing the Vitruvian Man (1487)[29] or painting The Last Supper (1498)[30] and Mona Lisa (1505)[31]. All three works readily reveal Leonardo da Vinci's attention to anatomical detail.

The Vitruvian Man, also known as the Canon of Proportions, offers the image of a man in two superimposed positions with arms and legs apart, inscribed within in a circle, and square. The original drawing is currently housed in the Gallerie del'Accademia, located in Venice, Italy and is displayed only occasionally. The Last Supper is currently on display in the rectory of the convent of the Santa Maria delle Grazie (Our Lady of Grace) church in Milan, Italy. The Mona Lisa is on display in the Louvre Museum, Paris, France. If you ever have an opportunity to travel Europe, it is well worth the experience to view these works in person.

Leonardo da Vinci receives formal training in anatomy, initially through his apprenticeship to Andrea del Verrocchio (1435-1488), an established Italian sculptor and painter. Verrocchio insists all of his students learn anatomy. Records reveal Leonardo da Vinci quickly becomes skilled in drawing surface anatomy and soon permitted to dissect human corpses. Working with physicians in several hospitals in Florence, Rome, and Milan, Leonardo da Vinci quickly compiles a substantial catalogue of hundreds of detailed drawing of anatomical structures, including muscles, tendons, bones, heart, and assorted internal organs. He is credited as being among the first to draw a human fetus in uterus with attention to scientific detail (1510)[32]. Many of his original anatomical drawings can be found today in the Biblioteca Ambrosiana, located in Milan; the Royal Library, located in Windsor, United Kingdom; the Biblioteca Reale located in Turin, Italy; and the Louvre Museum, located in Paris, France. Occasionally, his drawings are placed on tour and can be viewed in museums of major cities throughout the world.

Several of Leonardo da Vinci's detailed observations on human anatomy in his own words can be read online in "A Treaties on Painting" (1892)[33,34]. While this publication has been criticized by some, it provides you the medical student with insights into the contributions of professional artists of the period, their attention to anatomical detail, and their many contributions to advancing anatomy as an art form and scientific discipline.

Michelangelo (1475-1565) notable Italian sculptor, contributes to the continued advancement of anatomy as an artistic subject form and scientific discipline. Michelangelo and other period artists evidence attention to detail and ability to reproduce in drawing, paintings, and sculpture, anatomically detailed and anatomically correct surface and dissected structures. Consider now, for a moment Michelangelo's sculpture in marble of the Statue of David, currently located in the Galleria dell Academeia, located in Florence, Italy (1504)[35]. Inspection of the statue, immediately reveals Michelangelo's exquisite attention to anatomical detail and exceptional ability to reproduce the human anatomical form in three dimensions. Simply amazing.

Michelangelo and Leonardo da Vinci draw the human form in varying states, stationary, in movement, nude, and dissected. Both artists participate in human dissections. Michelangelo's drawing "Libyan Sybyl" (1510)[36] is used in the painting of the Sistine Chapel ceiling. This original drawing is currently housed in the Metropolitan Museum, located in New York City. A second notable and red chalk drawing is the "Study for Adam" (1510)[37]. This drawing too is used in his preparation for the painting of the Sistine Chapel ceiling. This original drawing is currently housed in the British Museum, located in London. Attention to the human form, from an artistic perspective, provides a new perspective of observation, with the artists noting shape, shadowing, coloring, and changes with movement.

Trivia: During the Renaissance, drawings are not considered a final art form but rather part of the process for a painting or sculpture.

Andreas Vesalius (1514-1564) Belgium anatomist uses professional artists of the period to provide the much needed illustrations to accompany his anatomical text. Imagine if you will, trying to learn medical human anatomy by reading text only and without illustrations. A very disturbing image, isn't it?

Andreas Vesalius participates in frequent, detailed human dissections. He uses his direct observations, gleamed from human dissections, to correct many of the anatomical errors, presented as dogma, since the publication of Galen's textbook, written over 1500 years earlier. Much of Andreas Vesalius' early career is devoted to correcting the errors of Galen anatomy. He publishes three substantive works, which challenge longstanding and prevailing medical anatomical dogma, and changes anatomy forever. Vesalius first publishes the "Tabluae Anatomicae Sex" [Six Anatomical Drawings] (1538)[38]. This is soon followed by his most comprehensive major work "De Humani Corporis Fabrica" [Concerning the Structure of the Human Body in Seven Books] (1543,1998,1999,2003,2008,2009)[39,40,41,42,43,44] and his "De Humani Corporis Fabrica Librorum Epitome" [Abridgment of the Structure of the Human Body] (1543)[45]. Each publication corrects errors in Galen anatomy.

Andreas Vesalius benefits from changing times, attitudes, and external influences. Human dissections are now permitted. During the time of Galen, human dissections are strictly prohibited. New information made available to investigators, as the direct result of human dissection, allows many errors to be corrected and allows anatomy to move forward once again.

The "Tabluae Anatomicae Sex" is Vesalius' first substantive challenge of anatomical dogma, offering six large, precise, professionally drawn images of human anatomy. This early work corrects only a few of Galan's errors. Not too unlike today, a person first beginning their professional career might think twice before openly challenging the dogma held by the established professional academic and medical communities. With the initial acceptance of the "Tabluae Anatomicae Sex", Vesalius appears comfortable in continuing with his challenges with his publication of "De Humani Corporis Fabrica", which is more commonly referred to as simply the "Fabrica" and his "De Humani Corporis Fabrica Librorum Epitome", more commonly referred to as the "Epitome".

The "Fabrica" contains over 200 detailed high quality human anatomical drawings and over 700 pages of encyclopedia text. This seven volume masterwork details specific anatomical systems in each volume and is divided as followed: first the skeleton, second the muscles (famous drawing of muscles with skin removed), third veins and arteries, fourth nerves and genitalia, fifth organs of the abdomen, six thorax, and seven the brain. The "Fabrica" corrects additional errors in Galen anatomy. Twelve years after his original publication of the "Fabrica", Vesalius issues a second edition, reorganizing the presentation of systems, correcting errors, and adding new information collected in the years following the original publication.

Specific errors of human anatomy corrected in the "Fabrica" and based upon human dissections are; the observations the mandible is one bone not two; the sternum consists of three major divisions not seven; the fibula and tibia are longer than the humerus; the inter-ventricular cardiac septum is impermeable not porous; ligaments, tendons, and aponeurosis are not nerves; nerves originate from the brain and spinal cord not the heart; nerves are solid not hollow; and man does not have one fewer ribs than a woman.

Sensitive to the needs of medical students, Vesalius publishes an abridged version of the "Fabrica" specifically for students. This abridged version of the "Fabrica" is commonly referred to as simply the "Epitome". The "Epitome" emphasizes illustrations rather than text. The "Fabrica" and "Epitome" both use professional artists for the illustrations and provide the first comprehensive collections of the human anatomical systems based upon human dissections to date.

Vesalius is a strong proponent of completing dissections oneself rather than delegating the task to others. As the result of his personal dissections, he identifies and names the mitral valve of the heart and offers the first professionally drawn, detailed and anatomically accurate, drawings of several major nuclei and white matter tracts within the central nervous system. Specific nuclei located deep inside of the brain identified and drawn are the thalamus, globus pallidus, putamen, and caudate. Specific white matter tracts identified and drawn are the corpus callosum connecting the two cerebral hemispheres and the cerebral peduncles (anterior midbrain) connecting the cerebral hemispheres with the brain stem.

Finally in regard to Vesalius, a note regarding his contributions beyond description and illustrations of human anatomical structures. Vesalius works represent a high standard, great attention to detail, a willingness and courage to challenge medical and scientific dogma, and an accepted willingness to suffer the potential professional consequences if wrong and enjoy the rewards if correct. The same standard and risks are in operation within the professional scientific and medical communities today.

Trivia: The original, incredibly detailed and accurate, hand carved wooden blocks used in the printing of the "Fabrica" survived for over 400 years, before being loss forever. The wooden blocks are destroyed by military conflict during the Second World War (1939-1945), when the Munich, Germany museum, in which the wooden blocks were being housed is destroyed.

Gabriele Falloppio (1523-1562) Italian anatomist, student of Vesalius, and perhaps remembered by medical students for his substantial contributions detailing the anatomy and functions of the female and reproductive systems, actually focuses most of his studies on the anatomy of the head. He details the middle and inner ears. Gabriele Falloppio is particularly interested in the study of the tympanic membrane, round and oval windows, and their relationship with the vestibular apparatus and cochlear. Additionally, Gabriele Falloppio provides detailed observations and descriptions on the development of bone. He pioneers and performs frequent dissections of human fetuses, new born infants, and children. He is responsible for naming numerous common anatomical structures e.g. the placenta (literally flat cake or pancake), ovaries, hymen, clitoris, vagina, and Fallopian tubes (1562)[46].

So ends the Greek, Alexandrian, and Galenian tradition of naming anatomical structures according to form and function and begins the popular professional practice in medicine and science of naming anatomical structures and diseases after oneself.

Bartolomeo Eustachio (1514-1574) Italian anatomist and contemporary of Falloppio makes contributions to anatomy with his studies of the middle and inner ears. He is first to publish observations of the anatomy of the pharyngo-tympanic tube connecting the middle ear and pharynx (1562)[47]. This structure will later bear his name. Less known, he describes in detail the anatomy of the dissected fetus and newborns, kidneys, venous systems, and teeth. He is credited with the discovery of the supra-adrenal glands and sympathetic ganglia. A stanch supporter of Galen dogma, Bartolomeo Eustachio spends much time and professional efforts directed to maintaining dogma and disproving the anti-Galen findings of Vesalius.

Eustachio compiles a remarkable series of engravings, detailing human anatomy however he refuses to publish the works in fear of excommunication by the Catholic Church. Some scholars argue, had he published his works, the field of anatomy would have been advanced by 200 years. The vast majority of his works are never published, even after his death. Some of his anatomical drawings survive as engraved copperplates and are published by the Italian anatomist and epidemiologist Giovanni Lansisi (1654-1720), approximately 125 years after Eustachio's death. Giovanni Lansisi provides his own text to accompany the engravings and publishes them as the "Tabulae Anatomicae Bartholomaei Eustachi" [Anatomical Illustrations of Bartolomeo Eustachio] (1714)[48]. Several of the Eustachio's engraved prints can be viewed today online (2009)[49].

Trivia: Eustatius did not assign his name to the pharyngo-tympanic tube he so elegantly describes in 1563. Rather the familiar term "Eustachian tube" is first assigned 130 years after Eustatius's death by the Italian anatomist Antonio Valsalva (1704)[50]. Yes, this is the same Italian anatomist, Antonio Valsalva (1666-1773) that gives us the Valsalva maneuver, you likely learned during your Physical Diagnostics course.

Italy remains the center for tremendous advances, throughout the Renaissance, in part due to advanced thinking and openness to new knowledge. Italy, unlike other Western European countries, permits dissection of women within the country's scholastic centers. This contributes enormously to understanding the differences in the internal anatomy of males and females. By the early-1600s, the English begin to contribute to the advancement of anatomy, as a science based discipline

William Harvey (1578-1657), English physician provides anatomy with several meaningful contributions. However, he is oftentimes credited with discoveries he never actually makes. So goes the too common and continuing practice of attributing discovery to individuals whom simply popularize or disseminate new information, rather than to the person actually making the discovery. So too is the case with many of the discoveries attributed to William Harvey. These misattributions, none the less, do not mitigate his actual contributions.

William Harvey is largely responsible for introducing Western Europe to the discovery of the cardio-pulmonary circulation, originally made by Ibn al-Nafis circa 1242 AD. Additionally and more original contributions are application of biometric calculations, coupled with keen observations and thoughtful analyses used to dispel longstanding medical dogma. For example; Harvey embraces the concept, blood circulates throughout the body and returns to the heart in a single closed vascular system. This is the model of Ibn al-Nafis and stands in stark contrast to the accepted Galen medical dogma of Western Europe. The dogma of the day simply states; blood moves from its source where it is produced in the liver (venous blood), moves to the heart (arterial blood), then on to other vital organs and tissues, were blood is simply consumed by tissues.

Based upon careful observation, numerous human dissections, synthesis of available information, and biometric calculations Harvey proposes an alternative. In a 1616 lecture he announces his conceptualization of the circulatory system, which is soon followed by a brief published manuscript, approximately 12 years later, titled "Exercitatio Anatomicia de Motu Cordis er Sanguinis et Sanguinis in Animalibus" [An Anatomical Exercise on the Motion of the Heart and Blood in Animals] (1628)[51]. This work is translated from Latin into English twenty-five years later (1653)[52]. In this 73 page publication, Harvey argues blood is pumped throughout the body by the heart, rather than simply moving down a pressure gradient from the source of its production to the point of consumption by tissues. He further suggests viewing the heart as a pump, emphasizing the heart can be studied and understood just as any mechanical device. This mechanistic view is consistent with the Renaissance mindset and rejection of the established vitalist view held by the Church.

Harvey is one of the first to apply biometric calculations in guiding his assessment of human anatomy and in particularly movement of blood through the body. Observing the heart pumps approximately two ounces of blood out of the left ventricle with every completed contraction, and the heart completes approximately 72 contractions every minute, the total result is approximately 1,620 gallons (sic) of blood needing to be produced by the heart and liver and subsequently consumed by body tissues every day!

Harvey's challenge to Galen dogma is met with much professional criticism. The most ardent of all is French anatomist Jean Riolan (1577-1657). Riolan is a vocal proponent of the traditional Galen school and challenges Harvey directly in "Opuscula Anatomica" [The Anatomical Works] (1649)[53]. Other noted anatomists and colleagues e.g. Thomas Willis, Thomas Wharton, and Thomas Sydenham all remain silent on Harvey's discovery, for over a decade after Harvey makes his initial presentation to the medical and scientific communities, circa 1628-1657 (1957)[54]. Withstanding the initial challenges and nonsupport from his colleagues and established scientific and medical communities, Harvey's conceptualization of a single, closed cardio-pulmonary and circulatory system for blood is accepted by the scientific and medical communities, during his lifetime.

True then and true today, many original ideas which challenge dogma of the day are met with considerable professional resistance, both active and passive, and can pose a substantial professional risk to the person daring to offer innovative and alternative explanations of established scientific and medical knowledge. Few take the risk and the few that do often contribute significant advances to their discipline's field of knowledge. Innovative challenges prove to be either correct or incorrect over time. If proven correct, the challenges provide a new way in which to understand old information and provide new directions for study. If proven incorrect, the challenges provide the necessary impetus for the professional communities to take time to re-evaluate their positions and re-accept current dogma or offer an alternative. In either event, thoughtful challenges to existing dogma are useful in advancing a discipline's knowledge base.

Marcello Malpighi (1628-1675) Italian anatomist, aided by advances in microscope technologies, reports his discovery of capillaries, three years after Harvey's death. Malpighi's report provides the anatomical evidence to corroborate the proposed anatomical connection between the arterial and venous systems (1661)[55].

Thomas Willis (1621-1675) English anatomist maintains particular interests in the brain and nervous systems. Most medical students will immediately recognize him for his description of the anastomoses of arterial blood vessels located at the base of the brain, which connects the anterior and posterior blood supplies of the cerebral hemispheres. Yes, the Circle of Willis. He publishes a detailed account of his anatomical observation of the Circle of Willis and nervous systems, in "De Anatome Cerebri" (1664)[56]. In addition to his anatomical descriptions of the circle of arteries, he provides detailed descriptions of white matter tracts connecting brain within and between cerebral hemispheres, and details much of the cerebellum. Willis further describes the brain as a gland capable of secretions, having effects on tissues at great distances from the brain itself. So begins the foundation of conceptual thought and reports of neuroendocrinology.

Unknown to many medical students, Willis introduces the term "mellitus", from the Latin meaning "honey", to differentiate it from diabetes insipidus (1670)[57]. For completeness and not attributed to Willis, "insipidus" is derived from the Latin meaning "without taste" and "diabetes" is derived from the Greek meaning "passing through". Diabetes mellitus is characterized by sweet tasting urine in contrast to diabetes insipidus which has no sweet taste.

Thomas Wharton (1614-1673) English anatomist is most remembered for his contributions offering detailed descriptions of glands, especially the pancreas, the anatomy of the submandibular salivary systems, and first to describe the Wharton jelly of the umbilical cord (1656)[58]. Although Wharton simply describes his Jelly and correctly associates function as a physiological clamp of umbilical vessel after separation of the umbilical cord from the placenta, today it is additionally recognized as a potential source of non-embryonic stem cells.

Antonio Valsalva (1666-1723) Italian anatomist, student of Marcello Malpighi, and professor to Giovanni Morgagni focuses much of his professional attention on the study of the ear. Antonio Valsalva details the anatomy, physiology and pathology of the human ear in "De Aure Humana" [The Human Ear] (1704)[59]. It is in this publication he offers his suggested subdivision of the ear into the external, middle, and inner ear. "De Aure Humana" remains the gold standard on the ear for over a century.

Valsalva is perhaps recognized by most medical students today as the individual who introduced the simple clinical maneuver which bears his name. This procedure, the Valsalva maneuver, continues to be used and is most often performed during the clinical assessment of cardiac functions.

Recall, the Valsalva maneuver is performed by having your patient forcibly exhale against resistance; for example closing their mouth and pinching off their nostrils to prevent exhaled air from leaving the body. The maneuver is used today to equalize pressure between the middle ear and sinuses, stimulate the parasympathetic innervation of the heart resulting in slowing of cardiac contractility rate, and to amplify cardiac murmurs on clinical auscultation examination. The same procedure is often used to equalize ear and ambient pressures when SCUBA diving, driving a car high in the mountains, or traveling in non-pressurized airplane cabins. Do you remember why the maneuver produces its desired effects?

Giovanni Morgagni (1682-1771) Italian anatomist, prosecter for Valsalva, and medical school lecturer to Antonio Scarpa (1742-1832). Morgagni assists Valsalva in the preparation of "De Aure Humana" early in his career. Yes, Giovanni Morgagni's medical student, Antonio Scarpa is the same Scarpa who later describes the deep thick membrane layer of the anterior abdominal wall, Scarpa fascia (1809)[60]. Giovanni Morgagni, at 79 years of age, publishes arguably his most important work; "De sedibus, et causis morborum per anatomen indagatis" [Seats and causes of disease investigated by means of anatomy] (1769)[61]. This massive, comprehensive and historically significant publication lays the foundation for modern anatomical pathology. The volumes report in detail 640 autopsy dissections and correlates anatomical pathological findings with clinical history and clinical findings. Among notable observations made in this publication, Morgagni describes the tetralogy of Fallot, pneumonia with consolidation, cerebral hemorrhages, and offers a detail descriptions of cerebral air embolisms, often associated with decompression sickness (the bends) (1769)[61]. He is a vocal proponent of using anatomical structure as the basis for all medical assessments, diagnosis, and treatments.

Trivia: French anatomist Etienne-Louis Arthur Fallot (1850-1911) (re)describes the condition, characterized by four congenital heart defects, originally described by Danish anatomist Nicolas Steno (1673)[62], Italian anatomist Giovanni Morgagni (1769)[61], and Dutch anatomist Edward Sandifort (1777)[63]. Fallot claims priority of discovery and assigns his name (1888)[64]. Today, the condition, the most common cause of blue baby syndrome, is simply termed the tetralogy of Fallot. So goes another example of physicians from the 1800s claiming priority for discovery of conditions previously discovered and assigning their name to the condition.

William Smellie (1697-1763) Scottish obstetrician is best remembered for his internal anatomical illustrations of the full term pregnant female (1754)[65]. A digitized copy of the original publication can be found online from the University of Madrid. Smellie's "Tables" are intended as a "birthing manual" and contain exquisite illustrations of fetus and mother in various positions, demonstrating internal forces during different stages of delivery.

Throughout William Smellie's writing, he emphasizes the importance of becoming a master of anatomy, for any who may choose to engage in the practice of delivering infants. He describes the mechanisms of labor and explains how an infant's head changes position during childbirth, as it passes through the pelvic canal. Among his many contributions, he makes and reports detailed measurements of the fetus in utero.

From an educational perspective, Smellie is credited with being first to incorporate a manikin into the training of obstetrics. A novel idea at the time and one which will be generalized to other medical specialties and soon becomes common place in medical education and training. Perhaps no other single figure in history has impacted the future of obstetrics as William Smellie.

William Hunter (1718-1783) Scottish anatomist and a medical student of William Smellie, offers internal illustrations of the full term pregnant female (1774)[66]. Two years later during 1776, he founds the Windmill Street School of Anatomy in the Soho district of London. William Hunter gives regular anatomy lectures, performs human dissections which are open to the general public, and trains many of the most talented anatomists and surgeon of the time. The School (a house, museum, and dissecting theater) continues to be used for anatomical dissections until 1832, fifty years following Hunter's death. The building remains standing today in London (Westminster) and is now used as part of the stage and dressing rooms of the performing arts, West End Lyric Theater.

William Hunter offers one of the first series of printing plates illustrating the pregnant female body with fetus (1774)[66].The plates are followed approximately 20 years later and after his death, by accompanying text (1794)[67]. The text provides a detailed anatomical description of each plate. Hunter's illustrations detailing the anatomy of the human gravid uterus complements well the work previously offered by his medical school professor William Smellie. Both publications are original and provide the first detailed and anatomically accurate illustrations of the pregnant female and internal anatomical processes of normal and abnormal birthing.

Anatomy continues to make advancements in Italy, France, and England, throughout the 1700s. It is not until the mid-1700s did anatomy, as an established medical discipline, make its way to the United States. The first formal combined course of human gross anatomy and human dissection, within the United States is taught at the University of Pennsylvania, circa 1745 (1958)[68]. Since its introduction into the medical education curriculum over 250 years ago, human dissection continues to be an integral part of the education and training of every first year medical student.

As reasonably expected, the religious, political, social, educational, and financial issues surrounding human dissection present in Europe for thousands of years come to the United States with the introduction of human dissection into the medical school curriculum. Established U.S. religious, political, social, medical, and educational institutions begin their struggle with the many and long standing issues always associated with conducting human dissections. Is it morally right? Morally wrong? Where will the cadavers be acquired? How will the cadavers be acquired? Is human dissection a useful educational experience for medical students?

The State of Massachusetts in 1784 passes state legislation in regard to human dissection. The legislation is passed as a hopeful, shocking deterrent, in efforts to reduce the practice of dueling within the State of Massachusetts. In brief, the Massachusetts law states "...a person hath been killed in fighting a duel...is to be buried without a coffin, with a stake drove through the body... or shall deliver the body to any surgeon or surgeons to be dissected and anatomized..." This legislation continues in Section 4 "...any person who shall slay or kill another in a duel...upon conviction shall...be dissected and anatomized..." (1784,1822)[69]. United States Federal legislation soon follows with similar deterrent objectives stating a Federal judge may add dissection to the sentence of death for any person convicted of murder (1790)[70]. So goes the early rationale and governmental regulations pertaining to human dissections in the USA.

In summary, the Early Modern Period (1400-1800 AD) witnesses the use of professional artists to illustrate internal and external human anatomies and to accompany anatomical text; Leonardo da Vinci completes the Vitruvian Man, emphasizing ratios between human anatomical structures; Michelangelo completes the Statue of David, emphasizing perspective and ratio between human anatomical structures; Vesalius offers his encyclopedic the "Fabrica"; Falloppio offers his descriptions and illustrations of the female reproductive system; Eustachio describes his tube, the ears, and pleas for a return to Galen dogma; Harvey applies biometrics and brings to Western Europe the conceptual matrix of a single, closed cardio-pulmonary and systemic circulatory system for blood; Malpighi observes the capillary connecting venous and arterial vessels; Willis gives us his Circle; Wharton his Jelly; Valsalva his maneuver; Steno, Morgagni, Sandifort the tetralogy of Fallot; Smellie and Hunter the anatomy of the pregnant human female; the University of Pennsylvania, the first required human dissection course in U.S. medical schools; and the U.S. Federal and State governments pass legislation permitting dissection of individuals, convicted of dueling or murder.

Middle Modern, 1800 AD - 1900 AD.

Anatomy, as a scientific and professional discipline, advances quickly during the 1800s.

Anatomists of the 1800s finalize the identification of gross internal human anatomical structures and offer new organizational systems, based upon an integration of structure, physiology, and function. Anatomy grows as a formal discipline, identifies new areas of investigation, and expands beyond gross anatomy. New areas of study are quickly established. Anatomy becomes more interdisciplinary, drawing upon and contributing to advances in embryology, developmental biology, histology, pathology, anthropology, and medicine. Legislation is enacted in an attempt to regulate the trafficking of human bodies for dissection purposes. The concept of evolution and the processes of natural selection are introduced, applied to biology, and immediately investigated by anatomists. Innovative imaging tools are introduced to better view the internal structures of the human body. Anatomy matures as a discipline, establishes standardized nomenclatures of anatomical structures, and establishes professional organizations.

Human dissection is incorporated into the training of most medical students in the USA and Europe. Human dissection is recognized and valued as an important and necessary component of the training curriculum of future physicians. Demand for human cadavers rapidly increases. By 1850, over half of the established medicals schools in the USA offer formal courses in human dissection. In Europe the demand for human cadavers is higher. The result of increased demand and limited supply begins the socially disturbing practice of trafficking in human bodies, for the purpose of medical education dissections, in both the USA and Europe (1874)[71].

Focusing for the moment on Europe and specifically the United Kingdom, for illustrative historical purposes, the only legal way to obtain a human body for medical or scientific dissection prior to 1832 is by court order and only then if a criminal has been condemned to death. Given the great emphasis placed upon the value of human dissection, for medical education purposes, the demand is very high and supply limited. When demand exceeds supply, motivated and enterprising individuals will devise a way to satisfy the demand. So too is the case in meeting the high demand for human bodies to be used in medical education dissections.

Robert Knox (1791-1862) Scottish anatomist and a much favored private lecturer of anatomy in Edinburgh, is most remembered for his efforts to maintain a sufficient supply of fresh human bodies for dissection instruction for his medical students. Limited supply and high demand, prior to 1832, result in the need and practice of purchasing fresh human bodies for dissection purposes. The practice of supplying fresh bodies to anatomists for dissection is soon recognized to be a financially profitable enterprise. Given the high demand, limited supply, and large financial gains at stake, some engage in questionable and sorted practices in efforts to meet the high demand. Practices of grave robbing, soon after a burial and occasionally murder are employed to meet the demand for fresh cadavers.

The practice becomes problematic in Edinburgh, during the late-1820s. Two notable and infamous figures, William Hare and William Burke, supply Robert Knox with a steady supply of fresh cadavers in exchange for payment. The acquisitions of the bodies are frequently by way of murder. Delivery to Robert Knox and payment are often made under the cloak of darkness. William Hare and William Burke are arrested and convicted of 17 serial murders, known as the West Port Murders of 1827-1828. William Burke is hanged and dissected for his participation. William Hare is released upon providing Kings' evidence against William Burke. Robert Knox remains silent and is not prosecuted. Five years later, Parliament addresses the pressing demand for human bodies need for medical education purposes and passes the Warburton Act (1832)[72], which increases the legal supply of fresh cadavers available to UK medical schools for dissection.

Recall, human dissections must be performed soon after death and before tissues begin to deteriorate, especially soft tissues. Prior to 1850 there is no formalin or other suitable fixative available to maintain and preserve the integrity of soft tissues. Hard tissues such as bone and teeth are easily prepared and studied long after the soft tissues has decomposed. The anatomist and medical student of this period and before require access to a recently deceased person, should they wish to investigate organs, muscles, vessels, glands, or other soft tissues.

Most of you remember the smell of formalin, from the many hours you spent in the gross anatomy dissection laboratory, during your first year of medical school. Imagine the smells experienced by medical students during the time before formalin and other tissue preservatives. See the Pathology chapter of this book for a discussion on the discovery and development of formalin and how it and other preservatives changed medical anatomy and medical pathology as scientific disciplines.

Charles Darwin (1809-1882) English naturalist and medical school drop-out, contributes to anatomy by opening new areas of investigation. His most recognized work, "On the Origin of Species by Means of Natural Selection", proposes a theory of evolution and identifies processes of natural selection (1859)[73]. The publication rekindles anatomists' interests in comparative anatomy and sparking anatomists' interests in evolutionary anatomy.

Charles Darwin, prior to embarking upon his historic voyage aboard the HMS Beagle in 1831 and to publishing his thoughts on evolution and natural selection, struggles as a student in medical school. At the insistence of his father, an established physician himself, Darwin completes only the first two years of his medical education, before focusing his attention on his passionate interest of natural history. A quick reading of a collection of letters between Charles Darwin and his family members, while attending the Basic Sciences portion of his medical education program, reveals his struggle with the subject material, medical school professors, family politics, and personal interests. As a current medical student, perhaps you recognize some of these stressors experienced by Charles Darwin and may experience them yourself today.

In a letter from Charles Darwin to his sister Caroline, in regard to his medical school anatomy class at Edinburgh University taught by Alexander Monro (tertius) (1773-1859), "…I dislike him & his lectures so much that I cannot speak with decency about them….he made his lectures on human anatomy as dull as he was himself…" (1826, letter January 6)[74]. Looks like a posting that might appear today on a current medical student's Facebook page. Right? In a subsequent letter from his sister Susan, she expresses the family's concern; "…I have a message from Papa to give you, which I am afraid you won't like, he desires me to say that he thinks your plan of picking and chusing (sic) which lectures you like to attend, not at all a good one, and as you cannot have enough information to know what may be of use to you, it is quite necessary for you to bear with a good deal of stupid and dry work…". (1826, letter March 27)[75]. It appears the standard line of reassurance from parents and occasional medical school faculty today has a long history of use by parents and medical school faculty. Soon after these letter exchanges, Charles Darwin drops out of medical school and pursues his joyful interests in natural history.

The history of medicine is filled with similar stories. If medicine is truly for you, great; follow your passions. If not, consider alternatives. The world is a big place filled with numerous alternative opportunities to medicine, with great personal and meaningful rewards. Something to consider if you too are struggling in medical school or even if you are succeeding as a medical student. OK…back to anatomy of the 1800s.

Charles Bell (1774-1842) Scottish anatomist and distinguished lecturer of anatomy maintains particular interests in the brain and nervous systems. He publishes numerous papers on the topic. Often the publications are co-authored with his elder brother John Bell (1763-1820), also an anatomist. Bell is an excellent artist and combining this talent with his writing, provides detailed illustrations of anatomical structures to accompany his texts. Bell frequently gives private lectures and demonstrations in anatomy to medical students and the general public in Edinburgh.

The established academic medical community at neighboring Edinburgh University is so annoyed by Charles Bell's success in private instruction, he is barred by the University's faculty from practicing in University affiliated hospitals or holding a University faculty position. So goes professional jealousies and politics then and today. Prohibited from practicing in Edinburgh, Charles Bell moves to London and continues private instruction of anatomy. He quickly proves to be students' favorite instructor of anatomy, at William Hunter's private Windmill School of Anatomy, during the period of 1812 and 1825.

Charles Bell self-publishes a brief pamphlet early in his career titled, "An Idea of a New Anatomy of the Brain", in which he describes the differences in form and function of the cerebrum and cerebellum (1811)[76]. He also describes his animal works, resulting in his identification and differentiation of neural fibers of the spinal nerve "…united in one bundle…", entering and exiting from the same side of the spinal cord. Bell describes the spinal rootlets as "…sensible and nonsensible…" with sensible fibers responsible for volitional and conscious actions, while nonsensible fibers are responsible for involuntary actions. He proposes sensible fibers have their origin and destination in the cerebral hemispheres, whereas nonsensible fibers have their origin and destination in the cerebellum. There are only 100 copies of this pamphlet printed and only distributed to close friends and colleagues.

Frequently and incorrectly this publication (1811)[76] is cited as Charles Bell's first report of the differentiation of the anterior motor and posterior sensory spinal rootlets. Actually, that distinction did not occur for another 10 years and first appears in Bell's landmark paper presented to the Royal Society (equivalent of the USA Academy of Science) titled "On the Nerves: Giving an account of some experiments on their structure and functions which lead to a new arrangement of the systeme" (1821)[77]. It is also within this presentation Bell first describes the selective loss of sensation and motor functions following the severing of branches of cranial nerves (CN) CN V and CN VII. His anatomical and clinical observations result in the accurate description of the clinical syndrome of unilateral paralysis of CN VII we term Bell's palsy.

Francois Magendie (1783-1855) French anatomist and physiologist, aware of Bell's 1821 report quickly duplicates Bell's finding. Magendie then applies the concept of independent sensory and motor function to the spinal rootlets. He selectively severs the anterior then the posterior rootlets, resulting in paralysis and loss of sensation respectively. He publishes his finding, confirming Bell's separation of sensory and motor functions in the cranial nerve systems, and offers his original findings of the separation of sensory and motor functions at the spinal rootlet level (1822a,1822b)[78,79]. In combination, these experimental studies into functional microanatomy provide the necessary information which will guide advances in neurophysiology for the next 195 years and beyond.

Francois Magendie, Charles Bell, and the professional community at large engage in much debate, as to whom should receive credit for this major discovery Bell or Magendie (1847)[80]. Did Bell make the original discovery? Did Magendie steal the idea and claim credit for himself? Did Magendie simply build on the findings of Bell and make an original contribution? Records reveal a politically acceptable compromise is reached within the profession; both men received credit for the differentiation of sensory and motor neural fibers. The professional community never resolves the debate, whether the observation should be called the Bell-Magendie law or Magendie-Bell law. So goes the struggle then and today for professional recognition for original contributions and the flurries of accusations of intellectual theft associated with major discoveries in science and medicine.

Frederich Gustav Jakob Henle (1809-1885) German anatomist describes the structure and function of the renal nephron (Henle's Loops) (1841)[81]. Additionally, he makes substantial contributions in describing the anatomy of the lymphatic systems, distribution of human epithelium, and is an early vocal proponent of the Germ theory of disease. He contributes an exceptionally well-illustrated textbook on anatomy in 1873 titled "Handbook of Systematic Anatomy" (1873)[82]. This textbook is recognized for completeness, detail descriptions, and masterfully well produced anatomical illustrations. The textbook stands as a landmark publication in anatomical knowledge of the late-1800s.

Henry Gray (1827-1861) English anatomist most remembered for his contribution of "Gray's Anatomy", a comprehensive yet relatively inexpensive textbook, originally designed for medical students in the UK. Gray publishes the first edition, "Anatomy of the Human Body" (Gray's Anatomy) during the late-1850s (1858)[83]. The edition contains approximately 750 pages, including over 360 illustrated figures. The illustrations are produced by English anatomist Henry Carter (1831-1897), who originally is assigned co-authorship with Gray by the publisher. However, upon much opposition by Gray, Carter is removed from authorship and noted only as the illustrator. So goes another example in history of medicine of professional competition and which is still common today. "Gray's Anatomy" has remained in print continuously for 150 years and is now in its current 41th edition (2016)[84].

By the mid-1800s anatomy shifts focus from identification of gross structure to microscopic investigations of normal and abnormal tissues. Microbiology becomes an active area of investigation with advances in the microscope and experimental works in support of the recently proposed Germ theory of disease.

Agostimo Bassi (1773-1856) Italian entomologist proposes Germ theory of disease (1835)[85,86]. The Germ theory simply states, disease is the result of microorganisms and not the product of spontaneous generation. Germ theory replaces the Aristotelian conceptualization of disease of spontaneous generation, which had guided medical diagnosis and treatment for over 2,000 years.

From the mid-1800s until the end of the century, anatomy continues to identify associations between anatomical structure and function. Anatomy is correlated with clinical findings and becomes common practice. Professional societies devoted to the advancement of the anatomical sciences are established in Europe and the United States. Anatomy nomenclature is standardized. New and innovative imaging technologies are introduced, making noninvasive visualization of internal human anatomical structures possible for the first time.

Two early professional societies are founded and devoted exclusively to the advancement of anatomy as a scientific and professional discipline. The Anatomische Gesellschaft [Anatomical Society] is founded in Germany in 1886 with 40 members. Albert Kolliker serves as the Society's first president, in 1876 (2018)[87]. The American Association of Anatomists is founded in the USA in 1888. American anatomist and parasitologist Joseph Leidy (1823-1891) (identification of trichinosis from undercooked pork fame) is the Association's first president, while American physician George Huntington (1850-1816) (Huntington disease fame) is the Association's fifth elected president (1891)[88].

By the end of the 1800s there are over 50,000 anatomical terms to name body parts. The large number and oftentimes confusing terms are the consequence of the same anatomical structure being named differently, based upon the use of Greek or Latin derivations, the anatomist's nationality, and the emerging popular use of eponyms beginning in the early-1800s, university politics, and more. This creates a confused vocabulary by the end of the 1800s which interferes with the effective communication between anatomists internationally. The solution and oftentimes the sign of a maturing discipline is standardization of the professional nomenclature. The first international system of anatomical terms is published in 1891, as the "Basle Nomina Anatomica" (BNA) (1891,1895)[89]. This publication provides the first attempt of an international standard for anatomical terms. Not without its very vocal critics and not without the customary political infighting among professionals (still occurring today) the publication reduces the number of terms from 50,000 to 5,528. Revisions and standardization of internationally accepted anatomical terms and nomenclature continues today.

Medical imaging technologies continue to advance throughout the 1800s, providing new and innovative methods to visualize human anatomical structures. Innovative imaging technologies open new areas of investigation and contribute to advancing the scientific study of human anatomy for medical purposes.

Phillip Bozzini (1773-1809) of Italy, introduces the Lichtleiter (light guiding instrument) to examine the urinary tract, rectum, and pharynx (1809) [90]. While written records demonstrate the ancient Greeks and Romans used instruments to explore internal structures of the human body, Bozzini's device serves as a reasonable approximation of the modern endoscope. Antoine Desormeaus (1815-1882) of France introduces his version of the instrument for the purpose of examining the urinary tract and bladder (1853)[91]. Antonie Desormeaus is credited with introducing the term "endoscope" into the professional literature. Antoine Desormeaus uses an open flame as the light source. Maximillian Nitze (1848-1906) of Germany, twenty three years later, uses Edison's new light bulb as a light source and introduces the cystoscope (1876,1879)[92,93].

Ludwig Turch (1810-1868) and Johann Czermak (1828-1873) introduce the laryngoscope, during the mid-1850s (1860,1863)[94,95]. The men engage in a much heated professional debate conducted over the course of several years, as to who should be awarded credit for its invention and development (1867)[96]. Actually, Manual Garcia, a singing teacher in London, had published a paper in 1855, "Physiological Observations of the Human Voice "(1855)[97], describes the laryngeal mirror and uses the mirror to successfully complete an examination of his own larynx. He describes its detailed anatomy and motion, years before Ludwig Turch or Johann Czermak publish their first papers. Garcia's significant contribution is often neglected in present day literature. Similar bitter professional battles for recognition, as evidenced between Turch and Czermak, continue to be fought today. See the battle between MRI developers Paul Lauderbaur, Peter Mansfield, and Raymond Damadian (2003) and which will be discussed later in this chapter.

Wilhelm Roentgen (1845-1923) German physicist changes imaging of anatomical structures forever, by introducing X-ray imaging in his original paper "Uber eine neue Art von Strahlen" [On A New Kind of Ray] (1898)[98]. While X- rays were known thirty years prior to Roentgen's first paper, it was Roentgen who studies the rays systematically and produces the first X-ray image of human structure, his wife's hand. Roentgen coins the term X-ray, simply indicating the unknown properties and applications of this electromagnetic energy. Roentgen is awarded the first Nobel Prize (1901) in the category of Physics "...in recognition of the extraordinary services he has rendered by the discovery of the remarkable rays ..." (1901)[99]. X-ray imaging is the most common form of anatomical imaging used today.

Trivia: German physicist Wilhelm Roentgen, French physicist Pierre Curie, and his wife Polish physicist Marie Curie share the 1903 Nobel Prize in Physics "...in recognition of the extraordinary services they have rendered by their joint researches on the radiation phenomena..." (1903)[100]. All three refuse to take out patents related to their discoveries, making the new technology available to all.

In summary, the Middle Modern period (1800-1900 AD) witnesses the finalization of identification of gross, internal human anatomical structures; anatomy becomes more interdisciplinary; human dissection becomes the standard in medical education curriculum within the US; Hare and Burke are prosecuted for providing human bodies for anatomical dissections by questionable means; Charles Darwin drops out of medical school to pursue his passions and introduces the ideas of evolution and natural selection; Bell and Magendie differentiate sensory and motor neural fibers; Henle describes his Loops; Gray publishes his anatomy textbook for medical students; professional societies are established in Europe and USA, for the purpose of advancing anatomy as a scientific discipline; Bozzini, Desormeaus, and Nitze visualize internal structures with new imaging tools the endoscope and cystoscope; and Roentgen successfully images internal anatomical structures with the X-ray.

Late Modern, 1900 AD - 2000 AD.

Anatomy progresses slowly during the 1900s compared to the advances during the previous 400 years. The discipline moves into a period of normal science, as conceptualized within Thomas Kuhn's developmental matrix on the history of science (1962)[101]. No particularly new or innovative contributions are made. Most of the 1900s is characterized by slowly adding to and building upon established knowledge.

Anatomy, establishes new professional associations devoted to clinical anatomy and other emerging subspecialties; rediscovers the value of professional artists in the preparation of anatomical illustrations; continues to emphasize clinical relevance of structure and function; continues the process of integrating anatomy with other disciplines e.g. physiology, neuroscience, and developmental biology; continues microscopic investigations of structures; searches for new ways to survive within the University successfully redirecting focus from gross anatomy to cell biology; and witnesses renewed interests and excitement by the end of the 1900s with the advent of non-invasive body imaging and digital computer technologies, which makes gross anatomy relevant once again to the routine daily practice of medicine.

Let us examine now a few specifics.

The 1900s witness a renewed appreciation of artists and their value in their contributions to medical illustrations.

Frank Netter (1906-1991) American medical illustrator contributes substantially to anatomy during the 1900s. As a young inspired art student in New York City, Frank Netter is dissuaded by his parents from continuing an art career and encourages him to enter medical school. In an effort to please his parents and maintain harmony within the family, he suspends his burgeoning passions and dreams of a successful art career and enters medical school. An all too familiar story throughout the history of medicine and one which remains too familiar today. Frank Netter completes medical school at the newly founded private New York University. Upon graduation he practices medicine for only a short period before abandoning clinical practice and returning to his true passion art.

Frank Netter secures initial successes as a medical illustrator, preparing anatomical illustrations for the pharmaceutical industry. His first notable commercial medical illustrations are prepared for the print marketing campaign of a new local anesthetic, Novocain (procaine). His anatomical illustrations are extremely well received by the professional community and are unlike any other available elsewhere. CIBA Pharmaceuticals, building upon the success of the Novocain sales, commission him to produce anatomical illustrations and pop-ups of the heart, to help sell the foxglove based compound used to increase cardiac contractility and control heart rate, Digitalis, circa 1936. His anatomical illustrations are so well received and generate such demand from practicing physicians and medical students, the CIBA Pharmaceutical Company collects the illustrations and releases them in a series of publications (CIBA Collection of Medical Illustration;

CIBA-Geigy Clinical Symposia Series) (1975)[102]. So begins Frank Netter contributions to anatomy as a medical illustrator.

Having crushed his parents' dream of ever becoming a successful clinical physician, he pursues his passion for art. Frank Netter becomes one of the most successful medical illustrators in the history of medicine. Frank Netter releases his colorful "Atlas of Human Anatomy" with over 4,000 illustrations to very appreciative medical students and practicing physicians throughout the world (1989)[103]. The "Atlas of Human Anatomy" becomes a familiar addition to every medical student's and practicing physician's bookshelf. Frank Netter is and will forever be linked with the time honored tradition of providing scientifically accurate and detailed anatomical illustrations which facilitate the understanding of the structure of the human body. The "Atlas of Human Anatomy" is now in its sixth edition and has been the gold standard for excellence for the past 25 years (2014)[104]. If you check the offices of any of your medical school professors or a practicing physicians, chances are high you will find a much used and well-worn copy of Frank Netter's "Atlas of Human Anatomy".

Charles Boileau Grant (1886-1973) Scottish anatomist provides one of the most successful lab manuals for the systematic step by step dissection of the human body, "Grant's Dissector". The first edition is released in 1940 and the manual is now in its 16th current edition (2016)[105]. "Grant's Dissector" has found a place on the dissecting tables of most medical students since 1940. It has served as the gold standard for human dissection manuals in medical schools for the past 78 years. A walk through the anatomy lab today reveals several copies of "Grant's Dissector" scattered around the lab. It remains very much a part of the first year medical students' education today.

Keith L. Moore (1925-2019) Canadian anatomist has contributed arguably one of the most popular English language textbooks on the topic of human anatomy for medical students. He continues the tradition of anatomical descriptions of systems and applies clinical relevance to structure for use in the practice of medicine. His immediately recognizable margin "blue boxes" are filled with relevant clinical applications for diagnosis, treatment, and management. A favorite among medical student is his very manageable "Essential Clinical Anatomy", provides a clearly written, well-illustrated, clinically relevant, and concise treatment of human anatomy for the medical student (1995)[106].

Human anatomy texts, atlases, and dissection manuals continue to improve throughout the 1900s. By the end of the century all published instructional materials are routinely accompanied by instructional, computerized compact disks, or digital video disks. The availability and affordability of digital computer technologies first introduced during the 1980s change the way medical students learn anatomy forever.

The mid and late-1900s witness tremendous advances with the invention and medical applications of innovative body imaging technologies.

George Ludwig (1922-1973) American medical researcher is credited with the first report of applying ultrasound frequency technologies, for the very specific purpose of imaging internal anatomical structures. His first released report by USA Department of Defense in the fall of 1949, "Device with Radar Principle Detects Foreign Objects in Body Tissue" describes the use of high frequency waves to image "stones" within the gallbladder (1949)[107]. Holding true to the tradition initiated by Roentgen fifty years earlier, Ludwig uses a family member, his daughter, as the test subject imaged. The technique provides an innovative and relatively safe method to image internal soft tissue structures which cannot be imaged by X-ray technologies. The technique continuously improves throughout the balance of the 1900s and today (2018) provides a familiar and frequently applied technology, in most medical settings.

Godfrey Hounsfield (1919-2004) English electrical engineer applies X-ray technology in the creation of his imaging machine which revolutionizes medical imaging in 1971. Godfrey Hounsfield invents the computerized axial tomography scanner (CAT). He first demonstrates its application on a patient in London who is suffering from a cerebral cyst. The successful machine (CT scanner) coupled with South African Alan Cormack's (1924-1998) calculations, soon offer an entirely new method for imaging the human body. Godfrey Hounsfield and Alan Cormack share the 1979 Nobel Prize in Medicine or Physiology for their invention of the CT scanner and associated technologies (1979)[108].

Paul Lauterbur (1929-2007) American chemist and Peter Mansfield (1932-2017) British physicist are frequently and incorrectly credited with the invention of nuclear magnetic resonance imaging (MRI) technology. It should be made clear, Paul Lauterbur and Peter Mansfield did not discover nuclear magnetic resonance imaging. Nuclear magnetic resonance (NMR) imaging had been discovered and established for uses in chemistry, for over thirty years before Paul Lauterbur and Peter Mansfield made their initial contributions, applying the technology to body imaging. Swiss physicists Felix Bloch (1931-1097) and Edward Purcell (1912- 1997) actually discovery NMR and are awarded the 1952 Nobel Prize in Physics for "...their development of new ways and methods for nuclear magnetic precision measurements..." (1952)[109].

Paul Lauterbur's and Peter Mansfield's contributions are no less important and arguably more important to the practice of medicine. They provide the necessary critical theoretical synthesis, formulation, and completion of the necessary formal calculations and produce the necessary hardware which will permit application of nuclear magnetic resonance technologies to non-invasive imaging of anatomical biological tissues. Paul Lauterbur and Peter Mansfield are awarded the 2003 Nobel Prize in Medicine or Physiology in recognition of "...their discovery of magnetic resonance imaging ... of human internal organs with exact and non-invasive methods..." (2003)[110]. The MRI technique differs significantly from the X-ray technologies used by the CT scanner and provide a new method of non-invasive imaging of soft and hard tissues with precision and clarity never seen before.

As with many significant contributions in medicine and science, spirited professional disputes regarding who should be credited with first introducing the contribution to the professional field are passionately waged. Politics of awards and recognition further fuel the flames of dispute. So too is the case with the magnetic resonance imaging (MRI) and medicine.

Raymond Damadian (1936-) American physician contributes significantly to the early development of the modern MRI scanner. His approach, while similar to Paul Lauterbur and Peter Mansfield, uses a different approach in the calculations necessary to generate an image. Lauterbur and Mansfield offers a "gradient" approach, whereas Damadian offers a "focused field" approach. Both approaches generate images. The professional and medical communities demonstrate a preference for the three dimensional imaging capabilities offered by Paul Lauterbur's and Peter Mansfield's approach. Raymond Damadian and others share a very public sense of resentment when Raymond Damadian is not recognized by the Nobel Prize Assembly for his contributions. Raymond Damadian expresses his outrage in a series of expensive, full page paid advertisements, in world newspapers e.g. the New York Times and Washington Post (2003)[111]. Another case of genuine, non-recognition for substantial contributions? Bias in favor of scientists and against physicians? Another case of professional politics? A case of self- promotion? Perhaps time and history will tell.

MRI technologies continues to advance throughout the balance of the late-1900s and introduce MRI based imaging of cerebral blood vessels (magnetic resonance angiography, MRA) and real time physiology (functional magnetic resonance imaging, fMRI). MRI remains one of the most commonly used non-invasive imaging tools in use today. In light of continuing professional disputes as to whom should receive professional credit for developing MRI technologies for medical imaging purposes, there is little disagreement MRI technologies have contributed substantially to the advancement of our ability to image internal human anatomical structures, has significantly advanced our understanding of normal and abnormal human anatomy, and provides essential and improved clinical care to patients.

By the end of the 1900s computers and innovative computer technologies are introduced to the world and applied to anatomy.

Personal computing expands exponentially during the late-1900s and changes anatomy forever. Internet availability and access to internet resources makes the study of human anatomy no longer the confines solely of scientists, physicians, and medical students. It becomes available to every elementary school child, with a home computer and internet access. Teaching of anatomy in medical schools changes. Attention is directed further away from students completing their own dissections of cadavers towards utilizing digital imaging and computer software to dissect a virtual body. As with any change, the new digital technology triggers a spirited professional debate. What is the best way to train medical students in the science of anatomy? Should medical education continue with medical students dissecting cadavers? Is virtual dissection a reasonable complement or substitution to physical dissection? Should time devoted to anatomical dissections be reassigned to other areas of study? With no clear consensus among medical educators today only time and history will reveal the most correct answers.

Digital technology advances during the late-1900s permit the initiation of the 1986 Visible Human Project (1986)[112]. The project, an online effort directed by the U.S. National Library of Medicine, applies recently developed CT and MRI technologies to provide a 3-dimentional, detailed, anatomically correct, computer generated image of a normal male and female human body. Images are digitally created from axial transverse one millimeter sections from the male and one third millimeter sections from the female. The project successfully completes the computer generated images in November 1994 for the male and November 1995 for the female. The Project provides a unique opportunity to correct errors appearing in modern textbooks of anatomy. The completed project is available for viewing at the National Museum of Health and Medicine in Washington, D.C.

Trivia: The male cadaver for the Visible Human project is that of a 38 year old male executed by the State of Texas by lethal injection in 1993. The female cadaver for the Project is that of a 59 year old female homemaker from the State of Maryland, who died from a lethal myocardial infarction.

As the 1900s comes to a close, the innovative process of Plastination is introduced to the world and anatomy.

Gunther Hagens (1945-) German anatomist introduces the most innovative technique of preserving anatomical tissues since formalin. The technique and process is termed Plastination (1979)[113]. In brief, the procedure replaces water and fat in tissues with plastics. The technique permits tissues to be handled without decay, without foul smell, while retaining most of the properties of the original unplastinated sample. Gunther Hagen introduces the technique first in 1977 after filing for patent protection. The technique is well accepted by anatomists, provides excellent specimens for educational purposes, and much appreciated by most medical students today.

Gunther Hagens successfully applies Plastination to medical specimens for over 20 years before developing the capability of plastinating the whole human body. Gunther Hagens first displays plastinated human bodies to the public in an art exhibit in Japan (1995)[114]. Subsequently and within two years, he establishes a traveling exhibit which displays approximately 25 human bodies, dissected, plastinated, and in life like poses, which dramatically illustrate the internal anatomy. Anatomical systems highlighted are the nervous systems, muscle systems, cardiovascular systems, and cardio-pulmonary systems (2005)[115]. The exhibit, while raising concerns by the public, governments, organized religions, scientists, and the medical community at large, have been viewed by over 25 million people of the world by the end of the 1900s. The exhibit originally titled Korperwelten [Body Worlds] continues to display the human form throughout the world, when not banned by government legislation, religious dictates, and local community protests. So continues the historic struggle whenever displaying the dissected human body to the general public.

In summary the Late Modern period 1900-2000 witnesses an approximate 70 year period of slow growth and normal science. The last 30 years witness a reawakening and renewed increased interests in anatomy. Anatomy moves away from the simple identification of gross structures and focuses on the interaction of structure and function. Microscopic anatomy (histology) offers significant advances with the advent of new microscopic imaging capabilities. The contributions of professional artists to anatomy are rediscovered, Frank Netter gives anatomy his Atlas; Charles Grant gives his step by step dissector manual; Keith Moore gives medical students his "blue boxes" and user friendly textbooks; George Ludwig his ultrasound; Godfrey Hounsfield and Alan Cormack give their CT scanner; Paul Lautenberg, Peter Mansfield, and Raymond Damadian give their MRI; U.S. National Museum of Medicine gives their virtual man and woman; Bill Gates his Windows; Steve Jobs his Apples; and Gunther Hagen his Plastination and shocks the world.

Anatomy once again becomes relevant to the daily practice of medicine.

Current Modern, 2000 AD - 2019 AD.

Medical imaging continues to improve its technologies and applications. CT and MRI imaging have become routine in the daily practice of medicine and whenever imaging of internal anatomical structures is required. Currently, radiology is one of the most coveted residencies among medical students.

Plastination exhibits continue to draw millions every year to view the dissected human body. Plastination provides a useful process for preserving internal organs and other soft tissues for subsequent inspection by medical students throughout the world and supplements use of virtual bodies and virtual dissections.

Standardization of international nomenclature for anatomical structures and terminologies continues with "Terminologia Anatomica", last updated in 1998 with approximately 7,500 structures (2000)[116]. "Terminologia Anatomicia" categorizes anatomical structures into 16 categories, based on major body systems as the primary organizational structure to define categories e.g. bones, muscles, respiratory, urinary, lymphatic, cardiovascular, and nervous systems. "Terminologia Anatomica" contains more than 9,200 terms replaces "Nomina Anatomica" 6th edition which contains over 6,400 terms (1998)[117]. "Terminology Anatomica" is available in several languages for free online (2018)[118].

Progress is being made in reference to U.S. Federal legislation regulating the donation and acquisition of human bodies for medical and research purposes. Federal legislation revises the Uniform Anatomy Gift Act of 1968, increasing the availability of human cadavers (1968, 2007)[119,120]. However, the availability of cadavers for medical school education continues to be limited. Digital anatomical dissections and virtual cadavers are being integrated into most medical school curriculum.

Medical education and the methods used in the teaching of anatomy to medical students are changing. Utilizing recent advances in computer technologies, most medical education programs today rely less on traditional textbooks and published atlases and more on rapid and quickly updated digital information available through the professional resource sites linked via the World Wide Web. Each year fewer and fewer medical schools offer students the opportunities for physical cadaver dissections and offer instead computer based digital virtual dissections. The debate continues today among medical educators and program administrators as to strengths and weaknesses of replacing educational practices which have been a part of every medical student's education for centuries with new practices only now made possible by advances in digital technologies. History will tell if the correct choices have been made.

In sum, recent years have evidenced a return of anatomy to a phase of normal science. Works continue in areas of cell biology, non-invasive medical body imaging, plastination, standardization of nomenclatures, virtual dissections, and the re-examination as to how to best teach and learn anatomy in medical school today.

References.

[1] Dirckx, J. (1997). Stedman's concise medical dictionary for the health professions. Third Edition. Baltimore: Williams and Wilkins.
[2] Scurlock, J. and Anderson, B. (2005). Diagnoses in Assyrian and Babylonian medicine: Ancient sources, Translations, and Modern Medical Analyses. Chicago: University of Illinois Press.
[3] Breasted, J. (1930). The Edwin Smith Surgical Papyrus, Volume 1: Hieroglyphic Transliteration, Translation, and Commentary; Volume 2: Facsimile Plates and Line for Line Hieroglyphic Transliteration. Chicago: University of Chicago Press.
[4] Edwin Smith Surgical Papyrus. [Online English translation]. Retrieved November 2009 from http://www.touregypt.net/edwinsmithsurgical.htm
[5] Joachim, H. (1890). Papyrus Ebers. Das alteste Buch uber Heilkunde [Translation from Egyptian into German]. Berlin: Druck und Verlag von George Reimer.
[6] Ebbell, B. (1937). The Papyrus Ebers: The greatest Egyptian medical document. English translation by B. Ebbell. Copenhagen: Levin & Munksgaar.
[7] Ebers Papyrus, Egypt (circa 1550 BC). Compendium of the whole Egyptian Medicine (Georg Ebers): Column 1-2. University of Leipzig Library, Special Collections. Leipzig, Germany.
[8] Bryan, C. (1974). Ancient Egyptian Medicine: The Papyrus Ebers. Translation from the German version by Cyril P. Byran. Ares Publishers: Chicago. Retrieved May 2018 from https://babel.hathitrust.org/cgi/pt?id=coo.31924073200077;view=1up;seq=6

[9] Griffith F. (1898). The Petrie papyri: Hieratic papyri from Kahun and Gurob. London: Benard Quartch.

[10] The Petrie Papyri: Petrie Papyri: Hieratic Papyri from Kahun and Gurob. [Online English translation]. Retrieved November 2009 from http://www.archive.org/stream/hieraticpapyrifr00grifuoft#page/n7/mode/2up.

[11] Wachtler, J. (1896). De Alcmaeone Crotoniata, Leipzig: B. Teubner.

[12] Diels, H. and Kranz, W. (1952). Die Fragmente der Vorsokratiker [The fragments of the Presocratic treaties] 6th edition. Dublin and Zürich: Weidmann.

[13] Huffman, C. (2008). Alcmaeon. In Stanford Encyclopedia of Philosophy. Retrieved November 2009 from http://plato.stanford.edu/entries/alcmaeon/

[14] Hippocratic Collection. [Digitized copies of the first printed editions (1525-1595) housed at the Biblioteque Interuniversitiarire de medicine of Paris]. Retrieved November 2009 from http://www.bium.univ-paris5.fr/histmed/medica/hipp_va.html

[15] Celsus, A. (circa 30 AD). De Medicina [On Medicine]. First printed 1478. Florence Nicolaus Laurentii. Rare Book Collection, Countway Medical Library, Boston.

[16] Celsus, A. (circa 30 AD). De Medicina [On Medicine]. Online English translation by W. Spencer (1935) Loeb Classical Library Edition. Retrieved November 2009 from http://penelope.uchicago.edu/Thayer/E/Roman/Texts/celsus/home.html

[17] Mondino de Luzzi. (1316 AD). Anathomia Mundini. First printed December 1478. Pavia: Antonio de Carchanno.

[18] Al-Razi, A. (circa 925 AD) Kitab al-Hawi fi al-tibb [The Comprehensive Book on Medicine]. National Library of Medicine, MS A17.

[19] Ali ibn Abbass al-Majusi (circa 980 AD). Kitab Kamil as-Sina'a at-Tibbiyya [The Complete Book of the Medical Arts]. Translated from Arabic into Latin by Constantine (980 AD). Later known as the Kitab al-Maliki [Royal Book].

[20] Ibn al-Nafis. (1242 AD). Sharh Tashrih al-Qanun Ibn Sina [A Commentary on the Anatomy in Avicenna's Canon].

[21] Ibn al-Nafis. (1242 AD). Sharh Tashrih al-Qanun Ibn Sina [A Commentary on the Anatomy in Avicenna's Canon]. Discovered by Muhyo Al-Deen Altawi (1924) Script No. 62243, Commentary on the Anatomy of Canon of Avicenna. In Keys, T, Watkin, K. Contributions of Arabs to medicine, Proceedings of the staff meeting. Mayo Clinic, 1953; 28:423-37.

[22] Sevetus, M. (1553). Christianismi restitutio [The Restoration of Christianity]. Book V, 168-173. [English translation by Christopher A Hoffman and Marian Hillar (2007).

[23] Colombo, R. (1559). De re Anatomica: Libri VII. Venice.

[24] Harvey, W. (1628). Exercitation anatomica de motu cordis et sanguinis in animalibus [On the motion of the heart and blood in animals]. English translation by Alex Bowie (1889) from Willis's translation. London: George Bell and Sons, York Street, Covent Garden.

[25] Mundini de'Luicci .(1316 AD). Anathomia Mudini - Emedata p doctore Melerstat [Mundini's Anatomy, edited by Dr. Mellrichstadt]. Manuscript (1316); printed in Leipzig (1493), edited by Dr. Martin Pollich von Mellrichstadt; digitized 11-19-2008 by Bayerische StaatsBibliothek (BSB); urn:nbn:de:bvb:12-bsb00M030125-2. Retrieved November 2009 from http://daten.digitale-sammlungen.de/~db/0003/bsb00030125/images

[26] Vesalius, A. and van Calcar, J. (1543). De humani corporis fabrica libri septem [On the Fabric of the Human body in seven books] Ex Officina Joannis Oporini, 1543. [English translation by Daniel Garrison and Malcom Hast (2003)] Retrieved November 2009 from http://vesalius.northwestern.edu/flash.html

[27] Vigevano, G. (1345 AD). Anathomia designata per figures. In Wickersheimer E: L'Anatomic de Guido de Vigevano, médecin de la reine Jeanne de Bourgogne (1345). [The Anatomy of Guido da Vigevano, physician to Queen Jeanne de Bourgogne]. Archiv für Geschichte der Medizin (1913), 7:1–25.

[28] Wickersheimer, E. (1926). Anatomies de Mondino dei Luzzi et de Guido de Vigevano. Paris: Droz F.

[29] Leonardo di Vinci. (1487). Vitruvian Man. Gallarie del'Accademia, Venice.

[30] Leonardo di Vinci. (1498). The Last Supper. Santa Maria delle Grazie, Milan.

[31] Leonardo di Vinci. (1505). Mona Lisa. Louvre Musem, Paris.

[32] Leonardo di Vinic. (1510). Drawing of human fetus. Windsor Castle Royal Library, sheets RL 19073v-19074v and RL 19102. London.

[33] Leonardo di Vinci, Rigaud, J., and Brown, J. (1892). Treaties on painting. London: George Bell & Sons, York Street, Covent Garden.

[34] Leonardo di Vinci, Rigaud, J., and Brown, J. (1892). Treaties on painting. [English translation by John Rigaud]. Retrieved from http://www.archive.org/stream/treatiseonpainti001974mbp#page/n5/mode/2up

[35] Michelangelo. (1504). David. Galleria dell Academeia, Florence.

[36] Micaelangelo. (1510). Libian Sybyl. Metropolitan Museum, New York.

[37] Micaelangelo. (1510). Libian Sybyl. Metropolitan Museum, New York.

[38] Vesalius, A. (1538). Tabulae anatomicae sex [Six anatomical drawings]. Venice: Imprimebat B. Vitalis. Facimilie located in the Royal Academy of Arts, Rare Book Collection, London: 1874 private printing for William Stirling Maxwell.

[39] Vesalius, A. (1543). De humani corporis fabrica [The structure of the human body]. Currently located in the Glasgow University Library, Special Collection Hunterian Z.1.8, Ce.1.18. Glasgow.

[40] Vesalius, A., Richardson, W. and Carman, J. (1998). On the fabric of the human body: Volume 1: The bones and cartilages. [English translation by William Richardson and John Burd Carman. San Francisco: Norman Publishing.

[41] Vesalius, A., Richardson, W. and Carman, J. (1999). On the fabric of the human body: A translation of de humana corporis fabrica libri septem. Volume 2, Book II: The ligaments and muscles. [English translation by William Richardson and John Carman]. San Francisco: Norman Publishing.

[42] Vesalius A., Richardson, W. and Carman, J. (2003). On the fabric of the human body: Volume 3. Book III: The veins and arteries; Book IV: The nerves [English translation by William Richardson and John Carman]. Novato, CA: Norman Publishing.

[42] Vesalius, A., Richardson, W. and Carman, J. (2008). On the fabric of the human body, Volume 4. Book V: The organs of nutrition and generation. [English translation by William Richardson and John Carman]. Novato, CA: Norman Publishing.

[44] Vesalius, A., Richardson, W. and Carman, J. (2009). On the fabric of the human body: Volume 5: Book VI The heart and associated organs, Book VII The brain. [English translation by William Richardson and John Carman]. Novato, CA: Norman Publishing.

[45] Vesalius, A. (1543). De humani corporis fabrica librorum epitome [Abrigment of the structure of the human body]. Currently located in the Glasgow University Library, Special Collection. Glasgow.

[46] Falloppio, G. (1562). Observationes anatomicae. Coloniae, Apud haeredes Arnoldi Birckmanni.

[47] Eustachio, B. (1562). Epistola de auditus organis. In Opuscula Anatomica (1564). Venetiis: V. Luchinus.

[48] Lancisi, G. (1714). Tabulae anatomicae Bartholomaei Eustachii quas e tenebris tandem vindicatas præfatione notisque illustravit, ac ipso suæ bibliothecæ dedicationis die publici juris fecit. [Anatomical Illustrations of Bartholmeo Eustachio]. Rome: Francesco Gonzaga.

[49] Historical Anatomies on the Web (2009). United States National Library of Medicine, National Institute of Health. Retrieved November 2009 from http://www.nlm.nih.gov/exhibition/historicalanatomies/eustachi_home.html

[50] Valslava, A. (1704). De aure humana tractatus. Page 184. Bononiae: C. Pissarii.

[51] Harvey, W. (1628). Exercitatio aatomicica de motu crdis et sanguinis et sanguinis in amimalibus" [An anatomical exercise on the motion of the heart and blood in animals]. Francofvrti, Sumptibus Gvlielmi Fitzeri. [Frankfurt-on-Main, Germany].

[52] Harvey, W. (1628). Exercitatio Anatomicica de Motu Cordis et Sanguinis et Sanguinis in Amimalibus" [An Anatomical Exercise on the Motion of the Heart and Blood in Animals].English translation from Latin (1653). London: Printed by Francis Leack for Richard Lowndes. (Original copy (1653) available from Bauman Rare Books from the library of the 8th Earl of Pembroke for $82,000.00 US.).

[53] Riolan, J. (1649). Ospuscula anatomica nova. Londoini: Typis Milonis Flesher.

[54] Weil, E. (1957). The echo of Harvey's de motu cordis (1628) 1628 to 1657. Journal of the History of Medicine and Allied Sciences, 12(2):167-174. Oxford University Press.

[55] Malpighi, M. (1661). De Pulmonibus observations anatomicae. Bononiae: Ferronius. [English translation by J. Young] (1929) Proceedings of the Royal Society of Medicine, 23:1-11. London

[56] Willis, T. (1664). Cerebri anatome: cui accessit nervorum descriptio et usus. [The Anatomy of the Brain and Nerves]. London. J. Flesher, J. Martyn & J. Allestry. [English translation by S. Pordage (1681)].

[57] Willis, T. (1674). Pharmaceutice rationali, sive diatriba de medicamentorum operationibus in humano corpore. 2 volumes. Oxford, 1674 and 1675. [English translation by S. Pordage (1683)].

[58] Willis, T. (1664). Cerebri anatome: cui accessit nervorum descriptio et usus. [The Anatomy of the Brain and Nerves]. London. J. Flesher, J. Martyn & J. Allestry. [English translation by S. Pordage (1681)].

[59] Valsalva, A. (1704). De aure humana tractatus: in quo integra ejusdem auris fabrica, multis novis inventis, & iconismis illustrata, describitur; omniumque ejus partium usus indagantur: quibus interposita est musculorum uvulae, atque pharyngis nova descriptio, et delineation. Bononiae: Constantini Pisari

[60] Scarpa, A. (1809). Sulli ernie: memorie anatomico-chirurgiche. Milano: D. Stamperia.

[61] Morgagni, G. (1769). De sedibus, et causis morborum per anatomen indagatis [The seats and causes of disease investigated by means of anatomy; English translation in 3 volumes by B. Alexander]. London: A. Milar and T. Cadell.

[62] Steno, N. (1673). Acta. Med. Phil. Hafniensia, 1:200.

[63] Sandifort, E. (1777). Observationes anatomicco-pathologicae. Book 1, Chapter 1. Leyden: P. Eyk & D. Vygh.

[64] Fallot, E. (1888). Contribution à l'anatomie pathologique de la maladie bleue (cyanose cardiaque). Marseille Medical: Barlatier et Feissat.

[65] Smellie, W. (1754). A set of anatomical tables and explanations, and an abridgement, of the practice of midwifery, with a view to illustrate a treatise on that subject, and collection of cases. London. Charles Elliot and Company.

[66] Hunter, W. (1774). The anatomy of the human gravid uterus, exhibited in figures. London: Joannes Baskerville.

[67] Hunter, W. (1794). An anatomical description of the human gravid uterus and its contents. London: J. Johnson, St. Paul's Church Yard and G. Nicol, Pall-Mall.

[68] Lassek A. (1958). Human dissection: Its drama and struggle. Springfield: Charles C Thomas. Retrieved November 2009 from htp://www.archive.org/details/humandissectioni00lassrich

[69] Lassek A. (1958). Human dissection: Its drama and struggle. Springfield: Charles C Thomas. Retrieved November 2009 from htp://www.archive.org/details/humandissectioni00lassrich.

[70] United States First Congress (1790). An Act for Punishment of Certain Crimes Against the United States. United States Statues at Large, Volume 1. United States Congress. Public Acts of the First Congress, 2nd Session, Chapter 9, Section 4. Passed April 30, 1790. New York City.

[71] Keen, W, (1874). A sketch of the early history of practical anatomy: The introductory address to the course of lectures on anatomy at the Philadelphia School of Anatomy. Philadelphia: J. B. Lippincott.

[72] Warburton Act. (1832). The Statutes of the United Kingdom and Ireland. Vol. XII: pp. 891–4 2 & 3 Gulielmi IV, Cap. 73–5. London: Eyre & Spottiswoode.

[73] Darwin, C. (1859). Origin of species by means of natural selection, or preservation of favoured races in the struggle for life. London: John Murray, Albemarle Street.

[74] Darwin, C. (1826). Letter January 6, Darwin C. R. to Darwin C. S. Correspondence Project. Retrieved November 2009 from http://www.darwinproject.ac.uk/darwinletters/calendar/entry-20. html

[75] Darwin, C. (1826). Letter March 27, Darwin, C. S. to Darwin C. R. Correspondence Project. Retrieved November 2009 from http://www.darwinproject.ac.uk/darwinletters/calendar/entry-20. html

[76] Bell, C. (1811). An idea of a new anatomy of the brain; submitted for the observations of his friends. A privately printed pamphlet. London: Strahan & Preston. Reproduced in Medical Classics, 1936, 1:105-120.

[77] Bell, C. (1821). On the Nerves; Giving an account of some experiments on their structure and function which lead to a new arrangement of the system. Paper presented at Royal Society. Philosophical Transactions of the Royal Society, p.398.

[78] Magendie, F. (1822). Expériences sur les fuctions des racines des nerfs rachidiens. Journal de Physiologie Experimentale et de Pathologie, 2:276-279.

[79] Magendie, F. (1822). Expériences sur les functions des racines des nerfs qui naissent de la moëlle épinière. Journal de Physiologie Expérimentale et de Pathologie, 2:366-371.

[80] Magendie, F. (1847). Comptes rendus hebdomadaires des seances de l'Académie des Sciences, [The Weekly Meetings of the Academy of Sciecnes], 24:320.

[81] Henle, F. (1841). Allgemeine Anatomie. Leipzig: L. Voss.

[82] Henle, F. (1873). Handbuch der Eingeweidelhre des menschen. Braunschweig: Druck und Verlad von Fredrich Wieweg und Sohn.

[83] Gray, H. (1858). Anatomy descriptive and surgical. London: John Parker and Son, West Strand.

[84] Standring, S. (2016). Gray's Anatomy. 41th Edition: The anatomical basis of clinical practice. Elsevier Health Sciences.

[85] Bassi, A. (1835). Del mal del segno, calcinaccio o moscardino, malattia che affigge ibachi da seta, e sul modo di liberarne le bigattaje anche le piui infestate. Tipografia Orcesi, Lodi.

[86] Bassi, A. (1835). Del mal del segno. Phytopathological Classic 10, 1958. American Phytopathological Society [Translated by into English P. Yarrow (1958). (Eds) Ainsworth, G. and Yarrow, P. Baltimore: Monumental Printing Company.

[87] Anatomische Gesellschaft [Anatomical Society] (2018). History. Retrieved May 2018 from http://anatomische-gesellschaft.de/index.php?id=geschichte-der-ag&lang=de

[88] American Association of American Anatomists (1891). History, Constitution, Membership, and the Titles and Abstracts of Papers, for the years 1888, 1889, 1890. Washington D.C. Beresford Printer, 617 E Street.

[89] His, W. (1895). Die anatomische Nomenklatur. Leipzig, Veit u. Co.

[90] Bozzini, P. (1809). Der Lichtleiter, oder, Beschreibung einer einfachen Vorrichtung und ihrer Anwendung zur Erleuchtung innerer Höhlen und Zwischenräume des lebenden animalischen Körpers. [The light guide, or description of a simple device and its application to enlightenment, inner cavities and interstices of the living animal body.]. Wiesbaden: Verlag des Landes Industrie Comptoirs.

[91] Desormeaux, A. (1853). Meeting of the Academy of Medicine. Paris 7-20-1853. In De l'endoscope et de ses applications au diagnositic et au traitement des affections de l'urethre et de la vessie.(1865). Paris: J. B. Bailliere et Fils.

[92] Nitze, M. (1876). Beitrage zur endoskopie.der mannlichen harblase. Langenbeck's Archive, bd. 36, heft 3.

[93] Nitze, M. (1879). Ueber eine neue Beleuchtugsmethode der hohlen des menschlichen korpers. Wien, med. Presse, 20:851-858.

[94] Turck, L. (1860). Beitrage zur Laryngoskopie un Rhinoskopie [Contributions to Laryngoscopy and Rhinoscopy]. Vienna.

[95] Czermak, J. (1863). Der kehlkopfspiegel und seine verwerthung für physiologie und medezin [The Laryngoscope, its application to physiology and Medicine]. 2nd edition, Leipzig: Verlag von Wilhelm Engelmann. The first edition, translated from the French, is published by the Sydenham Society Vol XI.

[96] Ruppaner, A. (1867). The practice of laryngoscopy and rhinoscopy: Survey of the history, discovery and development of practical laryngoscopy and rhinoscopy. The New York Medical Journal (1868), 6(1):1-14. New York: Moorhead, Simpson & Bond, 60 Duane Street.

[97] Garcia, M. (1855). Observations on the Human Voice. Philosophical and Journal of Science, Vol X and Gazette Hebdom. De Med. Et Chir., 16 Nov.

[98] Roentgen, W. (1898). Uber eine neue art von strahlen [On a new kind of ray]. Annalen. der Physik, 300 (1):1-11.

[99] Roentgen, W. (1901). Nobel Prize in Physics. Presentation speech by C. Odhner President of the Royal Swedish Academy of Sciences Dec 10, 1901. Nobel Foundation.

[100] Curie, P. and Curie, M. (1903). Nobel Prize in Physics. Presentation speech by H. Tornebladh President of the Royal Swedish Academy of Sciences on Dec 10, 1903. Nobel Foundation.

[101] Kuhn, T. (1970). The Structure of Scientific Revolutions. 2nd edition, enlarged. Volume I and II. Foundations of the Unity of Sciences Vol II, number 2. Chicago: University of Chicago Press.

[102] Netter, F. (1975). The CIBA collection of medical illustrations: Six volumes (Volumes 1-6). Saunders.

[103] Netter, F. (1989). Atlas of human anatomy. Summit, NJ: Ciba-Geigy Pharmaceutical Corporation.

[104] Netter, F. (2014). Atlas of Human Anatomy, 6th edition. Philadelphia: Saunders an Imprint of Elsevier Inc.

[105] Detton, A. (2016). Grant's Dissector. 16th edition. Philadelphia: Wolters Kluwer.

[106] Moore, K. and Agur, A. (1995). Essential clinical anatomy. Philadelphia: Lippincott, Williams & Wilkins.

[107] Ludwig, G. (1949). Device with radar principle detects foreign objects in body tissue. U.S. Department of Defense Office of Public Information, Washington DC. Release number 220-49, October 7.

[108] Hounsfield, G. and Cormack, A. (1979). Nobel Prize in physiology or medicine (1979). Nobel Prize Press Release. The Nobel Assembly at the Karlonska Institute October 11, 1979.

[109] Bloch, F. and Purcell, E. (1952). Nobel Prize in Physics. Presentation speech by E Hulthen, member of the Nobel Committee for Physics. Nobel Foundation.

[110] Lauterbur, P. and Mansfield, P. (2003). Nobel Prize in Physiology or Medicine. Nobel Prize Press Release October 6, 2003, The Nobel Assembly at Karolinska Institutet.

[111] Damadian, R. (2003, October 9, 10, 20; November 3, 11, 20, December 2, 9). The Shameful Wrong that must be righted. New York Times. Paid Advertisement by The Friends of Raymond Damadian.

[112] Visible Human Project (1986). US National Library of Medicine, Bethesda, MD, Retrieved November 2009 from www.nlm.nih.gov/research/visible/visible_human.html

[113] Hagens, G. (1979). Plastination. Retrieved November 2009 from http://www.bodyworlds.com/en/plastination/idea_plastination.html

[114] Hagens, G (1995). Korperwelten [Body Worlds] Exhibition, Tokyo, Japan. Retrieved from http://www.bodyworlds.com/en/exhibitions/current_exhibitions.htm

[115] Hagens, G. (2005). Body worlds. The original exhibition of real bodies -Catalog. Heidelberg: Arts and Sciences.

[116] Terminologia Anatomica (2000). International Federation Associations of Anatomists (IFAA), Federative International Committee on Anatomical Terminology. Terminologia Anatomica: Combination Book and CD-ROM: International Anatomical Terminology. Stuttgart: Georg Thieme Verlag.

[117] Federative Committee on Anatomical Terminology (FCAT). (1998). Terminologia Anatomica: International Anatomical Terminology. Stuttgart: Georg Thieme Verlag.

[118] Federal International Programme on Anatomical Terminologies. (1998). Terminologia Anatomica, 1998 online version. Retrieved May 2018 from https://www.unifr.ch/ifaa/Public/EntryPage/ShowTA98EN.html

[119] Uniform Anatomical Gift Act (1968). Uniform Anatomical Gift Act. National Conference of Commissioners on Uniform State Laws. Approved and recommended for enactment in all the States at its annual conference. 77th Annual Meeting, Philadelphia, Pennsylvania July 22-31-1968. Retrieved July 23, 2015, from www.uniformlaws.org/Act.aspx?title=Anatoical+Gift+(1968)

[120] Revised Uniform Anatomical Gift Act (2006). Last revised or amended in 2007, drafted by the Uniform Anatomy Gift Act 1968 revised (2007). The National Conference of Commissioners on Uniform State Laws. Chicago, IL. Retrieved November 2009 from www.nccusl.org

Chapter 3

Medical Physiology

Definition.

Physiology is "...the science concerned with the normal vital processes of animal and vegetable organisms, especially as to how things normally function in the living organism rather than to their anatomical structure, their biochemical composition, or how they are affected by drugs or disease..." (1997)[1]. The word physiology is derived from the ancient Greek "physis" meaning "nature" and "logia" the "study of a subject" (2018)[2].

The principle unit of study for physiology is the organ or organ system. This stands in contrast to histology, which holds the cell to be the principle unit of study or biochemistry which holds body chemistry to be the primary unit of study. The study of physiology also stands in contrast to gross anatomy. Gross anatomy and physiology both focus study upon organs and organ systems. However, physiology focuses study on function whereas, gross anatomy focuses study on form and structure. Understanding the function of organs and organ systems is essential to understanding the human body and the competent practice of medicine.

Introduction.

This chapter traces the history of human physiology and its application to the practice of clinical medicine. Plant physiology, while fascinating and with its own history will not be considered in this chapter. There will be no attempt to cover all contributions in detail. Rather, this chapter will provide an account of significant events, discoveries, influential people, and ideas which have shaped the field of medical physiology throughout time.

The chapter is organized chronologically for consistency with other chapters and to provide you, the first and second year medical student, an appreciation of significant contributions to the discipline, as a function of time. Specific individuals making substantive contributions are highlighted. Most of the people should be quickly recognized by you. If the person is unfamiliar, spend a little more time on that section. He or she is there for a reason. Understand their contribution.

Specific topics areas developed throughout the chapter include eight major systems, cardiovascular, respiratory, renal, gastrointestinal, endocrine, reproductive, skeletal-muscular, and neural, traditionally covered in most medical schools' Basic Science program.

This chapter additionally considers many of the factors producing change in medical dogma, professional rivalries, and the political, economic, religious, and social presses, which have influenced the advancement of medical physiology knowledge throughout time.

Finally, this chapter will present material in a contextual matrix of other commonly recognized world events, whenever it makes sense, in order to provide a more global perspective, from which to understand the people, events, and contributions.

History.

Early Records, 3500 BC - 500 BC.

There is a limited written record regarding the knowledge of human physiology and its application to medicine, during the period of the ancient civilizations. However, the Sumerians circa 3500 BC, ancient Egyptians circa 3200 BC, Babylonians circa 2000 BC, ancient Greeks circa 1100 BC, and ancient Romans 750 BC have left many clues.

Recently, thousands of ancient clay tablets, discovered primarily during the 1920s, are today in the process of being organized and translated. These tablets are quickly revealing a knowledge base of fundamental physiology with application to medicine previously unknown by modern man. The tablets reveal the ancient civilizations did indeed have a reasonable working knowledge of fundamental physiological relationships, including many which have stood the test of time (1923, 1951,1964,1976,2005)[3,4,5,6,7].

The dogma of modern academia which oftentimes portrays the knowledge of physiology by the ancient civilizations as limited, unsophisticated, and couched completely in non-empirical mysticism is proving to be incorrect and requires modification

Records reveal the Ancients applied an empirical-inductive approach to acquiring new information, including knowledge of function associated with organ systems. It is recorded in both the recently translated tablets, as well as several Egyptian papyri e.g. Edwin Smith papyrus (1600 BC,1930,2009)[8,9], Ebers papyrus (1550 BC,1890,1937)[10,11,12], and Brugsch papyrus, aka Berlin papyrus (1350 BC,1883,1893,1909)[13,14,15]. The ancient civilizations maintain not only an awareness of physiological organ systems, they study these systems.

For example, the cardiovascular system. The Ancients' records reveal not only do they have knowledge of the pulse; they are aware of its connection with the heart and attempt to measure it. The Ancients undoubtedly recognize the heart to be a life sustaining organ and when the heart stops so does physical life. Sounds like a fundamental association between organ and function to me. Yes, while perhaps less sophisticated than might be expected by modern standards, the elegance of the observation and association with function is undeniable. These are the very foundation upon which physiology is based.

Knowledge of physiology recorded by the ancient civilizations, derives almost exclusively from sensory experiences. The specific sensory experiences of many are combined to form a set of stable and recurring observations e.g. when the heart stops physical life stops. The set of combined observations is then subjected to inductive reasoning, which moves the set of specific observations to generalized conclusions. This empirical-inductive epistemological approach to knowledge provides the foundation upon which the ancient civilizations build and organize their understanding of nature.

The empirical-inductive epistemological approach stands in contrast to the rational-deductive process subsequently popularized by the Greek natural philosophers and mathematicians of Antiquity (500 BC- 500 AD), thousands of years later.

The rational-deductive approach of the Greeks minimizes experience in favor of careful intellectual reasoning and maintains the position, if well-reasoned premises are true, then the conclusions derived from the premises must be true. Deductive reasoning is applied to the intellectually derived premises to evaluate the truth of the premises and provides a method of establishing new knowledge, moving from the general to the specific.

Both epistemological approaches, the empirical-inductive applied by the ancient civilizations and the rational-deductive applied by the Greeks during Antiquity have advantages and disadvantages. Both methods expand and limit the base of new scientific knowledge.

In summary of the early records, modern academic dogma and popular beliefs portraying knowledge of physiology by ancient civilizations as limited, unsophisticated, and couched completely in non-empirical mysticism is proving to be incorrect and requires modification. Newly discovered evidence suggest many ancient civilizations, Sumerians circa 3500 BC, ancient Egyptians circa 3200 BC, Babylonians circa 2000 BC, ancient Greeks circa 1100 BC and ancient Romans 750 BC possess a fundamental understanding of physiology, a fundamental understanding of relationships between organs and function, and demonstrate interests in studying these relationships. The Ancients' knowledge of physiology is based largely upon sensory experiences and an empirical-inductive epistemological approach towards acquiring new knowledge. Many of the fundamental organ-function relationships established during this time remain true today. These early records punctuate the longstanding interests people have for understanding how the body works in both good health and disease.

Antiquity, 500 BC - 500 AD.

The cornerstones for the foundation of physiology are laid by the ancient Sumerians, Egyptians, Babylonians, Greeks, and Romans. The next phase in the development of physiology is evident during early-Antiquity. Physiology is recognized as essential in the training of future physicians and becomes a significant component of the education of physicians trained in the earliest medical schools.

The medical school, as a formal center for educating and training physicians, is founded by Greek natural philosopher Alcmaeon of Croton, circa 600 BC. The School emphasizes recognition of the relationships between anatomical structure and function, embraces a rational-empirical approach to acquiring knowledge, and proposes a Doctrine of balances, providing a theoretical matrix within which to organize knowledge of the human body and guide medical diagnosis and treatments.

Note: Croton is an ancient Greek colony founded circa 750 BC, located in southern Italy on the Ionian Sea coast, at the instep sole of the boot of Italy. The City is quickly recognized as a center of excellence in the training of physicians, during Antiquity.

Alcmaeon of Croton (510 BC- uncertain) pre-Socratic, Greek, natural philosopher provides physiology with the earliest known writings describing normal human body functions, within the matrix of physical processes. The few original fragments of his writings, which remain today [On Nature 470 BC, DKA2] and in combination with the written records of subsequent Greeks, specifically Greek historian Herodotus of Halicarnassus (484 BC-425 BC), Plato (428 BC-348 BC), Aristotle (384 BC-322 BC), and Galen (129 AD-200 AD), uniformly acknowledge Alcmaeon's fundamental contributions to physiology. His approach to acquiring new information is rational-deductive, standing in contrast to the empirical-inductive approach of the Ancients. He assigns function to every anatomical structure and offers a rational conceptual matrix to explain the mechanisms of the function, understand normal and abnormal function, and guide treatments.

Alcmaeon is first to propose balance, in human physiology, as necessary for normal and healthy functioning of the body. Imbalance results in impaired function. As stated by Alcmaeon, translated from Greek into English "… the qualities of the powers (wet, dry, cold, hot, bitter, sweet) maintain health and monarch among them produce disease…" (DK24B4) (1896,1903,1952,1958-1964, 1983)[16,17,18,19,20]. Alcmaeon proposes the balance doctrine, hundreds of years before a more recognizable Greek, itinerant physician, Hippocrates, proposes his now familiar balance doctrine of four humors.

Note: Much of the pre-Socratic written record has been lost to time. Almost all of what we know today of this period is traceable to the efforts and works of the German philologist Hermann Diels (1848-1922). Diels compiled known written fragments of pre-Socratic philosophers' works in a collection published first in 1903 (1903/1968)[17]. Additions and corrections are subsequently made to Diels volumes by German philologist Walther Kranz (1884-1960). The revised and corrected editions are known as the Diels-Kranz (DK) volumes and have become the academic record standard for pre-Socratic philosophic writings (1952)[18].

Pre-Socratic writings are commonly referred to by their Diels-Kranz "DK" number, e.g. DK24B4. Within the DK numbering system each pre-Socratic author is assigned a number; followed by the source of the writing coded by a letter A, B, or C; followed by the sequential number of individual fragments. More specifically, the letter code following the pre-Socratic author number "A" refers to a "Testimonia", an ancient account of the author's life and doctrines; a "B" signifies an "Ipsisima Verba", purportedly the exact words of the author; a "C" refers to an "Imitations", works not from the author themself but rather writings reflecting the philosophical positions of the author written by others. The final number represents the sequential number of a specific individual fragment. In the case of the example DK24B4, this references Alcmaeon (DK24), purported exact words written by Alcmaeon (B), and the fourth fragment to be sequenced by Diels (4).

Alcmaeon sets the agenda for Greek physiology and physiology for the next two thousand years. He describes numerous relationships between anatomical structures of the human body and associated functions. He provides the foundation for all sensory physiology, providing descriptions and conceptual explanatory models for the physiology underlying all five sensory modalities, olfactory, gustatory, auditory, visual, and tactile (DK24A5). He lays the foundation for all future research in sleep physiology, proposing the mechanism of action for sleep and wakefulness noting "…sleep is produced by the withdrawal of the blood away from the surface of the body to the larger vessels and that we awake when the blood diffuses throughout the body again. Death occurs when the blood withdraws entirely…" (DK24A18) (1952,1968)[18,17].

Not restricting himself to sensory physiology or the physiology of sleep, he makes contributions in the field of developmental embryology and reproductive physiology as well. He is first to challenge Greek dogma in human reproduction that states the father alone is responsible for the seed of new life. Alcmaeon proposes both mother and father contribute (DK24A13) and the child's sex is determined by the parent who contributes the most seed (DK24A14). Alcmaeon additionally proposes the brain to be responsible for thought and memory and challenges the more universally accepted cardio-centric position popular during this time (DK24A5,A8,A10). Alcmaeon is first to document the relationship between the eye, cranial nerve II, and the brain and offers a physiological explanation of vision, anchored securely within a conceptual matrix.

Trivia: Alcmaeon is the first to use analogies of plants and animals when writing about human physiology. This practice becomes a staple of Greek medical writings and continues to provide medical students today a useful learning tool, when appreciating and describing functional relationships within human physiology.

Hippocrates (460 BC- 370 BC) Greek, an itinerant practitioner of medicine, personally contributes very little if at all to physiology. However, the collection of multi-authored written documents detailing medical knowledge of the period, assembled in the City of Alexandria circa 300 BC and known today collectively as the Alexandrian Hippocratic Collection, includes several specific and notable contributions to physiology. Of the ten areas of medicine into which the Collection can be organized, physiology is one. Within the physiology grouping of books and treaties, primary attention is directed to the physiology of the cardiovascular system. Little or no attention is devoted to other organ based physiological systems. Inspection of the Collection reveals no record of systematic experimental investigations of physiological systems. The Collection does reveal a listing of diseases along with associated signs and symptoms, which can be interpreted loosely within the matrix of the balance of humors doctrine, popular during the period. The Collection provides a written record of contemporary knowledge of physiology and prior to 300 BC.

The first printed copies of the Hippocratic Collection (circa 1525AD) are housed in the Bibliotheque Interuniversitiariea de Medicine of Paris. Digitized images of these printed copies and accompanying English translations can also be found online (2009)[21].

Aristotle (384 BC-322 BC) applies an empirical-inductive approach to the study of physiological systems. While a student of Plato, Aristotle breaks from the rationalism advocated by his teacher Plato and advocates the alternative position of empiricism, embracing the belief that knowledge is best acquired through sensory experience and experiments. Aristotle systematically investigates body structures and associates function with each, in much the same manner as the Ancient civilizations discussed earlier. Today, over two thousand years after Aristotle and following in his footsteps, every medical student learns the value of associating anatomical structure with function and understanding the physiology responsible for the function.

The teleology of Aristotle rather than any specific experimental result proves over time to be the primary contribution of Aristotle to physiology. His influence upon Galen is apparent in "De uso partium" [On the Usefulness of the Parts of the Body] (circa 170 AD)[22] and countless additional publications. Aristotle offers a modification of the theoretical matrix originally proposed by Alcmaeon one hundred years earlier, which emphasizes the balance between conceptual dimensions hot, cold, wet, and dry.

The doctrine of balances and all of its many subtle modifications, including the one proposed by Aristotle is evident throughout the entire recorded history of medicine. The doctrine provides a theoretical matrix from which to organize and interpret knowledge. The specifics of any of the balance models e.g. Alcmaeon, Hippocrates, Aristotle, Four Elements, Four Humors, Four Temperaments, Four Basic Qualities, all emphasize the normal balance between and within physiological systems in maintaining good health and explaining disease. The strength is not in the specifics of each model but rather in the matrix of the conceptualization, thereby providing a way to organize knowledge, explain normal and abnormal function, and predict the effects of treatments based upon the diagnosis made within the given theoretical/conceptual matrix.

Herophilus (325 BC-280 BC) Greek physician, born in Chalcedon, present day Kadikoy, Turkey a suburb of Istanbul, co-founds the medical school at City of Alexandria with friend and colleague Erasistratus of Chios (304 BC-250 BC). He contributes to the foundation of physiology in providing systematic, experimental investigations into the relationship between human anatomical structure and basic vital physiological functions. He is credited with authoring nine texts, including "On Pulses" (300BC/1989)[23] which describes systemic arterial blood flow from the heart. Building upon the doctrine of balances, Herophilus proposes a substance in blood (pneuma) flows with blood from the heart to distant tissues and when the flow of pneuma is obstructed by an excess of any of the four humors, it fails to reach the brain, resulting in impaired vital bodily function. Herophilus provides experimental observations based upon systematic examination of the human anatomy and associated physiology of the reproductive systems. His approach to acquiring new knowledge and testing old knowledge is anchored in an organized, systematic assessment of functional systems through the use of experiment and observation. An Empiricist to be sure, he is often credited as one of the first to apply an approach to investigation, today we refer to as the scientific method.

Erasistratus (304 BC-250 BC) Greek natural philosopher, born on the Greek island of Chios, in the Aegean Sea just off the coast of Turkey and long-time resident, physician, and researcher in the City of Alexandria, is one of the many fathers of physiology. He with his friend and colleague Herophilus, co-found the medical school at the Greek City of Alexandria, located in northern Egypt (sic). Erasistratus embraces an Empiricist approach in acquiring new knowledge. Unlike Herophilus, who comfortably accepts the popular humors model, Erasistratus questions medical dogma and soon rejects the popular humors model as inadequate to explain his own observations and experimental results. He provides an alternative to the humors model, the Doctrine of atomic structure.

That is right; building upon the ideas of pre-Socratic Greek natural philosophers Leucippus of Miletus (400 BC- unknown) and Democritus (460 BC-379 BC), Erasistratus proposes the atomic structure model and offers a better matrix within which to organize and understand the physiological processes of the human body. The doctrine remains central to modern medicine today, over 2,500 years later.

Recall, the atomic structure hypothesis proposes all matter is composed of atoms and empty space between atoms. Atoms, within this model are the smallest unit of matter, too small to be seen and from which no further unit reduction can be made. The atomic model is not readily accepted by the contemporaries of Leucippus of Miletus, Democritus, or Erasistratus. The atomic structural model originally proposed during Antiquity proves to be the foundation upon which modern sciences come to understand all matter.

A lesson of wisdom here for you the medical student. Just because others around you think your ideas are too different from established medical dogma to make sense to them, it does not mean they are bad ideas. Seek out the medical school faculty member who is open to your new ideas and explore your ideas with them. Do not be easily dissuaded from an original and thoughtful idea that challenges existing dogma.

OK… back to contributions made by Erasistratus, during Antiquity, in his efforts to explain the physiology of the human body.

Specifics are provided here as an opportunity for you, the medical student, to begin to develop an appreciation of the historical foundations upon which physiology, as we know it today is built. Pay attention to two streams of information here. First, perhaps least important although interesting, note the differences and similarities in the understanding of physiological systems then and now. For example, during Antiquity the liver is considered the organ responsible for the production of blood. What is the function of the liver today? Second and more importantly, pay attention to the conceptual matrixes proposed by Erasistratus. The matrixes provide systematic and organized structure from which to understand, explain, and predict changes in normal physiological function. The matrixes allow systematic testing by observational and experimental procedures and provide the structure necessary to permit modification of the knowledge base as new or confirmatory information is discovered.

Erasistratus' approach to the study of physiological systems is original, innovative, productive, and open to modification. For example, Erasistratus' conceptual matrix of atomic structure explains old information in a new way, challenges the dogma of humoral balance theories, provides a new way to view physiological systems, and guides new research. Erasistratus and his contributions are notable milestones in the history of human physiology. Many of his investigation incorporate vivisection, permitting examination of organ systems as they function while the individual or animal is still alive. The amount of new knowledge obtained under such investigative conditions is exponential when compared to the static dissection investigations of organ systems, prior to and subsequent to Erasistratus. The City of Alexandria permits and encourages original and creative thought and investigative techniques, unlike many other centers of learning which suppressed originality and creativity in order to better conform to establish scientific, political, and religious dogma.

Erasistratus provides much of the foundational knowledge of human anatomy and associated human physiology. His integrated model of the human physiology is elegant and comprehensive. He accurately describes the valves of the heart; details the flow of blood through the heart; describes the irreversibility of flow through the valves; describes the flow of blood from the heart through the lungs and its return to the heart; recognizes the heart functions as a pump; and offers the first mechanical based explanation for the pulse. He is among the first to describe the differences between arteries and veins, both in structure and function. He correctly identifies the structure and function of gastric muscles and explains how nutrients from digestion are moved from the GI system to the liver and distributed throughout the body. He correctly details the differences between sensory and motor nerves, over one thousand years before Bell and Magendie argue over which one of them should be awarded credit for the discovery. Erasistratus correctly describes the four cerebrospinal fluid filled ventricles of the brain and describes and assigns function to the convoluted gyri of the cerebral and cerebellar hemispheres. He provides an integrated matrix from which to understand voluntary movement and provides the bases for all respiratory physiology. Erasistratus completes much of the early work in physiology recognizing and investigating pressure differences within the human body and the associated movement of substances such as air and blood, as a function of differences in pressures.

On a more applied front, Erasistratus is among the first to recognize the physiological benefits and associated good health benefits of exercise coupled with good diet, based upon experimental investigation, rather than simply anecdotal observations.

When thinking about Erasistratus, consider not only his specific contributions, consider the similarities and differences in the way we think about physiological systems then and today. Appreciate the differences in conceptual matrixes. See the elegance of his thought process and proposed conceptual matrix. Recognize the shift in paradigm taking place. Note the rejection of Aristotelian dogma; the invention and development of new procedures and techniques employed to challenge, test, and explain old, well-established ideas; and the resistance of many to new ideas.

Here are a few more specific examples of Erasistratus' many substantial contributions to physiology. Let's briefly examine three familiar systems: the cardio-pulmonary-vascular, neural, and respiratory systems. All three are proposed by Erasistratus around 275 BC and contribute to one of the first unified theories of multiple physiological systems working in unison, within the human body.

First, the cardio-pulmonary-vascular system. The heart is described as a four chambered muscle whose primary function is to pump a life giving substance from the left ventricle through a one way valve into the aorta (sic) and systemic arterial circulation. This substance circulates through the arterial system and provides the necessary substances to give and maintain life. The substance gives life to tissues, as it moves through an interwoven terminal network of arteries, veins, and nerves. After providing tissues with "life", the life giving substance is removed from the system, making room for new and fresh life giving substance. The substance is not returned to the heart but rather eliminated from the body through pores.

This life giving substance described by Erasistratus is not blood but rather "pneuma". The term is derived from ancient Greek meaning "breath" or more specifically "inspired air". Soon the Church and other organized religions offer a more mystic and religious synonym for the term, including "soul" and "spirit". Independent of the specific term used the concept remains the same. Pneuma is essential and necessary for life. Erasistratus describes it as a moist, warm, air like substance. Notice the terms moist and warm. Recall, the works of Alcmaeon and Aristotle over one hundred years before who describe the physical body within the matrix of balances between wet and dry, and hot and cold.

According to Erasistratus, pneuma is inhaled from the atmosphere into the lungs by way of negative pressure. The pneuma is mixed with blood in the lungs and moved to the left side of the heart through the blood filled pulmonary vein. In the left ventricle of the heart, pneuma is converted into "vital pneuma" (life giving pneuma). The "vital pneuma", not blood, is then pumped from the heart, through the aorta and arteries which are filled with air, not blood. Within this matrix, only veins are filled with blood. The "vital pneuma" moves to distant tissues through the arterial system, provides "life" to tissues, and is removed from the system through pores and never returns to the heart.

Erasistratus explains the pulse is the result of "vital pneuma" being pumped from the left ventricle during systole, resulting in cyclic distention of the arteries. During cardiac diastole "vitalized blood" moves from the lungs into the emptied left side of the heart, due to negative pressure left in the ventricle after pumping "vital pneuma" out of the heart and into the arterial system.

This new mechanical based explanation of cardio physiology stands in contrast to the dogma of the Aristotelian anatomical and five element functional models, which stood the test of time for over 100 years. Erasistratus further challenges medical dogma, that the heart is the organ responsible for the production of blood. He proposes the liver and not the heart is responsible for blood production. Within his model, the liver receives nutrients from the GI system through the portal vein. The nutrients are converted into blood in the liver. Blood then moves through the veins to all parts of the body, including the right side of the heart, where it nourishes the heart muscle. Blood then moves into the lungs where it provides nourishment to the lungs. Blood never leaves the lungs or returns to the heart. Only "non-vitalized pneuma" from the lungs are drawn into the left side of the heart as the result of negative pressure created when the heart contracts and moves "vitalized pneuma" into the arterial systems. Simply, an elegant system.

Again the important point here is not the correctness of the system but rather the integrated conceptual matrix of the system which permits experimental testing and revision of the systems based upon experimental results and an entirely new way of viewing the body.

Second example, the neural system. Erasistratus views the nervous system as central to all normal physiological function. Rejecting the current medical dogma which places the heart at the center of all physiological functions Erasistratus proposes the brain as a reasonable alternative, based upon anatomical and physiological conceptual matrixes and experimental findings. He soon challenges current medical dogma once again and proposes nerves emanate from the brain rather than the heart. He further provides an integrated anatomical-physiological matrix to understand nerves. Within his matrix, nerves are hollow vessels and filled with "psychic pneuma".

Psychic pneuma is a metabolic product of the more general pneuma contained in atmospheric air. Recall, pneuma is contained in atmospheric air which is inhaled into the lungs and moves to the left side of the heart where it is modified into "vital pneuma". The life giving "vital pneuma" is moved through bloodless arteries to the brain where the "vital pneuma" is further processed into "psychic pneuma". It is the "psychic pneuma" which is then moved from the brain, through hollow nerves, throughout the body to affect functional results such as movement.

Movement is dependent upon the amount of pneuma present in any muscle group at any point in time. As with "vital pneuma" within the arteries, "psychic pneuma" within the nerves is removed from the system through pores.

Erasistratus proposes function to the brain gyri and sulci. He proposes their function is simply to dissipated heat generated by the body, much in the same way heat is removed from a system by a radiator. More specifically, he views brain gyri and sulci as an essential part of a more complex cooling system whose purpose is to dissipate heat generated by heart muscles, generated during cardiac contractions.

The lungs are also an essential part of the cooling system for the heart. As pneuma is drawn from the lungs into the left side of the heart, residual air remains in the lungs. The residual air in the lung is the result of the limited volume capacity of the left side of the heart. It is the residual air in the lungs which acquires heat generated by the body, including the heart, and exhaled as a routine course of the respiratory and cardiac cycles. Simply an elegant system.

The third and final example is the respiratory system. Erasistratus states simply, air along with pneuma is inhaled into the lungs as the result of negative pressure in the thorax. The pneuma is extracted in the lungs and drawn into the heart as the left and right cardiac ventricles expand during diastole. Excess pneuma and air in the lungs acquires any heat which might be generated by the body and is simply removed from the system by exhaling. The system provides an efficient and integrated system to supply the heart and distant body tissues with necessary "vital pneuma" and a cooling-exhaust system to eliminate heat, generated by the pneuma consuming, heat producing tissues, such as cardiac and skeletal muscles.

Yes, the specifics of these systems are at odds with how we understand these three systems today, two thousand years later. However, the elegance of an integrated system which opens itself up to experimental examination and modifications is unique for its time and offers a much needed alternative to the current medical and religious dogma in both process and content.

Aulus Celsus (14 AD-37 AD), Roman encyclopedist offers his book "De Medicina" (30 AD) associating anatomical structure with function and offering treatments based upon accumulated knowledge to that time. "De Medicina" certainly can be argued to be one of the most influential medical texts of the period and continues to influence medical texts over two thousand years ago after its first publication. Celsus organizes "De Medicina" and knowledge into eight books; History of Medicine (A great choice don't you think?), General Pathology, Specific Diseases, Parts of the Body, Pharmacology, Surgery, and Orthopedics (30AD,1713,1814,2010)[24,25,26].

OK... for those of you counting, Books 5 and 6 are devoted to the topics of pharmacology. In addition to providing content, Celsus discusses the relevance of theory to the practice of medicine and the pros and cons of experimentation with animals and humans. He advocates a modified Hippocratic approach to treating patients. Basically, Celsus' position is to observe the patient and let nature work. Don't oppose it. He reassures practitioner and patient, fever is good and it is a sign the body is attempting to heal itself. Provide the patient with sound and comforting reassurance. A practice still applied by healthcare workers today, over two thousand years later.

"De Medicina" remains required reading for medical students for over one and half centuries. Some of what Celsus proposes in "De Medicina" is still taught in medical schools today. Remember the four cardinal signs of inflammation: calor (warmth), dolor (pain), tumor (swelling), and rubor (redness)? Yes, these are but a few of the bits of knowledge originally proposed in "De Medicina" which are as true today as they were when first written by Celsus two thousand years ago, circa 30 AD.

Caution: Don't make the mistake and confuse Aulus Celsus the encyclopedist with Anders Celsius (1701-1744) the Swedish astronomer who gave us the centigrade scale for measuring temperature.

Galen of Pergamum (129 AD-200 AD) physician and philosopher is arguably one of the most prolific medical investigators of Antiquity. The son of a wealthy architect, he contributes to anatomy, pharmacology, neurology, pathology and physiology. You may recognize him from the popular literature which oftentimes refers to him as the physician to the Roman gladiators. He is very much more. Actually, Galen is born in Turkey in the city of Pergamum. Pergamum is a Greek city (sic), located in Turkey and part of the Roman Empire. Today, Pergamum is the city of Bergama, Turkey. Recall, the Roman Empire encompasses most all of the coastal Mediterranean Sea during this period. Pergamum is a major cultural and intellectual center with its own impressive Library and second only to the City and Libraries of Alexandria.

Galen is independently wealthy, well-traveled, and educated. He lives for a brief period in the City of Alexandria where he is exposed to medical writings of such notables Erasistratus and Celsus, before settling in the city of Rome circa 161 AD. Today, in popular literature, Galen is often described as the physician to the gladiators. True enough, however he was physician to the gladiators of the Greek city of Pergamum, located in present day Turkey. There is no record of Galen ever being a physician to the gladiators of Rome. Physician to gladiators of the Roman Empire yes, but to Rome no. A subtle distinction perhaps, but one you as a future physician might want to know. Galen is never accepted by the physicians of Rome. Galen spends relatively little time in Rome, having been rejected by most of the practicing physicians of the City. He does return many years later to assist in the treatment of the City's population afflicted by the Antonine Plague. This plague ravages the City circa 166 AD and substantially reduces the City population. Galen's writings include descriptions of the clinical the signs and symptoms associated with this plague, which most people today will agree is consistent with smallpox.

Trivia: Gladiator is derived from the Latin "gladius" meaning "sword". Gladiator refers to a swordsman.

All of Galen's original writings are in Greek. Only later are they translated into Latin and Arabic, during the Eastern Roman Empire, aka Byzantine Empire of the Middle Ages. The translations are heavily influenced by and appear modified to be more consistent with the bourgeoning belief systems of the Christian Church and Islamic thought of the period. Recall, during the Middle Ages much of the financial support for scholars come from organized religion. Some if not all of the translations are influenced by organized religions, political, and social presses of the period.

Galen's contributions include an estimated 600 treaties. Approximately 200 of these treatises survive to date. A copy of Galen's first printed editions are housed in the Biliotheque Interuniversitaire de Medicine of Paris. Digitized copies of these texts are now available through the Bibliotheque Interuniversitaire de Medicine et d'Odontologie, Paris.

During the early-1800s, Carolus Kuhn (1754-1840) translates 122 of Galen's writings (1821-1833, 1821-1833,1829)[27,28,29]. His efforts include the original Greek text along with Latin translations. This extensive published collection of the majority of Galen's surviving treaties is over 20,000 pages in length, including 676 index pages, and bound in 22 volumes. John Coxe, an American physician, provides a less comprehensive treatment of Galen's treaties, which are devoted specifically to physiology, during the mid-1800s (1846)[30]. More recently, more complete English translations of Galen's works have become available (2002)[31].

Galen's contribution to physiology is found both in his empirical-experimental approach to acquiring knowledge, copious writings, ardent position every structure had a function, and he knew the function. If you disagree with him you simply fail to appreciate the truth. His writing shape medical dogma for over 1500 years.

Trivia: Galen is among the first to argue in favor of implementing a peer review system for medical publications, as a means to insure standards of excellence in all medical publications. The peer review system remains the standard today for all scholarly medical publications.

Notable examples of Galen's contributions to physiology are found in his treaties describing physiology of digestion, blood production, respiration, and blood distribution throughout the body for the purpose of tissue profusion. Galen's treaties on these subjects, written over three hundred years after Erasistratus, have an uncanny resemblance to the works of Erasistratus. Galen treaties describe the function of the gastrointestinal system as providing essential nutrients to the liver. The liver absorbs the nutrients and transforms them into purple colored venous blood, in the liver. The venous blood is moved through veins to the right side of the heart. The venous blood then moves through invisible pores in the cardiac septum and into the left side of the heart. It is here where blood is mixed with life generating "vital pneuma", which has been drawn into the heart by respiration. The life infused scarlet colored blood ebbs and flows through arteries from the heart to distant body parts, supplying the necessary "vital pneuma" to maintain life. Hummm… sounds a lot like a minor modification of the more complete physiological system presented by Erasistratus hundreds of years earlier. Another historical example of professional credit being awarded to a prolific writer rather than the original investigator? Which name do you most recognize, Erasistratus or Galen? You decide who most deserves credit for the original contribution.

In summary, Antiquity witnesses the founding of the first formal center for educating and training physicians. The center located in southern Italy, recognizes the value of the foundational principles of physiology associating function with anatomy and requires all future physicians be trained in these relationships. The first of many Doctrines of balances is introduced and provides a theoretical matrix within which to understand the functions of the human body. A rational epistemological approach displaces the empirical-inductive approach of the Ancients. The Hippocratic Collection is compiled in Alexandria circa 300 BC, with books and treaties on physiology, representing one of the ten major classifications of the Collection. Aristotle rejects his teacher's rationalism and advocates an empirical approach as the preferred approach whenever investigating sensory physiology. Aristotle offers his modification of the Doctrine of balances to explain good health and disease. The medical school at the City of Alexandria is founded and too emphasizes the importance of physiology investigations and application to all practicing physicians.

Specific systems e.g. cardio-vascular" are studied systematically. An alternative to the Doctrines of balances is proposed circa 420 BC, in the Doctrine of atomic structure and becomes the foundation upon which modern sciences come to understand all matter, over twenty five hundred years later. The physiology of traditional major systems e.g. cardio-vascular, respiratory, gastro-intestinal, neural, reproductive are investigated systematically using what will later be termed the scientific method and lay the foundation for understanding physiological systems. Celsus gives us "De Medicina" circa 30 AD and his four signs of inflammation: calor (warmth), dolor (pain), tumor (swelling), and rubor (redness). Galen is responsible for recording much of what is known about physiology and medicine of the period, applies an empirical experimental approach to his investigations, and takes credit for many works originally completed by others.

Middle Ages (Medieval Times), 500 AD - 1400 AD.

The Middle Ages witness few advances in physiology from Western Europe. The true advances are being made in the Middle East.

Ibn Sina (aka Avicenna when Latinized) (980 AD -1037 AD) Persian philosopher, physician, and scientist introduce experimentation and quantification to physiology in the 14 volume encyclopedia "Kitab al-Qanun fil al-Tibb" [The Canon of Medicine] in 1025 AD (1025AD,1632, 1999)[32,33,34]. The impact of this publication cannot be over emphasized in its importance in the history of medicine. It provides a systematic compilation and synthesis of medical knowledge, according to the principles of Galen and Hippocrates and proves to be the authoritative basis for training physicians in Western Europe for the next 500 years and in the Middle East for the next 800 years. The publication provides organized, theoretically based treatments, drawn from the basic sciences physiology, microbiology, pharmacology, and pathology. The publication addresses numerous specialized topics e.g. cardiology, endocrinology, bacteriology, gerontology, ophthalmology, neuropsychiatry and more.

Ibn Sina offers the first persuasive published arguments in support of the practice of evidenced based and experimental medicine. Many agree the "Canon of Medicine" is one of the most influential books in all of medical history.

Ibn al-Nafis (1213 AD-1288 AD) of Damascus, present day capital of Syria, is born approximately 300 years after Ibn Sina. As a physiologist he discredits much of the medical dogma which has been in place since the time of Galen. He correctly describes pulmonary circulation, displacing the thousand year old theory advanced by Galen. Ibn al-Nafis is first to correctly report blood from the right ventricle reaches the left ventricle by way of circulation first through the lungs, rather than through invisible pores in the intraventricular septum, as proposed by Galen and others. He correctly describes the function of the lungs as necessary for the mixing of air and blood. Ibn al-Nafis proposes the capillary and describes its function in pulmonary, coronary, and systemic circulation in 1242 AD (1924,1935,1953)[35,36,37]. His conceptualizations of circulation will not be significantly modified for the next 500 years. Ibn al-Nafis rejects Galenic theory regarding the pulse and offers an alternative. Ibn al-Nafis is first to correctly describe and explain the pulse as we understand it today (2006)[38].

Ibn al-Nafis, in addition to his highly influential "Commentary on the Anatomy of Avicenna's Canon" (1242AD)[39] offers a comprehensive encyclopedia of medical knowledge in a staggering 80 volume set titled "The Comprehensive Book on the Art of Medicine" (Kitab al-shamil fi al-tibb) (1275AD, 2000)[40,41]. He also provides a summary of the massive encyclopedia with an abbreviated version for the medical student and general practitioner, "The Epitome in Medicine" [Al-Mujaz fi al-Tibb] (2004)[42] and "A treatise on physiology" [Risalar al-aada] (1991)[43]. Through his publications Ibn-al-Nafis frequently and directly challenges the dogma of Galenian thought. He offers alternative explanations for many well established medical truths. Ibn al-Nafis' alternative explanations have stood the test of time for over 800 years and since he first dares to challenge the medical dogma of his day.

In summary, the Middle Ages witness few advancements in physiology within Western Europe. The greatest advancements are being made in the Middle East, where much of the knowledge from Antiquity is being examined, modified, reinterpreted, and often displaced by new knowledge. Ibn Sina offers his landmark 14 volume "Canon of Medicine", a compilation and synthesis of medical knowledge according to the principles of Galen and Hippocrates. His "Canon" provides a theoretically based matrix to guide medical treatments. Ibn Sina advocates the practice of evidenced based and experimental medicine. Towards the end of the Middle Ages, Ibn al-Nafis' experimental investigations and critical thought discredits much of the medical dogma accepted since Galan. The anatomy and function of cardio-pulmonary circulation is correctly described for the first time. Ibn al-Nafis offers his comprehensive 80 volume encyclopedia "The Comprehensive Book on Medicine" providing an authoritative and direct challenge to over one thousand years of medical dogma. As political, economic, and social stability returns to Western Europe, physiology is poised to continue its development as a science based discipline with clinical applications to medicine.

Early Modern, 1400 AD - 1800 AD.

Physiology matures as a discipline.

Physiology begins to establish itself distinct from anatomy. The term "physiology' first appears in scientific publications. Vitalism is replaced by laws of physics. The mechanisms of actions of organ systems are reinterpreted and conceptualized within the matrix of mechanical systems. Interests in the measurement of the intrinsic properties of biological systems (biometrics) increase rapidly and become a main stay of most physiological investigations. Physiological measurements blood pressures, pulse rates, and body temperatures, studied in the laboratory, move into the clinical setting and become routine measurements taken during the physical examination of patients. Research activities focus heavily upon the investigations of pulmonary, cardio, systemic circulations, and bioelectric properties of bodily tissues. Physiology continues to be recognized as necessary and essential knowledge for practicing physicians. Physiology becomes a familiar foundational course in the medical school curriculum, along with anatomy and pathology. By the end of the 1700s, the first scientific journal devoted specifically to the study of physiology begins publication.

Jean Fernel (1497-1558) notable French physician is first to use the term "physiology" in a printed publication to describe the study of function and the natural processes within the human body. Recall, "physis" is from the ancient Greek word meaning nature. The term first appears in 1542 in the introduction of Fernel's "Physiologia" (1567/2003)[44], which is the first book, in a three volume series, "Universa Medicinae" (1564)[45]. Fernel presents physiology, for the first time as an integrated study of body systems. However, resistant to change, Fernel organizes physiology within a Galenian matrix. He proposes physiology as the preferred methodology to understand organ system pathologies and to guide clinical therapeutics. He views physiology as necessary and essential knowledge to the practice of competent clinical medicine. In keeping with Fernel's proposals, over 500 years ago, physiology remains a foundations course, in every allopathic medical training program today.

Michael Servetus (1511-1553) Spanish physician and Realdo Colombo (1516-1569) Italian anatomist publish their observations regarding pulmonary circulation. Both reject the Galenian dogma which has dominated European thought for over 1,200 years. Recall, Galen states in his usual and customary authoritative manner, blood does not pass through the lungs but rather venous blood is moved from the liver, where it is made, into the right side of the heart. Blood is then moved directly through the cardiac septum into the left side of the heart, where it is mixed with "vital pneuma" supplied from the lungs. Blood is then moved to distant body tissues, where the blood is absorbed by the tissues.

Servetus (1546,1553)[46,47] and Colombo (1559)[48] in separate publications, propose an alternative to the Galenian model. Servetus and Colombo describe the pulmonary circulation as we understand it today. Blood moves from the right atrium into the right ventricle, through the lungs, then to the left atrium, into the left ventricle, then pumped into the systemic circulation and ultimately returning to the right atrium. Colombo further discoveries the main action of the heart is contraction rather than dilation, further challenging accepted medical knowledge of the period.

Michael Servetus and Realdo Colombo are frequently credited with the discovery of the correct pulmonary circulation, followed by additional credit to English physiologist William Harvey (1578-1657) (1628)[49]. It has recently been discovered the pulmonary circulation had been previously and correctly described in detail by Ibn al-Nafis, over 300 years earlier in his book "Sharh Tashrīh al-Qānūn" (1288AD). Certainly, Servetus, Colombo, and Harvey make substantial additional contributions in understanding pulmonary circulation and bring an increased understanding of pulmonary circulation to Western Europe. It is worthwhile to note many of Ibn al-Nafis writings on this topic are translated into Latin in 1547, approximately five years before Servetus, ten years before Colombo, and seventy years before Harvey, offer their first publications on this topic in Europe. Coincidence? You decide.

Santorio Santorio (sic) (1561-1636) Italian physiologist maintains interests in physiological systems responsible for temperature, respiration, and body weight. He is instrumental in inventing several of the medical instruments we routinely use today in clinical practice, including the numerically scaled thermometer "thermoscope" and an instrument for measuring the pulse "pulsilogium". Perhaps most will remember Santorio's famous experiment in which he empirically studies his own body metabolism, over the course of 30 years. He publishes his findings in "De Statica Medicina" [Concerning Static Medicine] (1614)[50]. Throughout the course of the experiment, Santorio carefully weights his solid and liquid intake and solid and liquid excretions. He weighs himself at regular intervals and following specific conditions e.g. eating and sleeping. Based upon careful calculations, he describes changes in total body weight as the result of metabolic processes and concludes the greatest part of loss in total body weight is due to perspiration. The experiment opens the doorway to metabolism physiology.

In addition to Santorio's empirical and quantitative methodologies, he offers a fundamental change in the philosophical conceptualization of the body. He rejects the Aristotelian and Galanean models which conceptualize the body in terms of elements and qualities. Santorio considers the fundamental properties of the human body to be best understood within a mathematical matrix, including number, form, and position. He proposes the body can best be understood as a biomechanical system of interlocking parts, similar to that of any mechanical device. Pathologies and treatments can be reasonably explained and directed by an appreciation of the independence and interdependencies of multiple functional systems interacting together.

William Harvey (1578-1657) English physiologist and foreign medical school graduate (Italian medical school in Padua) builds upon the works of Ibn al-Nafis, Servetus, and Colombo and details a closed system of blood circulation in his 72 page landmark publication titled "Exercitatio Anatomicia de Motu Cordis er Sanguinis ct Sanguinis in Animalibus" [An Anatomical Exercise on the Motion of the Heart and Blood in Animals] (1628)[49]. Twenty five years after the original publication, the paper is translated from Latin into English (1653)[51]. Harvey's "De Motus Cordis" challenges the dogma of Galen and incites controversy within the medical and scientific communities. Many of Harvey's contemporaries and colleagues, notably Thomas Willis (Circle of Willis), Thomas Wharton (Wharton Jelly), and Thomas Sydenham (Sydenham Chorea) all remain silent on Harvey's reported discovery for over a decade, perhaps fearing professional repercussions oftentimes associated in challenging scientific or medical dogma.

Harvey's conceptualization of the cardio-pulmonary and systemic-vascular system, as a closed anatomical system, best understood within the conceptual matrix of mechanistic and mathematical models is consistent with the Renaissance mindset of the period. Harvey's model of cardio-pulmonary and systemic-circulation challenges not only Galenian based scientific and medical dogma in place for over 1500 years, but also the Vitalist view held by the Church for over 1500 years.

This serves as another example to you, the medical student, of the resistance you may experience to any new and innovative ideas you might express, which challenge well established truths. I encourage you to exercise good professional/political judgement, but do not be easily discouraged by others around you when you present a well conceptualized idea, which challenges current dogma, and you fail to receive support from others around you. The history of medicine is filled with individuals who have made the most substantial contributions, yet were not supported and oftentimes ridiculed by individuals and institutions surrounding them. So is the nature of change.

Harvey further impacts physiology by his ardent support of the experimental method as the preferred method whenever studying human physiology and his application of biometric calculations in guiding his thoughts and experimental investigations. A biometric example will serve well here. Assuming the Galenian model is correct, the heart and liver produce blood; blood is distributed to body tissues through vessels; blood provides nutrients to body tissues; and blood is consumed by the tissues rather than recirculated; then applying Harvey's biometric calculations: the heart pumps approximately two ounces of blood out of the left ventricle with every contraction and the heart contracts approximately 72 times a minute, the result is approximately 1,620 gallons of blood needs to be produced by the heart and liver and subsequently consumed by body tissues every day. Hummm…

A priori biometric calculations remain a mainstay in the study of physiology today and continue to provide a methodology to assist in sound hypothesis generation and assessment.

Herman Boerhaave (1668-1738) Dutch physician and medical educator substantively influences medical school curricula and training of physicians in Europe. He is an ardent proponent and advocate of medical school curricula, requiring physicians in training, to complete an organized sequence of basic science education, including physics, chemistry, anatomy, physiology, and pathology, before allowing students to begin clinical training. Upon successful demonstration of a command of the basic sciences' content materials, students then and only then are moved into hospital based clinical training. Sound familiar? In addition to his commitment to the education and training of future physicians, Boerhaave summaries current knowledge of physiology in his most recognized publication, "Institutes Medicinae" (1708)[52].

As the Renaissance of Western Europe comes to a close, during the late-1600s, physiology establishes itself as a burgeoning academic discipline with methodologies based upon the scientific method and biometric quantification. Quantitative methodologies become evident and applied routinely in physiological investigations. Statistical based methodologies become relevant in the study of the normal and abnormal human body functions. The human body is viewed more like a mechanical device than ever before, offering new insights within and between organ systems. Physiology research, during the Renaissance period (1400s -1600s), focuses upon the study of cardio-pulmonary and systemic-circulations. The vitalist dogma of the Church and the medical dogma of Galen are challenged by observations and new discoveries. Movable type printing is invented and offers a new technology for disseminating scientific knowledge broadly throughout Western Europe. New methodologies continue to be applied to the systematic scientific investigations of the human body and yield good results. New methods of sharing scientific discoveries between investigators and medical practitioners are embraced, yielding advancements in scientific knowledge and improved medical care of patients.

The second half of the Early Modern Period (1700-1800) evidence much attention in two areas of physiological investigation. First, a there is continuation of interests in the cardio-pulmonary and systemic-circulations. Emphasis shifts from anatomy to the physics of blood flow. Second, there is much interest in the source and transmission properties of bioelectrical energy.

Stephen Hales (1677-1761) English physiologist invents a prototypical measuring device to objectively quantify arterial blood pressures. He first reports his device and quantitative measurement of arterial blood pressure in 1727 (1727)[53]. Soon after, he follows with two books, "Statistical Essays" (1731)[54] and "Haemastaticks" (1733)[55], in which he details his experiments on the force and flow rates of blood and the measured capacity and elasticity of a variety of blood vessels. One important observation Hales makes is that arteries have an elastic property and contribute to the transformation of the high pressure, pulsatile forces generated within the aorta during each cardiac contraction to much lower pressure and steady flow forces within peripheral vessels. His observations provide important advancements in the development of a more complete understanding of cardio-pulmonary-systemic circulations.

Daniel Bernoulli (1700-1782) Dutch mathematician develops and applies mathematical formula to the physiology of body fluid flow mechanics and dynamics. He proposes the Bernoulli Principle to explain the movement of fluids through body vessels. Recall, in brief the Bernoulli Principle states as the speed of a fluid increases, pressure decreases.

Bernoulli details the mathematics of the Principle in his book Hydrodynamica (1738)[56]. Applying the Principle to blood flow dynamics, in particular to the movement of blood through a vessel narrowed by plaque (stenosis of the vessel); blood flow through the constricted section of the vessel should increase in velocity due to the decrease in pressure. This makes sense if blood is inviscid. Blood, however is not inviscid. Additionally, the circulatory system does not meet the requirements of horizontal, non-turbulent, non-pulsatile, laminar flow, through uniform diameter vessels, thereby violating several assumptions upon which the Bernoulli Principle is based. While Bernoulli's application of hydrodynamic flow mathematics to the human vascular system goes wanting, it does provide an early attempt to integrate multidisciplinary knowledge, hydrodynamics, mathematics, physics, and statics and applies it to the study of physiology.

Trivia: Daniel Bernoulli completes the first epidemiological statistical analysis examining smallpox and vaccine effectiveness (1766)[57].

Jean Poiseuille (1797-1869) French physiologist, sorts out the viscosity problem and elaborates on the tremendous effect the radius of blood vessels play in blood flow dynamics, 100 years after Daniel Bernoulli introduced his principle of flow dynamics (1838)[58]. Perhaps you might recall Poiseuille's equation from your medical school's physiology class, $Q = \pi \Delta P r^4 / 8 \eta l$. Posiseuille's formulation of blood flow (Q) takes into consideration the additional factors; the differences in pressures between the ends of the vessel (ΔP), radius of the vessels (r), the viscosity of the blood (η), and the length of a vessel (l). Bottom line here is that Poiseuille's formulation is more appropriate to understanding and explaining the flow of blood through blood vessels than Bernoulli's Principle. Poiseuille's calculations can be further simplified for practical purposes by remembering blood flow equals 2x the radius of the vessel and vessel radius is the most important factor when determining blood flow.

OK… let us return to the mid-1700s.

Albrecht von Haller (1707-1777) Swiss physiologist, publishes the first textbook devoted specifically to physiology "Primae lineae physiologiae" (1747)[59]. Six years later he publishes his most important work "De partibus corporis humani sensibilibus et irritabilibus" in which he demonstrates two essential physiology principles (1753)[60]. First, only organs innervated by nerves are capable of generating conscious sensations. Second, tissues and organs independent of neural innervations are capable of responding to internal and external stimulations. Von Haller subsequently publishes a massive eight volume set describing the advances in physiology, during the past 130 years and since William Harvey's "De Motus Cordi", in "Elementa Physiologiae Corporis Humani" [Physiological Elements of the Human Body] (1757-1766)[61]. Von Haller's teachings and publications guide physiology, especially muscle physiology for the next 100 years.

Bioelectricity attracts a lot of attention during the mid and late-1700s. Luigi Galvani and Allessandro Volta make particularly important contributions in understanding bioelectricity.

Luigi Galvani (1737-1798) Italian physiologist is responsible the foundational work in electrophysiology. He is among the first to report biological tissues, specifically muscle, are influenced by electricity and more specifically bioelectricity. Galvani's theory is simple. A neuro-electrical fluid, an innate vital force, is secreted from the brain, conducted through nerves, and stored in muscles. When the negatively charged, "animal electricity" stored in tissue is pulled from tissue by means of positively charged fluid moving through nerves, the difference in charges result in the generation of an electrical arc. In the case of skeletal muscle, the discharge of the stored animal electricity produces contraction of muscle fibers and consequentially movement. He publishes his initial observations and experiments in a brief 55 page essay in 1791, titled "De Viribus Electricitatis in Motu Musculari Commentarius" [Commentary on the Effect of Electricity on Muscular Motion] (1791a,1791b)[62,63,64]. Galvani subsequently offers his physiological model as a potential explanation for common clinical disorders, tics, restlessness, and convulsive seizures. Galvani's explanations are consistent with the mechanistic models of fluids still popular within the scientific communities of the time. Galvani's experiments are soon replicated by Allessandro Volta. However, Volta challenges Galvani's explanation and offers an alternative.

Allessandro Volta (1745-1827) Italian physicist rejects Galvani's model of stored "animal electricity" and proposes an alternative explanation. Volta argues tissues e.g. skeletal muscle, do not store electricity but rather the tissue simply operates as a conductor and electricity is generated by the contact of two different metals. Volta argues an electrical potential must be applied to the tissue for the tissue to contract. Within Volta's model, tissues simply operate as an electrolyte.

Soon a heated professional debate between Galvani and Volta appears in the professional literature and professional conferences. Often described as the "Galvani-Volta debate", the "debate" in fact reflects a spirited discussion during the late-1800s by many scientists, as they struggle to assimilate their own observations into the polarizing positions of the vitalistic view of "animal electricity", the non-vitalistic view of "metallic electricity", and their role in explaining normal and abnormal physiology of the human body.

Trivia: The familiar, standardized unit of electromotive force "volt" is named in Volta's honor, forty-six years after his death (1873)[65]. The term "volt" is officially approved by the First International Congress of Electricians, eight years later, becoming an official international standard unit of measurement of electricity (1881)[66]. The Congress also approved four additional, now familiar measurements of electricity, ohm, ampere, coulomb, and farad (1881)[66].

Alexander von Humboldt (1769-1859) German scientist offers a synthesis of the two extreme position of Galvani and Volta suggesting both are correct and both wrong (1797)[67]. Recall, for

Galvani, electricity is generated directly from biological tissues. Contraction of a muscle results when the imbalance in electricity between the electric fluid secreted by the brain and transmitted within a nerve comes in contact with muscle tissues, discharging the stored electricity within the muscle tissues and restoring the electrical balance. The muscle contraction is the result of the electrical discharge in the muscle tissue. For Volta, the source of electricity must be applied externally. In light of von Humboldt's best conciliatory efforts to bring the positions of Galvani and Volta into a unified model, the polarizing positions of Galvani and Volta continue to be debated until the mid-1800s. The Galvani-Volta debate is finally resolved by the experimental works of German physiologist Emil du Bois-Reymond (1848)[68].

An incidental consequence of the passionate rivalry between Galvani and Volta is the development of an electrical cell battery capable of transmitting a continuous electrical current. In efforts to prove Galvani wrong and provide experimental data in support of his own position, Volta creates the voltic pile for use in his experiments. The pile provides the necessary hardware for Volta to complete repeated experiments in applying a controlled amount of electricity to various materials in his unrelenting efforts to prove Galvani wrong.

Less concerned with the scientific debate between Galvani and Volta, regarding the origin of the contraction of skeletal muscle and much more impressed by Volta's discovery of the chemical battery, Napoleon Bonaparte, in 1801 rewards Volta with the title of Count of Lombardy, in recognition of Volta's discovery. Recall, Lombardy is one of the twenty regions in Italy with its capital city Milan.

Trivia: The title "Count" is award by a European monarch, as an honorary Nobleman's title, to someone who has provided exceptional service to the state or territory.

Interests in electricity and in particularly bioelectricity during the late-1700s help to lay the foundations for early electrophysiology research and all future investigations during the next 200 years. The late-1700s also witness the first scholarly publication devoted exclusively to the exchange of information between investigators focusing investigations in the discipline of physiology.

Johannas Reil (1759-1813) German physiologist establishes in 1795 the first scientific journal devoted specifically to the study of physiology, the "Archives fur die Physiologie". The Journal represents the first attempt to provide investigators a regularly published, peer reviewed, scientific forum to report and discuss the science of physiology. The establishment of professional journals and organizations are signs a discipline is maturing. Reil advocates with great commitment, physiology should be the scientific foundation upon which all medicine should be based. He further advocates physiology should be grounded in the science of chemistry. Reil an advocate of the still popular concept of vitalism offers an early monograph describing vital "life forces" within the matrix of chemical and physiological function (1796)[69], serving as an example of the efforts of many to reconcile popular medical and organized religion's dogmatic beliefs of "life forces" with scientific advances in chemistry and physiology.

Reil maintains interests in the chemistry and physiology of mental illness. He publishes one of the first books devoted to the treatment of the mentally ill and advocates for the humane treatment of the mentally ill, including separate housing of psychiatric patients deemed curable from the incurable (1803)[70]. His interests in mental illness soon results in the establishment of two scientific journals devoted specifically to the study of mental illnesses and their treatment. Five years later,

Reil coins the term "psychiatry". The term first appears in the scientific literature in Reil's recently established journal "Beytrage zur Beforderung einer Kurmethode auf Psychischem Wege" [Contributions to the Advancement of a Treatment Method by Psychic Ways] in his 118 page paper titled "Uber den Begriff der Medizin und ihre Verzweigungen, besonders in Beziehung auf die Berichtigung der Topik in der Psychiaterie" [On the term of medicine and its branches, especially with regard to the rectification of the topic in psychiatry] (1808)[71]. The term remains in use today, defining the subfield in medicine devoted to the diagnosis and treatment of mental disorders.

In summary, the Early Modern Period (1400AD-1800AD) witness the maturation of physiology as a scientific discipline. The term "physiology" first appears in the scientific literature. Physics replaces vitalism. New and innovative conceptual thought slowly begins to replace Galenian dogma. Standardized measurements of physiological functions become more common. Blood pressure, pulse rate, body weight, body temperature become routine measurements. Biometric calculations become an important part of physiology. Cardio-pulmonary-systemic-circulation systems continue to be studied and refined. Interests in bioelectricity spark numerous investigations into the electrophysiology of major organ systems. The medical school education and training of future physicians is sequenced to insure a command of basics sciences before moving into hospital based clinical training.

Fernel gives us the term "physiology. Servetus and Colombo correctly describe cardio-pulmonary-systemic-circulation. Harvey refines cardio-pulmonary-systemic-circulation and is shun by his contemporaries. Boerhaave sequences medical school curriculums to ensure command of basic sciences prior to clinical training. Hale measures blood pressures. Bernoulli gives us the theoretical mathematics to describe the flow of fluids. Poiseuille describes and details factors most important in the flow of bodily fluids, modifies Bernoulli's formulations, and gives us the formula recognized by every medical student today, used whenever estimating blood flow, 2x the vessel's radius. Von Haller gives us the first textbook devoted specifically to physiology. Galvani and Volta debate the origin of muscle contractions and describe the important role of bioelectricity. Reil applies the study of physiology to mental illnesses and gives us "psychiatry".

Physiology is now well positioned for the explosion of interests, exponential increase in physiology research, and true maturation of physiology as a scientific discipline soon to occur.

Middle Modern, 1800 AD - 1900 AD.

Physiology having made some progress is still viewed as a nonexact science, at the beginning of the 1800s. Throughout the 1800s physiology matures as a scientific discipline. Physiology establishes itself separate from anatomy and chemistry. By the beginning of the 1900s physiology has made numerous and significant contributions to furthering the understanding of organ based systems unmatched by any period before.

Research continues in the traditional areas of GI, cardiovascular, respiratory, and muscle physiology. New areas of research focus upon the nervous systems, endocrine systems, intracellular and extracellular fluid systems, and bioelectrical systems, especially as bioelectricity relates to the heart and brain.

Magendie and Bell detail sensory and motor neural fibers. Purkinje details cerebellar systems, describes specialized electrical conducting fibers in the heart, and establishes the first university based Department of Physiology associated with a medical school. Beaumont directly observes digestion in real time, in the stomach through a gunshot wound to a patient's abdomen. Muller clarifies sensations as resulting from stimulation of specialized nerve endings. Volkmann describes the anatomy and physiology of the sympathetic nervous system. Du Bois-Reymond discovers the action potential. Bernard describes the importance of extracellular fluids, advocates the universal use of the "blind experimental" research design, and inclusion of physiology into medical school curricula. Physiology is declared essential for all physicians in training. Augustus V. Waller (the father) describes neural degeneration and regrowth following peripheral injuries. Duchenne describes his palsy, investigates the role of electricity in the diagnosis and treatment of many medical disorders, and applies photography to medicine. Lister studies blood coagulation, offers his antiseptic theory, and formulates an antiseptic mouth wash. Brown-Sequard describes his hemi-section spinal cord syndrome and the physiology of endocrine systems. Caton measures electrical potentials generated from the cerebral cortex.

The Physiological Society is founded in England. Gaskell introduces the concept of heart block and demonstrated the myogenic origin of the heartbeat. Ringer describes his isotonic electrolytic infusion solutions. Howell isolates thrombin and establishes its importance in the coagulation cascade. Mainkowski describes diabetes. The American Physiological Society is founded. Augustus D. Waller (the son) demonstrates the electrical current of the heart and lays the foundation for the development of the EKG. Kent and His, Jr. describe separate conducting fiber systems in the heart. Einthoven produces the first EKG record and describes 5 distinct waves P, Q, R, S, and T. Abel and Takamire isolate epinephrine from the adrenal gland. The American Physiology Society begins publication of their Journal. Yes, a busy 100 years for physiology.

Scholarly scientific publications in human physiology soar during the 1800s. No other time in history has the discipline of physiology enjoyed such attention and generated so many new publications.

Francois Magendie (1783-1855) French physiologist, while perhaps most recognized for his contributions to neuroanatomy, makes numerous contributions to the discipline of physiology. He provides much experimental evidence which challenges medical dogma. Very early in his professional career, he publishes a position paper rejecting the idea biological processes are governed by vital forces (1809)[72] and embraces the conceptual matrix physiological processes can best be explained through an understanding of chemistry and physics. Building upon the work of others, Magendie investigates digestion. He is first to demonstrate the passive role of the stomach in mechanisms of vomiting (1813)[73] and is first to establish dietary proteins are necessary nutrients to sustain life (1816,1816-1817)[74,75].

Among his many contributions, Francois Magendie is first to describe and detail cerebral spinal fluid (1825,1827)[76,77]. He founds the "Journal of Experimental Physiology" in 1821, providing one of the first scientific publications devoted specifically to the exchange of scientific knowledge in the field of experimental physiology (1821-1831)[78].

German physiologist Johannas Reil (psychiatry) and German physiologist John Merkel (1781-1833) (Merkel's diverticulum, 1809[79]) found two similar journals, committed to the advancement of physiology and before Magendie. Johannas Reil founds "Archiv fur die Physiologie" in 1795 and John Merkel founds "Deutsches Archiv fur die Physilogie" in 1815. These three new journals offer a much needed forum to share new knowledge among investigators and further signal physiology is maturing as an established scientific discipline.

In 1822 Magendie publishes his next landmark publication in which he experimentally differentiates and demonstrates the sensory and motor functions of the spinal rootlets as they enter and exit the spinal cord (1822a,1822b)[80,81]. The publication triggers a heated professional debate between himself and Scottish anatomist Charles Bell. The debate focuses upon which man should receive professional credit for differentiating the functions of the spinal rootlets (1847,1901)[82,83]. In fact, functional differentiation of the sensory and motor rootlets are first reported by Erasistratus in the City of Alexandria over 2,000 years before either Magendie or Bell ever publish their first papers.

In addition to contributions in anatomy and physiology Magendie contributes to experimental pharmacology and immunology. He describes and is first to explain the phenomenon of anaphylaxis, following a subsequent exposure to an antigen, in a series of experiments completed in 1839 (1839)[84]. Three years later he returns to his interests in anatomy and describes the anatomical structure for which medical students perhaps most remember him, the Foramen of Magendie (1842)[85].

Charles Bell (1774-1842) Scottish anatomist with interests in neural, muscle, and respiratory physiology is perhaps most remembered by medical students for his experimental investigations into the nerves and muscles of the face, leading to the first description in 1821 of a cranial nerve VII palsy, which continues to bear his name today, Bell's palsy (1821)[86]. His interest in these topics are evidenced early in his career with publication of an "Essay on the anatomy of expression in paintings" (1806)[87]. Charles Bell self publishes a brief pamphlet early in his career titled "An Idea of a New Anatomy of the Brain" (1811) in which he describes the anatomical and functional differences of the cerebrum and cerebellum.

Charles Bell is an accomplished medical illustrator and most of his writings are accompanied by detailed anatomical drawings. Another early publication by Bell is "The Dissertation on Gun-shot Wounds" (1814) in which he offers a series of drawings intended for medical professionals, illustrating visually the effects of gunshot trauma to the human body (1814)[88]. Two years later he publishes "The Anatomy and Physiology of the Brain and Nerves, the Organs of Senses, and Viscera", in a collected volume authored with his elder brother John Bell (1816)[89]. The book includes numerous medical illustrations and attempts to present an integrated synthesis of anatomical and medical physiological knowledge to date. The book is organized by organ systems and widely distributed throughout Europe.

Charles Bell becomes embroiled in a heated professional debate in 1821 with French physiologist Francois Magendie, over the award of rightful credit for first differentiating sensory and motor spinal rootlets. The spirited debate is reflected in the professional literature for years and continues well after the deaths of Bell in 1842 and Magendie in 1855 (1868,1868,1869)[90,91,92]. The debate includes biased and unbiased assessment of the timeline and content of published and presented works of both men; accusations and denials of intentional falsification of timelines; accusations and denials of what was known to each man and when; and accusations and denial of rewriting documents to support the claims of one side or the other. Does this type of behavior persists today? You decide. In an effort to satisfy both sides, the profession recommends both receive professional credit and will be termed the Bell-Magendie law. The controversy and debate, as to whom is most justified in receiving credit, is still debated by academics and medical students today (1974,1987,2008)[93,94,95].

The Bell-Magendie debate often overshadows Bell's other contributions to physiology. In his 1819 publication "An essay on the forces which circulate the blood; being an examination of the difference of the motions of fluids in living and dead vessels" he details fluid dynamics within the cardiovascular systems. Equally important as the anatomy and physiology content presented in the "Essay" is the way in which he presents the material and his words of caution offered to those who search out new knowledge. The publication details the anatomy and physiology of organ systems as they are understood at that time and offers a critical, thoughtful analysis of the dogma of anatomy and physiology. He provides confirmation, where the knowledge is supported by scientific investigations and reasoned thought, while providing criticism and caution, when the knowledge is unsupported by experimental findings or reasoned thought. He encourages those who are engaged in scientific investigation and clinical medical practice not to substitute authoritative dogma for independent and reasoned thought (1819)[96]. Certainly, good advice even today.

Johannes Purkinje (1787-1869) Czech physiologist is perhaps most remembered by medical students for his contribution in histology in identifying the Purkinje cells located in the cerebellar cortex between the molecular and granular cell layers and which inhibit cerebellar nuclei (1837)[97]. He also is instrumental in the early development of physiology as a discipline. In 1819 he publishes his dissertation on "Beobachtungen und Versuche zur Physiologie der Sinne" [Observations and experiments investigating the physiology of senses] (1819)[98] and six years later "Neue Beiträge zur Kenntnis des Sehens in subjectiver Hinsicht" [Contributions to the knowledge of vision from a subjective perspective] (1825)[99]. These two volumes are instrumental in the emergence of experimental psychology and experimental physiology.

Trivia: The Purkinje cells located in the cerebellar cortex, discovered by Johannes Purkinje, are named "Purkinje cells" by German physician Leopold Besser (1820-1906), 29 years after their discovery.

Purkinje investigates the underlying physiology responsible for vertigo and generates the Purkinje Law of vertigo (1827a)[100]. Briefly stated, the apparent direction of motion producing vertigo is determined by the position of the head during rotation. His early experiments on the physiology of the vestibular-ocular reflexes are conducted on swings and roundabouts in an amusement park in Prague (1820)[101]. In 1839, at the University of Breslau-Prussia, Purkinje establishes the first university based department of physiology. Three years later in 1842 he founds the Breslau Physiological Institute, the world's first official physiological laboratory. In 1845 he identifies the specialized electrical conducting muscle fibers of the inner ventricular walls of the heart which provide the electrical conduction pathway resulting in coordinated contraction of the ventricles (1845)[102].

Marie Flourens (1794-1867) French physiologist with interests in localization of brain function publishes numerous experiments investigating the physiology associated with specific regions of the brain. Through a series of celebrated lesion experiments in 1822 he demonstrates the localization of brain functions, including primary somato motor, somato sensory, special sensory e.g. vision, hearing, motor coordination, posture, balance, respiration, and more (1824)[103]. His attention to scientific detail and the experimental method adds much credibility to his work and rapid acceptance within the scientific community. His conceptual matrix, which emphasizes the localization of function within brain areas, stands in parallel with the work of German physiologist Franz Gall (1758-1828), who too advocates localization of mental functions, and uses alternative methodologies. Gall perhaps is most remembered for his association with the methods of "phrenology" for determining localization of brain functions.

Gall's methods are not based upon rigid experimental procedures as are Flourens and are the target of much ridicule in the scientific and popular press (1815,1823)[104,105]. Gall's conceptualization of the localization brain functions greatly disturbs the Roman Catholic Church, in that his ideas are contrary to established religious dogma. Revolutionary in his thoughts on localization of mental functions and restricted by his chosen methodologies, The Academy of Sciences of Paris, upon orders from Emperor Napoleon Bonaparte, enlists Marie Flourens to resolve the issue of localization of function within the brain. Flourens has little interests in localization of brain functions prior to Napoleon Bonaparte's executive order. A useful side note here. Bonaparte is at this time furious with Gall for political reasons. With much pressure and prejudice from Napoleon Bonaparte, Flourens soon publishes statements confirming localization of functions within specific brain areas, however denounces the methodologies of Gall as unscientific and should be dismissed by scientists and medical practitioners alike.

Here too are more examples, in the history of medicine, of governmental officials effecting influence upon investigators for reasons other than to advance scientific knowledge and the ridicule and rejection from colleagues experienced by investigators, when one's ideas depart too far from accepted scientific dogma. The investigation of localization of brain function also provides an example of the tremendous influence of the Church and organized religion have in guiding, if not controlling, scientific information, in order to ensure it conforms to religious doctrines and dogma. So to then, so to now, and so to in the future, government and organized religion will always be a part of the scientific process.

Trivia: The term "phrenology" is coined by English physician Thomas Forster (1813)[106] and popularized in Europe by Gall's anatomy dissection assistant German physician Johann Spurzheim (1815)[107]. Gall never refers to his methods or theoretical matrix used to determine personality and development of mental and moral faculties, based upon the external shape of the skull, as "phrenology".

William Beaumont (1785-1853) American Army surgeon systematically investigates the digestive process in the human stomach in real time, through a musket wound to the abdomen of a patient. Beaumont places food tied to string through the wound and observes the effect of the stomach on food. Beaumont is first to describe the digestive process directly observed in vivo. In addition to the mashing and squeezing of the stomach, Beaumont reports the importance and role of gastric juices in the digestive process. The wound of the musket shot patient never completely closes and allows Beaumont an opportunity to conduct a series of experiments exploring digestion over a period of years. He details his experiments in his landmark book on human digestion titled "Experiments and Observations on the Gastric Juice and the Physiology of Digestion" (1838)[108]. William Beaumont is today recognized as one of the many Fathers of American physiology.

Jean Poiseuille (1797-1869) French physiologist continues the efforts of Stephen Hales and others to develop measurement instruments, for the purpose of reliably measuring systemic blood pressures. Hales' method of measuring arterial pressures by a column of blood is limited and inconvenient due to the great height of the column necessary, large fluctuations, and rapid clotting. Poiseuille offers an alternative in 1828. He uses mercury, a metal 13.5 times heavier than blood, and thereby reduces the height of the column necessary and proportionally reduces the fluctuations in measurement (1828)[109].

Yes, this is the same Poiseuille discussed in an earlier section and who publishes his now familiar Poiseuille equation $\Delta P = 8\mu LQ/\pi\, r^4$ describing the physics of blood flow through body vessels (1840)[110]. Dispensing with a detailed discussion of the assumptions and specifics of the equation, which can be found in any medical physiology textbook, recall Poiseuille equation when reduced estimates blood flow through vessels to be approximately 2x the radius of the vessel. Stated differently, you need 16 tubes to pass as much fluid as one tube twice their diameter. Poiseuille's equation reflects well the interests in fluid dynamics popular during the late-1800s and application of measurements to the understanding of human physiology.

Johannes Muller (1801-1858) German physiologist discovers when a single sensory system is stimulated, the sensory systems gives rise to particular sensations and no other. The sensation a person experiences following stimulation does not depend on the mode of stimulation but upon the nature of the sensory system stimulated. Light, pressure, or mechanical stimulation of the retina or optic nerves invariably produces light and colors independent of the mode of stimulation. Stimulation of the auditory nerves results in the sensation of sounds and stimulation of the olfactory nerves results in the sensations of odors. Muller defines this phenomena as the Law of specific energies of the senses. His major work "Handbuch der Physiologie des Menschen für Vorlesungen" (1837)[111], is translated from German into English by William Baly and edited by John Bell (brother of Charles Bell) as "Elements of Physiology" (1843)[112]. Muller's work produces a renewed interest in physiology as an integrated scientific discipline, combining anatomy, physics, and chemistry in the study of physiological systems.

Alfred Volkmann (1801-1877) German physiologist provides experimental evidence in support of his discovery of the peripheral sensory and motor origins of sympathetic nervous system fibers. He reports the cell body of these fibers to be localized to the posterior root, paravertebral, and prevertebral ganglia (1842)[113]. Volkmann provides contributions to physiology in the areas of vision (1836)[114], hemodynamics, especially the measurement of blood flow (1850)[115], and sensory discrimination, especially from the skin (1858,1863)[116,117]. Perhaps most first year medical students recognize him from your histology course and remember him for his canals. Volkmann canals recall provide the blood supply from the periosteum to compact bone (1873)[118].

Emil Du Bois-Reymond (1818-1896) German physiologist provides the necessary experimental data to resolve the 50 year Galvani-Volta debate, discovers the "action potential", and demonstrates electric currents are involved in muscle contractions (1848,1849)[119,120].

In regard to the Galvani-Volta debate, Du Bois-Reymond is first to demonstrate muscular contraction are accompanied by chemical changes in the muscle. He demonstrates ions are formed within a nerve when a nerve is stimulated and nerves and muscles are not stimulated by a constant flow of bioelectrical current, but rather respond to sudden changes in current intensity. Du Bois-Reymond describes these small electrical potentials inherent in specific tissues and their effect on tissues as a function of change in the electrical potentials. Today, we know the electrical potentials "electric molecules" described by Du Bois-Reymond to be sodium, potassium, calcium, and chloride ions.

Du Bois-Reymond further describes a small voltage present in nerves and resting muscle he terms "action currents", which diminishes with the contraction of muscles (1848)[119]. He provides additional supporting evidence the following year with the publication of his second volume of "Studies on animal electricity" and introduces an instrument capable of measuring these small amounts of electricity "action currents", which today we term simply "action potentials" (1849)[120].

Hermann von Helmholtz (1821-1894) German physicist and close friend of Du Bois-Reymond successfully measures conduction velocity of the action potential two years later (1850a, 1850b)[121,122]. Prior to Helmholtz publication, it is universally held the speed of information passing through nerves travels at the speed of light. Given the short length of nerves, to and from the central nervous system, it is impossible to measure the conduction speed of neural transmission. This position is held too by one of the period's most respected physiologist Johannes Muller. So goes another lesson for you the medical student. Just because a professor or the medical community at large tells you it can't be done, keep an open mind. Perhaps all that is required is to think about the problem in a new and innovative way. Don't be lulled by the convenience of current dogma as a substitute for independent and innovative thought.

Von Helmholtz develops the three color theory of vision (1850c)[123], a theory originally proposed in 1802 by Thomas Young (1773-1829) (1802)[124]. Recall, the Young-Helmholtz Theory states vision depends on three different sets of retinal fibers responsible for the perception of red, green, and violet. Loss of any of these fibers results in an impairment in perception of primary colors or any color which is formed from the specific primary color (1850c)[123].

Von Helmholtz invents several measurement instruments, including the ophthalmoscope (1851)[125]. The ophthalmoscope remains one of the most frequently used instruments today by the practicing physician, over 100 years after it was first introduced and popularized in the medical community by von Helmholtz.

Claude Bernard (1813-1878) French physiologist and research assistant to Francois Magendie propels physiology into new areas of investigations which dominate physiological investigations for the balance of the 1800s. While maintaining interests in mainstream topics in physiology of the time e.g. digestion, respiration, skeletal muscle, and nervous systems, he moves forward with innovative investigations into bodily fluids, their origins, composition, and effects on organ systems. Bernard studies the liver and is first to outline its glycogenic functions (1843,1857)[126,127]. Six years later his attention focuses on the pancreas and the role of its fluids on the digestion and absorption of fats (1849)[128]. Two years later he publishes his observations and experimental finding detailing the vasodilator and vasoconstrictor motor systems (1851)[129]. Returning to his interests in body sugars he publishes his foundational work describing mechanisms of action and associated fluids of diabetes (1855-1856,1877)[130,131]. Soon thereafter Bernard releases studies describing the physiological effects of poisons especially carbon monoxide and curare on organ systems (1857)[132] and his observations on the importance of extra-cellular fluids in maintaining homeostasis within and between organ systems.

Bernard moves the discipline further forward with his major work "An Introduction to the Study of Experimental Medicine" (1865)[133]. He discusses the process of science and the role of the scientist, highlighting strengths, weaknesses, limitations, and providing thoughtful words of caution and guidance to all who participate in the scientific pursuit of new knowledge. Among the many topics addressed, Bernard advocates the use of "blind experimental" research designs; cautions against blind acceptance of scientific dogma; encourages openness to new and alternative explanations to even well-established theory; and cautions investigators to be aware of the limits of the methods applied in the pursuit of new knowledge.

Claude Bernard, Marie Bichat, Francois Magendie and others in France are instrumental in establishing the importance of physiology in the practice of medicine, particularly within the hospital setting.

Augustus V. Waller (1816-1870) English physiologist, not to be confused with Augustus D. Waller (1856-1922) his son, describes the infiltration of leukocytes from capillaries into tissues (1846)[134], degeneration of neural fibers (1850)[135]; and the effects of the sympathetic nervous system on vasoconstriction (1853)[136]. Perhaps his investigations into the degeneration of nerve fibers are most familiar to medical students. Recall, Wallerian degenerating is the result of degeneration of the distal segment of a neural fiber (axon) once it has been severed from the nutritive centers of the cell body (1852a,1852b,1857)[137,138,139].

By the mid-1800s physiology is well on its way to becoming a valued and respected scientific discipline. The second half of the 1800s insures physiology's position witnessing the applications of new technologies such as electricity and photography to the study of physiology; the invention, development, and medical applications of the electrocardiogram (EKG); electroencephalogram (EEG); blood oximetry; an understanding of intracellular and extracellular fluids; development of physiology societies in Europe and the United States of America; and the founding of new scientific journals devoted specifically to scientific studies and the advancement of physiology.

Guillaume Duchenne (1806-1875) French neurologist systemically investigates the application of electricity to biological tissues and details his thoughts and findings in "A treatise on localized electrization and its applications to pathology and therapeutics" (1855,1871)[140,141]. Duchenne maintains particular interests in muscle electrophysiology and completes landmark experiments in which he places electrodes subcutaneously on muscles of the face, stimulating the muscle with electricity, and observing changes in facial expressions (1862)[142]. He soon integrates the use of the recently invented camera to photograph the distorted facial expressions resulting from the electrical stimulations. The use of the camera in Duchenne's experiments establishes a landmark in the history of medical photography (1862,1867)[143,144].

Duchenne provides his first description of a familiar brachial plexus trauma in infants, resulting in paralysis of the arm with no sensory loss and later to be termed Duchenne-Erb palsy, in the second edition of "A treatise on localized electrization and its applications to pathology and therapeutics" (1862). Wilhelm Erb (1840-1921) German neurologist describes the exact same condition 12 years later (1874)[145]. Duchenne and Erb engage in a heated professional debate as to whom should receive credit for first describing the palsy we know today simply as Erb's palsy. In fact, Scottish obstetrician William Smellie describes the condition over 100 years earlier in his book titled "A collection of cases and observations in midwifery" (1754)[146]. Duchenne is today perhaps most recognized by medical students for his description of the X-linked, recessive muscular dystrophy which bears his name, Duchenne's muscular dystrophy (1868)[147].

Often lost in most discussions of Duchenne is his influence on physiology from his many studies into the application of electricity in the diagnosis, treatment, and management of numerous medical conditions (1883)[148]. In brief, Duchenne offers numerous case studies demonstrating the useful application of electricity in such conditions as muscle paralysis (1850)[149], muscle atrophy (1853)[150], disorders of muscle tone (1853)[151], motor coordination (1858)[152], neuro-sensory deafness (1858)[153], disorders of speech (1860)[154], disorders of respiration (1866)[155] and its effective use in cardio-pulmonary resuscitations (1876)[156]. That's right. Duchenne is responsible in large part in contributing to an understanding of the effective use of short bursts of electricity to reset the rhythms of the heart. A practice still used today in every hospital, over 135 years after Duchenne describes its effectiveness.

Charles Brown-Sequard (1817-1894) French physiologist is perhaps most remembered by medical students today for his works in spinal cord transections and hemi-section (1858)[157]. Recall, the Brown-Sequard syndrome is a constellation of sensory and motor signs and symptoms associated with the hemi-section of the spinal cord, characterized by loss of motor function at and below the level of the spinal lesion on the same side as the lesion and loss of pain and temperature sensations at and below the level of the spinal lesion on the side opposite the lesion. Perhaps less well known or unknown at all to many, two years earlier Brown-Sequard publishes a series of papers outlining causes and treatments of epilepsy (1856,1857)[158,159]. Brown-Sequard further contributes to physiology establishing three journals devoted to experimental physiology; "Journal de la Physiologie de l'Homme et des Animaux" (1858); "Archives de Physiologie Normale et Pathologique "(1868) with colleague French neurologist Jean Charcot (1825-1893); and later "Archives of Scientific and Practical Medicine" (1873).

Brown-Sequard is influenced by French physiologist Claude Bernard and maintains interests in endocrinology throughout his professional career. Early in his career he reports his observation that death occurs following the bilateral removal of the adrenal glands and concludes the adrenal glands are necessary for life (1856)[160]. Later in his career he returns to his interests in endocrinology. Brown-Sequard reports a sense of rejuvenation characterized by increased strength, improved cognition, relief from constipation, an increased arc of his urine, and additional clinical benefits, following self-injection of extracts from the testicles of dogs and guinea pigs (1889a,1889b)[161,162]. Later the same year he reports revitalization of women, following injection of ovary extracts into women (1889c)[163]. So begins the systematic investigation of clinical applications of hormone replacement treatments.

Brown-Sequard joins other investigators throughout the history of science and medicine who use themselves or family members as convenient experiment subjects.

Edwin Pfluger (1829-1910) German physiologist, assistant to Emil Du Bois-Reymond, founds the journal "Archiv für die Gesammte Physiologie" [Pfluger Archive: European Journal of Physiology] in 1868. The Journal is quickly recognized as the most influential journal of physiology in Germany. The Journal remains in continuous publication for over 145 years. It remains in publication today.

Establishment of professional scientific journal and societies mark maturational growth of any new scientific discipline. So too is the case of physiology during the second half of the 1800s.

Alexander Schmidt (1831-1894) Estonian physiologist moves his energies away from physiological systems currently being investigated by many others and towards exploring the biochemistry of physiological systems. Schmidt is first to demonstrate the enzymatic transformation of fibrinogen into fibrin. He terms the enzyme "thrombin" and its precursor "prothrombin" (1872)[164]. Schmidt's research into the enzymatic factors contributing to the coagulation cascade opens new avenues of research and further integrates the discipline of biochemistry with physiology.

The coagulation cascade is pieced together over the course of approximately 100 years with early contributions made during the middle and late-1800s by Johannas Muller (1801-1858) first in describing fibrin (1832), German pathologist Rudolf Virchow (1821-1902) first in describing fibrin's soluble precursor fibrinogen (1847)[165], French physiologist Nicolas Arthus (1862-1945) first in describing the essential role of calcium in the coagulation cascade (1890)[166], and Italian medical researcher Giulio Bizzozero (1846-1901) in identifying the role of platelets (1882)[167].

Richard Caton (1842-1926) English surgeon is first to report successful recordings of the electrical potentials generated from the brain (1875,1877)[168,169]. Recording from the exposed cerebral cortex of rabbits and monkeys, Caton reports changes in electrical brain activity associated with sensory stimulation, movement, and administration of anesthesia. He opens the door for the experimental study of electrical brain activity and associated functions for the next 130 years.

A review of regional differences in the development of physiology as a discipline reveals the discipline alive, well, and flourishing in France and Germany during the 1800s. However, physiology is virtually non-existent in England during the 1800s, especially during the early and middle-1800s. Not until the Physiology Society is founded in England during 1876 to promote the advancement of physiology, do scientists from Great Britain begin to contribute substantially to the new knowledge base of physiology.

The Physiology Society is founded quickly in response to a recently enacted Act of Parliament, requiring investigators using live animals in experimental research or engaging in dissection of live animals for demonstration purposes, be licensed by the government. The restrictions are enacted to ensure humane treatment of all animals, when animals are used in experimental research.

The Society is led by English physiologists, John Burdon-Sanderson (1828-1905) and Michael Foster (1836-1907) of London, authors of the "Handbook for the Physiological Laboratory" (1873,1911)[170,171] , which upon publication meets with much public outrage in England, fanning the flames of the Anti-Visection Movement. The Society is founded in a calculated effort to ensure physiologists are involved in the political decision making processes which potentially could restrict the advancement of scientific knowledge. The Physiology Society is initially restricted to male members only. Women are admitted as members 39 years later, in 1915. Michael Foster also founds the Society's journal, "Journal of Physiology", first published in 1878. The Physiology Society and the "Journal of Physiology" continue to remain active today, over 130 years since their founding.

Walter Gaskell (1847-1914) British cardiac physiologist provides evidence in support of a myogenic origin of the spontaneous heartbeat as opposed to the neurogenic origin popular at the time (1882)[172]; outlines the direction of electrical flow through the heart and sequence of cardiac contractions (1883)[173]; discovers the "natural pause" using his term to describe the delay in contraction as it passes over the AV groove and today recognize as the normal AV delay seen on the EKG as the PR interval (1883,1900)[173173,174]. Gaskell introduces the familiar terms today, "heart block", "fibrillation" and "gallop-rhythm" into the literature.

In addition to the many advances being made in the areas of electrophysiology, during the late-1800s, advances are being made in the area of body fluid physiology.

Sydney Ringer (1835-1910) English physiologist invents physiological saline. The solution, an isotonic electrolytic infusion solution known today in familiar terms simply as Ringer solution or the "drip" (1882a,1882b)[175,176]. The solution allows body tissues to function normally for a time even when isolated from their blood supply. Ringer is primarily a clinical investigator known to readily and frequently test his Solution and pharmacological substances on himself, as part of his investigations. He authors his major published work "Handbook of Therapeutics" (1869)[177], which soon becomes essential reading for all physicians. The Handbook sees 13 editions between 1869-1887 and establishes itself as a classic. Ringer's "Handbook of Therapeutics", in his words is designed "…for students and young practitioners…" and offers a systematic discussion of remedies for disease based upon established dogma of the period.

The "Handbook of Therapeutics" is organized by specific substances or procedure used to treat a disease or disorder rather than by the disease or disorder which is common today. For example, in the 11th edition, Ringer devotes a chapter to cannabis, recommending its chronic use as prophylaxis for migraine attacks. Today, the chapter is more likely to be organized not by treatment but by disorder e.g. a chapter on migraines with assorted treatments rather than the treatment with assorted disorders.

Ringer's now classic experiments resulting in the development of his Ringer's solution is noteworthy for any medical student. In brief, during 1882-1885 Ringer isolates frog hearts suspended in 0.75 percent solution of sodium chloride. Then introduces substances such as blood or albumin to the solution and observes the effect on the heart. He quickly recognizes prolonged ventricular dilation, induced by pure sodium chloride solution, can be reversed by blood or albumin and small amounts of calcium are necessary in the profusion solution to maintain a normal heartbeat (1880-1882,1883-1884)[178,179]. He perfects his physiological solution by adding small amounts of potassium, which when used, can keep isolated organs functional for extended periods of time (1895)[180]. More than 30 papers, on formulation of the Ringer Solution appear between 1875-1897, describing the effects of inorganic salts on living tissues. Ringer publishes most of his papers in the journal of the recently founded Physiology Society, the "Journal of Physiology".

Throughout the history of medicine, original, innovative, and landmark papers of a discipline are published in relatively new journals, rather than the well-established journals filled with the dogma of the time.

Physiological properties and chemical composition of bodily fluids are a primary focus of research during the late-1800s. Familiar names Bernard, Brown-Sequard, Virchow, Ringer and others all make substantial contributions to the understanding of body fluids. A less familiar name, Svante Arrhenius (1859-1927) Swedish physicist contributes in providing an understanding of the acid-base reaction you will immediately recognize as $H^+(aq) + OH^-(aq) \rightleftharpoons H_2O$, describing the formation of water from hydrogen and hydroxide ions, or hydrogen ions and hydroxide ions from the dissociation of an acid and base in an aqueous solution.

Svante Arrhenius investigates conductivities of electrolytes (1884)[181]. He details his experiments on the conductivities of electrolytes in a 150 page dissertation presented to the faculty of Uppsala in partial fulfilment of his doctorate degree. The faculty unimpressed, permits him to pass with a "low pass". Of the 56 theses Arrhenius puts forth in his 1884 dissertation, most are accepted today (2010). Five years after receiving the "low pass" on his dissertation, Arrhenius formulates the concept of activation energy, the energy barrier that must be overcome before two molecules will react (1889a,1889b)[182,183]. The work which so unimpressed his faculty and the concept of activation energy earns him the 1903 Nobel Prize in Chemistry "…in recognition of the extraordinary services he has rendered to the advancement of chemistry by his electrolytic theory of dissociation…" (1903)[184]. So goes another lesson for you the medical student.

William Howell (1860-1945) American physiologist and first Professor of Physiology at the new John Hopkins School of Medicine (1893) investigates the physiology of body fluids. He is among the first to suggest the anterior and posterior lobes of the pituitary are functionally distinct. Early in his career he contributes to the physiology of the nervous system, blood coagulation, blood complement, and blood circulatory systems. Howell is first to isolate and establish thrombin's importance in the clotting cascade (1884)[185]. Later, Howell isolates the powerful anticoagulant heparin, and names it for its abundance in the liver (1926)[186]. He writes an easily understandable textbook of physiology for medical students which is well received. Howell's textbook sees 14 editions between 1905 and 1940 (1905)[187] and represents the first American compendium of physiological knowledge derived from the new experimental method (1987)[188].

Oskar Minkowski (1858-1931) German physiologist recognizes the chemical basis of diabetes and suggests the disorder is the result of suppression of a substance released by the pancreas, which later is identified to be insulin (1884)[189]. Five years later he demonstrates diabetes can be produced by the removal of the pancreas (1889)[190]. In addition to his contributions to diabetes he investigates the physiology of other endocrine systems, being the first to report enlargement of the pituitary in acromegaly (1887)[191].

The American Physiological Society forms in New York in 1887 and restricts its membership to those who have published original research.

Augustus D. Waller (1856-1922) English physiologist, son of English physiologist Augustus V. Waller who first describes Wallerian nerve degeneration, demonstrates electrical current generated in the human heart can be recorded from surface electrodes (1887)[192]. He provides the physiology and prototype instrumentation resulting in the first electrocardiogram (EKG). The same year he improves the recording technique by immersing his own limbs into jars filled with saline and successfully recording a greater amplified electrical signal from the heart (1888)[193]. The EKG is still used regularly today, over 125 years after Augustus D. Waller first recorded subtle changes in electrical potentials from the skin and reflecting the electricity generated by the heart.

Albert Kent (1863-1958) English physiologist identifies an electrical conducting pathway between the atria and ventricles of the heart (1893)[194]. The pathway is composed primarily of modified muscle fibers (Purkinje fibers) originating in the AV node, continues through the interventricular septum, and divides into two large branches that pass to the left and right ventricles. Electricity passing through this pathway results in contraction of the ventricles. Kent names this pathway the "Bundle of Kent". Under certain conditions electrical signals bypass the regulation of the AV node and through the Bundle of Kent. This results in tachycardia and is the mechanism of action responsible for Wolf-Parkinson-White syndrome (1930)[195]. No this is not James Parkinson (1755-1924) associated with Parkinson's disease but rather cardiologist John Parkinson (1885-1976).

Wilhelm His, Jr. (1863-1934) Swiss cardiologist, son of Swiss anatomist Wilhelm His, Sr. discovers the "Bundle of His", the AV electrical conducting system which synchronizes the contraction of cardiac muscle (1893)[196]. Recall, disruption of normal electrical flow through the Bundle of His from the SA node to the ventricles produces heart block and associated arrhythmias.

Wilhelm Einthoven (1860-1927) Dutch physiologist completes his first major work into the physiology of respiration and the role of bronchial muscles in asthma (1892)[197]. He makes substantial contributions as the result of his experimental works into the electrophysiology of optical illusions (1898)[198], accommodation (1902)[199], and physiological responses associated with various intensities of light (1908)[200]. Einthoven is fascinated by the electricity of the body and devotes much energy to the investigation of body electricity, especially electricity generated by the heart.

Wilhelm Einthoven develops the first accurate EKG recording applicable to clinical assessment of cardio-electrical activities (1895)[201]. Einthoven describes the five distinct waves P, Q, R, S, and T. Why P, Q, R, S, T and not A, B, C, D, E you ask? It is mathematical convention dating back to the time of Descartes to use letters from the second half of the alphabet. The letter N already had meaning in mathematics and O already had meaning as the "origin" within the Cartesian coordinate system. P is simply the next available letter in the alphabet. Einthoven used letters O through X to note the different wave shapes and timelines in his original papers and only later adopts the more restricted P, Q, R, S, T labeling, as he refined his recording procedures.

Having established the electrophysiology of normal cardiac rhythms, Einthoven publishes his first reports of EKG tracing associated with specific pathologies of the heart; left and right ventricular hypertrophy, left and right atrial hypertrophy, atrial flutter, complete heart block, U wave, and notching of the QRS wave (1906)[202]. The value of objective, standardized, non-invasive physiological measurement with application in the clinical medicine setting is quickly recognized by the scientific and medical communities. Wilhelm Einthoven is awarded the 1924 Nobel Prize in Physiology or Medicine "…for his discovery of the mechanism of the electrocardiogram…" (1924)[203].

In addition to bioelectricity, hormones begin to be identified and soon become a major area of focus for physiologists, during the late-1800s.

Napoleon Cybulski (1854-1919) Polish physiologist discovers "nadnerczyna", later translated into "adrenaline". This represents the identification of one of the first naturally occurring hormones and opens the door to the physiology of a new field of investigations, endocrinology (1895)[211]. The same year Napoleon Cybulski releases the publication describing his invention, the "photohaemotachometre", a device to measure blood flow in vessels. He invents an instrument capable of measuring minute quantities of heat produced during muscle contractions. He demonstrates the excitability of body tissues are dependent upon the duration of electrical energy applied to the tissues. In collaboration with Austrian physiologist Adolf Beck (1863-1942), they discover the continuous oscillations of electrical potentials generated by the brain (1891)[204].

Cybulski's works, studying the physiology of the adrenal glands, registration of the speed of blood flow through vessels, and the nature of muscle and nerve electricity, earn him three separate nominations for the Nobel Prize in Physiology or Medicine, 1911, 1914, and 1918[205]. He is never awarded a Nobel Prize. Rather the Nobel Prize in Physiology or Medicine in these three years are awarded in 1911 to Swedish ophthalmologist Allvar Gullstand (1863-1930) "...for his work on the dioptrics of the eye…"; 1914 to Austro-Hungarian otologist Robert Barany (1876-1936) "…for his work on the physiology of the vestibular apparatus…"; and no Nobel Prize is awarded in 1918 (2010)[206].

George Oliver (1841-1915) and Edward Schafer (1850-1935) English physiologists describe the cardiovascular effects (constricts blood vessels and raises blood pressure) of an endogenous chemical produced by the adrenal glands, later identified as adrenaline, to the Physiology Society and opens further the doors to the scientific investigation of organ based endocrine systems (1894,1895a,1895b)[207,208,209].

Jokichi Takamire (1854-1922) Japanese chemist, while working for the Park-Davis Pharmaceutical Company in New York City, independently isolates adrenaline from the adrenal glands (1901)[210]. He makes his discovery approximately five years after Polish physiologist and endocrinologist Napoleon Cybulski discovers adrenaline (1895)[211] and one year following a visit with biochemist John Abel (1857-1938) at John Hopkins University, who also discovers adrenaline before Takamire (1898)[212]. Takamire and Park-Davis quickly file for United States patent protection, on November 5, 1900, under the name "Glandular extractive product" in their efforts to protect future financial interests. United States Patent number US730176 (1900)[213]. Takamire names the product "Adrenalin".

Trivia: Adrenaline is derived from the Latin roots "ad and renes" meaning "on the kidney", in reference to the anatomical location of the adrenal glands on top of the kidneys. Epinephrine is derived from the Greek "epi" and "nephros" having similar meaning. Because the Park-Davis patented trademark name Adrenalin (1900) is similar to the naturally occurring product adrenaline, and producing much confusion, the United States courts mandated the use of the alternative name "epinephrine" for Adrenalin generics within the USA.

Otto Frank (1865-1944) German cardiac physiologist, initially interested in fat absorption, makes his most lasting contribution to physiology when he describes the relationships between cardiac muscle fiber length and contractile force (1895)[214]. British physiologist Ernest Starling 20 years later extends Frank's original works which results in the now familiar Frank-Starling Law, which states simply within physiological limits, the isotonic or isometric contractile force generated by the heart is directly proportional to the initial length of its muscle fibers (1914,1918)[215,216].

The "American Journal of Physiology", associated with the newly founded American Physiological Society, publishes its first issue in 1898. America now has its own publication devoted to the scientific investigations of physiology and joins Europe in advancing new knowledge in the discipline. One of the first articles published in this new journal is authored by American physiologist William Howell, titled "The influence of high arterial pressures upon the blood flow through the brain" (1898)[217]. Yes, the same Howell responsible for the discovery of thrombin, heparin, and Howell-Jolly bodies. The Journal is still in print today, having split into seven sub-journals in 1976, each dealing with specific areas of physiology; cell, renal, gastrointestinal, circulatory, lung, comparative, and endocrine. Americans now begin to play a role in the development of physiology as a discipline, while the French, Germans, Polish, British, Russian, Danish, and Swiss continue to make the most substantial contributions.

In summary, the Middle Modern period (1800 AD-1900 AD) proves to be the most prolific period for physiology ever. Traditional areas of physiology investigations are expanded and new areas identified. New ideas and experimental data replace Galenian dogma. Vitalism continues to be challenged by experimental research findings. New and innovative conceptual matrixes provide the foundation upon which entirely new areas of physiology are built. Bodily fluids are investigated and reveal their extreme importance. Bioelectricity becomes a primary area of research interest for physiologists. The action potential is identified and explained, nerve conduction measured, EKG and EEG invented, and the electrophysiology of several major systems detailed. A demonstrated command of human physiology is deemed essential and is part of the basic science education of every allopathic medical school program. New professional societies and journals devoted specifically to the exchange of scientific information and the advancement of physiology as a discipline are founded and attract many of the brightest scientists of the time.

The first half of the 1800s in summary witness Magendie aggressively challenge medical dogma; proposes the body can best be understood within the matrix of chemistry and physics; demonstrates the passive role of the stomach during digestion; establishes dietary proteins are necessary to sustain life; founds two scientific journals, describes the foundations of anaphylaxis, identifies the structure and function of the Foramen of Magendie; and debates Bell, as to whom should receive professional credit for differentiating the functions of sensory and motor spinal rootlets. Bell describes his CN VII palsy; describes the different functions of the cerebrum and cerebellum; debates with Magendie over whom should receive credit for differentiating sensory and motor spinal rootlets; and is one of the first truly accomplished medical illustrators, to provide exquisite medical drawings, along with his published papers. Purkinje identifies the layer of inhibitory cells in the cerebellar cortex; explains the physiology of vertigo; establishes the first department of physiology associated with a medical school; and identifies specialized electrical conducting fibers in the heart. Flourens localizes brain functions and discredits Gall's methodologies under pressures from Emperor Napoleon Bonaparte. Beaumont studies digestion through a musket hole in a patient's stomach. Poiseuille offers his equation describing important factors effecting blood flow. Muller discovers the singularity of perception independent of the physical stimuli which initially stimulates the system. Volkmann identifies the origin of sympathetic nervous systems fibers; measures blood flow; describes his canals; and investigates the mechanisms responsible for sensory discrimination within and between sensory systems. Du Bois-Reymond discovers and explains the "action potential"; identifies and describes the role of "electric molecules", which today we know are sodium, potassium, calcium, and chloride ions; and resolves the Galvani-Volta debate.

The second half of the 1800s in summary witness Von Helmholtz measurement of nerve conductions; his expansion upon the three color theory of vision; and his invention of the ophthalmoscope. Bernard outlines glycogenic functions of the liver, digestive functions of the pancreas; describes the physiology of fat absorption; describes the physiology of fluids in diabetes; and details the importance of extracellular fluids in maintaining homeostasis within and between organ systems. Additionally, Bernard advocates the use of the "blinded" experimental design and offers caution to all investigators to be keenly aware of strengths, weakness, limitations, and influences, both internal and external, which effect the process of professional scientific investigations. Waller describes "Wallerian degeneration" of neuronal fibers following transection; effects of vasoconstriction resulting from sympathetic nervous system stimulation; and the movement of leukocytes from capillaries into tissues. Duchenne applies electricity to the treatments of a variety of medical condition; describes "Duchenne's muscular dystrophy"; argues with Erb over whom should receive professional credit for a palsy described 100 years before either Duchenne or Erb claim credit; and is first to apply the camera as a useful technology, in scientific study of medical investigations. Brown-Sequard identifies a syndrome associated with hemi-section of the spinal cord, the "Brown-Sequard syndrome"; offers his ideas on the causes and treatments of epilepsies; introduces hormone replacement therapies; and founds three journals devoted to the scientific study of physiology and medicine.

Pfluger issues the first issues of "Pfluger Archive: European Journal of Physiology". Schmidt offers a critical element to the blood coagulation cascade with his discovery and explanation of the mechanisms of action of thrombin, prothrombin, and calcium. Caton records the first EEG from the cerebral cortex. Burdon-Sanderson and Foster found the Physiology Society in London, in response to political and public pressures which threaten to regulate scientific investigations. Gaskell identifies myogenic rather than neurogenic origin of the spontaneous heart beat; describes flow of electricity through the heart; discovers the natural pause (AV delay); and introduces terms "heart block", "fibrillation", and "gallop rhythm". Ringer introduces his Solution and publishes his work in the newly founded "Journal of Physiology", the official journal of the new Physiology Society in London. Arrhenius describes the conductive properties of electrolytes and formulates the concept of activation energy. Howell identifies the functional differences between the anterior and posterior pituitary systems. Minkowski first describes the chemical basis of diabetes; identifies suppression of pancreas "insulin" as the probable cause; and recognizes pituitary enlargement to be associated with acromegaly. The American Physiology Society is founded in New York and restricts its membership to only men and those who have published original research.

The final decade of the 1800s in summary witness Waller develop the hardware for the first EKG; Kent identifies an electrical conducting system in the heart, he names the "Bundle of Kent"; His, Jr. identifies an electrical conducting system in the heart, he names the "Bundle of His"; Einthoven explains the role of bronchial muscles in asthma; explains accommodation; explains the electrophysiology of optical illusions; and develops the first accurate EKG recording, with descriptions of five clinically useful waves P,Q,R,S,T. Cybulski discovers "nadnerczyna" (adrenaline) and opens the door to the physiological investigations of hormones and the endocrine systems. Oliver and Schafer describe the effects of adrenaline upon the cardiovascular systems. Takamire and Park-Davis Pharmaceutical Company extend the development of Adrenalin and capitalize on the financial rewards. Frank describes the relationship between cardiac muscle fiber length and contractile force.

Yes, the 1800s prove to be a period filled with exciting and innovative advancements in physiology. The period establishes physiology as a respected and much valued discipline of scientific investigation.

Late Modern, 1900 AD - 2000 AD.

The first half of the 1900s witness rapid advances in physiology as a discipline and opens many new areas of investigation. The field has access to new and innovative technologies which provide investigators with the necessary tools to test new ideas.

Otto Loewi (1873-1961) German physiologist discovers "vagusstoff", the primary neurotransmitter released from the vagus nerve (CN X) and describes its role in neural transmission and effect on controlling the heart, when released from CN X (1921)[218]. Perhaps you recognize "vagusstoff" by its more familiar alternative name, acetylcholine. In the same article, Loewi additionally describes "acceleransstoff" ["accelcrans"] as the primary chemical substance released by sympathetic nervous system fibers onto their end organ (1921)[218]. You know this chemical as norepinephrine.

Henry Dale (1875-1968) English physiologist identifies acetylcholine to be a primary neurotransmitter used in the autonomic nervous systems (1918)[219]; identifies acetylcholine to be the primary transmitter of the neuromuscular junction (1936)[220]; and proposes a classification system of neuronal fibers based upon their primary neurotransmitters, cholinergic or adrenergic (1933)[221].

Loewi and Dale are the primary proponents of chemical synaptic transmission, during the early-1900s and collectively provide the clear conceptual thought and experimental findings necessary to establish chemical synaptic transmission as the primary mode of cell signaling within the central and peripheral nervous systems. Dale and Loewi receive the 1936 Nobel Prize in Physiology or Medicine "…for their discoveries relating to chemical transmission of nerve impulses…" (1936)[222].

Ernest Starling (1866-1927) British physiologist is remembered by most medical students for his contributions to the development of the Frank-Starling curve, plotting the relationship between cardiac muscle length and contractile force (1914,1918)[223,224]. However, he makes several additional contribution of equal or perhaps greater importance. Starling discovers the functional significance of serum proteins. He describes the "Starling sequence", detailing the exchange of fluids occurring at the level of the capillary (1896)[225]. Starling discovers the neural control mechanism responsible for the peristaltic wave of muscle contractions moving food through the intestines (1899)[226]. He demonstrates the importance of the gastrointestinal hormone secretin in the stimulation of pancreatic secretions, whenever the stomach empties (1902)[227]. Starling is first to use the term "hormone" to describe chemical messengers produced by endocrine glands (1905)[228]. He advances hypotheses proposing renal excretion of salts and water are dependent upon the volume of body fluids, especially blood volume (1909)[229] and details reabsorption of water and assorted electrolytes by the distal convoluted tubules of the kidney (1924)[230].

Hans Berger (1873-1941) German physiologist studies blood circulation in the brain (1901)[231]. He is particularly interested in the associations of brain pulsation with other measurable objective physiological measurements e.g. heartbeat, respiration, blood vessel diameter, brain temperature, and their correlations with subjective mental activities e.g. cognition and emotions (1910)[232]. His interests in "psychic energy" and its measurement are shared by many during the late-1800s and early-1900s. It is common belief the cerebral cortex converts metabolic energy into "psychic energy". He is disappointed with the results and soon turns to brain electricity. Berger reports his first measurements of brain electrical activity in 1902, replicating the early works of Richard Caton. His attempts in measuring evoked potentials are unsuccessful. He soon turns his studies to the spontaneously generated electrical brain potentials. Berger's landmark paper announcing variations in voltage can be recorded noninvasively from surface electrodes, through the intact cranium first appears in 1929 and is met with skepticism from the scientific and medical communities (1929)[233].

Berger is aware of Richard Caton experiments, recording electrical potentials from the exposed cortexes of animals (1875)[234] and credits him with discovering brain electrical activity. Berger is also aware of the work of Polish physiologist Adolf Beck (1863-1939) who reports recording electrical potentials from the cerebral cortex (1890,1891)[235,236] and Ukrainian physiologist Vladimir Prawdicz- Neminski (1879-1952) who provides the first photographic record of electrical activity recorded non-invasively from brain (1913)[237]. Berger's contributions can perhaps be most appreciated within the matrix of extension of electrical brain recordings to humans, using non-invasive technologies, and applying the procedure to the diagnosis and assessment of patients presenting with impaired brain function.

In the true spirit of many scientific investigators, Berger completes numerous electroencephalographic studies on himself and family members. He publishes a summary of these early investigations in a 1938 monograph (1938)[238]. Berger works are met with skepticism by the scientific and medical communities for over 25 years, dismissing the recorded signals simply as artifact. It is not until the mid-1930s and after numerous and careful publications do some in the professional community begin to accept his work (1934)[239]. The EEG never receives full recognition of its value until the mid-1950s and early-1960s, many years after Berger's death.

Today, the measurement of electrical brain activity is essential in the evaluation of seizure disorder patients.

Berger, as many others who have made substantial contributions to the advancement of science, is never awarded the Nobel Prize. A review of Nobel archives reveals he indeed is nominated in 1940, 1942, 1947, and 1950. No Prize in Physiology or Medicine is awarded in 1940. Berger's 1942 and 1947, 1950 nominations are not considered, due to his death. Nobel Prizes are not awarded to anyone deceased, unless the award is announced before the Laureate's death (2010)[240]. Frequent accounts found in current historical-medical publications stating Hitler forbid Berger from accepting the Prize in 1936 and subsequently denied the 1949 Prize are simply inconsistent with Nobel archival records (2005,2010)[241,242].

Trivia: Have you ever wondered why individuals awarded a Nobel Prize are called Nobel Laureates? The word "Laureate" refers to the laurel wreath. A laurel wreath is a circular crown made of branches and leaves of the bay laurel (In Latin: Laurus nobilis). In Ancient Greece, laurel wreaths are awarded to victors, as a sign of honor and to differentiate the most exceptional competitors in athletic competitions and poetic meets from all others (2010)[243].

Ivan Pavlov (1849-1936) Russian physiologists describes the relationships between learned and unlearned physiological responses. He presents his first paper on the topic and defines conditioned and unconditioned reflexes to the 14th International Medical Conference in Madrid and begins a new era in physiology (1903)[244].

Recall, Pavlov's now famous experiments in which he would ring a bell and a dog would have a physiological response, salivation, if the ringing of the bell had been previously and regularly presented to the dog, at the same time the dog was fed. This association results in a conditioned stimulus, ringing of the bell, which normally would not produce an unconditioned physiological response salivation, now produces the unconditioned response salivation, whenever the ringing of the bell is presented alone and without food. This fundamental paired association continues to be taught in universities and medical schools throughout the world still today.

The principles identified by Pavlov open doors for new areas of investigation into the impact environmental stimuli can have upon normal physiological functions. His work guides the direction of much research in both physiology and experimental psychology for the next 100 years. His work adheres closely to the scientific method in both design and execution, serving as an excellent model of investigative methodologies of the early-1900s. The scientific method remains the standard today in conceptualizing, designing, conducting, and reporting scientific based research.

Trivia: Pavlov's experiments are not limited to ringing a bell. He actually uses a wide variety of auditory, olfactory, and visual stimuli which prove equally effective in evoking an unconditioned response e.g. salivation when paired with unconditioned stimuli e.g. food.

Pavlov is not the first to use the term "conditioned reflex". This term first appears in print in a paper presented to the Congress of Natural Sciences in Helsinki (1903)[245]. The paper is presented by Pavlov's colleague Ivan Tolochinov, reporting on his own work completed in Pavlov's laboratory, completed two years earlier. Pavlov himself is ambivalent about the specific term used to describe what we today referred to as the "conditioned" and "unconditioned" reflexes. He offers several equally acceptable terms " acquired reflexes", "inborn reflexes", species reflexes", "individual reflexes", "conduction reflexes", connection reflexes" (1927)[246].

Pavlov is most remembered by the world for his experiments demonstrating "classical conditioning" and the conditioned reflex. However, few today remember the significant contributions he made in digestion physiology. His work focuses upon the role of salivation, demonstrating among many other dogmatic truths, saliva to be as important a stimulus for gastric secretions, as gastric secretions are stimuli for pancreas secretions. Pavlov completes his most influential work in the physiology of digestion years before embarking upon classical conditioning or the conditioned reflex. Pavlov summarizes 12 years of his most influential studies of the physiology of digestion at the end of the 1800s (1897)[247]. Pavlov is awarded the 1904 Nobel Prize in Physiology or Medicine, not for his work in classical conditioning but rather "…in recognition of his work on the physiology of digestion, through which knowledge on vital aspects of the subject has been transformed and enlarged…" (1904)[248].

Nikolai Korothov (1874-1920) Russian physiologist is first to report a new, non-invasive method to measure blood pressure. Korothov builds upon the work of Italian pediatrician Scipione Riva-Rocii (1863-1937) who describes a noninvasive method of recording systolic blood pressure. Riva-Rocii's procedure simply is to place a pressure cuff around the arm and inflating with air until the radial pulse is obliterated; then palpating the surface of the arm above the brachial artery until a pulse is detected (1896)[249]. Korothov modifies the procedure and makes his first report of a method of placing a pressure cuff around the arm, inflating the cuff with air, placing a stethoscope over the brachial artery, located just below the cuff, then listening to the onset and disappearance of pulsating sounds, as air within the cuff is slowly released. He introduces the concept of diastolic and systolic pressure measurements and proposes these two measurements in combination are more useful than the single blood pressure measurement of Riva-Rocii (1905,1906,1896)[250,251,249]. Korothov's procedure and the report of diastolic and systolic blood pressures are a routine part of ever physical examination today.

Few clinicians take time to reflect upon the origin of this or any other routine medical procedure. As a medical student you do have the time. Consider taking a few minutes and reflect upon the numerous routine procedures we use today, during the physical examination and consider the following: Why was the procedure developed? Who is responsible for its initial development? When was the procedure developed? And why does the procedure continue to be such a routine part of the physical examination of every patient?

Author Keith (1866-1955) Scottish anatomist and Martin Flack (1882-1931) English physiologist first observe and report the heartbeat originates from specialized cardiac muscle within the right atrium. They are first to report the anatomical location and pacemaker function of the sino-atrial node (SA) (1907)[252]. The AV node has already been identified by Japanese pathologist Sunano Tawara (1873-1952), one year earlier (1906)[253].

Martin Flack, after identifying the location and function of the SA node and detailing the effects of pharmacological agents, electrical stimulation, temperature, and mechanical compression have on the SA node (1910)[254], he returns to his primary interests, respiratory physiology. As one of the early medical directors of the recently established Medical Research Council of the Royal Air Force, he is responsible for the establishing the physiological basis, which require pilots to pass specific physical fitness examinations before flying (1918)[255]. His work provides the physiological basis, for supplying pilots flying at high attitudes, auxiliary oxygen (1928)[256].

John Haldane (1860-1936) Scottish physiologist, not to be confused with his son, population geneticist John B. Haldane (1892-1965), maintains interests in gases and their effects on biological tissues. Haldane, in the spirit of many special scientists, is known to frequently conduct experiments upon himself to test a hypothesis he may be working on at any given time. His interests in natural gases result in numerous self-experiments, during which he inhales various gases, at various concentrations, and records his own body's physiological responses.

Haldane in collaboration with John G. Priestley describe and demonstrate the key role of carbon dioxide in the regulation of breathing, which results in the discovery of the respiratory reflex, which is triggered by excess carbon dioxide rather than oxygen deficiency (1905)[257].

Haldane leads an expedition of respiratory physiologists to Pike's Peak in 1911 to study the effects of altitude on human breathing (1913)[258]. Findings revolutionize dogma concerning respiration. He is among the first to report deoxygenation of blood increases its ability to carry carbon dioxide and conversely oxygenated blood has a reduced capacity to carry carbon dioxide. The loss of oxygen from hemoglobin makes the hemoglobin more basic and enhances the absorption of carbon dioxide. This property of hemoglobin is termed the Haldane effect. He invents several apparatus to conduct blood gas analyses (1892,1900)[259,260]. He completes many studies which investigate the impact of oxygen deficiency and muscular exercise on breathing. Most notable contribution with John G. Priestly, demonstrates an excess of carbon dioxide in arterial blood, rather than a deficiency in oxygen, triggers the respiratory reflex, generated by the medulla (1922)[261].

Haldane continues his contributions during the early-1900s in the area of occupational medicine, helping to understand the effects of various gases on coal and metal miners, deep sea divers, and provides methods to detect potentially lethal exposures to various gases. He provides one of the first decompression tables used by divers and often credited with development of the early gas masks and respirators (1908)[262]. Haldane provides much of the original work and physiological foundations necessary to understand decompression sickness, also known as caisson disease or the bends.

Francis Bainbridge (1874-1921) English physiologist introduces the mechanism of lymph fluid formation (1900)[263]. His investigations reveal lymph fluid results from the local production of metabolites by cells, which results in a consequential rise in the osmotic tension in the tissue fluid, and which attracts additional fluid from blood vessels. He publishes a concise textbook on physiology for medical students, which is well received (1914)[264]. He describes the Bainbridge reflex, characterized by an increase in heart rate, resulting from increased central venous pressure and increased pressure in the right atrium, resulting in sympathetic stimulation and unopposed vagal inhibition of the heart (1915)[265]. Two years later, Bainbridge publishes his foundational work on exercise physiology and opens the door to a new area of investigations, for modern physiologists (1919)[266].

Trivia: Lymph is derived from the Latin "lympha" meaning "water".

Recall, lymphatic fluid is a clear fluid found between cells, which enter the interstitial space through the process of filtration from the walls of blood capillaries. The fluid is removed from the interstitial space by way of a network of lymph capillaries and vessels. Lymphatic fluid travels through vessels to lymph nodes, where it is filtered, moves into lymphatic collecting ducts, and ultimately reabsorbed into the venous blood system, at the left and right subclavian veins. Lymphatic fluid carries assorted toxins and waste, helping to rid the body of unwanted materials.

Walter Cannon (1871-1945) American physiologist applies newly discovered x-ray technologies to the study of digestion. He uses x-rays to image the process of swallowing and observing the motility of the stomach (1911)[267]. Perhaps more recognized by medical students, he coins the now familiar phase "flight or fight" to describe an animal's response to a threat. This phrase first appears in his 1915 publication "Bodily changes in pain, hunger, fear, rage: An account of recent research into the function of emotional excitement" (1915)[268]. He extends the ideas of Claude Bernard from the mid-1800s and investigates the body's continuous efforts to maintain an optimal biochemical environment. Walter Cannon popularizes the idea of the body maintaining an optimal biochemical environment and coins the term "homeostasis". The term, homeostasis, is first introduced by Walter Cannon in his 1932 book titled "The wisdom of the body" (1932)[269].

Otto Meyerhof (1884-1951) German cellular physiologist, building upon the works of English biochemist Fredrick Hopkins (1861-1947) and English physiologist Archibald Hill (1886-1977), details the glycogen-lactic acid cycles of skeletal muscle. Otto Meyerhof shares the 1922 Nobel Prize in Physiology or Medicine with Archibald Hill. Meyerhof is recognized "… for his discovery of the fixed relationship between the consumption of oxygen and the metabolism of lactic acid in the muscle…" and Hill is recognized "…for his discovery relating to the production of heat in the muscle…" (1922)[270]. Their works further integrate the disciplines of biochemistry and physiology and provide much of the foundation upon which subsequent investigations into muscle and exercise physiology over the next 100 years will build.

Frederick Banting (1891-1941) Canadian physiologist and American medical student Charles Best (1899-1978) at the University of Toronto, investigate and solve the problem of extracting insulin from the islet cells of Langerhans and inject the extract into patients suffering from diabetes, thereby providing an effective management of the endocrine disorder. Neither Banting nor Best discover insulin or diabetes as oftentimes reported. Lithuanian medical investigator Oscar Minkowski (1858-1931) and German medical investigator Josef von Mering (1849-1908) while working at the University of Strasbourg identify the hormone "insulin", its source the pancreas, and make the first connection with diabetes. Minkowski and von Mering publish their findings from their landmark experiments in 1889 and 1890, 30 years before Banting and Best initially address the problem (1889,1890)[271,272].

John Macleod (1876-1935) then Chair of the Physiology Department at the University of Toronto, whom provide Banting and Best with laboratory space and research funding, is awarded the 1923 Nobel Prize in Physiology or Medicine, along with Fredrick Banting, for "…the discovery of insulin…" (1923)[273]. Charles Best is not nominated and thereby never considered for the Prize. James Collip (1892-1965), Canadian biochemist who joins the Banting and Best research team late, yet makes critical contributions, is also never nominated. The omission of Best and Collip from the nominations and the inclusion of Macleod create a lively, oftentimes heated debate. The debate continues today.

In brief and following a review of the written statements from the Nobel Committee archives and only recently released to the scientific community, the Committee notes Banting came up with the original idea, however the idea may have never been effected without the help of Macleod's guidance and resources. Really?

Charles Best (1899-1978) medical student from Nova Scotia, so instrumental in the development of insulin extraction and applications to the management of diabetes, completes his medical degree and pursues a career in medical research physiology. He goes on to discover histaminase (enzyme that degrades histamine), recognizes choline as a dietary factor, and purifies heparin.

James Bertram Collip (1892-1965) physiologist/biochemist, also from the University of Toronto, with much experience in tissue extractions joins the team of Banting, Best, and Macleod and soon purifies the insulin extracts, sufficient for human testing. The team begins its first human trial with a 14 year old boy suffering from diabetes mellitus, January 11, 1922. The initial clinical trial with the boy results in failure. Collip subsequently modifies his extraction and "trapping" procedures and the clinical trial is repeated. This time the trial is successful. The results are presented in May 1922 at the Association of American Physicians in Washington D.C. Collip, instrumental in bringing to the team the necessary biochemical knowledge and technology permitting extraction and purification of insulin is accomplished within one month of joining the team. His contributions, essential in the success of the clinical trial moves the team forward and past the point where most other researchers have stalled.

In addition to his contribution with extraction techniques Collip is the one on the team to recognize the extracts do much more than simply reduce blood sugar. He recognizes the extracts reduce ketones in the urine and raise the glycogen storage capacity of the diabetic patient. His contributions are not readily acknowledged by Nobel recipients Banting or Macleod. Following much ill will between the original research team members Banting, Best, Collip, and Department Chair Macleod, James Collip successfully continues his career in the new area of investigative endocrinology and makes pioneering contribution through his innovative studies, especially adrenocorticotropic hormone (ACTH).

A brief note on the history of the discovery of insulin and diabetes. Before the discovery of insulin extracts, patients suffering from diabetes mellitus often die within a few months of diagnosis. Medical treatments are dependent upon diet control. The choice for the patient is simple, die soon or extend your life perhaps another few months by following a strict diet. Patients occasionally die from starvation as one consequence of the strict diet prescribed by their treating physician. Not until the work of Banting, Best, Collip, and Macleod in 1922 are alternative effective medical options available to diabetic patients.

Many investigators, working and reporting years before Banting, Best, Collip, and Macleod report their work, contribute substantially to the discovery of insulin and its role in diabetes mellitus. Paul Langerhans (1847-1888), German medical student in Berlin, at the age of 22 years, is first to recognize and report pancreatic tissues of patients whom have died from diabetes evidence damaged pancreas (1869)[274]. He identifies a cluster of previously unknown cells and with unknown function. The cell cluster is subsequently recognized by others to include the now familiar beta cells and are the source of the endocrine hormone insulin. Twenty years after Langerhans identifies the cell cluster, German physiologist Oskar Minkowski (1858-1931) and Josef von Mering (1849-1908) complete their landmark experiments in which they remove the pancreas of dogs and which then quickly results in an animal suffering diabetes (1889)[275]. Minkowski and Mering are first to identify the pancreas to have two functions, an exocrine function essential in the production of digestive juices and an endocrine function essential in the production of a substance that regulates blood sugar. Five years later, the pancreas cell cluster, first identified by Langerhans is named the "Islets of Langerhans" by French pathologist Gustave-

Edouard Laguesse (1861-1927) and whom ignores the endocrine function, reporting only the exocrine function of the cells in the regulation of digestion (1894)[276].

In addition to the investigators of the late-1800s described above, investigators of the early-1900s also contribute substantially to the understanding of insulin, years before Banting and Macleod. For example, Georg Zuelzer (1908)[277], Ernets Scott (1912)[278], John Murlin (1913)[279], Israel Kleiner (1919)[280], and Nicolae Paulescu (1921)[281] all publish findings, successfully reducing blood and urine sugar levels following injection of pancreas extracts, all before Banting's group report their discoveries in 1921. Of particular note are a series of four presentations made by Nicholae Paulescu to the Romanian Section of the Society of Biology, April through June 1921, followed by Paulescu's 1921 paper in which he details "pancreatin" and its ability to reduce blood sugar when administered intravenously (1921)[281]. Paulescu's paper appears eight months before Banting, Best, Macleod, and Collip report their "discovery". Hummm…..

The professional debate as to which individual or which group should receive credit for their contributions proves to be a hotly contested issues during it's time. Internal politics within the Banting, Best, Collip, and Macleod team soon disrupt the team's productivity and results in strained relationships for many years to come. In brief and at the risk of oversimplification to make the point clear, Banting believes he is solely responsible for the ideas leading to the breakthroughs in solving the long standing problem as to how to isolate and extract insulin from the pancreas. He also believes Macleod and Collip are attempting to take over the research project and take credit for work completed by himself and Best. Collip is suspicious of Banting and unwilling to disclose to him the revised extraction and "trapping" procedures he developed permitting sufficient purification of insulin extracts to be used with humans. Macleod sees himself as ultimately responsible for the success of the entire research team efforts, as the result of his administrative and advisory roles.

With the announcement of the Nobel Prize nominations and a flurry of internal University and professional politics Banting launches an aggressive campaign to the Canadian government and medical community to ensure he is the person recognized as responsible for insulin. Best is angered by the lack of recognition of his contributions and failure to receive the Prize nomination. Recall, the nominations went only to Banting and Macleod. The exclusion of Best and Collip from the Committee's consideration leads quickly to further strained relationships between the investigators. Seeing the success of Banting's campaign, Best launches his own successful campaign to ensure he too is recognized for his contributions and forever associated with the advancement of insulin research. And so it goes, then and now, in the professional scientific collaborative process.

One final note. Paulescu secures patient rights in his home country of Romanian for his method of manufacturing "insulin" in April 1922, one month before Banting, Best, Collip, and Macleod report results of their first successful clinical trial to the meeting of the Association of American Physicians, in Washington D.C, in May 1922. The team of Banting, Best, Collip, and Macleod subsequently secure U.S. and Canadian patent rights, which they soon give away to the University of Toronto. Monies generated from the U.S. and Canadian patents are used to support research at the University (2010)[282]. Eli Lilly starts full scale production of the insulin extract in 1923 (1982)[283]. Today, there is still no cure for diabetes and insulin remains the primary pharmaceutical agent used in the clinical management of diabetes mellitus.

Trivia: Insulin is derived from Latin "insula" meaning island, so named because it is secreted by the "Islets of Langerhans", located in the pancreas + "in" a noun ending for an organic compound. The term "insuline" enters the professional literature in 1909, introduced by French biologist de Meyer and subsequently modified spelling by British physiologist Edward Schafer in 1915 to "insulin". Romanian physiologist Nicolae Paulescu names his extract "pancreatine" (1916)[284]. Banting and Best originally name their extract "isletin". Macleod once involved, strongly suggests to Banting and Best the name be changed to "insulin" (Americanized spelling) as originally proposed by de Meyer 12 years earlier. Banting, Best, and Collip accept Macleod's suggestion and use the term "insulin" in their landmark presentation to the American Physiological Society, December 1921 and all subsequent publications. The term "insulin" receives uniform acceptance within the medical community and has been used ever since.

Carlo Monge-Medrano (1884-1970) Peruvian pathologist describes the physiology of mountain sickness, (high altitude sickness) in his now famous monograph "La Enfermedad de los Andes: syndromes eritremicos" [The Disease of the Andes: Erythema syndromes] (1928)[285]. He additionally describes the physiology underlying the ability of humans to adjust to high altitude environments. Monge-Medrano studies the indigenous practice of coca-leaf chewing by inhabitants of high altitude environments and details its role in aiding the metabolism (1946)[286]. High altitude sickness has been known for thousands of years, but not until Monge-Medrano is the physiology of high altitude sickness studied systematically.

Arman Quick (1894-1978) American physiologist investigates the physiology of the liver and reports its role in the production of blood clotting factors. Quick reports a one-step test for measuring the amount of prothrombin present in blood plasma and for determining prothrombin clotting times (1935)[287]. Recall, prothrombin clotting times measure the adequacy of the extrinsic and common pathways of the coagulation cascade. Quick demonstrates bleeding abnormalities can and do result from impairment of the liver e.g. obstructive jaundice (1935)[288]. Quick additionally identifies several now familiar coagulation deficiencies. Extending his studies, Quick is first to identify the anticoagulant effects of the Bayer Company's patented form of salicylic acid, acetylsalicylic acid, trademark name "Aspirin". Quick demonstrates Aspirin prolongs bleeding times and recognizes its potential role as an effective anticoagulant (1966)[289]. Quick's findings are met with much skepticism and ridicule from the scientific and medical communities. Only with time is the true value of his work recognized and accepted by the scientific and medical communities. Today, his work is regarded as foundational in the use of Aspirin as prophylactic for strokes and heart attacks.

Here lies another example of research efforts initially rejected and ridiculed by the established medical and scientific communities only later to be recognized and appreciated for their contributions to the advancement of scientific knowledge and application to the relief of suffering by patients in the care of physicians around the world.

James Danielli (1911-1984) English biologist and Hugh Davson (1909-1996) English physiologist propose their phospholipid bilayer-globular protein model of cell membranes (1935)[290]. Years before Danielli and Davson formulate their 1935 model, others had made substantial contributions. English biologist Ernest Overton describes a semi-permeable functional lipid layer surrounding cells but never refers to it as a structural component of the cell wall (1899)[291]. Twenty five years later, Dutch biologists E. Gorter (1881-1954) and F. Grendel (1897-1969) describe the now familiar phospholipid bilayer as a cell barrier consisting of two molecular layers of lipids rather than a single lipid layer (1925)[292]. Ten years later is when Danielli and Davson introduce their model of flanking proteins, proposing the phospholipid bilayer is coated on either side by globular proteins (1935)[290]. The Danielli and Davson model dominates for the next 40 years and until Seymore Singer (1924-2017) and Garth Nicolson (1943-) propose their fluid mosaic model (1972)[293].

Singer and Nicholson introduce the idea of transmembrane proteins embedded through the lipid bilayers and soon displace the flanking protein model. Singer and Nicholson's conceptualization of a permeable cell wall membrane and associated transmembrane transport mechanisms stimulate renewed interests and experimental investigations into the physiology of the cell wall and associated biological membrane structures. Their work energizes physiology for decades and opens a new focus in research physiology.

In summary, the first half of the 1990s witness many significant contributions to the advancement of physiology. Loewi and Dale describe chemical synaptic transmission, identify acetylcholine, and detail its role in neural transmission and at the neuromuscular junction. Starling first uses the term "hormone" to describe chemical messengers produced by endocrine glands, describes the Frank-Starling curves, and details reabsorption of water and electrolytes at the kidney. Berger develops the EEG and records spontaneous electrical brain activity from noninvasive scalp electrodes. Pavlov demonstrates the importance of saliva in digestion and introduces classical conditioning. Korothov introduces diastolic and systolic blood pressure measurements, recorded from inflation of a pressure cuff. Tawara, Keith, and Flack detail the roles of the AV and SA nodes in the heart. Flack details the flight physiology of pilots. Haldane identifies excess CO_2 to be responsible in triggering the respiratory reflex. Bainbridge describes the mechanisms of lymph fluid formation, gives us his reflex, and opens the door to exercise physiology. Cannon utilizes x-rays to study swallowing and introduces the phrase "fight or flight" and the term "homeostasis" into the professional literature. Meyerhof details the glycogen-lactic acid cycles of skeletal muscles. Banting, Best, Collip, and Macleod, advance the medical treatment of diabetes mellitus. Monge-Medrano details the physiology of high altitude sickness, building upon the works of Haldane from the Pike's Peak expedition. Quick identifies blood clotting factors and studies the anticoagulation effects of Bayer's Aspirin. Danielli and Davson propose and demonstrate the structure and physiology of the lipid bilayer of cell membranes.

The first half of the 1900s offers many of the fundamental concepts, physiological measurements, and terminologies still used in medicine today.

The second half of the 1900s witness important advancements in membrane physiology, cell signaling, muscle physiology, cardiac physiology, GI physiology, and acid-base physiology.

Walter Hess (1881-1973) Swiss physiologist investigates and establishes the importance of deep brain structures in the regulation of normal bodily functions (1948)[294]. He identifies the hypothalamus as the controller of autonomic nervous systems for functions such as blood supply to muscles and organs, heat regulation, activities of the GI systems, regulation of basal metabolism, sugar content in blood, and blood pressures (1956)[295]. He establishes anatomical and functional organization of brain respiratory centers (1931)[296], demonstrates the interdependence of sympathetic and parasympathetic nervous systems (1954)[297], and contributes to the understanding of the regulation of the circulatory systems (1930)[298]. Hess is awarded the 1947 Nobel Prize in Physiology or Medicine 1947 "… for his discovery of the functional organization of the interbrain as a coordinator of the activities of the internal organs…" (1949)[299].

Andrew Huxley (1917-2012) and Alan Hodgkin (1914-1998) English physiologists detail the physiology underlying action potentials and describe how the potentials allow communication between neurons (1952)[300]. They share the 1963 Nobel Prize in Physiology or Medicine with John Eccles. "…for their discoveries concerning the ionic mechanisms involved in excitation and inhibition in the peripheral and central portions of the nerve cell membrane" (1963)[301]. Their work with the action potential completes another important part of the physiological puzzle regarding the mechanisms of action of intra-body communication systems.

John Eccles (1903-1997) Australian neurophysiologist discovers the excitatory post synaptic potentials (EPSP) and the inhibitory post synaptic potentials (IPSP) (1953) [302]. Recall, these potential are both much smaller than action potentials and serve within the nervous systems to regulate the firing of an action potential in a neural fiber. Eccles studies the synaptic transmission believing it to be electrical in kind. The debate between electrical or chemical synaptic transmission, as the primary means of synaptic transmission, continues throughout the early-1900s and is hotly debated during the 1940s. The debate is settled for all intent and purposes when Eccles acknowledges chemical synaptic transmission is primary (1957)[303]. Eccles shares the 1963 Nobel Prize in Physiology or Medicine with Huxley and Hodgkin's "…for their discoveries concerning the ionic mechanisms involved in excitation and inhibition in the peripheral and central portions of the nerve cell membrane…" (1963)[301].

Hugh Huxley (1924-2013) British biologist, equipped with new technology the electron microscope, discovers sliding filaments within muscle and proposes the familiar model for muscle contraction sliding between actin and myosin filaments, in skeletal muscle (1954)[304]. The thick filaments defining the A-band, Z-line, and thin filaments extending from the Z-line through the I-band into the A-band are easily visible in the original electron microscope photograph (1957)[305]. Huxley's model defines the structural and physiological basis for muscle contractions for the next 50 years. His model is the foundation upon which our understanding of skeletal muscle contraction is built today.

Note: Hugh Huxley is not related to British physiologist, 1963 Nobel Prize Laureate in Physiology or Medicine, Andrew Huxley who details the "action potential" in 1952.

Jens Skou (1918-2018) Danish biophysicist discovers the Na+/K+ATPase pump (1957)[306]. Skou leaves out the term "sodium-potassium pump" from the title of his original paper and resists identifying the enzyme ATPase as essential in the movement of ions across the cell membrane. Shou soon discusses his work with American chemist Robert Post (1920-). Post is studying movement of potassium and sodium across the cell membrane of red blood cells and identifies three sodium ions are pumped out of the cell for every two potassium ions which move into the cell (1957)[307,308]. Both Shou and Post contribute substantially to the understanding of transport of ions across cell membranes. Skou is awarded the 1997 Nobel Prize in Chemistry "…for the first discovery of an ion-transporting enzyme, Na+, K+ ATPase…" (1997)[309].

Earl Sutherland (1915-1971) American physiologist discovers "second messenger" systems. Sutherland's discovery revolutionizes the understanding of inter and intra cell signaling. Studying the hormone epinephrine and its role in stimulating the liver to convert glycogen into glucose, Sutherland recognizes epinephrine does not convert glycogen to glucose directly; rather epinephrine triggers a "second messenger" system, cAMP. It is this "second messenger" system, stimulated by epinephrine, which initiates the necessary intracellular signaling required for the conversion of the energy rich storage molecule glycogen into the energy rich molecule glucose to be used by cells throughout the body (1956,1957)[310,311]. Sutherland is awarded the 1971 Nobel Prize in Physiology or Medicine "… for his discoveries concerning the mechanisms of the action of hormones…" (1971)[312]. Second messenger systems are today well established and very much a part of the understanding of cellular signaling and associated communications within and between organ-based physiological systems.

Arthur Guyton (1919-2003) American physiologist, thwarted cardiovascular surgery resident, polio patient, inventor of the "joy stick" controlled electrical wheel chair, long time Dean of University of Mississippi Medical School, author of over 600 professional articles and 40 books, including the "Textbook of Medical Physiology" familiar to most all medical students today, and scientist most responsible for the modern conceptualization and current understanding of cardiovascular regulation, greatly influences physiology throughout the second half of the 1900s.

Arthur Guyton provides original conceptualizations along with supportive evidence from thoughtful experimental investigations and frequently challenges medical dogma. One example is the mechanisms of control and regulation of cardiac output (1955a,1955b)[313,314]. Guyton's position in brief is simple; first, body tissues demand for oxygen is the ultimate regulator of cardiac output; second, cardiac output is dependent upon and proportional to venous return to the heart. He applies mathematical modeling derived from system engineering analyses to the study of the heart. Applying analytical models in combination with innovative computer modeling technologies Guyton is able to generate hypothetical models and test models using computer modeling technologies as an adjunct to laboratory based experimentation. His approach generates quantitative, objective, mathematical formulations which accurately detail the physiology of the cardiovascular system. He later applies newer technology and similar investigative methods to the study of renal, respiratory, gastrointestinal, and other physiological systems. His work, so familiar and basic to our current understanding of cardiac regulation today goes unchallenged and now is very much a part of modern medical dogma.

Guyton is perhaps most recognized by medical students today, as the likely author of your required textbook used in your medical school's physiology course. His textbook "Textbook of Medical Physiology" is popular among medical students and faculty alike. He releases his first edition in 1956 and the book remains very much in demand by medical students today, now in its 13th edition (2016)[315]. What is unique to Guyton's textbook is that he writes the first eight editions entirely on his own, providing a cohesion and easy flow of information across physiological systems. A single authored textbook in a complex area such as physiology is often unseen. Traditionally, this type of textbook is authored by 10 to 20 different people, with each writing a chapter on their particular area of expertise, and then ordered and edited by one or two editors.

John Hall (1946-) American cardiovascular and renal physiologist joins with Guyton to co-author editions 9 through 13. Guyton's textbook provides practicing physicians worldwide a common, shared reference and has become a familiar sight around the lecture halls, libraries, and study rooms of medical schools around the world.

Perhaps, less known to medical students, Arthur Guyton originally planned a career practicing cardiovascular surgery. However, during his residency he is infected with the polio virus, resulting in partial paralysis of his right leg, left arm, and both shoulders. Given the physical limitations he abandons his chosen career track and enters an alternative track in academic medicine. Soon after making the choice he invents the first motorized wheelchair with a "joy stick". He goes on to write over 600 academic papers and 40 books, makes legendary contributions to understanding cardiovascular physiology, and becomes the long term Dean of the University of Mississippi Medical School, making additional contributions to the education and training of thousands of medical students. Sometimes the "other" path taken results in the greatest contributions and rewards.

Seymour Singer (1954-2017) American biochemist and Garth Nicolson (1943-) American biochemist introduce their "fluid mosaic model" of the structure of cell membranes and revolutionize the understanding of cell membrane walls (1972)[316]. The model displaces the Danielli-Davson model, proposed during the mid-1930s and which serves as the dominant model throughout the mid-1900s. Both the Danielli-Davson (D-D) and Singer-Nicholson (S-N) models describe a lipid bilayer structure. However, the Singer-Nicholson model differs from the Danielli-Davson model in three basic features. First, S-N model introduces the idea of integrated membrane proteins in contrast to D-D idea of non-integrated, flanking proteins, located on either side of the lipid bilayer. Second, the integrated proteins are capable of lateral movement within the membrane. Third, there is an asymmetrical structure to the plasma membrane. Although the protein-lipid-protein sandwich model of biological membrane walls has been known for a long time and others recently proposed lateral motility of proteins components embedded in lipid bilayer membranes (1970)[317], the S-N landmark paper provides an integration of several important ideas related to the structure organization of the cell membrane, provides a reasonable molecular model alternative to all previous models, and is made available to a wide readership through its publication in the multidisciplinary journal "Science" (1972)[318]. The model is readily accepted by the scientific community and continues to serves as the most accepted model today.

Horace Davenport (1912-2005) American gastric physiologist revolutionizes the world of gastroenterology when he reports his discovery of carbonic anhydrase in the parietal cells of the stomach and offers his understanding of gastric mechanism which explain why the stomach does not digest itself. Davenport additionally explains the mechanism of action of Aspirin in relationship to how it breaches the gastric mucosal barrier and results in stomach ulcers. His research is foundational for the development of new generation pharmaceuticals designed to protect the gastric barriers, including histamine blockers and proton blockers. He writes extensively on acid-base relationships. Many medical students might be familiar with his textbook "The ABC of acid-base chemistry: The elements of physiological blood-gas chemistry for medical students and physicians" (1974)[319]. If you have never fallen asleep with this book clutched in your hands the night before your physiology course exam on acid-base you are the exception. Perhaps you might better remember him for his diagrams, the Davenport Diagrams, which visually describe the relationships between blood bicarbonate concentrations and blood pH following respiratory and/or metabolic acid base disturbances (1974)[319]. These diagrams provide a useful tool to quickly understand acid-base relationships and the resultant changes associated with physiological compensations in typical acid-base disturbances.

Erwin Neher (1944-) German biophysicist and Bert Sakmann (1942-) German physiologist develop the "patch clamp" technique which allows for the detection of movement of small amounts substances through the cell membrane (1978,1992)[320,321]. The technique provides the necessary procedures to identify ion channels, opening the door for more complete understanding of these specialized parts of the cell membrane, which permit movements of charged molecules into and out of the cell (1988)[322]. With an increased understanding of the normal physiology of ion channels, recent works have been directed to developing an understanding of a variety of disorders resulting in part from impairment in normal ion channel functions, now termed channelopathies. For example, multiple sclerosis is now known to result not only as the result of degeneration of the myelin sheathing around central neurons but also impairments in the channels of the effected cells. In recognition of their contributions Neher and Sakmann are awarded the 1991 Nobel Prize in Physiology or Medicine "… for their discoveries concerning the function of single ion channels in cells…" (1991)[323].

Dario DiFrancesco (1948-) Italian physiologist publishes his first paper introducing the "funny currents" (I_f) and explains their roles in contributing to the pacemaker function of cardiac muscle (1979)[324]. The "funny currents" are located in spontaneously active regions of the heart, especially the sino-atrial node (SA) and atrio-venticular node (AV). They are a mixed sodium-potassium current which regulates spontaneous activity of the SA node and consequently the rate of cardiac contractions (1980,1993)[325,326]. Over 100 years after Sunano Tawara (AV node), Author Keith, and Martin Flack (SA node) first report the anatomical locations and offer descriptions of the physiology of these specialized cardiac muscle tissues, details of SA and AV nodes continue to be investigated today. DiFrancesco reviews the role and physiology of the "funny current" as they relate to health, disease (2008)[327], and pacemaker activity (2010)[328], reminding all of us there is always more to learn from structures and systems we believe we already understand.

Robert Furchgott (1916-2009) American biochemist, Louis Ignarro (1941-) American pharmacologist, Ferid Murad (1936-) American pharmacologist, and Salvador Moncada (1944 -) Honduran pharmacologist describe the signaling and vasodilatation properties of nitric oxide, a major endothelium derived relaxing factor (1987,1987,1987)[329,330.331]. Furchgott, Ignarro, and Moncada focus on autocrine and paracrine signaling properties of nitric oxide. Murad focuses upon the mechanism of action responsible for vasodilatation and increased blood flow.

Furchgott, Ignarro, and Murad are awarded the 1998 Nobel Prize in Physiology or Medicine "…for their discoveries concerning nitric oxide as a signaling molecule in the cardiovascular system…" (1998)[332]. Salvador Moncada is not included in the award of the Nobel Prize to the surprise of the world's scientific community, sparking another heated debate as to who and how to recognize individuals making significant contributions to the advancement of scientific knowledge. The official reason(s) surrounding the failure of the Nobel Committee to recognize Moncada will remain sealed until the year 2048.

Trivia: Lists of Nobel Prizes nominations, investigations, and opinions concerning the award are kept secret for 50 years (2010)[333].

By the end of the 1900s, rapid advances enjoyed by physiology during the 1800s and 1900s slow. The discipline is now well established and entrenched in both the University and medical school settings. A command of medical physiology is mandated of all medical students enrolled in allopathic medical training programs throughout the world. Traditional departmental boundaries become blurred and physiology more than ever before embraces new opportunities for cooperative interdisciplinary investigations.

In summary, the Late Modern period (1900 AD-2000 AD) moves physiology from primary interests placed upon identification of functional relationships between organs and organ systems to interests of specific biochemical and physiological mechanisms responsible for the functional relationships, occurring at the cellular level. Hormones are identified, studied in detail, and result in clinical application for new treatments for several commonly occurring medical conditions. Interests in the physiology of bioelectricity results in clinical applications for the practicing physicians with development of the EEG and EKG. Physiological studies of blood pressures result in the development of now routine noninvasive measurements of diastolic and systolic pressures and an understanding of their clinical applications in medicine. The physiology of extreme conditions on the body e.g. high altitudes (high altitude sickness and high altitude flight); high pressures (mining and deep sea diving) are investigated and the physiology explained. Muscle contractions are explained within the matrix of actin and myosin sliding filaments. The structure and physiology of cell membranes are described and concepts such as phospholipid bilayers, single ion channels, and membrane pumps are introduced. Second messenger signaling is identified and explained. Acid-base disorders and associated physiological compensations are better understood. The blood coagulation cascade is pieced together. Normal science (1962)[334] clarifies subtleties in all major organ systems, cardiovascular, respiratory, gastrointestinal, renal, pancreas, liver, skin, skeletal-muscular, endocrine, and brain.

The first half of the 1900s sees Minkowski and von Mering extend and develop investigations following their discovery of "insulin". Starling details the exchange of fluids at the level of the capillary, discovers neural control of peristalsis, demonstrates the role of secretin, coins the term "hormone", details fluid reabsorption by the distal convoluted tubules of the kidney, and plots the relationship between cardiac muscle length and contractile force. Berger records electrical brain activity from surface electrodes and applies EEG technologies to the study of impaired brain functions. Pavlov details the role of salivation in digestion and introduces classical conditioning to the scientific communities. Korothov describes the value of diastolic and systolic measurements and a new, non-invasive method for taking blood pressures. Tawara, Keith, and Flack report the location and function of the AV and SA nodes in the heart. Flack additionally details the physiology of the pilot flying at high altitudes. Haldane and Priestly describe the role of carbon dioxide in triggering the respiratory reflex. Haldane leads an expedition of physiologists to Pike's Peak and details the relationship of oxygen and carbon dioxide carrying capacity of hemoglobin. He provides the first decompression tables for divers and describes the physiology of decompression sickness. Bainbridge describes lymph formation, change in rate with vagal nerve inhibition, and lays the foundation for exercise physiology. Cannon utilizes the newly discovered x-ray in the study of swallowing mechanics, coins the now familiar phrase "flight or fight" in association with sympathetic nervous system stimulation, and coins the term "homeostasis" to describe the optimal internal physiological environment between systems.

Meyerhof and Hill lay the foundation for muscle physiology. Dale and Loewi describe the mechanisms of chemical synaptic transmission and the role of acetylcholine at the neuromuscular junction. Banting, Best, Collip, and Macleod extract insulin and successfully provide a new medical management for diabetes mellitus. Monge-Medrano describes the physiology of mountain sickness. Quick describes the physiology of blood clotting factors and elucidates the anticoagulant properties of Bayer's Aspirin. Gorter and Grendel describe a lipid bilayer as part of the cellular wall membrane and Overton describe its semipermability properties. Danielli and Davison provide their phospholipid bilayer-globular protein model of cell wall membranes and lay the foundation for future understandings of membrane physiology. Hess identifies the hypothalamus as controller of autonomic functions, heat regulation, basal metabolism regulation, blood pressure and demonstrates the independence of the sympathetic and parasympathetic nervous systems.

The second half of the 1900s sees Huxley and Hodgkin discover and explain ionic mechanisms of neural transmission. Eccles discovers EPSPs and IPSPs. Huxley uses the new technology of the electron microscope to define A-bands, I-bands, Z-lines of skeletal muscles and proposes the sliding actin-myosin filament model to explain muscle contraction. Skou discovers the

Na+/K+ATPase pump and Post describes the familiar 3 Na+ in and 2 K+ out characteristics of this pump. Southerland discovers "second messengers". Guyton applies innovative computer modeling technologies as an adjunct to laboratory based experimentation and determines body tissue demand for oxygen is the ultimate regulator of cardiac output and cardiac output is dependent upon and proportional to venous return to the heart. Guyton publishes "Textbook of Medical Physiology". Singer and Nicholson introduce the "fluid mosaic model" of the phospholipid bilayer cell wall membrane and describe transmembrane transport mechanisms. Davenport discovers carbonic anhydrase in gastric parietal cells and explains why the stomach does not digest itself. He publishes his Davenport Diagrams, making acid-base disorders and the associated physiological compensations understandable for the medical student. Neher and Sakmann develop the "patch clamp" and provide the necessary techniques to detect movement of small amounts of substance through cell membranes and open the door for understanding single ion channels in the cell. DiFrancesco describe "funny currents" and explains their roles in pacemaker functions of cardiac muscle. Furchgott, Ignarro, Murad, and Moncada describe the signaling and vasodilatation properties of nitric oxide.

In addition to substantial advances in content knowledge, technology, and procedures, physiology during the 1900s is filled with its fair share of professional jealousies and political infighting among investigators, institutional politics, governmental, social, and religious influences, all effecting the scientific process and advancement of scientific knowledge. Recall, for example, the people and events associated with the development and release of insulin for the medical management of diabetes mellitus. And so it continues to go….

Current Modern, 2000 AD - 2019 AD.

The early beginning of the 2000s signals continuing changes in the direction of physiology as a discipline.

Equipped with new technologies and new innovative young minds, the discipline continues forward into exciting new territories of research. The traditional areas of physiology investigations; cardiovascular systems, respiratory systems, gastrointestinal systems, neural systems, renal systems, endocrine systems, and skeletal muscle systems continue to be investigated and refined. New technologies are being applied and more detailed understanding of the subtleties within each system continues to be evident. Traditional systems are being viewed in new ways. The discipline is becoming more integrated with other disciplines and boundaries of the past are becoming blurred. Capitalizing upon new technologies in molecular biology, physiology is being studied at the molecular level. There is much excitement in the field associated with recent advancements in the genetic sequencing of DNA and identification of specific structural and regulatory genes. Genes responsible for controlling cell cycles have been recently identified and manipulated. Genetic regulation of apoptosis has been recently identified and manipulated. Tissues are currently being modified through the manipulation of embryonic stem cells. In vitro fertilization is routine procedure today. The roles of chromosome telomeres and telomerases have been identified. Duplication of selected segments of human DNA is common.

A sample of specific recent advancements, current areas of activity, and future directions in physiology are briefly presented here.

Leland Hartwell (1939-) American cell biologist discovers cell "checkpoint" genes. Tim Hunt (1943-) English biochemist discovers proteins "cyclins" and the associated enzymes "cyclin dependent kinases". Paul Nurse (1949-) English cell biologist discovers specific genetic controls regulating the movement of the cell cycle from G1 phase to S phase and G2 phase to mitosis. Collectively, Hartwell, Hunt, and Nurse are awarded the 2001 Nobel Prize in Physiology or Medicine "… for their discoveries of key regulators of the cell cycle…" (2001)[335] .

Sydney Brenner (1927-2019) South African biologist, perhaps best known for his competing models as to how brain cells determine their neural function e.g. function of neighboring cells or genetic lineage; Robert Horvitz (1947-) American biologist known for his models of the mechanisms underlying neurodegenerative disease; and John Sulston (1942-) English biologist and passionate advocate for open access to genomic data, are awarded the 2002 Nobel Prize in Physiology or Medicine "…for their discoveries concerning genetic regulation of organ development and programmed cell death (apoptosis)…" (2002)[336].

Trivia: The term "apoptosis" is introduced into the scientific literature by John Kerr, Andrew Wyllie, and Alastair Currie, in order to differentiate naturally occurring cell death without inflammation from necrosis resulting from acute tissue injury with inflammation (1973)[337]. Apoptosis occurs naturally as part of the genetic program of every cell and is essential in normal organ development. The term is derived from the Greek "apo" meaning "away or apart from" and "ptosis" meaning "the process of falling". Medical students frequently pronounce apoptosis "a POP tuh sis" ignoring the origin of the word. A more correct pronunciation, which embraces the word's origin, is "APE oh TOE sis".

Mario Capecchi (1937-) Italian molecular geneticist perhaps best known for his methods for homologous recombination, Martin Evans (1941-) British scientist developer of the knockout mouse, and Oliver Smithies (1925-2017) British geneticist developer of gel electrophoresis are collectively awarded the 2007 Nobel Prize in Physiology or Medicine "…for their discoveries of principles for introducing specific gene modification in mice by the use of embryonic stem cells…" (2007)[338].

Elizabeth Blackburn (1948-) Australian molecular biologist known for the discovery of the enzyme telomerase, Carol Greider (1961-) American molecular biologist known for identifying the structure of telomeres and importance of telomeres in the physiology of normal aging and diseases, Jack Szostak (1952-) British biologist, known for his work in chromosome recombination are collectively awarded the 2009 Nobel Prize in Physiology or Medicine "…for discovery of how chromosomes are protected by telomeres and the enzyme telomerase…" (2009)[339].

Robert Edwards (1925-2013) British biologist, perhaps most recognized by medical students as first to report successful fertilization of a human egg in a cell culture dish in 1978 producing the first "test tube baby" [340] is awarded the 2010 Nobel Prize in Physiology or Medicine "…for the development of in vitro fertilization…" (2010)[341].

Jeffery Hall (1945-) American geneticist, Michael Robash (1944-) American geneticist, and Michael Young (1949-) American biologist and geneticist are awarded the 2017 Nobel Prize in Physiology or Medicine "…for their discoveries of molecular mechanisms controlling the circadian rhythm…" (2017)[342].

William Kaelin, Jr. (1957-), Peter Ratcliffe (1954-), and Gregg Semenza (1956-) are awarded the 2019 Nobel Prize in Physiology or Medicine "…for their discoveries of how cells sense and adapt to oxygen availability…" (2019)[343].

In summary, the Current Modern period 2000 -2019 moves physiology more and more towards molecular biology and further away from traditional investigations of organs and organ systems as its primary unit of study. New technologies are opening new and exciting areas of investigation for physiologists. The discipline is poised, once again, to capitalize upon recent technological advances and continue to move the discipline forward with the next wave of substantial advancements and displacement of comforting dogma.

References.

[1] Dirckx J. (1997). Stedman's concise medical dictionary for the health professions. Third Edition. Baltimore: Williams and Wilkins.

[2] Online Etymology Dictionary. (2018). Physiology. Retrieved June 2018 from https://www.etymonline.com/word/physiology

[3] Thompson, R. (1923). Assyrian medical texts from the originals in the British Museum. H. Milford, Oxford University Press.

[4] Labat. R. (1951). Traite akkadien de diagnostics et prognostics medicaux. Collection des travaux de l'Academie internationale d'histoire des sciences. Vol 7. Academie Internationale d'histoire des sciences. Wiesbaden: Franz Steiner Verlag.

[5] Kocher, F. (1964). Die babylonisch-assyrische medizin in testen und untersuchungen. Vols 1-6. Berlin: Walter de Gruyter.

[6] Hunger, H. (1976). Spaet babylonische text aus uruk. Vol 1. Berlin: Mann.

[7] Scurlock, J. and Andersen, B. (2005). Diagnoses in Assyrian and Babylonian medicine: Ancient sources, translation, and modern medical analyses. Chicago: University of Illinois Press.

[8] Breasted, J. (1930). The Edwin Smith Surgical Papyrus, Volume 1: Hieroglyphic Transliteration, Translation, and Commentary; Volume 2: Facsimile Plates and Line for Line Hieroglyphic Transliteration. Chicago: University of Chicago Press. Retrieved June 2018 from https://oi.uchicago.edu/sites/oi.uchicago.edu/files/uploads/shared/docs/oip3.pdf

[9] Edwin Smith Surgical Papyrus. [Online English translation]. Retrieved November 2009 from http://www.touregypt.net/edwinsmithsurgical.htm

[10] Ebers Papyrus, Egypt (circa 1550 BC). Compendium of the whole Egyptian Medicine (Georg Ebers): Column 1-2. University of Leipzig Library, Special Collections. Leipzig, Germany.

[11] Joachim, H. (1890). Papyrus Ebers. Das alteste Buch uber Heilkunde [Translation from Egyptian into German]. Berlin: Druck und Verlag von George Reimer.

[12] Ebbell, B. (1937). The Papyrus Ebers: The greatest Egyptian medical document. [English translation by B. Ebbell]. Copenhagen: Levin & Munksgaard.

[13] Reveil de Monuments Egyptians. (1883). Par le docteur Henri Brugsch, Deuxieme partie. PL lxxxvcvil, Leipzig.

[14] Finlayson, J. (1893). Ancient Egyptian Medicine: A bibliographical demonstration in the Library of the Faculty of Physicians and Surgeons, Glasgow, January 12th, 1893. The British Medical Journal, Vol 1 (1690): 1061-1064. Retrieved June 2018 from https://www.jstor.org/stable/20224516?readnow=1&loggedin=true&seq=1#page_scan_tab_contents

[15] Wreszinski, W. (1909). Der grosse medizinische Papyrus des Berliner Museums (Pap. Berl. 3038). J. C. Hinrichs.

[16] Wachtler, J. (1896). De Alcmaeone Crotoniata. Leipzig: Teubner. (The only full-scale commentary devoted to Alcmaeon. Greek texts of the fragments and testimonia with commentary in Latin).

[17] Diels, H. (1903, 1968). Die Fragmente der Vorsokratiker. Walther Kranz, editor. Weidmann Press, Dublin and Zurich.

[18] Diels, H. and Kranz, W. (1952), Die Fragmente der Vorsokratiker (in three volumes), 6th edition, Dublin and Zürich: Weidmann, Volume 1, Chapter 24, 210-216. Greek texts of the fragments and testimonia with translations in German. (Originally published 1903).

[19] Timpanaro-Cardini, M. (1958-64). Pitagorici, Testimonianze e frammenti, 3 vols., Firenze: La Nuova Italia, Vol. 1, 124-153 (Greek texts of the fragments and testimonia with translations and commentary in Italian).

[20] Freeman, K. (1983). Ancilla to the Pre-Socratic Philosophers. Cambridge: Harvard University Press. (Reprint edition). This book is a complete English translation of the 'B' passages–the so-called 'fragments'– from Die Fragmente der Vorsokratiker.

[21] Hippocratic Collection. [Digitized copies of the first printed editions (1525-1595) housed at the Biblioteque Interuniversitiarire de medicine of Paris]. Retrieved November 2009 from http://www.bium.univ-paris5.fr/histmed/medica/hipp_va.html

[22] Galen. (circa 170 AD). De usu partium.[Usefulness of the parts]. MS Urb. gr. 69 – Roll 8478; Anthony Grafton, ed. Rome Reborn: The Vatican Library and Renaissance Culture. Washington, D.C. 1993 in plate number order 132.

[23] Herophilus. (circa 300 BC/1969 AD). On Pulses, T21-T24, cf. Chapter VII, T144-T188, especially T148, T150, Fr162. from Herophilus: The art of medicine in early Alexandria, edition translation by Henrich Von Staden, Cambridge University Press 1989.

[24] Celsus, A. (1713). De medicina libri octo cum praefatione George Wolfgang Wedelius. Joannem Felicem Bielckius.

[25] Clesus, A. and Greive, J. (1814). Of medicine in eight books. Translated with notes critical and explanatory by James Greive. Edinburgh: University Press for Dickinson and Company, Infirmary Street.

[26] Daremberg, C. and Celsus, A. (2010). De Medicina Liri Octo. BibliBazaar.

[27] Kuhn, C. (1821-1833). Claudii Galeni Opera Omnia. Leipzig: C. Cnobloch, 1821-1833, rpt. Hildesheim: Georg Olms, 1964-5. (Greek, Latin translation.) Editio Kuchniana Lipsiae.

[28] Galen, Kuhn, C., Assmann, W., Nutton, V. (1821-1833). Claudii Galeni opera omnia. Vol 1-20. C. Cnobloch.

[29] Kuhn, C. (1829). Medicorum graecorum opera: quae exstant / editionem curauit D. Carolus Gottlob Kuhn: Lipsiae; Prostat in Officiana Libraaria Car. Cnoblochii.

[30] Coxe, J. (1846). The Writings of Hippocrates and Galen. Epitomized from the original Latin translations Philadelphia: Lindsay and Blakiston.

[31] Singer, P. (2002). Galen: Selected Works. Oxford University Press.

[32] Abu Ali al Husayn ibn Abd Allah Ibn Sina (aka Avicenna). Kitab al-Qanun fi al-tibb [The Canon of Medicine]. MS A 53, Islamic Medical Manuscripts at the National Library of Medicine.

[33] Ibn Sina (Avicenna). Kitab al-Qanun fi al-tibb (Canon on Medicine). London Welcome Library for the History and Understanding of Medicine, MS Arab. 155, copied in 1632 (1042 H).

[34] Avicenna. (1999). Canon of Medicine. (English.) Chicago: Kazi Publications.

[35] Tatawi, M. (1924). Der Lungenkreislauf nach Al-Koraschi. [The Pulmonary Circulation according to Al-Koraschi (Ibn al-Nafis)]. Doctoral dissertation, Freiburg.

[36] Meyerhof, M. (1935). Ibn an-Nafis and his theory of the lesser circulation. Isis, 23:100–120.

[37] Ibn al-Nafis. (1242). Sharh Tashrih al-Qanun Ibn Sina. (Commentary on the Anatomy of Canon of Avicenna). Script No, 62243. In Keys, T. and Wakim, K. (1953). Contributions of the Arabs to medicine, Proceedings of the staff meeting. Mayo Clinic, 28:423-37.

[38] Fancy, N. (2006). Pulmonary Transit and Bodily Resurrection: The Interaction of Medicine, Philosophy and Religion in the Works of Ibn al-Nafis (d. 1288). Electronic Theses and Dissertations, University of Notre Dame.

[39] Ibn al-Nafis. (1242). Sharh Qanun Ibn Sina [A commentary on Avivenna's Canon]. MS 2939. Bibilotheque Nationale. Paris. Retreived June 2018 from https://www.wdl.org/en/item/18199/view/1/1/

[40] Ibn al-Nafis. (2000). Al-shamel fi al-sinaa al-tibbiyyah. [The comphrehenisve book on the art of medicine, Vol 1 and 2. Y. Ziedan editor. United Arabic Emerates: Abu Ahabi. Al-Mujammaa al-Tjaaqfi.

[41] Ibn al-Nafis (circa 1275). [Comprehensive book of the art of medicine], 33:42-43. Fragment. Call number Z276. Special Collections: Arabic Oversize. Lane Medical Library, Stanford University Medical Center, Stanford, CA.

[42] Ibn al-Nafis. (2004). Al-Mujaz fi al tabb. A. Al-Ezbawy editor. 4th edition. Cairo: Islamic Heritage Revival Committee, Supreme Council for Islanic Affaires, Ministry of Endowments.

[43] Ibn al-Nafis. (1991). Risalat al-a'adaa. Y. Zicdan, editor. Cairo: Al dar al-Masriyas al Lubnaniya.

[44] Fernel, J. and Forrester, J. (1567/2003). The physiology of Jean Fernel (1567). Latin with English translation by John Forrester. American Philosophical Society Philadelphia.

[45] Fernel, J. (1564). Io. Fernelii Ambiana, Medicina. Ad Henricum II, Galliarum regcm Christianisimum. Apud Caesarem Farinam.

[46] Servetus, M. (1546). Christianismi Restitution, MS Latin 18212. Paris: Bibliotheque Nationale.

[47] Servetus, M. (1553). Christianismi Restitution. Vienna: Balthasar Arnoullet.

[48] Columbi, Realdi (1559). De re anatomica libri XV. Ex typographia Nicolai Builacquae. Biblioteca Digital Dioscorides. Original from Complutense University of Madrid.

[49] Harvey, W. (1628). Exercitatio anatomicica de motu cordis et sanguinis et sanguinis in amimalibus" [An anatomical exercise on the motion of the heart and blood in animals]. Frankfurt, Sumptibus Gvilielmi Fitzeri. [Frankfurt-on-Main, Germany].

[50] Santorio, S. and Obici, H. (1614). De statica medicina: Aphorismorum sectionibus septem comprehensa. G. Ritssch.

[51] Harvey, W. (1628). Exercitatio anatomicica de motu cordis et sanguinis et sanguinis in amimalibus. [An anatomical exercise on the motion of the heart and blood in animals]. English translation from Latin (1653). London: Printed by Francis Leack for Richard Lowndes. (Original copy (1653) available from Bauman Rare Books from the library of the 8th Earl of Pembroke, for $82,000.00 US.).

[52] Boerhaave, H. (1708). Institutiones medicae: in usus annuae exercitationis domesticos. Lugduni Batavorum, Apud Johannem vander Linden.

[53] Hales, S. (1727). Vegetable staticks: Or: an account of some statical experiments on the sap in vegetables: being an essay towards a natural history of vegetation. also a specimen to analyse the air by a great variety of chymico - statical experiments, Volume 1. London: Printed for W. Innys and T. Woodward.

[54] Hales, S. (1731). Statical essays containing vegetable staticks, or an account of some statical experiments on the sap in vegetables: being an essay towards a natural history of vegetation: also a specimen of an attempt to analyse the air, by a great variety of chymio-statical experiements, which were read at several meetings before the Royal Society. London: Printed for W. Innys, T. Woodward, and J. Peele. St. Dunstan's Church in Fleetstreet.

[55] Hales, S. (1733). Statical essays: Containing haemastaticks or an account of some hydraulick and hydrostatical experiments made on the blood and blood vessels of animals. Also an account of some experiments on stones in the kidney and bladder; with an enquiry into the nature of those anomalous concretions. To which is added an appendix containing observations and experiments relating to several subjects in the first Volume. London: Printed for W. Innys and R. Maney at the West End of St. Pauls.

[56] Bernoulli, D. (1738). Hydrodynamica sive de viribus et motibus fluidorum commentarii: Opus academicum ab auctore, dum petropoli ageret, congestum argentorati. Strasburgo: Sumptibus Johannis Reinholdi Dulseckeri. Typis Joh, Henr. Deckeri.

[57] Bernoulli, D. (1766). Essai d'une nouvelle analyse de la mortalite casusee par la petite verole. [Testing a new analysis of mortality caused by smallpox]. Mem. Math. Phys. Acad. Roy. Sci., Paris.

[58] Poiseuille, J. (1840). Recherches experimentales sur le movement des liquids dans les tubes de tres petits diameters. Comptes rendus hebdomadaires des séances de l'Academie des Sciences, 11:961-967; 1041-1048.

[59] Von Haller, A. (1747. Primae lineae physiologiae in usum praelectionum academicarvm Gottingae: A. Vandenhoeck. (English edition 1754).

[60] Von Haller, A. (1753). De partibus corporis humani sensilibus et irritabillibus. Commentarii Societatis Regiae Scientiarium Gottingensis, 2:114-158.

[61] Von Haller, A. (1757-1766). Elementa physiologiae corporis humani. 8 volumes. Volume 1-5 Lausanne, Vols. 6-8 Bern.

[62] Galvan, L. (1791a). De viribus electricitatis in motu musculari commentarius. Pars prima, Bononien. Sci. Art Instit. Acad., 7:363-418.

[63] Galvani, L. (1791b). De viribus electricitatis in motu musculari commentarius. Bologna: Ex typographia Instituti Scientiarum.

[64] Galvani, L. and Foley, M. (1953b). De viribus electricitatis in motu musculari commentarius. English. Commentary on the effects of electricity on muscular motion translated into English by Margaret Glover Foley, with notes and a critical introduction by Bernard Cohen. Together with a facsimile of Galvani's De vivibus electicitatis in motu musculari commentarius (1791) and a biography of the editions and translations of Galvani's book prepared by John Farquhar Fulton and Madeline E Stanton. Norwalk, Conn.: Burndy Library.

[65] Thomas, W. (1873). First report of the Committee for the Selection and Nomenclature of Dynamical and Electrical Units. 43rd meeting of the British Association for the Advancement of Science. Bradford.

[66] The Electrical Congress. (1881). General Meeting Minutes of The First Congress of Electricians, First section on Electrical Units, Paris. The Electrician, September 24:7:297.

[67] Von Humbolt, A. (1797). Versuche über die gereizte Muskel- und Nervenfaser. Berlin: Posen.

[68] Du Bois-Reymond, E. (1848). Untersuchungen uber thierische Elektricitat. Vol. I-II. Berlin: G. Reimer.

[69] Reil, J. (1796). Von der Lebenskraft. Archiv für die Physiologie, Halle, 1:8-162.

[70] Reil, J. (1803). Rhapsodieen über die anwendung der psychischen curmethode auf geisteszerrüttungen. [Rhapsodies on the use of psychological therapies for the mentally disturbed.] Dem Herrn Prediger Wagnitz zugeeignet. Halle in der Curtschen Buchhandlung.

[71] Reil, J. (1808). Ueber den begriff der medicin und ihre verzweigungen besonders in beziehung auf berichtigung der topik der psychiaterie. In: Johann Christian Reil and Johann Christoph Hoffbauer (1808). Beyträge zur beförderung einer curmethode auf psychischem wege. Halle in der Curtschen Buchhandlung.

[72] Magendie, F. (1809). Quelques idées générales sur les phénomènes particuliers aux corps vivants. (Some general ideas about the phenomena to living bodies) Bulletin des Sciences Médicales, 4:145-170.

[73] Magendie, F. (1813). Mémoire sur le vomissement. Paris: Crochard. English translation in Annals of Philosophy: or Magazine of chemistry, mineralogy, mechanics, natural history, agriculture, and the arts, London, 1813, 1:429-438.

[74] Magendie, F. (1816). Mémoire sur les propriétés nutritives des substances qui ne contiennent pas d'azote. Bulletin de la Société Philomatique, 4:137.

[75] Magendie, F. (1816-1817). Précis élémentaire de physiologie. 2 volumes. Paris, Méquignon-Marvis. A revised edition appears in French 1822. Italian translation, Napoli in 1819. German translation by Karl Friedrich Heusinger (1792-1883), Eisenach in 1820. American edition by John Revere: A Summary of Physiology. Baltimore, 1822. English translation, Edinburgh, 1826.

[76] Magendie, F. (1825). Mémoire sur un liquide qui se trouve dans le crâne et le canal vertébral de l'homme et des animaux mammifères. [Memory on a liquid found in the skull and vertebral canal of man and animal mammals]. Journal de Physiologie Expérimentale et Pathologie, Paris, 5:27-37.

[77] Magendie, F. (1827). Mémoire sur un liquide qui se trouve dans le crâne et le canal vertébral de l'homme et des animaux mammifères. (Memory on a liquid found in the skull and vertebral canal of man and animals mammals). Journal de Physiologie Expérimentale et Pathologie, Paris, 7:1-29; 66-82.

[78] Magendie, F. (1821-1831). Journal de Physiologie Expérimentale, 11 volumes; Paris.

[79] Meckel, J. (1809). Über die Divertikel am Darmkanal. Archiv für die Physiologie, Halle, 9:421-453.

[80] Magendie, F. (1822a). Expériences sur les fonctions des racines des nerfs rachidiens. Journal de Physiologie Expérimentale et Pathologie, 2:276-279.

[81] Magendie, F. (1822b). Expériences sur les fonctions des racines des nerfs qui naissent de la moëlle épinière. Journal de Physiologie Expérimentale et de Pathologie, 2:366-371.

[82] Magendie, F. (1847). Comptes rendus hebdomadaires des séances de l'Académie des Sciences, 24:320.

[83] Leyden, E. (1901). Eine historische studie uber die entdeckung des Magendie-Bell'schen lebrastzes. Von Dr. Adolf Bickel, (Aus der ersten medicinischen Universitatsklinki des Herrn Geh. Rath Professor Dr. E. v. Lyden zu Berlin. Pflüger's Archiv für die gesamte Physiologie des Menschen und der Tiere, [European Journal of Physiology] Berlin, 84:276-303.

[84] Magendie, F. (1839). Lectures on the blood; and on the changes which it undergoes during disease. Philadelphia: Harrington, Barrington & Haswell.

[85] Magendie, F. (1842). Recherches physiologiques et cliniques sur le liquide céphalo-rachidien ou cérébro-spinal. 1 volume and atlas. Paris: Méquignon-Marvis.

[86] Bell, C. (1821). On the nerves; giving an account of some experiments on their structure and functions, which lead to a new arrangement of the system .Philosophical Transactions of the Royal Society of London, 111:398-424.

[87] Bell, C. (1806). Essay on the anatomy of expression in painting. London: Longman, Hurst, Rees, and Orme.

[88] Bell, C. (1814). The dissertation on gun-shot wounds. London: Longman, Hurst, Rees, Orme, and Brown.

[89] Bell, C. (1816). The anatomy and physiology of the brain and nerves, the organs of the senses, and viscera by Charles Bell. In The Anatomy and Physiology of the human body (1816) John Bell and Charles Bell. 4th edition. Vol I. London: Longman, Hurst, Rees, Orme, and Brown, Paternoster-Row.

[90] Shaw, A. (1868). Magendie and Bell. Correspondence, The British Medical Journal, August 15, p 179.

[91] McDonnell, R. (1868). Magendie and Bell, Correspondences, British Medical Journal, 2:319 Sept 19.

[92] Hawkins, C. (1869). Sir Charles Bell and M. Magendie on the functions of the spinal nerves. British Medical Journal, Jan. 9, 1:21.

[93] Cranefield, P. (1974). The way in and the way out. François Magendie, Charles Bell and the roots of the spinal nerves. Mt. Kisco, NY: Futura Publishing.

[94] Rice, G. (1987). The Bell-Magendie-Walker controversy. Med. History, April 31(2):190-200.

[95] Jorgensen, C. (2003). Aspects of the History of the Nerves: Bells Theory, the Bell-Magendie Law and Controversy, and Two Forgotten Works by P.W. Lund and D.F. Eschricht. Journal of the History of the Neurosciences, 12(3):229-249.

[96] Bell, C. (1819). An essay on the forces which circulate the blood; being an examination of the difference of the notions of fluids in living and dead vessels. London: Printed for Messrs Longman & Co, Paternoster-Rowl and Burgess & Hill, 55, Great Windmill Street, Haymarket.

[97] Purkinjie, J. (1837). Versammlung der Naturforscher und Aertze zu Prag im September 1837 [Assembly of naturalists and doctors to Prauge, September 1837], Isis von Oken (1838), 7:581.

[98] Purkinje, J. (1819). Beobachtungen und Versuche zur Physiologie der Sinne, Volume 1. Prauge: Johann Gottfried Calve.

[99] Purkinje, J. (1825). Beobachtungen und Versuche zur Physiologie der Sinne: Neue Beiträge zur Kenntniss des Sehens in Subjectiver Hinsicht. Vol 2., Berlin: Reimer.

[100] Purkinje, J. (1827a). Ueber die physiologische Bedeutung des Schwindels und die Beziehung desselben zu den neuesten Versuchen śber die Hirnfunctionen. [On the physiological significance of vertigo and the relationship of the same to the experiments on brain functions] Ma~azin fiir die gesammte Heilkunde, 23:284-310.

[101] Purkinje, J. (1820). Beitrage zur naheren Kenntuiss des Schwindels aus heautognostischen Daten Medizinische Jahrbuch des kaiserlich-honiglichen oestereichischen Staates, 6:79-125.

[102] Purkinje, J. (1845). Archiv fur Anatomie, Physiologie und wissenschaftliche Medizin, p. 281.

[103] Flourens, M. (1824). Recherches expérimentales sur les propriétés et les fonctions du système nerveux, dans les animaux vertébrés (ed 1), 26:20. Paris, Chez Crevot.

[104] Spurzheim, J. (1815). The Physiognomical System of Doctors Gall and Spurzheim, founded on an anatomical and physiological examination of the nervous system in general, and of the brain in particular, and indicating the dispositions and manifestations of the mind. London: Baldwin, Cradock, and Joy.

[105] Anon. (1823). Introductory Statement. Phrenological Journal and Miscellany, Edinburg., 1:3-31.

[106] Foster, T. (1813). Paper presented to the Philosophical Society, Cambridge. See page v in Collection of Letters on early education and its influence in the prevention of crime. 2nd ed. London: Sherwood and Bowyer, Strand, and the Albion Library, No 37, on the Dyer, Bruges 1844 or Foster, T, (1815). Observations on a New System of Phrenology or the anatomy and physiology of the Brain of Dr. Gall and Spurzheim. Philosophical Magazine and Journal 45 (1815) 44-50.

[107] Spurzheim, J. (1815). The Physiognomical system of Drs. Gall and Spurzheim founded on an anatomical and physiological examination of the nervous system in general, and of the brain in particular; and indicating the dispositions and manifestations of the mind. 2nd edition, London: Printed for Baldwin, Cradock, and Hoy. 47 Paternoster Row.

[108] Beaumont, William (1838). Experiments and Observations on the Gastric Juice and the Physiology of Digestion. Edinburgh: Maclachlan and Stewart.

[109] Poiseuille, J. (1828). Recherches sur la force du Coeur aortique. Paris.

[110] Poiseuille, J. (1840). Recherches expérimentales sur le mouvement des liquides dans les tubes de très petits diameters. Comptes REndus Acad. Sci., 11:961-967.

[111] Muller, J. (1837). Handbuch der Physiologie des Menschen für Vorlesungen, Volumes 1-2. Verlag von J. Holscher.

[112] Muller, J. (1843). Elements of Physiology. Translated from German into English by William Baly and further edited by John Bell. Philadelphia: Lea and Blanchard.

[113] Volkmann, A. and Bidder, F. (1842). Die Selbständigkeit des sympathischen Nervensystems durch anatomische Untersuchungen nachgewiesen. Leipzig

[114] Volkmann, A. (1836). Neue Beiträge zur Physiologie des Gesichtssinnes. Leipzig: Breitkopf und Härtel.

[115] Volkmann, A. (1850). Die Hamodynamik. Leipzig. Druck und Verlag von Breitkopf und Hurtel.

[116] Volkmann, A. (1858). Ueber den Einfluss der Uebung, ect Leipzig Berichte, Math-Physi, Classe, x, p67.

[117] Volkmann, A. (1863). Physiologische Untersuchugen im Geniete der Optik: Vol 1. Leipzig. Druk und Verlag von Breitkoft und Hartel.

[118] Volkmann, A. (1873). Ueber die naheren Bestandtheile der menschlichen Knochen. Berichte über die Verhandlungen der königlichen sächsischen Gesellschaft der Wissenschaften zu Leipzig, Mathematisch Physikalische Klasse. 25: 275.

[119] Du Bois-Reymond, E. (1848). Untersuchungen über thierische Elektricität, Erster Band. (Studies on animal electricity. First Volume). Berlin: Georg Reimer.

[120] Du Bois-Reymond, E. (1849). Untersuchungen über thierische Elektricität, Zweiter Band, Erste Abtheilung. (Studies on animal electricity, Second Volume). Berlin: Georg Reimer.

[121] Helmholtz, H. (1850a). Vorläufiger Bericht über die Fortpflanzungs-Geschwindigkeit der Nervenreizung. In: Archiv für Anatomie, Physiologie und wissenschaftliche Medicin. Jg. 1850, Veit & Comp., Berlin, S. 71-73.

[122] Helmholtz, H. (1850b). Messungen über den zeitlichen Verlauf der Zuckung animalischer Muskeln und die Fortpflanzungsgeschwindigkeit der Reizung in den Nerven. In: Archiv für Anatomie, Physiologie und wissenschaftliche Medicin. Jg. 1850, Veit & Comp., Berlin, S. 276-364.

[123] Helmholtz, H. (1850c). Über die Theorie der zusammengesetzten Farben. (On the theory of compound colors). Archiv für Anatomie, Physiologie und wissenschaftliche Medizin, Berlin. 461-482.

[124] Young, T. (1802). On the theory of light and colours. Philosophical transactions of the Royal Society of London, 1802, 92:12-48.

[125] Helmholtz, H. (1851). Beschreibung eines Augen-Spiegels zur Untersuchung der Netzhaut im lebenden Auge. (Description of an eye mirror to examine the retina in the living eye) Berlin: Forstner.

[126] Bernard, C. (1843). Du sac gastrique et de son role dans la nutrition. Doctoral thesis, No. 242, v. 398. Paris.

[127] Bernard, C. (1857). Nouvelles recherches experimentales sur les phenomenes glycogeniques du foie. Comptes rendus de la Societe de biologie (Memoires), Paris, 2 ser. 4:1-7.

[128] Bernard, C. (1849). Du suc pancréatique et de son rôle dans les phénomènes de la digestion. Archives générales de médecine, Paris, 19: 60-81. Reprinted, with translation, in Medical Classics, 1919, 3:581-617.

[129] Bernard, C. (1851). Influence du grand sympathique sur la sensibilité et sur la calorification. Comptes rendus de la Société de biologie, Paris, 3:163-164.

[130] Bernard, C. (1855-1856). Leçons de physiologie expérimentale appliqué à la médecine. (2 volumes). Paris: J.B. Baillière.

[131] Bernard, C. (1877). Leçons sur le diabete et la glycogenèse animale. Paris: J. B. Baillière.

[132] Bernard, C. (1857). Leçons sur les effects des substances toxiques et médicamenteuses. Paris: J.B. Baillière et Fils.

[133] Bernard, C. (1865). Introduction a l'etude de la medecine experimentale [An Introduction to the Study of Experimental Medicine]. English translation by Henry Copley Greene, published by Macmillan & Co., Ltd., 1927; Reprinted Dover edition 1957; Dover Publications, Inc. New York, New York.

[134] Waller, A. (1846). Microscopic Observations on the Perforation of the Capillaries by the Corpuscles of the Blood and on the origin of mucus and pus globules. Philosophical Magazine, November; 29:397-405.

[135] Waller, A. (1850). Experiments on the section of the glossopharyngeal and hypoglossal nerves of the frog, and observations of the alterations produced thereby in the structure of their primitive fibers. Philosophical Transactions of the Royal Society of London, 140:423-429.

[136] Waller, A. (1853). Sur l'influence du grand sympathique sur la circulation. Comptes rendus hebdomadaires des séances de l'Académie des Sciences, 36:378-382.

[137] Waller, A. (1852a). Observations sur les effects de la section des racines spinales et du nerf pneumogastrique au dessus de son ganglion inférieur chez les mammifères. Comptes rendus hebdomadaires des seances de l'Académie des Sciences, Paris, 34:582-587.

[138] Waller, A. (1852b). Sur la reproduction des nerfs et sur la structure et les fonctions des ganglions spinaux. Archiv für Anatomie, Physiologie und wissenschaftliche Medicin, Leipzig, 392.

[139] Waller, A. (1857). Experience sur les sections des nerfs et les alterations. Comptes-rendus de la Societe de biologie, Paris, 2 (3): 6.

[140] Duchenne, G. (1855). De l'électrisation localisee et de son application a la pathologie et a la thérapeutique. Paris J. B. Bailliere et Fils.

[141] Duchenne, G. (1871). A Treatise on Localized Electrization, and its applications to pathology and therapeutics (1855, 1871). Translated from the third edition of the original by Herbert Tibbits. London: Robert Hardwicke, 192 Piccadilly.

[142] Duchenne, G. (1862), Mécanisme de la physionomie humaine, ou analyse électro-physiologique de ses différents modes de l'expression. Archives générales de médecine, P. Asselin; vol. 1:29-47; 152-174.

[143] Duchenne, G. (1862). Album de photographies pathologiques complémentaire du livre intitulé de l'électrisation localisée. Paris: Ballière et Fils.

[144] Duchenne, G. (1867). Physiologie des mouvements démontrée à l'aide de l'expérimentation électrique et de l'observation clinique, et applicable à l'étude des paralysies et des déformation. Paris, Ballière et Fils.

[145] Erb, W. (1874). Ueber eine eigenthümliche Localisation von Lähmungen im Plexus brachialis. Verhandlungen des naturhistorisch-medicinischen Vereins zu Heidelberg, Neue Folge, 1:130-137.

[146] Smellie, W. (1754). A collection of cases and observations in midwifery. London.

[147] Duchenne, G. (1868). Recherches sur la parslysie musculaire pseudohypertophique ou paralysie myosclerosique. Arch Gen, de, Med, 6 s, xi. 5, 179, 305, 421, 552.

[148] Duchenne, G. (1883). Selections from the Clinical works of Dr. Duchhenne de Boulogne. Translated, edited, and condensed by G. Poore. London: The New Sydenham Society.

[149] Duchenne, G. (1850). A Critical Investigation by the help of electricity on the state of contractility and sensibility of the muscles in paralysis of the upper limbs.

[150] Duchenne, G. (1853), On the use of localized electrisation in progressive muscular atrophy.

[151] Duchenne, G. (1853). On the special action of induction currents on muscular tone.

[152] Duchenne, G. (1858). Investigation of Locomotor Ataxy: A disease specially marked by general troubles of motor coordination. Compte rendu de l'Academ des Sciences; Bullet de l'Academ de Medcc., 59 t. 24:210.

[153] Duchenne, G. (1858). Faradisation of the chorda tympani and muscles of the ossicles applied to the treatment of nervous deafness.

[154] Duchenne, G. (1860). Progressive muscular paralysis of the tongue, soft palate, and lips. A disease not before described. Arch. Gen. de Med., Sept. and Oct.

[155] Duchenne, G. (1866). The movements of respiration. Paris.

[156] Duchenne, G. (1871) A Treatise on Localized Electrization, and its applications to pathology and therapeutics (1855, 1871). Translated form the third edition of the original by Herbert Tibbits. London: Robert Hardwicke, 192 Piccadilly.

[157] Brown-Sequard, C. (1860). Course of lectures on the physiology and pathology of the central nervous system. Series of 12 lectures presented to the Royal College of Surgeons of England, May 1858. Philadelphia, J. B. Lippincott & Company.

[158] Brown-Sequard, C. (1856). Recherches expérimentales sur la production d'une affection convulsive epileptiforme, a la suite de lésions de la moëlle epinière. Archives Generales de Médecine, Paris, 1856, 5 sér., 7:143-149.

[159] Brown-Sequard, C. (1857). Researches on epilepsy: its artificial production in animals, and its etiology, nature and treatment in man. First part of a new series of experimental and clinical researches applied to physiology and pathology. Boston. Printed by David Clapp.

[160] Brown-Sequard, C. (1856). Recherches experimentales sur la physiologie et la pathologie des capsules surrénales. Comptes rendus hebdomadaires des séances de l'Académie des sciences. Paris, 8: 422-425.

[161] Brown-Sequard, C. (1889a). Experience demontrant la puissance dynamogenique chez l'homme d'un liquide extrait de testicule d'animaux. Archives de physiologie normale et pathologique, Paris, 5, ser. 1:651-658.

[162] Brown-Sequad, C. (1889b). The effects produced on man by subcutaneous injections of a liquid obtained from the testicles of animals. Lancet, 2:105-107.

[163] Brown-Sequard, C. (1889c). Archives de physiologie normale et pathologique, Paris, 5 sér., 1: 739-746.

[164] Schmidt, A. (1872). Neue Untersuchungen ueber die Fasserstoffesgerinnung. Pflüger's Archiv für die gesamte Physiologie, 6:413–538.

[165] Virchow, R. (1847). Zur pathologischen Physiologie des Blutes. 1. Veränderungen des Blutplasma's. 2. Weisses Blut. 3. Faserstoffarten und fibrinogene Substanze. [The pathological physiology of the blood. 1. Changes in blood plasma. 2. White blood. 3. fiber types and fibrinogen substance] Virchows Archiv, 1.

[166] Arthus, N. and Pages, C. (1890). Nouvelle théorie chimique de la coagulation du sang with calixte pages. Archives de physiologie normale et pathologique, Paris, 5th ser., 2:739-746.

[167] Bizzozero, J. (1882a). Ueber einen neuen Forrnbestandteil des Blutes und dessen Rolle bei der Thrombose und Blutgerinnung. Archiv für pathologische Anatomie und Physiologie und für klinische Medicin., 90:261–332.

[168] Caton, R. (1875). The electric currents of the brain. British Medical Journal, 2: 278.

[169] Caton, R (1877). Interim report on investigation of the electric currents of the brain. Brit. Med. J., (1), Supp. 62:7.

[170] Sanderson, J., Klein, E., Foster, M., and Brunton, T. (1873). Handbook for the Physiological Laboratory. Lindsay & Blankiston.

[171] Sanderson, J. (1911). Sir John Burton-Sanderson A memoir by the late Lady Burton Sanderson completed and edited by his nephew and niece with a selection from his papers and addresses. London: Clarendon Press. Henry Frowde publisher to the University of Oxford.

[172] Gaskell, W. (1882). On the rhythm of the heart of the frog, and on the nature of the action of the vagus nerve: The Croonian Lecture, Royal Society. Philosophical Transactions, 993-1033.

[173] Gaskell, W. (1883). On the innervation of the heart, with special reference to the heart of the tortoise. J. Physiol., 4:43–127.

[174] Gaskell, W. (1900). The contraction of cardiac muscle. In Schäfer, E. Textbook of Physiology. Edinburgh and London: Young J Pentland, 169–227 2.

[175] Ringer, S. (1882a). Regarding the action of hydrate of soda, hydrate of ammonia, and hydrate of potash on the frog's heart. J. Physiol., 3:195-202.

[176] Ringer, S. (1882b). Concerning the influence exerted by each of the constituents of the blood on the contraction of the ventricle. J. Physiology, 3:380-393.

[177] Ringer, S. (1869). A Handbook of Therapeutics. London: H. K. Lewis, 136 Gower Street.

[178] Ringer, S. (1880-1882). Concerning the Influence Exerted by Each of the Constituents of the Blood on the Contraction of the Ventricle. Journal of Physiology, Cambridge, 3:380-393.

[179] Ringer, S. (1883-1884). Concerning the Influence Exerted by Each of the Constituents of the Blood on the Contraction of the Ventricle. Journal of Physiology, Cambridge, 4:29-42, 222-225.

[180] Ringer, S. (1895). Further Observations Regarding the Antagonism Between Calcium Salts and Sodium, Potassium and Ammonium Salts. Journal of Physiology, Cambridge, 18: 425-429.

[181] Arrhenius, S. (1884). Recherches sur la conductivité galvanique des électrolytes. Doctoral dissertation, Stockholm: Royal Publishing House, P.A. Norstedt & Soner.

[182] Arrhenius, S. (1889a). Uber die Gleichgewichts verhaltnisse zwischen elektrolyten. [On the equilibrium relationships between electrolytes]. Zeitschr. F. physical Chem., Bd. V, S. 1-22.

[183] Arrhenius, S. (1889b). Über die Dissociationswärme und den Einfluss der Temperatur auf den Dissociationsgrad der Elektrolyte (About dissociation and the influences of temperature on the degree of dissociation of electrolytes). Wilhelm Engelmann.

[184] Nobel Prize in Chemistry 1903. Nobelprize.org. Retrieved 12-23-2010.

[185] Howell. W. (1884). The Origin of the Fibrin Formed in the Coagulation of Blood. Studies from the Biological Laboratory, Johns Hopkins University, 3:63-71.

[186] Howell, W. (1926). The Purification of Heparin and its Presence in Blood. American Journal of Physiology, Bethesda, Maryland, 71: 553-562.

[187] Howell, W. (1905). Textbook of Physiology for Medical Students and Physicians. Philadelphia: W. B. Saunders.

[188] National Institute of Health (1987). A century of American Physiology. Bethesda Maryland: National Library of Medicine.

[189] Minkoski, O. (1884). Ueber das Vorkommen von Oxybuttersäure im Harne bei Diabetes mellitus. Centralblatt für die medicinischen Wissenschaften, 22:242-243.

[190] Mering, J. and Minkowski, O. (1889). Diabetes mellitus nach Pankreasextirpation. Centralblatt für klinische Medicin, Leipzig, 10 (23): 393-394.

[191] Minkowski, O. (1887). Ueber einen Fall von Akromegalie. Berliner klinische Wochenschrift, 24:371-374.

[192] Waller, A. D. (1887). A demonstration on man of electromotive changes accompanying the hearts beat. Journal of Physiology, 8:229-234.

[193] Waller, A. D. (1888). Introductory address on the electromotive properties of the human heart beat. British Medical Journal, 2:751-754.

[194] Kent, A. (1893). Researches on the structure and function of the mammalian heart. The Journal of Physiology, London, 14:233-254.

[195] Wolff, L., Parkinson, J., and White, P. (1930). Bundle-branch block with short P-R interval in healthy young people prone to paroxysmal tachycardia. Am. Heart J., 5:685.

[196] His, W. (1893). Die Thätigkeit des embryonalen Herzens und deren Bedeutung für die Lehre von der Herzbewegung beim Erwachsenen. Arbeiten aus der medizinischen Klinik zu Leipzig, Jena, 14-50. English translation in F. A. Willis and T. E. Keys: Cardiac Classics, 1941: 695.

[197] Einthoven, W. (1892). Uber die Wirkung der bronchialmuskeln nach einer neuen methode untersucht, und uber asthma nervosum. [On the function of the bronchial muscles investigated by a new method and on nervous asthma].

[198] Eithoven, W. (1898). Eine einfache physiologische Erklarung fur verschiedene geometrisch-optische Tauschungen. [A simple physiological explanation for various geometric-optical illusions].

[199] Einthoven, W. (1902). Die Accomodation des menschlichen Auges. [The accommodation of the human eye].

[200] Einthoven, W. and Jolly W. (1908). The form and magnitude of the electric response of the eye to stimulation by light at various intensities. Experimental Physiology, 1(4):373-416. Retrieved 10-26-2019 from https://physoc.onlinelibrary.wiley.com/doi/pdf/10.1113/expphysiol.1908.sp000026

[201] Einthoven, W. (1895). Uber die form des menschlichen electrocardiogramus. Acrh. F. d. ges. physiol,. 60:101-123.

[202] Einthoven, W. (1906). Le telecardiogramme. Arch. Int. de Physiol., 4:132–64 (Translated into English, Am. Heart J., 1957; 53:602-15).

[203] Einthoven, W. (1924). Nobel Prize 1924. Nobelprize.org. retrieved 11/01/2010.

[204] Beck, A. and Cybulski, N. (1891). Weitere Untersuchungen über die Electrischen Erscheinungen des Hirnrinde der Affen und Hunde. (Futher studies on the phenonmena of electricity of the cerebral cortex of monkeys and dogs). Separat-Abdruck aus dem Anzeiger der Akademie der Wissenschaffen in Krakau.

[205] Nobelprize.org. Nomination Data Base for the Noel Prize in Physiology or Medicine 1901-1952.

[206] Nobelprize.org. The Nobel Prize in Physiology or Medicine. Retrieved December 7, 2010.

[207] Oliver, G. and Schafer, E (1894). The physiological action of the suprarenal capsules. J. Physiology (Lond), 16:1.

[208] Oliver, G. (1895a). On the therapeutic employment of the suprarenal glands. Brist. Med. J II, 451.

[209] Oliver, G. (1895b). Pulse-gauging, London: H. K. Lewis.

[210] Takamine, J. (1901). The isolation of the active principle of the suprarenal gland. J. Physiol Lond. 27:29-30.

[211] Cybulski, N. (1895). O funkeji nadnercza. [About the adrenal gland]. Gaz. Lek., 12:299-308.

[212] Abel, J. (1898). On epinephrine, the active constituent of the suprarenal capsule and its compounds. Proc Am Phys Soc, 3-4:3-5.

[213] United States Patent Office. (1900). United States Patent number US730176. Glandular extractive product. Inventor Jokichi Takamine of New York, N.Y. Retrieved June 2018 from https://patents.google.com/patent/US730176A/en

[214] Frank, O. (1895). Zur Dynamik des Herzmuskels, (On the dynamics of the heart muscle) Z Biol 32 (1895) 370.

[215] Starling, E. (1918). Linance Lecture on the law of the heart. Presented at Cambridge University 1915. London: Longmans, Green, and Co.

[216] Patterson, S. and Starling, E. (1914). On the mechanical factors which determine the output of the ventricles. J. Physiol. (Lond). 48:357–379.

[217] Howell, W. (1898). The influence of high arterial pressures upon the blood flow through the brain. Am. J. Physiology, 1: 57-70.

[218] Loewi, O. (1921). Uber humorale Ubertragbarkeit der Herznervenwirkung. I. Pflügers Archiv., 189:239-242.

[219] Dale, H, (1918). The action of certain esters and ethers of choline and their relation to muscarine. J. Pharmacol. Exp. Ther., 6:147-190.

[220] Dale, H., Feldberg, W., and Vogt, M. (1936). Release of acetylcholine at motor nerve endings. J. Physiology, May 4; 86(4):353-380.

[221] Dale, H. (1933). Nomenclature of fibers in the autonomic system and their effects. J. Physiology. 80:10-11.

[222] Nobel Prize Physiology or Medicine 1936. Nobelprize.org. Retrieved December 2010.

[223] Starling, E. and Patterson, S. (1914). On the Mechanical Factors Which Determine the Output of the Ventricles. Journal of Physiology, Cambridge, September 8, 48:357-379.

[224] Starling, E. (1918). The Linacre Lecture on the Law of the Heart. Delivered at St. John's College, Cambridge, London, Longmans, Green & Co.

[225] Starling, E. (1896). On the absorption of fluids from the connective tissue spaces. Journal of Physiology, Cambridge, 19: 312-326.

[226] Bayliss, W. and Starling, E. (1899). The movements and innervation of the small intestine. J. Physiology. Vol 24(2), 11 May.

[227] Starling, E. (1902). The Mechanism of Pancreatic Secretion. Journal of Physiology, Cambridge, September, 28: 325-353.

[228] Starling, E. (1905). The Croonian Lectures on the chemical correlation of the functions of the body. Lancet, 2: 339-341, 423-425, 501-503, 578-583.

[229] Starling, E. (1909). The Fluids of the Body. London: Constable.

[230] Starling, E. and Verney, E. (1924). The secretion of urine as studied on the isolated kidney. Proceedings of the Royal Society of London. Series B, 1924-1925, 97:321-363.

[231] Berger, H. (1901). Zur Lehre von der Blutzirkulation in der Schädelhöhle des Menschen namentlich unter dem Einfluss von Medikamenten; experimentelle Untersuchungen, von Hans Berger. Jena, G. Fischer.

[232] Berger, H. (1910). Untersuchungen uber die temperature des gehirns. Jena: Gustav Fischer.

[233] Berger, H. (1929). Ueber das Elektroenkephalogramm des Menschen. Archiv für Psychiatrie und Nervenkrankheiten, Berlin, 87:527-570.

[234] Caton, R. (1875). The electric currents of the brain. British Medical Journal, 2:278.

[235] Beck, A. (1890). Die Bestimmung der Localisation des Gehirn- und Rückenmarksfunctionen Vermittelst der Electrischen Erscheinungen. [The determination of the localization of the brain and spinal cord functions by means of electrical phenomena]. Cbl. Physiol. 4:18, 473-476.

[236] Beck, A. and Cybulski, N. (1891). Weitere Untersuchungen über die Electrischen Erscheinungen des Hirnrinde der Affen und Hunde. [Further studied on the phenomena of electricity of the cerebral cortex of monkeys and dogs].

[237] Neminski, W. (1913). Ein Vesuch der Registrierung der elektrischen Gehirnerscheinungen. Zentralblatt für Physiologie, 27:951-960.

[238] Berger, H. (1938). Das elektrenkephalogramm des menschen. Nova Acta Leopoldina. Halle, 6:173-309.

[239] Adrian, E. and Matthews, B. (1934). The Berger rythmns: Potential changes from the occipital lobes in man. Brain. 57:356-385.

[240] Manual for the Nomination Database for the Nobel Prize in Physiology or Medicine, 1901-1951 (2010). Nobelprize.org, Retrieved December 2010.

[241] Gerhard, U., Schonberg, A., and Blanz, B. (2005). [If Berger had survived the Second World War, he certainly would have been a candidate for the Nobel Prize. Hans Berger and the legend of the Nobel Prize. Fortschr Neurol Psychiatr., March, 73(3):156-60.

[242] Nominations Database - Physiology or Medicine, 1901-1951 (2010). Hans Berger. Nobelprize.org. Retrieved December 2010.

[243] Nobel Prize Facts. (2010). Retrieved from Nobelprize.org December 2010.

[244] Pavlov, I. (1903). The experimental psychology and psychopathology of animals. Proceedings of the 14th International Medical Congress, Madrid, Spain.

[245] Tolochinov, I. (1903). Contributions a l'etude de la physiologie et de la psychologies des glandes salivaires. Torhandlinger vid Nord. Naturforscara-och Loveremot, Helsingfors. Preceedings of the Congress of Nauralists and Physicians of the North. Helsinki (1902).

[246] Pavlov, I. and Anrep, G. (1927). Conditioned Reflexes: An investigation of the physiological activities of the cerebral cortex. London: Oxford University Press. Translated into English and edited by G. Anrep 2003. Mineola, New York: Dover Publications, Inc.

[247] Pavlov, I. (1902). The work of the digestive glands. London: Charles Griffin and Company.

[248] Pavlov, I. (1904). Nobel Prize for Physiology or Medicine 1904. Nobelprize.org.

[249] Riva-Rocci, S. (1896). Un sfigmomanometro nuovo. Gazetta Medica di Torino, 47:981-986.

[250] Korothov, N. (1905). To the question of methods of determining the blood pressure. Reports of the Imperial Military Academy St Petersburg, 11:365-367.

[251] Korothov, N. (1906). On methods of studying blood pressure: second presentation. Izv Imper Voen-Med Acad., 12:254-257.

[252] Keith, A. and Flack, M. (1907). The form and nature of the muscular connections between the primary divisions of the vertebrate heart. Journal of Anatomy and Physiology, London, 41:172-189.

[253] Tawara, S. (1906). Das Reizleitungssystem des Säugetierherzens. Eine anatomische Studie über das atrioventrikuläre Bündel und die Purkinjeschen Fäden. Mit einem Vorwort von L. Aschoff. [The conduction system of the mammalian heart, An anatomical study of the atrioventricular bundle and Purkinje fibers]. Jena: G. Fischer.

[254] Flack. M. (1910). An investigation of the sino-auricular node of the mammalian heart. J. Physiology, October 11; 41(1-2):64-77.

[255] Flack, M. (1918). Scientific tests for the selection of pilots for the Air Force. Nature Publishing Group. Nature Publishing Group Metadata Repository. Zurich, Switzerland.

[256] Flack, M. (1928). The physiological effects of flying. Nature Publishing Group. Nature Publishing Group Metadata Repository Zurich, Switzerland.

[257] Haldane J. and Priestley, J (1905). The regulation of lung ventilation. Journal of Physiology, 32:225-66.

[258] Douglas, C., Haldane, J., Henderson, Y., and Schneider, E. (1913). Physiological Observations made on Pike's Peak, Colorado with special reference to adaptation to low barometric pressure. Phil. Trans. Royal Society B., 203:185-318.

[259] Haldane, J. (1892). A new form of apparatus for measuring the respiratory exchange of animals. The Journal of Physiology Society. July 13(5):419-430.

[260] Haldane, J. (1900). Some improved methods of gas analysis. The Journal of Physiology.25: 295, 331-332.

[261] Haldane, J. (1922). Respiration. New Haven, CT: Yale University Press.

[262] Boycott, A., Damant, G., and Haldane, J. (1908). The prevention of compressed air illness. Journal of Hygeiene, 8:342-443.

[263] Brainbridge, F. (1900). Observations on the lymph flow from the submaxillary gland of the dog. Journal of Physiology, December 26(1-2):79-91.

[264] Bainbridge, F. and Menzies, J. (1914). Essentials of physiology. London, 1914.

[265] Bainbridge, F. (1915). The influence of venous filling upon the rate of the heart. Journal of Physiology, Cambridge, 50:65-84.

[266] Bainbridge, F. (1919). The physiology of muscular exercise. New York: Longmans, Green, and Company.

[267] Cannon, W. (1911). The Mechanical Factors of Digestion, New York: Longmans, Green, and Company.

[268] Cannon, W. (1915). Bodily Changes in Pain, Hunger, Fear and Rage: An Account of Recent Researches into the Function of Emotional Excitement. New York: Appleton and Company.

[269] Cannon, W. (1932). The wisdom of the body. New York: W.W. Norton and Company.

[270] The Nobel Prize in Physiology or Medicine 1922 Nobelprize.org 8 Nov 2010.

[271] Mering, J. and Minkowski, O. (1889). Diabetes mellitus nach Pankreasextirpation. Centralblatt für klinische Medicin, Leipzig, 10 (23):393-394.

[272] Mering, J. and Minkowski, O. (1890). Archiv für experimentelle Patholgie und Pharmakologie, Leipzig, 26: 37.

[273] The Nobel Prize in Physiology or Medicine 1923. (2018). Nobelprize.org. Nobel Media AB 2014. Web 14 Jun 2018. <http://www.nobelprize.org/nobel_prizes/medicine/laureates/1923/>

[274] Langerhans, P. (1869). Beitrag zur mikroskopischen Anatomie der Bauchspeicheldrüse.Dissertation. Berlin, Gustav Lange.

[275] Mering, J. and Minkowski, O. (1889). Diabeted mellitus nach pancreas extirpation. Arch. f Exper. Path. u Pharmakol., 26:371.

[276] Laguesse, E. (1894). Structure et developpement du pancreas d'apres les travaux recent. Paris: Balliere.

[277] Zuelzer G. (1908). Ueber Versuche einer specifischen Fermenttherapie de Diabetes. Zeitschrift fur experimentelle Pathologie und Therapie, 5:307 318.

[278] Scott, E. (1912). On the influence of intravenous injections of an extract of the pancreas on experimental pancreatic diabetes. Am J Physiol., 29:306-10.

[279] Murlin, J. and Kramer, B. (1913). The influence of pancreatic and duodenal extracts on the glycosuria and the respiratory metabolism of depancreatized dogs. J. Biol. Chem., 15:365-383.

[280] Kleiner, I. (1919). The action of intravenous injections of pancreas emulsions in experimental diabetes. J. Biol. Chem., 40:153-170.

[281] Paulescu, N. (1921). Action de l'extrait pancreatique injecte dans le sang, chez un animal diabetique. Comptes Rendus des Seances de la Societe de Biologie, 85:555-559.

[282] The Discovery of Insulin. Nobelprize.org. 6 Nov 2010.

[283] Bliss, M. (1982). The discovery of insulin, Chicago: University of Chicago Press.

[284] Paulescu, N. (1921). Action de l'extrait pancreatique injecte dans le sang, chez un animal diabetique. (In French). Comptes Rendus des Seances de la Societe de Biologie, 85:555-559.

[285] Monge, C. (1928). La enfermedad de los Andes (syndromes eritremicos). Facultad de Medicina. Lima.

[286] Monge, C. (1946). El problema de la coca en el Peru. An. Fac. Med. Univ. Nac. Mayor San Marcos Lima Peru 29:312-315.

[287] Quick, J., Stanley-Brown, M., Bancroft, F. (1935). A study of the coagulation defect in hemophilia and in jaundice. American Journal of the Medical Sciences, Thorofare, N.J., 190:501-511.

[288] Quick, J. (1935). The prothrombin in hemophilia and in obstructive jaundice. Journal of Biological Chemistry, Baltimore, 109:73-74.

[289] Quick, A. (1966). Salicylates and bleeding: the aspirin tolerance test. Am. J. Med. Sci. Sept, 252(3):265-9.

[290] Danielli, J. and Davson, H. (1935). A contribution to the theory of permeability of thin films. J. Cell. Comp. Phys., 5(4): 495.

[291] Overton, E. (1899). Uber die allgemeinen osmotischern eigenschaften der zelle ihre vermutliche ursachen und ihre bedeutung fur die physiologie. Vierteljahrschr. Naturforsch Ges, Zurich, 44:88-114.

[292] Gorter, E. and Grendel, F. (1925). On bimolecular layers of lipoids on the chromocytes of the blood. JEM, 41:493.

[293] Singer, S. and Nicolson, G. (1992). The Fluid Mosaic Model of the Structure of Cell Membranes. Science 175: 720-731.

[294] Hess, W. (1948). Die funktionelle organization des vegetativen nervensystems. Basel: Schwabe.

[295] Hess, W. (1956). Thalamus and Hypothalamus, Stuttgart: Thieme.

[296] Hess, W. (1931). Die Regulierung der Atmung. (The Regulation of Respiration). Leipzig: Thieme.

[297] Hess, W. (1954). Diencephalon. Autonomic and Extrapyramidal Functions. New York: Grune & Stratton.

[298] Hess, W. (1930). Die Regulierung des Blutkreislaufes. [The regulation of blood circulation]. Leipzig: Thieme.

[299] Nobel Prize in Physiology or Medicine 1949. Nobelprize.org.

[300] Hodgkin, A. and Huxley, A. (1952). A quantitative description of membrane current and its application to conduction and excitation in nerve. J. Physiol., 117:500-544.

[301] Nobel Prize in Physiology or Medicine 1963. Nobelprize.org. Retrieved December 25, 2010.

[302] Eccles, J. (1953). The Neurophysiological Basis of Mind: The Principles of Neurophysiology. Clarendon Press.

[303] Eccles, J. (1957). The Physiology of Nerve Cells. John Hopkins Press.

[304] Huxley, H. and Hanson, J. (1954). Changes in the cross-striations of muscle contractions and their structural interpretation. Nature, 173:973-977.

[305] Huxley, H. (1957). The double array of filaments in cross-striated muscle. J. Biophys. & Biochem. Cytol. 3:631.

[306] Skou, J. (1957). The influence of some cations on an adenosine triphosphatease from peripheral nerves. Biochimica et Biophysica Acta, 23:394-401.

[307] Post, R. and Jolly, D. (1957). The linkage of sodium, potassium, and ammonium ative transport across the human erythrocyte membrane. Biochimica et Biophysica. Acta, 25:118-28.

[308] Post, R., Merritt, C., Kinsolving, C., and Albright, C. (1960). Membrane Adenosine triphosphatase as a participant in the active transport of sodium and potassium in the human erythrocyte. Journal of Biological Chemistry, Vol. 235, No. 6, June.

[309] Skou, J. (1997). Nobel Prize Chemistry 1997. Nobelprize.org.

[310] Sutherland, E. and Wosilait, W. (1955). Inactivation and activation of liver phosphorylase. Nature. 175(4447):169-70 Jan 22.

[311] Rall, T., Sutherland, E., Berthet, J. (1957). The relationship of epinephrine and glucagon to liver phosphorylase. IV. Effect of epinephrine and glucagon on the reactivation of phosphorylase in liver homogenates. Journal of Biological Chemistry, 224(1):463-75 Jan.

[312] Nobel Prize in Physiology or Medicine 1971. Nobelprize.org.

[313] Guyton, A., Lindsey, A., and Kaufmann, B. (1955a). Effect of mean circulatory filling pressure and other peripheral circulatory factors on cardiac output. Am. J. Physiol., 180:463–468.

[314] Guyton, A. (1955b). Determination of cardiac output by equating venous return curves with cardiac output responses. Physiology Rev., 35:123–129.

[315] Hall, J. (2016). Guyton and Hall Textbook of Medical Physiology. Sanders.

[316] Singer, S. and G. Nicolson. (1972). The fluid mosaic model of the structure of cell membranes. Science, 175:720-731.

[317] Frye, L. and Edidin, M. (1970). The rapid intermixing of cell surgace antigens ager formation of mouse-human hererokaryons. Journal of Cell Science, 7:319-35.

[318] Singer, S. and Nicolson, G. (1972). The fluid mosaic model of the structure of cell membranes. Science, 175(4023):720-731.

[319] Davenport, H. (1974). The ABC of Acid-Base Chemistry. Chicago: The University of Chicago Press.

[320] Neher, E. and Sakmann, B., and Steinbach, J. (1978). The extracellular patch clamp: a method for resolving currents through individual open channels in biological membranes. Pflügers Archiv., 375 July (2):219–228.

[321] Neher, E. and Sakmann, B. (1992). The patch clamp technique. Scientific American. 266 March (3):44–51.

[322] Neher, E. (1988). The use of the patch clamp technique to study second messenger-mediated cellular events. Neuroscience, 26 (3):727–34.

[323] The Nobel Prize in Physiology or Medicine 1991. Nobelprize.org 10 Nov 2010.

[324] Brown, H., DiFrancesco, D., Nobel, S. (1979). How does adrenaline accelerate the heart? Nature. 280:235–236.

[325] DiFrancesco, D. and Ojeda, C. (1980). Properties of the current i_f in the sino-atrial node of the rabbit compared with those of the current iK, in Purkinje fibres. Journal of Physiology, 308:353-367.

[326] DiFrancesco, D. (1993). Pacemaker mechanisms in cardiac tissue. Annual Review of Physiology, 55:455–472.

[327] Barbuti, A. and DiFrancesco, D. (2008). Control of cardiac rate by "funny" channels in health and disease. Annals of the New York Academy of Sciences, 1123:213-23.

[328] DiFrancesco, D. (2010). The role of the funny current in pacemaker activity. Cir. Res., Feb 19; 106(3):434-46.

[329] Furchgott, R. (1987). Mechanisms of vasodilation. Ed. P.M. Vanhoutte. New York: Raven.

[330] Ignarro, L., Buga, G., Wood, K., Byrns, R., Chaudhuri, G. (1987). Endothelium-derived relaxing factor produced and released from artery and vein is nitric oxide. Proc Natl. Acad. Sci. USA, Dec 84:9265-9269.

[331] Palmer, R., Ferrige, A., Moncada, S. (1987). Nitric oxide release accounts for the biological activity of endothelium-derived relaxing factor. Nature, 327:524-526.

[332] The Nobel Prize in Physiology or Medicine 1998. Nobelprize.org.

[333] "Nomination Facts". Nobelprize.org. 11 Nov 2010.

[334] Kuhn, T. (1962). The Structure of Scientific Revolutions. Chicago: Chicago Unvierstiy Press.

[335] The Nobel Prize in Physiology or Medicine 2001. Nobelprize.org.

[336] The Nobel Prize in Physiology or Medicine 2002. Nobelprize.org.

[337] Kerr, J., Wyllie, A., Currie, A. (Aug 1972). Apoptosis: a basic biological phenomenon with wide ranging implications in issue kinetics. Br. J. Cancer., 26 (4):239–57.

[338] The Nobel Prize in Physiology or Medicine 2007. Nobelprize.org.

[339] The Nobel Prize in Physiology or Medicine 2009. Press Release 10-04-2010. Nobelprize.org.

[340] Steptoe, P. and Edwards, R. (1978). Birth after the reimplantation of a human embryo. Lancet, 2:366.

[341] The Nobel Prize in Physiology or Medicine 2010. Nobelprize.org.

[342] The Nobel Prize in Physiology or Medicine 2017. Nobelprize.org.

[343] The Nobel Prize in Physiology or Medicine 2019. Nobelprize.org.

Chapter 4

Medical Biochemistry

Definition.

Biochemistry is "…the chemistry of living organisms and of the chemical, molecular, and physical changes occurring therein…" (1997)[1]. Medical biochemistry "…is the formal study of biochemical exchanges that occur within the human body in the context of medicine, usually in terms of drug interactions or cellular responses to disease or stimulation…" (2014)[2].

Introduction.

Medical biochemistry reveals a relatively short, formal, and written recorded history, spanning less than 400 years.

This chapter traces the history of human biochemistry and its application to the practice of medicine. There is no attempt to cover all contributions in detail. Rather, this chapter provides an account of significant events, discoveries, influential people, and ideas which have shaped the field of medical biochemistry throughout time.

The chapter is organized chronologically for consistency with other chapters and provides you, the first and second year medical student, with an opportunity to begin to understand and appreciate significant contributions to the discipline; how the contributions are made; the factors influencing discovery; important individuals making significant contributions; and how the discipline has changed over time.

Topic areas, familiar to you as a medical student are examined from a historical perspective and placed along a developmental timeline to provide context and perspective. Specific topic areas discussed are amino acids; protein structure and function; enzymes; intermediate metabolism; carbohydrates; glycolysis; TCA cycle; gluconeogenesis; glycogen metabolism; sugar metabolism; lipid metabolism; amino acid synthesis and degradation; nitrogen metabolism; nucleotides; vitamins; and nutrition.

In addition, this chapter will identify and discuss factors influencing significant changes in medical biochemistry; biochemistry contributions resulting in significant change to long standing medical dogma; notable professional rivalries; and the many political, economic, religious, and social influences which have facilitated and hindered advancement of medical biochemistry, as a scientific discipline throughout time.

History.

Early Records, 3500 BC - 500 BC.

There is a limited written record, regarding the knowledge of biochemical processes as they relate to life and medicine known to the ancient civilizations. The Sumerians circa 3500 BC, ancient Egyptians circa 3200 BC, Babylonians circa 2000 BC, ancient Greeks circa 1100 BC, and ancient Romans 750 BC have however left many clues. Recently, thousands of ancient clay tablets, discovered primarily during the 1920s, are today in the process of being organized and translated. These tablets are quickly revealing a knowledge base of chemistry previously unknown and unimagined by modern man. The tablets reveal the ancient civilizations did indeed have a good working knowledge of many chemical relationships and applied their knowledge within a matrix of functional applications. The dogma of modern academia which often portrays the biochemical knowledge of the ancient civilizations as limited, unsophisticated, and couched completely in nonempirical mysticism is proving to be incorrect and requires modification (2005,1976,1964, 1951,1923)[3,4,5,6,7].

Records reveal the Ancients did apply an empirical-inductive approach to acquiring new knowledge, including knowledge of chemistry. Their knowledge base is derived almost exclusively from combined personal sensory experiences. Personal sensory experiences are combined to form a set of observations. The set of observations are then subjected to inductive reasoning, which moves the set of specific observations to generalized conclusions. This empirical-inductive epistemological approach to knowledge provides the foundation upon which the ancient civilizations build and organized their understanding of nature and chemistry.

The Ancients' knowledge of biochemistry and their manipulation of biochemical systems are derived from and focused upon maintaining good health and treating illness. Their knowledge base is built largely upon the experiential use of plants and plant extracts, ingestion or topical application of organic and inorganic compounds, and the use of temperatures, heat and cold. The oldest known ancient Mesopotamian medical text is a therapeutic manual written in Sumerian, which dates circa 2112 BC- 2004 BC. Mesopotamia therapeutic texts, circa 1894 BC- 1595 BC, begin to include descriptions of signs and symptoms, diagnosis, and instructions for administering medicines (2005,1976,1964,1951,1923)[3,4,5,6,7].

The Ancients are aware of the medicinal properties of mineral spring waters, oils, creams, herbal plasters, and alcohol. Their biochemical knowledge, as applied to medical treatments, is based on empirical observations e.g. if you do this, then this happens and if you do or don't do this, then this happens rather than an understanding of the underlying biochemistry properties responsible for the medicinal effects. The empirical-inductive epistemological approach of the Ancients stands in mark contrast to the rational-deductive process popularized by the subsequent Greek philosophers and mathematicians, during Antiquity (500 BC- 500 AD).

The rational-deductive approach of the Greeks, in contrast to the Ancients, minimize experience in favor of careful intellectual reasoning, maintaining if well-reasoned premises are true, then conclusions derived from the premises must be true. Deductive reasoning is applied to evaluate the truth of intellectually generated premises and provides a specific method for establishing new knowledge, by moving from the general to the specific. Recall, the Ancients established new knowledge by moving from the specific to the general.

While our knowledge today is limited in understanding the extent and specifics of biochemical knowledge of these Ancient civilizations, it is well established these civilizations maintained a good understanding of inorganic chemical systems. Historical written records reveal metals were extracted from ore as early as 9000 BC, mortars were used regularly in construction during 4000 BC, and assorted glasses were manufactured during 1500 BC. These are three of many examples offering insight into the sophistication of chemical knowledge known and applied by the Ancient civilizations.

There is a growing body of scientific evidence accumulating, confirming inorganic chemistry, with its immediate practical application to daily life is studied and findings recorded by the Ancient civilizations. The knowledge base is periodically modified and carefully passed on to subsequent generations. The most specific example can be found in the processing of ores at extremely high temperatures to produce glass and metal alloys. The Ancients lay the foundation, upon which much of the fundamental knowledge and principles of present day inorganic chemistry is based.

Trivia: Copper, one of the few uncompounded metals occurring in nature is discovered by the early Ancients circa 9000 BC. The metal is heavily mined on the island of Cyprus giving the metal one of its earliest names, Cyprium (the metal of Cyprus). Cyprium is later shortened to the Latin translation "Cuprum" and is the origin of the chemical symbol for copper "Cu".

In sum, the written record of Ancient civilizations, during the period of 3500 BC-500 BC, reveals a fundamental knowledge of chemistry and biochemistry, generated largely by way of empirical sensory experiences and inductive reasoning. The acquisition, modification, and transmission of their knowledge base is governed by survival, maintaining good physical health, and effectively treating injury and disease. Written records of accumulated biochemical knowledge are organized and collected into applied medical therapeutic manuals. The value of chemistry and biochemistry is appreciated and applied for medical purposes, although it is not yet completely understood by the Ancients.

Antiquity, 500 BC - 500 AD.

Antiquity witnesses a fundamental change in the general approach to acquiring new knowledge of the natural world, including chemistry. The empirical-inductive approach of the Ancients is replaced by the rational-deductive approach popularized by the Greek philosophers. This new approach results in continued and substantial advances in the knowledge of chemistry, not from careful observation and experimental analysis, but rather from examining nature as a whole and searching for patterns.

A lesson to be appreciated by modern investigators here; new knowledge can and is generated when methods change radically from a conventional, well established paradigm. Be open to conceptualizing and applying new investigative methods to study old and new ideas.

In the developmental history of chemistry, early Greek pre-Socratic natural philosophers, focus upon fundamental questions such as "...what is matter?...", "...what is the origin of matter?...", "...how is matter maintained?...", and "...how is matter changed?..." (1898)[8]. They reject mythology as acceptable explanations of the natural world and seek to explain the natural world within a matrix of rules and laws of nature (physics). Their process is that of reasoned discourse, formulating conclusions based upon assumptions and premises, which are then tested by simple logic and without need for empirical experiences. This epistemological approach stands in mark contrast to the sensory based, empirical-inductive process applied by the Ancients.

Thales of Miletus (624 BC-546 BC) from the ancient Greek city of Miletus, now a part of the western coast of Turkey, is one of the first pre-Socratic philosophers to address these fundamental questions of nature, within the matrix of a rational–deductive epistemology. Simply stated, Thales questions "…What is the origin of all matter?...". The answer then and today continues to be the same and has tremendous implications for understanding biochemistry. The answer is water. That's right, water. H_2O.

Today, we recognize approximately 60% of the adult human body is composed of water. Water is an essential component of most all biochemical systems within the human body. Adequate amounts and sophisticated regulation of intake and elimination are essential to all human body biochemical processes and good physical health.

Thales of Miletus gives biochemistry and science more than a reasoned solution to the fundamental question as to the essential composition of matter. He introduces an epistemological process, which has proven to be a corner stone in the foundation of scientific investigation and has sustained the test of time. Posing a question, providing a method to systematically evaluate the question, and if the method is followed by others, the resultant answer will be the same no matter how many times the question is posed and answered. Thales of Miletus lays the foundation for the present day scientific method.

Thales of Miletus' monistic view, everything is one and that water is the fundamental basis of all matter, quickly becomes accepted dogma of the time and is maintained well into the Middle Ages, 500 AD-1400 AD.

Anaximander (610 BC-546 BC) also from Miletus, a pre-Socratic natural philosopher, and student of Thales, offers similar monistic conceptualizations of the fundamental composition of all matter in nature. In contrast to his teacher Thales of Miletus, Anaximander postulates air to be the most basic substance from which all other substances originate and eventually return. He formulates his conceptualization upon the principles of rarefaction (reduction of a medium's density) and condensation.

In brief, Anaximander's position is as follows. When air condenses it becomes visible as mist; with additional condensation it becomes precipitation e.g. rain, sleet, or snow, which falls to earth and becomes earth. Water then evaporates from the earth into the air and with additional rarefaction produces fire. While others had previously advocated cyclic transitions of states of matter, Anaximander is responsible for first introducing the concept of changes in density associated with temperature of a single material. A concept which will prove to be fundamental to the development of modern-day biochemistry.

Empedocles of Agrigento (490 BC-430 BC) pre-Socratic natural philosopher from the Greek city of Agrigentum, located in Sicily (sic). Empedocles offers a modified and extended version of Thales' conceptualization of the fundamental composition of matter. He proposes four distinct elements Water, Air, Fire, and Earth, from which all known substances are composed in varying proportions and which are held together, mixed, and separated by opposing natural forces, Love and Strife. Love explains the attraction of different forms of matter, whereas Strife accounts for the separation. This four element theory with minor modifications becomes dogma for the next two thousand years.

Aristotle (384 BC-322 BC) Greek philosopher, student of Plato (428 BC-328 BC) and perhaps as a medical student, the only person you recognize so far, offers his own conceptualization of the nature of matter. Building upon the two dimensional model of Empedocles (4 elements x 2 energy forces) and integrating the concepts of temperature and density, as proposed by Anaximander, Aristotle offers his conceptual matrix of nature. Aristotle's conceptualization, while perhaps having received much greater recognition throughout the course of time than others, is essentially a restatement and superficial modification of the matrix presented by Empedocles 100 years earlier.

Although lesser known men contribute more substantially and with much more originality to the advancement of new knowledge, Aristotle integrates and synthesizes preexisting information and receives a lion's share of perhaps misplaced recognition. So goes another example of the unheralded works of many original contributors and recognition awarded to a single person.

Leucippus of Miletus (400 BC- unknown) and his pupil Democritus (460 BC- 370 BC) pre-Socratic Greek natural philosophers offer an alternative to the contemporary monistic views that everything is one, as proposed by Thales and Anaximander over 180 years earlier. Applying the rational-deductive approach to scientific investigation, the preferred approach in Miletus, Leucippus and Democritus offer an alternative conceptualization of matter, the Atomic hypothesis.

In brief, the Atomic hypothesis proposes all matter is composed of atoms and the empty space between atoms. Atoms within this model are the smallest unit of matter, too small to be seen, and from which no further unit reduction can be made. While not readily accepted by Leucippus's contemporaries, the Atomic hypothesis, formulated during Antiquity, will prove to be the foundation upon which modern sciences, over two thousand years later, will come to conceptualize and understand matter.

A lesson of wisdom here. Just because others around you think your ideas are too different, fail to conform to established dogma, and makes no sense to them, does not mean the ideas are bad ideas. Just be prepared to deal with a lot of pushback from those around you whom are invested in establish dogma.

Trivia: The term "atom" is derived from the Greek prefix "a" meaning "not" and the Greek word "tomos" meaning "to cut". The term is based upon the original idea, an atom is the smallest unit of matter and cannot be divided (cut) into smaller units.

During Antiquity, efforts are made by world leaders, initiated, organized, and led under the direction of self-proclaimed King of Egypt (King Ptolemy I) to collect, consolidate, and organize records of human knowledge. Much of the Western world's recorded knowledge is brought to one Greek city, the City of Alexandria, located on the western end of the Nile delta, in northern Egypt. By all accounts, the City of Alexandria is one of the world's most recognized cities of scholarship, knowledge, and new learning, during Antiquity. The corpus of all Western scientific knowledge is soon carried to Alexandria, compiled, translated, evaluated, interpreted, and reinterpreted within both historical and current period contexts. The fertile intellectual environment and innovative scholastic investigations of Alexandria help lay the foundation of modern chemistry and many other modern scientific disciplines.

The City of Alexandria and its associated Libraries flourish during Antiquity, as places of scholarship and new learning. Natural philosophers and other thoughtful people, from near and far, are invited to the City. They are instructed to bring with them innovative ideas, new thoughts, and written records of established knowledge from their places of origins. The City of Alexandria and Libraries quickly attract the brightest and most innovative. The City and Libraries are established as the principal repository for all Western knowledge circa 323 BC and thrive as places of intellectual curiosity, innovation, open mindedness, and scientific discovery. Individuals with courage to think differently and explore new possibilities are readily accepted and embraced by a dynamic and rapidly growing scientific community.

The City and Libraries thrive as centers of new learning and scholarship for approximately 275 years and until 47 BC. At this time, the City and Libraries are burned by invading military forces, led by Roman general Julius Caesar (110 BC- 44 BC). The City and Libraries soon rebuild and continue as centers of new learning for the next 340 years. Circa 292 AD, the City and Libraries are once again destroyed, by orders of the Roman Empire to eliminate all non-Christian temples and non-Christian contents within. Much of the Western world's collected and recorded knowledge is intentionally purged. So begins the influence of organized religion and government upon determining for all what knowledge is acceptable, what knowledge needs to be retained, what knowledge needs to be purged, and in which direction new discovery need to be guided.

Trivia: The word "library" is derived from the Greek "bibilotheca" meaning a collection of books. The word "museum" is derived from the Greek "mouseoin" meaning a place of study.

The City and Libraries of Alexandria offer a stimulating intellectual center, during Antiquity for more than 600 years. Within the City and Libraries the Greeks examine the record of chemical knowledge accumulated by the ancient civilizations, especially ancient Egypt. Applying the "newer" rational-deductive approach preferred by the Greeks to the empirical-inductive derived knowledge base of the ancient civilizations, the Greeks reinterpret knowledge within this "newer" epistemological paradigm. The process results in a simple logical deduction and greatly influences the development of chemistry for the next two thousand years. If the difference between substances is simply a matter of balance between elements, then one should be able to change the balance among the elements and change the substance. Applying this logic, copper might become gold. So begins the practice of alchemy in the City of Alexandria, circa 330 BC.

Alchemy, the art of transmuting metals has its early beginnings not in the City of Alexandria but rather in ancient Egypt, circa 5000 BC. Alchemy is considered a serious science in Europe until the 1700s. The best-known goals of the alchemists are transmutation of common base metals into precious metals such as gold or silver. The lesser known goal of alchemy, plant alchemy, focuses upon the creation of a panacea which can cure all disease and provide eternal life.

The first known written records of Western alchemy can be traced to the Stockholm papyrus (circa 300 AD, 1926)[9], Leyden papyrus X (circa 250 AD,1926)[10], and the Greek Magical papyri (circa 300 AD,1928)[11]. All three original papyri are in existence today. Thousands of other papyri housed in the Alexandrian Libraries are destroyed by fire when the Libraries are burned circa 47 BC by the Romans. Subsequently, Roman Emperor Diocletius (244 AD-311 AD) ordered all alchemy books, including ones in the Alexandrian Libraries to be burned in 292 AD, as part of his efforts to maintain political, social, economic, and religious stability in the region. Many of the ancient clay tablets survived the fire and now serve as a useful historical record of chemical knowledge of not only the ancient civilizations but Greek Antiquity as well.

In summary, Antiquity introduces a fundamental change in the approach to acquiring new knowledge, replacing the careful observations of the experiential-inductive approach of the Ancients with the intellectual, rational-deductive approach of the Greek philosophers. Secondly, the conceptualization and understanding of physical nature moves from the atheoretical collections of observations of the Ancients to the organized, philosophical matrix of the Greek philosophers. Thales introduces a monistic view of nature and identifies water as the substance from which all matter originates, including biological matter. Empedocles expands Thales monistic view into a two dimensional theoretical matrix, which includes four elements on one dimension, Water, Air, Fire, and Earth and forces which combine and separate the elements along the second dimension, Love the forces of attraction of elements and Strife the forces of separation of elements. Leucippus and Democritus introduce the conceptualization that matter is composed of atoms and empty space between atoms. The City and Libraries of Alexandria are established as a center of scholarly activity and repository of world knowledge. The City and Libraries of Alexandria, centers of original thought, creativity, and new scientific discovery are twice destroyed and much of the recorded knowledge is purged by organized religion and state government. So goes another example of the influence of Church and State in modifying scientific knowledge.

Middle Ages (Medieval Times), 500 AD - 1400 AD.

Chemistry during the Middle Ages witness few advancements in Europe. Most scholastic thought and investigative efforts are heavily influenced by organized religion, especially the Catholic Church. Original scholarship and scientific thought, characteristic of the ancient civilizations and Antiquity is replaced by translation and transcription of the existing known knowledge of ancient civilizations and Antiquity. This knowledge is translated from the original records into the approved official language of the Church, Latin. The translations reflect the great influence the Church has during the period, often resulting in not only a translation of the original material, rather a translation modified by religious dogma. Scientific knowledge of the ancient civilizations and Antiquity is modified to conform to faith based beliefs of organized religion, especially the Catholic Church. So goes another example in the history of medicine, when an institution which controls funding determines areas of science to investigate, what will be acceptable findings, and how findings need to be interpreted to ensure continued financial funding support.

Advances in chemistry, during the Middle Ages, especially 700 AD-1100 AD, come not from Western Europe, rather from the Middle East, most notably Persia (present day Iran).

Abu Musa Jābir ibn Hayyān al Azdi (721 AD-815 AD) (aka "Jibir"or "Geber") an Arabic/ Persian chemist emphasizes the use of systematic experimentation as the preferred method for understanding and acquiring new knowledge of chemical substances and their combinations. He is credited with founding many of the chemical processes still used today in the chemistry labs across the world, including distillation and crystallization. He conducts much of the foundational work on acids and bases. He introduces the term alkali from the Arabic "al-qaly". Today, in its adjective form, alkaline is still used to denote compounds with pH greater than 7.0 e.g. bases. Many of his works are translated into Latin during the Middle Ages and become the standard texts in Europe for alchemy.

Alchemy flourishes in Western Europe as the interests in transmuting base metals into gold and silver is encouraged by formal religious organizations. Organized religion requires more and more financial resources to support their efforts to spread religious beliefs throughout Europe. For example, the financial costs of the series of military campaigns waged by England against the

Muslims in the Middle East, circa 1076 AD-1276 AD, "The Crusades", generate staggering expenses for the Church. Alchemy offers a hopeful solution as a potential income source for the Church.

In order to ensure teaching of the Church's philosophical views, the Church founds and provides financial support to many schools, academies, and universities throughout Europe. Most of the Universities, including Bologna, Paris, Salamanca, Oxford, and Coimbria are founded in the 1200s of the Middle Ages and receive funding from organized religion. Organized religion, as the principle source of funding, continues to greatly influence the areas of investigation, methods used to acquire new information, and encourages modification of new and old information to be consistent with the faith based beliefs of the Church.

Saint Albertus Magnus (1193 AD-1280 AD) German, Dominican scholar, philosopher, and frequent arbitrator between organized religion and science, advocates the peaceful coexistence of science and religion. Albertus Magnus scholarly efforts are largely committed to the translation of Aristotle's model of nature, into a matrix more palatable to the Church (1210)[12]. He devotes considerable energies organizing theory and the knowledge of minerals. Albertus Magnus contributes substantially to advancing the Western world's understanding of inorganic chemistry. Albertus Magnus coins the term "affinity" to qualify the forces of chemical actions, which result in the combination of substances (1250 AD/1967)[13]. Affinity, the force that causes a chemical reaction, is replaced approximately 700 years later with the familiar modern term "free energy" (1923)[14]. Recall, free energy (G) predicts the direction in which a reaction will spontaneously proceed (2005)[15].

Plant alchemy, the lesser heralded branch of alchemy, focuses not upon transmutation of base metals into gold and silver, but rather finding a combination of substances which will produce a cure for all disease, contributes significantly and directly to medicine, during the 1300s-1400s. With repeated outbreaks of the plague and unsatisfactory explanations from organized religion as to the cause and cure e.g. punishment from God as the cause and prayer to God as the treatment, the general public is open to alternatives, including plant alchemy. So begins a renewed interest in the properties of medicinal biochemistry.

In brief sum, the Middle Ages produce little new knowledge in the area of chemistry. Most all new knowledge originates in the Middle East, including the fundamental understanding of acids and bases. Western Europe scholarship is influenced tremendously by organized religions, especially the Church. The influence results in the translation of the knowledge of the ancient civilizations and Greek antiquity from their original language into the language of the Church, Latin. The translations include conscious reinterpretations of the world's cumulative knowledge of the natural world to be more consistent with the dogma of the Church. The Church founds many universities and provides much funding to universities and investigators offering support of Church doctrine. Alchemy flourishes and is encouraged by the Church, viewing transmutation of base metals into precious metals as a reasonable and potentially financially useful mechanism to support the tremendous financial debt incurred by the Church, during the Crusades and religious expansionism throughout Europe and the Middle East. Saint Albertus Magnus coins the term "affinity" to qualify the forces of chemical actions which result in the combination of substances. Plant alchemy witnesses resurgence in interests when the Church provides unsatisfactory explanations for the source and treatment of the plague. The plague is estimated to have killed 30-60% of the entire population of Europe and in effect reducing the world population from an estimated 450 million to approximately 350 million in 1400 AD. Plant alchemy and its search for finding the combination of substances which would produce a cure for disease is reawakened during the Middle Ages. The end of the Middle Ages witness biochemistry taking a deep breath of fresh air, as it prepares for the many advances to be made during the Early Modern period.

Early Modern, 1400 AD - 1800 AD.

Early Modern Period provides much of the foundations of modern biochemistry. The period witnesses a gradual movement in chemistry away from alchemy and towards a more analytical analysis of the chemical structure of matter, both inorganic and organic. Processes such as photosynthesis are beginning to be understood by the mid-1600s. The well accepted Earth, Air, Fire, and Water conceptual matrix, used to understand the fundamental composition of the nature for more than two thousand years is challenged. Investigators begin reexamining scientific dogma and offer new ideas, methods, and conceptualizations, based upon experimental methods. By the mid-1700s investigators have well established the foundation for the scientific study of the chemistry of biological systems. The late-1700s witness the discovery of oxygen, nitrogen, hydrogen, and carbon dioxide.

Let us take a brief look at some of the most influential people and their unique contributions, whom substantially guide the course and advancement of biochemistry as a scientific discipline, during the Early Modern Period (1400 AD-1800 AD).

Theophrastus Phillippus Aureolus Bombastus von Hohenheim (aka Paracelsus) (1492-1541) Swiss physician and alchemist is born, one year after Christopher Columbus's first voyage to the New World. Paracelsus is a contemporary of perhaps more familiar notables, mathematician and astronomer Nicholas Copernicus (1473-1543), polymath Leonardo da Vinci (1452-1519), explorer Ferdinand Magellan (1480-1521), Protestant Reformation leader Martin Luther (1483-1546), and artist and sculptor Michelangelo (1475-1564). Collectively these men and others shatter medieval thought and ignite the Renaissance.

The Renaissance, largely a cultural movement defines the rebirth of scholarly learning based upon the classical sources and a period of intellectual revitalization. Paracelsus' contributions to medicine are many with over two hundred publications. As his work relates to biochemistry, he is one of the first to emphatically advocate the position; life is essentially a chemical process (1633)[16].

Paracelsus views illness and disease to result from an imbalance of chemicals and minerals in the body. While embracing the general conceptual framework of the balance theories of health and illness set forth during Antiquity by the Greeks and Romans e.g. the Four Humors theories posited circa 400 BC, Paracelsus emphasizes chemicals and minerals rather than fluid humors. He advocates the use and manipulation of chemicals and minerals to restore good health by correcting the body's imbalances believed to be responsible for the illness or disease. A practice still followed in most Western medical hospitals and clinics today.

For those of you in allopathic medical school training programs, does this approach to understanding, diagnosing, and treating disease sound familiar? It should. It is the fundamental principle upon which allopathic medicine is based.

Francious Bacon (1561-1626) English philosopher, scientist, statesman, author, and advocate of scientific revolution and the scientific method, popularizes deductive methodologies and offers words of caution to those who teach, investigate, and heal the human body. He offers his words of caution in his major work "Novum Organum" (1620)[17]. His contributions to biochemistry are less in specific knowledge to the field and rather in advocating an approach to acquiring new knowledge, through the use of the scientific method and his thoughtful words of caution, whenever one accepts knowledge as dogma.

> "…They who presume to dogmatize on Nature, as on some well-investigated subject, either from self-conceit or arrogance, and in the professional style, have inflicted the greatest injury on philosophy and learning. For they have tended to stifle and interrupt inquiry exactly in proportion, as they have prevailed in bringing others to their opinion and their own activity has not counterbalanced the mischief they have occasioned by corrupting and destroying that of others...". (Novum Organum, (1620), page 343)[17].

Jan Baptist van Helmont (1579-1644) Belgian chemist and founder of pneumatic chemistry, a branch of scientific investigation during the 1600s, 1700s, and early-1800s, which focuses upon the experimental investigation of the physical properties of gases and how they relate to chemical reactions. Helmont coins the term "gas", from the Dutch "gheest" (breath, vapor, spirit), and introduces "gas" as one of the three classical states of matter to the scientific community. He discovers carbon dioxide and terms it "gas sylvestre" or "wild spirit", noting this new substance "…could not be contained by vessels nor reduced into a visible body…" (1821)[18].

Van Helmont writes extensively on the physiology and the chemistry of digestion. He offers six stages of digestion and which are facilitated by chemical reactions, which today we describe as specific enzymatic reactions (1648)[19]. Van Helmont provides the early scientific based experiments into photosynthesis and provides innovative, although later proven incorrect, explanations for the growth of plants and trees, when nourished only by soil, sun, and water.

A brief and frequently repeated account of one of Jan Baptist van Helmont's famous experiments provides an useful demonstration of the approach to knowledge utilized by van Helmont and others of the period. In questioning the dogma of the time in regard to nature, which was then couched heavily in mysticism and religion, he applies an experimental research design and qualitative measures in an investigation of the chemical nutritional value of water. In brief, he plants a young willow plant (weight 5 lbs.) in a container filled with soil (weight 200 lbs.) and waters the plant for five years. No additional nutrients are added to the soil. After five years, the willow plant weights 169 lbs. 3 ounces. He concludes the increase in mass and weight of the tree is the result of the water and not the soil nutrients, given there is no significant change in the weight of the soil after five years and no substance other than water had been added to the soil (1662)[20]. So goes another experiment well executed and findings incorrectly interpreted by the investigator, resulting in incorrect conclusions. So is the nature and progress of science.

Many of van Helmont's scientific publications challenge academic and Church dogma. As the result, van Helmont is condemned for heresy by the General Inquisition of Spain (a special committee established to punish those whom contradict the Catholic Church), placed under house arrest, and denounced by his University's medical school faculties (University of Louvain). Given his experience with the Spanish Inquisition he refrains from further publishing during his lifetime and passed his academic papers on to his son for publication after his death (1648,1662)[19,20]. So goes another example of political and religious factors affecting the course of scientific discovery.

Robert Boyle (1627-1691) Irish-English chemist is perhaps most recognized by medical students for his Law describing the inverse relationship between pressure and the volume of gases. In fact, "Boyle's Law" had been previously described by English mathematician Richard Towneley (1629-1707). After viewing an early draft of Richard Towneley and Henry Power's (1623-1668) book series, "Experimental Philosophy" (1664)[21], in which they describe the relationship between pressure and volume of gases, Boyle, without authorization from either Towneley or Power, includes the formulation in his own book "The Sceptical Chymist: or cheymico-physical doubts and paradoxes; touching the spagyrist's principles commonly called hypostatical, as they are wont to be proposed and defended by the generality of alchymists" (1661)[22]. Now that's a book title!

Boyle's "Sceptical Chymist" reaches press before Richard Towneley and Henry Power's "Experimental Philosophy". Robert Boyle, with nothing more than a few passing words, does refer to "…Mr. Towneley's hypothesis…", in describing the relationship between pressure and volume of gases, yet the relationship is soon remembered then and today simply as "Boyle's Law". So goes another lesson to be learned in timely publication of one's work. It also serves as another example in the history of science of some individuals very willing to accept credit for the innovative and original works of others.

Robert Boyle's most notable contribution, "The Sceptical Chymist", advocates the use of the experimental method in all investigations of chemistry and reflects the increasing value placed upon use of experimental methods (1620,1680)[22,23]. In 1670 Boyle applies principles and methods of chemistry to physiology and provides one of the first descriptions of bubbles forming in biological tissues when ambient pressures are lowered, offering one of the first physiological reports which will later explain decompression sickness (1670,1676)[24,25].

Boyle applies his acquired knowledge of biochemistry, publishing a popular collection of medicinal remedies, which according to the collection can be easily prepared in the home, for "…families and fitted for the service of country people…" (1693)[26]. Translational medicine is alive and well in England, during the late-1600s.

Carl Scheele (1742-1786) German-Swedish chemist is credited among several contemporaries, Antoine Lavoisier, Joseph Priestly, and Henry Cavendish, as the person who discovers oxygen. Scheele writes an account of this discovery in his manuscript titled "Treatise on Air and Fire", which he sends to his publisher in 1775. However, that document is not published until 1777 (1777a,1777b)[27,28]. Consequently, Joseph Priestly rather than Carl Scheele is most often arguably credited with the discovery of oxygen, based upon being first to publish his observations and before Scheele. Another lesson learned in the importance of timely professional publication of ones findings.

Joseph Priestly (1733-1804) English theologian, teacher, occasional chemistry experimenter announces his discovery of the gas oxygen to the Royal Society in 1775. His paper titled "An account of further discoveries in air" is immediately published in the Society's journal "Philosophical Transactions" (1775)[29]. This landmark paper is republished with revisions in the second volume of Priestley's six volume comprehensive work, "Experiments and Observations on Different Kinds of Air" (1774,1775,1790)[30,31,32].

The controversy between Joseph Priestly and Carl Scheele in securing professional credit for the discovery of oxygen is typical of professional science and medicine. Similar controversies continue today. One need not look far to find similar controversies throughout the entire course of the history of science or medicine.

Trivia: The journal "Philosophical Transactions" is the oldest printed scientific journal in the English speaking world. It has remained in continuous publication since March 6, 1665.

Joseph Priestly deserves additional historical recognition in that he is responsible for the discovery of carbonated water. That's right; he discovers soda water and publishes his discovery in a 1772 pamphlet prepared for the British Navy, John Earl of Sandwich, First Lord Commissioner of the Admiralty, proposing its potential medicinal use "...in long voyages, by preventing or curing the sea-scurvy..." (1772)[33]. Although water "...impregnated with fixed air..." fails to prove useful in the prevention or cure of scurvy, the publication articulates a position shared by several scientists of the period and much less so today; in that "...if this discovery (though it doth not deserve that name) be of any use to my countrymen, and to mankind at large, I shall have my reward... (and)... expressing my wishes, that all persons, who discover anything that promises to be generally useful, would adopt the same method..." (1772)[33]. Something to think about, when in class and your lecturing medical school professor strays off topic and onto a long tangent.

Antoine Lavoisier (1743-1794) noted French chemist claimed to have independently discovered and named oxygen (1776,1778)[34,35]. However, historical records suggest Antoine Lavoisier's claim of independent discovery may not have been as independent as he claimed. Records reveal Joseph Priestley visited Antoine Lavoisier in October of 1774 and told him about his "gas" experiments. Joseph Priestly later that year and while on tour with Lord Shelburne, demonstrated his oxygen experiments in Paris to Antoine Lavoisier and others. Records further reveal Carl Scheele (remember Carl Scheele?) posted a letter to Antoine Lavoisier on September 30, 1774, in which he describes to Antoine Lavoisier his work and his discovery of oxygen. Antoine Lavoisier never publicly acknowledged receiving Carl Scheele's letter. A copy of the letter was found in Scheele's belongings, after his death in 1786.

Historical records reveal Antoine Lavoisier frequently assigns himself credit for discoveries and works completed by others and without acknowledging their contributions. In addition to the controversy regarding the discovery of oxygen discussed above, Lavoisier claims to have discovered hydrogen (1783)[36]. However, British scientist Henry Cavendish (1731-1810) reports his discovery of hydrogen, in 1766, which he terms "inflammable air", in his paper "On factitious air" (1766)[37], seventeen years before Antoine Lavoisier's claim appears in the scientific literature. Antoine Lavoisier appears to have simply replicated Cavendish's experiments and to have coined the term "hydrogen" and without acknowledging Cavendish's contributions.

Another example is found in Lavoisier's claim for the discovery and demonstration of the Law of Conservation of Mass (1789)[38]. The Law of Conservation of Mass had been published prior to Lavoisier's claim by Russian chemist Mikhail Lomonosov (1711-1765) in his paper titled "Meditations on the solidity and liquidity of bodies", thirty years before Lavoisier's claim (1760,1760)[39,40]. So goes more examples in history of some investigators seizing professional credit for the work of others.

Lavoisier is not without original contributions. Lavoisier's experiments demonstrate how oxygen can rust metals and proposes a model in which oxygen serves an essential and necessary component in cellular respiration in plants and animals. Lavoisier conceptualizes cellular respiration to be a slow combustion of organic material, dependent upon inhaled oxygen. He additionally offers one of the first modern chemistry textbooks, which includes a new system of chemical nomenclature still used today and provides a unified view of new theories in chemistry during the late-1700s (1789)[38].

In summary, biochemistry of the Early Modern period (1400-1800) provides the foundation of modern biochemistry. Mystical and religious explanations of the composition of matter begin to be replaced by systematic, experimental, analytical, chemical deconstruction of matter. Dogma regarding the very nature of matter and which has been in place for over two thousand years is challenged by new discoveries. Paracelsus emphatically proposes life to be essentially a chemical process, viewing illness and disease as the result of imbalance in body chemicals and minerals. Bacon cautions the academic and medical communities of the dangers associated with dogma. Van Helmont founds pneumatic chemistry and opens the doors for the discovery and study of gases. He discovers carbon dioxide, advances the understanding of the biochemical processes of photosynthesis, and offers his willow experiment, ousted by a medical school faculty, condemned for heresy by the Church, and imprisoned for innovative thought and scientific investigations which challenged scientific and religious dogma of the period. Towneley and Boyle gives us Boyle's Law. Scheele gives us oxygen and a lesson in timely publication. Priestly gives us his carbonated water and a consciousness for sharing knowledge for the betterment of all mankind. Lavoisier gives us his oxygen for cellular respiration and a lesson on the temptation to represent the work of others as your own. By the end of the Early Modern period, biochemistry is well positioned for rapid and substantial advances to be made during the Middle Modern period.

Middle Modern, 1800 AD - 1900 AD.

The Middle Modern Period witness biochemistry establishing itself as a separate discipline. Biochemistry enjoys rapid and substantial advancements in knowledge as it quickly develops as a professional discipline.

The term "biochemistry" is coined and introduced into the professional literatures. Professional journals are founded and devoted to the advancement and understanding of biochemistry. Early in the 1800s biochemistry is dominated by investigations into physiological chemistry, especially digestion and the digestive juices. Amino acids are first identified, enzymes isolated and begin to be understood, organic substances are produced from inorganic substances and the dogma of vitalism is challenged. A system for standardized notation of chemical formula is introduced. During the mid-1800s, focus slowly shifts from understanding digestion to the chemical study of proteins and sugars. Glycogen is identified as an energy store for animals, isomeric structure of proteins is identified, reversible oxygen binding of the globular protein hemoglobin begins to be understood, the understanding of the chemistry and structure of glucose is clarified, fermentation is accomplished without "vital forces", peptide bonds are discovered, and purines are identified and linked to the storage of genetic information.

Let us take a brief look at some of the most influential people, their unique contributions, and whom substantially guide the course and advancement of biochemistry, as a scientific discipline during the Middle Modern period (1800 AD-1900 AD).

Louis Nicolas Vauquelin (1763-1829) French chemist and his student assistant Pierre Jean Robiquet (1780-1840) isolate and describe the first amino acid (asparagine) in 1806. The amino acid is isolated from asparagus shoots (1805,1806)[41,42]. Cystine, the second amino acid discovered is described four years later by English chemist William Wollaston (1766-1828) in 1810 and isolated from urinary calculus (kidney stones) (1810)[43]. Other amino acids are slowly identified for example glycine (1820)[44] from gelatin by French chemist Henri Braconnot (1780-1855) and glutamate (1866)[45] is isolated from gluten, a wheat protein by German agricultural chemist Heinrich Ritthausen (1826-1912). The fundamental building blocks of all proteins are slowly being identified, isolated, and understood. Of the 500 plus amino acids known today, only 20 kinds are constituents of body proteins. Of these 20, only 9 are essential amino acids and must be taken into the body through diet.

Trivia: Pierre Jean Robiquet goes on to discover, isolate, and describes the chemistry of codeine (1832)[46]. Codeine with its analgesic, anti-tussive, and anti-diarrhea properties remains one of the most used drugs in the world today.

William Prout (1785-1850) English biochemist and vitalist studies numerous biological secretions, which he believes to be the result of the physical breakdown of biological tissues. He discovers stomach juices contain hydrochloric acid and provides the chemical analyses in 1827 which leads to the classification of food substances, which we are all familiar today, saccharides (carbohydrates), oleaginous (fats), and albunious (proteins) (1827)[47].

Friedrich Wohler (1800-1882) German biochemist and pioneer of organic chemistry demonstrates organic compounds can be produced from inorganic materials. His revolutionary work challenges scientific dogma which had remained securely in place for centuries. His work shakes the very foundation upon which the doctrine of vitalism is built.

Recall, the theory of vitalism is first proposed during the early-1600s and provides an explanation for the differences between organic and inorganic compounds. Simply stated, organic materials contain the "vital force" of life and inorganic materials do not. Many of the most respected scientists of the period held tenaciously to the vitalism doctrine. For example, Louis Pasteur (1822-1895) held tightly to the vitalist doctrine and frequently offered scientific evidence in its support (1858,1863)[48,49].

Friedrich Wohler is first to recognize cyanic acid possesses the identical elemental composition as fulminic acid, although their properties are very different. Welcome the discovery of isomers. The concept two or more compounds with the same chemical formula, can exist in more than one functional or chemical form, based upon the arrangements of the atoms within the molecule, is novel at this time (1824)[50]. Four years later he discovers urea has the same atomic composition as ammonium cyanate (1828)[51]. Friedrich Wohler publishes his 1828 landmark, four page paper "On artificial formation of urea" and describes the synthesis of an organic compound urea from inorganic materials (1828)[51]. Prior to this, urea is dogmatically held to be the sole product of "vital forces" and only produced within the bodies of living animals.

Although Wohler's findings send shock waves through the scientific community, challenging the core foundation of the vitalist doctrine, challenging long standing scientific dogma, and challenging the conclusions of respected scientists, Wohler appears to be more interested in the chemical consequences of isomerism rather than the philosophical implications of his contributions. So begins science's understanding of isomeric chemical structure and the need to reevaluate the well-established dogma of the time, chemical compounds can only be different if they have different elemental compositions. Scientific truths change as new information is discovered. In recognition of his exceptional contribution to biochemistry, Friedrich Wohler is quickly promoted to full professor.

Jons Jakob Berzelius (1779-1848) Swedish biochemist, perhaps most remembered in chemistry for his recognition of the Law of Proportions, is also responsible for another milestone in the history of biochemistry. He introduces the modern chemical notation system used for chemical formula (1811)[52]. His notation system uses simple letters to represent elements e.g. O for oxygen, H for hydrogen and he adds a superscript denoting proportions of each element e.g. H^2O (1814)[53]. Today, we have modified the notation and use subscripts rather than the superscript to denote proportions, H_2O.

Early in his professional career Jons Berzelius writes a chemistry textbook specifically for medical students, "Larobok i Kemien" [Textbook of Chemistry] (1818,1819)[54,55]. Jons Berzelius coins many of the terms, familiar to every medical student today, "protein", "polymer", "isomer", "allotrope" and "catalyst". The term "protein" is derived from the Greek meaning "of primary importance"; the term "isomer" is from the Greek word meaning "equal parts"; the term "catalyst" also from the Greek, meaning "to speed up" (1836)[56].

Jons Berzelius rejects the doctrine of vitalism in favor of a biochemical explanation of life. Rejecting scientific dogma and challenging established scientists early in one's career is always a risky career decision and one which holds great reward if you are right and great consequences if you are wrong. In the case of Berzelius, things worked out well for him. Of lesser note, while in medical school and for his medical school thesis Jons Berzelius systematically studies the effects of electrical shock on patients with different diseases. He terms the treatment "Galvano therapy" and reports no obvious effects on patient's conditions, as the result of applying electrical shocks (1802)[57]. The basis of his thesis is couched in the idea of electrochemical dualism. That is, compounds can be decomposed by application of an electric current, with acidic components being attracted to one electrically charge pole and basic components being attracted to the opposite electrically charged pole. The theory is popular during the early-1800s and replaced around 1830 by radical theory.

Thomas Schwann (1810-1882), yes, the same German physiologist who discovers the myelin producing Schwann cell, makes additional significant contributions in the area of digestion physiology. More specifically, Schwann studies the biochemistry of digestion and coins familiar terms, such as the enzyme "pepsin" from the Greek meaning "digestion" (1836a,1836b)[58,59]. Recall, pepsin is secreted by the serous cells of the stomach as an inactive zymogen (proenzyme) pepsinogen and is activated by HCl in the stomach, which results in the release of peptides and amino acids from dietary proteins. Schwann joins the growing ranks of scientists of the early-1800s who begin to offer a biochemical matrix, from which to study and understand life, as an alternative to the dogma of vitalism.

Anselme Payen (1795-1871) French chemist, a student of Louis Vauquelin and Michel Chevreul, is most remembered for his co-discovery of the enzyme distase, with Swiss chemist and colleague Francious Persoz (1805-1868) (1833)[60]. Distase, today is termed amylase. Payen and Persoz identify distase while working on processes to accelerate the conversion of grain starches into sugar. They further observe the enzyme can be deactivated by heat. A property recognized today of any enzyme. Distase is derived from Greek meaning "to separate". The suffix "ase" has it origin in the term distase and is the standard suffix used today whenever naming an enzyme.

Gerardus Johannes Mulder (1802-1880) Dutch organic chemist describes the chemical composition of proteins and first to use the term, coined by Jons Berzelius "protein", in a professional publication. The term appears in the 1839 paper "On the composition of some animal substances" (1839)[61]. Gerardus Mulder maintains an interest in the chemistry of wine and beer, as do many of the early biochemists. His interests results in two books on the subjects, titled "The Chemistry of Wine" (1856,1857)[62,63]. The English translation of Mulder's book detailing the chemistry of wine is edited by Bence Jones (1857)[64]. Yes, the same Henry Bence Jones (1813-1873) of Bence Jones protein fame who identifies the light chain of immunoglobulin molecules in 1848 and which is frequently evident in patients today, suspected to suffer cancer formed by malignant plasma cells, multiple myeloma (1848)[65].

Friederich Wilhelm Kuhne (1837-1900) German physiologist adds to the chemical study of digestion, so popular during the early-1800s. Kuhne identifies the digestive enzyme trypsins, which recall breaks down peptides into amino acids in the duodenum (1877)[66]. The peptides in the duodenum are the result of Thomas Schwann's enzyme pepsin, which have broken down food stuff proteins in the stomach. Friederich Kuhne also identifies the contractile protein myosin (1859)[67]. The relationship between myosin and actin in muscle contraction however will not be described until 94 years later by Huxley and Niedergerke (1954)[68] and Huxley and Hanson (1954)[69]. Perhaps one of Kuhne's most notable contributions is in the area of histology rather than biochemistry. Friederich Kuhne is first to identify the neuromuscular junction (1862)[70].

Claude Bernard (1813-1878) French physiologist and student of French experimental physiologist Francois Magendie studies digestion. In 1857 he identifies a starch like substance in the liver which he named "…la matiete glycogene…", glycogen (1857,1858)[71,72]. He demonstrates small molecules are taken from the blood and combined in the liver to form a larger molecule glycogen, which serves as a carbohydrate energy store for the body. He successfully demonstrates as blood glucose levels decrease, glycogen is broken down into smaller molecules and released into the blood stream, restoring the sugar level. Carl and Gerty Corti (of Cori cycle fame) detail the specific metabolic pathway responsible for the metabolism of glycogen 83 years later (1929)[73].

Claude Bernard is responsible for additional significant contributions in the area of physiology. He correctly describes the neural innervation of blood vessels and their roles in constricting and dilating the vessels (1851,1853)[74,75]. He recognizes and reports erythrocytes are responsible for carrying oxygen from the lungs to body tissues (1857)[76]. He is among the first to recognize and describe the body's continuous attempt to maintain a stable internal environment to optimize routine biochemical reactions, essential to normal bodily functions, which he terms "milieu interieur" (the environment within) (1865,1878)[77,78] and later termed homeostasis by Walter Cannon (1926)[79].

By the mid-1800s, biochemistry as a discipline enjoys a series of notable advancements and contributions. The field remains focused upon the chemistry of digestion and fermentation. The first amino acids are identified. Enzymes are identified and their roles in catalyzing biochemical reactions are beginning to be understood. Organic substances once believed to only be produced by living animals and the "vital forces" contained within the animal are produced in the laboratory from inorganic materials. Biochemical evidence is mounting which challenges the foundation of vitalism and scientific dogma which has prevailed thousands of years. The understanding of composition of biological substances now includes isomeric chemical structure. A uniform notation system is introduced for writing chemical formulas. New proteins including the contractile protein myosin are discovered. Glycogen is discovered and the biochemical processes of glycogenesis and glycogenolysis are outlined.

Biochemistry flourishes during the second half of the 1800s.

The Periodic Table of Elements is established, governments turn to biochemists for answers, biochemists are granted patents on their discoveries and engage in commercial ventures, hemoglobin as a reversible oxygen transport system is understood, sugars including glucose are investigated and understood in detail, carbohydrates are recognized to store genetic information, the bonds which hold amino acids together are discovered, fermentation is established to occur without vital forces, and professional organizations and journals devoted to the exchange of scientific information between biochemists are established.

Dmitri Ivanovich Mendeleev (1834-1907) Russian chemist recognizes relationships between known elements and generates his first version of the periodic table of elements. He presents his Table and observations to the Russian Chemical Society in March of 1869. The Table and eight noted comments explaining how to use the Table is published in the Society's journal's first volume, "Zeitschrift fur Chemie" (1869)[80]. While several others offer similar periodic tables of elements, during the 1860s, Mendeleev's Table provides clarity, consistency, a relative simple organization structure, and correctly accommodates most knowledge of the time period. Relationships within and between elements can be quickly recognized upon examining the Table's rows, columns, and diagonals. A copy of the manuscript draft is located online, located at the Chemical Achievers Chemical Heritage Foundation's website (1869)[81].

Trivia: In 1906, Mendeleev came within one vote of being awarded the Nobel Prize for his works. The Prize instead is awarded that year to Henri Mossian (1852-1907) "...in recognition of the great services rendered by him in his investigation and isolation of the element fluorine, and for the adoption in the service of science of the electric furnace called after him..." (1906)[82]. Exactly ...who? So goes the politics of professional science and the Nobel Prize Selection Committee.

Hippolyte Mege-Mouries (1817-1880) French chemist responds to Charles-Louis Napoleon Bonaparte III (1808-1852) Emperor of the French, offer of a prize to anyone who can develop a suitable substitute for butter, for use by the military armed forces and lower classes. Mege-Mouries builds upon the work of Michel Eugene Chevereul (1786-1889) whom identified margaric acid (1813)[83]. While employed to complete chemical research on dairy products, on a dairy farm owned by the Emperor, Hippolyte Mege-Mouries quickly completes his efforts, combining approximately 80% vegetable oils with 20% milk, creating the product we know today as oleo-margarine. A great substitute for the much more expensive dairy product butter. Mege-Mouries quickly claims the Emperor's prize for his efforts in 1869. He patents the product and two years later sells the patent to a Dutch soap manufacturing company Jurgens, following a failed business venture to market the product himself.

Trivia: The word margarine is derived from the Greek word "margaron" meaning pearl (the color of fatty acids) and "oleo" from the Latin "oleum" meaning oil. Today, margarine is very much a part of the typical American diet. The United States of American imports over ten billion pounds of margarine annually.

Felix Hoppe-Seyler (1825-1895) German chemist and physiologist is perhaps most remembered for his recognition and report in 1866 of the role of the globular protein hemoglobin, in reversibility binding oxygen. While hemoglobin is known and reported earlier by Friedrich Hunefeld (1840)[84], its role and mechanism of action for carrying oxygen to tissues is not made clear until the work of Felix Hoppe-Seyler (1866)[85]. Hoppe-Seyler identifies iron in hemoglobin and outlines its chemical contributions to reversible oxygen binding. The familiar sigmoid shaped oxygen-hemoglobin dissociation curve describing this relationship however will have to wait another 65 years and will first appear in 1904 due to the efforts of Christian Bohr (1855-1911) (Bohr Effect), Karl Hasselbalch (1874-1962) (Henderson-Hasselbalch equation) and August Krogh (1874-1949) (Nobel Prize laureate, describes blood flow control regulation at the level of capillaries) (1904)[86].

Felix Hoppe-Seyler makes broader professional contributions, which identify biochemistry as an emerging and distinct discipline. He founds the professional journal "Der Zeitschrift fur Physiologische Chemie" [Journal of Physiological Chemistry] in 1877. The Journal provides a necessary forum for early biochemists to share their thoughts and findings with others. The Journal, while having gone through a few name changes is still in publication today and continues to provide a highly respected forum for biochemists and others to share their contributions. The term "biochemistry" first appears in the professional literature in volume one of "Der Zeitschrift fur Physiologische Chemie" and stands as a landmark in the professional development of biochemistry as a scientific and professional discipline (1877)[87].

Hermann E. Fischer (1852-1919) German chemist and Nobel Prize Laureate, works perhaps best exemplifies the rapid advances being made in biochemistry, during the late-1800s. Hermann Fischer is largely responsible for providing an understanding of the chemical and molecular structure of glucose. He introduces an organizational system of sugars based upon chemical and molecular structures. The system identifies the now familiar monosaccharides, disaccharides, and polysaccharides. His extensive work investigating sugar metabolism and thoughtful integration of both new and old chemical knowledge provides a foundation in biochemistry upon which much work today continues to build.

Hermann Fischer is first to recognize carbohydrates as a store of genetic information and coins the term "purine" (1884)[88]. He clearly outlines the relationships between glucose, fructose and mannose (1888)[89] and introduces the "lock and key" visualization used to understand the mechanism of action of enzymes (1894)[90]. His interests and studies changes to proteins during the late-1890s and results in his discovery of the unique amino acid proline. Recall, proline contains an imino group rather than an amino group and provides the unique structural geometry important in the formation of the fibrous structure of collagen. Hermann Fischer is responsible for the discovery of the peptide bond, which holds amino acids together. Hermann Fischer is awarded the 1902 Nobel Prize in Chemistry "…in recognition of the extraordinary services he has rendered by his work on sugar and purine syntheses …" (1902)[91].

Eduard Buchner (1860-1917). German chemist persuasively demonstrates fermentation is a metabolic pathway and not dependent upon microorganisms and "vital forces", as reported by Louis Pasteur (1897,1858,1863)[92,48,49]. Eduard Buchner is first to isolate a zymase (an enzyme complex which ferments sugar into ethanol and CO_2) to ferment sugar in the lab, without use of living cells. His work strikes another powerful blow to the dogma of vitalism. Buchner's work moves fermentation from the providence of microbiology to chemistry. He is awarded the 1907 Nobel Prize in Chemistry "…for his biochemical researches and his discovery of cell-free fermentation..." (1907)[93].

In summary, the 1800s witness the identification of the first amino acids by Vanquelin and Robiquet. Prout's chemical analysis of food gives us the familiar classification system of fats, carbohydrates, and proteins. Wohler synthesizes organic substances from inorganic substances, striking a staggering scientific blow to the dogma of vitalism, and identifies isomeric structures of proteins. Berzelius offers his standardized notation system we still use today, in writing chemical formula. Payen, Chevreul, and Persoz discover distase and provide the foundational basis for enzyme research to follow. Mulder describes the chemistry of proteins. Kuhne isolates the contractile muscle protein myosin. Bernard isolates the energy storage molecule glycogen and emphasizes the body's continuous attempt to maintain a stable internal environment to optimize biochemical reactions essential to normal bodily functions. Mendeleev gives us his periodic table of elements. Hoppe-Seyler describes the chemistry of reversible oxygen binding in hemoglobin and publishes one of the first professional journals devoted to biochemistry. Fischer explains sugar metabolism, introduces the "lock and key" visualization to understand enzymatic actions, coins the term "purine", and is first to recognize the role of carbohydrates as a store of genetic information. Buchner describes fermentation as a metabolic pathway, moving fermentation from the providence of microbiology to that of biochemistry. So goes the 1800s.

Late Modern, 1900 AD - 2000 AD.

A shift in biochemistry is evident during the Late Modern period and the discipline enjoys tremendous and rapid advancements in the knowledge base. Biochemistry rapidly develops into a separate scientific discipline and demonstrates value to the practice of clinical medicine.

The early-1900s witness a change in focus from physiology based biochemistry to the physics of biochemistry. Biochemistry establishes itself as a legitimate scientific discipline, establishing specialized journals, founding specialized professional societies, identifying areas of research, focusing resources, establishing preferred research methodologies, developing a consensus within the discipline regarding accepted scientific facts and dogma, establishing training and educational programs for new investigators, and integrating specialized biochemistry course work into academic and medical curricula. Biochemistry is now recognized as necessary and essential to understanding the healthy and unhealthy human body and essential to providing high quality medical care.

Biochemistry enjoys significant advancement, as a specialized discipline during the very early-1900s, with the release of the Flexner Report, which revolutionizes medical education training in the United States and Canada (1910)[94]. The Flexner Report, commissioned by the Carnegie Foundation and in cooperation with the American Medical Association's Council on Medical Education, includes in their final recommendations, all medical school curriculum should include "biological chemistry" as a significant component of the training of all future physicians. Biochemistry soon becomes required for all medical students and continues today as a core foundation of all modern allopathic medical training programs.

Biochemistry shifts away from the chemistry of digestion physiology so popular during the 1800s, to interests in the physics of chemistry and its applications to the practice of medicine, during the 1900s.

Let us once again take a brief look at some of the most influential people, their unique contributions, and whom substantially guide the course and advancement of biochemistry as a scientific discipline, during the Late Modern period (1900 AD - 2000 AD).

Jacobus van Hoff (1852-1911) Dutch organic and physical chemist contributes to the burgeoning field of biochemistry through his contributions in describing the physical properties of one of the most important physical properties in biology, "osmotic pressure". Yes, he is responsible for first describing the forces which stops the flow of solute molecules from crossing a semi-permeable membrane (1887,1888)[95,96]. Van Hoff is also responsible for providing the first papers which propose a new and revolutionary formula for describing 3-dimensional chemical structures. He presents his revolutionary formula simply in a twelve page pamphlet with one page of diagrams (1874)[97]. Van Hoff's notation for three dimensional chemical structures is the familiar graphic representations of chemical compounds we know today, with the atoms and bonds represented for the molecule or compound being described. His chemical formula predates other systems, including Fischer's projections (1891)[98], Lewis structures (1916)[99], Haworth projections (1926)[100], or Newman projections (1952,1955)[101,102].

The very early beginnings of stereochemistry can be quickly traced to the imaginative and innovative original works of Jacobus van Hoff. He is awarded the first Nobel Prize in Chemistry in 1901 "…in recognition of the extraordinary services he has rendered by the discovery of the laws of chemical dynamics and osmotic pressure in solutions…" (1901)[103].

Karl Landsteiner (1868-1943) Austrian biologist and student of Hermann Fischer applies biochemistry to establishing the familiar modern classification system for blood types (1901)[104,105]. His discovery, with application for blood transfusion, revolutionizes surgery. Based upon identification of aggultins in serum, Landsteiner categorizes blood into three primary categories A, B, C (today we classify C as O). He soon recognizes transfusion of human blood between patients, with the same blood type, does not result in lysis of erythrocytes. His discovery is soon applied in medicine and surgery. Routine blood transfusions between patients begin in 1907. Prior to 1907, blood transfusion between patients is outlawed in many European countries due to the unpredictable and oftentimes fatal consequence of the practice. Blood transfusions continue to be a familiar and routine practice in medicine and surgery throughout the 1900s. Karl Landsteiner is awarded the 1930 Nobel Prize in Physiology or Medicine for "…his discovery of blood groups…" (1930)[106].

Ten years after receiving the Nobel Prize, Karl Landsteiner discovers a surface protein antigen on erythrocytes and introduces the "Rh factor" to the scientific and medical communities (1940)[107]. Landsteiner coins the term "Rh factor" to indicate the specific cell surface protein that stimulates the body's immune system and production of antibodies. The Rh factor antigen is first recognized on the surface of erythrocytes of the Rhesus macaque, explaining the factor's familiar name, "Rh" or "Rhesus" factor" (1941)[108]. The Rh blood group classification system remains one of the most important clinical blood group classifications today. Karl Landsteiner's discovery has immediate medical and surgical applications. Recognition of the presence or absence of the Rh factor (Rh+ or Rh-) in blood has tremendous implications for organ transplants and pregnancies.

In between his discovery of the A, B, O, blood groups and receipt of the Nobel Prize, Karl Landsteiner in collaboration with Austrian physician Erwin Popper (1879-1955) finds time to successfully identify and detail the polio virus (1909)[109]. What have you done with your time this year?

Benjamin Moore (1867-1922) British biochemist advances the discipline in founding one of the first and most influential professional journals devoted specially to biochemistry, the "Biochemistry Journal" (1906)[110]. Moore founds one of the first professional societies devoted specifically to the advancement of biochemistry as a recognized scientific discipline, the Biochemical (Club) Society, March 4, 1911, in London, England (1949)[111]. The Society is very much alive and well today. The Society continues to be a highly respected lead organization in the professional advancement of biochemistry and other molecular life sciences. Take note of Moore's choice of the term "biochemistry" for his new journal and society. His choice is deliberate choosing to emphasize the separation from physiological chemistry.

Biochemistry is now on its way to a period of normal science, as defined by Thomas Kuhn, in "The Structure of Scientific Revolutions" (1962)[112], establishing itself as a distinct scientific community with its own journals, societies, accepted methods of research, accepted areas of research, and core knowledge shared by all.

Lenor Michaelis (1847-1945) German biochemist and Maud Menten (1876-1960) Canadian medical scientist formulate a formula to express the relationship between an enzyme and its substrate. Specifically, they are interested in the rate of the interaction as a function of substrate concentration. Their findings reveal a nonlinear, hyperbolic relationship. Recall, if you add additional substrate to a substrate-enzyme mix, then the rate of reaction increases quickly until such point that adding more substrate appears to make no difference at all in changing the speed of the reaction. The relationship is described in their formula you most certainly read in your medical school's biochemistry course and perhaps struggled to understand its application to clinical medicine and patient care.

Yes, Lenor Michaelis and Maud Menten are responsible for the Michaelis-Menten Equation (1913)[113], describing the relationship between the rate of an enzyme catalyzed reaction, as a function of the substrate concentration; $V_0 = V_{max}[S]/K_m+[S]$; where V_0=initial reaction velocity (as soon as the enzyme and substrate are mixed), V_{max}=maximal velocity (the maximum speed the reaction can occur), K_m=Michaelis constant (the point at which the substrate concentration is equal to one half of V_{max}), and [S]=substrate concentration (concentration of the substance being catalyzed by an enzyme). While you may still be struggling with the clinical value of Michaelis-Menten equation (Hint: it provides a quick indicator of affinity, important for pharmacological therapeutic dosing), from a historical perspective their findings, graphical representation, and Equation provide a summary of our fundamental understanding of enzyme kinetics for the past 100 years.

Trivia: Menten of the Michaelis-Menten equation is female. As such she is prohibited from conducting research in her homeland of Canada. Consequently, Menten leaves Canada to conduct her research in the USA and Germany.

Lawrence Henderson (1878-1942) American chemist discovers the regulation of acid-base balances within the body are regulated by blood based buffer systems (1909)[114]. He develops the buffer equation (1908a,1908b)[115,116] and is soon modified by Karl Hasselbalch (1916)[117]. Henderson's investigations during the early-1900s provide the fundamental biochemical foundations of blood and specifically gas transport systems (1928)[118].

Karl Hasselbalch (1874-1962) Danish chemist describes how the affinity for oxygen in blood is dependent upon blood level concentrations of carbon dioxide. He converts the Henderson formula into a log scale and is known today to all medical students as the Henderson-Hasselbalch equation, $pH=pK_a + \log [A-]/[HA]$. The Equation describes the derivation of pH as a function of acidity using the dissociation constant pK_a, a measure of the strength of acid in solution. Recall, it is useful for estimating pH of a buffered solution and finding the equilibrium pH in an acid–base reaction.

Stated differently and with application to medicine, the Henderson-Hasselbalch equation can and is used to quickly understand at which pH level in the body a medication will pass most readily through a cell membrane. Recall, molecules pass through membranes when they are uncharged, so a base such as an amphetamine with a pK=8 will require a base environment pH greater than 8 to be quickly absorbed and become more quickly bioavailable. An acid such as Aspirin with a pK=4 will be absorbed more quickly through biologic membranes in an acidic environment, when the pH is less than 4. The point when pK= pH, half of the hydrogen ions of the molecule have been dissociated (removed) from the carboxyl group the rate of movement of the molecules across the membranes and into tissue becomes neutral. As the pH environment of the tissue changes from the neutral point, (pK=pH) and in the direction which makes more of the molecule more uncharged, more of the molecule will pass through the cell membranes and increase the bioavailability of the chemical to the tissues.

The bottom line with the Henderson-Hasselbalch equation and its associated graphic representation is the information can quickly reveal under which conditions a medication or toxin will be absorbed by the body or eliminated from the body. Useful information whenever you are prescribing medications, giving patient instructions e.g. "take this after a meal (produces a more basic environment with weak acidic medications less likely to be absorbed and weak basic medications more likely to be absorbed) or don't take this after drinking grapefruit juice (produces a more acidic environments with weak acidic medications more likely to be absorbed and weak basic medications less likely to be absorbed) or treating toxic overdoses. Understanding the relationship expressed by Henderson-Hasselbalch over 100 years ago provides the knowledge for you to improve medication treatments or save someone's life.

OK…enough biochemistry… this chapter is about history.

Soren Sorenson (1868-1939) Danish biochemist introduces pH as unit of measurement in 1909 as a convenient way of expressing acidity. We know pH ("power of hydrogen") is the negative log of hydrogen ion concentration, right? Actually, his 1909 paper never expressed pH as a log scale (1909)[119]. It was modified to a log scale later (1924)[120]. Sorensen's scale ranges from 0 -14, with a pH less than 7.0 defined an acid and greater than 7.0 defined a base, with 7.0 being neutral. Water has a pH of 7.0; battery acid has a pH of 0.3, beer 4.5, blood 7.4, sea water 8.0, and bleach 12.5. Sorenson invented the measurement while working on amino acids, proteins, and enzymes at the Carlsberg Laboratories. Yes, the Carlsberg Laboratory in Copenhagen Demark established in 1875 by J. C. Jacobsen to increase the scientific understanding of malting, brewing, and fermenting processes. The pH measure used today in medicine was invented by a man making and studying beer! Soren Sorenson while working in the brewery, discovers acids release hydrogen when combined with water, whereas; alkaline compounds combine with water. Once again beer and wine help shape the future of clinical medical practice.

Wilhelm Ostwald (1853-1932) German chemist, 1909 Nobel Prize Laureate in Chemistry, person responsible for introducing the mole measurement (1893)[121] invents the electrical conduction equipment, necessary to measure the quantity of hydrogen ions in solution 19 years before Sorenson applies the instrumentation to the development of pH measurements. Wilhelm Ostwald's instrumentation measures hydrogen concentration by measuring the electrical current generated in an electrochemical cell, when ions migrate to oppositely charged electrodes. Measurements of pH are performed routinely today on bodily fluids, including urine and blood, becoming an indispensable part of modern-day clinical medicine.

Christian Eijkman (1858-1930) Dutch, Professor of Physiology describes the biochemistry of vitamins. Christian Eijkman initially discovers these compounds while conducting investigations into the etiology of beriberi. Beriberi, an acquired biochemical disorder affecting the breakdown of energy molecules, had reached epidemic proportions in the Dutch East Indies colonies during the late-1800s and early-1900s. Working initially for the Dutch army in Batavia, Java (modern-day Jakarta, Indonesia) and having recently suffered the death of his wife, Eijkman is eager to find the bacterium responsible for beriberi.

Prior to Eijkman's investigations, beriberi is believed to be the result of a microbial infection. Christian Eijkman notices the link between chickens consuming polished white rice soon develop beriberi and chickens consuming brown rice do not develop beriberi (1897a,1897b)[122,123]. Recall, polished rice has the outside of the grain removed which improves taste, while unpolished rice maintains the outer covering of the grain. Christian Eijkman quickly begins to unravel the biochemistry responsible for the now identified water soluble, essential dietary nutrient deficiency of thiamine (vitamin B1) which produces the beriberi patient. This opens the door for all future investigations into the biochemistry of vitamins.

During the 1800s it is well established people require proteins, carbohydrates, salts, and fats to remain healthy. Not until the work of Christian Eijkman's beriberi investigations did the scientific community begins to recognize and appreciate the important contribution of vitamins in maintaining good health. Vitamins are soon recognized as essential to several normal biochemical processes within the human body. Christian Eijkman shares the 1929 Nobel Prize in Physiology or Medicine "…for his discovery of the antineuritic vitamin…" with English biochemist Frederick Hopkins (1861-1947) for "…his discovery of the growth stimulating vitamins…" (1929)[124]. Fredrick Hopkins discovers the amino acid tryptophan, 28 years before being recognized by the Nobel Committee for his contributions in vitamin research (1901a,1901b)[125,126].

Kazimierz Funk (1884-1967) Polish biochemist coins the term "vital amine", which is shorten to "vitamine", to describe a complex of micronutrients he identifies the same year (1912,1922)[127,128]. However, the Japanese biochemist Umetaro Suzuki (1874-1943) former student of Hermann Fischer, had presented a report on the identical micronutrient complex to the Tokyo Chemical Society two years earlier in 1910. Umetaro Suzuki publishes his findings in the Japanese journal "Tokyo Kagaku Kaishi" one year before Funk's paper appears in the scientific literature (1911)[129]. Kazimierz Funk's paper did not appear in the literature until after Suzuki's paper is translated into German earlier the same year and two years after Suzuki made his initial report to the professional biochemical community (1912)[130]. Hummm….coincidence?

Biochemistry continues to establish itself as a clearly identifiable academic discipline, distinct from physiology during the early-1900s. Professional journals, professional organizations and their associated scientific meetings devoted to the advancement of biochemistry are founded and begin to attract some of the brightest minds in chemistry. The discipline supports the 1919 efforts of the recently founded International Union of Pure and Applied Chemistry (IUPAC), an international association of chemistry societies, academies, and associations, in efforts to establish a standardized nomenclature for use within the discipline. The standardized nomenclature will include weights, measures, symbols, and terminology.

Prior to the IUPAC efforts, there exist tremendous variability in biochemical terminologies and no universally agreed nomenclature system. Chemical terminology varied dependent upon which country or university the work was completed (1782,1787,1789,1798,1811,1870,1892)[131,132,133,]

[134,135,136,137]. As with all newly developing discipline the lack of standardized nomenclature quickly leads to impaired communications between biochemistry professionals. In 1921 the IUPAC appoints a Commission charged with the international standardization of nomenclature of inorganic, organic, and biochemistry (1921)[138]. Working cooperatively with the international chemistry societies and with the usual amount of internal political fighting, the Commission establishes a nomenclature acceptable to most (1940,1940,1941)[139,140,141]. The IUPAC continues its work today with frequent revisions and continues as the world's authority on chemical nomenclature among scientists and applied chemists (1992,2010)[142,143].

Standardization of a discipline's nomenclature is another important developmental milestone and sign indicating the discipline is maturing. Standardization of the nomenclature did not come easily or without its fair share of heated interdisciplinary political bickering. At the time of the IUPAC's first publication on the topic, two distinct and competing factions have developed in chemistry in Europe, the "French School" comprised primarily of the French and English chemists and the "German School". Both lobby aggressively for acceptance of their particular nomenclature to become the standard. Today, the IUPAC continues to move forward with its efforts in standardizing the nomenclature of chemistry and biochemistry in order to keep pace with the rapid advances in technology and knowledge. The internal, regional, and institutional politics evident in the early-1900s are very much alive and well today in regard to efforts to introduce new or modify old nomenclature of biochemistry. So it goes.

Otto Meyerhof (1884-1951) German biochemist is most recognized for his contributions to understanding intermediate metabolism. He is first to recognize and describe the cyclic nature of energy transformation in living cells. His work details how glycogen is converted into lactic acid in the absence of oxygen and then reconverted back into glycogen. He is responsible for recognizing less glycogen is consumed in muscles in the presence of oxygen than in the absence of oxygen (1920)[144]. Otto Meyerhof is awarded the 1922 Nobel Prize in Chemistry for his works in intermediate metabolism and "...for his discovery of the fixed relationship between the consumption of oxygen and the metabolism of lactic acid in the muscle..." (1922). Five years later he discovers hexokinase (1927)[145], which is subsequently recognized as the necessary enzyme to catalyze the first step of glycolysis by transferring a phosphate group from ATP to glucose in order to form glucose-6-phosphate (1935)[146]. Otto Meyerhof is responsible for ultimately correctly sequencing the multistep metabolic pathway of glycolysis.

David Keilin (1887-1963) Soviet biochemist outlines the steps of the electron transport chain and coins the term "cytochrome' for the membrane bound protein which carries out electron transport (1925)[147]. Keilin recognizes a series of chemical reactions are necessary to transfer electrons from high energy molecules to low energy molecules and provides the initial outline of the chemical pathway necessary to produce the high energy molecule adenosine triphosphate (ATP), essential to most biochemical reactions.

Karl Lohmann (1898-1978) German biochemist isolates ATP from muscle and liver extracts (1929)[148] and correctly describes the structure of ATP (1932)[149]. By 1934 Lohmann provides direct evidence that ATP synthesis is the by-product of glucose metabolism (1935)[150]. Today we now recognize ATP is widely utilized in reactions involving energy transfer in all cells and is the essential bio molecule for normal cell function.

Hans Lineweaver (1907-2009) American physical chemist and Dean Burke (1904-1988) American biochemist straighten out the Michaelis-Mention Curve with their introduction of the Lineweaver-

Burke double reciprocal plot (1934)[151]. The Lineweaver-Burke Plot in essence transforms the Michalelis-Menton Plot into a straight line and makes the determination of Vmax easier, especially at high substrate concentrations. Both curves, the Michaelis-Menten and the Lineweaver-Burke, are used to determine important and specific terms in enzyme kinetics, Km and Vmax. Today, these terms are rapidly and precisely calculated using nonlinear equations and digital computer technologies. Both curves are still taught in medical schools for their value in helping to understand the basic foundations of enzyme kinetics and quickly determining the type of enzyme inhibition present; competitive, non-competitive, or uncompetitive. The Lineweaver-Burke Plot is currently preferred in that this straight line plot makes it easy and quick to identify when Vmax is achieved and to quickly identify the type of enzyme inhibition. Given this, the Lineweaver-Burke Plot remains a true pain in the #@* for most medical students, since it plots the reciprocals (1/Vo=Km/Vmax{S} + 1/Vmax) rather than Vmax and Km directly. As a result the Lineweaver- Burke Plot is often misread and consequently misinterpreted by medical students today.

Fritz Lipmann (1899-1986) German biochemist focuses his professional life upon the investigation of cellular conversion of food stuffs into energy. He contributes to understanding the role and biochemical mechanisms for the synthesis and oxidation of fatty acids and pyruvate, in the TCA cycle (1941)[152]. Fritz Lipmann is commonly credited with coining the familiar term "energy currency" when referring to the energy rich phosphate molecule ATP although the term "energy currency" never appears in any of his writings, including his landmark publication of 1939 "Metabolic Generation and Utilization of Phosphate Bond Energy", in which he describes the role of ATP (1939-1941)[153]. He shares the 1953 Nobel Prize in Physiology or Medicine "…for his discovery of co-enzyme A and its importance in intermediary metabolism…" (1953)[154].

Hans Adolf Krebs (1900-1981) German biochemist identifies two important intermediate metabolic cycles, the urea cycle (1932)[155] and citric acid cycle (1937)[156]. Recall, the urea cycle is the sequence of biochemical reactions that produce the less toxic waste product urea from ammonia produced by cells, during normal cellular metabolism. The urea cycle is completed primarily in the liver and secondarily in the kidneys. The citric acid cycle is a sequence of chemical reactions within human cells required to release stored energy in the form of ATP and produces precursors of several amino acids as well as the reducing agent NADH used in many biochemical reactions. The citric acid cycle as described by Krebs is also known to medical students as the Krebs cycle or tricarboxylic acid cycle (TCA cycle). Hans Krebs shares the 1953 Nobel Prize in Physiology or Medicine "…for his discovery of the citric acid cycle…" (1953)[157].

Carl Cori (1896-1984) and his wife Gerty Cori (1896-1957) Czechoslovakian biochemists are most noted for their work detailing the metabolism of glycogen. Their research into carbohydrate metabolism result in our current understanding of the biochemical processes used by the body to reversibly coverts glucose to glycogen. Their work explains how carbohydrates supply energy to muscles during exercise and how carbohydrates are regenerated and stored, until needed again by exercising muscles. Their work into the regulation of blood glucose concentrations and sugar metabolism result in the now familiar Cori Cycle (1929)[158].

Building upon work of Claude Bernard (1856)[159] and others, the Coris recognize muscle glycogen does not contribute to blood glucose levels. Muscle glycogen must form an intermediate that circulates in blood. This intermediate (lactate) is then converted into glucose within the liver and then the glucose is moved into the systemic blood circulation. The Coris were jointly awarded the 1947 Nobel Prize in Physiology or Medicine "…for their discovery of the course of the catalysis conversion of glycogen…" (1947)[160]. Their research provides the foundation for all future research into glycogen metabolism.

Trivia: Gerty Cori is repeatedly denied academic posts in the USA due to being female. After her husband Carl Cori was promoted to Department Head at Washington University in St. Louis, his wife Gerty was awarded an academic position and soon promoted to the level of professor. Her research efforts are recognized by the world academic community and shares the 1947 Nobel Prize in Chemistry with her husband Carl Corti. Gerty Cori is the third woman to receive the Prize. The first is Marie Curie in 1911 "…in recognition of her services to the advancement of chemistry by the discovery of the elements radium and polonium, by the isolation of radium and the study of the nature and compounds of this remarkable element…" (1911)[161]. The second is Marie Curie's daughter, Irene Curie in 1935 "…in recognition of their synthesis of new radioactive elements…" (1935)[162].

Albert Lehninger (1917-1986) American biochemist and pioneer in the field of bioenergetics contributes to a more complete understanding of metabolism at a molecular level. In 1947 he discovers mitochondria to be the site of oxidative phosphorylation in eukaryotic cells. That's right; he is the one, along with Eugene Kennedy (1919-2011), to localize the biochemical synthesis of ATP to the mitochondria (1947)[163]. Albert Lehninger pioneers the field of bioenergetics, providing biochemical insights into how nutrients derived from food are oxidized and converted into biochemical forms. He offers three classic textbooks; "Mitochondrion" (1964)[164], "Bioenergetics" (1965)[165], and "Biochemistry" (1978)[166], in addition to numerous professional articles. He is embroiled in a heated professional controversy, when British biochemist Peter Mitchell (1920-1992) is awarded the 1978 Nobel Prize in Chemistry "...for his contribution to the understanding of biological energy transfer through the formulation of the chemiosmotic theory…" rather than being awarded to Lehninger for his many contributions (1978)[167]. Another case of significant scientific contributions going unrecognized due to professional politics or something else? You decide.

The early-1900s prove to be a rewarding time for biochemistry. The knowledge base of the discipline is recognized as essential for medical practice; research focus is redirected from simple digestion physiology to the physics of biochemical structures and processes; osmotic pressure is introduced and understood; blood groups are identified using agglutination procedures, making blood transfusions possible; the Rh factor is identified in blood and contributes to advancements in immunology; the "Biochemistry Journal" begins publication emphasizing a separation from physiological chemistry; enzyme kinetics are investigated resulting in simple equations explaining relationships between enzymes and substrate; acid-base relationships are described along with buffering systems leading to simple formula to understand which medications will move across biological membranes and become bioavailable (therapeutically active); pH is introduced as a useful and easily obtained measure of acidity, important to every biochemical reaction; the discipline standardizes nomenclature to facilitate communication between investigators; intermediate metabolism is studied intensely generating our understanding of such basic biochemical systems as glycolysis, the electron transport chain, TCA cycle, and urea cycle; the structure of ATP is detailed; the biochemical importance of vitamins are recognized and studied; and mitochondria is identified as the site of oxidative phosphorylation and the source of cellular energy. Yes, the early-1900s proves to be good for biochemistry.

The second half of the 1900s demonstrates continued progress with identification of cAMP and its role in second messenger cell communication systems; new imaging techniques permit the visualization of protein structures; advances in understanding fatty acids and cholesterol metabolism are made; DNA is imaged; G protein systems are recognized; the polymerase chain reaction (PCR) for rapidly producing specific segments of genetic materials is introduced; ion-transporting enzymes are discovered; intrinsic cell signaling between proteins is discovered; biochemistry emerges as essential in understanding and manipulating genetic materials; and biochemistry reestablishes itself as necessary and essential to the medical education of practicing physicians.

Let's now take a brief look at the second half of the 1900s.

Earl Sutherland (1915-1974) American biochemist isolates cAMP and demonstrates its role within the second messenger systems and in response to hormones (1957,1957,1958,1958)[168,169,170,171]. Working with the Coris, he details the mechanisms of action, responsible in epinephrine's regulation of the degradation of glycogen into glucose (1951)[172]. Recall, epinephrine activates membrane bound adrenergic receptors which activate adenylyl cyclase and results in cAMP, which in turn activate a cAMP dependent kinase inside of the cell and activates glycogen phosphorylase kinase A, which then activates glycogen phosphorylase A, which degrades glycogen and makes glucose, for entry into the blood or muscle, as an immediate energy source. Truly a remarkable biochemical system. Sutherland's isolation of cAMP and his conceptualization of the role of cAMP, in hormonal and intracellular signaling, are initially and quickly rejected by scientists as too simple and unlikely. Years later and after the work of Martin Rodbell (1969)[173] and others which confirm Sutherland's postulated second messenger systems, do Sutherland's contributions become fully appreciated by the scientific community. Karl Sutherland is awarded the 1971 Nobel Prize in Physiology or Medicine "…for his discoveries concerning the mechanisms of action of hormones…" (1971)[174].

Max Perutz (1914-2002) Austrian molecular biologist offers the first x-ray images of the globular protein hemoglobin and provide images of its physical structure (1959)[175]. This breakthrough application of imaging technology in biochemistry provides further understanding as to how oxygen is transported. His discovery recognizing hemoglobin structure changes when it picks up and releases oxygen, provides the necessary technology and data to understand the molecular mechanisms responsible for oxygen transport throughout the body.

Trivia: Max Perutz (1914-2002) supervises the doctoral work of Francis Crick (1916-2004) and James Watson (1928-), whom later image the structure of deoxyribonucleic acid (DNA) (1953). Max Perutz is a vocal critic of Thomas Kuhn's philosophical position that advances in science and changes in scientific paradigms, respond to social and cultural presses of the time (1970, 1994)[176,177].

Jon Kendrew (1917-1997) English biochemist also focuses his efforts on applying imaging technologies in new and innovative ways to reveal the physical structures of proteins. Kendrew studies myoglobin, a molecule one quarter the size of hemoglobin. He successfully images and describes its structure (1957)[178]. Jon Kendrew and Max Perutz share the 1962 Nobel Prize in Chemistry "…for their work on the globular structure of proteins…" (1962)[179].

Konrad Bloch (1912-2000) German biochemist is responsible for much of what we know today about cholesterol. Prior to Bloch's work, little was known of cholesterol other than a speculation that fats in the diet might be associated with buildup of cholesterol and lipid deposits inside of arteries and this may be associated with arteriosclerosis. Bloch recognizes the essential role of cholesterol in stabilizing cell membranes and discovers all steroid molecules in the body e.g. hormones are derived from cholesterol. He describes the 36 biochemical steps necessary to transform acetate into cholesterol (1950a,1950b)[180,181]. He utilizes innovative radioisotope tagging technologies to tag acetic acid and determines acetic acid to be a major component of all cholesterols. Konrad Bloch's work detailing the biochemical pathway from acetic acid to cholesterol proves essential to the discovery of the satin drugs, which interfere with cholesterol synthesis. Konrad Bloch shares the 1962 Nobel Prize in Physiology or Medicine with Feodor Lynen (1911- 1979) "…for discoveries concerning the mechanism and regulation of cholesterol and fatty acids metabolism…" (1962)[182].

By the end of the 1900s biochemistry turns much of its attention to the biochemistry of genetic materials. Biochemists however continue to play critical roles in understanding basic chemical structures and mechanisms of action of fundamental biological systems throughout the remaining half of the century. The following investigators provide a representative, although brief and incomplete, listing of biochemistry's contributions to medicine, during final years of the 1900s.

Paul Berg (1926-) American biochemist is awarded the 1980 Nobel Prize in Chemistry "…for his fundamental studies of the biochemistry of nucleic acids, with particular regard to recombinant-DNA…" (1980)[183]. The same year American biochemist Walter Gilbert (1932 -) and English biochemist Fredrick Sanger (1918-2013) share in the 1980 Nobel Prize in Chemistry "…for their contributions concerning the determination of base sequences in nucleic acids…" (1980)[183]. Fredrick Sanger had been awarded a previous Nobel Prize in 1958 "…for his work on the structure of proteins, especially that of insulin…", which prove to have immediate and tremendous impact and effect in clinical medicine (1958)[184].

Pamela Champe (1945-2008) American microbiologist and biochemist Richard Harvey (unknown -) offer perhaps the most welcomed contribution to biochemistry for medical students, their first edition of "Lippincott's Illustrated Reviews: Biochemistry" (1987)[185]. The text provides a brief, straight forward, comprehensible presentation of relevant biochemical topics for medical students. It has helped thousands of students make it through their medical school's basic sciences program's biochemistry course. The text is currently in its seventh edition (2017)[186] and continues to be the gold standard for most current medical students worldwide.

Kary Mullis (1944-2019) American biochemist is awarded the 1993 Nobel Prize in Chemistry "…for his invention of the polymerase chain reaction (PCR) method…" (1993)[187].

Alfred Gilman (1941-2015) American biochemist and Martin Rodbell (1925-1998) American biochemist are awarded the 1994 Nobel Prize in Physiology or Medicine "…for their discovery of G-proteins and the role of these proteins in signal transduction in cells…" (1994)[188].

Paul Boyer (1918-2018) American biochemist and English biochemist John Walker (1941-) share the 1997 Nobel Prize in Chemistry "…for their elucidation of the enzymatic mechanism underlying the synthesis of adenosine triphosphate (ATP)…" with Danish biochemist Jens Skou (1918- 2018) "…for the first discovery of an ion-transporting enzyme, Na+, K+ -ATPase…" (1997)[189].

Gunter Blobel (1936-2018) German biochemist details the biochemistry of intracellular protein signaling and is awarded the 1999 Nobel Prize in Physiology or Medicine "…for the discovery

that proteins have intrinsic signals that govern their transport and localization in the cell..."
(1999)[190].

In summary, the 1900s is quite a century for biochemistry. Flexner gives us his Report; van Hoff osmotic pressure and notation system for chemical structural formula; Landsteiner his blood groups; Moore the biochemistry Journal and Society; Michaelis and Menten their equation; Henderson his acid and base buffered regulation; Hasselbalch his affinity for oxygen and CO_2 and modifies Henderson's equation; Sorenson gives us his pH; IUPAC their standardized nomenclature; Meyerhof gives us glycolysis and hexokinase; Keilin his electron transport chain; Lohmann his ATP; Hopkins and Eljkman their vitamins; Lineweaver and Burke their Plot; Lipmann coenzyme A and "energy currency"; Krebs his cycle; Coris their cycles; Lehninger bioenergetics; Sutherland cAMP; Perutz images of hemoglobin; Kendrew images of myoglobin; Crick and Watson images of DNA; Bloch his cholesterol; Berg his recombinant DNA; Sanger his base sequences; Champe and Harvey their illustrated review; Mullis his PCR; Gilman and Rodbell their G-proteins; Boyer and Walker their synthesis of ATP; Skou his ion transporting enzymes; and Blobel his intrinsic signals. Yes, quite an impressive time in the history of biochemistry.

Current Modern, 2000 AD - 2019 AD.

Currently exciting areas and contributions from the fields of biochemistry continue to emerge rapidly. The disciplinary boundaries between molecular biology, genetics, and biochemistry are less clear today than ever. Biochemistry continues its lead in the understanding of genetic materials and its applications to modern medicine.

Examples of current areas of rapid development and advancements are exemplified by recent Nobel Prize in Chemistry recipients. Peter Agres "...for discovery of water channels" (2003) [191]; Robert Kornberg "...for his studies of the molecular basis of eukaryotic transcription..." (2006) [192]; Venkatraman Ramakrishnan, Thomas Steitz, and Ada Yonath "... for studies of the structure and function of the ribosome..." (2009) [193]; Robert Lefkowitz and Brian Kobilka "...for their studies of G-protein coupled receptors..." (2012)[194], Tomas Lindahl, Paul Modrich, and Anziz Sancar "...for mechanistic studies of DNA repair..." (2015)[195], Frances Arnold "...for the directed evolution of enzymes" and George Smith and George Winter "...for the phage display of peptides and antibodies..." (2018)[196].

Medical education continues to emphasize biochemistry as important and necessary in the education and training of every future allopathic physician and remains a required, core, basic science program course, in most medical training programs today. Recent advances in digital technologies facilitate the learning of medical biochemistry by medical students and challenges their imaginations. Lippincott, William, and Wilkins publishing continues to provide a much welcomed aid for medical students around the world with the recent release of their very readable, revised, seventh edition of "Lippincott's Illustrated Reviews: Biochemistry".

Yes, these are exciting times for biochemistry in general and especially exciting times for medical biochemistry.

References.

---

[1] Dirckx, J. (1997). Stedman's concise medical dictionary for the health professions. Third Edition. Baltimore: Williams and Wilkins.

[2] Furr, C. (2014). What is medical biochemistry? Wise GEEK. Revised by C. Mitchell and edited by C. Wilborn. Modified 22 September 2016. Retrieved 9-28-2016 from www.wisegeek.org/what -is-medical-biochemistry.htm

[3] Scurlock, J. and Anderson, B. (2005). Diagnoses in Assyrian and Babylonian medicine: Ancient sources, translation, and modern medical analyses. Chicago: University of Illinois Press.

[4] Hunger, H. (1976). Spaet babylonische text aus uruk. Vol 1. Berlin: Mann.

[5] Kocher, F. (1964) Die babylonisch-assyrische medizin in testen und untersuchungen. Vols 1-6. Berlin: Walter de Gruyter.

[6] Labat. R. (1951). Traite akkadien de diagnostics et prognostics medicaux. Collection des travaux de l'Academie internationale d'histoire des sciences. vol 7. Academie Internationale d'histoire des sciences. Wiesbaden: Franz Steiner Verlag.

[7] Thompson, R. 1923). Assyrian medical texts from the originals in the British Museum. H. Milford, Oxford University Press.

[8] Fairbanks, A. (1898). The first philosophers of Greece: An edition and translation of the remaining fragments of the pre-Socratic philosophers together with a translation of more important accounts of their opinions contained in the early epitomes of their works. London: Kegan Paul, Trench, Trubner, and Company, Ltd.

[9] Caley, E. (1926). The Stockholm Papyrus: An English Translation with brief notes. Journal of Chemical Education, 4(8):979-1002.

[10] Caley, E. (1926). The Leiden Papyrus X: An English translation with brief notes. Journal of Chemical Education, 3:1149-1166.

[11] Preisendanz, K., Abt, A., Eitrem, S., Fahz, L., Jacoby, A., Moller, G., and Wunsch, R. (1928) Papyri Graecae Magicae Die Griechischen Zauberpapyri. Leipzig: Verlang Und Druck von B.G. Teubner.

[12] Magnus, A. (1210). De animalibus. English translation by Irven Resnick and Kenneth Kitchell. (1999). Albertus Magnus. On Animals: A medieval "Summa Zollogica". Foundations of Natural History. vol. 1-2. Baltimore: John Hopkins University Press.

[13] Magnus A. (1250). De mineralibus. English translation by Dorothy Wyckoff, (1967). Oxford: Claredon Press.

[14] Lewis, G. and Randall, M. (1923). Thermodynamics and the free energy of chemical substances. New York: McGraw Hill.

[15] Champe, P., Harvey, R., Ferrier, D. (2005). Lippincott's Illustrated Reviews: Biochemistry. (3rd edition). Philadelphia: Lippincott, Williams, and Wilkins.

[16] Hohenheim, P. (Paracelsis). (1633). A storehouse of physical and philosophical secrets. London: Thomas Harper.

[17] Bacon, F. (1620). Novum Organum. Basil Montague, editor and translator. The Works, 3 vols. (1854). Philadelphia: Parry and MacMillan.

[18] Helmont, J. (1621). De magnetica vulnerum naturali et legitima curatione contra. Paris: R.P. Joannem Roberti.

[19] Helmont, J. (1648). Ortus Medicinae, id est, initia physicae inaudita progressus medicinae novus, in morborum ultionem, ad vitam longam. Edited by Francisco Mercurio van Helmont. Amsterdam: Louis Elzevir.

[20] Helmont, J. (1662). Ortus medicinae, vel opera et opuscula omnia; In Oriatrike or Physics Refined. The common errors therein refuted, and the whole art rectified: being a new rise and progress of philosophy and medicine, for the destruction of diseases and prolongation of life. English translation by John Chandler. London: Lodowick Loyd.

[21] Power, H. (1664). Experimental Philosophy: In Three Books: Containing New Experiments Microscopical, Mercurial, Magnetical; with some deductions, and probable hypotheses, raised from them, in avouchment and illustration of the now famous Atomical Hypothesis. Martin and Allestry.

[22] Boyle, R. (1661). The Sceptical Chymist: or chymico-physical doubts and paradoxes;.touching the spagyrist's principles commonly called hypostatical, as they are wont to be proposed and defended by the generality of alchymists. London: Printed by F. Cadwell for F. Crooke and are to be sold at the Ship in St. Pauls Church Yard.

[23] Boyle, R. (1680). The sceptical chymist: or chymico-physical doubts and paradoxes;.touching the experiments whereby vulgar spagirists are wont to endeavour to evince their salt, sulphur, and mercury, to be the true principles of things. 2nd Edition. London: Oxford, printed by Henry Hall for R. Davis and B. Took. St. Pauls Church Yard.

[24] Boyle, R. (1670). New pneumatical experiments about respiration. Phil. Trans. R. Society, 5:2011-2058.

[25] Boyle, R. (1676). Experiments and notes about the mechanical origine or production of divers particular qualities: among which is inserted a discourse of the imperfection of the chymist's doctrine of qualities; together with some reflections upon the hypothesis of alcali and acidum. Oxford: E. Flesher.

[26] Boyle, R. (1693). Medicinal experiments or a collection of choice and safe remedies for the most part simple and easily prepared: very useful in families and fitted for the service of country people.3rd edition. London: Printed for Samuel Smithand B. Walford, Printers to the Royal Society at Prince's Armes in St. Pauls Church Yard.

[27] Scheele, C. (1777a). Chemische Abhandlung con der luft und dem feuer. Upsala und Leipzig.

[28] Scheele, C. (1777b). Chemical treatise on air and fire. In Alembic Club Reprints, No 8. Edinburgh. E and S. Livingstone Ltd 1952. Translated into English by Bibliolife.com. The Discovery of oxygen 2009, Discovery of Oxygen, Part 2: Experiments 2009.

[29] Priestley, J. (1775). An Account of Further Discoveries in Air. Philosophical Transactions, 65:384–94.

[30] Priestley, J. (1774). Experiments and Observations on Different Kinds of Air. London: W. Bowyer and J. Nichols.

[31] Priestley, J. (1775). Experiments and Observations on Different Kinds of Air. Vol. 2. London: Printed for J. Johnson.

[32] Priestley, J. (1790). Experiments and observations on different kinds of air [electronic resource]: and other branches of natural philosophy, connected with the subject. In three volumes; being the former six volumes abridged and methodized with many additions. London: printed by Thomas Pearson; and sold by J. Johnson.

[33] Priestly, J. (1772). Impregnating water with fixed air; in order to communicate to it the peculiar spirit and virtues of pyrmont water, and other mineral waters of a similar nature. London: J. Johnson.

[34] Lavoisier, M. (1776). Essays Physical and Chemical by M. Lavoisier, translated from the French with notes and an appendix by Thomas Henry. London. Printed for Joseph Johnson No. 72. St Pauls Church Yard.

[35] Lavoisier, M. (1778) Considerations generales sur la nature des acides, et sur les principes dout ils sont composes: Présenté le 5 Septemb. 1777. Lu le 23 Nov. 1779. Paris: Académie des Sciences.

[36] Lavoisier, M. (1783). Essays on the effects produced by various processes of air; with a particular view to an investigation of the constitution of the acids. Translated from the French into English by Thomas Henry. London: printed by W. Eyers for J. Johnson No. 72. St. Pauls Church Yard.

[37] Cavendish, H. (1766). Three papers containing experiments on factitious air. Philosophical Transactions, 56:141-184.

[38] Lavoisier, A. (1789). Traite elementaire de chimie, présenté dans un ordre nouveau et d'après les decouvertes modernes: avec figures, 2 vols. Paris: Chez Cuchet.

[39] Lomonosov, M. (1760). Meditations on the solidity and liquidity of bodies. Paper presented to the Russian Academy of Sciences, September 6, 1760. St. Petersburg.

[40] Lomonosov, M. (1760). Mikhail Vasilyevivh Lomonosov on the Corpuscular Theory. Translated, with an introduction by Henry M. Leicester, (1970).Cambridge Massachusetts: Harvard University Press.

[41] Robiquet, P. (1805). Essai analytique des asperges Annales de Chimie., 55:152–171.

[42] Vauquelin, L. and Robiquet, P. (1806). La decouverte d'un nouveau principe vegetal dans le suc des asperges. Annales de Chimie, 57:88–93.

[43] Wollaston, W. (1810). On cystic oxide, a new species of urinary calculus Phil. Trans .Royal Society London, 2:223-230.

[44] Braconnot, H. (1820). Annals de Chimie et de Physique, 2(13):114.

[45] Ritthausen, H. (1866). Ueber die Glutaminsaure. Journal fur Praktische Chememie, 99:454-462.

[46] Robiquet, P. (1832). Nouvelles observations sur les principaux produits de l'opium. Annales de Chimie et de Physique, 51:225–267.

[47] Proust, W. (1827). On the Ultimate Analysis of Simple Alimentary Substances, with some Preliminary Remarks on Organic Analysis'. Read to the Royal Society on I4 June 1827. Phil. Trans., 355-88.

[48] Pasteur, L. (1858). Memoire sur la fermentation appelee lactique. Annales de Chimie Ser., 52: 404-18.

[49] Pasteur, L. (1863). Recherches sur la putre´faction. Compt Rend, 56:1189–1194.

[50] Wohler, F. (1824). Recherches analytiques sur l'acide cyanique. Ann. Chim. Phys., 27(2):196-200.

[51] Wohler, F. (1828). Ueber kubstliche bildung des harnstoff. [On artifical formation of urea]. Annalen der Physik und Chemie, 88(2):253-256.

[52] Berzelius, J. (1811). J. Phys., de Chimie, et d'Histore Naturelle., 73:248.

[53] Berzelius, J. (1814). Essay on the cause of chemical proportions, and on some circumstances relating to them: together with a short and easy method of expressing them. Annals of Philosophy, 3:51-52. [Preliminary note on the subject had appeared in Annals of Philosophy, 2:359 (1813)].

[54] Berzelius, J. (1818). Larobok i kemien. Stockholm.

[55] Berzelius, J. (1819). Essai sur la theorie des proportions chimiques et sur l'influence chimique de l'electricite. (French translation of the 3rd volume of Larobok i Kemien). Paris: Mequignon-Marvis.

[56] Berzelius, J. (1836). Einige Ideen über bei der Bildung organischer Verbindungen in die lebenden Natur wirksame ober bisher nicht bemerkte Kraft. (Organic and inorganic processes differ only in complexity.), Jahres-Berkcht über die physichem Wissenschaften., 5:237–45.

[57] Berelius, J. (1802). De electricitatis galvanicæ apparatu cel. volta excitæ in corpora organica effectu quæ notavit venia experientiss. Facult. Medic. Upsal. praeside Petro Afzelio ... pro gradu medico examini defert Jacobus Berzelius ... Ostrogothus, in auditorio Gustav. maj. d. I Maji MDCCCI.

[58] Schwann, T. (1836a). Uber das wesen des verdauungsprocesses, [About the essence of the digestive processes] Archive fur Anatomic, Physilogie und Wissenschaftliche Medicine, 90-183

[59] Schawann, T. (1836b). Ueber das Wesen des Verdauugsprocesses. Annalen der Physik und Chemie, 38:358-364.

[60] Payen, A. and Persoz F. (1833). Memoire sur la diastase, les principaux produits de ses reactions et leurs applications aux arts industriels. Annales de Chimie et de Physique, 2 e série., 53:73-92.

[61] Mulder, G. (1839). Bulletin des Sciences Physiques et Naturelles en Neerlande on July 30, 1838, stated (in French) [On the composition of some animal substances (1839)].

[62] Mulder, G. (1856). Die Chemie des Weines [The chemistry of wine]. Leipzig: Verlagsbuchhandlung von J.J. Beber.

[63] Mulder, G. (1857). Le guide du brasseur ou L'art de faire la biere: Sa composition chimique et practique. [The brewers guide or the art of brewing: Its chemical and practical composition]. L.F. Dubiet Translator. Paris: J. Hetzel and Cie.

[64] Mulder, G. (1857). The chemistry of wine. London: John Churchill.

[65] Jones, B. (1848). On a new substance occurring in the urine of a patient with mollities ossium. Phil Trans Royal Society London, 138:55-62.

[66] Kuhne, T. (1877). Uber das Trypsin (Enzym Des Pankreas), in Verhandlungen des naturahistorisch - medizinischen Verieins zu Heidelberg, 1:94–198.

[67] Kuhne, T. (1859) Untersuchungen über bewegungen und veränderungen der contractilen substanzen. Arch. f. Anat. Physiol. u. Wissensch. Med., 748.

[68] Huxley, A. and Neidergerke, R. (1954). Structural changes in muscle during contraction; interference microscopy of living muscle fibres. Nature, May 22; 173 (4412):971-3.

[69] Huxley, H. and Hanson, J. (1954). Changes in the cross-striations of muscle during contraction and stretch and their structural interpretation. Nature, 173(4412):973-976.

[70] Kuhne, T. (1862). Über die peripherischen endorgane der motorischen nerven. Leipzig.

[71] Bernard, C. (1857a). Nouvelles recherches experimentales sur les phénomenes glycogeniques du foie. Comptes rendus de la Societe de biologie (Memoires), Paris, 2 sér., 4:1-7.

[72] Bernard, C. (1857b). Discovery of glycogen. Comptes rendus hebdomadaires des séances de l'Académie des Sciences, Paris, 44:578-586, 1325-1331.

[73] Cori, C. and Cori, G. (1929). Glycogen formation in the liver with d- and l-lactic acid. Journal of Biological Chemistry, 81:402.

[74] Bernard, C. (1851). Influence du grand sympathique sur la sensibilite et sur la calorification. Comptes rendus de la Societe de biologie. Paris, 3:163-164.

[75] Bernard, C. (1853). Recherches experimentales sur le grand sympathique et specialement sur l'influnce que la section de ce nerf exerce sur la chaleur animal. Comptes rendus de la Societe de boologie (Memoires) Paris, 5:77-107.

[76] Bernard, C. (1857). Lecons sur les effects des substances toxiques et medicamenteuses. Paris: J. B. Baillere.

[77] Bernard, C. (1865). Introduction a l'etude de la Medecine Experimentale. Paris: J. B. Bailliere et Fils; English translation by H. C. Greene (1957), Dover Publications, Inc. New York.

[78] Bernard, C. (1878). Leçons sur les phénomènes de la vie communs aux animaux et aux vegetaux. Paris: J. B. Bailliere.

[79] Cannon, W. (1926). Physiological regulation of normal states: some tentative postulates concerning biological homeostatics. In A. Pettit (ed.). A Charles Richet: ses amis, ses collègues, ses élèves (in French). Paris: Les Éditions Médicales. p. 91.

[80] Mendeleev, D. (1869). On the relationship of the properties of the elements to their atomic weights. Zeitscrift für Chemic., 12:405-406.

[81] Mendeleev, D. (1869). Draft for first version of Mendeleev's periodic table (17 February 1869). Courtesy Oesper Collection, University of Cincinnati. Retrieved from image bank of the Chemical Achivers Chemical Heritage Foundation. http://www.chemheritage.org/classroom/chemach/pop/04periodic/meyer1.html

[82] Nobel Prize Foundation (1906). The Nobel Prize in Chemistry 1906. Royal Swedish Academy of Sciences. Stockholm. Retrieved May 2010 from www.nobelprize.org

[83] Chevereul, M. (1813). Recherches chimiques sur plusieurs corps gras, et particulièrement sur leurs combinaisons avec les alcalis. Mémoire 1 - Sur une substance nouvelle obtenue du savon de graisse et de potasse, Ann. Chim., 88:225-261.

[84] Hünefeld, F. (1840). Die Chemismus in der thierischen Organization. Leipzig.

[85] Hoppe-Seyler, F. (1866). Über die oxydation in lebendem blute. Med-chem. Untersuch Lab, 1:133–140.

[86] Bohr, C., Hasselbalch, K., and Krogh, A. (1904). Ueber einen in biologischer beziehung wichtigen einfluss, den die kohlensäurespannung des blutes auf dessen sauerstoffbindung übt. (Concerning a biologically important relationship-the influence of carbon dioxide conent of blood on its oxygen binding). Skand. Arch. Physiol.,16:402-12.

[87] Hoppe-Seyler, F. (1877-78). Vorwort zur Zeitschrift für physiologische Chemie (Preface to he Journal of Physiological Chemistry). Zeitschrift für Physiologische Chemie, 1:1-3.

[88] Fischer, E. (1884). Verbindungen des Phenylhydrazins mit den Zuckerarten. Berichte der Deutschen Chemischen Gesellschaft, 17:579–584.

[89] Fischer, E. and Hirschberger, J. (1888). Ueber Mannose. Ber. Dtsch. Chem. Ges., 21:1805-1809.

[90] Fischer, E. (1894a). Einfluss der Configuration auf die Wirkung der Enzyme. Ber. Dtsch. Chem. Ges., 27:2985–2993.

[91] Nobel Prize Foundation. (1902). The Nobel Prize in Chemistry 1902. Royal Swedish Academy of Sciences. Stockholm. Retrieved May 2010 from www.nobelprize.org

[92] Buchner, H. (1897). Die Bedeutung der aktiven lo"slichen Zellprodukte fur den Chemismus der Zelle. Munchener, Medizinische Wochenschrift, 44:299–302, 321–322.

[93] Nobel Prize Foundation. (1907). The Nobel Prize in Chemistry 1907. Royal Swedish Academy of Sciences. Stockholm. Retrieved May 2010 from www.nobelprize.org

[94] Flexner A. (1910). Medical Education in the United States and Canada: A Report to the Carnegie Foundation for the Advancement of Teaching. Bulletin No. 4. Boston, Mass: Updyke.

[95] Hoff, J. (1887). Die rolle osmotischen drucks in der analogiezwischen losungen und gasen. Zeirschrift fur Physikalische Chemie, 1:481-508.

[96] Hoff, J (1888). The function of osmotic pressure in the analogy between solutions and gases. Translated by W. Ramsay, Philosophical Magazine, S.5, 26(159):81-105.

[97] Hoff, J. (1874). Voorstel tot Uitbreiding der Tegenwoordige in de Scheikunde gebruikte Structuurformules in de Ruimte; benevens een daarmee samenhangende ompmerkung omtrent het verband tusschen optisch actief Vermogen en Chemische Constitutie van Organische Verbindingen. (Proposal for extending the currently employed structural formulae in chemistry in space, together with a related remark on the relationship between optical activating power and chemical constitution of organic compounds.), Utrecht, Greven.

[98] Fischer, E. (1891). Uber die Konfiguration des Traubenzuckers und seiner Isomeren', I & II, Berichte der Deutschen Chemischen Gesellschaft, 24:2683-2687.

[99] Lewis, G. (1916). The Atom and the Molecule. J. Am. Chem. Soc., 38:762-785.

[100] Haworth, W. (1926). J. Chem. Soc., 2303.

[101] Newman, M. (1952). Record. Chem. Progr. (Kresge-Hooker Sci. Lib.), 13:111.

[102] Newman, M. (1955). A notation for the study of certain stereochemical problems. J. Chem. Educ,. 32:344-347.

[103] Nobel Prize Foundation (1901). The Nobel Prize in Chemistry 1901. Royal Swedish Academy of Sciences. Stockholm. Retrieved May 2010 from www.nobelprize.org

[104] Landsteiner, K. (1900). Zur Kenntnis der antifermentativen, lytischen und agglutinierenden Wirkungen des Blutserums und der Lymphe. Zentbl. Bakt. Orig., 27:357-362.

[105] Landsteiner, K. (1901). Ueber Agglutinationserscheinungen normalen menschlichen Blutes. Wien. Klin. Wochenschr. 14: 1132–1134. [Translation: On agglutination phenomena of normal human blood, in S. H. Boyer (Editor), 1963, Papers on Human Genetics, 27–31. Prentice-Hall, Englewood Cliffs, NJ.]

[106] Nobel Prize Foundation. (1930). The Nobel Prize in Physiology or Medicine 1930. Royal Swedish Academy of Sciences. Stockholm. Retrieved May 2010 from www.nobelprize.org

[107] Landsteiner, K. (1940). An agglutinable factor in human blood recognized by immune sera for rhesus blood. Proc. Soc. Exp. Biol. Med., 43:223–4.

[108] Landsteiner K. and Wiener A. (1941). Studies on an agglutinogen (Rh) in human blood reacting with anti-rhesus sera and with human isoantibodies. J. Exp. Med., 74(4):309–320.

[109] Landsteiner, K. and Popper, E. (1909). Übertragung der Poliomyelitis acuta auf Affen in Zeitschrift für Immunitätsforschung und experimentelle Therapie, 2:377-390.

[110] Moore, B. and Whitely, E (1906). The Bio-Chemical Journal (editors). Liverpool: University Press. Agent for America: New York City: G. E. Stechert & Company, West 20th Street.

[111] Pllimmer, R. (1949). The Foundation, 4 March 1911. In The History of the Biochemical Society 1911-1949. University Press: Cambridge. Retrieved June 2018 from http://www.biochemistry.org/Portals/0/About%20Us/Docs/History%20of%20Biochem%20Soc%201911-1949%20by%20Plimmer2.pdf

[112] Kuhn, T. (1962). The Structure of Scientific Revolutions, 1st. ed., Chicago: University of Chicago Press.

[113] Michaelis, L. and Menten, M. (1913). Die Kinetik der Invertinwirkung. Biochemische Zeitschrift, 49:334–336.

[114] Henderson, L. and Spiro, K. (1909-10). Zur Kenntnis des Ionengleichgewichts im Organismus, Series Part I-III, Biochemische Zeitschrift.

[115] Henderson, L. (1908a). Concerning the relationship between the strength of acids and their capacity to preserve neutrality. Am. J. Physiology, 21(4):173–179.

[116] Herderson, L. (1908b). The Theory of Neutrality Regulation in the Animal Organism. American Journal of Physiology, 21:427-48.

[117] Hasselbalch, K. (1916). Die berechnung der Wasserstoffzahl des blutes auf ders freien und gebundenen Kohlensaure desselben, und die Sauerstoffbindung des Blutes als Funktion der Wasserstoffzahl. Biochem. Z., 78:112–144.

[118] Henderson, L. (1928). Blood: A Study in General Physiology. Yale University Press.

[119] Sørensen, S. (1909). Enzymstudien. II: Mitteilung. Über die Messung und die Bedeutung der Wasserstoffionenkoncentration bei enzymatischen Prozessen. Biochemische Zeitschrift, 21:131–304.

[120] Sørensen, S. and Linderstrøm-Lang, K. (1924). Compt. Rend. Trav. Lab. Carlsberg, 15:6.

[121] Ostwald, W. (1893). Hand- und Hilfsbuch zur ausführung physiko-chemischer Messungen. Leipzig.

[122] Eijkman, C. (1897a) Note on the prophylaxis of beriberi. Janus., 2:23.

[123] Eijkman, C. (1897b). Ein Versuch sur bekampfung der beriberi. [An attempt to control beriberi]. Arch. Path. Anat. (Virchow's), 149:187.

[124] Nobel Prize Foundation. (1929). The Nobel Prize in Chemistry 1929. Royal Swedish Academy of Sciences. Stockholm. Retrieved May 2010 from www.nobelprize.org

[125] Hopkins, F. and Cole, S. (1901a). On the protcid reaction of Adamkiewicz with contributions to the chemistry of glyoxylic acid. Proc. Roy. Soc., 68:21-23.

[126] Hopkins, F. and Cole, S. (1901b). A hitherto undescribed product of tryptic digestion. J. Physiol., 27:418-28.

[127] Funk, C. (1912). The etiology of the deficiency diseases. J. State Med June.

[128] Funk C. (1922). The Vitamines. Authorized translation from second German edition by Harry E. Dubin. Baltimore: Waverly Press by Williams and Wilkins Company.

[129] Suzuki, U. (1911). On the one active ingredient in rice bran. Tokyo Kagaku Kaishi, 32(1):4-17.

[130] Suzuki, U., Shimamura, and Odake (1912). Ueber oryzanin, ein bestandteil der reiskleie und seine physiolgische bedeutung. Bio. Z., 43:89.

[131] Guyton de Morveau, L. (1782). J. Phys., 19:310.

[132] Guyton de Morveau, L, Lavoisier, A., Berthollet, C., Fourcroy, A. (1787). Methode de nomenclature Chimique. Paris: Cuchet.

[133] Lavoisier, A. (1789). Traite elementaire de chimie, presented an un ordre nouveau et d'apres les de couverates modernes, avec figures. Paris: Chez Cuchet.

[134] Guyton de Morveau, L. (1798). Am. Chim. Phys., 1:24.

[135] Berzelius, J. (1811). J.. Phys. de Chimie, et d'Histore Naturelle, 73:248.

[136] Madan, H. (1870). Report on Chemical Nomenclature. Journ. Chem. Soc., 23:22.

[137] Congres de Nomenclature Chimique, Geneve. (1892). Bull. Soc. Chim. Paris, 37:13-24.

[138] IUPAC Commission on Nomenclature. (1921). International Union of Pure and Applied Chemistry (IUPAC) 2nd International Conference. June 25-30. Brussels, Belgium.

[139] Jorissen, W., Bassett, H., Damiens, A., Fichter, F., and Remy, H. (1940). Ber. Dtsch. Chem. Ges. A., 73:53–70.

[140] Jorissen, W., Bassett, H., Damiens, A., Fichter, F., and Remy, H. (1940). J. Chem. Soc., 1404-1415.

[141] Jorissen, W., Bassett, H., Damiens, A., Fichter, F., and Remy, H. (1941). Rules for naming inorganic compounds: Report of the Committee of the International Union of Chemistry for the reform of inorganic chemical nomenclature, 1940. J. Am. Chem. Soc., 63:889-897.

[142] Liefecq, C. (1992). Biochemical Nomenclature and Related Documents for IUBMB (International Union of Pure and Applied Chemistry), "The White Book". London: Portland Press.

[143] IUPAC and Moss, P. (2010). IUPAC Nomenclature Books Series. Online resources to current IUPAC nomenclature and proposed recommended changes. Retrieved from http:// www.chem.qmw.ac.uk/ iupac/bibliog/books.html

[144] Meyerhof, O. (1920). Pflügers Arch. Gesamte. Physiol. Menschen. Tiere., 185:11–32.

[145] Meyerhof, O. (1927). Biochem. Z., 183:176.

[146] Meyerhof, O. (1935). Naturwissenschaften. (Natural Sciences), 23:850.

[147] Keilin D. (1925). On cytochrome, a respiratory pigment common to animals, yeast and higher plants. Proc. R. Soc. Lond. B. Biol. Sci., 98:312-229.

[148] Lohmann, K. (1929). Uber die pyrophosphatfranktion im muskel. Naturwissenschaften, 17(31):624–5.

[149] Lohmann, K. (1932). Untersuchungen zur konstitution der adenylphosphoraure. Biochem. Z., 254:381.

[150] Lohmann, K. (1935). Konstitution der adenlypryophosphoraure and adeninediphosphorasure. Biochem. Z., 282:120.

[151] Lineweaver, H. and Burke, D. (1934). The Determination of Enzyme Dissociation Constants. Journal of the American Chemical Society, 56:658–666.

[152] Lipmann, F. (1941). Metabolic Generation and Utilization of Phosphate Bond Energy, Advances in Enzymology and Related Subjects, 1: 99-162. New York: Intersciences Publishers.

[153] Lipmann, F. (1941). Metabolic generation and utilization of phosphate bond energy. Adv. Enzymol. Relat. Areas Mol. Biol., 1:99-162.

[154] Nobel Prize Foundation. (1953). The Nobel Prize in Physiology or Medicine 1953. Royal Swedish Academy of Sciences. Stockholm. Retrieved May 2010 from www.nobelprize.org

[155] Krebs, H. and Henseleit, K. (1932). Studies on urea formation in the animal organism. Hoppe-Seylers Z. Physiol. Chem., 210:33-66.

[156] Krebs, H. and Johnson, A. (1937). Metabolism of ketonic acids in animal tissues. Biochem. J., 31:645-660.

157 Nobel Prize Foundation. (1953). The Nobel Prize in Chemistry 1953. Royal Swedish Academy of Sciences. Stockholm. Retrieved May 2010 from www.nobelprize.org

158 Cori, C. and Cori, G. (1929). Glycogen formation in the liver with d- and l-lactic acid. Journal of Biological Chemistry, 81:402.

159 Bernard, C. (1855-1856). Leçons de physiologie expérimentale appliqué à la médicine. 2 volumes. Paris, J. B. Baillière.

160 Nobel Prize Foundation (1947). The Nobel Prize in Physiology or Medicine 1947. Royal Swedish Academy of Sciences. Stockholm. Retrieved May 2010 from www.nobelprize.org

161 Nobel Prize in Chemistry. (1911). Nobelprize.org. Nobel Media AB 2014. Web. 7 Jun 2018. http://www.nobelprize.org/nobel_prizes/chemistry/laureates/1911/index.html

162 Nobel Prize in Chemistry. (1935). Nobelprize.org. Nobel Media AB 2014. Web. 7 Jun 2018. http://www.nobelprize.org/nobel_prizes/chemistry/laureates/1935/

163 Kennedy, E. and Lehninger, A. (1947). Oxidation of fatty acids and tricarboxylic acid cyclic intermediates by isolated rat liver rnitochondria. J. Biol. Chem., 172:847-848.

164 Lehninger, A. (1964). The mitochondrion: molecular basis of structure and function. New York: W.A. Benjamin, Inc.

165 Lehninger, A. (1965). Bioenergetics: the molecular basis of biological energy transformations. New York: W.A. Benjamin, Inc.

166 Lehninger, A. (1978). Biochemistry: the molecular basis of cell structure and function. New York: Worth Publishers.

167 Royal Swedish Academy of Sciences (1978). Press Release October 17, 1978. The Nobel Prize in Chemistry 1978. Stockholm: Sweden. Retrieved May 2010 from www.nobelprize.org.

168 Rall, T, Sutherland, E., and Berthet, J. (1957). The relationship of epinephrine and glucagon to liver phosphorylase. IV. Effect of epinephrine and glucagon on the reactivation of phosphorylase in liver homogenates. Journal of Biological Chemistry, 224(1):463-75.

169 Sutherland, E. and Rall, T. (1957). The properties of an adenine ribonucleotide produced with cellular particles, ATP, Mg+++, and epinephrine or glucagon. Journal of the American Chemical Society, 79:3608.

170 Rall, T. and Sutherland, E. (1958). Formation of a cyclic adenine ribonucleotide by tissue particles. Journal of Biological Chemistry, 232(2):1065-76.

171 Sutherland, E. and Rall, T. (1958). Fractionation and characterization of a cyclic adenine ribonucleotide formed by tissue particles. Journal of Biological Chemistry, 232(2):1077-91.

172 Sutherland, E. and Cori, C. (1951). Effect of hyperglycemic-glycogenolytic factor and epinephrine on liver phosphorylase. Journal of Biological Chemistry, 188(2):531-43.

173 Rodbell, M., Birnbaumer, L., and Pohl, S. (1969). Hormones, receptors, and adenylcyclase activity in mammalian cells, in: The Role of Adenyl Cyclase and Cyclic 3'5'-AMP in Biological Systems (T. W. Rail, M. Rodbell, and P. Condliffe, eds.), Fogarty International Center Washington, 59-76.

174 Nobel Prize Foundation. (1971). The Nobel Prize in Physiology or Medicine 1971. Royal Swedish Academy of Sciences. Stockholm. Retrieved May 2010 from www.nobelprize.org

175 Perutz, M., Rossmann, M., Cullis, A., Muirhead, H., Will, G., and North, A. (1960). Structure of myoglobin: A three-dimensional Fourier synthesis at 5.5 angstromresolution, obtained by x-ray analysis. Nature, 185:416–422.

176 Kuhn, T. (1970. The Structure of Scientific Revolutions. 2nd Edition. Chicago: University of Chicago Press.

177 Perutz, M. (1994). Living molecules. Address at Cambridge University November 24, 1994. Cambridge, UK.

178 Kendrew, J., Dickerson, R., Strandberg, B., Hart, R., Davies, D., Phillips, D., and Shore, V. (1960). Structure of myoglobin: A three-dimensional Fourier synthesis at 2 angstrom resolution. Nature, 185:422–427.

179 Nobel Prize Foundation. (1962). The Nobel Prize in Chemistry 1962. Royal Swedish Academy of Sciences. Stockholm. Retrieved May 2010 from www.nobelprize.org

180 Bloch, K. (1950a). The intermediary metabolism of cholesterol. Circulation, 1:214-219.

181 Bloch, K. (1950b). The biological conversion of cholesterol to prenanediol. J. Biol. Chem., 157:661-666.

182 Nobel Prize Foundation (1962). The Nobel Prize in Chemistry 1962. Royal Swedish Academy of Sciences. Stockholm. Retrieved May 2010 from www.nobelprize.org

183 Nobel Prize Foundation (1980). The Nobel Prize in Chemistry 1980. Royal Swedish Academy of Sciences. Stockholm. Retrieved May 2010 from www.nobelprize.org

184 Nobel Prize Foundation (1958). The Nobel Prize in Chemistry 1958. Royal Swedish Academy of Sciences. Stockholm. Retrieved May 2010 from www.nobelprize.org

185 Champe. P. and Harvey, R. (1987). Lippincott's Illustrated Review in Biochemistry. Philadelphia: Lippincott, Williams and Wilkins.

186 Ferrier, D. (2017). Lippincott's Illustrated Reviews: Biochemistry (7th edition). Philadelphia: Lippincott, Williams, and Wilkins.

[187] Nobel Prize Foundation. (1993. The Nobel Prize in Chemistry 1993. Royal Swedish Academy of Sciences. Stockholm. Retrieved May 2010 from www.nobelprize.org

[188] Nobel Prize Foundation. (1994). The Nobel Prize in Physiology or Medicine 1994. Royal Swedish Academy of Sciences. Stockholm. Retrieved May 2010 from www.nobelprize.org

[189] Nobel Prize Foundation. (1997). The Nobel Prize in Chemistry 1997. Royal Swedish Academy of Sciences. Stockholm. Retrieved May 2010 from www.nobelprize.org

[190] Nobel Prize Foundation. (1999). The Nobel Prize in Chemistry 1999. Royal Swedish Academy of Sciences. Stockholm. Retrieved May 2010 from www.nobelprize.org

[191] Nobel Prize Foundation. (2003). The Nobel Prize in Chemistry 2003. Royal Swedish Academy of Sciences. Stockholm. Retrieved May 2010 from www.nobelprize.org

[192] Nobel Prize Foundation. (2006). The Nobel Prize in Chemistry 2006. Royal Swedish Academy of Sciences. Stockholm. Retrieved May 2010 from www.nobelprize.org

[193] Nobel Prize Foundation. (2009). The Nobel Prize in Chemistry 2009. Royal Swedish Academy of Sciences. Stockholm. Retrieved May 2010 from www.nobelprize.org

[194] The Nobel Prize in Chemistry 2012. Nobelprize.org. Nobel Media AB 2014. 8 Jun 2018. Retrieved from http://www.nobelprize.org/nobel_prizes/chemistry/laureates/2012/

[195] The Nobel Prize in Chemistry 2015. Nobelprize.org. Retrieved from https://www.nobelprize.org/prizes/chemistry/2018/prize-announcement/

[196] The Nobel Prize in Chemistry 2018. Nobelprize.org. Retrieved from https://www.nobelprize.org/prizes/chemistry/2018/summary/

Chapter 5

Medical Psychology

Definition.

Medical psychology is the "… application of psychological principles to the practice of medicine for both physical and mental disorders…" (2013)[1]. Others define medical psychology simply as "… the branch of medicine dealing with the diagnosis and treatment of mental disorders…" (2013)[2].

Most accredited medical schools located within the United States, Canada, Caribbean, and Europe extend the definition. In addition to instruction in the diagnosis and treatment of mental disorders, many medical schools now include instruction in bioethics, medico-legal issues, biostatistics, epidemiology, normal human growth and development, and more, all under the rubrics of medical psychology.

The medical psychology course is typically taught during the first two years of medical school, during the Basic Sciences phase of a student's medical education and is often termed Behavioral Sciences. This general and broadly encompassing term allows flexibility within the curriculum and provides faculty more leeway in regard to specific content material they choose to emphasize during a semester. No matter what it is called in the curriculum, the course content remains similar and recognition of the importance of content and process knowledge in these areas remain essential to the education and training of every well prepared physician. Today, more than ever, medical schools are placing increased emphasis on medical students learning, understanding, and applying fundamental clinical content knowledge and concepts of medical psychology.

Introduction.

This chapter explores the historical development of medical psychology from its earliest beginnings as practiced by the ancient civilizations of Mesopotamia, Egypt, and Greece to its current state today, as practiced by modern Western medicine. Emphasis is placed upon the development of medical psychology as a professional and scientific discipline. Particular attention is devoted to developing an understanding of the fluid conceptual matrix used across time to think about, diagnosis, treat, and manage the conditions today we described as mental illness. Influential people whom have shaped the discipline throughout history are briefly presented, along with milestone discoveries, and changes in conceptual matrixes which have led us to our current knowledge base and the way in which we understand and practice medical psychology today.

History.

Early Records, 3500 BC - 500 BC.

The written records of the ancient civilizations of Mesopotamia (circa 3500 BC), ancient Egypt (circa 3200 BC), Babylonia - present day Iraq (circa 2000 BC), and ancient Greece (circa 500 BC) reveal a rich history of the early beginnings of medical psychology (circa 1500 BC,1923, 2005)[3,4,5].

The earliest written records contain evidence of man's long standing interest in the relationships between mental processes and behavior. Of particular interests to most and perhaps surprisingly well documented, are when normal relationships between mental processes and behavior become disordered. Since the beginning of recorded history, man has observed, documented, and explained conditions in which people think, feel, and relate to others in ways very different from most people.

The ancient civilizations of Mesopotamia, Egypt, and Greece are aware of mental disorders, attempt to understand the underlying etiologies, and provide treatment to individuals whom present with impairments of thought, mood, affect, or behavior (circa 1500 BC,1923,2005)[3,4,5].

Impairments are thoughtfully recorded into the written records of each ancient civilization and preserved in the form of fired clay tablets, stone tablets, steles, and papyri. The recordings attest to the importance placed upon these conditions by the Ancients and allows for the passing of knowledge to successive generations. Entries typically include a brief description of the clinical presentation, recommended treatment, and a prognosis. Occasionally, a brief statement regarding the suspected underlying etiology is appended to the brief descriptions.

Signs and symptoms are interpreted within the matrix of physical (natural) and deity/spirt (supranatural) models. All abnormal signs and symptoms are interpreted to be the result of impaired physical body functions and impaired physical body functions are the result of supranatural interventions. No distinction is made between mental, physical, or behavioral disorders. Individuals present either with normal (healthy) function or impaired (disordered) function. This is a truly an elegant system. The system eliminates the artificial dualism (functional vs organic) subsequently imposed by modern systems.

Translation of cuneiform inscribed, medical clay tablets, dated circa 3500 BC to 1600 BC reveal the ancient civilizations are aware of and differentiate between normal and abnormal functions. The written record is replete with entries describing impairments in the form, content, and processes of thought (thought disorders); impairments in the range, duration, intensity, reactivity, and context of mood or affect (mood and affect disorders); impairments in sensation and perception (hallucinations and illusions); in behavior (compulsions, impulsiveness, self-mutilation, suicide); in cognition (delirium, dementias, amnesias); and in substance use (dependency, abuse, withdrawal). Each is considered within a conceptual matrix which identifies the condition as functionally debilitating, significant deviation from normal, resulting from impaired physical body function, and attributed to supranatural entities (gods, ghosts) intervention. Recommended management and treatments are empirically based and conceptualized within a rational matrix which attributes all disturbances in body health to supranatural forces (2005)[5].

Ebers Papyrus (circa 1550 BC) an approximate 110 page scroll, measuring in length of approximately 20 meters, written in hieratic Egyptian (a cursive writing system which develops alongside the hieroglyphic system), is currently housed in the library at the University of Leipzig, Germany and offers one of the oldest records describing depression, anxiety, and dementia. Specific examples are found within the Papyrus's Book of Hearts; "…when his heart is afflicted and has tasted sadness, behold his heart is closed in and darkness is in his body because of anger…"; "…when the heart is sad…vessels of the heart are closed…" (circa 1550 BC/1930)[6].

The heart throughout history always plays a central role in understanding and explaining emotional reactions. Still today, you are likely to hear such colloquial expressions as "…he suffers from a broken heart….", "…he carries a heavy heart…", "…he died from a broken heart…", "…his heart is filled with sadness…", "…she tore his heart apart…", "…her heart is filled with joy and happiness…", "…he has a big heart…". Similarly, the heart throughout history is colloquially referenced to be involved in specific cognitive functions, such as "…she knows the lyrics to this song by heart…" or "... she has memorized and can recall all of the bones in the hand and wrist by heart…". These colloquial references have their basis in the early beliefs of the ancient civilizations which pair emotions and cognitive processes with the heart.

The historical written records reveal the Ancients consider the heart to be a vital reservoir from which the body draws life sustaining substances e.g. moisture, air, nutrients. These vital substances are distributed from the heart throughout the body by way of a unidirectional complex of vessels. Within this conceptual matrix, impairment of the central vital reservoir (heart) or its distribution system (vessels) readily explains most all signs and symptoms associated with impaired physical body functions, including disorders in cognition, thought, mood, affect, and behavior.

The ancient Egyptian civilization (circa 1500 BC) considers the heart essential for life and good health, in the physical world and is equally important and necessary in the afterlife, following physical death of the body. Unlike other essential body organs typically removed during the ritualistic preparation of the body for burial and commonly placed in four canopic jars carved from limestone or clay and buried alongside the body e.g. stomach, intestines, lungs, and liver, the heart is left intact inside of the body. Organs considered less important and less necessary in the afterlife e.g. the brain, are removed and discarded before burial.

Kahun Papyrus (circa 1800 BC) actually a collection of Egyptian texts rather than a single papyrus, offers an additional and perhaps earlier written record of knowledge of the ancient Egyptian civilization. Similar to the Ebers Papyrus, the Kahun Papyrus reveals impairments of cognition, thought, mood, affect, and behavior are considered to be signs and symptoms of underlying physical pathology within the physical body. Relief from these signs and symptoms necessitates identifying the physical pathology within the body and subsequently treating the pathology with a recommended course of interventions, which oftentimes includes a combination of topical application and ingestion of herbals, modification of the person's physical environment, and a recitation of a recommended incantation to complement physical treatments.

Ebers Papyrus (circa 1550 BC) reveals the ancient Egyptians share a common belief with the Ancients of Mesopotamia, in that both civilizations recognize, identify, conceptualize, diagnose, and treat "mental disorders" as physical disorders. Signs and symptoms characterizing impairments in cognition, thought, mood, affect, and behavior are viewed as just another manifestation of impaired physical body function and are conceptualized within matrix of impaired physical body function. Effectively treat the underlying physical pathology, signs and symptoms will resolve and the person will return to a state of good physical health without impairments in cognition, thought, mood, affect, or behavior. Ineffectively treat the underlying physical pathology, signs and symptoms will not resolve and the person will require continuing compassionate management (circa 1550 BC,1930 AD)[6].

Ancient civilizations keenly recognize the therapeutic value of combining physical treatments with non-physical treatments (e.g. incantations). Additionally, these civilizations recognize the positive therapeutic value of administering interventions within the matrix of culturally defined belief systems. There is no evidence from the written historical record, impairments in cognition, thought, mood, affect, or behavior are ever associated with social stigma, during the period of the ancient civilizations. This mind set, stigma associated with mental impairments, must await the founding and development of organized religions.

The ancient Greeks introduce a conceptual model which explains impaired physical health and associated signs and symptoms of impaired cognition, thought, mood, affect, and behavior circa 525 BC. The model embraces the mathematical relationships, observed and proposed, which exist between diametrically opposing forces. The model reflects the philosophical conceptualization proposed by several pre-Socratic Greek philosophers, emphasizing physical nature and society exists within the matrix of opposites e.g. single-plural, movement-motionless, male-female, straight-crooked, dark-light, healthy-unhealthy, hot-cold, wet-dry, left-right, love-hate, peace-war, good-bad. Illness results from an imbalance of opposing natural forces. The ratio between physical forces can be measured and treatments prescribed to return ratios to their normal balances. The same conceptual model is used to explain variability among people and their personalities.

Trivia: The term "pre-Socratic" describes the Greek based belief systems of natural (physical) philosophers, first described prior to the birth of Socrates (470 BC), emphasizing a rejection of mystical explanations in favor of natural (physical) explanations for disease and illness. The term is popularized by Herman Diels (1848-1922) in his scholarly publication, "Die Fragmente der Vorsokratiker" [The Fragments of the pre-Socratics] (1903,1948)[7,8].

Let's take a brief look at two influential people, during the pre-Socratic period circa 550 BC, whom are instrumental in establishing early conceptual matrixes and shaping the history of medical psychology for the next 2,500 years.

Pythagoras (582 BC-510 BC) of Samos (Greek island located in the eastern Aegean Sea) exemplifies the pre-Socratic philosophers and conceptualizes nature within the matrix of dynamic balances of opposing forces. He is among the first to offer a rational conceptual matrix which attributes disturbances in mental functions and behavior to be the result of imbalances in natural (physical) forces. The Pythagorean model offers guidance as to how one might prevent illness by modifying one's lifestyle to incorporate a vegetarian diet, daily meditation, daily physical exercise, organized and structured daily routines, residence in a healthy climate, and maintain belief systems which positively resolve imbalances in social, legal, and political systems which impact the individual.

Pythagoras emphasizes the natural (physical) basis of impaired mental functions; offers a rational conceptual matrix within which to understand normal and impaired mental functions; searches to identify mathematical relationships present within impaired health e.g. periodicity of fevers and associated impairment in mental functions accompanying malaria and the ratio of body fluids necessary for good physical health; applies number theory to medicine whenever possible; and is tremendously influential in guiding the philosophical perspective of medicine, as medicine is being taught at the medical school in Croton, Italy. Croton is a much respected Greek colony and international center of learning.

In regard to treatment for individuals presenting with impairment of mental functions e.g. impairment in cognition, thought, mood, affect, or behavior, the intervention is driven rationally by the conceptual matrix outline above. Simply stated, the goal of treatment is to restore balance. Specific treatments incorporate practices to reduce stress by establishing a calming, relaxing environment, often incorporating calming music, complemented with ingestion of calming herbs. Building upon the mathematical relationships between musical tones and their recognized calming effect upon people, Pythagoras encourages the use of music to help restore disordered harmonies within a person. Notice Pythagoras recommends the use of music as a therapeutic intervention not based solely upon empirical observation that music can be calming, but rather upon a rational application of mathematic ratios, designed to restore proposed disordered harmonies existing within the individual.

Alcmaeon of Croton (southern coastal Italy) (557 BC-491 BC) pre-Socratic natural philosopher, contemporary of Pythagoras, and proponent of the Pythagorean model expands the fundamentals of this conceptual matrix. Alcmaeon believes, as do most others of the period, impairment in cognition, thought, mood, affect, or behavior is the result of physical impairments, centered within the physical body, and are to be understood and treated just as any other physical disorder. Impairment in the physical body can best be understood within a conceptual matrix of disordered harmonies present within the body. Disease is the result of imbalance or disharmony of opposing physical forces, within the body e.g. hot-cold, wet-dry. The goal of treatment is to restore the equilibrium of internal harmonies. If successfully accomplished, the body will return to good physical and emotional health.

Alcmaeon of Croton, born approximately 25 years after Pythagoras, embraces the Pythagorean model of mental functions. He develops the conceptual matrix which considers mental functions to be of natural (physical) origins and best understood within a model of movement and balance of body fluids. Body fluid and associated forces can be mathematically calculated and adjusted as necessary, whenever impairment in mental functions present. He openly challenges medical dogma, proposing the brain rather than the heart to be the physical center controlling balances between opposing physical forces; introduces the concept and emphasizes the importance of inter-individual variability whenever providing treatment; and advocates the use of empirical investigations to evaluate all rationally generated conceptual models in order to ensure a solid foundation of new knowledge. Alcmaeon like Pythagoras is influential in guiding the philosophical perspective of medicine, as medicine is being taught at the medical school in Croton, Italy.

Alcmaeon builds upon the Pythagorean model, develops it further, and introduces his own unique ideas. Alcmaeon's new ideas challenge medical and scientific dogma. Three of Alcmaeon's ideas particularly impact medical psychology for the next 2,500 years.

Specifically, Alcmaeon is first to introduce the conceptual idea of individual variability. That is, while everyone possesses natural, opposing forces within the body and these forces need to remain in balance to maintain good physical health, there exists natural variability between people. Medical interventions must be adjusted to accommodate the individual variability which naturally exists between people. This is a nontrivial observation. All people are not the same. Any intervention therefore necessitates consideration of natural (physical) variability between individuals (circa 500 BC,1952)[9].

Second, Alcmaeon directly challenges existing dogma that the heart is the physical center of life. He proposes instead, the brain. He offers new and compelling empirical evidence to substantiate his claim, offering anatomical dissection evidence, demonstrating the physical connection between brain and body. He rationally applies this empirical anatomical evidence to support his contention the brain is the governing faculty of the body, the anatomical location for balancing natural (physical) opposing forces, and the anatomical location and source of conditions today we refer to categorically as mental disorders e.g. disorders in thought, cognition, mood, affect, or behavior (circa 500 BC,1879,1983)[10,11].

Third, Alcmaeon is influential in establishing investigative methodologies which impact most Greek sciences. He advocates the use of empirical investigations, as essential and necessary complements to all rational conceptual models, to insure a solid foundation of new knowledge (circa 500 BC,1965,1965)[12,13].

In sum, since the time of the first written record, there is persuasive evidence civilizations are aware some individuals experience impairments in cognition, thought, mood, affect, and behavior. These individuals require the attention of society. Civilizations have always acknowledged a social responsibility to provide assistance to individuals unable to care for themselves, as a consequence of illness or disease. So too is the case for individuals whom suffer from impairments in cognition, thought, mood, affect or behavior. Given early civilization conceptualize "mental disorders" as constellations of signs and symptoms of physical illness or disease, society establishes policies and procedures to manage individuals unable to normally participate in society as a consequence of illness or disease.

Abnormalities observed in cognition, thought, mood, affect, and behavior are routinely recorded into the written record, acknowledging their importance in the presentation of impaired physical health. Organized conceptual matrixes are proposed and refined. Early models offer structural organization to repeated empirical observations, a rationally derived theoretical framework from which to understand suspected causes, and offer rational, theory driven guidance for treatments. Ancient civilizations recognize the therapeutic value of combining physical treatments (eat this herb and drink this potion), with management of the individuals physical environment (spend time in a relaxing, healthy, stress free environment, with good air, good food, and good climate), and complementing physical treatments and environmental controls with therapeutic incantations or instructions drawn from a familiarity with the individual's culturally defined belief system.

By mid-500s BC models emphasize mathematical relationships between opposing physical forces which occur naturally in nature. When the normally balanced ratio between two opposing forces becomes unbalanced impaired health is the result. Physical forces are measured and ratios calculated. Treatments are designed to return harmony and balance to unbalanced natural forces.

Commonalities shared among early models are summarized by understanding observed impairments in cognition, thought, mood, affect, or behavior to be the resultant product of impaired physical bodily functions. Impairments in cognition, thought, mood, affect, or behavior are interpreted as signs and symptoms, just like fevers, chills, sweats, aches, and pains. Impairments of mental functions are rationally treated by treating the underlying physical impairment. Notice here, these early models do not differentiate between mental and physical disorders, they are one of the same.

The ancient civilizations of Mesopotamia, Egypt, and Greece and pre-Socratic Greek natural philosophers lay the foundations upon which all future understanding of normal and abnormal cognition, thought, mood, affect, and behavior will build. Their models are simply elegant and provide insight into how they conceptualize and treat "mental disorders".

Do their models seem similar to models used today, now over 5,000 years later? Is it useful to conceptualize "mental disorders" as signs and symptoms of underlying physical disorders? Did the ancient civilizations and pre-Socratic natural philosophers have it right from the very beginning?

Antiquity, 500 BC - 500 AD.

Antiquity witnesses radical changes in the conceptual matrixes within which mental disorders are understood, diagnosed, and treated. Early models emphasize natural (physical) causes and treatments, which remain consistent with the models of the ancient civilizations of Mesopotamia, Egypt, Babylonia, and Greece. Later models of Antiquity reject and displace traditional early models and instead emphasize supranatural (deity) causes and treatments. The two models build their conceptual matrix upon two diametrically opposite suppositional and anchoring foundations. They share in common the use of an organized, conceptual, theoretical matrix. Each conceptual matrix explains the primary cause, maintenance, guides diagnosis, treatment, and management.

Early-Antiquity models emphasize a physical (natural) cause for impairments in thought, cognition, mood, affect, and behavior. Diagnostic and prognostic statements are based upon empirical observations, systematically documented, and integrated over time. Treatments are rational, guided by conceptual matrixes and emphasize restoring the physical body to balanced natural forces and good physical health.

Models of early-Antiquity emphasize balance of opposing natural physical forces e.g. the balance of the four fundamental elements, Earth, Air, Water, and Fire as proposed by Empedocles; the balance of body humors e.g. blood, phlegm, black bile, yellow bile as extended by Hippocrates; or the flow of atoms through the body as proposed by Leucippus and developed by Democritus.

Mid-Antiquity models build upon the models of early-Antiquity and introduce abstract constructs such as the immortal soul and God into the equations. Additionally, social, economic, cultural, and environmental factors are introduced into the models, by influential Greek philosophers Socrates, Plato, and Aristotle. These abstract constructs explain much of the unexplained variance unaccounted for in the balance of natural forces, balance of humors, or atomic models alone. Their introduction begin to slow progress in understanding the physical and more specifically the biological foundations of impairments in thought, cognition, mood, affect, and behavior.

Late-Antiquity models embrace newly organized religions e.g. Judaism and Christianity. Organized religions emphasize divine (supranatural) causes rather than physical (natural) causes. Mental disorders are understood to be the product of divine interventions. Type and severity of the disorder are selected and sent by an angered supranatural entity (God). Mental disorders are considered to be punishment imposed upon an individual, often as the result for failing to follow the rules, beliefs, and teachings of organized religion. Treatments are based upon appeasing the angered deity. Most often treatments necessitate public acknowledgment and acceptance of the teachings, beliefs, and governing rules of the organized religion, before God will return the individual to good mental health. Physical (natural) models are relegated to a secondary position in favor of deity (supranatural) models.

Existing in parallel with the three dominant models outlined above is an additional model embraced by the Asclepiad temples. This is a hybrid model emphasizing physical (natural), divine (supranatural), and socio-economical-cultural-environmental explanations of mental disorders. Treatments are rational, multifaceted, and directed to returning a person's physical and mental health to harmony. This model first appears during early-Antiquity and remains popular throughout all Antiquity.

Let's now take a look at a few specifics.

Empedocles (495 BC-435 BC) of Agrigento (southern coastal Sicily), Greek pre-Socratic natural philosopher, builds upon the Pythagorean and Alcmaeonean models presented earlier. Empedocles also explains mental disorders within the conceptual matrix of impaired equilibrium between naturally opposing forces. More specifically, Empedocles introduces his conceptual matrix of four permanent, indestructible, unchangeable elements, termed Earth, Air, Fire, and Water, which are periodically united and then again separated by opposing physical forces termed Love and Strife. It is the interaction of these four essential elements and two modulating physical forces which determines normal and abnormal thought, cognition, mood, affect, and behavior. Imbalance among the elements or forces produce pathology. Treatment is directed to restoring balance and harmony among the elements and modulating forces within the physical body.

Unique to Empedocles' model is emphasis upon the ratio of elements and modulating forces rather than upon their absolute quantity, quality, or anatomical location. Mental disorders are the natural physical product of disordered ratios occurring among the four elements and two modulating forces. Empedocles commits much time, energy, and other resources to the measurement and calculation of these ratios in efforts to better understand and explain impaired physical functions which result in the presentation of impairments in thought, cognition, mood, affect, and behavior.

Incorporating into his model the concept of "pneuma", the life giving breath of air inhaled by all living organisms, which according to period dogma moves through the body via blood and provides the vital energy necessary for life, leads Empedocles to focus his investigations on blood. Empedocles argues blood contains the perfect balance of elements Earth, Air, Fire, and Water. Any individual presenting with impaired function e.g. impairments in thought, cognition, mood, affect, or behavior should reveal impaired ratios found within the blood. Similarly, impaired ratios found in blood should be associated with impaired function. Hummm…is it possible to identify impairment in normal body function and explain clinical signs and symptoms through thoughtful inspection of blood? Is Empedocles on to something valuable and useful here?

Trivia: Empedocles offers an early model of selective advantage for survival, based upon differences in blood types. Simply stated, individuals presenting with particular blood types, as defined by specific ratios of the constituent elements Earth, Air, Fire, and Water in blood are more likely to survive than others. Particular blood types offer a biological selective advantage for survival. Empedocles model of biological selective advantage predates Charles Darwin's much more familiar model of Natural Selection by more than 2,300 years (1859)[14].

Hippocrates (460 BC-377 BC) of Cos (Greek island located in the Aegean Sea between Greece and Turkey), Greek itinerate physician and founder of the Hippocratic (Coan) School of medicine, offers a modified version of the established balance models to conceptualize mental disorders. Hippocrates conceptualizes mental disorders as having natural (physical) rather than supranatural (deity) etiologies. He emphasizes the need to understand the relationships of four body humors, specifically blood, phlegm, yellow bile, and black bile, in order to explain pathologies and rationally guide treatments. When humors are imbalanced, pathologies will appear. When humors are returned to balance, good health returns (circa 400 BC,1839-1861,1849)[15,16].

Specifically in regard to mental disorders, Hippocrates considers mental disorders to be the result of excess bile. Within the conceptual matrix of Hippocrates and period dogma, biles are normal body fluids and essential for good health. The spleen produces black bile and the liver produces yellow bile. When biles are produced in excess or when they become unbalanced pathologies develop. The physical excess and imbalance produce the observed impairments in thought, cognition, mood, affect, or behavior. Excess and unbalanced bile disrupts the normal flow of the body's pneuma carried by blood. The disruption prevents sufficient pneuma from reaching the brain and consequently disrupts normal brain functions.

Bad dreams and anxiety result from sudden, transient, unregulated flow of bile to the brain. Excessive amounts, imbalances, or shifts in the quantity and quality of black bile are responsible for the chronic mental disorder Hippocrates terms "melancholia". Excessive amounts, imbalances, or shifts in the quantity and quality of yellow bile are responsible for the acute mental condition Hippocrates terms "frenzy" or "mania".

Treatments are rational, designed to restore balance among the four humors and harmony between patient and their physical surrounding environment. Treatments are based upon the defining presupposition of the Hippocratic (Coan) school of medicine, that nature maintains strong healing forces which will heal the body naturally. The process can be facilitated if equilibrium among the four humors and harmony with the surrounding environment can be restored. Procedures for restoring balance are multiple. For example, modifying diet, increasing daily exercise, residing in more favorable weather locations, and thoughtful use of compounded natural herbs and ingredients, rationally derived and with empirically demonstrated efficacy all assist the body in returning to a state of internal and external balanced harmony. The objective of the physician providing care is to treat the entire individual and not the disease. Restore balance in the patient's physical body and surrounding environment and then the body will heal itself.

Hippocrates and the Coan School of medicine are responsible for identifying, describing, and systematically classifying several conditions, labeled mental disorders. Each condition is interpreted within a rational conceptual matrix. All conditions are described by presenting clinical signs and symptoms, followed by a brief description of the observed course of the condition, followed by recommended treatment and management options, and finally a statement regarding prognosis. All conditions are interpreted within a conceptual matrix emphasizing the natural (physical) rather than supranatural (deity) origin of the disorder, balance of body fluids (e.g. phlegm, blood, black bile, yellow bile), innate opposing physical qualities (e.g. hot-cold, wet-dry), and an holistic assessment of the patient's overall physical, emotional, and environmental condition. Focus is placed upon providing a holistic assessment and treatment of the patient's condition.

Specific conditions committed to the written record by Hippocrates and the period schools are 1) phrenitis (delirium with fever), 2) mania (delirium without fever), 3) melancholia (chronic mental impairment), 4) epilepsy (seizure disorders), 5) hysteria (excess emotion evidenced by women), 6) Scythian disease (transvestitism; a practice common among the Scythians located north of Greece), and 7) insanity following child birth (postpartum depression) (circa 400 BC,1839-1861, 1849)[15,17].

Trivia: The term "hysteria" is derived from an ancient Greek word meaning "uterus" or "womb".

Of the seven specific conditions described, four receive particular attention, are routinely associated with "…madness…", and characterized by impairments in thought, cognition, mood, affect and behavior. These four conditions, phrenitis, mania, melancholia, and epilepsy are briefly presented below by way of example to demonstrate the conceptual matrix applied by Hippocrates and the Coan School, during early-Antiquity, to understand and treat "mental disorders".

Phrenitis (acute; delirium associated with fever) according to the Hippocratic Collections is an illness of the brain (circa 400 BC,1839-1861,1849)[15,18], producing madness (circa 400 BC,1839-1861,1849)[15,19], characterized by confusion (circa 400 BC,1839-1861,1849)[15,20], fever (circa 400 BC,1839-1861,1849)[15,21,22], trembling (circa 400 BC,1839-1861,1849)[15,23], convulsions (circa 400 BC,1839-1861,1849)[15,24], sleeplessness (circa 400 BC,1839-1861,1849)[15,25], wandering speech (circa 400 BC,1839-1861,1849)[15,26], impairment in rational thought (circa 400 BC/1839-1861, 1849)[15,27,28,29] and this condition is typically fatal (circa 400 BC,1839-1861,1849)[15,30,31]. The condition is the result of imbalance in bodily humors, especially bile. Specifically, when bile settles in the upper abdomen next to the phren, this is the source of phrenitis (circa 400 BC,1839-1861,1849)[15,32,33].

Note: "Phren" is an ambiguous anatomical site located in the lower chest, possibly including the lungs, diaphragm, or heart. During early-Antiquity, this anatomical area is considered important in regulating human emotions.

An alternative period explanation for phrenitis is the condition produced when bile and phlegm are made too hot, especially by weather, diet, or internal heat. Heating bile or phlegm makes blood watery, which consequently compromises thought, cognition, mood, affect, and behavior, as compromised blood effects the brain. Patients become deranged and are no longer themselves (circa 400 BC,1839-1861,1849)[15,34].

Trivia: The term "phrenitis" is commonly used in the field of medicine from its earliest use during the Hippocratic period of early-Antiquity (circa 400 BC,1839-1861,1849)[15,41] and well into the mid-1800s AD (1840)[35]. The term then gives way to the now more familiar and substituted terms, "delirium" or "confusion".

Important to the Hippocratic and Coan School models of mental disorders is the idea of causal external forces. For example weather, climate, seasons of the year, and direction of blowing winds all have tremendous impact upon bodily humors balances and consequently health (circa 400 BC/1839-1861,1849)[15,36]. So too in the case of phrenitis. Winter and early spring are periods of the year when phrenitis is most common (circa 400 BC,1839-1861,1849)[15,37].

Prognostic statements consider age and individual constitution of patients important in phrenitis. If your patient is older than 40 years of age and does not recover quickly, the condition is almost always fatal (circa 400 BC,1839-1861,1849)[15,38]. "…Delirium attended with laughter is less dangerous than delirium attended with a serious mood…" (circa 400 BC,1839-1861,1849)[15,39].

Treatments are directed to assisting the body to return to its normal, healthy balance of internal bodily humors and balance with environmental surroundings e.g. weather, seasons of the year, living conditions. Treatments are multi-pronged, often using emetics, diuretics, bloodletting, diet, exercise, and warm soothing baths. All are directed to reducing imbalance of body humors and restoring harmony of the physical body with its physical surroundings (circa 400 BC,1839-1861, 1849)[15,40].

Mania (acute; delirium without fever) results when brain is corrupted by phlegm or bile. Two forms of mania are identified and described. In one form of mania the person is silent and calm (circa 400 BC,1839-1861,1849)[15,41]. This form is attributed to an imbalance in phlegm. In a second form of mania the patient becomes angry, impatient, noisy, restless, excited, cries out during the night and behaves inappropriately (circa 400 BC,1839-1861,1849)[15,42]. This form is attributed to bile, which has been heated, abnormally heating the brain. More specifically, "…those who are mad from phlegm are quite, and do not cry out nor make a noise; but those from bile are vociferous, malignant, and will not be quite, but are always doing something improper…" (circa 400 BC,1849)[43].

Treatments for mania are the same as for phrenitis. Assist the body in returning to its normal, healthy balance of body humors and balance with environmental surroundings e.g. weather, seasons of the year, living conditions. Treatments are administered in combinations, using emetics, diuretics, bloodletting, diet, exercise, mild cooling procedures, and soothing baths.

Trivia: The term "mania" is derived from the Greek word "mainesthai" meaning "to be mad".

Melancholia (chronic; general "madness") is characterized by signs and symptoms similar to and more severe than phrenitis (circa 400 BC,1839-1861,1849)[15,44]. While profound sadness, fear, and anxiety are part of the constellation of signs and symptoms, the writing of Hippocrates focus upon the chronic nature of the condition and its associated "madness", rather than sadness, fear, and anxiety. Additional symptoms noted are aversion to food, sleeplessness, irritability (and) restlessness (circa 400 BC,1839-1861,1849)[15,45]. The condition results when bile and phlegm mix with blood. The person becomes deranged in their thinking and becomes mad; this is melancholia (circa 400 BC,1839-1861,1849)[15,46]. Spring is the time of year melancholia is most common (circa 400 BC,1839-1861,1849)[15,47].

Treatments are directed to assisting the body's return to its normal, healthy, balance of body humors and balance with its environmental surroundings e.g. weather, seasons of the year, living conditions. Treatments are exactly the same as treatments for mania and phrenitis described above. Emetics, diuretics, bloodletting, diet, exercise, mild cooling procedures, and soothing baths are primary to returning the body to internal harmony and harmony with the environment.

Specific recommended treatments for melancholia, useful in reducing surplus black bile, are to have the patient maintain a regular and tranquil life, abstain from excess in all areas of behavior, initiate a vegetarian diet, daily exercise to the point short of fatigue, abstain from all sexual activity, "…purge them freely downward…", and if necessary remove the patient from living with family members (circa 400 BC,1839-1861,1849)[15,48]. Once balance and harmony is achieved, the body's natural healing forces will return the patient to good health, free from impairment in thought, cognition, mood, affect, or behavior.

Trivia: The term "melancholia" is derived from the Greek "melaina" meaning "black" and "chole" meaning bile.

Epilepsy (chronic; seizure disorders) presents in many ways; some "…lose his speech, and chokes, and foam by the mouth, the teeth are fixed, the hands are contracted, the eyes distorted, he comes insensible, and in some cases the bowels are evacuated…the body immediately shivers…" (circa 400 BC,1839-1861,1849)[15,49]. In the case of children, the condition often becomes "…habitual and even increasing if not treated by suitable remedies…the greater part die…" (circa 400 BC, 1839-1861,1849)[15,50].

According to period dogma, epilepsy is a disease sent by the gods. Hippocrates rejects this dogma. He argues epilepsies are the result of natural (physical origins) not supernatural (deity origins), they are specifically the result of impaired brain function, and impaired brain function is the result of blockage of blood vessels by phlegm, which interfere with pneuma (air) reaching the brain, thereby producing seizures and associated symptoms (circa 400 BC,1992)[51]. More specially, the brain is responsible for intelligence, cognition, and movement. Air is inhaled from the surrounding atmosphere, enters the body and travels immediately to the brain, carrying information from the surrounding environment to be interpreted by the brain. The air then moves to the lungs, abdomen, and all part of the body via veins, allowing body parts to move (circa 400 BC,1839-1861, 1849)[15,52]. Epilepsy occurs when the passage of air through the body is blocked. The location of the blockage determines the specific signs and symptoms of clinical presentation (circa 400 BC, 1839-1861,1849)[15,53].

Seizures can be triggered by rapid changes in body temperatures e.g. when the body has "…been heated at the great fire and then the person is brought into cold…or from cold he comes into warmth, and sits at the fire, he is apt to suffer in the same way, and thus he is seized…" (1839-1861,1849)[15,43]. Similarly, in individuals whom have a history of previous seizures "…such a person usually suffers attacks, and is seized with them, in changes of the winds, especially in south winds…" (1839-1861,1849)[15,43]. Each of these risk factors are easily explained from the conceptual matrix emphasizing changes in bodily humors density, balance, and movement thorough the body. Heat decreases density, increase moisture content, and increases flow, whereas cold increases density, decreases moisture content, and obstructs normal flow.

Wind directions also have importance in understanding seizure disorders when considered within the Hippocratic conceptual matrix. In brief, northern winds are favored to southern winds. Southern winds warm and moisten the body, oftentimes changes body temperatures and set into motion the physical conditions which produce seizure activity.

Hippocrates emphasizes hereditary in the presentation of epilepsy. Individuals whom have parents characterize as having "…phlegmatic constitution…" are much more likely to present with epilepsy than individuals having parents with a "…bilious constitution…" (circa 400 BC,1839-1861,1849)[15,43].

Treatment for epilepsy follows the Hippocratic (Coan School) rational models and argues the use of regimen to cure this disease. Physicians must attend to diet, climate, weather, risk factors, and balance of body humors. The principle of opposites is important and applied here. Recall the principle of opposites as applied to treatment simply states; if it is hot cool it; if is cold heat it; if it is dry moisten it; and if it is moist dry it.

Prognosis for the treatment of epilepsy is dependent in part upon the age of the patient. Prognosis for a favorable outcome is best if the seizure disorder first appears during adulthood especially after the age of 40 years. Prognosis for a favorable outcome is worst if the seizure disorder first appears during childhood (circa 400 BC,1839-1861,1849)[15,54].

Hippocrates believes epilepsies are treatable, if the proper regimen is administered. All treatments are based upon an understanding of the physical (natural) body and contributing environmental factors which effect normal body function. The goal is to restore balance of bodily humors and harmony with the surrounding environment. Once balance and harmony are restored, the body's natural healing forces can once again function normally and the patient will return to good health, free from the signs and symptoms of impaired brain functions.

Recommended regimens specifically discourage the use of "…purification, spells, and all other illiberal practice of a like kind…", based upon supranatural (deity) models of disease. For Hippocrates, the underlying causes of epilepsies can best be found in the physical world. Treatments too are best found in the physical world and with emphasis on regimens which best restore the physical body to its normal physical balance.

All four conditions presented above, phrenitis (acute delirium with fever), mania (acute delirium without fever), melancholia (chronic, general "madness"), and epilepsy (chronic seizure disorders) are considered by Hippocrates and the Coan school to result from physical disorders of natural, earthly origins. Hippocrates and the Coan School further argue the observed impairments in thought, cognition, mood, affect, and behavior result ultimately from impairments of brain function. "…Men ought to know that from the brain and the brain only arrive our pleasures, joys, laughter, and jests, as well as our sorrows, pains, griefs, and tears…" (400 BC/1992)[55]. Phrenitis, mania, melancholia, and epilepsy are all conceptualized as brain disorders. Treatments and management are directed to restoring normal brain functions.

Hippocrates extends the balance of four humors model to explain personality traits and associated behavioral characteristics. Knowing an individual's personality type provides useful information helpful to understanding the constellation of signs and symptoms presenting as impaired thought, cognition, mood, affect, or behavior. Knowing the personality type additionally provides useful information which can be used to fine tune treatment interventions and improve prognostic statements.

Hippocrates identifies four principle personality types, based upon careful observations and attributes differences between personality types to differences in the natural (physical) constitutions between people. Specifically, the Choleric personality is characterized as angry and hostile, resulting from an excess increase in yellow bile; the Melancholic personality is characterized as pessimistic and depressed, resulting from an excess increase in black bile; the Sanguine personality is opportunistic and cheerful, resulting from an excess increase in blood; and the Phlegmatic personality is apathetic and indifferent, resulting from an excess increase in phlegm.

Hippocrates' efforts to understand relationships between personality traits and underlying physical differences provide the foundation upon which medical psychology and biological psychiatry will build.

The balance of humors models, in their various permutations, serve as the dominant models from which to investigate and treat mental disorders for the next 2,000 years.

Two notable models are proposed as alternatives to the balance of humors model, during early-Antiquity and receive much attention and support from within the scientific and medical communities. The first model to be discussed is the Atomic model which enjoys brief popularity. The second model to be discussed is the Asclepian model which maintains sustained popularity throughout Antiquity.

Leucippus of Avdera (480 BC-420 BC) (coastal city of Thrace, Greece) and his student Democritus of Avdera (460 BC-370 BC) both natural philosophers and physicists, propose and develop the Atomic model, as an alternative to the balance of physical force models offered by Pythagoras of Samos, Alcmaeon of Croton, Empedocles of Sicily, and Hippocrates of Cos. The Atomic model emphasizes the natural (physical) rather than the supranatural (deity) origin and maintenance of mental disorders. This emphasis is shared by the balance of physical force models. However, the physical processes underlying the development and maintenance of mental disorders are very different.

The Atomic model, as it relates to biology simply states the body is composed of atoms and space between atoms. Atoms are the smallest unit of matter, invisible, solid, and remain in constant motion. Atoms have differing physical properties e.g. shape, smoothness, volume, and weight which determine specific characteristics of all matter e.g. the human body. Recall, the term "atom" literally means "what cannot be cut further". Disease results from the physical obstruction of normal circulation of atoms through pores in the human body (1958,2004,2013)[56,57,58].

The Atomic model introduces the concept of soul. The concept of soul here differs radically from the more familiar conceptualization of soul taught by organized religions towards the end of Antiquity. In the Atomic model, soul is defined as a physical part of the body comprised of fine, smooth, round atoms distributed throughout the body. The function of these atoms, termed the soul, is to put into motion the other atoms inside of the body. Atoms of the soul are constantly renewed by the process of inhalation. In conditions where expiration exceeds inhalation, the atoms of the soul are lost to the atmosphere and death occurs. Atoms of the soul are mortal and are subject to consumption and decay just as any other part of the human body. Changes in mental functions occur as the result extreme changes in body temperature e.g. hot or cold. Excessive heat excites movement of atoms, whereas cold temperatures inhibit movement. Both effect the normal functioning of the body to process sensory information, maintain normal levels of consciousness, and maintain normal cognition.

Treatments of impaired mental functioning are directed to restoring the movement of atoms to normal. Given there is no supranatural (deity) factor in the Atomic model to explain the presence of mental disorders e.g. punishment sent from God or guide treatment e.g. "beat the devil out" of the person to purify the body; treatments are humane in kind and typically characterized by changes to healthier diets, engaging in passive exercises, frequent body massage, and moderate ingestion of wine. Notice all treatments are designed to restore to normal the physical movement of atoms. The Atomic model embraces the concept the body possesses all the power and all necessary elements to heal itself.

The second model introduced during early-Antiquity, as an alternative to the balance of forces model, is the Asclepiad model. The model gains rapid acceptance and remains popular for the next thousand years. The model is first introduced and later developed by lay practitioners, whom offer treatments to the ill and diseased, from remotely located temples of healing. More specifically, these sites are collectively termed Asclepiad temples, in recognition of Greek mythology's god of healing, the son of Apollo, Asclepius and Asclepius' three daughters, Hygieia goddess of health, Iaso goddess of recuperation from illness, and Aceso goddess of the healing process.

Trivia: Asclepius is deified in the Greek culture circa 500 BC.

The Asclepiad model is complex, multi-dimensional, and fluid. It is founded upon the basic premise all illness and associated impairment in function are the result of divine (supranatural, deity) cause and cured by a combination of divine (supranatural) and physical (natural) treatment interventions. More specifically and in regard to impaired function of thought, cognition, mood, affect, or behavior the Asclepiad model attributes cause and cure to the gods of Greek mythology. Maintaining its initial commitment to divine processes the model is modified across time and incorporates many of the dominant principles of contemporary physical (natural) models e.g. Atomic and Balance of humors models.

By the end of Antiquity and before being razed by organized religion e.g. Christianity, Asclepiad temples are well established, enjoy much popularity among the general public, and are readily present throughout the eastern Mediterranean. Often Asclepiads coexist in close proximity with Greek centers of medical learning, such as found at Pergamum (450 BC), Cnidus (420 BC), Cos (420 BC), Athens (420 BC), and Epidaurus (420 BC).

Asclepiad treatments emphasize purification rituals, incorporate psychological techniques of faith healing, and dream interpretations. Individuals suffering signs and symptoms of impairment in thought, cognition, mood, affect, and behavior are routinely treated within the temple compound. Asclepiad temples are typically located in remote regions, away from family, trade, war, commerce, and the stresses of life. They are characteristically located in the most beautiful of country sides, often near mineral springs. Compounds typically contain buildings devoted to thoughtful reflection, deity worship, exercise, performing arts, sports, and dreaming. Throughout Antiquity, Asclepiad compounds are recognized sites of universal asylum.

Trivia: The term "asylum" is derived from the Greek "asylos", meaning that which cannot be seized ("a"= without and "sulon"= right of seizure) (2013)[59]. Any person seeking sanctuary at a site of asylum, places themselves under the protection of the gods and out of secular control.

Individuals seeking treatment at an Asclepiad are comforted, fed well, bathed, massaged, given hypnotic plant based medication, and surrounded by calming music. Individuals are encouraged to exercise moderately during the day, participate in the performing arts theater productions when possible, relax in the stress free environment, and sleep. Sleep plays an important role in the Asclepiad model. It provides opportunity for the body to begin to restore physical health and to dream. Dreaming has much significance and oftentimes is facilitated by opioids (e.g. poppy extracts) and augmented by hallucinogens (e.g. mandrake). Dreams are discussed and interpreted by attending practitioners. Dreams contain tremendous prognostic value and offer the opportunity for divine intervention to effect a cure. Individuals whom seek care and treatment from the Asclepiad are permitted to stay as long as necessary.

Treatments are directed by resident lay practitioners of healing. The practitioners are neither priests nor trained physicians (1921)[60]. One practice, typical of the Asclepiads, which carries symbolic significance to the practice of medicine, is their routine use of non-poisonous snakes. Often snakes are left to crawl the floors of the sleeping rooms of individual seeking treatments. Snakes are additionally handled and part of many of the treatment rituals.

Recall from ancient Greek mythology, snakes symbolize rebirth, transformation, regeneration, and healing. All very positive. This symbolization stands in marked contrast to the symbolism assigned to snakes much later by formal organized religions e.g. Judaism and Christianity. Within these religions, snakes symbolize cunning deception, evil, and Satan (Genesis 3:4-5, 3:22; Revelations 12:9, 20:2). Arguably less positive. The power and positive symbolism of the snake within the Asclepiads are used oftentimes quite effectively in addition to physical interventions to facilitate recovery of function.

Trivia: The Rod of Asclepius is a serpent, entwining a single staff, and carried by the Greek god Asclepius. It is the symbol, historically, most associated with medicine and health care throughout the world. This symbol should not to be confused with the caduceus. The caduceus is the symbol displaying two intertwined serpents, on a single staff, surmounted with wings, and carried by the Greek god Hermes. The caduceus is well recognized as a symbol associated with medicine and health care within the USA. The caduceus is popularized as a symbol of medical practice since the U.S. Army Medical Corp adopts it as its insignia in 1902. These two symbols are oftentimes confused. As a future physician, take time now and know the difference.

The Asclepiad at Epidaurus, located on the east coast of southern Greece, offers additional reassurance to all seeking treatments and cures. The Asclepiad displays engraved tablets and steles for all to see within the compound, chronicling the case histories of individuals whom have sought treatments and have been healed. Perhaps the most representative of these are 70 case histories recorded in engraved marble tablets, and steles recovered from the Asclepiad at Epidaurus, dated circa 400 BC. Each case history list the name of the man or woman seeking treatment, presenting signs and symptoms, and the manner in which the treatment interventions effected a successful cure.

Recent reviews of the engraving strongly suggest they reflect more advertisement of temple healing services and reassuring the hopeful expectations of those seeking treatment than verbatim recordings of successful case histories (1931)[61]. The displayed case histories offer individuals seeking treatment, guided expectations they too will have success in their own treatments. The power of expectation coupled with resources to realize the expectation is well known to those providing care within the Asclepiad model. This construct is effectively integrated into the intervention strategies utilized by the Asclepiad practitioner, often with positive result.

Before leaving our discussion of the Asclepiad model, one note of caution; throughout Greek Antiquity several medical practitioners preface their name with the title Asclepiades. This is a self-assigned, honorary title, implying direct hereditary decent from the Greek god of medicine, Asclepius. Over 20 separate physicians of this period claim the title e.g. Asclepiades of Bithynia (circa 120 BC) and Asclepiades Pharmacion (circa 100 AD)[62,63]. Few if any whom claim the title actually provide services within an Asclepiad temple or embrace the fundamental supranatural tenet of divine intervention as primary to the cause and recovery of illness or disease.

By mid-Antiquity the emphasis upon understanding impairments in thought, cognition, mood, affect, and behavior shifts from physical (natural) bodily processes to a combination of physical (natural) processes, divine (supranatural) interventions, and socio-economical-cultural factors. The soul, previously considered a part of the physical body and intermixed with body humors, is separated from the physical body and assigned immortal status. Greek philosophers, Socrates, Plato, and Aristotle expand the concept of the immortal soul and introduce the foundational framework for a dualistic division between body and soul. Signs and symptoms of impaired mental functioning are now interpreted within the conceptual matrix of a disordered body, soul, or body and soul.

Let's take a closer look at three of the most influential Greek natural philosophers, Socrates, Plato, Aristotle, one oftentimes unrecognized influential Greek physician Asclepiades of Bithynia, and two influential Roman scholars Marcus Tullius Cicero and Galen of Pergamum. All six men contribute to the dynamic conceptualization of impaired mental functions, offer theories within which to organize one's thinking, understand the etiology of mental disorders, and guide treatments, during Antiquity 500 BC-500 AD.

Socrates (470 BC-399 BC) of Athens, Greek, master stonecutter and subsequent philosopher views mental disorders to be gifts from the gods. He argues these gifts should be embraced. No treatment or interventions are necessary or required.

As a philosopher, he offers valuable guidance to all future physicians. Question all truths, especially those which are held as dogma. He embraces the use of rational, critical thinking, and use of questioning to examine that which others tell you to be true or is widely accepted to be true by most others. Reality can be lost in acceptance of commonly held misbeliefs. Socrates offers a word of caution to all who challenge medical dogma. If one challenges the established beliefs of the many, there is oftentimes a weighty professional, political, and personal price to pay. Be prepared to weather much opposition to your novel ideas and never allow opposition to quash well-reasoned ideas (360 BC)[64].

Trivia: The term "philosopher" is derived from the Greek word "phliosophos", meaning sage or one who speculates on truths. Literally "one who loves knowledge"; "philo"= loving, "sophia"= "knowledge or wisdom" (2013)[65]. The exact time period and first person to introduce the term is still debated. Many suggest Pythagoras is first to use the term. Other suggest Socrates or Plato are first. The term first appears in the written record of early-Antiquity, in the writings of Socrates and Plato (circa 360 BC to 380 BC)[66,67].

Plato (429 BC-347 BC) Greek philosopher and student of Socrates, offers an elegant integrated conceptual model to explain impairments in thought, cognition, mood, affect, and behavior. The model incorporates divine intervention, body anatomy, physical forces, balance of humors, and introduces the importance of the contributory influences of social, cultural, and economical factors. He is among the first to propose social, cultural, and economic factors to be important in the development of mental disorders

Plato introduces the concept of the immortal soul as a complement to the mortal soul and offers an early tripartite model of impaired internal control as primary to development of specific mental and behavioral disorders. He is among the first to explore social issues of accountability and responsibility for individuals presenting with impaired mental functions and in particular reference to criminal behavior.

Plato divides the soul into two separate souls (360 BC,1892,1925)[68,69]. One soul is immortal, rational, and is located in the brain. A second soul is mortal, irrational, and located in assorted regions of the body e.g. heart in the case love, passion, fear, and anger. Mental disorders appear when the rational soul of the brain becomes disconnected from the irrational soul located in other regions of the body e.g. heart, liver, stomach, diaphragm, thighs (sic). The disconnection results in excessive sadness, happiness, or uninhibited pleasure seeking behaviors.

Plato explains his logic behind the need for physical anatomical separation of the rational soul (brain) from the irrational soul (heart, liver, stomach, diaphragm, thighs (sic)). The rational soul needs to be segregated from the irrational soul in order to maintain its rule of reason and control. Physical segregation minimizes the powerful forces of emotions spurred by the irrational soul.

Similarly, Plato offers his explanation for the anatomical placement of the lungs and their function. Noting during periods of excited emotions, such as anger, passion, or fear, the heart beats more quickly and forcefully than usual and respiration increases in depth and rate. The lungs are "…placed about the heart as a soft spring, that when passion is rife within, the heart beating against a yielding body might be cooled and suffer less and might thus become more ready to join with passion in the service of reason…" (360 BC/2009)[70]. Physical proximity produces reciprocal influence. In the case of the mortal soul and the immortal soul, independent physical locations and balanced functions are essential to normal emotional and cognitive functioning.

Plato initially accepts the popular balance of four humors model and then proposes a modification. Plato proposes a modified two dimensional model, which offers a physical (natural) dimension to explain impaired mental functions, consistent with Hippocratic dogma, and a divine intervention (supranatural) dimension to explain the original source of all impaired mental impairments. Mental disorders are sent from deities (gods). The specific mental disorder is manifested in a disturbances in the quantity or quality of the four fundamental body humors, which disrupts the normal flow of the humors and consequently the normal flow and movement of the souls through the body. Treatments are directed to restoring balance among the body humors and restoring normal movement of the souls.

Plato subsequently modifies his model again to emphasize the importance of social, economic, and cultural factors, in contributing to the development of mental disorders. He is among the first to emphasize the importance of social, economic, and cultural factors in contributing to the development and maintenance of mental disorders and other physical disorders of the body. He is among the first to associate changes in physical body functions with irrational thoughts and emotions. Thoughts and emotions influence the physical body and the physical body influences thoughts and emotions.

Plato offers one of the first tripartite models based upon balance and control of internal processes as being primary to the development of mental disorders. In brief his model proposes a hierarchical model of control and regulation between "…logical, spirited, and appetitive…" internal forces. The "logical" force offers thoughtfulness and good judgment. The "appetitive" force offers primal urges directed towards maintaining survival e.g. eating, drinking, and sexual reproduction. The "spirited" force works in cooperation with the "logical" force to keep the "appetitive" force in check. The dynamic balance between forces is responsible for normal mental functions. Disruption in the usual healthy dynamic balance results in internal conflict and associated mental distress.

Similar tripartite models appear over 2,000 years later in the history of medical psychology e.g. the psychodynamic model of Freud with the Id, Ego, and Super Ego proposed during the late-1800s and the neuroanatomical models with the cerebral cortex systems, limbic systems, and brainstem systems proposed during the late-1900s. Dynamic balance and controlled regulation are fundamental to all three models. Disturbance in the balance results in impaired mental functions.

Plato maintains a special interest in the study of mental disorders and their role in criminal behavior. Specifically, do patients evidencing signs and symptoms of impaired thought, cognition, mood, or affect commit more crimes against society than other patients? What are the responsibilities of society to people evidencing impaired mental functions? Should society hold these people to the same standards as others who do not evidence signs or symptoms of mental impairment? Should individuals with mental impairments and whom commit crimes be punished similarly to individuals without mental impairments whom commit crimes? Does presence of impaired mental function negate responsibility? These and similar questions continue to be debated today and have no universally agreed answers, over 2,000 years after originally proposed and investigated by Plato.

From a treatment perspective, Plato is a proponent of a combined natural, supranatural, environmental, and humane treatment approach to the treatment of mental disorders. He argues the importance of restoring balance among and within the four bodily humors, attending to the mortal and immortal souls, and use of talk based cognitive therapies. The cognitive therapies are directed to assisting the individual in understanding how thoughts, beliefs, cultural influences, and superstitions can and do contribute to development and maintenance of some mental disorders. Plato offers guidance as to how these beliefs systems might be altered to improve mental and behavioral functioning. Modifying the way one thinks about problems can assist in reducing the intensity and contribute to resolving the emotional and physical distress experienced by some presenting with impairments in thought, cognition, mood, affect, or behavior. According to Plato's model, dream interpretation is another useful treatment tool and is important in complementing physical (natural), divine (supranatural), and environmental treatment regimes. "...The great error of our day in the treatment of human beings is that some physicians separate treatment of soul from treatment of body..." (circa 347 BC/1961)[71].

Trivia: Plato's given birth name is Aristocles. The name is chosen in honor of his grandfather. "Plato" is a nickname, assigned to him as a young wrestler in Athens by his wrestling coach. Plato means "broad" in Greek and perhaps refers to his broad shoulders developed while competing in gymnastic and wrestling competitions (225 AD/1925)[72].

Aristotle (384 BC-322 BC) Greek philosopher and student of Plato offers nothing particularly new or innovative here, with a single important exception; mental disorders only occur within a contextual frame.

Aristotle presents an integrated model, to explain mental disorders, based upon previously proposed popular models, especially models proposed by Alcmaeon, Hippocrates, and Plato. Aristotle's integrated model incorporates both physical (natural) and deity (supranatural) factors as important to the cause, presentation, maintenance, and resolution of all mental disorders. He accepts and incorporates Plato's conceptualization of two souls, one immortal rational and therefore immune from physical disease and one mortal irrational and subject to disease of the physical body. He accepts and incorporates the popular balance of four humors to explain signs and symptoms of impaired mental function. He places particular emphasis on the role of the biles. He accepts and incorporates Plato's ideas regarding the importance of social, economic, and cultural factors in the onset and effective treatment of mental disorders.

Aristotle's model rejects Plato's ideas regarding the conceptualization of three internal forces, logistic, spirited, appetitive and that mental disorders result from internal conflict between emotion and reason mediated by these three internal forces. Aristotle proposes mental disorders can be sufficiently explained by his integrative model and without the unnecessary introduction of the additional tripartite internal forces proposed by Plato.

Aristotle's model does offer one unique element of original contribution. Aristotle introduces the idea mental disorders only occur within a contextual matrix. For example, human cannibalism is reasonably considered a deviant behavior when evaluated against conventional societal norms. A person whom engages in cannibalism, within the social matrix of most civilized societies, can reasonably be argued to be experiencing impairment in mental functions. However, does the exact same behavior, cannibalism, in a different contextual matrix, constitute impairment in mental function, when it is the only option for life survival?

For a dramatic, concrete example demonstrating the fundamental premise of Aristotle's proposition and extracted from the mid-1800s American history, think of the Donner Party. In the winter of 1846-1847 AD a wagon train of Irish-American pioneers from Illinois, on their way to California by way of a new, untested route find themselves trapped by severe weather and snow in the Sierra Nevada. After many members perish from starvation, some members reportedly resort to cannibalism as their only means of survival (1847 AD)[73]. This demonstrates the fundamental point made by Aristotle. Can a behavior within one context be considered irrational and abnormal, while the exact same behavior embedded within a different context be considered rational and reasonable?

What do you think? If you struggle with your answer, be assured you are not alone. The question is still debated over 2,200 years later, in the halls of academia throughout the world today.

Treatments from Aristotle's model are based upon its fundamental premise, mental disorders result from excess emotional excitement. Treatments are directed to releasing excess emotions and controlling the physical environment to reduce exposure to extreme presses and stressors of life. Specific treatments procedures release excess emotions by purging and calming residual emotions by ingestion of moderate amounts of wine and relaxing botanicals. As with Plato, Aristotle embraces the use of talk therapy, directed to modifying cognitions held by individuals seeking treatment and controlling the external environment to produce less stressful surroundings.

Asclepiades of Bithynia (modern-day Bursa, Turkey) (124 BC-40 BC) accepts the Greek fundamental premise mental disorders are the result of physical (natural) processes and are not the result of divine (supranatural) intervention. He directly and passionately rejects the popular balance of four body humors models and offers an alternative based upon atomic models. He is among the first to distinguish between acute and chronic mental conditions, offering a physical explanation for each. He is first to differentiate symptoms of hallucinations, illusions, and delusions. He proposes sub-typing of disorders based upon presumed underlying physical processes responsible for the generation of observed signs and symptoms. He is among the first to advocate for equal access to care for women. Treatments are humane and directed to restoring normal balance and flow of atoms within the body.

Working within his atomic model, Asclepiades of Bithynia conceptualizes acute disease and its associated signs and symptoms of impaired mental functions to result from obstruction of the normal flow of atoms through the body. Obstruction results from either constriction or excess atoms. Chronic disease and associated signs and symptoms of impaired mental function result from relaxation or insufficient numbers of atoms.

Asclepiades explains the underlying physical processes for two conditions, phrenitis and catatonia. Both conditions are the product of impaired flow of atoms through the body resulting from constriction. In the case of phrenitis, it is the constriction of the meninges surrounding the brain responsible. In the case of catatonia, it is the constriction of the skeletal muscles responsible. Impaired flow of atoms to the brain disrupts normal thought, cognition, mood, affect, and behavior.

Treatments are directed to restoring normal atom flow and restoring harmony within the physical body. Specific procedures used to accomplish this are exercise, massage, diet, bathing, exposure to fresh air, exposure to sunlight, use of selected botanicals, herbs, minerals, chemicals, and wine, listening to calming music, and physical manipulation of the immediate surroundings to reduce stresses and demands placed upon the individual. Treatments are offered with kindness and compassion.

Asclepiades specifically rejects use of confinement, physical restraints, or punishment. He rejects the popular Hippocratic premises, nature is benevolent and the role of a physician is to only observe and support, while the body heals itself.

Marcus Tullius Cicero (106 BC-43 BC) philosopher resident of Athens and Rome is often neglected in the history of medical psychology. He writes an influential series of dialogues concerning his personal insights into the origins and treatments of mood disorders. He specifically addresses depression and grief. Rejecting Greek models emphasizing balance of body humors, Cicero proposes mood disorders result from disordered thoughts. He emphasizes the importance of how one thinks about life events, in determining whether a person experience extreme debilitating moods. Cicero is among the first to state explicitly cognitions and mood directly impact physical health. Impaired cognitions and moods contribute to impaired physical health. Cicero proposes any effective treatment of individuals suffering severe impairment in mood necessitates a cognitive based intervention. Change the way in which a person thinks about their life's events and change their mood (45 BC/1877)[74].

The following excerpts are taken directly from Marcus Tullius Cisero's dialogues. In reference to the prevalence and severity of mental disorders of the period, "…there are more disorders of the mind than of the body, and they are of a more dangerous nature…" (45 BC/1877)[75]. In reference the origins of mental disorders and in particularly mood disorders, "…all the disorders and perturbations of the mind precede from a neglect of reason…" (45 BC/1877)[74]. In reference to the prognosis of mental disorders, "…sicknesses and diseases of the mind are thought to be harder to eradicate…" than sicknesses and diseases of the body (45 BC/1877)[74]. Finally, in reference to his recommended cognitive based treatments, "…the emotions of the mind, all griefs and anxieties are assuaged by forgetting them, and turning thoughts to pleasure…" (45 BC/1824)[76].

Times are changing. As the Greek Empire falls and the Roman Empire begins, the conceptual matrix within which mental disorders are understood and treated change. Gone are emphasis on the physical body and empirical investigations. New and revised models, emphasizing supranatural forces, faith based religions, and deity models soon displace the natural (physical) Greek conceptualizations of mental disorders. Conceptualizations and treatments are reinterpreted or changed to accommodate the political influences of the new governing powers, governmental and religious. By mid-Antiquity, society establishes formalized legal and social responsibility guidelines with reference to individuals presenting with impaired mental functions.

Aulus Cornelius Celsus (25 BC-50 AD) Roman encyclopedist, contemporary of Jesus Christ (5 BC-30 AD) summarizes the current state of knowledge of mental disorders, in "De Medicina" (circa 30 AD,1478)[77]. He focuses attention on the Greek balance of humor models and offers modifications to make the models more acceptable to the new Roman Empire. He dogmatically states mental disorders originate from supranatural deities (gods) and specific mental disorders represent a deity's chosen punishment for an individual's transgression(s). Notice Celsus' modification emphasizing supranatural deities. At the time of Celsus' writings, supranatural deities are no longer an element of the Greek models. The Greeks modified their models hundreds of years earlier and removed supranatural causes and replaced them with natural (physical) causes for the origin of all physical and mental impairments.

Trivia: The use of the term "encyclopedist" first appears in 1651 AD (2013)[78].

Consist with the Greek models of the times, impairments in thoughts, cognition, mood, affect and behavior result from impairment in physical body functions. Subtypes of insanity are differentiated upon whether impairments in thought, cognition, mood, or behaviors result during episodes of fever or intoxication (acute confusional states) or as the result of excessive black bile produced by the body (chronic conditions). Second order subtypes are based upon based upon the quality of mood impairment (e.g. depressed, fearful, or anxious), immediate management issues (e.g. easily controlled), and tendency to engage in violent or harmful behaviors. There are "…several sorts of insanity; for some among insane persons are sad, others hilarious; some more easily controlled and rave in words, others are rebellious and act with violence and of these only some do harm…" (circa 30 AD/1935)[79].

Inconsistent with the Greek models, Celsus incorrectly reports the usual and customary treatments employed by the Greeks, in the treatment or management of individuals suffering impairments in mental functions, emphasize punishment. Again, a misrepresentation of the current Greek models and much more in line with the new Roman Empire belief systems.

> "…if it is the mind that deceives the madman, he is best treated by certain tortures. When he says or does anything wrong, he is to be coerced by starvation, fetters, and flogging…to be thoroughly frightened is beneficial in this illness…it also makes a difference if whether from time to time the patient laughs, or is saddened, dejected: for hilarity of madness is better treated by those terrors I have mentioned above. If there is excessive depression, light and prolonged rubbing twice a day is beneficial as well as cold water poured over the head and immersion of the body in water and oils… The following a general rule: the insane should be put to fatiguing exercises, and submitted to prolonged rubbing, and given neither fat meat nor wine; after clearance the lightest food of the middle class is to be used; they should not be left alone or among those they do not know, or among those whom

either they despise or disrespect; they ought to have a change of scene and if the mind returns they should undergo the tossing to travel..." (circa 30 AD/1935)[80].

Areteus of Cappadocia (central Turkey) (30 AD-90 AD) practicing Greek physician, providing care principally in Rome and Alexandria, more correctly describes the conceptual matrix embraced by most practicing physicians and their usual and customary treatments of mental disorders of the period, than is reported by his contemporary, encyclopedist Aulus Celsus, in "De Medicina".

Areteus accepts the traditional Greek balance of humors model; believes mental disorders originate from physical (natural) processes rather than sent from deities (supranatural); is an advocate of the pneumatic school ascribing to the premise a life giving vital force (pneuma) moves through the body by way of the four body humors; is among the first to suggest mental disorders are not localized to specific body organs or body regions; clearly defines mania as a chronic mental disorder separate from acute confessional states (delirium) or acquired impairments of intellectual and cognitive functions of the elderly (dementia); identifies specific risk factors typically associated with mania; is among the first to suggest there are specific subtypes of mania necessitating different treatment interventions based upon the specific subtype; is among the first to note depression frequently appears in the course of mania; recognizes premorbid personality characteristics are often predictive of the subtype of mania; and recognizes premorbid personality characteristics are typically exacerbated and amplified with onset of mania (circa 200 AD/1856)[81].

The following extract from Areteus of Cappadocia writings "On Madness" offer details and exemplifies his fundamental conceptualization of mania and how it differs from delirium and dementia. Mania is

> "...a chronic derangement of the mind, without fever. For if fever at any time should come on, it would not owe its peculiarity to the mania, but to some other incident. Thus wine inflames to delirium in drunkenness, and certain edibles, such as mandragora and hyoscyamus, induce madness, but these affections are never called mania; for springing from a temporary cause, they quickly subside, but madness had something confirmed in it. To this mania there is no resemblance in the dotage which is the calamity of old age, for it is a torpor of the senses, and a stupefaction of the gnostic and intellectual faculties by coldness of the system. But mania is something hot and dry in cause, and tumultuous in its acts. And, indeed, dotage commencing with old age never intermits, but accompanies the patient until death; while mania intermits, and with care ceases altogether..." (circa 200 AD/1856)[81].

Areteus identifies specific risk factors for chronic mental conditions (mania);

> "...those prone to the disease, such as are naturally passionate, irritable, of active habit, of an easy disposition, joyous, puerile; likewise those whoses disposition inclines to the opposite condition, namely, such as are sluggish, sorrowful, slow to learn, but patient in labor, and who when they learn anything, soon forget it; those likewise are more prone to melancholy, who have formerly been in a mad condition...persons are more given to mania, namely thoses about puberty, young men...those in whom heat is enkindled by black bile and whoses from of constitution is inclined to dryness, most readily pass into a state of melancholy..." (circa 200 AD/1856)[81].

Arteaus reports common signs and symptoms of mania;

> "...they are of changeable temper, their senses acute, they are suspicious, irritable without cause...given to insomnolency...very slow in judgment...some cut their limbs in a holy phantasy..." (circa 200 AD/1856)[81].

Treatments of mania follow traditional Greek models emphasizing adjusting diet, participation in moderate exercise, improve personal hygiene, smoothing baths, massage, elimination of excess in behavior, (e.g. sex, eating, drinking) and rational use of herbals, botanicals, minerals, chemicals, and oils. Treatments are compassionate and humane. Similarly, treatments of delirium and dementia follow the traditional Greek models emphasizing humane, compassionate interventions directed to restoring balance of body humors within the body and balance of the body with the surrounding physical environment.

Galen of Pergamum (129 AD-200 AD) arguably one of the most influential figures in medicine, offers little new to the development and understanding of mental disorders. His writings are largely restatements of existing knowledge with little new or original. His writings on mental disorders are fragmented. In light of these limitations, he is a prolific writer on topics of medicine and has tremendous influence in guiding the future of Western European medicine and preferred models used to understand impaired mental function.

Galen offers two primary models within which he explains mental disorders. Both models are essentially restatements of earlier models proposed by other investigators during the past 700 years.

The first model, perhaps most recognized and influential is his balance model. The model is built upon the original ideas of Empedocles (Sicily, circa 460 BC), Hippocrates (Cos, circa 400 BC), Herophilus (Alexandria, circa 300 BC), and Erasistratus (Alexandria, circa 275 BC). This model states impaired mental function is the product of natural (physical) rather than supranatural (deity) cause and process. Impaired mental function is explained based upon anatomy and physiology. Impaired mental function is the result of physical imbalance within or among four body humors; blood, phlegm, black bile, and yellow bile. These four humors are modified by four opposite qualities; hot-cold, wet-dry. Dependent upon which humor is over or under expressed and knowing its associated qualities; signs and symptoms can be understood and appropriate treatments provided.

For example, excess black bile produced by the gall bladder will result in signs and symptoms of melancholia; while excess yellow bile produced by the liver will result in mania. By conceptualizing mental impairments within the matrix of humors' quantity and quality the model guides treatment. For example, melancholia results from excess amounts of black bile (humor) and has the quality of cold and wet (qualities). Treatments follow the rule of opposites. Melancholia necessitates the removal of excess black bile, usually by purging, and warming and drying the body, usually by medications, diet, or manipulation of the immediate physical environment. Mania on the other hand results from excess yellow bile and has the qualities of hot and dry. Mania therefore necessitates the removal of yellow bile and cooling and wetting the body. Again this is accomplished primarily by medication, diet, bathes, and manipulating the immediate physical environment. Again, nothing original or particularly innovative found here. This model is essentially a restatement of the Hippocratic balance of humors model.

The second model, much less recognized and less influential is his two souls model. The model is built upon the original ideas of Plato (Athens, circa 375 BC) that the body contains two souls; one mortal and rational with residence in the brain and another immortal and irrational with residence in the heart or liver. Incorporating the concept of pneuma, originally proposed by Empedocles (Sicily, circa 485 BC), Galen explains impaired mental functions as the result of impaired movement of the souls and pneuma throughout the body via blood and in particular their movement to the brain. This model explains movement of the souls and pneuma by way of a rational, organ system based physiology originally proposed by the influential Alexandrian investigators Herophilus and Erasistratus approximately 500 years earlier.

The model states pneuma (air) is inhaled from the external environment and into the lungs. It moves first into the heart and from there into the liver and brain. Once in the brain, pneuma mixes with the rational soul and provides the essential ingredient necessary for normal brain functions. All mental impairments are the product of brain disorders, resulting either from impaired movement of the souls or pneuma to brain. Treatments are directed to restoring normal brain function by restoring normal flow of the souls and pneuma throughout the body and to the brain.

Galen, one of the most prolific science writers in history, never writes a single treatise devoted exclusively to mental disorders. Our knowledge of Galen's views on this topic are scattered and poorly organized. However, he does comment on several specific disorders common to the period. His comments are largely restatements of known information.

By way of example and summary, Galen acknowledges the need to separate impaired mental functions resulting from fever (phrenitis, aka delirium) from those presenting without fever (mania). He acknowledges severity of mental impairment occurs along a continuum and individuals presenting with the same categorical condition often evidence different signs and symptoms e.g. "…some melancholics want to die…some love solitude…others are convinced they have been turned into animals…" (circa 200 AD)[82]. He comments on the decline in cognitive functions associated with advance age. He offers an alternative to the Hippocratic dogma of a wandering uterus to explain the cause of hysteria. Galen proposes hysteria is the result of toxicity from stagnant semen and is best treated by regular sexual intercourse (circa 200 AD)[82].

Note: The Hippocratic concept of a "…wandering uterus…", frequently reported as the cause of hysteria in women, may have been misinterpreted in translations. Perhaps the translation of a "wandering uterus" is better interpreted as a "moving uterus". This alternative translation might be applied to the observation of a prolapsed uterus. Women presenting with a prolapsed uterus often experience concomitant changes in hormones. Changes in hormones are associated with notable changes in thought, cognition, mood, affect, and behavior. This proposed alternative translation makes sense from an anatomical, physiological, endocrine, and behavioral perspective and is consistent with the observational methodologies applied by investigators of the period.

Galen's recommended treatments for individuals presenting to medical practitioners with disorders of impaired thoughts, cognition, mood, affect, or behavior, offers nothing really new. He recommends, most all which has been recommended during the previous 500 years; a regime to improve diet, improve personal sanitation and hygiene, engage in moderate physical exercise, elimination of extremes and excesses in life, purging as indicated, and thoughtful use of medications. His guiding rule, with regard to rational, theory driven treatments is the application of the Rule of Opposites; e.g. if it is wet dry it, if it is dry wet it, if it is hot cool it, if it is cool heat it. The ultimate goal is to restore balance and flow within the body.

Galen offers little new to understanding mental disorders. However, his prolific writings, authoritative, dogmatic presentation influence the development of medical psychology and treatment of mental disorders for the next 1,500 years. It is only with the critical examination of old ideas, during the European Renaissance, are Galen's conceptual matrixes and dogma seriously challenged by the scientific and medical communities. Perhaps no single individual slows progress in the advancement of medical psychology and the understanding and effective treatments of mental disorders more than Galen.

There is always a price to pay, often a huge price, whenever science or medicine become too confident and dogmatic about its knowledge base. I encourage you as future physicians to continue to thoughtfully question all dogma presented to you by any authority. What are the consequences to science and medicine for not challenging established truths? What are the personal and professional potential consequences and benefits for challenging established truths? Are you willing to accept the consequences?

Antiquity comes to a close with the fall of the Roman Empire. There is a major shift in the conceptual matrix within which mental disorders are understood and treated. Emphasis and popularity quickly moves away from the physical (natural) models embraced by the ancient Greeks and Romans and to the deity (supranatural) models embraced by newly organized religions e.g. Judaism, Christianity, and Catholicism. The role of treating mental disorders shifts from physician to rabbi, minister, and priest.

Organized religions initially struggle with the issue of mental disorders. Having rejected the physical models of the Greeks and Romans, in favor of deity models and effectively shifting the point of control from science and medicine to religion, it is incumbent upon organized religion to offer nonsecular explanations for mental disorders. This proves to be a problem and a point of much debate within the leadership of the Christian based organized religions, from approximately 100 AD to 600 AD.

For example, Christianity initially questions whether those whom hear voices or see visions are communicating with God or Devil. By the early-600s AD the answer is decreed by Church leadership. Mental disorders are sent by God, as the consequence of sinful transgressions committed against God or the Church. The Devil is responsible for all deviant behavior. Marks on the skin are left by the Devil. Cures are effected only by organized religion's intervention, typically in the form of acknowledging sinful transgressions, prayer to supranatural deity, and participating in ritualistic behaviors e.g. wearing amulets, confessing sins to church leaders, and offerings gifts (donations) to the Church.

Progress in the scientific advancement and effective treatment of mental disorders comes to an abrupt pause with the rapid acceptance of organized religions.

In brief sum, Antiquity witnesses an important shift in the way mental disorders are conceptualized and treated. Early models emphasize the natural (physical) influences as most responsible for impaired mental functioning, whereas models appearing by the middle and end of Antiquity emphasize supranatural (deity) influences.

Early models emphasize balance of natural opposing forces such as Earth, Air, Wind, and Fire as proposed by Empedocles; balance of internal body humors blood, yellow bile, black bile, and phlegm as proposed by Hippocrates; and movement of atoms through the physical body as proposed by Leucippus and Democritus. Later models, introduce the concept of soul and moderator variables such as socioeconomics factors, culture, and environment, all which function synergistically with the physical body as proposed by Socrates, Plato, Aristotle, and Galen.

By the end of Antiquity, models which emphasize the natural (physical) basis of impaired mental functioning are displaced by newly founded organized religions, such as Christianity and Catholicism, emphasizing supranatural (deity) models. Throughout all of Antiquity one hybrid model thrives, the model embraced by the Asclepiad temples. Drawing upon a fluid interpretation of both natural and supranatural processes, offering asylum to all suffering, and guidance from the mythical Greek Gods and Goddesses, the model proves extremely influential in the development of the future of medical psychology and psychiatry.

Each of the principal models of Antiquity, while seemingly polar, actually share much in common. They all provide a conceptual matrix within which to understand the origin of mental disturbances; offer a treatment and management approach based upon their preferred conceptual model; and acknowledge the complex interaction of multiple factors contributing to the onset, maintenance, and relief from debilitating impairments in mental functions.

Completion of Antiquity sets the stage for the turbulent times of the Middle Ages to come.

Organized religions soon exert tremendous influence upon the future direction of medical psychology and psychiatry. Conceptual matrixes, methods of investigation, and content of investigations are dictated by the Church. Investigators unwilling to accept the new Church dogma with regard to impaired mental functioning and embrace a supernatural (deity) model are punished. Scientific study of mental processes and associated mental impairments for all intent and purposes stops. Science in Europe is displaced by faith based religion for the next 1,000 years.

Middle Ages (Medieval Times), 500 AD - 1400 AD.

The Middle Ages introduce significant change in the direction and development of medical psychology.

Geopolitical, economic, social, and religious factors have tremendous influences upon the course and development of medical psychology during this period. New geopolitical borders are being drawn, form and organization of government is changing, and newly founded organized religions exert tremendous influence upon the development of new governing bodies, and establish the rules and guidelines upon which European society is based. Organized religion establishes itself as the exclusive authority in identifying and treating all mental disorders. Mental disorders are no longer understood or treated within the matrix of natural (physical) biological systems, but rather in faith based, supranatural deity models defined by organized religion. Science is displaced by religion.

Recall, the Middle Ages are defined by tremendous and chaotic change throughout Europe. The Roman Empire has fallen, eliminating structure and order in society. In absence of structure, people actively seek new structure from almost any available source. Structure provides order, reassurance, confidence, and a sense that all will be well. Organized religions offers the much needed structure and quickly establishes its powerful influence. Organized religions now effectively controls government, the general population, how new knowledge is acquired, and how old knowledge should be understood.

Trivia: The term "Middle Ages" is first introduced approximately 69 years after the end of the Middle Ages and during the early part of the European Renaissance by Giavani Andrea Bussi (1417-1475) Catholic bishop, Italian Renaissance humanist (1469)[83]. The term is subsequently popularized by Georg Horn (1620-1670) German, Professor of History, as one of the three distinct and now familiar primary divisions of time in history; Antiquity, Middle Ages, and Modern Age (1666)[84].

The Middle Ages are often referred to as the "Dark Ages". This term actually appears before the term Middle Ages is introduced. The conceptualization of the "Dark Ages" and subsequently coining the term, is proposed and developed by Italian humanist scholar Francesco Petrarca (1304 AD-1374 AD). He originally proposes the conceptualization of the "Dark Ages" to refer to the period of time immediately following the fall of the Western Roman Empire at the end of Antiquity and before the beginning of the Italian Renaissance (1372)[85]. The "Dark Ages" occurs roughly between 500 AD and 1400 AD. He offers the term "Dark Ages" to emphasize his perception that very few intellectual advances are made during the period relative to the many made during Antiquity.

In fact, only the first half of the Middle Ages is characterized by few intellectual advancements. The second half of the Middle Ages are characterized by many advancements, such as the founding of many early influential universities, medical schools, and centers of learning throughout Western Europe. The term Dark Ages is misleading and fails to accurately describe the totality of this period of time.

The Middle Ages are also frequently referred to as the "Medieval period". This term has its origin in Latin "medium aevum", which simply translates to the "middle ages". This term is first introduced during the 1800s. As future physicians, do take note of the spelling Medieval. A common mistake among the poorly informed is to refer to this period as the Midevil (sic) period. Don't make this common mistake yourself.

OK, back to the history of medical psychology.

Organized religions, Judaism, Christianity, Catholicism, and Islam exert tremendous influence upon how mental disorders are conceptualized and understood. Their influence upon the direction and future development of medical psychology cannot be overstated. Fundamental conceptual matrixes, emphasizing the biological basis of mental impairments and treatments are displaced. New faith based models are substituted in their place. Empirical, systematic, rational investigation of nature (science) is displaced by faith based dogma. Religion replaces science. Mental disorders are aggressively explored from the unique perspectives of the four most influential organized religions of Europe, Middle East, and North Africa. Impaired functions of thought, cognition, mood, affect, and behavior are once again understood within the conceptual matrix emphasizing supranatural deities. Treatment of mental disorders change radically. New treatments reflect the new change in conceptual matrixes. No longer is treatment based upon the secular biological origin of impaired mental function. New treatments are based upon nonsecular origin and religious dogma. The role of physician as primary treatment providers is displaced. This role now becomes the exclusionary domain of rabbi, priests, minsters, and imams of organized religion.

Two distinct courses are charted early for medical psychology during the early Middle Ages. One course begins in Europe and travels into the Middle East and North Africa before returning to Europe, approximately 500 to 1000 years later. The other course begins in Europe and ends in

Europe, during the same 500 to 1000 year time period. Both contribute and have tremendous influence upon the development of medical psychology as a professional discipline and the ways in which mental disorders are conceptualized and treated today, over 1000 years later.

The first track begins with the fall of the Roman Empire and associated mass exit of academics and scholars from established centers of learning. These academics embrace traditional physical models of health e.g. balance of humors models, leave Europe and take refuge in the centers of learning found in the Middle East and North Africa. They take with them many of the original records of ancient Greek knowledge e.g. tablets and papyri. In the Middle East and North Africa, they continue their intellectual pursuits to understand the physical body and associated disorders of thought, cognition, mood, affect, and behavior within the established conceptual matrixes of physical (natural) rather than the new deity (supranatural) models which are quickly gaining acceptance and popularity in Europe. The natural scholars have significant impact upon the development of Middle East and Arabic medicine. After approximately 1,000 years, many of the academics return to Europe, as Europe returns to a more stable political, economic, social, and intellectual place. They bring with them the influences of the Middle East and North Africa and are influential in the scientific development of medicine in Europe.

The second track also begins with the fall of the Roman Empire and academics and scholars whom choose to stay in Europe. While many academics seek intellectual refuge in the Middle East and North Africa in order to maintain their pursuit of physical models to understand and treat the human body, many others remain in Europe. The ones who remain in Europe are heavily influenced by the rapid expansion, popularity, and influence of the new organized religions. Organized religions reject or minimize knowledge generated from physical models in favor of knowledge generated from the organized religions' own, faith-based, supranatural models. The deity, faith-based (supranatural) models dominate Europe throughout most all of the Middle Ages. These models and resultant dogma only begin to be seriously challenged after approximately 1,500 years of use and limited success.

Let's now examine a representative sample of a few of the most influential people of this period, their contributions, major shifts in conceptual matrixes, and how European society defines its responsibilities to any and all presenting with impaired function, attributed to impaired intellectual ability, thought, cognition, mood, affect, or behavior.

First, let us examine the first track which leads academics out of Europe and into the Middle East and North Africa. Ibn Sina and Constantine the African will be discussed specifically as representative of the many who follow this track. Second, let us examine the second track of those whom elect to remain in Europe. Albertus Magnus and Thomas Aquinas will be discussed specifically, as representative of the many who follow this second track.

Ibn Sina (980 AD-1037 AD) Persian encyclopedist, authors a comprehensive summary of medicine, in his five volume encyclopedia titled "Kitab al-Qanun fi al-tibb" [Canon of Medicine] (1025 AD/1930)[86]. There is nothing new here. He essentially restates the knowledge of the ancient Greeks and Galen's Roman modifications with regard to mental disorders, emphasizing the conceptual matrix of balance of elements (earth, wind, fire, water), humors (phlegm, blood, yellow bile, black bile), and qualities (hot, cold, wet, dry), from which to understand cause and treatment of mental disorders. He notes the knowledge base is most supportive of a physical (natural) rather than the alternative deity (supranatural) models of origin. The brain is identified as the primary organ effected and treatments are based upon the Rule of Opposites e.g. if the patient is hot, cool them; if the patient is cold, warm them; if the patient is dry, moisten them; if the patient is wet, dry them. He further notes specific medicinal herbs, botanicals, minerals, and metals have beneficial and therapeutic effects when thoughtfully administer to individuals presenting with impaired mental function. Mental disorders are viewed as signs and symptoms of physical disorders of the body and treated accordingly. Specific symptoms such as delirium, paranoia, melancholia, psychosis, and phobias are specifically addressed. Humane treatment of the insane is specifically recommended.

Ibn Sina offers a second and much less well known manuscript titled "De Anima", in which he describes and discusses the relationship between body and soul (circa 1020 AD/1959)[87]. This treatise is largely a restatement of Aristotle's position and offers nothing new.

Ibn Sina does however make a notable original contribution. He recognizes and documents the relationships between emotional states and the body's predictable physiological responses e.g. change in pulse rate (circa 1035 AD/1951)[88]. His writings on the topic form an early foundation for subspecialty physiological psychology.

Constantine the African (1020 AD-1067 AD) of Carthage (North Africa), further preserves the classic Greek and Roman conceptualizations and writings emphasizing the physical nature of mental disorders. He is perhaps most remembered for his translation of several influential Greek writings e.g. Hippocratic and Galen corpus, originally translated into Arabic after being carried by Greek and Roman scholars into the Middle East upon the fall of the Roman Empire, into Latin and reintroducing the writings back into Europe. He also is influential in establishing the first medical school in Salerno, Italy and contributing to its early curriculum development, emphasizing the natural (physical) rather than supranatural basis of impaired functions.

In regard to mental disorders he embraces the traditional balance of humors model, offers his own detailed description of melancholia, details delusional thinking associated with melancholia, notes acute, reactive episodes of melancholia are much more amenable to treatments than chronic longstanding episodes, and reiterates impairments of thought, cognition, mood, affect, or behavior result from impairment of the brain (De Melancholia). Constantine the African conceptualizes mental disorders as brain disorders.

Ibn Sina and Constantine the African represent the scholars instrumental in preserving traditional Greek and Roman conceptual models from which to understand impaired function. They and their writings are representative of the first track of development, scholars and academics whom leave Europe seeking intellectual refuge in the Middle East and North Africa and later return to Europe.

Scholars choosing to remain in Europe, following the fall of the Roman Empire and whom follow the second track, are greatly influenced by the rapidly expanding and powerful Catholic Church. The Church bases its foundational position on the cause and treatment of mental disorders from faith-based beliefs, described in the writings contained within the Christian Bible.

The Church considers mental disorders to be punishment imposed by the Christian deity (God) and directed against individuals whom fail to follow the rules and teaching of the newly organized Christian religion. By way of example, in the book of Deuteronomy, the prophet Moses (1391 BC-1271 BC) perhaps most remembered for authoring the Torah (first five books of the Hebrew Bible) and delivering the two tablets reportedly inscribed by God containing ten guiding principles of Christianity (Ten Commandments e.g. "…thou shall not kill…thou shall not steal…thou shall have no other gods before me...") (Deuteronomy 5:4-21), warns in the event a person fails to adhere to the instructions contained in the Ten Commandments, "...the Lord will strike you with madness, blindness, and panic..." (Deuteronomy 28:28). The Bible contains numerous reports of punishment sent by God, often in the form of debilitating mental disorders, as consequence for disobedience to the instructions of God (Samuel 1:31). The concept of demonic possession, as punishment, is additionally reported in the Bible, as is the ability of those whom embrace the Church's teachings to cast out the Devil and other demons from the physical body, thereby effecting a cure (Luke 6:18, 9:1, 10:17; Mathew 8:16, 10:1-8,17:14-17; Mark 6:7).

The Church considers mental disorders to be disorders of the soul, not the physical body and as such assumes authority over persons presenting with impairments of thought, cognition, mood, affect, or behavior. According to period Church beliefs, treatment of mental disorders is best provided by priests not physicians. This Church dogma is modified and tempered with time.

The classic Greek and Roman models of Antiquity, emphasizing the natural (physical) cause of impaired mental function are eventually integrated into the belief systems of the Church. With time and much debate within the Church leadership the idea of natural (physical) cause contributing to mental disorders is no longer completely rejected. The Church successfully modifies natural models to accommodate supranatural beliefs upon which the Church is founded and maintained. Simultaneously the Church establishes its authority and primacy in the care and treatment of individuals presenting with any and all mental disorders. According to Church doctrine, the Church and only the Church is equipped to offer a rational conceptual matrix to explain impaired mental function and offer effective treatments to treat the disordered soul, thereby providing relief from impaired mental functions.

Reinforcing its absolute certainty, Pope Innocent III (1160 AD-1216 AD) decrees any challenge to the Church's position on this matter is to be considered heresy and punishable by excommunication from the Church and or death (1199 AD)[89]. So if you choose to disagree with the Church on this matter you can expect rather severe consequences. Certainly, this is a modifying influence upon scholars and academics choosing to remain in Europe.

Representative of the academic and scholastic communities whom remain in Europe, rather than taking refuge in the Middle East and North African, after the fall of the Roman Empire and reflecting the tremendous influence organized religions has upon framing the conceptual matrix within which mental disorders are understood and treated are found in the writings of Albertus Magnus and Thomas Aquinas.

Albertus Magnus (1193 AD-1289 AD) German Dominican friar and Catholic Saint attempts to reconcile the two extreme positions which attribute mental disorders to the exclusive domains of the natural or the supranatural. He offers interpretations of mental disorders which find common ground. He explains mental disorders within both the conceptual matrix of classic balance of humors models proposed by Greeks and Roman academics during Antiquity and demonic possession as proposed by organized religions and specifically the Church (circa 1250 AD/1891, 1933)[90,91].

Thomas Aquinas (1225 AD-1274 AD) Italian Dominican friar and Catholic Saint draws upon an old idea separating the soul from the physical body and argues the soul cannot become sick; therefore only disorders of the physical body can cause madness (1274)[92]. He further differentiates madness into several dichotomies. For example, impairments present since birth verse impairments acquired during life; impairments which occur with lucid intervals verse impairments which occur without lucid intervals. Independent of the age of onset, specific mental impairment, or underlying cause, Thomas Aquinas argues care for the mentally impaired is the responsibility of the Church.

Residential care is oftentimes necessary in the treatment and management of individuals suffering mental disorders. At the onset of the Middle Ages, this role is fulfilled by immediate family members. Recall, at this time the signs and symptoms of impaired mental function e.g. thought, mood, affect, or behavior are considered simply another sign or symptom of physical illness or disease, much like a cough, fever, or sweating. There is no stigma associated with mental disorders. As organized religions become increasing successful in shifting the belief mental disorders are the result of punishment from a supranatural deity (God), social stigma is soon associated with these conditions. Family members respond to the presses of the Church and local community by relinquishing care to the Church. Individuals suffering mental disorders are quickly segregated from the local community and placed in Church or government controlled facilities.

As governments enact statutes to restrict civil rights and liberties of individuals suffering impaired mental functioning, organized religions assume more responsibilities in guardianship and custodial care of these individuals. Assumption of responsibility is not all together altruistic. Newly enacted laws provide opportunity for organized religions e.g. the Church, to permanently acquire real and personal properties originally held by impaired individuals in exchange for guardianship. Now an individual's property and wealth can legally be taken by the Church in exchange for proving care and guardianship to people evidencing mental impairments. Similar statutes are enacted and applied to newly formed governments. If the government assumes guardianship, then the individual's wealth and property can be seized and converted to government ownership. Acquisition of wealth and property by these means further establishes the ruling powers and tremendous influence of both Church and government. Organized religions do offer needed care to individuals experiencing impaired mental functions and during a period when few treatment and care alternatives are available. However, the motives may not have been as altruistic or as pure as some would like others to believe.

Early custodial care facilities are established throughout Europe for a few suffering mental disorders. These facilities arise in part from the change in thought regarding the cause of mental disturbances and out of necessity, once organized religions successfully associate sigma with impaired mental functioning. Families and friends, once the primary custodians are less willing to accept this responsibility now that it is known the source of the mental impairments are punishment from God and oftentimes includes demonic possession. No longer are mental disorders considered signs and symptoms of physical disease. Disorders are the consequence of immorality, as defined by organized religion. Family members and friends distance themselves from custodial care responsibilities in concern that they too might be judged.

Notable early facilities established in Europe during the Middle Ages to provide custodial care to individuals suffering mental impairment are found at Metz, France (1100 AD), Milan, Italy (1111 AD), Uppsala, Sweden (1305 AD), Bergamo, Italy (1325 AD), Hamburg, Germany (1375 AD), and Florence, Italy (1385 AD). These facilities are representative of the prevailing shift in residential custodial care from family and friends to government and Church. Although none of these facilities are dedicated exclusively to the care of individuals suffering mental impairments, they all offer facilities as alternatives to family and friends care, wandering the streets, or imprisonment. There is no evidence to suggest these facilities provided specialized treatments or care. They are all primary custodial care facilities. These facilities are initially established to care for only the wealthy.

Custodial care facilities are much less available to individuals with restricted financial resources. The poor whom evidence impaired intellectual abilities since birth (Natural Fool), experience transient periods of impaired function in thought, cognition, mood, affect, or behavior, and deemed nonviolent are often driven out of town and left to roam the country sides. Some find sustenance living as the "village idiot". Individuals whom are violent are segregated from society and isolated alongside criminals in prisons and dungeons.

Note: The term "Natural Fool" is a legal term first introduced during the Middle Ages and refers to individuals evidencing impaired intellectual ability since birth, as defined in the Statute de Prerogativa Regis [The Statute of the King's Prerogative] (1339 AD)[94]. Today, American Psychiatric Association's Diagnostic and Statistical Manual of Mental Disorders (DSM-5) refers to this condition as an "Intellectual Developmental Disorder" (2013)[93].

As European society restructures itself during the Middle Ages, land and other wealth are redistributed by the new ruling governments. Governments actively restrict the legal rights of individuals suffering mental impairments. In short, any person deemed to be insane as established by law is not allowed to inherit real property, is not allowed to enter into legally binding contractual agreements, is deemed by law incapable of making rational decisions or participating meaningfully in business and commerce, and by law as the consequence of diminished mental capacity are exempt from criminal responsibility or punishment by the State (1255 AD-1290 AD)[94]. These statutes are based in ancient Greek and Roman law (450 BC)[95].

Treatments of mental disorders are also changing. Physical treatments characteristic of the ancient Greeks and Romans e.g. improved diet, improved hygiene, residing in more favorable climates, residing in more stress free settings, moderate exercise, massage, mineral baths, use of empirically derived herbs and minerals, are all based upon the conceptual understanding mental disorders result from natural (physical) disorders of normal body functions. Treatments now shift to accommodate the conceptual matrixes of organize religions. Mental disorders are no longer understood as physical disorders but rather viewed as punishment, imposed by a supranatural deity (God) upon an individual for their transgressions against the beliefs of the organized religion. Given the conceptual matrix, individuals suffering impairment in thought, cognition, mood, affect, or behavior are believed to be possessed by demons, especially the Devil (Christian belief) and which needs to be driven out of the body to restore mental functions. Individuals are segregated and brutally punished. Specific treatments are detailed by the Church's leaderships e.g. beatings, flogging, starvation, burnings, exorcism, and prayer (Proverbs 26:3).

Organized religion more than any other single factor is responsible for changing the way individuals suffering mental disorders are treated. The impact of organized religion continues to impact the treatments of individuals suffering mental disorders for the next 1,500 years. The Middle Ages are especially brutal times for individuals suffering any mental disorder.

In summary, the Middle Ages witness a Europe in chaos, following the fall of the Roman Empire. Organized religions offer structure and guidance and quickly establish tremendous powers, which impact the future development of medical psychology and psychiatry. Two dichotomous lines of thought and investigative processes evolve. The first is committed to traditional Greek and Galen modified Roman models, emphasizing the physical, biological (natural) bases of mental impairments. The second is the newer, faith based models of organized religions, and emphasizing the supranatural (deity) based models of mental impairment. Influential and notable individuals representative of the physical (natural) approach are Ibn Sina and Constantine the African. Influential and notable individuals representative of the supranatural (deity) approach are Albertus Magnus and Thomas Aquinas. Organized religion and the supranatural (deity) model is predominate in Europe, while the physical biological (natural) models are predominant in the Middle East and Northern Africa. In Europe, the primary care of individuals suffering impairments in mental functioning shift from family and physicians to the leadership of organized religions. Organized religions, especially the Church establishes residential care facilities for individuals suffering mental impairments, which segregates them from society. Simultaneously, newly established governments, heavily influenced by organized religion pass statutes which permit the irrevocable conveyance of real and personal properties of individuals suffering mental impairments to the Church and State, without the individual's consent. Governmental statutes are passed, based upon ancient Greek and Roman law, which exempt individuals suffering mental impairments from criminal culpability and responsibility. Treatments arise from the conceptual matrix within which mental disorders are understood by the Church e.g. punishment from a deity (God), resulting in typically brutal treatments, such as beatings, flogging, burnings, and prayer. These are especially brutal times for any individual suffering impairments in mental functions.

Early Modern, 1400 AD - 1800 AD.

The Early Modern Age witness the changes of the European Renaissance and many fundamental changes, effecting the historical development of medical psychology.

The Church continues its dogma in regard to mental disorders as outlined during the Middle Ages. Mental disorders continue to be conceptualized as disorders of the soul, sent as punishment by an angered deity (God), and as such fall within the exclusive domain of the Church. Effective treatments can only be provided by the Church. Physicians have little to no role in the treatment of mental disorders. Academics whom disagree with Church dogma e.g. argue in favor of secular rather than non-secular origins of mental disorders, are subject to excommunication from the Church, branded as heretics, and suffer associated devastating, financial, social, and professional consequences.

The Church exerts powerful influence upon the development of medical psychology throughout the Early Modern Age. Science is replaced by religion. Efforts to understand the physical basis of impairments of mental functions is replaced by efforts to understand them within the matrix of organized religions' faith-based beliefs. Within this matrix, many individuals evidencing signs and symptoms of impaired mental functions are understood to be possessed by demons or the devil. Treatments oftentimes necessitate exorcism of the demons or devil from the physical body and often utilize extreme, brutal, inhumane procedures. Individuals associated with or in other ways in contact with an individual suffering mental impairment are oftentimes identified to be secular agents of the demons or devil (witches) and subjected to Church sanctioned trials, cruel brutal punishments, and even executions. There is great, self-serving, self-righteous intolerance of any person who challenges Church dogma or Church sanctioned actions.

The Church provides moral and written guidance to any faithful believer who might encounter a person suffering impaired mental functions or behaving in an odd or unusual manner. Given the Church's fundamental belief that impaired mental functioning and odd, unusual, or amoral behavior result from demon possession, the Church offers an extremely popular "How to Manual" to identify, torture, and execute all suspected secular agents of the Devil (i.e. witches). It is believed through witches and demons, the Devil is able to effect possessions of the physical body.

Given individuals suffering impairments in thought, cognition, mood, affect, and behavior oftentimes appear odd or unusual to others, many are soon identified as witches and subjected to the horrible fates prescribed by the Church. Hundreds of thousands of people are falsely identified, falsely accused, brutally punished, and executed as witches throughout Europe and beyond. This is all done in accordance with the guidelines published in the Church's "How to Manual", "Malleus Maleficarum" [The Witch's Hammer] (1484,1487)[96,97]. These are truly horrific times for all individuals suffering mental disorders.

The care and treatments available to individuals suffering impairments of mental function and behavior change radically throughout the Early Modern Age. Early during this period, care is typically provided by family and friends. As the Church introduces new explanations as to the origin and maintenance of mental disorders, families and friends provide less care. The role of treatment and management shifts from family and friends to the Church. The Church introduces and offers specialized care facilities, segregating individuals who need care, from the general population. Treatments, if provided, no longer focuses on treating the physical body, rather focus is directed to treating a disordered soul.

Many of the early care facilities are founded by the Church. Most are located in Spain and provide an operations model for new facilities soon to be founded across Europe. Complementing the efforts of the Church and responding to the rapidly increasing demand for segregated care facilities for the mentally impaired, governments of Europe slowly begin to found new facilities, specifically to provide custodial care for the individuals evidencing congenital or acquired mental impairments. Unable to meet the increase demand, created in large part by beliefs regarding mental impairment popularized by the Church, and coupled with an assured sense of righteousness, governments begin committing large numbers of individuals evidencing mental impairments to prisons, workhouses, and poor houses, for the purposes of providing custodial care. These facilities provide no treatment.

By the mid-1500s, King Henry VIII of England, orders the repurposing of a priory outside of London to provide custodial care exclusively to individuals suffering mental disorders. This marks the beginning of housing large numbers of individuals in specialized care facilities, soon termed collectively as insane asylums. Quickly, the asylums are overcrowded and necessitates a reevaluation as to how to house large numbers of individuals requiring specialized care and services. Each country responds with its own approach, from building more asylums and placing restriction on admissions; encouraging the private sector to build for-profit "retreats" and "madhouses"; establishing county hospitals which provide short term hospital based care to limited numbers of individuals evidencing impaired mental functions; to doing nothing at all.

By the end of the 1700s, faith based Church dogma is boldly challenged by a handful. These few individuals alter the future course, study, and understandings of mental disorders. Investigations and understanding begin to shift away from religion and return to science and scientific methods.

Governments struggle with how to best manage individuals suffering mental impairments. Individuals suffering mental impairments continue to be segregated from the general population and warehoused into prisons, workhouses, poorhouses, large asylums, and financially lucrative for profit madhouses. Governments attempt to legislate the care and treatment of the mentally impaired.

From an academic and medical perspective, emphasis is now placed once again upon the examination of mental impairments within the matrix of the natural (physical) rather than supranatural, religion based (deity) models. Mental impairments are dissected and examined. Detailed treaties are written discussing specific disorders and impairments e.g. melancholia and hysteria. Physical origins of mental impairments are offered along with new, rational treatments based upon new conceptual matrixes. Mental disorders are associated with specific disease conditions e.g. syphilis. The epidemiology of mental disorders is described and reported with increasing frequency. Institutional care of individuals begins to change, as the conceptual matrix within which mental disorders are understood changes.

Let us examine a few specifics.

In light of organized religions' emphasis upon the supranatural (deity) origins of mental disorders and horrific prescribed treatments, the Church is largely responsible for establishing early care facilities which accept individuals suffering the effects of impaired mental functions. Restricting ourselves to Europe, the preponderance of these facilities are located not in England, France, Germany, or Italy as might reasonably be expected, but rather Spain.

Spain and her many Church affiliated care facilities prove to be early leaders in providing custodial, nursing, and faith based care to individuals evidencing mental disorders. Of particular note are the Hospital de la Santa Cruz de Barcelona [Hospital of the Holy Cross] located in Barcelona, Spain (1401) and El Hospital de los Lunaticos, Orates e Inocentes [The Hospital for Lunatics, the Insane, and Innocents] also known as The Hospital de Nuestra Senora Maria de los Inocentes [The Hospital of Our Lady of the Innocents] located in Valcencia, Spain (1409-1410). These two facilities are devoted exclusively to the care of individuals suffering impairments of thought, cognition, mood, affect, or behavior.

A notable and oftentimes unrecognized facility important to the development and advancement in the care of individuals experiencing impairment of normal mental functions is the Hospital General de Nuestra Senora de Gracia [General Hospital of Our Lady of Grace] founded in Zaragoza, Spain (1425). Additional notable specialized facilities of Spain are founded at Saragossa (1435), Seville (1436), Toledo (1483), Granada (1507), and Madrid (1540). High costs associated with the operation of so many specialized facilities necessitates expanding care beyond the mentally impaired to include general hospital care. Several of the early specialized care facilities transition into providing general hospital care by the end of the 1400s e.g. the asylum located at Valencia, Spain.

Trivia: The term "lunatic" is based upon the belief episodic insanity is associated with changes in moon phases. Alignment of planets, stars, and other physical heavenly bodies are frequently used to understand and explain the onset, duration, and resolution of medical conditions throughout the early history of medicine. The term originates from the old French word "lunatique" simply meaning "moon-struck" (2013)[98]. The term "innocents" is applied to individuals of limited intellectual abilities and resources, typically present since birth. Today in 2018, we would term "innocents" to be individuals meeting diagnostic criteria for Intellectual Developmental Disorders (DSM-5)[93].

While the Church is instrumental in establishing many specialized care facilities across Europe during the 1400s, recall the conceptual matrix used by the Church to understand mental disorders, during this period. Prescribed and oftentimes brutal treatments follow the conceptual matrix embraced by The Church. Mental disorders are believed to result when a supranatural deity (God) becomes angered and decides to punishment an individual. Typically, the deity imposed punishment results when an individual fails to accept or adheres to the specific beliefs of an organized religion e.g. Christianity.

Mental disorders present in a wide assortment of clinical presentations and many are considered to be the result of demonic or Devil possession. Possession is facilitated by the assistance of secular agents of these demons and Devil (witches). Prescribed treatments necessitate prayer to the deity asking forgiveness, physical segregation from the faithful, physical starvation, physical beatings, public humiliation, physical torture, and yes even death. These are horrific times for individuals suffering impaired mental functions.

In the Church's efforts to assist the faithful in identifying individuals possessed by demons or the Devil or functioning as secular agents of demons and the Devil (witches), Pope Innocent XIII commissions two Dominican theologians, Jacob Sprenger (1436-1495) of the University of Cologne, Germany and Heinrich Kramer (1430-1505) of the University of Salzburg, Austria to write a "How to Manual" (1484)[96]. Their manual, "Malleus Maleficarum" [The Witch's Hammer], offers direction and guidance to the faithful, as to how to identify those whom have been possessed and how to identify, interrogate, bring to trial, and punish the secular agents of demons or the Devil (witches) (1487)[97]. Perhaps no other single, period publication does more harm to individuals suffering mental disorders than the "Malleus Maleficarum".

Given the tremendous historical influence the "Malleus Maleficarum" has in shaping the course and development of religious and popular beliefs towards individuals suffering mental impairment during the late-1400s through the early-1600s, let us examine this publication in brief.

The "Malleus Maleficarum" is divided into three major sections. Each section addresses a series of specific questions and details the Church's position with regard to each question. Section One argues the existence of the Devil, identifies witches as secular agents of the Devil, and discusses assorted issues such as whether Incubi and Succubi are able to obtain semen from one body and pass it on to another body. Section Two defines the methods for identifying witches, details their many powers, and offers prescribed remedies for individuals bewitched. Section Three describes legal and procedural issues, offers a step by step instruction guide as to how to conduct a witch trial, from accusation, interrogation (torture), through disposition (execution), details specific tortures and devices, details signs by which to recognize a witch, and discusses acceptable trial by ordeal procedures.

"Malleus Maleficarum" offers guidance for practicing physicians; if a doctor cannot find a physical cause for a patient's disease or the patient fails to respond to traditional treatments, de facto this condition is caused by the Devil. The idea is extended to all individuals suffering mental impairments. According to the "Malleus Maleficarum", "…lunatics…" are possessed by the Devil. In accordance with Church dogma and given possession by the Devil, individuals are to be tortured and/or executed in accordance with guidelines and procedures detailed in the "Malleus Maleficarum". If the prescribed torture proves ineffective in returning the individual to a normal mental state, execution is one Church approved option. Burning a possessed individual at the stake is one recommended, popular, and acceptable practice of execution.

Exact numbers of individuals executed in accordance with the "Malleus Maleficarum" during its period of its high popularity 1400s-1600s remains unclear. Estimates place the numbers in the hundreds of thousands in France alone, during the reign of King Francis I, 1515-1547. Given the book's extreme popularity throughout Europe, coupled with the explicit support of the Church, and the willingness of the masses to be led by others without independent thought, one can only imagine the total number of individuals executed across Europe, during the late-1400s-1800s, who suffered impairments in thought, cognition, mood, affect, and/or behavior.

The Church in creating the need for segregated facilities for individuals suffering mental impairments, offers partial solutions. The Church establishes residential care facilities across Europe for the mentally impaired. Most early facilities are founded in Spain as described earlier, however one facility located on the outskirts of London, England, founded in 1247 AD originally as a monastery, housing the priory of the New Order of Saint Mary of Bethlem is notable. Founded for purposes of collecting alms to support the Christian Crusades and providing housing to the poor and visiting Church officials, the facility is repurposed in 1547 by order of King Henry VIII, to provide custodial care, exclusively to individuals suffering mental disorders. The facility continues in operations today, as the Bethlem Royal Hospital. Today, this facility stands as a world class research, training, and treatment facility, devoted to understanding and treating mental disorders (2018)[99].

Trivia: The term "insane" is derived from the Latin word "insanus" meaning "not well", (in = "not" + sanus = "well"). The term first gains popularity during the mid-1500s (2014)[100].

Bethlem Royal Hospital is recognized as Europe's oldest hospital providing care and treatment to individuals suffering impaired mental functions. The first documented admission of the insane appears in 1403. At this time the facility offers care and treatment to only a handful of mentally impaired patients. Exclusive admissions of the mentally impaired does not occur until 144 years later (1547). With a history of operations spanning over 600 years and providing care to mentally impaired patients, the facility exemplifies the best and worst in care and treatment. During its history patients are treated and managed according to period dogma. Patients have been shackled, beaten, made to live in overcrowded, filthy conditions, inside of buildings in disrepair, and displayed to the general public as a paid amusement attraction. You may recognize this facility by its colloquial name which first appears during the 1300s AD, Bedlam.

Trivia: The English term "bedlam" is introduced circa 1377 AD, referring to the noisy chaotic confusion observed by visitors to the Bethlem Royal Hospital. The term is still used today to refer to "…a place or situation of noisy uproar and confusion…an insane asylum…" (2018)[101].

Few challenge the powerful Church and its dogma in respect to the origins and treatments of mental disorders. Two who do, Dutch psychiatrist Johnann Weyer and Swiss alchemist Paracelsus, alter the direction of the care and treatment of individuals presenting with mental disorders forever. Their challenges force the scientific and medical communities to reevaluate their thinking in respect to the way impaired mental functioning is conceptualized and treated. Collectively, both challenge the Church's dogma of supranatural origins of mental disorders and propose instead natural (physical) origins. The challenges are made in complete awareness of the potential severe consequences likely to be imposed by the Church e.g. execution for heresy.

Jacob Weyer (1515-1588) Dutch psychiatrist offers his 479 page, landmark publication "De Pragestigiis Daemonun et Incantationibus ac Veneficiis" [On the Deceptions of the Demons and on Enchantments and Poisonings] (1563)[102]. It is here he argues madness results from natural rather than supranatural causes; many individuals identified by the Church as mad, possessed by demons, or bewitched are actually evidencing signs and symptoms of impaired mental functions due to disordered bodily functions, not disorders of the soul; and any person identified as bewitched, mad, or possessed should be evaluated by a physician.

Additionally, he unapologetically challenges the Church's "Malleus Maleficarum", referring to its contents as "…silly and often godless absurdities of the theologians Heinrich Kramer and Johann Sprenger… Any man who is not completely dull-witted will easy conclude that these things…are absurd and unworthy of belief…" (1563)[102].

"On the Deception of Demons and on Enchantments, and Poisonings" sees four editions; in Latin 1563-1568, into German and French in 1579, and subsequently into English, offering a wide readership. The Catholic Church quickly places the book on the Catholic Church's Index Librorum Prohibitorum [List of Prohibited Books], books not to be read and under penalty of excommunication. The book remains on the prohibited lists of readings well into the 1800s when it is removed.

Paracelsus, aka Theophratus Aureolus Bombastus von Hahenhiem (1493-1541) Swiss physician, alchemist, Professor of Medicine at Basal University, contemporary of Leonardo da Vinci and Nicolas Copernicus, openly rejects Church and Galenian dogma regarding the origins of mental disorders and prescribed treatments. He offers one of the first books devoted specifically to the topic of mental disorders, "The diseases that deprive man of his reason, such as St. Vitus' Dance, falling sickness, melancholy, and insanity, and their correct treatments" (1567)[103]. Paracelsus prepares this book when he is approximately 30 years of age and it is published post humously 26 years after his death. Here he argues mental disorders are the sole result of natural processes and not "…ghostly beings…" as claimed by the Church.

Paracelsus further offers an early classification of mental disorders based upon clinical descriptions of their presentations and hypothesized natural processes underlying each disorder. He organizes mental disorders into four categories; lunatic, insane, melancholic, and vesani (1567)[103]. Briefly, lunatics evidence impaired mental abilities and behaviors as a function of the differing physical forces occurring during the natural phases of the moon. Insanes evidence impairments in thought, cognition, mood, affect, and behavior since birth and are associated with family inheritance. Melancholics evidence impairments in thought, cognition, mood, affect, and behaviors as the result of impaired reasoning abilities. Vesanies evidence psychotic impairment due to poisons or contaminated food or drink. Notice here how his conceptualization of mental disorders differ from Galenian models based upon humor imbalances and the Church models based upon disorders of the soul and demon possessions. Paracelsus' categorizations anticipate the organization systems used today, over 600 years later to classify, understand, and treat mental disorders.

By the mid-1600s there is much interests within the academic and medical community in understanding mental disorders within the matrix of impaired nervous system function. Two men you most likely associate with neurology, Thomas Willis (Circle of Willis) and Thomas Sydenham (Sydenham chorea), exemplify the types of contributions being made with regard to the suspected neural origins of mental disorders.

Thomas Willis (1621-1675) English physiologist challenges much of the medical dogma regarding origins and medical treatments of mental disorders. He is an ardent, outspoken proponent of the physical (natural) origins of mental disorders and argues these disorders can best be understood by better understanding human anatomy, human biochemistry, and human physiology.

By way of specific example, Thomas Willis rejects the Church's belief hysteria has its origin in an angered supranatural deity who has sent it to punish an individual for their transgressions against Church doctrine. He argues hysteria is the result of impaired brain functions. Additionally, he provides autopsy findings which dispel the long held belief, hysteria results from structural changes occurring within the uterus and is among the first to acknowledge hysteria is not restricted to women, as commonly believed, reporting the condition also appears in men (1664,1666,1667, 1670,1671)[104,105,106,107,108].

Thomas Willis argues mental disorders are the result of impaired brain structure and function. He details the anatomy, biochemistry, and physiology of several mental disorders. He offers extensive discussions on melancholia, congenital intellectual impairment, and epilepsies, addressing issues of origins, causes, and treatments (1661-1664,1667,1672,1672,1683)[109,106,110,111,112]. His writings on melancholia additionally offer a cautionary note to medical practitioners; melancholia "…being long time protracted, passes oftentimes into stupidity, or foolishness, and sometimes also into madness…" (1672)[112]. His writings on congenital intellectual impairments offers insight into the conceptualization and management of these disabilities during the mid-1600s (1672)[110,111]. His writings on epilepsy are unmatched by any other of the period (1667,1681)[106,113].

Always emphasizing the natural (physical) basis of hysteria, melancholia, and other mental disorders, Thomas Willis readily acknowledges his observed reciprocal relationship between emotions, cognitions, and physiology. He notes, thoughts which originate in the brain generate emotions such as fear and sadness. These thoughts and emotions effect body physiology. Similarly, physiology effects an individual's thoughts and emotions. Over 345 years ago, Thomas Willis proposes mental disorder can best be understood within a conceptual matrix of disordered physiology.

Thomas Sydenham (1624-1689) English physician and contemporary of Thomas Willis is perhaps most recognized for his description of Saint Vitus' Dance, which today we commonly term Sydenham chorea (1686)[114]. Among his many notable contributions, he carefully describes the clinical course of hysteria and describes its presence in men (1681-1682,1693,1850)[115,116,117]. He emphasizes the clinical fluidity of the disorder and stresses it to be much more common that originally believed. He and Thomas Willis are instrumental in refining the diagnostic criteria of hysteria, by efforts to remove confounding conditions which might better be diagnosed as melancholia. Sydenham provides an explanation as to why hysteria appears more frequently in women than men; "…women are more frequently affected with this disease than men, because they have received from nature a finer and more delicate constitution of body, being designed for an easier life and the pleasure of men…" (1681,1743)[118,119].

As the 1600s come to a close, attitudes in Europe are slowly changing within the academic and medical communities regarding the origins of mental disorders. Consequently, methods used to treat mental disorders are also changing. Greater emphasis is being placed upon the investigation and understanding of the biological basis of common mental disorders. However, in the New World, British colonies e.g. Salem, Massachusetts, hold fast to old ideas and Church dogma of the 1400s, 1500s, and early-1600s. Mental disorders are considered to be the consequence of immorality and the work of demons, devils, and witches. As late as 1692, Church faithful in Salem, Massachusetts continue to execute members of their community, as witches and those possessed by demons or Devil (1693)[120].

By the early-1700s, large and increasing numbers of individuals evidencing debilitating impairments of mental functions necessitate most European governments to reevaluate their roles and responsibilities in the social management of these individuals. Most governments view their responsibilities as limited. Individuals evidencing impairments of thought, cognition, mood, affect, or behavior who cannot be effectively managed by family, friends, Church, or community, and pose a nuisance to the general population are simply segregated from the general population and confined in government prisons, workhouses, and poor houses. Few national laws or local statutes specially address the social management of individuals evidencing mental impairments. Fewer still address issues of treatment, reasonable care, safety, and protection for those confined. Early legislation does little to improve conditions for the mentally and emotionally impaired.

The United Kingdom (UK) pioneers modern legislation which address the management of individuals evidencing impaired mental functions with enactment of the Vagrancy Act of 1714 (1714)[121]. In general this legislation provides guidance to Justices in reference to the social management of rouges, vagabonds, beggars, vagrants, and "…poor lunatics and mad persons…". Specifically, this legislation states the government is permitted to arrest, detain, and confine a person evidencing signs and symptoms of impaired mental function, for as long there is evidence of impaired mental functions, as determined by a Justice. Perhaps the exact words will be of value here; "…Persons…who by lunacy…are furiously mad… (are to) be apprehended and locked up, and if the Justices think fit, to be chained…without whipping, and there to be kept (in the county of their arrest)…during lunacy…" (1714)[121]. That is right; individuals can now be held by statute, against their will, confined by the government for as long as the government chooses, having committed no crime, and simply because they evidence signs and symptoms of impaired mental functioning.

The Vagrancy Act of 1714 is amended and modified 30 years later by the Vagrancy Act of 1744, which imposes an additional requirement; any "…lunatic…" confined by the government, as the result of impaired mental function, must receive treatment during their confinement (1744)[122]. Nothing is specified within the Act as to what constitutes treatment.

British Parliament enacts additional legislation the same year, known as the Act of 1744 for Regulating Madhouses. This Act establishes physicians the powers to certify an individual to be "…a lunatic…" and for the first time gives physicians the power to commit individuals against their will to facilities, for the purposes of confinement and treatment, when demonstrating impaired mental functions (1744)[123].

It soon becomes clear; governments are poorly equipped and resourced to provide the necessary care and treatment to adequately service the large numbers of individuals requiring housing, care, and treatment. The solution in the UK is to establish a network of short term and long term care facilities, established in cooperation between the government, Church, and private sector, offering housing and care to individuals unable to care for themselves, due to impairments of intellectual resources, cognitive abilities, emotions, or behavior.

These facilities take many forms. Some facilities are publicly funded and others privately funded. Some are charitable, non-profits and others for-profit. Some are large State asylums, housing hundreds of individuals and other are small, private "…madhouses…", housing only a few individuals. Some are county asylums providing long term custodial care while others provide short term acute care. Some general medical hospitals offer specialized wards inside of the hospital for the "…mad and insane…". Some facilities provide housing and care for only "…curables…" and separate facilities provide housing and care for "…uncurables…". Some facilities have less than Spartan accommodations while others offer elaborate trappings of the most wealthy country manors. Some facilities are operated by ruthless, debased individuals and others operated by compassionate individuals insisting upon the highest levels of care. Some facilities are licensed by the government and others operate independent of government regulations. Some facilities accommodate only the very wealthy while others accommodate only the poor. The variability between facilities is tremendous.

The UK witnesses a rapid proliferation of facilities during the 1700s. The State continues its support of a few established State facilities and founds new additional custodial care and treatment facilities, specifically for individuals evidencing "…madness or insanity…".

For example, facilities of historical note are the infamous Bethlem Royal Hospital (Bedlam), located outside of London, is first to provide exclusive admissions to the "…mad and insane…" (1547). It remains in continuous operation from the 1700s and now into 2020. Bethel Hospital located at Norwich, is founded as the first asylum in the UK specifically for the "…benefit of distrest Lunaticks …" and "…is not to be alienated or employed to any other use or purpose whatsoever…" (1713)[124]. Guy's Hospital, located in central London is founded by the wealthy English publisher Thomas Guy (1644-1724), as a charitable hospital to treat "…incurables discharged from St. Thomas Hospital…". Guy's Hospital establishes a ward specifically for "…chronic lunatics…" in 1728. Saint Luke's Hospital for Lunatics located in London is founded in 1751. Saint Lukes' operates under the initial direction of chief physician William Battie and is among the first to advocate a preferred non-restraint policy. Manchester Lunatic Hospital is founded in 1766 and too advocates humane treatments.

York Asylum is founded in 1772 and is designed as an institution "…where the patients might expect to meet with the most humane and disinterested treatment; and where they might have a chance of being restored to their health…" (1772)[125]. Leicester County Lunatic Asylum is founded in 1794, under the leadership of physician Thomas Arnold and gives physicians much more control in the care of patients and management of the asylum and advocates humane treatments (1782,1806,1809)[126,127,128]. York Retreat, not to be confused with the York Asylum, is founded in 1796 and prohibits the admission of individuals who have been discharged from other asylums as "…incurable…", as well as "… epileptics, idiots, pregnant women, and those suffering from venereal disease…" (1815)[129].

The facilities above characterized the rapid expansion of State and privately funded asylums, specialized hospital wards, and restrictions placed upon facilitates, providing services during the 1700s. Most of the larger asylums e.g. Bethlem Royal Hospital (Bedlam) provide housing and care to approximately 200-300 patients. The smaller ward facilities e.g. Guy's Hospital provide housing and care to only a few.

Private madhouses complement care provided by large asylums. By definition madhouses are privately owned, for profit facilities, which provide housing and care to the mentally impaired. Conditions vary considerably between madhouses. Some offer horrific accommodations and care, characterized by brutal physical and sexual abuses, indiscriminate, long term use of physical restraints e.g. chaining to walls, brutal, forced feedings, filthy, overcrowded, poorly ventilated, squalor living conditions, and continuous fiduciary abuses. Thomas Warburton's Red House and Whites House, located in Bethnal Green (East London) and Jonathan Miles' Hoxton House, located in Hoxton (East London) exemplifies these infamous madhouses (1815,1816)[130,131]. In contrast other madhouses typically catering only to the very wealthy, offer accommodations of luxury and comfort characteristic of the finest country manor of the period. Samuel Newington's Ticehurst House, located in East Sussex (southeast England) exemplifies a madhouse for the very wealthy.

Perhaps one of the most recognized private asylums is the York Retreat, founded in 1796 by William Tuke (1732-1822). York Retreat is located in the countryside outside the city of York in North Yorkshire, England and is founded upon the fundamental religious beliefs of the Quakers. It is established in reaction to harsh and brutal treatments well recognized to exist at State funded asylums and many for profit madhouses across England. The York Retreat embraces humane treatment of individuals suffering mental disorders and applies an approach to treatment which later will be termed Moral Therapy. No physical punishment, no manacles, no chains. Treatments focus upon restoring self-esteem, self-confidence, and self-control. Specific therapies incorporate personalized attention, benevolence, kindness, early forms of occupational therapies, handicrafts, therapeutic farming, and religious prayer. The roles of physicians and the use of medications are limited. This facility soon provides a new model of care, which stands in marked contrast to the State asylums and for profit madhouses, providing residential care to individuals suffering mental impairments. The Retreat has remained in operation for more than 220 years and continues today as a charitable, not-for-profit facility offering specialized care to individuals experiencing impairments in thought, mood, affect, or behavior (2018)[132]

Many people during the 1700s and early-1800s decry the horrific living conditions and quality of care provided by the for-profit madhouses. However, the majority of madhouses provide reasonable living conditions, care for their residents, and provide a much needed alternative to confinement in workhouses, poorhouses, prisons, and government asylums.

The British Parliament in response to public outcry introduces and passes new legislation regulating the operations of madhouses (1774)[133]. In brief, the legislation requires all madhouses to be licensed by the Royal College of Physicians; the license must be reviewed and renewed each year; all houses must be inspected once a year by a physician appointed from within the Royal College of Physicians or a local Justices of the Peace; a license permits the holder to maintain a single house for accommodating "…lunatics…(or) person of unsound mind…"; all residents require certification by a physician, surgeon, or apothecary that the resident "…is proper to be received to such house or place as a lunatic…"; all new admissions require an order from a physician; and substantial fines are to be imposed upon owners and operators of madhouses when failing to comply with the provisions detailed in the 1774 Act for Regulating Private Madhouses (1774)[133].

Elsewhere in Europe, slower progress is being made with regard to the housing, care, and treatment of individuals evidencing impaired mental functions. For example, in Vienna, Austria, a new government funded facility is constructed in 1784, five stories high, circular building with a center courtyard, consisting of 139 rooms with lattice barred doors, designed to house 250 patients identified to suffer assorted mental disorders (1845)[134]. The new facility is constructed adjacent to the Vienna General Hospital and is popularly known as the Narrenthurm (aka Lunatic's Tower or Tower of Fools). Care and management inside of the facility soon becomes reminiscent of the infamous days of Bethlem Royal Hospital (Bedlam), located outside of London, England. Patients are subjected to overcrowding, generally poor living conditions, physical restraint by "… strong jackets, bed straps, iron manacles and anklets, or chains…", and outdated approaches to treatment and management practices (1845)[134]. Patients are displayed to the general public for amusement, often presented in cages much like zoo animals (1845)[134].

By the end of the 1700s the UK has established a network of care facilities, large government funded asylums, smaller government funded county asylums, large and small for profit madhouses and retreats, to address the growing demand for housing, care, and treatment of individuals suffering debilitating impairments of thought, cognition, mood, affect, or behavior.

Having established an extensive network of care facilities, at the national and local level, with the best intentions of providing humane treatments, in healthy, uncrowded, supportive environments, without the use of physical restraints, or physical, sexual, or fiduciary abuse, the system is soon challenged. Many facilities soon address allegations of corruption, scandal, claims of abuse, neglect, and cruelty, all which play out in the public press e.g. York Asylum, Bethlem Royal Hospital (Bedlam), Thomas Warburton's Red and White Houses, and Jonathan Miles' Hoxton House (1815,1816)[135,136].

Public reaction is so great in the UK to these allegations, a special Committee is assembled by the British Parliament House of Commons to investigate charges of abuse within asylums and madhouses. Committee records of the investigations and final recommendations are made readily available to the public. The findings reveal shocking evidence, supporting claims of horrific living conditions and brutal mistreatment of individuals housed in these care facilities (1815,1816)[135,136]. The Committee's findings lead to substantial reform, within Britain, in the housing, care, and treatment of individuals experiencing debilitating impairments of thought, cognition, mood, affect, or behavior.

Many of the claims of overcrowding and abuse, within residential care facilities providing services to the mentally impaired, producing public outcry and demand for change now over 200 years ago, unfortunately continue to periodically appear today, throughout Europe, USA, Canada, and many other countries of the world. What do you think about this issue as a medical student? Can we do better? If so, what are your suggestions and recommendations? Are you willing to take a leadership role and make change happen?

Trivia: The "strait jacket" is invented in France by an upholsterer for the Bicetre Asylum for insane men, during 1790. The term is derived from the word "straiten" meaning to restrict. The strait jacket is considered a more humane method to control violent patients than chains. The strait jacket is still in use today in facilities throughout the world, as a method to control patients who may be in danger of harming themselves or others, now over 225 years since first introduced in Paris.

For a moment, stop reading and think about this. You are providing medical care in one of the many facilities during the 1700s e.g. asylum, madhouse, or retreat and your patient becomes violent and poses an immediate potential danger to themselves and others. The patient is in a delirious or psychotic state and does not respond to you or the staff's efforts to calm them. Would you use physical restraints to control this patient? Remember, the resources available to you during this time period e.g. no Haloperidol. What would you do? It is important to keep in mind resources available, before being too self-righteous in judgement of methods and procedures used by others whom have come before you. Think about it. What would you do and why?

OK, back to the history.

Progress is being made in Europe during the 1700s in response to the demands to provide housing, care, and treatment to individuals living with impaired mental functions. While progress is slow and not without problems, progress is being made. This stands in contrast to European colonies being established in the New World of North America. The leadership of the colonies hold fast to old ideas and Church dogma in respect to the origins of mental disorders and methods of treatment.

The first hospital in the American Colonies providing care to individuals evidencing mental disorders is the Pennsylvania Hospital for the Insane. This facility is founded in 1751 as a general medical hospital with special provisions to house, care for, and treat the mentally impaired. It is located in Philadelphia, Pennsylvania. Benjamin Franklin (1706-1790) born in Boston, Massachusetts drafts the original petition to the Colonial Assembly proposing the founding of this new facility. In the proposal he makes specific his request the hospital in addition to providing care to the sick poor of the Providence provide "… for the reception and care of lunaticks…". The first "…lunaticks…" are to be admitted during the first year of operation and housed in the basement (1751,1895)[137,138].

The first asylum in the American Colonies providing exclusive care to individuals evidencing mental disorders is The Publick Hospital for Persons of Insane and Disordered Minds, located in Williamsburg, Virginia. The facility subsequently changes its name to The Eastern Lunatic Asylum and again to the Eastern State Hospital. Founded in 1773 as legislated by the House of Burgesses of Virginia, the facility is chartered to provide "…for the support and maintenance of idiots, lunatics, and other persons of unsound mind…so unhappy to be deprived of their reason…" (1766,1769)[139,140]. Initially, admissions are restricted to the "…curable…" and those considered a danger to themselves, others, or society.

The fundamental conceptual matrix adopted by this asylum is to view impaired mental functions as the result of physical (natural) causes and with no connection to moral responsibilities or the soul. Treatments are rational, based upon acceptance of a physical origin of mental disorders and the additional belief some mental disorders appear as a conscious choice made by the individual. Specific treatments administered during the 1700s and early-1800s are typical of treatments being used in Europe; liberal use of physical restraints, plunge baths via dunking chairs, potent medications, blistering salves, bloodletting, electrostatic stimulation, and intimidation.

By 1836 the asylum modifies its treatment approaches to align with popular new treatments being used in Europe. Physical restraints and treatments are replaced by the popular Moral Treatments, emphasizing non-medical interventions, characterized by kindness, empathy, firm but gentle encouragements for more self-control, participation in work therapy, and increased time in leisure activities (1846)[141]. The facility known today as Eastern State Hospital has remained in continuous operation since its founding over 245 years ago, continues to provide mental care services to the residents of Virginia.

The second half of the 1700s, while struggling with how to best segregate individuals with mental disorders from the general population; how to provide necessary housing and care; how government can best socially manage these individuals; a few clinicians propose revised models from which to better understand, define, manage, and treat mental disorders. Four investigators provide a representative sample of the prevailing thoughts of the period and whom offer revised conceptualizations as to the origin of mental disorders, classification, and recommended treatments. Let us briefly examine their contributions.

William Battie (1703-1776) English physician and whom the term "batty" originates, offers an elegant new classification system and rational treatments based upon his many years providing direct clinical services to patients of the Bethlem Royal Hospital (Bedlam), the new Saint Luke's Hospital for Lunatics, and his privately owned for-profit madhouse. He presents his conceptual matrix in his "Treatise on Madness" (1758)[142].

In brief, William Battie ascribes to the natural (physical) origins for all mental disorder. He organizes mental disorders into two primary categories, Original Madness and Consequential Madness. Original Madness is due to deficits present since birth or as the result of heredity. Original madness is incurable and "…is not removable by any method which the science of Physick in its present imperfect state is able to suggest…" (1758)[142]. Consequential Madness is due to an acquired impairment of "…nervous substances…" of brain and nerves. Consequential Madness most typically results from head trauma, infections or obstructions producing inflammation of the brain and surrounding tissues, intoxication by drugs or alcoholic beverages, sudden excitement of "…tumultuous passions of joy and anger…", or other external events which modify "…nervous substances…". Consequential Madness is curable (1758)[142].

Treatment recommendations are largely management of the individual's living conditions and daily routines. The individual should be placed in confinement some distance from their home; receive no visits from friends, family, enemies, or the impertinent curious; the patient's body and place of residence should be kept clean; the air he breathes should be fresh and dry; his food simple and easily digested; amusements not too long or engaging; exercise should be moderate, his employment not too demanding and about things he is rather indifferent. Treatment recommendations are to be based upon rational science and if that is wanting, empirically established treatments derived from years of clinical practice (1758)[142].

William Battie in no uncertain terms directly challenges medical dogma and encourages young physicians to take a new, critical, and fresh look at madness. He proclaims madness is poorly understood, poorly defined, and poorly conceptualized. He rejects all prior popular conceptual models of madness e.g. Balance of humors, supranatural deity (organized religions) models. He proposes a precise definition of madness to replace the current definition which is so encompassing that it has little value. He further encourages physicians to question all they have been taught in regard to madness. Finally, he is one of the first to actively encourage physicians to seek supervised training and experience firsthand in the diagnosis and treatment of individuals suffering mental disorders. Unlike other large facilities e.g. Bethlem Royal Hospital, William Battie is instrumental in establishing training opportunities for physicians at St. Luke's Hospital for Lunatics, in order that physicians have a formal opportunity to learn how to more effectively diagnose, treat, and manage individuals suffering mental disorders (1758)[142].

As with most whom challenge medical dogma, William Battie's ideas are met with much resistance from the established medical community. The criticism is nowhere better exemplified than in John Monro's paper titled "Remarks on Dr. Battie's Treatise on Madness" (1758)[143]. John Monro (1718-1791) physician at the Bethlem Royal Hospital, systematically rejects each point made by William Battie in the "Treatise on Madness", offering medical dogma as his primary reasons for his rejections of Battie's ideas.

Trivia: The term "neurosis" is coined by William Cullen (1710-1790) Scottish, Professor of Medicine at Edinburg and introduced into the medical literature in 1769. The term is selected to emphasize the new belief, within the medical community, mental disorders result from impairment of the nervous system (1769,1786)[144,145].

Thomas Arnold (1742-1816) English physician and owner/medical director of the Lancaster County Lunatic Asylum, offers his new classification system and rational treatments based upon his many years of providing direct clinical services to patients of the Lancaster County Lunatic Asylum. He presents his new classification system of mental disorders and thoughts on madness in three volumes; "Observations on the nature, kinds, causes, and prevention of insanity" (1787, 1806)[146,147] and "Observations on the management of the insane and particularly on the agency and importance of humane and kind treatment in effecting their cure" (1809)[148]. Volume one addresses the definition and epidemiology of insanity; volume two the causes of insanity; and volume three the treatments of insanity.

In brief, Thomas Arnold ascribes to a natural (physical) origin of mental disorders. He organizes mental disorders into two primary categories, Ideal insanities and Notional insanities. He defines Ideal insanities as "… that state of mind in which a person imagines he sees, hears or otherwise perceives or converses with, persons or things, which have no external existence…" (1787)[146]. Within this broad category he identifies four subtypes: phrenic, incoherent, maniacal, and sensitive. He defines Notional insanities as "…that state of mind in which a person sees, hears or otherwise perceives external objects as they really exist, as objects of sense; yet conceives such notions of the powers, properties, design, state, definition, importance, manner of existence, or the like, of things and person, of himself and others, as appear obviously, and grossly erroneous, or unreasonable, to the common sense of the sober and judicious part of mankind. It is of considerable duration; is never accompanied with any great degree of fever, and very often without fever at all…" (1787)[146]. He identifies nine subtypes within the Notional insanities: delusive, fanciful, whimsical, impulsive, scheming, vain or self-important, hypochondriacal, pathetic, and appetitive (1787)[146]. What is most important here is not his classification system, rather how he constructs his categories. Each subtype is based upon observations of clinical presentations rather than the traditional classifications based upon suspected underlying etiologies e.g. imbalance of humors (Galen), demonic possession (Church).

Treatments recommendations are largely management of the individuals' living conditions and daily routines. Management of the individual should consist of firm management, without the use of chains; "…care should be taken that they (lunatics) neither injure themselves nor others nor be subjected to any probable means of injury…" (1809)[148]; temperance in food, drink, exercise, recreation, amusements, and sleep; regulation of passions, and a rational view of God and religion is to be encouraged. Similar in many ways to the recommendations of William Battie, Thomas Arnold encourages humane treatment of the insane, primarily by way of management techniques. He discourages use of medicines and popular medical procedures such as bleeding, purging, dunking into cold shock baths, and blistering, in the treatment of the insane.

Thomas Arnold argues too the current definition of insanity necessitates significant revisions to make it meaningful. He specifically draws attention to the many physical conditions which produce transient episodes of impaired mental functions, such as seen associated with violent fevers, canine madness, frequent intoxications, constant use of narcotics, and habitual convulsions. He recommends the following restricted definition; "…a real unequivocal mania or madness, such a mania as characterizes itself by an alienation of reason, a deprivation of intellectual powers, and an ungovernable impetuosity of disconnected ideas and irrational conduct. That is the kind of madness and that alone which deserves the name of insanity…" (1787)[146,146].

Andrew Harper (unknown-1790) English military surgeon offers an innovative alternative to understanding mental disorders in his book titled "A treatise on the real cause and cure of insanity in which the nature and distinction of this disease are fully explained and the treatments established on new principles" (1789)[149]. It is here, he first argues against the popular dogma that insanity results from heredity, disordered brain anatomy, or numerous other physical conditions commonly used to explain impaired mental functions e.g. violent fevers, bites from a mad dog (canine madness- rabies), epileptic fits, head trauma, intoxications by opium abuse, alcoholic beverages, or medicinal remedies e.g. mercury poisoning associated with the medical treatment of venereal disease, brain irritations (encephalitis, meningitis, or mechanical compression), impairment in profusion of blood to brain, obstructions of the liver or spleen, infarction of the uterus. He argues these conditions do unquestionably alter mental functions, typically are transient, circumstantial, and mental functions improve when the primary cause is removed. These disorders although very real and debilitating are distinctly different from insanity, although they produce impairments in normal mental functions yet "…have really no share whatsoever, in producing that disease (insanity)…" (1789)[149]. He further differentiates melancholic and hypochondriacal states from true insanity,

Insanity as defined by Andrew Harper is "…a disease of the mind, independent of any corporal existing cause…" (1789)[149]. This perspective sets him apart from others of the period whom argue insanity is the product of heredity, structural lesions evident in a person's anatomy, or chemical lesions evident in disorders of metabolism and physiology.

Andrew Harper offers a new model from which to understand insanity and to guide treatment. In brief, his model is based upon an imbalance of ideas occurring within the mind. An ordered system that is balanced in the healthy mind and disordered in the insane. For Andrew Harper, ideas within the mind have specific characteristics, note, pitch, and modulation, which define an idea or experience. Opposing ideas and experiences, for example pain and pleasure, happiness and sadness, goodness and badness occur in reciprocal proportions and are balanced in the healthy individual. In the case of insanity, the order and balance of ideas is disordered or destroyed. What is important here is not his specific model, rather to understand the model directly challenges medical dogma and proposes a new, innovative model of insanity based not upon anatomy or physiology, rather upon abstract constructs operating within the mind (1789)[149].

Treatment recommendations are rational and follow the conceptual matrix. Given insanity is a disease of the mind and not the body, treatments must be designed to restore the normal balance and order of ideas within the mind. Before a disordered mind can be effectively treated, the physical body needs to be as healthy as possible. The usual and customary, popular physical interventions are recommended and prescribed according to the physical malady. Once the physical body is attended then attention is directed to the physical environment and to include fresh dry air, clean living conditions. Once this is established, attention is directed to restoring balance within the disordered mind.

This is to be achieved by coordinating interventions and designing patient specific regimens to ease the mind. Specifically, encourage the patient to sleep "…because the longer it continues, the more is the mental tranquility established, as well as with respect to its effects, because the incongruous tumult of ideas being calmed…"; encourage relaxing warm baths, listening to soothing music, and take a "… plain and slender…" diet with the "…quantity of animal…to be less proportion than that of vegetables…" ; avoid astringent medicines, unnecessary coercion, and "…the custom of immediately consigning the unfortunate victims of insanity to the cells of Bedlam, or the dreary mansions of some private confinement, is certainly big with ignorance and absurdity. This practice, 'tis true, may answer the purpose of private interest, and domestic conveniency, but at the same time destroys all the obligations of humanity, robs the suffer of every advantage, and deprives him of all the favorable circumstances which might tend to his recovery…" (1789)[149]. Patients are further encouraged to discuss with their attending physician odd, unusual, distressing, or disturbing ideas, in order that the physician might, through talk therapy, assist the patient to restore balance within the disordered mind.

John Haslam (1764-1844) English apothecary (pharmacist) specializes in the treatment and study of the insane, while practicing at Bethlem Royal Hospital (Bedlam). He is an advocate of period medical dogma, believing insanity is the result of multiple potential causes such as heredity and observable anatomical changes in the brain; occurs more frequently in women than men; and best treated by a combination of medical treatments e.g. bleeding, purging, cold baths and behavior management e.g. confinement, "time outs" in darkened rooms, and thoughtful use of physical restraints.

He offers a non-selected collection and descriptions of 29 brains autopsied from his personal case load of insane patients to whom he provided services at Bethlem Royal Hospital, during the late-1790s. He presents his findings in his book titled "Observations on insanity, with practical remarks on the disease, and account of the morbid appearances on dissection" (1798)[150]. The brains are harvested from individuals ranging in age from 28 years of age to 78 years of age. This series contains 19 males and 10 females. Durations of signs and symptoms, length of hospitalizations, primary clinical pathologies, and post mortem findings are heterogeneous. Duration of signs and symptoms and associated hospitalized range from 3 weeks to 20 years. Primary clinical pathologies contained in the series are melancholia, mania, paranoid delusions, delusions of grandeur, dementia, complicated bereavement, immediate suicide risk with recent attempt, aphasia, delirium, strokes, and more. Post mortem findings range from normal to assorted, now recognizable lesions, such as meningitis, meningioma, brain abscess, enlarged ventricles, cerebral hemorrhage, cerebral infarctions, and more. This brain series exemplifies the type and level of sophistication used during the late-1700s to identify underlying anatomical origins of mental disorders.

By the end of the 1700s, the study of the insane becomes popular in Britain.

English physician William Pargeter (1760-1810) offers his "Observation on maniacal disorders" (1792)[151]. Here he encourages the use of behavioral management practices rather than medical intervention, whenever treating individuals with impaired mental functions.

Alexander Crichton (1763-1856) Scottish physician offers his "Inquiry into the nature and origin of mental derangement, comprehending a concise system of the physiology and pathology of the human mind, and a history of the passions and their effects, in two volumes" (1798a,1798b)[152,153]. Here he offers his views and conceptualizations of impaired mental functioning based upon his synthesis of current knowledge available from the UK, France, and Germany. He emphasizes the point mental disorders arise from impaired brain functions. Causes responsible for these impaired functions are attributed to physical impairments within the brain itself, impairment of other physical body systems secondarily impairing brain function, or impairments generated by the mind. His conceptual matrix proposes disordered brains produce mental disorders and disordered minds can produce disordered brains. This sets him apart from most describing the causes of impaired mental functions during the late-1700s. He further offers a simple classification system of mental disorders based upon clinical signs and symptoms rather than suspected underlying cause.

Interest in mental impairments is now rapidly gaining in popularity. Scientific and medical journals devoted to its study begin to appear e.g. the new German journal, "Magazin zur Erfahrungsseelenkunde" [Journal for Empirical Psychology] (1783-1793)[154]. This early journal contains primarily case studies and is used heavily by Alexander Crichton in developing his synthesis of mental impairments. More familiar journals devoted to understanding impaired mental functions do not appear until the mid-1800s.

In summary, the period of 1400-1800 witness much change in the conceptual matrix within which mental disorders are understood and individuals suffering the disorders are cared for and treated. Organized religion and its associated faith-based belief systems, rather than science, continue to dominant most thinking towards individuals suffering mental impairments. However, movement is slowly being made away from the acceptance mental disorders have a supranatural origins and towards understanding mental disorders as having natural (physical) origins. Medical psychology as a scientific discipline, further differentiates itself from philosophy and religion. As a developing new profession, it makes its first advances by establishing professional journals and interest groups devoted specifically to the scientific and professional understanding of impaired mental functions. Exchange of scientific and clinical information flows freely between investigators. New organizational systems appear for mental disorders based upon clinical presentations of signs and symptoms rather than suspected underlying secular and non-secular pathologies. Governments struggle with its responsibilities in caring for individuals suffering impaired mental functions and attempt to legislate the care and treatment of the mentally impaired with variable success. Physicians once again become relevant in the treatment and management of the mentally impaired. Specialized clinical training is offered to physicians choosing to specialize in the care and treatment of the mentally impaired. Notable figures Johann Weyer, Paracelsus, Thomas Willis, Thomas Sydenham, William Battie, Thomas Arnold, Andrew Harper, John Haslam, and Alexander Crichton guide medical psychology into a new period by challenging dogma, seeing things differently from all others around them, and taking actions to effect meaningful change.

Middle Modern, 1800 AD - 1900 AD.

The 1800s witness a rapid maturation of medical psychology and psychiatry as scientific disciplines. New academic and professional associations and their associated journals are founded, and devoted specifically to the scientific advancement of our understanding of impaired mental functions. Two predominant models are established. One emphasizes brain anatomy, brain physiology, and brain chemistry. The second emphasizes abstract constructs of mental functions and mental development. Moderator variables e.g. age, sex, heredity, social stressors are explored to further explain the variability in mental functions, both normal and disordered. Residential asylum based care and treatments become more humane in response to public activism demanding change. New classification systems are introduced and refined. New terms and vocabulary are introduced into the scientific and medical literatures.

Influential notables e.g. Jean-Baptiste Pussin, Phillipe Pinel, Johannas Reil, Franz Gall, Benjamin Rush, Thomas Sutton, Johann Heinroth, Jean-Estienne Esquirol, Dorthea Dix, Benedict Morel, Emil Kraepelin, Wilhelm Wundt, James Cattell, Paul Mobius, Josef Breuer, and Sigmund Freud make many of their major contributions which guide medical psychology and psychiatry for the next 200 years.

Jean-Baptiste Pussin (1745-1811) French, senior administrator for the Paris based insane asylum for incurable men at Bicetre Hospital and later the insane asylum for incurable women at Salpetriere Hospital, pioneers asylum reform. He is instrumental in effecting meaningful changes within these two premier asylums, greatly improving the living conditions and treatments for patients suffering mental impairments. Following years of empirical observation and detailed record keeping at both asylums, Jean-Baptiste Pussin abandons the traditional practices of long term physical restraint by chains, manacles, and shackles, housing patients in dark isolated rooms, public display of patients for amusement purposes, indiscriminate beating of patients by staff, and many of the harsh conventional medical treatments of the time e.g. bleeding, purging, blistering. He replaces these with more humane approaches to care, treatments, and management practices.

Jean-Baptiste Pussin implements a moral therapy model at both facilities, emphasizing clean living conditions, good personal hygiene, healthy diet, emotional support, kindness, respect, moderate exercise, therapeutic voluntary work, and strict policy of nonviolence for patients and staff (1800)[155]. He first implements these changes at the Bicetre asylum for men in 1797 and within ten years effects these same changes at the Salpetriere asylum for women. The changes prove to be extremely successful and provide a catalysis for change in many asylums throughout France and beyond. Jean-Baptiste Pussin additionally introduces a crude classification system for new admissions, based upon the patient's history and current temperament. The classification is used to make appropriate housing assignments and too is successful.

Jean-Baptiste Pussin contributions in the reformation of practices within large asylums, charged with the care and treatment of individuals suffering mental impairments, are often unrecognized. His empirical observational methods, commitment to detailed record keeping of patient progress or non-progress while hospitalized, rejection of dogmatic institutional management practices, and ineffective medical procedures contribute significantly to the change in the care and treatment of patients suffering mental impairments confined to institutional facilities.

Note: The word "moral" as in "Moral therapy" or "Moral treatment" when correctly and best translated from French into English, does not mean "moral" but rather "psychological". This is oftentimes a point of confusion for many medical students.

Phillipe Pinel (1745-1826) French internist, proves instrumental in influencing the way in which mental impairments are understood and treated in France. He rejects Church dogma as to the origins of mental impairments and unequivocally states the origins of mental impairment is multifactorial with principle factors identified to be heredity, impaired physiology, social and psychological stresses (1798)[156]. He rejects traditional medical treatments and encourages the use of humane treatment and management models (1801,1806)[157,158]. He proves instrumental in the reform of the treatment of patients suffering mental impairments confined to asylums.

Phillipe Pinel introduces a classification system of mental disorders, while working with Jean-Baptiste Pussin, based largely upon his observations of patients made at the Bicetre asylum for men. The system categorizes mental impairments "…for the time being…" into five principle groups: melancholia (depressions), mania without delirium, mania with delirium, dementia, and idiotism (1798,1801)[156,157]. Pinel is aware of the limits of his classification system and attributes the limitations to the paucity of knowledge within medicine regarding mental disorders. It is here he first differentiates various types of psychoses and offers the first description of dementia praecox (schizophrenia) (1798,1801,1806)[156,157,158]. Pinel advocates the use of empirical observation and descriptive categorization of mental disorders, rather than suspected underlying causes.

From a treatment perspective, he discourages the use of popular medical treatments for patients suffering mental impairment e.g. bleeding, purging, blistering, medications, and long term physical restraints. He encourages the use of moral (psychological) therapies, as practiced by Jean-Baptiste Pussin at the Bicetre asylum for men. Jean-Baptiste Pussin's moral therapies emphasize mutual respect between physician and patient, kindness, emotional support, encouraging patients to discuss problems with their treating physician, fostering social skills and self-control, encouraging friendly contact between patients and staff, healthy diet, moderate exercise, good personal hygiene, clean living conditions, and limited use of physical restraints (1798,1801, 1806)[156,157,158].

Perhaps no single person has more influence upon Phillipe Pinel's thoughts on the care and management of individuals suffering mental impairments than Jean-Baptiste Pussin. The two men work together at the Bicetre asylum for men during 1793-1795 and again at the Salpetriere asylum for women a few years later. Jean-Baptiste Pussin's practice of daily observation of patients, documenting patient response to treatments, documenting patient progress or lack of progress throughout hospitalization, noting dramatic improvements in many patient's conditions when moral (psychological) therapies are implemented in contrast to traditional medical interventions, and compiling complete patient case histories for educational and training purposes have a great impact upon Pinel. His thinking and approach to the treatment of patient suffering mental impairments change forever, as the direct result of his two years spent with Jean-Baptiste Pussin and the many patients of the Bicetre and Salpetriere asylums in Paris.

Historically, the lion's share of credit for effecting meaningful reform within the asylums of France during the late-1700s and early-1800s is assigned to Phillipe Pinel. However, Pinel readily and frequently acknowledges the influence, great respect, and many contributions made by Jean-Baptiste Pussin; "…he lived among the insane night and day, studied their ways, their character, and their tastes, the course of their derangements…" (1801)[157].

Trivia: Phillipe Pinel, as a graduate of the medical school in Toulouse (1773), is initially prohibited from practicing medicine in Paris as a licensed physician. He subsidizes his income as an unlicensed physician by conducting private lectures on human anatomy and translating documents such as "The Philosophical Transactions of the Royal Society of London" into French.

Johannas Reil (1759-1813) German, Professor of Medicine at the Universities of Halle (central Germany) and Berlin makes numerous contributions to the fields of anatomy, histology, physiology, neurology, and psychiatry. He founds the first journal in Germany devoted to the scientific study of physiology, chemistry, biology, histology, and comparative anatomy, "Archives fur die Physiologie" with the intent to make these disciplines the scientific foundation of medicine

(1796a)[159]. An ardent proponent of Vitalism, he argues life force results from a chemical expression of normal physiological processes (1796b)[160]. Disease and disease processes are simply the consequence of disorders of body chemistry and physiology.

In regard to mental impairments, Johannas Reil is impressed by marked changes in mental functions evidenced by patients suffering fever (1802)[161]. He soon expands his interest to patients suffering impaired mental functions in the absence of fever. He quickly concludes all mental impairments result from an interaction of mental, chemical, and physical processes, with no single factor responsible (1803)[162].

He develops conceptual matrixes which explain impaired mental functions within the matrix of anatomy and physiology and later in more abstract terms of a fragmentation of self (1807-1808,1812)[163,164]. In both matrixes his fundamental belief is mental disorders appear when the physical or more abstract "common sense" forces which hold mental processes together become disordered (1808,1812)[163,164]. Johannas Reil founds the German journal, "Magazin fur die Psychische Heilkunde" [Journal of Psychiatric Medicine], devoted to the scientific understanding of the processes responsible for mental impairments (1805)[165].

From a treatment perspective, he advocates humane treatment approaches. He emphasizes the value of talk based psychotherapies, which he terms "…psychic therapy…" to be equally important as medications or surgical interventions. He further proposes using the whole atmosphere of the asylum as a treatment tool (1803)[162]. His treatise, "Rhapsodieen uber die Anwendung der Psychischen Curemethode aug Geisteszerruttung" [Reflections on the Application of the Psychological Method of Treatment for Mental Disorders], triggers a reform in Germany as to how mental disorders are conceptualized and treated (1803)[162]. He is active in efforts to eliminate the stigma currently associated with impaired mental functions. He is among the early proponents advocating the need for specialized training for physicians seeking to offer treatment to individuals suffering mental disorders.

Johannas Reil is perhaps most recognized by medical students as the person who coins the term "psychiatry" (1808)[166]. The term "psychiatry" first appears in Johannas Reil's 118 page paper titled "Uber den bergriff der medizin und ihre verzweigungen, bsesonders in beziehung auf die berichtigung der topik in der psychiaterie" [On the concept of medicine and its branches, especially with regard to the justification of the topic of psychiatry]. This paper appears in the short lived German journal "Beytrage zur Bedorderung einer Kurmethode auf Psychischem Wege" [Contributions to the Advancement of a Treatment Method by the Psychic Ways] (1808)[166].

The term "psychiatry" is carefully selected by Johannas Reil. The first half of the term "psych" is derived from the Greek meaning "mind/soul". The second half of the term "iartry" is derived from the Greek meaning "healing". Literally, the translation of the term "psychiatry" is "healing of the mind/soul". Johannas Reil deliberately and mindfully incorporates "iartry" into the term to emphasize the proposed new discipline's commitment to healing (treatment) and differentiate the newly proposed discipline from philosophy or theology. The term is not initially embraced by the medical or scientific communities and only over the course of time becomes an accepted term.

Johann Reil further offers detailed anatomical descriptions of nerve structure (1796)[167], the ascending neural fibers of the lateral lemniscus ("lemniscus" means ribbon) located in the brain stem, an essential neural pathway for hearing (1796)[167], and the insula located deep inside the lateral fissures of the brain's cerebral hemispheres (1796,1809)[167,168.]

Trivia: The anatomical brain structure known to every first year medical student, as the "Island of Reil" (aka insular cerebral cortex) is described by Reil in 1796 and 1809. The term "Island of Reil" first appears approximately 50 years later. The term is offered by English anatomist Henry Gray and appears in the first edition of "Gray's Anatomy" (1858)[169].

By the late-1700s and early-1800s, the brain is aggressively investigated with regard to its role and contribution to impaired mental functions. Models emphasizing brain chemistry and brain physiology are investigated with the same enthusiasm as alternative models emphasizing abstract conceptualizations of mental processes.

Franz Gall (1758-1828) Austrian neuroanatomist and physiologist proposes a conceptual model which states the brain is the organ of mental activities, emotions, and all human behavior. He first publishes his model in a letter sent from Gall to a Viennese censorship official, Joseph von Retzer (1798)[170]. The model changes very little over time and identifies 27 specific "...fundamental faculties..." (innate personality traits and innate abilities) e.g. instinct for reproduction, love of one's offspring, vanity, pride, guile, memory for words, people, and places, mechanical ability, talent for poetry, sense of satire and witticism, compassion, moral sense, benevolence, which all can be localized to 27 distinct, yet connected areas of the brain. It is the interaction of these fundamental faculties which is responsible for normal mental function and human behavior. When brain areas are disordered, the result is "... different kinds of insanity...", characterized by impairments in thought, cognition, mood, affect, and behavior (1798,1807a,1807b)[170,171,172].

Gall's model embraces a naturalistic approach to understanding mental processes. His conceptual model is based upon his medical training as an anatomist and physiologist, coupled with personal observations of hundreds of individuals suffering impairments of mental functions and behavior. These observations are made of individuals confined in asylums, hospitals, prisons, and houses of correction throughout Berlin. Gall is interested in the association of physical surface anatomy with localization of mental processes. He collects hundreds of skulls and plaster casts of heads, then carefully measures each. He then associates abnormal head and skull measurements with abnormal mental functioning and deviant human behavior. Initial findings prove promising. For example, several individuals evidencing impaired intellectual abilities and cognitive function since birth reveal enlarged skulls, which Gall attributes to sustained internal pressure on the skull, compromising brain tissues responsible for intellectual abilities and cognitive function. It is reasonable to assume these patients suffered congenital and uncorrected hydrocephalus and offers support of Gall's hypothesis, abnormalities in skull measurements are associated with impaired intellectual ability and cognitive function (1817)[173].

Most medical students associate Franz Gall with the practice of "phrenology". A theory and practice which purports to identify innate abilities and personality traits through an analysis of changes in skull contour. Changes in contour are detected by the physician simply feeling the patient's head and noting areas of relative contour differences. Contour changes (bumps) are interpreted within the matrix of assigned brain functions underlying the bumps. This practice is based upon Gall's belief "...the surface of the skull is determined by the external form of the brain..." and thereby reflects the specific, localized brain faculties located immediately below (1798)[170]. Abnormalities in skull contours are associated with abnormalities of specific faculties (1822,1835)[174,175]. Be aware, while this part of Gall's model receives tremendous attention it represents only a fraction of the much larger and often neglected conceptual matrix offered by Gall's model (1798)[170].

Franz Gall and his student Johann Spurzheim (1776-1832) German anatomist and ardent proponent of the Gall model, part ways over professional differences by 1812. Gall relocates to Paris and continues his research and teachings, focusing upon his studies of localized brain functions. Spurzheim embarks on financially lucrative lecture tours across Europe and the USA, promoting the practice of phrenology to the general public. Gall's original theory is soon distorted by many, physicians included, by over interpretations and extension to the point of losing its scientific value. By the end of the 1800s the system is so popularized by the lay public it becomes little more than a parlor game.

Trivia: Gall himself never uses or approves of the term "phrenology". Gall's preferred terms for his model of localization of brain function are "schadellehre" (doctrine of the skull), "organology" (referring to the areas of localized brain functions, he terms "organs"), and "the physiology of the brain". It is the English naturalist Thomas Forster (1789-1860) who first coins the term "phrenology", 17 years after Gall first introduces the system (1815)[176]. The term "phrenology" is popularized by Johann Spurzheim during lecture tours across Europe, especially in Britain, and gains widespread use by the early-1820s.

It is of historical value and instructive to all students today to note Franz Gall prepares a large, multi-volume collection detailing his theory in 1801. He is forbidden from publishing this work due to political pressures exerted by the Church. The Church cites their reasons for prohibiting publication, to be the content of the work challenges "…the first principles of morality and religion…" (1801,1801)[177,178]. So goes another example of organized religion controlling the distribution of new ideas and scientific thought.

In many ways Gall's theory and conceptual matrix emphasizing localization of brain function and belief impairments in localized brain regions produce specific impairments in mental abilities, emotions, and behavior are accepted scientific and medical dogma today, over 220 years after he first proposes the idea to the scientific and medical communities.

Trivia: Upon Gall's death in 1828 his skull is added to his own scientific collections of skulls. It can be viewed today in Paris, at the Musee de l'Homme [Museum of Man], catalogue number 19216.

Investigations and study of mental disorders flourish in Europe during the early 1800s. Significant advancements are being made in Germany, France, and England. At the same time, there is little interests in the investigation of mental disorders in the USA or Canada.

Benjamin Rush (1745-1813) American, Professor of Chemistry at the College of Philadelphia and later Professor of Medical Theory at the University of Pennsylvania offers his textbook "Medical Inquires and Observations upon the Disease of the Mind" (1812)[179]. This is the first attempt by an American to organize and synthesize the rapidly growing body of new information regarding mental impairments and their associated epidemiology, origin, cause, course, management, and treatment. He offers information dogmatically from a theoretical perspective with little interest in scientific empiricism.

In brief, he argues mental impairments result when normal body systems are unbalanced. The imbalances produce impaired brain functions and consequently disorders of thought, cognition, mood, affect, and behavior. He is heavily influenced by Scottish physician William Cullen's model of mental disorders, which emphasizes the balance of energy within the nervous system. Excess stimulation necessitates therapeutic depletion, whereas a deficit of energy necessitates stimulation. He proposes the usual and customary medical treatments of purging, emetics, and bleeding as most effective when depletion of energy is required and wine, aromatic warm baths, and body massage when stimulation is required. Diet changes are recommended in the treatment of both imbalanced energy state (1812)[179].

As part of his recommended treatments of mental disorders Benjamin Rush introduces the "tranquilizing chair". This apparatus is essentially a chair to which the patient's arms, legs, and head are bound. The head is placed inside of a shielded hood which minimizes auditory and visual sensory input into the nervous system. Binding to the chair restricts patient movement. The fundamental idea here is to eliminate sensory input and body movement, thereby reducing stimulation of the nervous system and calming the patient. He objects to the use of traditional physical restraints (chains and manacles), physical punishment, and coercion as methods for managing the mentally impaired. He is a proponent of humane treatments such as occupational therapies, work therapies, and is instrumental in establishing treatment facilities for the mentally impaired at the new Pennsylvania Hospital. He pioneers work into the medical treatments of alcohol abuse (1785)[180].

Trivia: Benjamin Rush is one of the 56 signatures appearing on the United States Declaration of Independence (1776)[181]. His image is incorporated into the official medallion seal of the American Psychiatric Association (APA) with 13 stars above his image representing the 13 original founding members of the organization. The seal first appears, on the cover of the publication Semi-Centennial Proceedings of the American Medico-Psychological Association, at the 50th annual meeting in Philadelphia in 1894 (1895,1998)[182,183].

In Europe, issues of differential diagnosis and new treatment methods are debated and new ideas challenge medical dogma. Scientific and professional advancements being made during this period shape the discipline of medical psychology for the next 200 years.

Thomas Sutton (1767-1835) English physician first describes the signs and symptoms of delirium tremens (DTs), coins the term, and differentiates the syndrome from phrenitis and mania. He reviews current literature, offers 16 case histories from his personal case load, and offers keys to identifying delirium tremens both as an independent disease entity and as a syndrome embedded within other disease conditions. He emphasizes the need for practicing physicians to be aware of this commonly occurring condition, understand how the syndrome can be embedded within the clinical presentation of primary mental disorders, and encourages the use of opium as an effective treatment, based upon empirical observations. Sutton concludes DTs are the result of an acquired brain impairment, caused by chronic consumption of "…fermented liquors, and more especially spirits…" and presents most commonly in "…those who confessedly indulged in the use of spirits to excess…" (1813)[184].

From a treatment approach perspective with regard to DTs, Thomas Sutton discourages the use of the popular medical treatments of bleedings, purging, emetics, and blistering, noting his personal observations of their repeated failures to improve patient conditions from both his personal case load, as well as other physicians reporting in the professional literature. He proposes the use of large doses of opium as an effective treatment for DTs. He recognizes opium may be a substitute for the alcohol, providing a tranquil feeling to the patient and not rendering a cure, yet prefers this to the horrors experienced by the patient by this disease, in the absence of opium. He justifies the use of opium upon empirical grounds; it relieves "…the urgent symptoms of the disease…" and "…the horrors which follow…" (1813)[184].

Governments in Europe are now becoming more involved in the oversight of institutional care facilities and influencing where and how patients suffering mental disorders are managed within the social matrix of society and treated within institutional care facilities. Specific government interests focus upon improving living conditions within institutions, eliminating neglect and brutality, and improving overall care in general in response to public outcry of reported horrific conditions within several government funded and private for profit institutional care facilities of the period (1815)[185].

The academic and medical communities debate whether medicine has any role in the treatment or management of patients suffering mental disorders beyond relieving physical symptoms associated with mental disorders. There is a rapidly growing consensus among both communities, mental disorders result primarily from impaired brain structure and function. However, there are few studies which have revealed specific brain lesions beyond generalized inflammation of the brain and brain meninges. Most conventional physical treatments of bleeding, purging, emetics, and blistering are proving to be of little value in the treatment of most mental disorders. The growing consensus at this time is management is much more useful and effective than medical treatments, in the care of the mentally impaired patient (1817)[186].

Johann Heinroth (1773-1843) German, Professor of Psychiatry at Leipzig University challenges and rejects the idea, mental disorders result from impaired brain or other body functions. Rather he attributes the cause of mental disorders to be solely the result of moral weakness. Sin, selfishness, and associated guilt are the definitive causes of mental disorders. By the patient's life choices or life circumstances the soul is deranged and unable to function normally. The consequential result is appearance of mental impairments. Physical signs and symptoms associated with impaired mental functions appear as the consequence of a disordered soul and not the cause. His model should be familiar to you now. This is the view embraced by the Christian Church, separating body and soul. The body is "…the carrier, supporter, and tool of the soul…". Mental disorders only result when the soul is disordered (1823,1825)[187,188].

Effective treatments need to address the soul and not the body alone. Heinroth proposes use of "…a special building for the physical treatment of the mentally disturbed…a special correction and punishment room with all the necessary equipment…" to effect a successful treatment of the disordered soul. The room is to include "…immersion vessels…punishment chair…Langermann's cell (isolation cell)…Cox swing (swing used to spin patients until they vomit or convulse)… and Johannas Reil's fly-wheel (much like a hamster exercise wheel for humans)…" (1818)[189]. He justifies the use of each device and punishment procedure as necessary and essential to effect a cure. He dismisses all criticisms his physical methods are inhumane with self-assured self-righteousness.

Perhaps less remembered is Johann Heinroth's conceptualization of the interaction between body and soul. He introduces the term "psychisch-somatisch" [psychosomatic] into medicine to emphasize internal psychological conflict can and does produce very real and potentially debilitating physical symptoms (1818)[190]. He extends the idea and encourages physicians to treat not only the body but treat the soul too; "…the person is more than just the mere body as well as more than the mere soul; it is the whole human being…" (1825)[188]. Yes, this is the same guidance offered by the early Greek philosophers during 300 BC.

Johann Heinroth conceptualizes mental disorders as debilitating internal psychological conflict. He encourages, in addition to brutal physical punishment procedures discussed above, exploration of the benefits of an early form of retrospective life analysis, predating Sigmund Freud by 80 years, "…if we… make a detailed study of the past life of the patient, prior to the complete derangement of his psyche, we would perhaps find the key…" (1818)[189].

Jean-Etienne Esquirol (1772-1840). French psychiatrist passionately continues the works of Jean-Baptiste Pussin and Phillipe Pinel in reforming the asylums of France. He offers medical services at the Salpetriere asylum for women, aside fellow reformers Jean-Baptiste Pussin and Phillipe Pinel. He shares a common belief with Phillipe Pinel, the origins of mental disorders can best be found in the passions of the soul. He publishes his medical doctoral thesis titled "Des passions considerees comme causes, symptômes et moyens de traitement de l'alienation mentale" [The passions considered as causes, symptoms, and means of cure in cases of insanity], in which he outlines his model to understand and treat mental disorders (1805)[191]. He joins Phillipe Pinel at the Salaptriere asylum for women and provides medical services to those suffering impairments in thought, cognition, mood, affect, and behavior. During the period of 1810-1817 he tours the asylums for the insane across France and reports horrific living conditions (1814)[192].

Based upon empirical observations and influence of mentors Jean-Baptiste Pussin and Phillipe Pinel, Jean-Etienne Esquirol encourages specialized training for all physicians choosing to treat mental disorders. He advocates treatment of mental disorders be provided within the milieu of the specialized psychiatric hospital rather than the general medical hospital, noting the hospital itself can be an important instrument in the comprehensive integrated treatment of patients suffering mental disorders. He encourages hospital administrators to acknowledge the physician as the supreme authority within specialized hospitals for the insane. He encourages recent advances made in the large medical centers regarding new or more effective treatments of the insane be more effectively communicated to practitioners providing services in rural communities.

Etienne Esquirol offers influential new definitions for hallucinations and illusions. Given hallucinations and illusions have been described and documented for thousands of years before Esquirol offers his definitions, he is among the first to describe a conceptual matrix which interprets hallucinations and illusions to be the result of impaired biological systems.

In brief, he dismisses definitions based upon clinical descriptions. He provides criteria which clearly differentiate hallucinations from illusions. He introduces a new conceptual matrix within which to understand hallucinations, defining hallucinations to be physical symptoms. This new definition and conceptualization allows hallucinations to be readily interpreted within the matrix of anatomical-clinical correlations, a framework gaining rapid popularity in France during the early-1800s (1817)[193]. He emphasizes a "…hallucination is a cerebral or psychic phenomenon which operates independently of the senses…everything happens in the brain…"; whereas in the case of illusions "…the sensitivity of the nervous extremities is altered…the impression produced on them by external objects will be modified; if the transmission nerves are damaged and, at the same time, the brain is in a pathological state, the latter will be incapable of remedying the error or the senses: hence the illusions…(1838)[194].

Additional notable contributions offered by Jean-Estienne Esquirol are his early descriptions of congenital, generalized cognitive-intellectual impairments as a separate and distinct entity from insanity; proposes a new and much simplified classification system of mental impairments, identifying five "...general forms of madness..."; proposes mental disorders can result equally from emotional disturbances as from brain disorders; and identifies specific contributory factors leading to onset, frequency, duration, and type of mental disorder most likely to present clinically and their contribution to the probability of a successful cure. Specifically, Jean-Estienne Esquirol identifies age, sex, temperaments (personality), profession, and life style to be the most influential contributory factors (1838,1845)[194,195]. His ideas are detailed in his textbook "Mental Maladies: Treatise on Insanity" (1838,1845)[194,195]. This textbook is used as a primary text and source of information in psychiatry throughout Europe and the USA for more than 50 years.

In addition to the development of meaningful classification systems and continued debate regarding the underlying etiology responsible for impaired mental function, this period witnesses the founding of professional organizations and societies devoted specifically to the scientific advancement of knowledge and understanding of mental impairments. Attention is additionally directed to establishing more humane treatment and physical care of individuals suffering debilitating impairments in thought, cognition, mood, affect, and behavior.

Dorthea Dix (1802-1887) American activist reforms horrific living conditions and physical treatments of individuals suffering mental disorders throughout the USA. During the period of 1841-1842 she visits jails, prisons, almshouses, work houses, asylums, and private homes documenting horrific living conditions and appalling abuse. She describes brutal, physical and sexual abuse by keepers, floggings, starvation, chaining, with individuals "...confined in closets, cellars, stalls, pens...lashed into obedience...", without clothing, sanitation, furniture, light, or heat. Initially, she conducts visits in the state of Massachusetts and submits her findings to the state legislature with a call for action (1843)[196]. As the result of her efforts conditions begin to change and improve.

She continues her political activism on behalf of individuals suffering mental disorders over the course of the next 40 years. She effectively generates meaningful change in the care and treatment of patients suffering mental impairments in no less than 15 USA states, Canada (Nova Scotia), and Europe. She advocates construction of specialized care facilities, staffed with specially trained staff, utilizing the preferred and popular moral treatment model, humane approach to care, treatment, and management.

Reform is now occurring in the care and treatment of individuals suffering mental disorders, in the USA, Europe, and Canada. Medical dogma is being challenged and replaced by new conceptual matrixes within which to understand and treat mental disorders. Emphasis is now being focused upon the brain as the organ most responsible for impaired mental function. Modifying influences such as heredity, age, sex, occupation, economic advantage, personality, and life style choices receive greater attention and are recognized to be important factors in contributing to the appearance of mental disorders and their effective treatments. Specialized training become more available to physicians choosing to provide medical services to patients suffering mental impairments. Professionals committed to the care and treatment of individuals suffering mental disorders join together to share new information. Professional societies committed to the advancement of scientific knowledge and professional development are founded in the USA, Europe, and Canada. Scientific and professional journals are founded to further facilitate the exchange of new information. Medical psychology and psychiatry enter a new phase of professional development, as recognized professional, scientific, and valued disciplines.

The first professional association in Europe founded and committed specifically to improving the care and treatments of the mentally impaired patient is the Association of Medical Officers of Asylums and Hospitals for the Insane. The Association is founded in Nottingham, England November 4, 1841. The purpose of the Association is to bring together medical practitioners providing services or administering public and private facilities for the insane, in England, Scotland, and Ireland; freely communicating their experiences; and assisting each other in improving the care and treatment of the insane within the United Kingdom. This organization changes names several times since its founding in 1841 and is known today simply as the Royal College of Psychiatrists. The organization is the main professional organization for psychiatrists in the UK today (2018)[197].

As part of the Association's commitment to freely disseminate information among professionals committed to the scientific and professional advancement of understanding mental disorders; providing medical treatments and administering care facilities, it publishes an official Association journal. Originally titled the "Asylum Journal" (1853-1858), it too witnesses name changes over time. It is known as the "Journal of Mental Sciences" (1858-1963) and today as the "British Journal of Psychiatry" (1963-present). Archive issues are readily available online (2018)[198].

The first professional association in the USA founded and committed specifically to improving the care and treatments of the mentally impaired patient is the Association of Medical Superintendents of American Institutions for the Insane. The Association is founded in Philadelphia, Pennsylvania in October 1844. The stated objectives of the Association are "…to communicate their experiences to each other, to cooperate in collecting statistical information relating to insanity and assisting each other in improving the treatment of the insane…" (1844)[199]. This organization changes its name in 1892 to the American Medico-Psychological Association and again in 1921 to its present name the American Psychiatric Association.

The Association founds its official journal, the "American Journal of Insanity", first published in June 1844 (1844)[200]. The Journal changes names several times since its first publication and is known today by the name adopted in 1921, the "American Journal of Psychiatry".

Newly organized professional associations and journals mark the continued maturation of medical psychology and psychiatry as science based disciplines. Interests within the academic and medical communities continues to grow as new information and recent advances into understanding mental disorders appear in the professional literature and presented at annual association meetings.

Similar activities are occurring in Europe.

All major advancements and contributions being made to the discipline of medical psychology and psychiatry are occurring in Europe, during the second half of the 1800s, with the exceptions of the works by American psychology professor James Cattell and founding of the American Psychological Association in the USA. Let us now take a look at a few of the most influential men making contributions during the mid and late-1800s.

Benedict Morel (1809-1873) Austrian born, French physician is active in asylum reform during the mid-1800s. Greatly influenced by his work at the Salpetriere asylum for women in Paris during 1841 and tours of lunatic asylums in Switzerland, Germany, Netherlands, and Italy during 1843-1845, he makes meaningful changes in how asylums provide care and treatments to patients suffering mental impairments. He offers summaries of his travels and observations, describing the state of psychiatry, incidence of "…lunacy…", prominent conceptual matrixes, and overall state of asylums outside of France in a series of seven letters he publishes in the newly founded journal "Annales Medico-Psychologiques" (1845-1846)[201].

As superintendent of the Asilie d'Alienes de Mareville [Asylum for Lunatics at Mareville], located outside of Nancy (north-eastern France), he eliminates the use of physical restraints as a course of management of patients, much in the manner accomplished previously by Jean-Baptiste Pussin and Phillipe Pinel at the Salpetriere asylum in Paris. He directly challenges the medical or administrative justification for continued use of physical restraints and coercive methods by asylums throughout Europe in his notable book, titled "Le no-restraint ou de l'abolition des moyens coercitifs dans le traitement de la folie: Suivi de considerations sur les causes de la progression dans le nombre des alienes admis dans les asiles" [Non-restraint and the abolition of coercive means in the treatment of insanity: Followed by considerations on the causes of the increase in the number of insane asylums.] (1860)[202].

Benedict Morel, in addition to his influential roles in the reform of "…asylums for the insane…", offers a new theory and conceptual matrix to account for the cause, nature, and course of mental disorders across the life span (1857)[203].

In brief, the model extends Charles Darwin's model of evolution. It is based upon a biological origin of mental impairment which is modified by environmental factors. The model emphasizes heredity as a principle factor to impairments. Environmental factors, such as alcohol and drug abuse, poor nutrition, poor living conditions, poor sanitation, and physical illness modify biology. These modifications are passed from parents to child, having deleterious effects on successive generations. The effects are cumulative from generation to generation (think genetic anticipation). Mental disorders are the consequence of mental de-evolution across an individual's life span and subsequent generations. Benedict Morel's model of heredity mental degeneration is well received by the academic and medical communities (1867)[204]. The model significantly influences conceptual thought within psychiatry and medical psychology, especially in France, for the next 100 years.

Benedict Morel introduces the term "demence precoce" (dementia praecox) into the medical literature, referring to a condition of mental and emotional degeneration, beginning during puberty (1857,1860)[205,206]. Decades later, German psychiatrist Emil Kraepelin (1856-1926) and Swiss psychiatrist Eugene Bleuler (1857-1939) usurp and modify the term to refer to a newly proposed grouping of mental disorders, "schizophrenia" (1893,1908,1911)[207,208,209].

Benedict Morel offers several investigations into intellectual developmental disorders (mental retardation) conducted at the Mareville asylum and publishes findings supporting his model of mental degeneration across successive generations. He emphasizes the role of environmental factors acting upon biology and demonstrates their cumulative effects, passed from parent to child, across generations. He describes how environmental pollutants first effect parents, place the second generation at high risk for mental impairments, such as epilepsy, hysteria, and neurasthenia (mechanical weakness of the nerves, resulting in symptoms of fatigue, anxiety, headache, and depressed mood), place the third generation at high risk for insanity, and the fourth generation at high risk for congenital idiocy (1860)[210].

Trivia: Benedict Morel's model of hereditary mental degeneration is the origin for the popular derogatory lay term "degenerate" to refer to an individual evidencing compromised mental functions.

In addition to advances being made in public awareness, improved care, and understanding of impaired mental functioning, advances are now being made organizing mental impairments into diagnostic taxonomies.

Emil Kraepelin (1856-1926) German psychiatrist proposes a new and influential classification system for the mental disorders. Traditionally, mental disorders have been classified based upon suspected underlying cause e.g. imbalance of humors or primary presenting symptom e.g. melancholia (depression). Emil Kraepelin proposes a system based upon syndromes i.e. constellations of multiple signs and symptoms. The system avoids dependency upon any one sign or symptom or underlying pathology as criteria. Classifications are based upon patterns of signs and symptoms. This multivariate, pattern recognition approach forms the basis of most modern diagnostic classification systems used today, such as the DSM-5 (2013)[211].

Emil Kraepelin introduces his classification of mental disorders in 1883 (1883)[212]. The system is continuously refined and proves to be popular within the academic and medical communities. The system avoids many of the criticisms arising from investigator biases as to origins and causes of mental disorders by remaining focused upon observable clinical signs and symptoms, without attention to the many and oftentimes competing theories as to the origins of mental disorders e.g. brain pathologies, psychosocial factors, intra-psychic conflict. The system, with all of its strengths and weaknesses, brings order to an area of medical psychology and psychiatry (diagnosis) fast moving into a state of professional chaos.

Notable refinements made by Emil Kraepelin to his system across time (1883-1926) are reflected in his rejection of the popular classification of psychosis as a unitary disorder. He introduces a separation of psychosis into two distinctively different clinical presentations, "manic-depressive psychosis" and "dementia praecox" (schizophrenia) (1899)[213]. Subsequently, he further sub-classifies dementia praecox into three clinical subtypes: "catatonia" in which motor activity is substantially increased or more commonly decreased; "hebephrenic" in which affect is characterized by uncontrolled affect such as laughing; and "paranoia" characterized by delusions of persecution or grandeur. The classification systems influences conceptual thought within clinical psychiatry and medical psychology for the next 100 years.

Equally and arguably more important than his classification system are his many other contributions to the advancement of medical psychology. He is among the first to apply laboratory based experimental psychology procedures and methodologies to the study of mental disorders. His objective is to quantify fundamental mental processes and apply this information to assist in the differentiation of mental disorders, for the purposes of diagnosis and treatment. He investigates the effects of intoxicants e.g. alcohol, morphine, and tobacco, documenting their effects on mental processes (1883c)[214]. He investigates body fatigue and sleep, quantifying changes in assorted mental processes (1886e,1903b)[215,216]. He investigates the epidemiology of mental disorders outside of Europe e.g. Java, Dutch East Indies (Indonesia) (1904b,1904c,1904g)[217,218,219]. His cross cultural studies find dementia praecox (schizophrenia) to be present in all non-European societies; the prevalence of mania and melancholia to be extremely low in Java relative to European society; and the prevalence of alcohol psychosis also to be extremely low in Java

(1904b,1904g,1907e,1909)[217,219,220,221]. He concludes mental disorders occur in similar forms in all cultures, while specific symptoms are modified by cultural factors.

Trivia: Many notable and recognizable figures train in and conduct seminal investigations at Emil Kraepelin's clinic in Munich, Germany. For example, Alois Alzheimer conducts histological experiments, investigating histological changes in brain associated with general loss of memory, decreased reasoning abilities, and decreased comprehension. He reports a particularly interesting case to the 37th Conference of the South-West German Psychiatrist in 1906. The title of the paper is "Ueber einen eigenartigen, schweren erkrankungsprozess der hirnrinde" [A study on a particular, serious process of the cerebral cortex] (1906)[222]. This is the first description of "presenile dementia", a condition which generates much scientific study for the next 110 years. Emil Kraepelin coins the clinical condition, "Alzheimer's disease" four years later (1910)[223].

Wilhelm Wundt (1832-1920) German professor, physiologist, and psychologist establishes the first psychology lab for the study of psychological research at the University of Leipzig, Germany in 1879. He is first to define psychology as an independent field of scientific study, separate from biology and philosophy (1874,1897)[224,225]. He approaches the understanding of mental processes by breaking down each mental process into its most basic components. It is his belief the way to understand complex processes, such as the totality of any single human's life experiences, is to understand separate individual components which have contributed to the overall life experience. Once each component is identified and described the task is to understand how each component contributes to the overall human experience. He terms this approach Structuralism. Wilhelm Wundt investigates the structural components of human sensations, thoughts, ideas, volition, moods, cognition, and feelings, resulting in over 223 separate publications on these and related topics between 1858 -1908 (1908)[226].

Trivia: Emil Kraepelin completes post-doctoral training in the psychology research laboratories of Wilhelm Wundt. It is here Kraepelin embraces the rigors of experimental investigations and applies the techniques used by Wundt, in the study of sensation and perception, and applies these lessons to his own investigations of mental processes and mental disorders.

Influential, pioneering American researchers receive training in the newly established experimental research laboratories of Europe, before establishing their own and similar laboratories within the USA.

James Cattell (1860-1944) American, Professor of Psychology, a doctoral student of Wilhelm Wundt and while working at the University of Pennsylvania and Columbia University, applies Wilhelm Wundt's experimental methods to the study of sensation, perception, and cognitive processes. He applies a heavily weighted quantitative approach to investigations of basic mental processes. His investigations typically deconstruct complex mental processes into their most basic components. He measures and quantifies performance on each basic component of a complex mental process using tests based paradigms (1886,1890,1895)[227,228,229]. He introduces the term "mental tests" into the vocabulary of psychology (1890)[228]. Much of his research establishes the scientific foundation for psychometric testing widely used today.

James Cattell is active in the professional development of psychology, as a scientific discipline. He is a founding member of the American Psychological Association (1892) and outspoken proponent of academic freedom. He firmly believes university professors need protection from university administrators in order to engage in the process of creative scientific investigations. He passionately argues professors should by necessity have an effective voice in university governance and administrative decisions effecting research, teaching, and curriculum (1913)[230].

Perhaps lesser known than his many contributions to scientific investigations into mental processes and mental testing, he purchases a financially troubled scientific journal from Alexander Graham Bell for $500.00 (1894)[231]. Cattell assumes role of chief editor and soon guides the journal into profitability and an affiliation with the recently founded American Association for the Advancement of Science. Perhaps you recognize the journal today, as the internationally highly respected journal, "Science".

James Cattell co-founds the journal "Psychology Review", a journal dedicated to the advancement of scientific based theories within the rapidly emerging discipline of psychology (1894)[232]. The Journal continues publication today as a prominent and influential journal focusing upon "…important theoretical contributions to any area of scientific psychology, including systematic evaluation of alternative theories…" (2014)[233].

James Cattell as a proponent of the value of standardized psychometric assessment, uses monies collected from a wrongful termination lawsuit filed against Columbia University to begin and develop The Psychological Corporation, the soon to be preeminent publisher of psychological testing materials (1921)[234]. Perhaps you recognize a few of their psychological tests, Wechsler Intelligence Scales, Minnesota Multiphasic Personality Inventory (MMPI), and Beck Depression Inventories. Upon founding the Corporation, Cattell ensures "…all profits that accrues from the work of the Corporation must be used for psychological research…" (1923)[235].

As a side note, the basis for Cattell's successful litigation against Columbia University claiming wrongful termination stems from his dismissal from the University's faculty for his vocal and very public opposition to the military draft, during World War I. So goes another example in the history of medicine where political powers challenge academic freedoms within the university setting and effect the scientific advancement of knowledge.

The American Psychological Association is founded July 1892 at Clark University, located in Worcester, Massachusetts. The Association's stated objective "…is the advancement of psychology as a science…" (1894)[236]. The first official meeting of the Association is held December 1892 at the University of Pennsylvania and attended by 31 members. The Association soon adopts the "American Journal of Psychology", originally founded in 1876 by American psychologist and university professor Stanley Hall (1844-1924), as the official journal of the Association. Today, over 120 years later the Association is alive and well continuing to represent and promote the scientific and professional interests of psychology. Currently it is the largest scientific and professional psychology organization within the USA and a world leader in the profession, currently boasting more than 77,500 members (2018)[237].

Returning now to Europe, medical psychology and psychiatry witness rapid advances. Conceptual models building upon traditional anatomical matrixes are developed and refined and new, abstract models are introduced, in order to better understand disturbances in mental functions and behavior. Many of the most influential advances and developments are made by neurologists e.g. Paul Mobis, Sigmund Freud, and Josef Breuer.

Paul Mobius (1853-1907) German neurologist introduces a simple conceptualization of mental disorders which has immediate clinical relevance with regard to treatment and management decisions. The simplicity and clinical utility of the classification matrix makes it a popular system which continues to be used well into the late-1900s. Paul Mobius organizes mental disorders into endogenous and exogenous disorders. Endogenous mental disorders are those in which "...the principle condition must lie in the individual, in a congenital disposition...". Mobius offers specific examples of endogenous mental disorders to be neurasthenia, hysteria, epilepsy, and migraines. Exogenous mental disorders are those produced by identifiable toxins and infections "...engendered from without...". Specific examples are thyroid disease, multiple sclerosis, and Parkinson's disease (1892,1893)[238,239]. With time, Paul Mobius' dichotomous classification system becomes confused by misinterpretations and over extension (1896,1913,1915)[240,241,242]. In brief, Mobius never intends "endogenous" to refer to "organic" factors or "exogenous" to refer to "environmental" factors.

Paul Mobius offers an early model of hysteria. He proposes the condition results from degeneration of mental faculties, a thought consistent with Benedict Morel's popular degeneration theory. Mobius notes the condition to be more common in women, given women are intellectually inferior to men and minimally developed, placing women's mental capacities halfway between the child and the adult male (1900,1908)[243,244]. His words not mine.

Sigmund Freud (1856-1939) Austrian neurologist is perhaps most remembered by medical students for his contributions and development of a personality theory based upon three fundamental constructs (Id, Ego, Super Ego) and five successive stages of psychosexual development (Oral, Anal, Phallic, Latent, Genital) or perhaps his psychoanalytical treatment methods (Psychoanalysis). Of relevance here is his early conceptualization of hysteria, which is uniquely distinct from most popular models of the period. He publishes his thoughts, findings, and conclusions in "Studies on Hysteria" (1895)[245].

In brief, Sigmund Freud challenges popular models of hysteria for the period, such as the "...degeneracy..." and "...physical inefficiency..." models (1893,1895)[246,247]. He challenges popular models which propose mental disorders are the product of identifiable anatomical lesions within the central nervous system, as suggested by French neurologist Jean-Marie Charcot (1825-1893) (1889)[248]. He notes no such lesions have been identified in cases of hysteria. He additionally notes hysteria is a condition to the period and signs and symptoms appear and disappear seemingly at random. In "Studies of Hysteria" Sigmund Freud offers five case studies of patients diagnosed to be suffering the mental disorder hysteria; reports the clinical presentation of signs and symptoms; proposes a new comprehensive theoretical matrix within which to understand hysteria; explains the underlying physical mechanics of hysteria; and introduces the treatment technique of psychoanalysis.

This historical collection of case histories is compiled by Sigmund Freud and Austrian neurophysiologist physician Josef Breuer (1842-1925). Actually, Josef Breuer is the first author on this paper and Sigmund Freud is second author. You might remember Josef Breuer from his earlier seminal contributions in which he identifies and details the autonomic nervous system's contribution to the respiratory reflex (1868) [249] or perhaps his investigations in which he describes the physiology of balance, detailing the physiology of the semi-circular canals, utricle, and saccule (1873,1874,1875)[250,251,252].

Trivia: The Nobel Prize in Physiology or Medicine 1914 is awarded to Robert Barany "… for his work on the physiology and pathology of the vestibular apparatus…" (2015)[253]. Two years later Robert Barany is denied academic advancement, by the Academic Faculty Senate of the

University of Vienna, for failing to give sufficient credit to earlier researchers on this subject, specifically Josef Breuer. Here is another example of many, in the history of medicine, where an individual claims priority for discovery without acknowledging the contributions of other investigators whom lay the foundations for new discovery.

Given the historical influence, "Studies on Hysteria" has on the future development and direction of medical psychology, especially in terms of introducing a new conceptual understanding of mental disorders and new treatment methods, let us briefly review two of its most notable case histories here.

Case #1 is the now famous case of 21 year old Anna O. The patient is a patient of Josef Breuer to whom he provides medical treatments between 1880-1882. Josef Breuer describes the primary presenting signs and symptoms as "…A psychosis of a peculiar kind, paraphasia (language disorder), convergent squint (diplopia), severe disturbances of vision, paralyses complete in the right upper and both lower extremities (spastic with contractures), partial in the left upper extremity, paresis of the neck muscles…(and) period of persisting somnambulism (sleepiness or self-induced hypnotic state)…". Initial onset of debilitating signs and symptoms are sudden and first appear while caring for her ill father who is suffering a "...peripleuritic abscess…" and whom she is passionately fond. During the one year period in which Josef Breuer provides treatment to Anna O., she reveals regular and frequent episodes of "…day-dreaming…" described by Anna O. and Josef Breuer as her own "… private theater…", "...auto-hypnotic absences…" without memory recall, and "…visual hallucinations…" (1895a)[254].

Given the demonstrated poor success rate of medical treatments for hysteria, during the late-1800s, Josef Breuer investigates a new treatment approach, in search of a more effective treatment. The new approach is rational, based upon a new conceptual matrix, and focuses heavily upon the patient actively engaging in the treatment process. Josef Breuer refers to the new approach as the "…talking cure…" and in particular emphasizes use of the cathartic method.

In brief, the model proposed by Josef Breuer and Sigmund Freud to explain hysteria and upon which their new "…talking cure…" is based, states the experience of traumatic events in a person's life produces the pathology of hysteria and it is the memory of the traumatic event that is far more debilitating than the physical trauma itself. Treatment is based upon having the patient recall the memory of the event. The patient is to describe "…the event in the greatest possible detail and put the affect into words. Recollection without affect almost invariably produces no result…". This process "…discharges…" the physical energy stored and associated with the emotional event, thereby removing the pathological hysterical signs and symptoms. In the case of Anna O, following treatment "…she regained her mental balance entirely…" (1895a)[254].

Case # 2, 40 year old Emmy von N. is the first patient Sigmund Freud contributes to the case series collection on hysteria and which he applies the "…talking cure…" using primarily the cathartic method. Sigmund Freud provides treatment to Emmy von N. for approximately one year between 1888 and 1889. Primary presenting signs and symptoms are depression, anxiety, horrifying visual hallucinations, tormenting somatic pains, insomnia, tics, stammering speech, and multiple phobias. Signs and symptoms are of sudden onset, first appearing when the patient is approximately 26 years of age and associated with the sudden death of her husband. From a treatment perspective, at this time, Freud is still using hypnosis and the introduction of therapeutic suggestions as a component of his treatment interventions. He applies this approach in the case of Emmy von N. He additionally explores numerous traumatic childhood memories, recalled by the patient while under hypnosis. Soon he begins to incorporate the "…talk therapy…" and utilization of the cathartic method described earlier in efforts to "…discharge…" the physical energy stored and associated with emotionally traumatic events. "…The therapeutic success on the whole was considerable; but it was not a lasting one. The patient's tendency to fall ill in a similar way under the impact of fresh traumas was not got rid of. Anyone who wanted to undertake the definitive cure of a case of hysteria such as this would have to enter more thoroughly into the complex of phenomena that I attempted to do…" (1895a)[254].

At his point Freud is in the process of moving from a physiological to a psychological explanation of psycho-pathologies. The year he publishes "Studies on Hysteria", he publishes two papers discussing the chemical explanation of neuroses (1895b,1895f)[255,256] and two papers discussing neurosis solely within a matrix of psychological defenses and repression (1894a,1896b)[257,258]. This is a period of maturation and transition in Freud's thinking. He is beginning to question the medical dogma of the period and all that he has been taught in medical school, regarding the etiologies and treatment of mental disorders. He is beginning to think more independently and begins to explore alternative conceptualizations and treatment approaches to mental disorders.

In brief summary the 1800s witness continuing growth and maturation of medical psychology as a scientific based academic and professional discipline.

Many academic and professional organizations recognizable today, such as the Royal College of Psychiatrist, American Psychiatric Association, and American Psychological Association are founded and provide a forum for exchange of new information regarding the rapidly expanding knowledge base related to the understanding and treatment of individuals suffering impairments of thought, cognition, mood, and affect. New professional and scientific journals devoted to understanding impaired mental functioning are founded and begin publication, such as the "British Journal of Psychiatry", "American Journal of Psychiatry", "American Journal of Psychology", and "Psychology Review".

Two models dominate the thinking during the 1800s about impairments of thought, cognition, mood, and affect. The first model emphasizes changes in brain chemistry, physiology, and anatomy. The second model emphasizes abstract constructs of mental functions and mental development. Moderator variables, such as age, sex, heredity, social stressors are being introduced to further explain impairments of mental function.

Treatment modalities are changing to accommodate changes in conceptual matrixes. Moral (psychological) humane behavioral/environmental treatments become mainstream and slowly displace physical restraints, physical punishment, and traditional medical interventions e.g. bleeding, purging, and blistering as the preferred modality of treatment interventions. Talk therapies become popular. The value and role of physicians in the treatment of individuals suffering impairments of thought, cognition, mood, and affect is hotly debated.

Asylum based treatments and management of individuals suffering impairments of thought, cognition, mood, and affect is revolutionized through the passionate commitment and sustained efforts of activist practitioners and lay public. Exemplary models of change first appear in France during the early-1800s followed by the USA by the mid-1800s. Changes reflect changes in the conceptual understanding of the underlying causes of impaired functions in thought, cognition, mood, and affect. In general, humane approaches replace harsh punishment and exploitation.

New classification systems are introduced to organize the increasing large and varied clinical presentations of individuals suffering impairments of thought, cognition, mood, and affect. The new classification systems emphasize clinical presentations of signs and symptoms and place much less emphasis upon suspected underlying cause than earlier classification systems.

New terms are introduced into the academic and medical literature, which are familiar to most medical students today, such as psycho-somatic disorder, endogenous vs exogenous disorder, manic-depressive psychosis, dementia praecox (schizophrenia), delirium tremens, catatonia, paranoia, and psychiatry.

Notable figures making substantial contributions and guiding the continuing development of medical psychology, as a maturing, scientific based, academic and professional discipline, during the 1800s are Jean-Baptiste Pussin, Phillipe Pinel, Johannas Reil, Franz Gall, Benjamin Rush, Thomas Sutton, Johann Heinroth, Jean-Etienne Esquirol, Dorthea Dix, Benedict Morel, Emil Kraepelin, Wilhelm Wundt, James Cattell, Paul Mobius, Josef Breuer, and Sigmund Freud.

Medical psychology is establishing itself as a new respected academic and professional discipline. Criteria defining a new discipline are quickly being satisfied. Medical psychology is establishing a shared knowledge base; establishing shared methodologies and technologies; research investigations are beginning to produce a cohesive body of scientific literature; new terms and a new vocabulary are introduced to describe new concepts and methodologies; specialized training standards are defined for those choosing to enter into the profession; discipline specific professional organizations and societies are founded; and new journals committed to the exchange of ideas and scientific investigation begin publication and gain increasing readership. Medical psychology is well positioned to continue its rapid development and maturation during the next 100 years. Hold on; things begin to happen quickly.

Late Modern, 1900 AD - 2000 AD.

The 1900s witness the development and maturation of medical psychology as a scientific discipline and profession. Scientific and professional organizations committed to the advancement of medical psychology witness a continuing rise in membership. Popular models used to explain impaired thought, cognition, mood, and affect are modified to accommodate new research and clinical findings. Conceptual matrixes are honed and become more sophisticated.

Three dominant schools of thought emerge early in the 1900s. One, exemplified by prominent leaders Sigmund Freud, Carl Jung, and Alfred Adler, whom focus on abstract conceptualizations of personality structure, development, and internal psychic energies. This school of thought will become termed the Psychoanalytic school. Psychopathologies result when balance between hypothetical constructs become disordered.

The second school of thought is exemplified by prominent leaders Ivan Pavlov, John Watson, and B. F. Skinner, whom focus on empirical observations of behaviors and embrace the belief all behaviors, normal and abnormal can best be explained by learning theory, with no need for abstract conceptualizations of personality structure, development or internal energies. This school of thought will become termed Behaviorism. Psychopathologies result when individual learn the pathology.

The third school of thought is exemplified by founders and leaders Carl Rogers and Abraham Maslow. This model is first introduced during the late-1930s as an alternative to the psychoanalytic and behaviorism models and gains increasing popularity. In brief, this model emphasizes the role of free will, responsibility for choices, and a progressive development of a sense of an ideal self which is determined in large part by societal expectations. Psychopathologies develop and are maintained when there is incongruence between an individual's perceived sense of self (how one perceives oneself) and their sense of their ideal self (how they and society would like for them to be). This school of thought will be termed Humanistic Psychology.

All three schools gain popularity during the first half of the 1900s and slowly begin to lose popularity by the end of the 1900s. Each in their own right make substantial contributions to the advancement of medical psychology as an academic and professional discipline, offering models which explain normal behaviors, psychopathologies, and a conceptual matrix from which to design and implement treatments. More on these later.

By the mid-1900s interests is renewed in models which conceptualize impairments in thought, cognition, mood, and affect to be best understood and treated by way of direct physical, electrical, or chemical intervention at the organ responsible, the brain. Psychosurgeries typified by frontal lobe brain leucotomies are a popular treatment strategy. Electroconvulsive therapy (ECT) introduces short burst of moderate voltage electricity to the brain and soon proves to be a popular treatment intervention. Chemical pharmacological treatments produce good results when administered to specific subpopulations of individuals suffering impairments in thought, cognition, mood, or affect.

Psychosurgeries, electroconvulsive, and psychopharmacological treatments are administered independent of well-reasoned conceptual matrixes, such as offered by the psychoanalytical, behaviorism, or humanistic Schools. The approaches are founded primarily upon empirical evidence, oftentimes unexpected. However, explanatory models begin to be introduced post facto and contribute to the further development of the scientific knowledge base used to treat impairments in thought, cognition, mood, affect, and behavior.

Psychometric assessment becomes an important part of medical psychology early in the 1900s and remains throughout all of the 1900s. It offers quantitative, standardized assessments of abstract constructs such as intelligence, aptitude, and personality. Psychometric assessment quickly proves to be a valuable tool in understanding thought, cognition, mood, and affect. Psychometrics generates new and valuable knowledge in both the research laboratory and applied clinical settings.

The second half of the 1900s witness an explosion of chemical pharmaceutical treatments of mental disorders and gains wide acceptance. Pharmaceuticals quickly become a predominant treatment tool. New theoretical models of brain function and brain dysfunction are offered based upon the success or failure of specific pharmaceuticals to produce clinical improvement.

New classification systems are introduced for use specifically with individuals evidencing impairments of intellectual resources, thought, cognition, mood, affect, or behaviors. The most notable system is presented in the American Psychiatric Association's "Diagnostic Statistical Manuals of Mental Disorders" e.g. DSM-I, DSM-II, DSM-III, DSM-IV, DSM-IV-TR. These manuals provide a system of classification which brings order and an attempt at standardization to diagnostic categories and nomenclature whenever applied to disordered mental functioning.

Legislation at the national level (USA) mandates financial reimbursements paid by insurance companies for the diagnosis and treatment of impairments of intellectual resources, thought, cognition, mood, affect, or behavior be paid in parity to all other disorders of anatomy or physiology. Legislation at the national level (Italy) mandates closure of all large state supported psychiatric hospitals and moves to community based psychiatric treatment models.

The 1900s prove extremely influential in the development and advancement of fundamental concepts in regard to the diagnosis, classification, assessment, and treatment of mental disorders. No other time in the history of medical psychology and psychiatry have so many resources been committed to understanding and improving mental disorders.

Let's now look at a few specifics.

Sigmund Freud continues to develop and refine his thinking, during the early-1900s, with respect to the origin, maintenance, and treatment of mental disorders. He moves away from his initial interest in the neurological basis of mental impairments and towards the development of a conceptual matrix based upon abstract constructs, emphasizing the importance of personality structure, personality development, and internal psychic energies. Psychopathologies result whenever an individual fails to progress normally through universal stages of personality development. Treatments are based upon assisting the individual in identifying events which have occurred in their life which have contributed to an arrest in normal personality development. Identification of these events and discharge of psychic energies associated with the events are primary in this model and necessary to effect a successful treatment outcome and resolve the specific psychopathology. Treatment uses talk therapy as its primary modality of intervention.

Given the tremendous influence of Freud's conceptual matrix to the development of medical psychology, a brief summary of his most salient contributions will provide you, the first or second year medical student, an opportunity to understand his basic model and allow you to better appreciate the impact his model has upon the development of medical psychology throughout the 1900s.

First, Freud is among the first in modern times, to introduce the concept of the conscious and unconscious, with regard to levels of mental activities and personality dynamics. He proposes all mental processes and associated resultant behaviors can be organized into two fundamental groupings, those of which the individual is aware (conscious) and those of which the individual is unaware (unconscious) (1900,1915c)[259,260].

Second, innate, dynamic, opposing internal psychic energies are driving forces which underlie all mental processes and behavior. Freud identifies two primary internal psychic energies. He assigns the name Eros to that internal energy responsible for preserving and perpetuating life. He assigns the name Thanatos to that energy responsible for one's self destruction and terminating life (1920)[261]. Psychopathologies result when the dynamic balance between these two opposing forces become disordered and become unbalanced. The goal of treatment is to restore balance.

Third, individuals normally pass through five stages of personality development (1905)[262]. These stages are loosely defined by chronological age and specific developmental challenges occurring at each stage of development. The movement through the five stages is normally completed by 5 years of age. Failure to move consecutively through these developmental stages or unsuccessful resolution of specific developmental challenges at any stage, termed fixation, results in abnormal personality development and increased probability of the individual evidencing impairments of thought, cognition, mood, affect, or behavior.

Freud terms these five stages of development Oral, Anal, Phallic, Latent, and Genital. Movement through these stages is propelled by an internal psychic energy. Freud terms this internal psychic energy sexual drive. Freud identifies sexual drive to be the most important factor in driving and determining normal personality development. This fundamental belief, sexual drive is primary to personal development, leads Freud to term his five stages of psychosexual development.

Fourth, Freud proposes an elegant, structured, tripartite model of personality. He offers his conceptualization of the Id, Ego, and Super-Ego (1923b)[263].

The Id is an unorganized component of the personality, present since birth, responsible for basic instinctual drives, wants, and needs, such as engaging in sex. The Id operates on immediate gratification and is not concerned with consequences or societal values of right and wrong. It wants what it wants and wants it now.

The Super-Ego is an organized component of personality that incorporates and reflects societal values for the standards for right and wrong. It strives to follow accepted rules defining good and appropriate social behavior. It is the Super-Ego that controls an individual's sense of right and wrong. Think of the Super-Ego as a person's conscience. When social norms are violated it is the Super-Ego which is responsible for the moods characterized by a sense of guilt, shame, and contrition.

The Ego is at birth an unorganized component of the personality which differentiates and becomes organized and structured with time and maturation. The Ego functions as that part of the personality which mediates the uncontrolled, immediate demands and wants of the Id with the Super-Ego's ideals reflecting society's rules and laws governing acceptable and proper thoughts, moods, and behaviors. The Ego operates typically on the principle of delayed gratification, in order to successfully mediate the competing and frequently oppositional demands of the Id and Super-Ego. When the Ego continually fails to be successful in mediation, psychopathologies result.

Fifth and finally in regard to selected influential contributions made by Freud to the development of medical psychology is the concept of psychological defense mechanisms (1915)[264]. These are techniques employed by individuals, at the unconscious level, to manipulate, deny, or distort reality in order to reduce feelings of internal emotional discomfort. Examples of specific defense mechanisms are repression, regression, projection, reaction formation, sublimation.

In brief, Repression is characterized by forcing socially unacceptable feelings or thoughts into the unconscious. Regression is characterized by returning to an earlier and safer stage of psychosexual development. Projection is characterized by projecting socially unacceptable ideas or urges one may have onto others around you. Reaction formation is simply behaving in the opposite way from which the unconscious would choose one to behave. Sublimation is the process of expressing socially unacceptable behavior in socially acceptable ways.

All defense mechanisms are used by the Ego to resolve internal conflicts between the Id and Super-Ego and to dissipate disruptive internal psychic energies. Sigmund Freud's daughter Anna Freud (1895-1982) and others subsequently further develop Sigmund Freud's conceptualization of defense mechanisms, adding many more to the list (1936)[265]. Sigmund Freud emphasizes only a few defense mechanisms in his original conceptual matrix, focusing initially and principally upon Repression (1915)[264].

Sigmund Freud founds several regional and international professional associations along with each associations' official journal. Specifically, he is instrumental in the creation of the Wednesday Psychological Society (1902)[266], meeting initially in Freud's apartment and which later changes its name to the more recognizable Vienna Psychoanalytic Society (1908)[267]. He founds the International Psychoanalytical Association two years later (1910)[266]. He founds the "International Journal for Psychology" (1913) and the "International Journal of Psychoanalysis" (1919)[266]. Associations and journals are committed to the lively and oftentimes heated exchange of information and ideas related to the new and rapidly developing psychoanalytic model.

Carl Jung (1875-1961) Swiss psychiatrist embraces the new theoretical matrix which emphasizes abstract constructs of personality, the importance of the unconscious with regard to normal and abnormal thoughts, cognition, mood, affect, and behaviors (1912)[268]. He is active in the early development of Sigmund Freud's psychodynamic models of personality development and underlying cause of impaired mental functions and behavior. By 1917 he breaks away from the psychodynamic model and offers his own modified model of personality structure.

Carl Jung identifies three primary components of personality, which he terms Ego, Personal Unconscious, and Collective Unconscious.

In brief, the Ego is that component of personality capable of conscious thought; the Personal Unconscious is that component of personality which holds suppressed memories; while the Collective Unconscious is that component of personality which is a reservoir of all memories, experiences, and knowledge assimilated across time by the entire human species and inherited from ancestors. It is the dynamic interaction between these three components of personality, modified by the influence of socialization, which determines thoughts, cognitions, mood, affect, and behavior. Impairment within and between components of personality results in psychopathologies. Treatment interventions are based upon efforts to bring the Personal Unconscious and Collective Unconscious into conscious awareness and differentiate the individual from the inherited Collective Unconscious. Specific techniques applied to achieve the treatment objective rely heavily upon Dream Analysis, Symbol Analysis, and Fantasies Analysis. Carl Jung terms his modified psychodynamic model, which deemphasizes psychosexual stages of development and emphasizes developmental stages of differentiation of the individual from the Collective Unconscious, Analytical Psychology (1916,1917)[269,270].

Carl Jung's conceptual matrix leads to the identification of personality subtypes e.g. introverted personality, extroverted personality. Perhaps you might recognize examples of the many personality characteristics which he attributes to inheritance and which he terms archetypes (1921)[271]. The fundamental idea here is much of that which determines an individual's personality i.e. how he or she interacts with the world around them is largely inherited and subsequently modified by society.

Alfred Adler (1870-1937) Austrian ophthalmologist embraces the Freudian psychodynamic model, abstract constructs to define personality, and importance of the unconscious. He is a member of the Wednesday Psychological Society, meeting regularly in Sigmund Freud's apartment, and a vocal, outspoken member of the International Psychoanalytical Association. He soon breaks away from the Freudian psychodynamic model and its professional associations, and offers an alternative model (1907,1917)[272].

Alfred Adler rejects the Freudian model emphasizing internal driving forces of sexual intrinsic energies and proposes a modified model, emphasizing the tremendous external influence society has upon the development of an individual's personality. Alder's model emphasizes the role society plays in the development and maintenance of many psychopathologies. Alfred Adler chooses the term Individual Psychology to define his new conceptual matrix (1912,1913, 1921)[273,274,275].

The term Individual Psychology does not refer to the individual as a person, but rather to an individual person as a complete, total, and whole element functioning within a dynamic and influential social matrix.

In brief, Alfred Adler's model proposes society defines standards and expectations for each individual participating in the society. Each individual compares himself or herself to the standard or expectation. When the individual fails to meet the ideal "...fictional final goal..." he or she internalizes these failures, which manifest as personality traits, altered perception of self, and behaviors. The individual internalizes into the unconscious a sense of "...inferiority...". Alfred Adler introduces the term "...inferiority complex..." to describe an individual's exaggerated expectation of failure in the tasks of life, leading to a pessimistic resignation with associated impairments in cognition, thought, mood, affect, and behavior (1907,1912)[272,276]. Treatment interventions are directed to the process of examining the validity of the perceived inferiority and when necessary, such as in the case of psychopathologies, assisting the individual to overcome perceived senses of inferiority by challenging their distorted perception of self by external reality testing or offering more effective methods to deal effectively with life tasks.

The Adlerian model further differentiates itself from the Freudian psychodynamic model in that it encourages proactive treatment intervention rather than retroactive intervention and focuses on the individual as an element of a more complex social matrix rather than a single and independent element. Similar to the Freudian model, the Adlerian model incorporates the abstract construct of the unconscious, as essential to its conceptual matrix and structure of personality. Strategies characteristically uses by individuals to deal with the world around them are entrenched by 5 years of age. Both the Adlerian and Freudian models emphasize a single driving force as responsible for personality development and ultimately the potential to produce psychopathologies. In the Freudian model, it is the internal force (drive) generated by sexual energies. In the Adlerian model, it is the internal force (drive) to achieve the perceived ideal self (1908)[277]. Both models gain popularity and support from the medical and academic communities and have significant influence upon the direction of medical psychology throughout all of the 1900s.

As a side note, it is Alfred Adler whom is among the first to introduce the idea birth order is important in determining personality characteristics (1928)[278]. Briefly, he proposes the eldest child is socially dominant, highly intellectual and extremely conscientious. The middle child is most competitive, diplomatic, and eager to please others. The youngest child tend to be dependent and selfish and often the life of any party. The only child is "...pampered and spoiled..." and experience difficulties when they don't get their way, especially when dealing with others around them. The birth order model is aggressively investigated throughout the 1900s producing variable findings. What is most important here is the concept of birth order effecting personality development and contribution to normal and abnormal thought, cognition, mood, affect, and behavior. It highlights Alder's emphasis on the social context within which an individual develops and functions greatly influences how the individual perceives and interacts with the world.

Sigmund Freud, Carl Jung, and Alfred Adler psychoanalytic conceptual matrixes are tremendously influential in the development of medical psychology and psychiatry throughout all of the 1900s.

The early-1900s witness the introduction and development of a second tremendously influential school of thought and offers an alternative conceptual matrix to the models offered by the psychoanalytic school. This alternative conceptual matrix will become termed Behaviorism. Unlike the psychoanalytical models which emphasize abstract constructs such as personality and the unconscious, pioneers of Behaviorism emphasize empirical, systematic observation of behavior and conceptualize impairments of thought, cognition, mood, affect, and behavior within the conceptual matrix of learning theory, with no need for abstract construct such as personality, the unconscious, or internal energies. Psychopathologies result as a consequence of impaired learning or are simply learned in the same way normal behavior is learned.

Three influential investigators, Ivan Pavlov, John Watson, and B. F. Skinner pioneer the application of learning theory to understanding and treating impairments of thought, cognition, mood, affect, and behavior. Behaviorism receives and maintains high popularity throughout all of the 1900s.

Let's look at a few specifics pertaining to Behaviorism, as a conceptual matrix, and the influential investigators most responsible for its tremendous influence on medical psychology during the 1900s.

Ivan Pavlov (1849-1936) Russian physiologist establishes an influential experimental laboratory paradigm which permits the quantitative evaluation of internal mental processing, specifically learning (1903)[279]. The terms assigned to define the paradigm change with time and today are simply termed classical conditioning. The conceptual matrix and associated experimental paradigm, originally developed in the animal laboratory, is extended to the assessment of human learning. It offers a new, organized, scientific based, testable model, which can explain the development of normal and abnormal thoughts, cognitions, moods, affects, and behaviors (1927,1928)[280,281]. The paradigm stands in marked contrast to the psychoanalytical models which rely heavily upon subjective reporting from individuals and abstract constructs such as personality and the unconscious (1906)[282].

In brief, the classical conditioning model states individuals learn through the process of paired associations. When a person experiences an event in their life (event A) and has an emotional or cognitive reaction to the event (reaction A), the person soon learns when event A occurs they experience the emotional or cognitive reaction A. Event A is associated with reaction A. The unique contribution made by Ivan Pavlov is that he recognizes when a second event B occurs, which does not by itself generate any emotional or cognitive reaction, and is paired in time with event A, presentation of event B alone will result in the same emotional or cognitive reaction as if event A occurred.

Ivan Pavlov and proponents of the classical conditioning model introduce new vocabulary to define the elements of their new paradigm. Perhaps you recognize some of the terms, unconditioned stimulus, unconditioned response, neutral stimulus, conditioned stimulus, and conditioned response. The necessity to introduce new vocabulary to define new constructs is characteristic of all new and developing conceptual matrixes. So too is the case with the introduction of classical conditioning.

Classical conditioning models place the sight of learning and paired associations to occur in the brain, specifically the cortex of the cerebral hemispheres (1927)[283]. This stands in contrast to the psychoanalytic models which deemphasize the brain in favor of the abstract construct the unconscious mind. Classical conditioning models gain popularity and acceptance from both academic and medical communities and prove influential throughout the entire 1900s.

Trivia: Ivan Pavlov is awarded the Nobel Prize in Physiology or Medicine 1904 "…in recognition of his work on the physiology of digestion, through which knowledge on vital aspects of the subject have been transformed and enlarged…" (1904)[284]. This work investigates the reflex of salivation and demonstrates the phenomenon of eliciting a salivation reflex in the absence of the presentation of food (conditioned reflex) (1903)[285]. He is subsequently nominated three additional times for the Nobel Prize in Physiology or Medicine, 1925, 1927, and 1929, for his work on the "… function of the central nervous system, especially conditioned responses…" (2014)[286]. Ivan Pavlov does not receive the Prize during these years.

John Watson (1878-1958) American behavioral psychologist embraces Ivan Pavlov's model of classical conditioning, extends its fundamental premise of associative learning, and applies it to humans. Watson is instrumental in establishing Behaviorism in the USA. He publishes "Psychology as the Behaviorist Views It" (aka The Behaviorist Manifesto), which outlines the fundamental conceptual matrix of behaviorism (1913)[287].

In brief, John Watson defines behaviorism as an objective experimental branch of the natural sciences with its primary objective to predict and control behavior. Behaviorism emphasizes external, observable behaviors and rejects internal constructs such as the unconscious, as areas of investigation. He argues medical psychology should no longer focus efforts on the investigation of the mind and instead should focus on behavior (1916,1919)[288,289]. This proposed change in the focus of study for the discipline represents a significant shift in the fundamental conceptual matrix used to understand normal and abnormal behaviors.

John Watson knowingly overstates his position, in his influential book Behaviorism, to make his point "…Give me a dozen healthy infants, well formed, and my own specified world to bring them up in and I'll guarantee to take any one at random and train him to become any type of specialist I might select - doctor, lawyer, artist, merchant, chief, and yes, even beggar man and thief, regardless of his talents, penchants, tendencies, abilities, vocations, and race of his ancestors…." (1924)[290].

John Watson and graduate student assistant Rosalie Rayner dramatically demonstrate the tremendous influence classical conditioning paradigms can play in the development of disordered cognitions, thoughts, mood, affect, and behavior with publication of the intensely controversial experiment known to most simply as the case of Little Albert. (1920)[291].

In brief, the experiment is designed to test the classical conditioning principle of stimulus generalization. John Watson and his wife select a 9 month old, healthy, infant, reared in The Harriet Lane Home for Invalid Children, located in Baltimore Maryland and associated with Johns Hopkins University School of Medicine, as their test subject. The infant is suddenly exposed to a series of neutral stimuli e.g. rabbit, dog, white rat, monkey, masks, cotton. The infant's reactions to each of these neutral stimuli are recorded. No evidence of fear or rage is observed. Later, the infant is exposed to a series of loud, unexpected noises, produced by striking a steel bar with a hammer. This elicits the expected startle reflex and crying from the child. The child is then exposed to both the neutral stimuli e.g. white rat, at the same time the steel bar is struck loudly by the hammer. The infant reacts by a rapid violent jerk, falls forward, and begins to whimper.

Approximately one week later, a white rat is suddenly introduced to the infant, without the loud sound produced from striking the steel bar. The infant responses immediately by crying, falling over, quickly picking himself up, and rapidly crawling away. Similar intense emotional and behavioral reactions are observed whenever any of the other neutral stimuli e.g. rabbit, mask, cotton, are introduced to the infant (1920)[291].

The experiment findings are interpreted to reveal an associated pairing of an intense emotional and behavioral reaction to an otherwise neutral stimulus. The findings offer support for the behaviorist models, which conceptualized psychopathologies within the matrix of learning theory. The experiment of Little Albert impacts the future of Behaviorism for the balance of the 1900s. It additionally raises the issue of ethics in research whenever human subjects are being investigated. Do you see any ethical issues which concern you about this investigative study?

Trivia: Whatever happens to Little Albert? He dies at 6 years of age, from complications associated with hydrocephalus (2009)[292].

B. F. Skinner (1904-1990) American behavioral psychologist introduces the conceptual matrix of radical behaviorism. Central to this model is the idea all human behavior is the result of environment and reinforcements an individual encounters during life. Like John Watson and other behaviorists of the 1900s, B. F. Skinner rejects the abstract constructs of the unconscious and similar constructs central to psychoanalytical models. Simply stated, all behavior is learned through interaction with a person's environment and brought into existence, maintained, or extinguished as the result of reinforcement schedules. Normal behaviors as well as psychopathologies result from exposure of the individual to environmental conditions, which either increase or decrease the frequency of the behavior. B.F. Skinner and proponents of his conceptual matrix reject the idea of free will.

New vocabulary is necessary and introduced to define the specific elements and constructs of his model. The model is heavily dependent upon the construct of reinforcement schedules. All behavior, past, present, and future can be explained within the matrix of reinforcement schedules.

In brief, reinforcement schedules determine whether a behavior will continue or be eliminated. Dependent upon the specific reinforcement schedule operating e.g. fixed, variable, continuous, intermittent, the frequency of engaging in any particular behavior can be determine with reasonable certainty. The term operant conditioning is introduced to explain the relationship between a behavior and the probability of that behavior reappearing. Perhaps you are familiar with the idea of positive reinforcement, negative reinforcement, punishment, and extinction. These too are specific schedules operating in a person's external environment which increase or decrease the probabilities of engaging in any specific behavior.

Ivan Pavlov, John Watson, and B. F. Skinner's behavioristic conceptual matrixes tremendously influence the development of medical psychology throughout all of the 1900s.

By the early-1930s a third school of thought is developing in medical psychology. It offers an alternative to the psychoanalytical and behaviorism models. This new school is termed humanistic psychology. Its fundamental conceptual premise focuses upon the belief individuals have free will, responsibility for choices, and personality is the result of a progressive development of a sense of an ideal self, termed differentiation, which is determined in large part by societal expectations. Psychopathologies develop and are maintained when there is incongruence between an individual's perceived sense of self (how one perceives oneself) and their sense of an ideal self (how they and society would like for them to be). New terms are introduced to describe the pathological condition. In the parlance of humanistic psychology, the perceived sense of self is incongruent with the idealized self. Treatment is talk based and directed to assisting the individual, in a supportive, empathetic, nonjudgmental approach, in reconciling the differences between the perceived self with the idealized self. Leaders of the humanistic school are exemplified by Carl Rogers and Abraham Maslow.

Carl Rogers (1902-1987) American psychologist offers a theory of personality termed phenomenal field theory. In essence, it states an individual exist in a continually changing world around them (phenomenal field) and the individual reacts to the field. The individual's perception of the field is reality for that individual. As the individual is exposed to and experiences the phenomenal field, the individual begins to differentiate themself from the field. The individual begins to develop a sense of self (who they are and who they are not) and develops a sense of an ideal self (how they and society would like to see them in an ideal state), and a sense of self-worth (or self-esteem., what a person thinks about themselves). Incongruence between sense of self and ideal self-results in psychopathologies. Treatment is directed to restoring congruency between perceived self and perceived ideal self. This process is accomplished through empathetic, nonjudgmental, supportive listening, which creates a non-threatening environment, permits the individual to discover for themself the incongruences and make the necessary adjustments in self-perception or the environmental field to bring into congruence the real self and ideal self (1951,1952,1959)[293,294,295].

You have heard of the phrases "…unconditional acceptance…" in regard to providing a safe and supportive environment within which to allow a person to pursue their dreams and goals in life; or perhaps the phrase "…self-actualization…" an idealized state to which all humans strive (1946,1959)[296]. These terms and ideas are offered by Carl Rogers.

Abraham Maslow (1908-1970) American humanistic psychologist offers his influential conceptual model of hierarchy of needs. In brief, the model states every person has a need to realize their fullest potential as a human being. Each person moves through life in pursuit of reaching an idealized state of existence, later termed self-actualization. A pyramid structure defines specific needs, which need to be met in order to obtain the highest state of existence, self-actualization. At the base of the pyramid are basic Physiological needs required for survival e.g. food, water, sleep. The next higher level identifies the need for Safety e.g. shelter. The next higher level identifies the need for Love and Belonging e.g. family, friends, and sexually intimate relationships. The next higher level identifies the need for Esteem e.g. sense of accomplishment, respect for self and others. The highest level within the hierarchy of needs model pyramid is the idealized state of Self-Actualization, a state of existence characterized by understanding, harmony with self, others, and with the environment in which one lives.

The hierarchy of needs model is introduced as a humanistic model alternative to the predominant models of the period, psychoanalysis and behaviorism (1943)[297]. The humanistic models recall, reject biological determinism and internal psych energies, as proposed by the psychoanalytic models, and reject social determinism and sole reliance upon classical and operant learning theories, as proposed by the behaviorist models. The humanistic models embraces the concept of free will, while living in an ever changing environment which effects life choices, and a driving motivational force for each individual to be all they can be.

Humanistic models deemphasize the need for diagnosis in the case of impaired mental function, which focuses upon impairments (psychopathologies). Humanistic models choose, in the case of impaired mental function, instead to emphasize an individual's positive strengths as a human being; assist the individual in recognizing they are affected by an ever changing world around them; their perceptions of self and reality can be incongruent, which can contribute to the current level of functioning; and treatments offered focus upon assisting the individual in recognizing debilitating incongruences between self (reality) and ideal self and attempt to move the individual from a state of potentially debilitating functioning to their highest level of functioning possible, by providing a supportive, non- judgmental, empathetic therapeutic environment. Although influential in the development of medical psychology, the humanistic models never achieve the same popularity in the academic and medical communities as do the psychoanalytic and behaviorist models.

OK…perhaps a little too much personality theory here. Back to the history of medical psychology.

At the same time the psychoanalytic, behaviorist, and humanistic models are introduced and gaining popularity during the first half of the 1900s, another influential movement is taking place. Investigators begin to investigate the value of psychometric assessment as a potentially useful tool in understanding human behavior. Using standardized testing protocols, first introduced and developed in the experimental psychology research laboratory, are soon incorporated into the clinical practice of medical psychology.

Psychometric testing finds its roots in the works of experimental psychologist Sir Francis Galton (1822-1911), completed in Great Britain during the late-1800s (1883)[298]. He is among the first to attempt to quantitatively measure the abstract constructs of intelligence and personality. Francis Galton's measurements are heavily dependent upon reaction time and sensory discrimination performance (1924)[299]. Faster reaction times are believed to measure faster thought processing. His efforts to objectively and quantitatively measure external behavioral performance, as correlates of internal psychological processes, lay the foundation upon which all future psychometric assessment will build.

Given the tremendous influence psychometric testing and testing in general has upon the development of medical psychology throughout the 1900s, let's now look at a few specific individuals and associated concepts which shape the development of medical psychology.

James McKeen Cattell (1860-1944) American experimental psychologist extends the works of Europeans Francis Galton and Wilhelm Wundt in the use of objective, quantitative physical measurements to assess internal intellectual resources and cognitive processing. He proposes all mental processes can be reduced to fundamental elemental tasks which can be reliably measured, quantified, and used to describe complex internal psychological processes. It is his belief physical energies cannot be separated from mental energies. Good performance on a measure of physical strength e.g. hand dynamometer is associated with good mental strength. He assembles a series of 10 tasks e.g. reaction time, hand strength, sensory discrimination, line bisection, judgement, which can be administered to the general public and used to quantify an individual's mental abilities (1890)[300]. So begins psychometric assessment in the USA.

One of the first attempts to associate mental test performance with academic performance is conducted by one of James McKeen Cattell's graduate students, Clark Wissler (1870-1947) as part of the student's doctoral dissertation, at Columbia University. In brief, Wissler administers the Cattell battery to 300 college students and applies the recently developed Pearson product moment correlation coefficient (1902)[301] to explore the relationship between performances on each mental test in the Cattell battery with students' undergraduate academic grades.

Virtually no correlation between mental test performance and academic grade performance is demonstrated (1901)[302]. Is it possible the mental tests are not measuring mental performance or ability as suspected? Is it possible mental tests cannot measure intellectual resources or cognitive abilities? Is there a flaw in methodologies or interpretation of the findings, you can recognize? The findings shake the academic community and testing of mental abilities and mental processes is called into question as a potentially invalid methodology for assessing mental abilities and processes. For all intent and purposes the use of reaction time and sensory discrimination measurements are abandoned in the assessment of mental processes for the next 70 years.

As investigators in the USA rethink their approach of assessing mental processes, in France, Alfred Binet (1857-1911) French psychologist introduces an alternative approach. He suggests intelligence is better measured by evaluating higher order psychological processes rather than their elemental components (1896)[303]. This approach stands in contrast to the approaches of influential German investigator Wilhelm Wundt and American investigator James McKeen Cattell, whom argue intelligence is best measured by evaluating the most basic, elemental components of mental processes, such as measured by reaction times and sensory discrimination tasks.

Alfred Binet joins with Theodore Simon (1872-1961) a French psychologist who is investigating the relationship between physical development and intellectual capacity in children, at the asylum of Vaucluse, France (1900a,1900b)[304,305]. Together they compose a simple battery of brief tests, which assesses 10 areas of primarily higher order psychological processes. Specific areas assessed are memory, attention, imagination, understanding, moral sense, mental imagery, suggestibility, motor adaptability, motor strength, and aesthetic sensibility. The entire battery can be administered within 1.5 hours and without elaborate equipment. The original battery is refined and results in the battery of 30 brief tests, which range along a continuum from simple sensory and motor tasks to complex abstract reasoning tasks. The revised battery is offered as a useful instrument to assist with the classification of children within the Paris public schools whom will benefit or fail to benefit from current public school curriculum (1905)[306].

The battery, soon to be known simply as the Binet-Simon Scales, is further refined over the next six years resulting in two substantial published revisions (1908,1911)[307,308]. The revised versions introduce the new term "mental age" to describe an individual's assessed level of functioning relative to age controls and extend the scales to permit the assessment of adults (1908,1911)[307,308]. The Binet-Simon Scales gain quick acceptance from the education community and prove successful in meeting the recent governmental mandate to classify public school children. The Scales are modified again by Lewis Terman (1877-1956) an American educational psychologist and colleagues at Stanford University, resulting in the popular Stanford-Binet Scales, used throughout the United States. Lewis Terman and colleagues modify the calculation of the now familiar term "intelligence quotient" (IQ) by multiplying the IQ by 100 to move the decimal point over two places which allow IQ to now be expressed as a whole number (1916)[309].

Trivia: The term "intelligence quotient" (IQ) is first introduced by William Stern (1871-1938) German psychologist, working with the Binet-Simon Scales, in an attempt to provide a way to compare an individual's assessed level of functioning with others in the same age group. IQ = mental age/chronological age (1912)[310].

Lewis Terman's interests in the Stanford-Binet Scales of Intelligence have little to do with the goals upon which Alfred Binet and Theodore Simon founded the battery. Lewis Terman is interested in using the instrument to advance his beliefs in eugenics. Eugenics recall is the term used to define the belief and practices with aims to improve the genetic quality of the human population. Specifically, Terman is interested in the brightest of the brightest students. The Stanford-Binet scales offer a quick and reliable measurement which allow for segregation of the brightest children from the average and below average. He believes intelligence is inherited and high IQ children will be the leaders of tomorrow and should receive special attention. He is influential in having the Stanford-Binet administered in public schools across the USA. Few school children, during the past 90 years in the USA, have not been tested by the Stanford-Binet or similar intelligence test, for classification for educational purposes. Every parent believes their child possesses above average intelligence and cognitive skills. The reality, oftentimes difficult for parents to accept, is most children are average or below average. Think about it.

David Wechsler (1896-1981) Romania born and influential American psychologist rejects the Binet-Simon concept of a single score and unitary concept of intelligence. He is advocates additional factors contribute to intelligent behavior beyond intellectual ability. Critical of Stanford-Binet Scales as being too heavily weighted on verbal skills, such as vocabulary skills, David Wechsler introduces tasks which he considers nonverbal, such as assembling puzzles, copying geometric symbols, pointing to missing details in a picture drawing. The introduction of nonverbal tasks is an attempt to overcome language, cultural, and education biases.

He publishes a series of Wechsler Intelligence Scales e.g. the Wechsler Adult Intelligence Scale (WAIS) (1939), WAIS-R (1981), WAIS-III (1997), WAIS-IV (2008); Wechsler Intelligence Scales for Children (WISC) (1949), WISC-R (1974), WISC-III (1991), WISC-IV (2003), WISC-V (2014); and Wechsler Preschool and Primary Scale of Intelligence (WPPSI) (1967), WPPSI-R (1989), WPPSI-III (2002). Each composite battery of subtests of the Wechsler Scales results in a report of an overall IQ, a Verbal IQ, and a Non-verbal IQ. The average IQ for age is set at 100 and with the standard deviation set at 15. Comparative norms for each instrument are reviewed, revised, and updated as necessary with each new released revision. These instruments are the gold standard for assessment of intelligence across the lifespan and extensively used today, over 75 years since being introduced to the academic and medical communities.

Standardized intellectual testing and quantification of individuals' intellectual resources and cognitive skills are now an established, routine component of most every comprehensive psychological assessment of individuals presenting with impairments of thought, cognition, mood, affect, or behaviors.

Most standardized assessments of intelligence assess the integrity of primary sensory and motor functions (Can the person see, hear, feel, and move normally?); attention and concentration skills and ability (Can the person focus on tasks over time without being distracted); intellectual resources (Has the person acquired age and education appropriate knowledge e.g. vocabulary words, fund of general information); and cognitive skills (Can the person use intellectual resources to think, solve problems, and make good judgements?). Intelligence testing, such as accomplished by the Wechsler Scales, permits a properly trained individual e.g. licensed clinical psychologist, to evaluate these four fundamental components of intelligence in isolation and in combination, providing useful information to be used in the diagnosis, treatment, and management of individuals presenting with impaired thought, cognition, mood, affect, or behaviors.

Projective techniques, such as the Jung's Word Association Test (1910)[311], Rorschach Inkblots (1921)[312], Morgan and Murray's Thematic Apperception Tests (1935)[313], and Rotter's Incomplete Sentence Tests (1950)[314], gain popularity and offer an alternative approach and complement standardized intellectual/cognitive assessment procedures. In brief, these test procedures introduce an ambiguous image to an individual e.g. ink blot, and the person verbally responds to the image with the first thing that comes to mind. Responses are recorded and later interpreted within a conceptual matrix, providing information as to personality structure and organization, primary defenses, and areas of emotional conflict.

The projective techniques are embraced and utilized primarily by practitioners using the psychodynamic, psychoanalytical models which emphasize the role of the unconscious in the development, maintenance, and resolution of impairments of thought, cognition, mood, affect, and behaviors.

Complementing the projective techniques being applied to assess personality during the first half of the 1900s, investigators at the University of Minnesota offer a new, alternative, quantitative, approach. Starke Hathaway and Charnley McKinley introduce the Minnesota Multiphasic Personality Inventory (MMPI) (1943)[315]. This instrument consists of 504 items, presented in the form of short statements e.g. I cry easily; I always tell the truth. The individual reads each statement and responds simply by answering true or false. Responses are then compared to normal and patient groups resulting in a multifactorial profile, which when interpreted by a properly trained practitioner e.g. licensed clinical psychologist, meaningful information regarding the patient's thought, cognition, mood, affect, and behaviors is collected and can be used in the diagnosis, treatment, and management of the individual seeking treatment. The MMPI is routinely revised throughout the 1900s and proves to be a gold standard in the assessment of personality.

The MMPI and similar inventory assessment instruments are embraced and utilized primarily by practitioners using empirically driven models to understand and treat impairments of thought, cognition, mood, affect, and behaviors.

In combination, the psychometric and projective techniques applied during the 1900s, in efforts to understand intelligence, cognition, mood, affect, and personality, contribute greatly to advancing our understanding of both normal and abnormal processes. These tools prove tremendously useful to clinicians, assisting in the effective, high quality of care offered to individuals seeking treatment for debilitating impairments in thought, cognition, mood, affect, or behavior.

Treatments available to individuals experiencing impairment of thought, cognition, mood, affect or behavior during the 1900s are organized into three broad categories; approaches emphasizing self-awareness e.g. psychoanalysis and humanistic psychology; approaches emphasizing behavior e.g. behaviorism; and approaches emphasizing direct physical manipulation of the brain e.g. psychosurgery, electroconvulsive treatments (ECT) and psychopharmacology.

Psychoanalytic and behavioral treatment approaches are couched in strong theoretical matrixes which guide treatment. Direct brain manipulation approaches are offered with much less theoretical foundation and are established principally upon empirical findings. Each approach finds its place in relieving suffering, experienced by many individuals presenting for medical treatment as the consequence of impaired functioning.

Treatments guided by the psychoanalytical and behavioral models have already been discussed. Let us now briefly examine direct brain manipulation procedures which gain popularity during the early-1900s and generate much support from within the academic and medical communities throughout all of 1900s.

Egas Moniz (1874-1955) Portuguese neurologist introduces procedures which chemically and structurally alter brain tissue and provide an alternative to the popular psychoanalytic and behavioralist treatments, currently being offered by the medical profession to individuals experiencing impaired mental functions (1935,1936b)[316]. He is instrumental in reawakening interests in the longstanding conceptual model which states the brain is the source and mediator of all intellectual, cognitive, emotional, and behavioral activities. As such, the most reasonable point of treatment intervention is the organ responsible for these activities, the brain.

Building upon the works of Swiss psychiatrist Gottllieb Burkhardt (1836-1907) whom successfully removes brain cerebral cortex in treatment of auditory hallucinations and schizophrenia during the late-1800s, while working as director of the asylum for the insane, located at Prefargier on the banks of Lake Neuchatel, Switzerland (1891)[317] and American neurophysiologists Carlyle Jacobsen (1902-1974) and John Fulton (1899-1960) investigating the behavioral calming effects of bilateral ablation of the prefrontal cortex in chimpanzees and monkeys, while working at Yale University. Egas Moniz investigates the treatment benefit of chemically and surgically disrupting neural transmission within the brain's frontal lobes in humans experiencing severe mental impairments, while working at the University of Lisbon, Portugal (1931,1935,1935,1935,1936)[318,319,320,321,322].

Egas Moniz suggests mental disorders result directly from abnormal neural transmission within the brain. He suggests the primary source responsible for abnormal transmission is an abnormal stickiness of brain cells, found in individuals experiencing impaired mental function. Abnormal stickiness causes neural impulses to become disrupted (stuck), causing the individual to repeatedly experience impairments of thoughts e.g. rumination, cognition, mood, affect, and behavior (1936a,1936b,1949a)[323,324,325]. Destroying brain pathways which have become "stuck" should improve the patient's debilitating mental and behavioral condition. There is no empirical evidence to support this model; however it provides Moniz with the foundation of a conceptual matrix to guide his scientific investigations.

He presents his first series of patients (n=4) treated with this approach, to the scientific and communities, reporting significant improvement observed in all patients. More specifically, this series presents two individuals diagnosed as experiencing chronic depression and two individuals experiencing paranoid schizophrenia. Ethyl alcohol is injected directly and bilaterally into the white matter tracts of the brain frontal lobes of each patient. Neural transmission is disrupted. Subsequent to this procedure, each patient evidences a reported significant transient improvement (1936a)[323]. Encouraged by the initial results, Egas Moniz modifies the procedure to induce a permanent result, switching from alcohol injections into the white matter tracts of the brain frontal lobes to surgically severing the white matter tracts.

He soon completes a second patient series. The second series reports 20 patients, suffering severe mental impairments, with half of the patients (n=10) treated with the alcohol injection only and half of the patients (n=10) treated surgically using the modified leucotomy procedure. Egas Moniz and colleague Diogo Furtado (1906-1964) declare seven individuals cured, seven individuals significantly improved, and six individuals unchanged (1936b)[324].

The news of a potentially new and effective treatment for use with severely mentally impaired individuals and which additionally produces significant calming effects in violent behavior patients, receives much attention within the medical and scientific communities and general public at large.

The next 15 years witness a worldwide and hopeful use of the new psychosurgery procedure, in efforts to effectively treat individuals suffering severe mental and behavioral impairments. Thousands of patients undergo the procedure worldwide, which Egas Moniz terms "prefrontal leucotomy". Particularly aggressive use and study of this procedure are completed in the countries of Portugal, Italy, France, UK, and USA (1936b,1937,1938,1942,1949,1950)[324,326,327,328,329,330].

Overall, results confirm, individuals experiencing severe impairments in thought, cognition, mood, affect, or behavior more often than not evidence improvement in function following the completion of the procedure. These findings have tremendous impact on the treatment of severely, mentally impaired individuals worldwide. Recall, at this time, effective psychopharmacological agents for use in the effective treatment and management of severe mental disorders e.g. psychosis and severe depression have yet to be introduced. These psychopharmacological agents are introduced during the late-1940s and 1950s e.g. lithium for manic-depressive disorders; chlorpromazine (Thorazine), dopamine receptor blocker for psychosis; imipramine (Tofranil), tricyclic antidepressant for depression; and iproniazid (Marsilid), nonselective monoamine oxidase inhibitor for depression.

The scientific and medical communities acknowledge Egas Moniz contributions and is awarded the Nobel Prize in Physiology or Medicine in 1949 "...for his discovery of the therapeutic value of leucotomy in certain psychoses..." (1949)[331].

Trivia: Egas Moniz introduces and develops the now familiar procedure cerebral angiography. Combining recent advances in X-ray imaging technologies and utilizing opaque dyes which he injects into the carotid arteries, he is first to successfully images cerebral blood vessels without the need of opening the head (1927,1931,1934)[332,333,334]. His innovative contribution and work in cerebral angiography results in four separate nominations for the Nobel Prize in Physiology or Medicine; 1928, 1933, 1937, and 1944. He is never awarded the Prize for his contributions for the discovery and development of cerebral angiography (2014)[335].

Walter Freeman (1895-1972) an American neurologist modifies the Moniz procedure to enter the brain via a trans-orbital approach, using an "ice pick" like instrument to section brain prefrontal lobe white matter tracts. In brief, the modified procedure is completed by inserting an "ice pick" like instrument through a small hole in the superior orbit (roof of the eye-socket) and into the white matter tracts of the brain prefrontal lobes, bilaterally and swishing the instrument around severing white matter tracts in the process, especially connections between the prefrontal lobes and the thalamus. The modified procedure eliminates the need for general anesthesia, is completed within minutes and typically results in an impressive calming effect on patients (1942,1942)[336,337]. Walter Freeman meets the need of overcrowded and understaffed psychiatric hospitals across the

USA traveling to these facilities and completing thousands of trans-orbital leucotomies (aka pre-frontal lobotomies) from the mid-1930s to the early-1950s.

Introduction of the first wave of effective antipsychotic and antidepressant medications during the 1950s displace the widespread and popular use of psychosurgical procedures. Effective medications such as lithium carbonate (bipolar mood disorders), chlorpromazine (antipsychotic), and iproniazid (antidepressant) become the first line of treatment intervention reserving psychosurgical procedures for the most severe and medication resistant patients. However, before effective antipsychotic and antidepressant medications are introduced, another procedural approach is aggressively investigated as a potential treatment, shock therapy.

Shock therapies, popular during the first half of the 1900s are based upon the fundamental belief impairments in thought, cognition, mood, affect, or behavior result as a consequence of abnormal brain activity. Procedures are introduced to disrupt the suspected abnormal brain activity responsible for observed impaired mental and behavioral functions. Procedures can be organized into two categories; ones which use assorted chemical agents or hormones to shock the brain and ones which use external application of repeated bursts of electricity delivered to the head and brain.

Given the popularity of these two approaches, their influential role in the treatment of severe mental impairments, and their impact upon the developing course of medical psychology, let's now briefly examine the historical roots of these two treatment approaches.

Constance Pascal (1877-1937) Romanian-French psychiatrist is among the first to advocate the therapeutic benefits of shocking the brain, in cases of severe impairment of mental functions. Proposing dementia praecox (schizophrenia) to be the consequential product of a "…mental anaphylactic reaction…", she proposes the brain can be shocked into a state of equilibrium through the administration of assorted chemical agents (1926)[338].

Manfried Sakel (1900-1957) Polish neurophysiologist, working at the private psychiatric Lichierielde Hospital in Berlin and attending to patients undergoing morphine addiction withdrawal, proposes a similar shock treatment. He makes the observation many patients presenting with morphine addiction evidence impaired mental function and many experience seizures during the course of physical withdrawal. Upon completion of the physical withdrawal phase of treatment many patients demonstrate marked improvements in their mental abilities and function. Manfried Sakel reasons, given seizures are associated with improvements in mental function in the morphine withdrawal patient, perhaps inducing seizures in other patient groups whom are experiencing severely impaired mental functions such as schizophrenia, will too demonstrate improved mental functions (1933)[339].

Manfried Sakel's approach to induce seizures and shock the brain is accomplished by inducing an extreme hypoglycemic state, through injection of large dosages of insulin. Dosage amounts are administered in sufficiently large amounts to induce reversible comas. Injected individuals are removed from coma by pumping glucose into the patient's stomach allowing the body to return to its normal state of equilibrium. The procedure is repeated daily resulting in approximately 30-50 shocks or until the patient demonstrates improvement (1933,1934,1937)[340,341,342]. The physiology underlying the reported treatment effect, as offered by Manfried Sakel, is the "…insulin puts a barrier between the cell and external stimuli, thus putting the cell at rest and enabling it to recuperate…" (1938)[343]. The procedure, Insulin Shock Therapy, remains popular well into the 1950s, falling out of favor with introduction of effective antipsychotic medications e.g. Thorazine.

Ugo Cerletti (1877-1963) an Italian neurologist and Lucio Bini (1908-1964) an Italian psychiatrist introduce Electroconvulsive Therapy (ECT) to the scientific and medical communities, as a treatment approach which too intervenes directly at the point of suspected organ dysfunction, responsible for severe disturbances in thought, cognition, mood, affect, and behavior, the brain (1938,1940)[344,345]. The procedure is founded in part on the observation seizure disorders, especially epilepsies, rarely coexist with schizophrenia.

In brief, ECT is offered as another early shock procedure, designed to induce seizures by applying brief bursts of electrical currents to the brain with the explicit intent to disrupt brain electrical activity.

Ugo Cerlette reports in his original paper, two electrodes are secured to the patient's head positioned over the left and right temporal bones. Brief bursts of electricity at 80-110 volts for duration of approximately 250 ms are applied until the patient seizes. The first patient to undergo the ECT procedure by Cerlette presents with a diagnosis of longstanding, severe, paranoid schizophrenia. The procedure is completed at the Clinic for Nervous and Mental Diseases in Rome, where Ugo Cerletti provides medical care and serves as the Clinic's senior administrator.

The first patient to undergo the ECT procedure is patient "S.E.". He is an adult male admitted to the Clinic having been found by police, wandering the local train station in a confused state. Patient S.E. undergoes one incomplete and 11 completed ECT treatments before his mental state is declared significantly improved and ready for discharge from the Clinic. The ECT procedure is modified over time and is the source of much debate within the medical, academic, and lay public regarding its clinical effectiveness and ethical use. The procedure continues to be used today in modified forms, over 80 years after its introduction (2018)[346].

Treatment and management approaches change significantly for individuals experiencing impairments in thought, cognition, mood, affect, and behavior by the mid-1900s. Chemical agents and new pharmaceuticals with demonstrated effectiveness in relieving psychiatric signs and symptoms are introduced and quickly displace other treatment modalities. Many of the new pharmaceuticals are introduced without a clear understanding as to why or how they produce their clinical effects. Recognition of their effectiveness in relieving psychiatric symptoms is oftentimes a serendipitous empirical observation made by an observant and knowledgeable practitioner when using a pharmaceutical for an entirely different and unrelated purpose. For example, iproniazid (Marsilid), one of the first monoamine oxidase inhibitors used to effectively treat depression, is initially marketed as a treatment for tuberculosis (TB) and only later recognized for its antidepressant properties.

Pharmaceuticals gain rapid popularity as an effective treatment and management tool. The idea of manipulating brain chemistries for the treatment of impaired mental functioning is not new and has been practiced for thousands of years. See the beginning of this chapter for details.

During the mid-1900s emphasis is placed upon the brain as the target organ responsible for normal and abnormal mental processing. Treatment approaches directed to altering brain physiology with the use of pharmaceuticals are congruent with medical dogma of the period. New and effective chemical agents and pharmaceuticals are aggressively investigated. These investigations result in many of the early, identified pharmaceuticals effective in the treatment and management of impaired mental functions. Many of these identified compounds establish the foundation for many pharmaceutical still used today in 2020, over 100 years since their first introduction.

Let us now briefly examine, by way of example, a few of the most influential chemical agents and pharmaceuticals which significantly influence the development of medical psychology and psychiatry.

Lithium carbonate is first introduced into medicine as an effective treatment for gout (1859)[347]. Recall, gout is a disorder characterized by deposition of urate deposits in cartilage and associated with increased uric acid, a breakdown product of urea in blood. By the late-1800s, it is popularly believed, individuals evidencing increased body uric acid, suffer a urate imbalance, placing the individual at high risk for medical conditions such as gout, rheumatoid disorders, cardiac disease, and mental disorders. Given, lithium carbonate has the chemical property to dissolve urate crystals and high urate levels are suspected to produce mental disorders, it is investigated as a chemical agent in the treatment of mental disorders and proves most effective in the treatment of mania and depression (1871,1896)[348, 349]. However, given the toxicity of lithium and lack of technologies necessary to monitor blood levels, this agent soon loses popularity within the clinical medical community.

Lithium carbonate is rediscovered in the mid-1900s as an effective pharmacological treatment for bipolar mood disorders presenting with psychosis (1949)[350]. Systematic assessment of lithium carbonate, as an effective pharmaceutical is completed in the 1950s and confirms its value in the treatment and management of bipolar mood disorders (1954)[351]. Lithium continues to be used today, over 70 years since its rediscovery.

Trivia: The term lithium is derived from the Greek "lithos" meaning stone. The term is coined by Jons Berzelius (1779-1848) Swedish physician turned chemist while investigating and classifying minerals. Remember, lithium is a soft, silver-white metal. Lithium carbonate (Li_2CO_3) is the form used in medicine. Yes, Jons Berzelius is the same person responsible for introducing the system for chemical notation we use today where elements are abbreviated and portions between elements are denoted by numbers e.g. H_2O. In Berzelius's original chemical notation system, numbers are written as superscript (H^2O) rather than our current system writing numbers as subscripts.

The 1950s witness the introduction of the first effective phenothiazine antipsychotic to gain widespread popularity, chlorpromazine (Thorazine). Introduced in France, initially as an agent to potentiate general anesthesia, clinical observation and prepared minds soon recognize the medication's potential use for individuals suffering severe impairments of thought, cognition, mood, affect, and behavior (1952,1952b,1952)[352,353.354]. Chlorpromazine remains one of the most commonly used medications in the treatment and management of schizophrenia worldwide today, now over 70 years since its recognition as a potent and effective antipsychotic medication. Chlorpromazine continues to be used as the benchmark antipsychotic medication against which all others are compared.

The 1950s also witness the introduction of the first monoamine oxidase inhibitor (MAOI) as an effective antidepressant, iproniazid (Marsilid). This medication is designed and used successfully in the treatment of pulmonary tuberculosis (TB) and later investigated as a potential antidepressant when some TB patients taking the medication appear euphoric and unusually happy (1952)[355]. Recall, monoamine oxidases normally degrade serotonin and norepinephrine in the brain.

Recognizing inhibition of monoamine oxidases result in increased levels of serotonin and norepinephrine in brain and associated improvements in thought, cognition, mood, affect, and behaviors, the popularity of models which conceptualize mental disorders to be the consequence of disordered brain chemistry quickly rise in the medical and scientific communities (1958)[356]. Pharmaceuticals directed to restoring balances in brain chemistries gain popularity.

The late-1950s witness the introduction of the first tricyclic antidepressant, imipramine (Tofranil) (1957)[357]. Initially introduced in Switzerland by the powerful pharmaceutical company Geigy, as a medication to compete with chlorpromazine for the market in treatment of schizophrenia, the medication proves unsuccessful as an antipsychotic. However, by way of serendipitous discovery, the medication is soon recognized to be an effective antidepressant (1958)[358]. Unlike the rapid acceptance of chlorpromazine, the academic and medical communities are initially and passionately resistant to use of imipramine for the treatment of depression. Recall, at this time medical dogma states depression is the result of disordered psychodynamic processes. Soon, repeated demonstrations of Imipramine's effectiveness for the treatment of depression allow the medication to be embraced by both academic and medical communities (1959)[359]. New models emphasizing the role of brain monoamines to explain depression slowly begin to gain acceptance and compete with popular psychodynamic models to explain the etiology of depression and guide clinical treatments.

The early-1960s witness the introduction and widespread marketing of the tranquilizing anti-anxiety medications chlordiazepoxide (Librium) (1960) and diazepam (Valium) (1963). These two benzodiazepines are designed and developed in the USA by the Switzerland based Hoffman-La Roche pharmaceutical company. Diazepam quickly becomes the top selling pharmaceutical in the USA between 1969 and 1982, reflecting the rapidly growing acceptance of pharmaceuticals as a primary mode of treatment for individuals suffering impairments of thought, cognition, mood, affect, and behavior. Medical psychology and the treatment of psychiatric conditions are now becoming more dependent upon pharmaceuticals than ever before in the history of medicine.

The late-1960s witness the FDA approval of a new antipsychotic medication, originally designed at the Janssen Pharmaceutical Laboratories located in Beerse, Belgium and clinically tested with severely impaired psychiatric patients under treatment at the University of Liege Hospital; haloperidol (1958,1967)[360,361]. Haldol quickly proves useful in the treatment and management of schizophrenia, allowing many patients to be released from inpatient hospital care.

Trivia: The term "psychopharmacology" is first introduced into the academic and medical literature in a paper published in 1920 describing the analgesic effects of opium, opium alkaloids (morphine, codeine, papaverine, narcotin, narceine, thebaine) and antipyretic drugs (quinine, acetanilide, phenacetin, antipyrine, saldol, pyramidon, aspirin) to alter pain thresholds, when subjects are subjected to painful electrical shocks applied to back of the hand, tip of the nose, tip of the tongue, and lips. The investigators, Drs. Bollinger and Johnson serve as research subjects in many of their painful electrical shock experiments. The 1920 study additionally investigates the effects of these analgesics on simple motor reaction times and complex reaction times (requiring mental calculations), as well as tasks of neuromuscular speed and coordination (tapping tasks), field of vision, and hearing acuity (1920)[362].

The 1970s through the end of the 1900s witnesses refinement of psychiatric medications, reducing unwanted side effects, becoming more specific to brain receptor targets, and contribute to the development of new models of brain neurochemistry believed to underlie debilitating impairments of thought, cognition, mood, affect, and behavior. New medications are introduced such as the atypical antipsychotic clozapine (Clozaril) (1971); the non-tricyclic, non MAOI antidepressant trazodone (Desyrel), a serotonin reuptake inhibitor, originally designed and clinically tested in Italy during the 1960s is later approved by the FDA for use in the USA (1981); alprazolam (Xanax) a short acting benzodiazepine (1981); fluoxetine (Prozac) a selective serotonin reuptake inhibitor (SSRI) antidepressant (1988); donepezil hydrochloride (Aricept) an acetylcholine esterase inhibitor marketed for the used in early dementia of the Alzheimer's type to slow cognitive impairment (1993); and Adderall an amphetamine for use in the treatment of Attention Deficit Hyperactivity Disorder (ADHD) (1996).

The introduction and acceptance of pharmaceuticals, directed for use with patients suffering impairments in thought, cognition, mood, affect, and behavior, during the mid-1900s through the end of the 1900s, revolutionize the care and primary treatment modality used by the medical community in the treatment and management of psychiatric patients. Psychiatry, based upon biological models of brain function and associated imbalances in brain chemistries, displace psychodynamic models as the predominant models guiding the development of medical psychology in the USA, Canada, Europe, and most countries throughout the world.

As much as conceptual models and treatments reflect the mind set underlying the medical care provided to individuals suffering impairments in thought, cognition, mood, affect, and behavior, so do classification systems. Let us now briefly examine the historical development of now familiar classification systems, as they apply to the diagnostic organization of impaired mental and behavioral functions. Building upon Emil Kraepelin's early classification system which proposes mental disorders be classified categorically into "…curable…" and "…incurable…" (1883)[363], the second half of the 1900s witnesses directed attention into developing a standardized nosology for organizing impairments of thought, cognition, mood, affect, and behavior.

Two classification systems develop in parallel. The International Classification of Disease and Related Health Problems (ICD) system used by most countries in the world and the Diagnostic Statistical Manual (DSM) system used by the USA. Both systems undergo substantial revisions in their diagnostic categories related to impairments of thought, cognition, mood, affect, and behavior since their introduction during the mid-1900s, ICD (1949), DSM (1952).

The ICD system is the international standard for classification of diseases. Designed originally as a manual to assist in worldwide epidemiology research, diseases are assigned diagnostic codes. The ICD is the officially recognized diagnostic manual for diseases by the World Health Organization. The first manual to include diagnostic codes for mental disorders appears in the ICD-6, published in 1949. The ICD manual is updated approximately every 10 years and to date has undergone five revisions (ICD-6 1947, ICD-7 1955, ICD-8 1968, ICD-9 1979, ICD-10 1999). Each revision reveals a progressive change in the way mental disorders are conceptualized and categorized based upon prevailing medical dogma. The system continues to emphasize etiologies responsible for mental disorders, as opposed to their clinical manifestation.

The DSM system is a standardized system of classification specific to mental disorders and used principally in the United States of America. The DSM is the official diagnostic manual for the American Psychiatric Association. Similar to the ICD, the DSM undergoes periodic revisions which reflect the prevailing medical dogma. The first DSM is published in 1952 and contains 134 pages and identifies 182 mental disorders. This manual is now in its 6th revision (DSM-I 1952, DSM-II 1968, DSM-III 1980, III-R 1987, DSN-IV 1994, DSM-IV-TR 2000, DSM-5 (sic) 2013).

The DSM-5 contains 947 pages and identifies more than 300 mental disorders. Unlike the ICD which emphasize etiology of mental disorder the DSM-5 places emphasis on clinical manifestations of mental disorders. The recent release of the DSM-5 has reignited the passionate debate inside and outside the medical community as to what are mental disorders; what are their underlying etiologies; and how can individuals suffering impairment of thought, cognition, mood, affect, or behavior best be managed, treated, and cared for by mental health care professionals and society at large.

Governments throughout history have contributed to the way in which individuals suffering mental disorders are managed, treated, and cared for by society. So too is the case during the late-1900s. In Italy, by way of legislative action, all new admissions to psychiatric institutions are uniformly prohibited and impose directives to close all psychiatric hospitals in Italy. This law is termed the Italian Mental Health Act of 1978 or simply the Basaglia Law in recognition of the psychiatrist who wrote much of the legislation and promoted its passage (1978)[364]. The legislation reflects the changing mind set within Italy to move away from long term State psychiatric institutions and towards community based psychiatric services.

In the USA. President William J. Clinton signs into law the Mental Health Parity Act which mandates all impairments of thought, cognition, mood, affect, and behavior be considered on parity with all other medical or surgical conditions necessitating diagnosis and intervention by mental health professionals, with respect to health insurance reimbursement payments to the health care provider (1996)[365]. Prior to this legislation health care insurance companies within the Unites States routinely deny payment for services provided to individuals who suffer impairments in thought, cognition, mood, affect, or behavior. These examples characterize the many reforms being made during the late-1900s in attempting to improve services and care to individuals suffering mental impairments.

The second half of the 1900s comes to a close with continuing progress being made in the scientific based understanding of impaired mental function and behavior. Rapid advancements are being made into the exploration of genetic material and its association with impaired mental function and behaviors. The predominant model applied in the clinical treatment of severe mental disorders in most countries throughout the world continues to be based upon pharmaceutical intervention. Society at large is more aware of mental disorders and treatments than ever before. More individuals today are receiving medical treatments for disordered mental functioning than ever before in history. However, the specific underlying causes, clinical manifestations, and specific treatments for mental and behavioral disorders continue to remain elusive and passionately debated within the academic and medical communities, with no clear, definitive answers visible on the horizon. So it goes….

In summary, the 1900s witness continuing progress in the development of medical psychology as an important professional discipline. The early-1900s witness the introduction and development of three predominant conceptual matrixes which greatly influence the direction of medical psychology. The psychoanalytic schools, the behaviorist schools, and the humanistic schools. Psychometric assessment of intellectual resources, cognitive abilities, and personality is introduced and proves valuable in advancing the knowledge base as to the fundamental constructs underlying thought, cognition, mood, affect, and behavior. Psychometric assessment becomes an essential component in diagnosis and assessment of individuals presenting with both normal and abnormal mental functions. Treatment modalities focusing upon direct, physical intervention at the organ of all mental processes, the brain, gain popularity. Brain leucotomies and chemical agent induced, insulin induced, and electroconvulsive shock treatments exemplify the direct physical interventions. Pharmacological treatments displace most treatments as the preferred choice of treatment by the second half of the 1900s. Psychopharmacology remains the most popular and dominant intervention approach through the end of the 1900s. Commercial pharmaceutical companies generate billions of dollars in revenue from the production, distribution, and demand for psychopharmacological agents. More people than ever before in the history of medicine access medical care for treatment of impairments of thought, cognition, mood, affect, and behavior.

Current Modern, 2000 AD - 2019 AD.

Awareness of the historical and current treatment practices of individuals experiencing mental impairments are once again brought to the attention of the public at large with the publication "Mad in America" (2002,2010)[366,367]. The book offers an unforgiving and fair indictment of medicine and society's attempts to deal effectively with the care and treatment of individuals presenting to medical care with severe impairments in thought, cognition, mood, affect, and behaviors.

Medical schools in the USA respond favorably to recommendations generated by a joint committee of the National Academy of Sciences Institute of Medicine and National Research Council, upon the request of the National Institutes of Health, to improve medical education by modifying existing medical school curricula to include additional and formalized training in the behavioral sciences for all medical students (2004)[368]. Medical schools recognize the need and modify their curricula, to better train medical students in the behavioral sciences, to meet the rapidly growing demands of a society accessing health care for treatment of impairments in thought, cognition, mood, affect, and behavior at rising and unprecedented rates. Initial reports indicate the additional training in medical school is indeed improving the awareness of physicians to the many unique skills and knowledge base required to effectively and responsibly diagnose and treat individuals suffering impairments in thought, cognition, mood, affect, and behaviors.

The American Psychiatric Association releases its newest and 5th edition of the "Diagnostic Statistical Manual (DSM-5)" (2013)[93]. The debate as to what actually is a mental disorder, the underlying etiologies responsible, and what are the most effective treatments continue. Efforts continue to establish a standard nomenclature and nosology for mental disorders.

Clinical psychologists are granted prescription privileges and permitted by law to prescribe medications for the treatment of mental disorders. Three states currently grant prescription privileges to psychologists; New Mexico (2002), Louisiana (2004), Illinois (2014). The legislative decision to grant appropriately trained psychologists prescription privileges to prescribe psychiatric medications comes at tremendous expense. These and similar legislative initiatives to increase the availability of clinical services to individuals suffering impairment in mental functions is passionately contested and opposed by the American Medical Association and equally passionately advocated by the American Psychological Association.

Opposition to granting prescription privileges, to qualified psychologists, have been and continue to be based more in professional turf issues than reasonable objections based upon training, knowledge, or best interests of the patient. Discussions and heated debates continue within and among clinical service providers and the professional organizations representing the special and focused interests of their members e.g. American Medical Association and the American Psychological Association. Perhaps the future will witness a more cooperative and less confrontational environment with passions redirected to providing high quality clinical services to those in need of psychiatric and medical psychology services.

The future of medical psychology and psychiatry is going to be exciting. The field is in need of bright, energetic, and thoughtful young professionals to lead the discipline into the next phase of development. Are you one?

References.

[1] Medical Psychology. (2013). Wikipedia. Retrieved 6-21-2013. http://en.wikipedia.org/wiki/Medical_psychology
[2] Medical Psychology. (2013). The Free Dictionary. Retrieved 6-21-2013 from http://www.thefreedictionary.com/psychological+medicine
[3] Ebers papyrus (circa 1550 BC). Compendium of the whole Egyptian medicine (Georg Ebers), Columns 1-2. University of Leipzig Library, Special Collections. Leipzig, Germany.
[4] Thompson, R. (1923). Assyrian medical texts from the originals in the British Museum. London: H. Milford, Oxford University Press.
[5] Scurlock, J. and Anderson, B. (2005). Diagnoses in Assyrian and Babylonian medicine: Ancient sources, translations, and modern medical analyses. Chicago: University of Illinois Press.
[6] Bryan, C. (1930). The Papyrus Ebers. Translated from the German version by Cyril P. Bryan with an introduction by Professor G. Elliot Smith. London: Geoffrey Bles.
[7] Diels, H. (1903). Die fragmente der Vorsokratiker griechissch und deutsch. Berlin: Widenmannsche Buchhandlung.
[8] Freeman, K. (1948). Ancilla to the Pre-Socratic Philosopher: A Complete Translation of the Fragments in Diels' "Fragmente der Vorsokratiker". Cambridge: Harvard University Press.
[9] Diels, H. and Kranz, W. (1952) Die Fragmente der Vorsokratiker, 6th edition. Berlin: Weidmann.
[10] Diels, H. (1879). Doxographi Graeci, Editio Iterata. Lipsiae: G. Reimer.
[11] Freeman, K. (1983). Ancilla to the Pre-Socratic Philosophers: A complete translation of the Fragments in Diels, Fragment der Vorsokratiker. Cambridge, MA: Harvard University Press.
[12] Lanza, D. (1965). Un nuovo frammento di Alcmeone, Maia, 17:278-280.
[13] Taran, L. (1965). Paramenides: A text with translation, commentary, and critical essays. Princeton: Princeton University Press.
[14] Darwin, C. (1859). On the origins of species by means of natural selection or the preservation of favoured races in the struggle for life. London: John Murray.
[15] Littre, E. (1839-61). Oeuvres completes d'Hippocarates, 10 volumes. Paris: Bailliere.
[16] Hippocrates (circa 400 BC), Adams, F. (1849). Affections 1 (6.208 Littre). The genuine works of Hippocrates, translated from the Greek with a preliminary discourse and annotations. London: Sydenham Society; New York: William Woods (1891).
[17] Hippocrates (circa 400 BC), Adams, F. (1849). Epidemics. The genuine works of Hippocrates, translated from the Greek with a preliminary discourse and annotations. London: Sydenham Society; New York: William Woods (1891).
[18] Hippocrates (circa 400 BC), Adams, F. (1849). Regimen in Acute Disease 5 (2.232 Littre). The genuine works of Hippocrates, translated from the Greek with a preliminary discourse and annotations. London: Sydenham Society; New York: William Woods (1891).
[19] Hippocrates (circa 400 BC), Adams, F. (1849). Morbus, 1.30 (6.200 Littre). The genuine works of Hippocrates, translated from the Greek with a preliminary discourse and annotations. London: Sydenham Society; New York: William Woods (1891).
[20] Hippocrates (circa 400 BC), Adams, F. (1849). Affections, 10 (6.216 Littre). The genuine works of Hippocrates, translated from the Greek with a preliminary discourse and annotations. London: Sydenham Society; New York: William Woods (1891).
[21] Hippocrates (circa 400 BC), Adams, F. (1849). Affections, 10 (6.216 Littre). The genuine works of Hippocrates, translated from the Greek with a preliminary discourse and annotations. London: Sydenham Society; New York: William Woods (1891).
[22] Hippocrates (circa 400 BC), Adams, F. (1849). Prorrhetics, 1.15 (5.514 Littre). The genuine works of Hippocrates, translated from the Greek with a preliminary discourse and annotations. London: Sydenham Society; New York: William Woods (1891).
[23] Hippocrates (circa 400 BC), Adams, F. (1849). Epidemics, 7.79 (5.434 Littre. Epidemics 1.2.9 (2.650-652 Littre). The genuine works of Hippocrates, translated from the Greek with a preliminary discourse and annotations. London: Sydenham Society; New York: William Woods (1891).

[24] Hippocrates (circa 400 BC), Adams, F. (1849). Epidemics, 1.2.6 (2.636 Littre). The genuine works of Hippocrates, translated from the Greek with a preliminary discourse and annotations. London: Sydenham Society; New York: William Woods (1891).

[25] Hippocrates (circa 400 BC), Adams, F. (1849). Prognostics, 10 (2.134 Littre). The genuine works of Hippocrates, translated from the Greek with a preliminary discourse and annotations. London: Sydenham Society; New York: William Woods (1891).

[26] Hippocrates (circa 400 BC), Adams, F. (1849). Epidemics, 1.2.9 (2.652 Littre). The genuine works of Hippocrates, translated from the Greek with a preliminary discourse and annotations. London: Sydenham Society; New York: William Woods (1891).

[27] Hippocrates (circa 400 BC), Adams, F. (1849). Affections, 10 (6.216-218 Littre). The genuine works of Hippocrates, translated from the Greek with a preliminary discourse and annotations. London: Sydenham Society; New York: William Woods (1891).

[28] Hippocrates (circa 400 BC), Adams, F. (1949). The genuine works of Hippocrates, translated from the Greek with a preliminary discourse and annotations. London: Sydenham Society (1849); New York: William Woods (1891).

[29] Hippocrates (circa 400 BC), Adams, F. (1849). Coan Prenotions 93 (5.602 Littre), 94 (5.602 Littre). The genuine works of Hippocrates, translated from the Greek with a preliminary discourse and annotations. London: Sydenham Society; New York: William Woods (1891).

[30] Hippocrates (circa 400 BC), Adams, F. (1849). Epidemics, 3.3.17(4) (3.116-118 Littre), 5.52 (5.236-238 Littre), 7.71(5.432 Littre), 7.112 (5.460 Littre), 5.52, 7.71, 7.79 Littre). The genuine works of Hippocrates, translated from the Greek with a preliminary discourse and annotations. London: Sydenham Society; New York: William Woods (1891).

[31] Hippocrates (circa 400 BC), Adams, F. (1849). Affections, 10 (6.218 Littre). The genuine works of Hippocrates, translated from the Greek with a preliminary discourse and annotations. London: Sydenham Society; New York: William Woods (1891).

[32] Hippocrates (circa 400 BC), Adams, F. (1849). Affections, 12 (6.220). The genuine works of Hippocrates, translated from the Greek with a preliminary discourse and annotations. London: Sydenham Society; New York: William Woods (1891).

[33] Hippocrates (circa 400 BC), Adams, F. (1849). Affections, 10 (6.216-218 Littre). The genuine works of Hippocrates, translated from the Greek with a preliminary discourse and annotations. London: Sydenham Society; New York: William Woods (1891).

[34] Hippocrates (circa 400 BC), Adams, F. (1849). Morbus, 1.30 (6.200 Littre). The genuine works of Hippocrates, translated from the Greek with a preliminary discourse and annotations. London: Sydenham Society; New York: William Woods (1891).

[35] Tweedie, A. (1840). A system of practical medicine comprised in a series of original dissertation and arranged and edited by Alexander Tweedie. Diseases of the nervous systems. Philadelphia: Lea and Blanchard.

[36] Hippocrates (circa 400 BC), Adams, F. (1849). Aphorism. 3.1 (4.486 Littre). The genuine works of Hippocrates, translated from the Greek with a preliminary discourse and annotations. London: Sydenham Society; New York: William Woods (1891).

[37] Hippocrates (circa 400 BC), Adams, F. (1849). Epidemics, 1.2.9 (2.650 Littre). The genuine works of Hippocrates, translated from the Greek with a preliminary discourse and annotations. London: Sydenham Society (1849), New York: William Woods (1891).

[38] Hippocrates (circa 400 BC), Adams, F. (1849). Aphorism, 7.82 (4.606 Littre). The genuine works of Hippocrates, translated from the Greek with a preliminary discourse and annotations. London: Sydenham Society (1849), New York: William Woods (1891).

[39] Hippocrates, Aphorism. 8.53. The Genuine works of Hippocrates vol 2. The genuine works of Hippocrates, translated from the Greek with a preliminary discourse and annotations. London: Sydenham Society; New York: William Woods (1891).

[40] McDonald, G. (2009). Concepts and treatments of Phrenitis in Ancient Medicine. Doctoral dissertation, Newcastle University.

[41] Hippocrates (circa 400 BC), Adams, F. (1849). Morbus Sacred, 18 (6.388 Littre). The genuine works of Hippocrates, translated from the Greek with a preliminary discourse and annotations. London: Sydenham Society; New York: William Woods (1891).

[42] Hippocrates (circa 400 BC), Adams, F. (1849). Morbus Sacred, 18 (6.388-390 Littre). The genuine works of Hippocrates, translated from the Greek with a preliminary discourse and annotations. London: Sydenham Society; New York: William Woods (1891).

[43] Hippocrates, (400 BC). On the sacred disease. Translated by Francis Adams. The Internet Classics, http://classics.mit.edu/Hippocrates/sacred.html

[44] Hippocrates (circa 400 BC), Adams, F. (1849). Morbus, 1.30 (6.200 Littre). The genuine works of Hippocrates, translated from the Greek with a preliminary discourse and annotations. London: Sydenham Society; New York: William Woods (1891).

[45] Hippocrates (circa 400 BC), Adams, F. (1849). Epidemics, 346-7. The genuine works of Hippocrates, translated from the Greek with a preliminary discourse and annotations. London: Sydenham Society; New York: William Woods (1891).

[46] Hippocrates (circa 400 BC), Adams, F. (1849). Affections, 10 (6.216-218 Littre). The genuine works of Hippocrates, translated from the Greek with a preliminary discourse and annotations. London: Sydenham Society; New York: William Woods (1891).

[47] Hippocrates (circa 400 BC), Adams, F. (1849). Aphorisms, Section III, no 20, 22. Library of Alexander. Translation by Francis Adams. The genuine works of Hippocrates, translated from the Greek with a preliminary discourse and annotations. London: Sydenham Society; New York: William Woods (1891).

[48] Hippocrates (circa 400 BC), Adams, F. (1849). Aphorism, Section IV, no 9. Translation by Francis Adams. Library of Alexanders. The genuine works of Hippocrates, translated from the Greek with a preliminary discourse and annotations. London: Sydenham Society; New York: William Woods (1891).

[49] Hippocrates (circa 400 BC), Adams, F (1849). The Genuine Works of Hippocrates, Translated from the Greek with a preliminary discourse and annotations by Francis Adam. Volume 2. 843- 858. The Sacred Disease. Sydenham Society, London: C. and J. Adlard, Printers. http://books.google.com/books?id=GIJIAAAAYAAJ&printsec=frontcover&source=gbs_ge_summary_r&cad=0#v=onepage&q&f=false

[50] Hippocrates (400 BC). On the sacred disease. Translated by Francis Adams. The Internet Classics, http://classics.mit.edu/Hippocrates/sacred.html

[51] Hippocrates. (400 BC). The sacred disease, Translation by W.H.S. Jones, Vol. II. 1992 fragments of text selected from pages 139-183.Cambridge MA: Harvard University Press.

[52] Hippocrates (circa 400 BC), Adams, F. (1849). Morbus Sacred, (6.352-397 Littre). The genuine works of Hippocrates, translated from the Greek with a preliminary discourse and annotations. London: Sydenham Society: New York: William Woods (1891).

[53] Hippocrates (circa 400 BC), Adams, F. (1849). Morbus Sacred, 9-12 (6.370-374 Littre). The genuine works of Hippocrates, translated from the Greek with a preliminary discourse and annotations. London: Sydenham Society; New York: William Woods (1891).

[54] Hippocrates (circa 400 BC), Adams, F. (1849). The genuine works of Hippocrates. Volume 2 (google e-book). Aphorisms, 7, 738. Retrieved 5-27-2015 from https://books.google.com.jm/books?id=GIJIAAAAYAAJ&pg=PA685&source=gbs_toc_r&cad=3#v=onepage&q&f=false

[55] Hippocrates (circa 400 BC). The sacred disease. Translated by WHS Jones, Volume II. Harvard University Press, Cambridge MA, 1992, fragments of text selected from pages 139-183.

[56] Diels, H. (1958). Doxographi Graeci. p 590. Berolini, Gruyter et Socios.

[57] Nutton, V. (2004). Ancient Medicine. London and New York: Routledge.

[58] Tsoucalas, G. (2013). The "atomic theory" of Leucippus, and its impact on medicine before Hippocrates. Hellenic Journal Nuclear Medicine, 16(1):68-69.

[59] Online Etymology Dictionary (2013). http://www.etymonline.com/index.php?term=asylum

[60] Withington, E. (1921). In Studies in the history and method of science. Ed. Singer, Oxford: Clarendon Press.

[61] Herzog, R. (1931). Die Wunderheilungem von Epidauros, Philologus Supplementband 22, Hft. 3, Lepzig.

[62] Gumpert, C. (1794). Asclepiadis Bithyni Fragmenta. Vinariae: Industrie-Comptoir.

[63] Harless, C. (1828). De Medicis Veteribus Asclepiades Dietis. Bonn.

[64] Plato. (360 BC). Apology. English translation by Benjamin Jowet. The Internet Classic Archives. Retrieved 9-20-2013 http://classics.mit.edu/Plato/apology.html

[65] Online Etymology Dictionary. Philosophy. Retrieved 7-7-2013. http://etymonline.com/?term=philosophy

[66] Plato. (circa 360 BC). Plato Dialogues, Volume 1, Phaedrus. Translation by Benjamin Jowett. The Internet Classic Archives. Retrieved 7-9-2013. http://classics.mit.edu/Plato/phaedrus.html

[67] Plato. (circa 380 BC). Plato Dialogues, Volume 1, Protgaoras. Translation by Benjamin Jowett. The Internet Classic Archives. Retrieved 7-9-2013. http://classics.mit.edu/Plato/protagoras.html

[68] Plato. (circa 350 BC,1892). Plato Dialogues, Volume 2. Phaedo. Translation by Benjamin Jowett. The Dialogues of Plato translated into English with Analyses and Introduction by Benjamin Jowett, in five volumes, 3rd edition and corrected. Oxford University Press (1892).

[69] Plato. (circa 350 BC, 1925). Plato, Phaedo, Section 64c. Plato in Twelve Volumes, Volume 1. Translated by Harold North Fowler; Introduction by W.R.M. Lamb. Cambridge, MA, Harvard University Press; London, William Heinemann Ltd. 1966. 1925: full text (English & Greek).

[70] Plato. (circa 360 BC). Timaeus. Translated by Benjamin Jowett. The Internet Classic Archives. Retrieved November 2009 from http://classics.mit.edu/Plato/timaeus.html

[71] Plato. (circa 347 BC, 1961). Plato: The collected dialogues including letters. Edited by Edith Hamilton and Huntington Cairns. Translated by Lane Cooper (1961). Charmides, p103. Princeton: Princeton University Press.

[72] Diongenes Laertius (circa 225 AD, 1925). Lives of the Eminent Philosophers. Translated by Robert Drew Hicks Book III, Plato, paragraph 4, Loeb Classical Library 1925.

[73] Breen, P. (1847), Diary of Patrick Breen, One of the Donner Party. Edited by Frederick J. Teggart. Published by Academy of Pacific Coast History, Volume 1, No 6; University of California, Berkley: The University Press.

[74] Cicero, T. (45 BC, 1877). Tusculan Disputations. On other perturbations of the mind. Book IV, sec XIV, p140. Translated by C. D. Yonge, New York: Harper & Brothers Publishers. http://www.gutenberg.org/files/14988/14988-h/14988-h.htm

[75] Cicero, T. (45 BC, 1877). Tusculan Disputations. On grief of mind. Book III, Sec III, p93. Translated by C. D. Yonge (1877), New York: Harper & Brothers Publishers. http://www.gutenberg.org/files/14988/14988-h/14988-h.htm

[76] Cicero, T. (45 BC, 1824). The Tusculan Disputations of Cicero. A new edition, revised and corrected by W.H. Main. P 280. London: W. Pickering.

[77] Celsus, A. (circa 30 AD). De Medicina [On Medicine]. First printed 1478 Florence Nicolaus Laurentii, Rare. Book Collection, Countway Medical Library, Boston.

[78] Merriam-Webster Online Dictionary and Thesaurus. Retrieved 9-21-2013 from www,merriam-webster.com

[79] Celsus, A. (circa 30 AD). De Medicina [On Medicine]. Online English translation by W. Spencer (1935). Loeb Classical Library Edition, Retrieved November 2009 from hhtp://penelope.uchicago.edu/Thayer/E/Roman/Texts/celsus/home.html

[80] Celsus, A. (circa 30 AD). De Medicina [On Medicine]. Book III 17-21.Online English translation by W. Spencer (1935). Loeb Classical Library Edition, Retrieved November 2009 from hhtp://penelope.uchicago.edu/Thayer/E/Roman/Texts/celsus/home.html

[81] Aretaeus. (circa 200 AD). The Extant works of Aretaeus, The Cappadocian. Edited and translated by Francis Adams. On the causes and symptoms of chronic disease. Book I, Chapter VI on Madness. London: Sydenham Society (1856). Digital Hippocratic Collection. Retrieved 9-23-2013. http://www.chlt.org/sandbox/dh/aretaeusEnglish/page.55.a.php?size=240x320.

[82] Galan (circa 200 AD). De locis affectis. 3:10. (8,190-191 Kuhn= S 93).

[83] Bussi, G. (1469). Letter of introduction to Apuleius. Dated November 28, 1469). Reprinted in T. Ricklin. Giovanni Andrea Bussi und die media tempestas oder was die Geschichte von einem Esel lehrt'. Internatinal Zeitschrift fur Philosophie, 2 (2004), p 5-47.

[84] Horn, G. (1666). Arca Noae: Sive historia imperiorum et regnorum a condito orbe ad nostra tempora. Lugd, Batau, et Roterod. Ex Officina Hackiana.

[85] Petracra, F. (circa 1372). Medieval Sourcebook: Francesco Petrarch: Letters. Letter to Posterity. Translated by James Robinson and Henry Rolf (1909). New York: Putnam's Sons. Retrieved from Fordham University 5-29-2015. http://legacy.fordham.edu/halsall/source/petrarch1.asp

[86] Ibn Sina (Avicenna). (circa 1025 AD,1930). Kitab al-Qanun fi al-tibb [Canon of Medicine]. Translated by O. Cameron Gruner. London: AMS Press.

[87] Ibn Sina (Avicenna) (circa 1020 AD,1959). De anima, Arabic text: being the psychological part of Kitab al-shifa. University of Durham publications. Oxford University Press.

[88] Ibn Sina. (circa 1035 AD,1951). Rag Shenasi ya Resaleh dar Nabz [Pulsology or treatise on pulse]. In S.M. Meshkal (Ed.) Tehran Selsele Intisharat-e Anjomane Asare Melli:

[89] Pope Innocent III (1199). Vergentis in senium.. March 25, 1199. Letter sent from Innocent to the city Viterbo, Italy.

[90] Magnus, A. (circa 1250 AD, 1891). Alberti Magni opera omnia. Ed, A. Borguet (1891). Paris: 35 Babne.

[91] Kopp, P. (1933). Psychiatrisches bei Albertus Magnus, Beitrage zur psychiatrie der scholaskic I. Aus der Deutschen Forschungsanstalt fur psychiatrie. Kaier Wilhelm Institue, Munchen. Eingegangen am 17, Mai 1933. Zeitschrift fur die gesamte Neurologie und Psychiatrie. Springer.

[92] Aquinas, T. (1274). Summa Theologia. English translation retrieved 12-26-2013 from http://www.basilica.org/pages/ebooks/St.%20Thomas%20Aquinas-Summa%20Theologica.pdf

[93] American Psychiatric Association (2013). Diagnostic and Statistical Manual of Mental Disorders (DSM-5). 5th edition. American Psychiatric Publishing

[94] De Praerogativa Regis 1255-1290. [The Statute of the King's Prerogative] Sections 11 and 12, which deals with mentally ill, "Natural Fools" congenital intellectual subnormal and "non compos mentis" tempory psychiatric d/o and mared lucid intervals.

[95] Roman Law (449 BC). Law of the Twelve Tablets. "…excused children and the insane from crimes, gave guardianship for fools…".

[96] Pope Innocent VIII (1484). Summis desiderantes affectibus. Papal Bull December 9, 1484.

[97] Kramer, H. and Sprenger, J. (1487). Malleus Maleficarum. Approved by the Theology Faculty of the University of Cologne May 9, 1487.

[98] Online Etymology Dictionary. (2013). Lunatic. Retrieved 10-10-2013 from https://www.etymonline.com/word/lunatic

[99] Bethlem Royal Hospital (2018). Bethlem Royal Hospital. History. Retrieved 6-23-2018 from http://www.slam.nhs.uk/about-us/art-and-history/our-history/prior-to-1600

[100] Online Etymology Dictionary (2014). Insane. Retrieved 1-26-2014 from http://www.etymonline.com/index.php?term=insane

[101] The Free Dictionary (2018). Bedlam. Retrieved 6-23-2018 from http://www.thefreedictionary.com/bedlam

[102] Weyer, J. (1563). De praestigiis daemonnum et incantationibus, ac veneficiis. Basel: Johnannes Oporinus.

[103] Paracelsus (1567, 1941) Von den Krankheiten, so die vernufft berauben [On diseases depriving man of his reason, such as St. Vitus' dance, falling sickness, melancholy, and insanity, and their correct treatment. Basel: Adam of Bodenstein; [Four treaties of Theophrastus von Hohenheim allied Paracelsus] (Henry Sigerist Ed and Gregory Zilboog, Trans) Baltimore: John Hopkins University Press.

[104] Willis, T. (1664). Cerebri antome: cul accessit nervorum descriptio et usus. Londini: Typis Flesher, Impernsis Martyn & Allestry apud insigne Campaanae in Coemeterio D. Pauli.

[105] Willis, T. (1666). Cerebri anatome: cul accessit nervorum descriptio et usus. Amstelodame: Gerbrandum Schagen. Retrieved 12-31-2013 from http://books.google.com/books?id=3FKI0ZVLEsAC&pg=PA21&dq=willis,+thomas+Cerebri+anatome&hl=en&sa=X&ei=Xs_CUpHEOJPwkQeEiYCAAQ&ved=0CCwQ6AEwAA#v=onepage&q=willis%2C%20thomas%20Cerebri%20anatome&f=false

[106] Willis, T. (1667). Pathologie cerebri et nervosi generis specimen. In quo agitur de morbis convulsivis, et de scorbuto [An essay of the pathology of the brain and nervous stock: In which convulsive diseases are treated]. Oxford: Guil and Hall, printed for J. Allestry. English translation from Latin into English by Samuel Pordage (1681). London: Dring.

[107] Willis, T. (1670). Affectionum quae dicuntur hystericae et hypochondriacae pathologia spasmodica vindicata. Accesserunt exercitationes medico-physicae duae de sanguinis accensione et de motu musculari. [Spasm of pathology which are called affections hypochondriacae hystericae and she was vindicated. Medico-physical exercises, and of the two came to the movement from blood which ignites muscle movement]. London: Jacob Allestry.

[108] Willis, T. (1671). Affectionum quæ dicuntur hystericæ et hypochondriacæ pathologia spasmodica vindicata, contra responsionem epistolarem Nathanael. Highmori [Spasm of things that are said to have been punished pathology of hysterical and hypochondriac afflections]. Cui accesserunt exercitationes medico-physicae duae. 1. de sanguinis accensione [The blood ignition]; 2, De motu musculari [The muscular movement]. Lugd. Bat., Driehuysen et Lopez.

[109] Willis, T. (1661-1664) Oxford Lecture Series. In Dewhurst, K. (1980). Thomas Willis Oxford Lectures, Oxford: Sandfor Publications.

[110] Willis, T. (1672). De anima brutorum quae hominis vitalis ac sensitiva est, excertitationes duae; prior physiologica ejusdem naturam, partes, potentias et affectiones tradit; altera pathologicca morbos qui ipsam, et sedem ejus primarium, nempe cerebrum et nervosum genus atticiunt, explicat, eorumque therapeias insituit. Oxford: R. Davis. English translation by Samuel Pordage, London, 1683.

[111] Willis, T. (1672). Instructions and precepts for the cure of stupidity or folly. In De Anima Brutorum (Of the Souls of Brutes). In London Practive of Physick, translated by Samuel Pordage. London: Printed for Thomas Basset and William Crooke.

[112] Willis, T. (1683). Two discourses concerning the soul of brutes, which is that of the vital and sensitive man. Translated into English by Samuel Pordage. London: Dring, Harper, and Leight.

[113] Willis, T. (1681). An Essay on the pathology of the brain and nervous stock; in which convulsive diseases are treated. London: T. Dring.

[114] Sydenham, T. (1686). On Saint Vitus'Dance. In Schedula monitoria de novae febris ingressu. Chapter XVI. Londini: Kettiby.

[115] Sydenham, T. (1681-1682). Epistolary Dissertation to Dr. Cole. Presentation copy in the College of Physicians dated March 21.

[116] Sydenham, T. (1693). Processus integri in mobrbis fere omnibus curandis: a do Thoma Sydenham, M.D. conscripti. Quibus accessit graphica symptomatum delineatio. Londini: Impensis Samuel Smith, and Benjami. Walford, ad insignia Principis, and Jason. Knapton, ad insigne Coronaw in Coemeterio D. Pauli.

[117] Lathan, R. (1850). The works of Thomas Sydenham, MD. Translated from Latin edition of Dr. Greenhill with a life of the author by R.G. Latham. In two volumes. London: C. and J. Adlard, printers.

[118] Sydenham, T. (1682). Epistolary dissertation. Letter to William Cole of Worcester, dated January 20, 1681-2.

[119] Swan, J. (1742). The entire works of Dr. Thomas Sydenham, Newly made English from the originals: wherein the history of acute and chronic diseases, and the safest and most effectual methods of treating them, are faithfully, clearly, and accurately delivered. p. 376. London: Edward Cave at St John's Gate.

[120] Massachusetts Archives: Superior Court of Judicature Witch Trials (January – May 1693). Cases Heard. Salem Witch Trials, Documentary Archive and Transcription Project. Retrieved 6-24-2018 from http://salem.lib.virginia.edu/archives/SCJ.xml

[121] Middlesex Sessions. (1713). Vagrancy Act of 1714. Session Papers- Justices' working documents. Section 22. 1st August 1714. Original held at the London Metropolitan Archives. LL ref: LMSMPS501360028.

[122] The Vagrancy Act of 1744. (1744). 17 George II, Chapter 5, Section 20.

[123] An Act for Regulating Madhouses. (1744). 14 George III, Chapter 49.

[124] Norwich HEART-Heritage Economic and Regeneration Trust (circa 1713). Research Centere, Social Innovation, The Bethel Hospital (2015). Retrieved 6-18-2015 www.heritagecity.org/research-centre/social-innovation/the-bethle-hospitla.htm

[125] York Courant (newspaper), 5 September 1772. York, England. LCCN: sn88063447. Retrieved from https://www.loc.gov/item/sn88063447/

[126] Arnold, T. (1782). Observations on the nature, kinds, causes, and prevention of insanity, lunacy, or madness. Vol 1. Containing observations on the nature, and various kinds of insanity. Leicester: Printed by G. Ireland for G. Robinson, in Paternoster Row and T. Cadwell in the Strand, London.

[127] Arnold, T. (1806). Observations on the nature, kinds, causes, and prevention of insanity: In two volumes, Volume II containing observations on the causes and prevention of insanity. 2nd edition corrected and improved. London: Richard Phillips.

[128] Arnold, T. (1809). Observations on the management of the insane, and particularly on the agency and importance of humane and kind treatment in effecting their cure. London: Richard Philips.

[129] Gray, J. (1815). The York Retreat from Jonathan Gray, A history of the York Lunatic asylum with an appendix containing evidence of the cases of abuse lately inquired into by a Committee. Printed by W. Hargrove and Company. Institute of Psychiatry Historical Collection.

[130] Rogers, J. (1815). A statement of the cruelties, abuses and frauds which are practiced in madhouses. London: E. Justins.

[131] Select Committee Inquiry into the State of Madhouses (1815-16). First report: Minutes of Evidence, taken before The Select Committee, appointed to consider of Provision being made for the better Regulation of Madhouses, in England. Ordered by the House of Commons, to be printed 26 April 1816. Retrieved from https://books.google.com/books?id=aiESAAAAYAAJ&dq=private%20madhouse&pg=RA2-PA1#v=onepage&q=private%20madhouse&f=false

[132] The Retreat-York (2018). The Retreat - York. Who we are; about us; History. Retrieved 6-24-2018 from https://www.theretreatyork.org.uk

[133] Parliament of Great Britain (1774). Madhouse Act 1774. 14 George 3 c49.

[134] Viszanik, M. (1845). Die Irren Heil- und Pflegeanstalten Deutschland, Frankreichs, samt der Cretinen-Anstalt auf dem Abendberge in der Schweiz, mit eigenen Bemerkungen. Wien. [The insane healing and nursing homes Germany, France, along with the cretins' institution on the mountains in Switzerland, with my own observations. Vienna].

[135] Gray, J. (1815). A history of the York Lunatic Asylum with an Appendix containing minutes of the evidence of the cases of abuse lately inquired into by the Committee of the House of Commons and addressed to William Wilberforce, Esquire. York: W. Hargrove and Company.

[136] Great Britain, Parliament House of Commons, Committee on Mad-Houses in England. (1816). The First annual report on madhouses, made in the year 1816, ordered by the House of Commons to be printed April 26, 1816: Singular and shocking details, consisting of the important minutes of evidence, two letters, and appendix. London: W. J. Clement. Retrieved 1-3-2014 from https://archive.org/details/39002086342426.med.yale.edu

[137] Franklin, B. (1751). Some accounts of the Pennsylvania Hospital; From its first rise, to the beginning of the fifth month, called May, 1754. Philadelphia: Printed by B. Franklin and D. Hall. Printed in facsimile, with an introduction by I. Bernard Cohen. Baltimore: John Hopkins Press.

[138] Morton, T. (1895). The history of the Pennsylvania Hospital, 1751-1895. Philadelphia: Times Printing House.

[139] Journal of the House of Burgesses of Virginia, Session of November 20, 1766. In JHBV 1766-69, p33.

[140] Journal of the House of Burgesses of Virginia, 1766-1769, p259.

[141] Galt, J. (1846). The treatment of insanity. New York: Harper and Brothers. Retrieved 1-20-2014 from https://archive.org/stream/treatmentofinsan00galtuoft#page/n5/mode/2up

[142] Battie, W. (1758). A treatise on Madness. London: Printed for J. Whiston and B. White in Fleet Street Retrieved 1-1-2014 from http://books.google.com/books?id=F6JbAAAAQAAJ&pg=PA1&source=gbs_toc_r&cad=4#v=onepage&q&f=false

[143] Monro, J. (1758). Remarks on Dr. Battie's Treatise on Madness. London: Printed for John Clarke Retrieved 1-10-2014 from
http://books.google.com/books?id=KYSLJIb6W8IC&printsec=frontcover&dq=Remarks+on+Dr.+Battie's+Treatise+of+Madness&hl=en&sa=X&ei=WP_PUr-9NLHnsATDpoDQBg&ved=0CDAQ6AEwAA#v=onepage&q=Remarks%20on%20Dr.%20Battie's%20Treatise%20of%20Madness&f=false

[144] Cullen, W. (1769). Synopsis nosologiae methodicae. Edinburgh. English translation, N. Palten (1792). Synopsis and nosology. Hartford, Connecticut. N. Palten.

[145] Cullen, W. (1786). Kurzer Inbegriff der Medizinischen Nosologie: Oder Systematische Einteilung der Krankheiten von Cullen, Pinne, Sauvages, Vogel und Saga, after 3rd ed, 2 vols, Leipzig.

[146] Arnold, T. (1787). Observations on the nature, kinds, causes, and prevention of insanity, lunacy, or madness. Volume I. Leicester: Printed by G. Ireland for G. Robinson, in Paternoster Row, and T. Cadell, in the Strand, London. Retrieved 1-10-2014 from
http://books.google.com/books?id=lOgVD2rMFgsC&printsec=frontcover&dq=inauthor:%22Thomas+Arnold%22&hl=en&sa=X&ei=LhbQUsajL6XMsQTZ64CICg&ved=0CEEQ6AEwAw#v=onepage&q&f=false

[147] Arnold, T. (1806). Observations on the nature, kinds, causes, and prevention, of insanity. Volume II. London: Printed for Richard Phillips, Bridge Street, Blackfriars. Retrieved 1-10-2014 from
http://books.google.com/books?id=LoIUAAAAQAAJ&pg=PA11&source=gbs_toc_r&cad=4#v=onepage&q=imagines%20he%20sees&f=false

[148] Arnold, T. (1809). Observations on the management of the insane and particularly on the agency and importance of humane and kind treatment in effecting their cure. London: Phillips.

[149] Harper, A. (1789). A treatise on the real cause and cure of insanity in which the nature and distinction of this disease are fully explained and the treatments established on new principles. London: Printed for C. Stalker, Stationers Court, Ludgate Street and J. Walter, Opposite Bond Street, Piccadilly. Retrieved 1-10-2014 from
http://books.google.com/books?id=lntZAAAAcAAJ&printsec=frontcover&dq=inauthor:%22Andrew+Harper%22&hl=en&sa=X&ei=xCrQUsryMovJsATD94DwCw&ved=0CEEQ6AEwAw#v=onepage&q&f=false

[150] Haslem, J. (1798). Observations on insanity, with practical remarks on the disease, and account of the morbid appearances on dissection. Printed for F. and C. Rivington, No 62, St Paul's Church-Yard: London. Retrieved from
https://archive.org/stream/observationsonin00hasl#page/10/mode/2up

[151] Pargeter, W. (1792). Observations on maniacal disorders. Murray, London.

[152] Crichton, A. (1798a). An inquiry into the nature and origin of mental derangement. Comprehending a concise system of the physiology and pathology of the human mind and a history of the passions and their effects. Volume I. Printed for T. Cadwell, Junior, and W. Davies, in the Strand. London Retrieved 1-15-2014 from
http://books.google.com/books?id=XlRJAAAAYAAJ&pg=PP7&source=gbs_selected_pages&cad=3#v=onepage&q&f=false

[153] Chichton, A. (1798b). An inquiry into the nature and origin of mental derangement. Comprehending a concise system of the physiology and pathology of the human mind and a history of the passions and their effects. Volume II. Printed for T. Cadwell, Junior, and W. Davies, in the Strand. London. Retrieved 1-19-2014 from
http://books.google.com/books?id=xHVJAAAAYAAJ&printsec=frontcover&dq=inauthor:%22Sir+Alexander+Crichton%22&hl=en&sa=X&ei=--XbUqPiF-ahsQSQ5YCIDw&ved=0CC0Q6AEwAA#v=onepage&q&f=false

[154] Journal of Empirical Psychology (1783-1793). Edited by K. Moritz, K. Pockels, S. Maimon. Table of contents and full text articles. Berlin. Retrieved 1-19-2014 from http://www.ub.uni-bielefeld.de/diglib/aufkl/magerfahrgsseelenkd/index.htm

[155] Pussin, J. and Pinel, P. (1800). Observations du citoyen Pussin sur les fous. Written by J. Pussin and transmitted by Pinel to the Miniser of Internal Affairs. Manuscript in Archives Nationales, Paris, 27 AP 8 (doc2). [Observations of citizen Pussin on the Insane]. English translation by D.B. Weiner (1979). The apprenticeship of Philippe Pinel: A new document, "observations of Citizen Pussin on the Insane". American Journal of Psychiatry 136:1128-1134.

[156] Pinel, P. (1798). Nosographie philosophique ou méthode de l'analyse appliquee a la médecine. [Philosophical Classification of Diseases]. Paris.

[157] Pinel, P. (1801). Traite medico-philosphique sur l'aleniation mentale ou la manie. Paris: Richard, Caille and Ravier, an IX, (1801). A Treatise on Insanity. Translated from French by D. D. Davis. New York: Published under the Auspices of the Library of the New York Academy of Medicine by Hafner Publishing Co., 1962.

[158] Pinel, P. (1806). A treatise on insanity. Translation by D. D. Davis, facsimile reprint of 1806 edition, New York, Haftner, 1962, p 1iv-v.

[159] Reil, J. (1796a). Archiv fur die physiologie. Halle, in der curtschen buchnandlung. Vol. 1. Halle, Germany.

[160] Reil, J. (1796b). Von der Lebebskraft. [On the vital force]. Archiv fur die Physiologie, 1: 8-162. Halle, Germany.

[161] Reil, J. (1802). Fieberhafte Nervenkrankheiten [Feverish nervous illness]. Vol 4. In Ueber die Erkenntniss und cur der fieber, 5 vols. (1799-1815). Halle: Curtschen Buchhandlung.

[162] Reil J. (1803). Rhapsodieen über die Anwendung der psychischen Curmethode auf Geisteszerrüttungen. [Reflections on the application of psychic (psychological) methods of cure in mental disorders]. Halle: Curtschen Buchhandlung.

[163] Reil, J. (1807-1808). Fragmente uber die bildung des kleinen gehirms im menschen. Archi fur die Physiologie, Halle an der Saale. 8:1-58, 273-304, 385-426.

[164] Reil, J. and Hoffbauer, J. (1812). Beytrage zur beforderung einer kurmethode auf psychischem wege. [Contributions to the advancement of a psychiatric treatment method]. Erster band. Halle.

[165] Reil, J. and Kayssler, A. (1805). Magazin dur die psychische heilkunde. Berlin: Reil und Kayssler.

[166] Reil, J. and Hoffbauer, J. (1808). Ueber den Begriff der Medicin und ihre Verweigungen, besonders in Beziehung auf die Berichtigung der Topik der Psychiaterie. Beyträge zur Beförderung einer Kurmethode auf psychischem Wege. [Contributions to the Advancement of Psychiatric Treatment Method]. 161-279. Curtsche Buchhandlung.

[167] Reil, J. (1796). Exercitationum anatomicarum fascicles primus. De structura nervorum. In Anatomical Practice: On the structure of nerves. Vol. 1. Halle: Venalis.

[168] Reil, J. (1809). Die Sylvische grube oder das thal, das gestreifte gorsse hirnganglium, dessen kapsel und die seitentheile des grossen gehirns. Archiv. fur die Physiologie., 9:195-208.

[169] Gray, H. (1858). Gray's Anatomy. London: J.W. Parker and Sons.

[170] Gall, F. (1798). Schreiben uber seinen bereits geendigten Prodromus über die Verichtungen des Gehirns der Menschen und der Thiere an Herrn Jos. Fr. von Retzer. [Letter from Dr. F.J. Gall to Joseph Freiherr von Retzer, upon the functions of the brain in man and animals]. Der neue Teutsche Merkur, [The new German Mercery], 3, Dec 311-332.

[171] Gall, F. (1807a). Doktor Gall uber irrenanstalten. Allgemeine Zeitung, Ulm 10, No 21, Supplement 81-83. Beilage.

[172] Gall, F. (1807b). Beantwortung der Ackermann'schen Beurtheilung und Wiederlegung der Gall'schen Hirn-Schedel- und Organenlehre, vom Gesichtspuncte der Erfahrung aus. Von einigen Schülern des Dr. Gall und von ihm selbst berichtigt. Halle.

[173] Spurzheim, J. (1817). Observations on the deranged manifestations of the mind, or insanity. London: Baldwin, Cradock, and Joy.

[174] Gall, F. (1825). Sur les fonctions du cerveau et sur celles de chacune de ses parties, avec des observations sur la possibilité de reconnoitre les instincts, les penchans, les talens, ou les dispositions morales et intellectuelles des hommes et des animaux, par la configuration de leur cerveau et de leur tête. 6 volumes. Paris: J. B. Ballière.

[175] Gall, F. (1835). On the Functions of the Brain and of Each of Its parts: With Observations on the Possibility of Determining the Instincts, Propensities, and Talents, Or the Moral and Intellectual Dispositions of Men and Animals, by the Configuration of the Brain and Head. Six volumes. Boston: Marsh, Capen & Lyon.

[176] Forster, T. (1815). Observations on a new system of phrenology, or the anatomy and physiology of the brain, of Drs. Gall and Spurzheim. Philosophical Magazine, 45.

[177] Gall, F. (1801). Lehre über die Verrichtungen des Hirns, und über die Möglichkeit, die Anlagen mehrerer Geistes und Gemuthseigenschaften aus dem Bau des Kopfes, und des Schedels des Menschen und der Thiere zu erkennen [Doctrine of the Functions of the Brain, and the possibility of recognizing the tendency of several properties of mind from the structure of the heads and skulls of humans and animals]. Unpublished work.

[178] Franz II, Holy Roman Emperor. (1801). Decree issued December.

[179] Rush, B. (1812). Medical Inquires and observations, upon the diseases of the mind. Philadelphia: Kimber and Richardson, no 237 Market Street; Merritt, printer, no 9, Watkins Alley. Retrieved 1-21-2014 from http://deila.dickinson.edu/cdm/pageflip/collection/ownwords/id/20236/type/compoundobject/show/18168/cpdtype/monograph/pftype/image#page/1/mode/2up

[180] Rush, B. (1823). An Inquiry into the effects of ardent spirits on the human mind and body: with an account of the means of prevention and the remedies for curing them. 8th edition. Boston: James Loring. Retrieved 2-2-2014 from http://books.google.com/books?id=-6UoAAAAYAAJ&pg=PA1&source=gbs_selected_pages&cad=3#v=onepage&q&f=false

[181] Jefferson, T., Adam, J., Franklin, B., et. al. (1776). Declaration of Independence. Continental Congress. Philadelphia, July 4, 1776. Retrieved 2-1-2014 from http://www.archives.gov/exhibits/charters/declaration_transcript.html

[182] American Medico-Psychological Association. (1895). Semi-Centennial Proceedings of the American Medico-Psychological Association at the Fiftieth Annual Meeting held in Philadelphia, May 15-18, 1894. Utica, New York: American Medico-Psychological Association.

[183] Ozarin, L. (1998). The Official Seal of APA. History Notes. Psychiatric News. Retrieved 2-3-2014 from http://www.psychiatricnews.org/pnews/98-04-17/hx.html

[184] Sutton, T. (1813). Tracts on delirium tremens, on peritonitis and on some other internal inflammatory affections and on the gout. London: Printed by James Moyes, Greville Street for Thomas Underwood, Fleet Street. Retrieved 1-21-2014 from https://archive.org/stream/tractsondelirium00sutt#page/76/mode/2up

[185] Report of Committee for better Regulation of Madhouses, London, Baldwin, Cradock, and Joy. 1815. Great Britain, Parliament House of Commons, Committee on Mad-Houses in England. (1816). The First annual report on madhouses, made in the year 1816, ordered by the House of Commons to be printed April 26, 1816: Singular and Shocking Details, consisting of the important minutes of evidence, two letters, and appendix. London: W. J. Clement. Retrieved 1-3-2014 from https://archive.org/details/39002086342426.med.yale.edu

[186] Haslam, J. (1817). Consideration on the moral management of insane persons, London.

[187] Heinroth, J. (1823). Lehrbuch der seelen gesundheitskunde: zum behuf academischer vortrage und zum privatstudium. Theorie un lehre von der leibespflege [Textbook of the souls of healthy clients: for the purpose of academic lectures and private study. Theory and teaching of the care of the physical body] Leipzig: Vogel.

[188] Heinroth, J. (1825). Anweisung fur angehende Irrenärzte sur richtigen Behandlung ihrer kranken. [Instructions for the psychiatrist in training and proper treatments for their sick]. Leipzig: Vogel.

[189] Heinroth, J. (1818). Textbook of disturbances on mental life or disturbances of the soul and their treatment. Translated by J. Schmorak. 2 volumes (1975). John Hopkins Press.

[190] Heinroth, J. (1818). Lehrbuch der storungen des Seelenlebens oder der seelen-storungen und threr Behandlung. [Textbook of disturbances of mental life or disturbances of the soul and their treatment]. Leipzig: Vogel.

[191] Esquirol, E. (1805). Des passions considerees comme causes, symptômes et moyens de traitement de l'alienation mentale; These presented et soutenue a l'Escole de Medicine de Paris. Doctoral thesis.

[192] Esquirol, E. (1814). Dictionnaire des sciences médicales, par une société de médecins et de chirurgiens. Paris: Panckoucke.

[193] Esquirol, E. (1817). Hallucination. In Adelon et al (Eds). Dictionarie des Sciences Medicales par une socitete de medcins et de chirurgiens. Vol XX. Paris: Panckoucke.

[194] Esquirol, E. (1838). Des maladies mentales: considerees sous les rapports medical, hygiénique, et medico-legal Vol. 1 and 2. Bruxelles: Libraire Medicale et Scientifique de J.B. Tircher. Paris: Chez-Bailliere.

[195] Esquirol, E. (1845). Mental maladies, treatise on insanity. Translation into English by E.K. Hunt. Philadelphia: Lea and Blanchard. Retrieved 1-21-2014 from https://archive.org/stream/mentalmaladiestr00esqu#page/n7/mode/2up

[196] Dix, D. (1843). Memorial to the Legislature of Massachusetts 1843. Retrieved 1-22-2014 from https://archive.org/stream/memorialtolegisl00dixd#page/n3/mode/2up

[197] Royal College of Psychiatrist. (2018). College history and archives. Retrieved 6-24-2018 from http://www.rcpsych.ac.uk/usefulresources/thecollegearchives.aspx

[198] British Journal of Psychiatry (2018). Archive of All Online Issues, October 1855 - present. Retrieved 6-24-2018 from http://bjp.rcpsych.org/content/by/year

[199] Association of Medical Superintendents of American Institutions for the Insane. (1844). American Psychiatric Association, History. Retrieved 1-22-2014 from http://www.psychiatry.org/about-apa--psychiatry/more-about-apa/history-of-the-apa

[200] The American Journal of Insanity. (1844). The American Journal of Insanity. The Officers of the New York State Lunatic Asylum, Utica (Eds.). Vol 1. Utica: Bennett, Backus, & Hawley.

[201] Morel, B. (1845-1846). Pathologies mentale in Belgique, en Hollande et en Allemagne. Annals medico-psychologiques. Paris.

[202] Morel, B. (1860). Le no-restraint ou de l'abolition des moyens coercitifs dans le traitement de la folie suivi de considerations sur les causes de la progression dans le nombre des alienes admis dans les asiles. [Non-restraint and the abolition of coercive means in the treatment of insanity: Followed by considerations on the causes of the increase in the number of insane asylums]. Paris: Victor Masson et Fils. Retrieved 2-6-2014 from http://books.google.com/books?id=IYBaAAAAcAAJ&pg=PA34&lpg=PA34&dq=Le+no-restraint+ou+de+l'abolition+des+moyes+coercitifs+dans+le+traitement+de+la+folie.&source=bl&ots=SuPOf7ptE2&sig=aN780eKR7jfzk3OV9mTS7j1bFGg&hl=en&sa=X&ei=797zUp-CPMXokQeX_YGoBQ&ved=0CEIQ6AEwAw#v=onepage&q=morel&f=false

[203] Morel, B.(1857). Traite des degenerescences physiques, intellectuelles et morales de l'espece humaine. Vol 1. with Atlas. Paris: Bailliere.

[204] Maudsley, H. (1867). The physiology and pathology of the mind.New York: D. Appleton and Company. Retrieved 1-23-2014 from https://archive.org/stream/physiologyandpa03maudgoog#page/n8/mode/2up

[205] Morel, B. (1852-53). Traite des maladies mentales. 2 vols. volumes. Paris: J. B. Balliere.

[206] Morel, B. (1857). Traite des degenerescences physiques, intellectuelles et morales de l'espèce humaine.: et des causes qui produisent ces variétés maladives. Paris: J.B. Balliere. Retrieved 1-23-2014 from http://books.google.com/books?id=dD36WlUtypUC&printsec=frontcover&dq=morel+traite+des+degenerescences&hl=en&sa=X&ei=V0DhUom4EaXMsQSvxYKwCQ&ved=0CCoQ6AEwAA#v=snippet&q=demence%20precoce&f=false

[207] Kraepelin, E. (1893). Psychiatrie: En lehrbuch fur studirende und aerzte. 4th edition. Leipzig: Barth.

[208] Bleuler, E. (1908). Die Prognose der dementia praecox (Schizophreniengruppe). Allgemeine Zeitschrift fur Psychiatrie un psychischgerichtliche Medizin. 65:436-464.

[209] Bleuler, E. (1911). Dementia Pracecox or the Group of Schizophrenias. Translated by J. Zinkin. New York: International Universities Press (1950).

[210] Morel, B. (1860). Traites des maladies mentales. 2 vols, Paris (1852-1853), 2nd ed..

[211] Statistical Manual of Mental American Psychiatric Association (2013). Diagnostic and Disorders. 5th edition. (DSM-5). Washington, D.C.: American Psychiatric Publishing.

[212] Kraepelin, E. (1883). Compendium der Psychiatrie. Vol 1. Leipzig: A. Abel.

[213] Kraepelin, E. (1899). Psychiatrie: Enin lehrbuch fur studierende und artze. 6th edition. Leipzig: A. Able.

[214] Kraepelin, E. (1883c). Ueber die Einwirkung einiger medicamentoser Stoffe auf Dauer einfacher psychischer Vorgange. Wilhelm Wundt (Hg.): Phiolosophische Studien, [As to the influence of some medicated substances to the duration of simple mental processes. Wilhelm Wundt (ed): Philosophical Studies, Vol 1, 417-462, 573-605.

[215] Kraepelin, E. (1886e).Schlaflosigkeit und deren Behandlung durch die neueren Schlafmittel. Jahresberichte der Gesellschaft für Natur- und Heilkunde in Dresden [Insomnia and their treatments by the newer sleeping pills. Annual reports of the Society for Nature and Medicine in Dresden]. 153-155.

[216] Kraeplelin, E. (1903d). Uber Ermundungsmessungen. Archiv fur die gesamte Pschologie. [About fatigue measurements. Archive for the whole of psychology], 1: 9-30.

[217] Kraepelin, E. (1904b). Psychiatrisches aus Java.[Psychiatry from Java]. Allgemeine Zeitschrift fur Psychiatrie und Psychischgerichtliche Medizin, 61:882-4.

[218] Kraepelin, E. (1904c). Vergleichende Psychiatrie. Centralblatt fur Nervenheilkunde und Psychiatrie, [Comparative Psychiatry. Central Journal of Neurology and Psychiatry]. Vol 27, New Series Vol.15, 433-7.

[219] Kraepelin, E. (1904g). Psychiatrisches aus Java. Centralblatt fur Nervheilkunde und Psychiatrie [Psychiatitry from Java. Central Journal of Neurology and Psychiatry], vol 27, New Series vol 15:468-469.

[220] Kraepelin, E. (1907e). Alkoholische Geistesstörungen. Jahresbericht uber die Königliche Psychiatrische Klinik in München für 1904 und 1905. Alcoholic mental disorders. Annual Report on the Royal Psychiatric Clinic in Munich for 1904 and 1905. 22-28. Munich: Lehmann Verlag.

[221] Kraepelin, E. (1909). Psychiatrie. Ein Lehrbuch für Studierende und Ärzte. Achte, vollständig umgearbeitete Auflage. I. Band. Allgemeine Psychiatrie. Leipzig: Barth Verlag 8th completely revised edition.

[222] Alzheimer, A. (1906). Ueber einen eigenartigen, schweren erkrankungsprozess der hirnrinde. 37th Tagung der Suedwestdeutschen Irrenaerzte. [Study on a particular, serious disease process of the cerebral cortex. 37th Conference of the South-West German Psychiatrist].

[223] Kraepelin, E. (1910a). Psychiatrie. Ein Lehrbuch für Studierende und Ärzte. Achte, vollständig umgearbeitete Auflage. II. Band. Klinische Psychiatrie. I. Teil. Barth Verlag, Leipzig 1909.

[224] Wundt, W. (1874). Grundzuge der physiologischen psychologie, 2 volumes. [Principles of Physiological Psychology]. Leipzig: W. Engelmann.

[225] Wundt, W. (1896). Grundriss der Psychologie [Outlines of Psychology]. Leipzig: W. Engelmann. Translated by Charles Judd (1897).

[226] Titchener, E. and Grissler, L. (1908). A bibliography of the Scientific Writings of Wilhelm Wundt (October 1, 1908). Retrieved 2-9-2014 from https://archive.org/details/jstor-1413398

[227] Cattell, J. (1886). The time it takes to see and name objects. Mind, 11:63-65.

[228] Cattell, J. (1890). Mental tests and measurements. Mind, 15:373-381.

[229] Cattell, J. (1895). Measurements of the accuracy of recollection. Science, 2,761-766.

[230] Cattell, J. (1913). University control. New York: The Science Press. Retrieved 1-23-2014 from https://archive.org/stream/universitycontr00cattgoog#page/n8/mode/2up

[231] American Association Advancement of Sciences (AAAS). (2015). 150 years of advancing science: A history of AAAS origins: 1848-1899. AAAS Archives and Records Center. Retrieved 6-15-2015. http://archives.aaas.org/exhibit/origins4.php.

[232] Psychological Review. (1894). Volume 1. J. Cattell and J. Baldwin (Eds). New York: Macmillan and Company. Retrieved from https://babel.hathitrust.org/cgi/pt?id=uc1.b4270585;view=1up;seq=7

[233] Psychology Review. (2014). Psychology Review. An official journal publication of the American Psychological Association. Description. Retrieved 2-10-2014 from http://www.apa.org/pubs/journals/rev/index.aspx

[234] Achilles, P. (1937). The role of the Psychological Corporation in applied psychology. The American Journal of Psychology, 50(1-4) Golden Jubilee Volume 1887-1937. Nov., 229-247.

[235] Cattell, J. (1923). The Psychological Corporation. Annals of the American Academy of Political and Social Science. Vol 110. Psychology in Business. Nov. 1923. p165. Retrieved from https://www.jstor.org/stable/1015081?seq=1#page_scan_tab_contents

[236] American Psychological Association (1894). American Psychological Association Constitution, Article 1, Objectives. Adopted by the APA membership 1894.

[237] American Psychological Association (2018). American Psychological Association - About APA. Retrieved 6-24-2018 from http://www.apa.org/about/

[238] Mobius, P. (1892). Uber die einteilung der krankheiten. Centralblatt fur die gesamte neurologie in wissenschaft und praxis mit besonderer beriicksichtgung der degenerations-anthropologie, 15:289-301.

[239] Mobius, P. (1893). Abriss der lehre von den Nervenkrankheiten. [Demolition of the doctrine of the nervous system].Leipzig: Abel.

[240] Kraepelin, E. (1896). Psychiatrie. 5th edition. Leipzig: Barth.

[241] Jasper, K. (1913). Allgemeine Psychopathologie.Ein leitfaden fur Studierende Artze und pscyhologen. 1st edition. Berlin: Julius Springer.

[242] Aschaffenburg, G. (1915). Die Einteilung der pschosen. Leipzig: Franz Deuticke.

[243] Mobius, P. (1903). Beitrage zur lehre von den geschlechtsuntersxchieden [Contributipons to the theory of gender differences]. Halle: Carl Marhold.

[244] Mobius, P. (1900). Uber den physiologischen schwachsinn des weibes [About the physiological idiocy of the woman]/Halle: Carl Marhold. Retrieved 2-11-2014 from https://archive.org/details/ueberdenphysiolo00mb2

[245] Breuer, J. and Freud, S. (1895d). Studies on hysteria. Translated from the German and edited by James Strachey in collaboration with Anna Freud. New York: Basic Books. Retrieved 1-24-2014 from https://archive.org/stream/studiesonhysteri037649mbp#page/n115/mode/2up

[246] Breuer, J. and Freud, S. (1893). On the psychical mechanism of hysterical phenomena: A preliminary communication. In Strachey, J. translated edition (1955), The Standard Edition of the Complete Psychological Works of Sigmund Freud, Vol 3. 53-59. London: Hogarth Press.

[247] Magnan, V. and Legrain, M. (1895). Les degenere: etat mental et syndromes espisodiques. Paris: Rueff et Cie.

[248] Charcot. J. (1889). Lectures on the diseases of the nervous system. Vol 128 of the New Sydenham Society. New Sydenham Society Publisher.

[249] Breuer, J. (1868). Die selbstseuerung der athmung durch den nervus vagus. Sitzungsberichte der kaiserlichen Akademe der Wissenschaften. Mathematisch naturwissenschaftliche classes, Wien. 58 Band II, Abtheilung: 909-937 [The self-control of respiration through the vagus nerve. Proceedings of the Imperial Academy of Sciences. Mathematics and Natural Sciences Classe, Vienna. 58 band II, Division. 909-937.].

[250] Breuer, J. (1873). Uber bogengange des labyrinths. In: Allg. Wein. Med. Ztg., 18, S. 598, 606.

[251] Breuer, J. (1875). Hering-Breuer reflex. Ueber die function der bogengange des ohrenllabyrinths. Medizinische Jahrbucher, Wein, 2nd series, 4:72-124. [Hering-Breuer reflex. As to the function of the semicircular canals of the ear labyrinth.].

[252] Breuer, J. (1875). Beitrage zur lehre vom statischen sinne (gleichgewichtsorgan, vestibularapparat des ohrenlabyrinths). Medizinische Jahrbucher, 2nd series, 65:87-156. [Contributions to the theory of the static sense (organ of balance, vestibular apparatus of the ear labyrinth].

[253] All Nobel Prizes in Physiology or Medicine, Nobelprize.org, Nobel Medcia AB 2014. Web 14 Jun 2015. Retrieved 6-15-2015. http://www.nobelprize.org/nobel_prizes/medicine/laureates/.

[254] Breuer, J. and Freud, S. (1895a). Studien en Hysterie. Leipzig und Wien: Franz Deuticke. Translation by A. Brill (1937). Nervous and mental disease monograph series no. 61. New York: Nervous and Mental Disease Publishing.

[255] Freud, S. (1895b). Uber die Berechtigung, von der Neurasthenie einen bestimmten symptomenkomplex als "Angstneurose" abzutrennen. In Gesammelte.Schriften (12 volumes), Vienna.1:306. [On the Grounds for detaching a particular syndrome from neuroasthenia under the description of "Anxiety Neurosis"]. Standard edition 3:85-117. London: Hogarth.

[256] Freud, S. (1895f). Zur Kritik der "Angstneurose", Gesammeleete Schriften (12 vols). 1, 343. Vienna. [A reply to criticisms of my paper on Anxiety Neurosis. Collected Papers (5 vols) 1, 107. London.]

[257] Freud, S. (1894a). Die abwehr-neuropsychosen. Gesammeleete Schriften (12 vols) 1,290, Vienna; Gesammelte Werks, (18 vols.) 1:59. London. [The neuro-psychoses of defense.] Collected Papers, (5 vols.), 1:59. London: Hogarth.

[258] Freud, S. (1896b). Weitere bemerkungen uber die abwehr-neuropsychosen. Gesammelte Schriften (12 vols), 1,363, Vienna; Gesammelte Werke (18 vols 1,379. London. [Heredity and the Aetiology of the Neuroses.].

[259] Freud, S. (1900). Die Traumdeutung. [The Interpretation of Dreams.]. Translated by James Strachey. London: Hogarth Press.

[260] Freud, S. (1915c). The Unconscious. Standard Edition, 14:178. London: Hogarth.

[261] Freud, S. (1920g). Beyond the pleasure principle. Standard Edition, 18:7-64. London: Hagarth.

[262] Freud, S. (1905). Drei Abhandiungen zur sexualtheorie. [Three essays on the theory of sexuality]. Studienausgabe, Bd. III. Frankfurt: Fischer.

[263] Freud, S. (1923b). The Ego and the Id. Translated by James Strachey. Standard Edition, 19:12-66. London: Hogarth Press.

[264] Freud, S. (1915d) Repression. Standard Edition, 14:141. London: Hogarth.

[265] Freud, A. (1936). The Ego and the Mechanisms of Defense. New York: International Universities Press.

[266] International Psychoanalytical Association. (2018). History of the International Psychoanalytical Association. Retrieved 6-26-2018 from http://www.ipa.world/en/De/IPA1/ipa_history/history_of_the_ipa.aspx

[267] Vienna Psychoanalytic Society. (1908,1962). Minutes of the Vienna Psychoanalytic Society, Vol 1, 1906-1908. Herman Nunberg & Ernst Federn (Eds.). New York: International Universities Press.

[268] Jung, C. G. (1912). Psychology of the unconscious: a study of the transformations and symbolisms of the libido, a contribution to the history of the evolution of thought. Translated Hinkle, B. M. (1916), London: Kegan, Paul, Trench, and Trubner.

[269] Jung, C. (1916). Analytical Psychology. Editor Constance Ellen Long. Moffat, Yard.

[270] Jung, C. (1917). Collected papers on Analytical Psychology. Translation by Constance Long. 2nd edition. New York: Moffat Yard and Company.

[271] Jung, C. and Baynes, H. (1921). Psychological Types or the Psychology of Individuation. London: Kegan Paul Trench Trubner.

[272] Adler, A. (1907,1917). Study of organ inferiority and its psychical compensation: A contribution to clinical medicine. Translation by Smith Ely Jelliffe. New York: The Nervous and Mental Disease Publishing Company.

[273] Adler, A., Glueck, B., and Lind, J. (1921). The Neurotic Constitution. Translated by Bernard Glueck and John Lind. Kegan, Paul, and Company.

[274] Adler. A. (1913a). Nervenkrankheiten: individual-psychologische Behandlung der Neurosen [Nervous diseases: Individual psychological treatment of neuroses]. Munich: Lehmann.

[275] Adler, A. (1912a). Uber den nervosen Charakter: Grundzuge einer vergleichenden Individual Psychologie und Psychotherapie. [The nervous character: Outline of comparative Individual Psychology and psychotherapy]/ Weisbaden Germany: J. F. Bergman.

[276] Adler, A. (1907). Studie uber Minderwertigkeit von Organen. Vienna: Urban and Schwarzenberg.

[277] Adler, A. (1908). Der aggressionstrieb im leben und in der neurose. [The aggressive drive in life and neurosis]. Germany: Fortschritte des Medizin., 26:577-584.

[278] Adler, A. (1928). Characteristics of the first, second, third child. Children, the Magazine for Parents, 3(5):14-52.

[279] Pavlov, I. (1903). The experimental psychology and psychopathology of animals. Paper presented to the 14th International Medical Congress. Madrid, Spain.

[280] Pavlov, I (1927). A physiological study of the types of the nervous systems, i.e. of temperaments.. Paper presented to the the Pirogov Surgical Society, December 1927.

[281] Pavlov, I. (1928). How psychiatry may help us to understand the physiology of the cerebral hemispheres. In Lectures on conditioned reflexes: Twenty five years of objective study of the higher nervous activity (behavior) of animals. Translated by W. Horsley. New York: Liverwright Publishing Company.

[282] Pavlov, I. (1906). The scientific investigation of the physical facilities or processes in the higher animals. Science 16, November, 24(620):613-619.

[283] Pavlov, I. (1927). Conditioned reflexes: An investigation of the physiological activity of the cerebral cortex. Translated by G. V. Anrep. London: Oxford University.

[284] The Nobel Prize in Physiology or Medicine 1904. (2014). The Nobel Prize in Physiology or Medicine 1904. Retrieved from www.nobelprize.org July 25, 2014.

[285] Pavlov, I. (1903). The experimental psychology and psychopathology of Animals. Paper presented to the 14th International Medical Congress in Madrid.

[286] Nomination Database - Physiology or Medicine. Nobelprize.org. Nobel Media. Retrieved July 25, 2014.

[287] Watson, J. (1913). Psychology as the Behaviorist Views it. Psychological Review, 20:158-177.

[288] Watson, J. B. (1916). Behavior and the concept of mental disease. Journal of Philosophy 13:589-597.

[289] Watson, J. (1919). Psychology from the standpoint of a behaviorist, Philadelphia: Lippincott.

[290] Watson, J. (1924). Behaviorism. p82. New York: Norton.

[291] Watson, J. and Rayner, R. (1920). Conditioned emotional reactions. Journal of Experimental Psychology, 3(1): 1-14.

[292] Beck, H. P., Levinson, S., & Irons, G. (2009). Finding Little Albert: A journey to John B. Watson's infant laboratory. American Psychologist, 605-614.

[293] Rogers, C. (1951) Client-centered therapy. Boston: Houghton Mifflin.

[294] Rogers, C. (1952). Client centered psychotherapy. Scientific American, 187:1-7.

[295] Rogers, C. (1959). A theory of therapy, personality, and interpersonal relationships: As developed in the Client-centered framework. In Psychology, A study of science. Vol. III. Formulations of the person and the social content. Ed. Sigmund Koch. New York: McGraw Hill.

[296] Rogers, C. (1946). Significant aspects of client-centered therapy. American Psychologist, 1:415-422.

[297] Maslow, A. (1943). A theory of human motivation. Psychology Review 50(4):370-396.

[298] Galton, F. (1883). Inquiries into human faculties and its development. London: Macmillan.

[299] Pearson, K. (1924). The life, letters and labours of Francis Galton. Volume II, Researches of middle life. London: Oxford University Press.

[300] Cattell, J. (1890). Mental tests and measurements. Mind, 15: 393, July.

[301] Pearson, K. (1902). On the systematic fitting of curves to observation and measurements. Biometrika, 1(3):265-303.

[302] Wissler, C. (1901). The correlation of mental and physical tests. Doctoral Dissertation, Department of Psychology, Columbia University. New York: Macmillan Company.

[303] Binet, A., & Henri, V. (1896). La psychologie individuelle [Individual psychology].L'Annee Psychologique, 2:411-465.

[304] Simon, T. (1900a). Documents relatifs a la correlation entre le developement physique et la capacite intellectuelle. Paris: G. Carre & C. Naud.

[305] Simon, T. (1900b). Recherches antropometriques sur 223 garcons anormaux ages de 8 a 23 ans. L'Annee Psychologique, 6:191-247.

[306] Binet, A., & Simon, T. (1905). Methodes nouvelles pour le diagnostic des états inférieures de l'intelligence. L'Annee Psychologique, 11:161–190.

[307] Binet, A. and Simon, T. (1908). The development of intelligence in the child. In H.H. Goddard (ed.) Development of intelligence in children (the Binet-Simon scales). Translated by E.S. Kite (1916), 182-272. Baltimore: Williams and Williams.

[308] Binet, A. and Simon, T. (1911). Nouvelle recherches sur la mesure du niveau intellectual chez les enfants d'ecole. L'annee Psychologique, 17(17):145-201.

[309] Terman, L. (1916). The measurement of intelligence: An explanation of and a complete guide for the use of the Stanford revision and extension of the Binet-Simon Intelligence Scales. Boston: Houghton Mifflin Company.

[310] Stern, William (1912). Psychologische methoden der intelligenczprufung. Paper presented at the Fifth Conference of the Society of Experimental Psychology, April 16-20, 1912. Berlin. Published as Die psycholgischen methoden der intelligenzprufing und deren anwedung an schulkindern (1912). Leipzig:Barth.

[311] Jung, C. (1910). The association method. The American Journal of Psychology, 21(2) (April 10): 219-269.

[312] Rorschach. H. (1921). Psychodiagnostik. Bern: Huber.

[313] Morgan, C. and Murray, H. (1935). A method of investigating fantasies: The Thematic Apperception Test. Archives of Neurology and Psychiatry, 34: 289-306.

[314] Rotter, J. and Rafferty, J. (1950). Manual. The Rotter Incomplete Sentences Blank: College Form. New York: Psychological Corporation.

[315] Hathaway, S. and McKinley, J. (1943). The Minnesota Multiphasic Personality Schedule. Minneapolis: University of Minnesota Press.

[316] Moniz, E. (1936b). Essai d'un traitement chirurgical de certaines psychoses. Bulletin de l'Academie de Medecine. 115(9):385-392.

[317] Burckhardt, Gottlieb (1891). Ueber rindenexcisionen, als beitrag zur operativen therapie der psychosen.[About cortical excision, as a contribution to surgical treatment of psychosis]. Allgemeine Zeitsschift fur Psychiatrie, 47: 463–548.

[318] Jacobsen, C. (1931). A study of cerebral functioning in learning. The prefrontal lobes. Journal of Comparative Neurology, 52:271-340.

[319] Jacobsen, C. (1935). Functions of frontal association areas in primates. Archives of Neurology and Psychiatry, 33, 558-569.

[320] Jacobsen, C., Wolf, J., and Jackson, T. (1935). An experimental analysis of the functions of the frontal association areas in primates. Journal of Nervous and Mental Disease, 82:1-14.

[321] Fulton, J. and Jacobsen, C. (1935). Functions des lobes frontaux: Etude comparee chez l'homme et les singes chimpanzes. Paper presented at the 2nd International Neurological Congress, London. August.

[322] Jacobsen, C. (1936). Studies on cerebral functions in primates. The function of the frontal association areas in monkeys. Comp Psychol. Mono., 13:1-60.

[323] Moniz, E. (1936a). Tenatives operatoires dans le traitement de certaines psychoses. Paris.

[324] Moniz, E. and Furtado, D. (1936b). Essais de traitement de la schizophrenie par leucotomie pre-frontale. Paper presented to the Societe Medico-Psychogique, 26 July 1936.

[325] Moniz, E. (1949a). Confidencias de um Investigador Ciientifico. Lisboa.

[326] Moniz, E. and Furtado, D. (1937). Essais de traitement de la schizophrenie par la leucotomie prefrontale. Annals Medico-Psychologiques II, 298-309.

[327] Rizzatti, E. (1938). L'operazione frontale bilaterale di Egas Moniz nelle psicosi postencefaliche. Schizophrenie, 6: 203.

[328] Freeman, W. and Watts, J. (1942). Psychosurgery. Springfield.

[329] Furtado, D. (1949). Results of leucotomy: A twelve year follow up. Psychosurgery. First International Congress. Lisbon.

[330] Meyer, A. (1950). Anatomical lessons from prefrontal leucotomy A report on the investigation of 122 brains. Congress International de Psychiatrie. Paris. 107-141.

[331] Moniz. E. (2014). Egas Moniz. Nobel Prize in Physiology or Medicine. Retrieved 21 August 2014 from nobelprize.org

[332] Moniz, E. (1927). Radiografia das arterias cerebrais. J. Soc. Ciencias Med. Lisbosa, XCL.

[333] Moniz, E. (1931). Diagnositic de tumeurs cerebeles et epreuve de l'encephalographie arterielle. Paris.

[334] Moniz, E. (1934). L'angiographie cerebrale. Ses applications et resultats en anatomie, physiologie et clinique. Paris.

[335] Nobelprize.org (2014). Nomination database - Physiology or Medicine. Retrieved 21 August 2014 from http://www.nobelprize.org/nomination/archive/medicine/nomination.php?string=Moniz&action=simplesearch&submit.x=-485&submit.y=-750&submit=submit

[336] Watts, J. and Freeman, W. (1942). Surgical aspects of prefrontal lobotomy. Journal of International College of Surg. 5:233.

[337] Freeman, W. and Watts, J. (1942). Prefrontal lobotomy: the surgical relief of mental pain. Bulletin of the New York Academy of Medicine, Dec. 18(12):794-812.

[338] Pascal, C. and Davesnes, J. (1926). Le traitment des maladies mentales par les chocs. Paris: Masson.

[339] Sakel, M. (1933). Neue behandlung der Morphinsucht [New treatment of morphine addition]. Zeitschrift fur die gesamte Neurologie und Psychiatrie [International Journal of Neurology and Psychiatry]. Springer.

[340] Sakel, M. (1933). Neue Behandlungsart Schiophreniker und verwirrter Erreger [New type of treatment of schizophrenia and confused manic]. Weiner Kliniscke Wochenschrift.

[341] Sakel, M. (1934). Schizophreniebehandlung mittels insulin-hypoglykamie sowie hypoglykamischer schock [Schizophrenia treatment with insulin-hypoglycemia and hypogylcemia shock]. Wiener med Wochenschrift.

[342] Sakel, M. (1937). The origin and nature of the hypoglycemic therapy of the psychoses. Bull. New York Academy of Medicine, 13:97.

[343] Easton, N. (1938). The insulin shock treatment of schizophrenia. The Canadian Medical Association Journal, Sept: 229-236.

[344] Cerletti. U. and Bini, L. (1938). L'Electroshock. Archive General Neurology, Psychiatry, Psicoanal., 19:266.

[345] Cerletti, U. (1940). L'electroshock. Rivista Sperimentale di Freniatria, 64:209-310.

[346] Mayo Clinic. (2018). Electroconvulsive therapy (ECT). Retrieved 6-26-2018 from https://www.mayoclinic.org/tests-procedures/electroconvulsive-therapy/about/pac-20393894

[347] Garrod, A. (1859). Gout and Rheumatic Gout. London, UK: Walton and Maberly. 438.

[348] Hammond, W. (1871). A treatise on the disease of the nervous system. New York, New York: D. Appleton and Company, p 381.

[349] Lange, C. (1886). Om oeriodiske depressiostilstande og deres, Patagonese Copenhagen, Denmark: Jacob Lunds Forlag.

[350] Cade J. (1949). Lithium salts in the treatment of psychotic excitement. Med. J. Aust. 2:349–352.

[351] Schou, M., Juel-Nielsen, N., Stromgren, E., Voldby, H. (1954). The treatment of mania psychosis by the administration of lithium salts. J. Neurol. Neurosurg, Psychiatry, 17:250-260.

[352] Laborit, H, Huguenard, P, Alluaume, R. (1952).Un noveau stabilisateur végétatif (le 4560 RP) La Presse Médicale. 60:206–8.

[353] Delay, J. and Deniker, P. (1952b). 38 cas de psychoses traitèes par la cure prolongèe et continuè de 4560 RP. CR Congr. Méd. Alién. Neurol. (France), 50:503–13.

[354] Follin, S. (1952). Discussion. Annales Médico-psychologiques, 110:126–7.

[355] Selikoff, U., Robitzck, E., and Orenstein, G. (1952). Treatment of pulmonary tuberculosis with hydrazine derivatives of isonicotinic acid. JAMA, 150:973-980.

[356] Spector, S., Prockop, D., and Brodie, B. (1958). Effect of Iproniazid on brain levels of norepinephrine and serotonin. Science, 127(704) March.

[357] Kuhn, R. (1957). Uber die Behandlung depressiver Zustande mit einem Iminodibenzyl derivat (G 22 355). Schweizerische Medizinische Wochenschrift. 87:1135-1140.

[358] Kuhn, R. (1958). The treatment of depressive states with G 22355 (imipramine hydrochloride). Am. J. Psychiatry, 115:459-464.

[359] Ball, J. and Kiloh, L. (1959). A controlled trial of impiramine in the treatment of depressive states. British Medical Journal, 2:1052-5.

[360] Divry, P., Bobon, J., Collard, J. (1958). Le R-1625: nouvelle therapeutique symtpmatique de l'agitation psychomotrice. [R-1625: a new drug for the symptomatic treatment of psychomotor excitation]. Acta. Neuol. Psychiatry Belg., October 58(10):878-88.

[361] FDA (1967). FDA approved Drug Products; Haldol, FDA Application No. (NDA) 015921, Company Ortho McNeil, Active ingredient Haloperidol; FDA approved April 12, 1967.

[362] Macht, D. (1920). Contributions to psychopharmacology. Johns Hopkins Hospital Bulletin. 31:167-73.

[363] Krapelin, E. (1893). Compendium der Psychiatrie: Zum Gebrauche fur Studirende und Aerzte 1st edition. Leipzig: Verlag von Ambr. Abel.

[364] Legge 13 maggio 1978, n.180. (1978). Legge 13 maggio 1978, n. 180; Accertainmenti e trattamenti sanitari volontari e obbligatori. Pubblicata nella Gazzetta Ufficiale 16 maggio 1978, n. 133. Retrieved 9-26-2014 from http://www.salute.gov.it/imgs/C_17_normativa_888_allegato.pdf

[365] Mental Health Parity Act of 1996. 110 Stat. 2874. Public Law 104-204; September 26, 1996. United States Government Printing Office.

[366] Whitaker, R. (2002). Mad in America: Bad science, bad medicine, and the enduring mistreatment of the mentally ill. Cambridge, MA: Perseus Publishers.

[367] Whitaker, R. (2010). Mad in America: Bad Science, Bad Medicine, and the Enduring Mistreatment of the Mentally Ill. Basic Books, 2nd edition May 25, 2010.

[368] National Academy of Sciences. (2004). Improving medical education, enhancing the behavioral and social science content of medical school curricula. Report prepared by the Committee on Behavioral and Social Sciences in Medical School Curricula. Patricia Cuff and Neil Vanselow, editors. Institute of Medicine of the National Academies. Washington, D.C.: The National Academy Press.

Chapter 6

Medical Microbiology

Definition.

Microbiology is "…the science concerned with microorganisms, including fungi, protozoa, bacteria, and viruses…" (1997)[1]. Medical microbiology is concerned with the importance of these four classes of microorganisms as they are capable of causing diseases in human beings. The term "microbiology" is derived from the Greek "micro" meaning small, "bio" meaning life, and "logia" meaning the study of a subject.

Introduction.

This chapter traces the history of medical microbiology. Emphasis is placed upon the development of microbiology as a scientific discipline. Particular attention is devoted to developing an understanding of the most influential people who have shaped the discipline throughout history, milestone discoveries, and recognition of changes in the conceptual matrixes which have led us to our current knowledge base in microbiology today.

The chapter is organized chronologically for consistency with other chapters and to provide you, the first and second year medical student, with an opportunity for an appreciation of the many significant contributions to the discipline, as a function of time.

Specific topic areas developed within this chapter are familiar to you as a medical student and represent major areas of instruction appearing in most all medical school microbiology courses today; parasitology, mycology, bacteriology, and virology. Immunology, while oftentimes integrated into the microbiology course of most medical schools today, will not be developed within this chapter. Immunology is introduced and developed in its own chapter, elsewhere in this book.

Upon completion of this chapter you will have had the opportunity to develop an appreciation of the exciting history of medical microbiology; begin to understand the historical foundations of modern-day medical microbiology; and begin to understand why and how microbiology has influenced the practice of medicine past, present, and future.

Much of the history of microbiology traditionally taught to medical students today begins with the invention of the microscope during the late-1600s, followed by a superficial treatment of the contributions of Antonie van Leeuwenhoek, Edward Jenner, Louis Pasteur, Ignaz Semmelweis, and Joseph Lister, during the 1800s. The history of medical microbiology is much richer than that and has it beginning in the ancient civilizations of Mesopotamia, Egypt, and the early written records of 3500 BC- 500 BC.

History.

Early records, 3500 BC - 500 BC.

The written records of the ancient civilizations of Mesopotamia and ancient Egypt, as well as many additional archeological significant artifacts, are beginning to reveal a rich history in the foundations and development of medical microbiology (1800 BC/1898 AD,1550 BC,1500 BC,1923,2003,2005)[2,3,4,5,6,7].

The early written records reveal vivid descriptions of familiar parasites of Mesopotamia, Egypt, and surrounding regions; provide listings of clinical signs and symptoms evidenced by and experienced by individuals infected by various parasites; and oftentimes include suggested recommended treatments directed towards eliminating the parasite or providing symptom relief. Specific human parasites which reside inside of the human body and recorded in the ancient written records remain familiar to practicing physicians today e.g. Guinea worms (Dracunculus medinensis) a roundworm; Ascaris (Ascaris lumbricoides) a roundworm; pinworm (Enterobius vermicularis) a round worm; hookworm (Ancylostoma duodenale) a nematode; and Schistosomes (Schitosomes haematocbium) blood flukes. Similarly, parasites which live outside of the human body and have an adverse effect on good physical health documented in the early written records are familiar to practicing physicians today e.g. Pthirus pubis - pubic lice ("the crabs"); Pediculus humanus capitis - head lice; Pediculus humanus - body lice; and bed bugs (Cimex lectularius).

In addition to written records, artifacts reveal people of these ancient civilizations maintain an awareness of parasites, an awareness of the parasites' adverse impact upon good physical health, and an awareness as to how to rid the body of parasites. Treatment and management efforts of parasitic infestations, as practiced by the Ancients, can be grouped into four general categories; medical (treatment with herbs, salves, elixirs, and compounds); surgical (physical removal); environmental (manipulation of the physical environment); and religious (faith based interventions).

The parasites reported in the earliest of written records are easily observable with the naked eye or with minimal magnification. No need for a microscope here. Notice too the knowledge base is built upon empirical observations. For example, if this worm is inside of a person's body it will generate these observable signs and the person will experience these symptoms. If you do this to the worm, then the person's condition will improve. If you don't do this then the person's condition will deteriorate. There is no evidence of systematic study of these parasites beyond recording observations and compiling similar observations between people and across generations. The process leads however to a rather stable knowledge base regarding specific parasites.

Yes, many of the parasitic infestations you will be asked to recognized and treat as you begin your clinical training in medical school today are first described and similar treatments offered over 5,000 years ago.

Bacterial infections are also recognized by the Ancients and have an ancient written history. Similar to the recordings of parasites, bacterial infections are described based upon clinical presentation of signs and symptoms followed by listings of potentially effective treatments. There is no written record to suggest the Ancients systematically studied bacteria, bacterial infections, or recognized the potential of bacteria to produce infection or disease. The written record does reveal bacterial infections are common in the regions of Mesopotamia, Ancient Egypt, and surrounding areas. Clear and specific treatments are prescribed for patients, primary caregivers, and all individuals having contact with the infected patient.

Fungi in their many forms, mushrooms, molds, yeast, lichen, and truffles have a well-documented recorded history. Many have proven pivotal in understanding disease, infection, and offer foundations for many effective medical treatments used today. Given fungi lack immune systems, it is necessary for them to create and secrete antibacterial, antiviral, antifungal, and antimicrobial compounds in order to survive in nature. While there is no recorded evidence ancient civilizations systematically studied fungi for medicinal purposes, there is evidence they are aware and use fungi to treat infection and disease. The knowledge base regarding fungi and their effect upon the health of the human body is accumulated by way of repeated empirical observation, between people, and across multiple generations. There is no conceptual matrix to organize observations or guide systematic study. Simply stated, the ancient written records state; if you eat this, drink this, or rub this into the body, then this will happen.

Viruses are unrecognized as a source of infection or disease, however; physical clinical manifestations of viral infections can be found in the written records of ancient Mesopotamia and Ancient Egypt. Records reveal viral infections such as polio, smallpox, measles, and shingles are known, produce specific clinical signs and symptoms, and respond to specific recommended treatments (circa 800 BC/1951)[8]. There is no record these or other viral infections are studied in a systematic way. Most typically, clinical signs and symptoms are listed along with recommended treatments without regard to the microorganism ultimately responsible. Recent archeological evidence, in the form of physical examination and DNA analyses of mummified remains, add additional support of viral infections of many and certainly posed diagnostic and treatment challenges to the medical practitioners of the ancient Mesopotamia, Egypt, and surrounding regions.

Parasitic, bacterial, fungal, and viral etiologies resulting in impaired health are conceptualized and explained within the matrix of external, supranatural forces. The reason any person is in poor health is due to an angered deity (god). Different deities hold responsibilities for the clinical manifestation of signs and symptoms of particular disease. This organizational structure begins to provide a matrix within which to organize and understand poor health. Notice, if you substitute any recognized parasite, bacterium, fungus, or virus known to modern medicine today with the associated ancient "deity", you will quickly recognize much similarity between the conceptual matrix used by the Ancient civilizations and that used in modern medicine of today, over four thousand years later. Both systems provide organization of information and offer a logical course of treatment given the presumed etiology.

Trivia: The term "etiology" is derived from the Greek word "aitologia"; with the combination of "aitia" meaning "cause " and "logia" meaning "the study of a subject". The concept predates written history, while the term first enters the English language circa 1555.

In sum, medical microbiology reveals a rich history dating back to the earliest known written record. Parasites and fungi are easily seen with the unaided eye and associated with a person's health. Specific treatments are associated with specific parasites and fungi. Several of the treatments remain essentially unchanged during the past 5,000 years e.g. treatment for removal of a Guinea worm continues to be wrapping the worm around a stick and pulling it out of the body. Associations between clinical signs and symptoms are made with parasites and fungi on an empirical experiential basis. Associations are recorded in a listing format. Pathogenic bacteria and viruses have devastating impact upon a person's health. Unseen by the unaided eye, infection and disease produced by bacteria or viruses are recorded as listings of clinical signs and symptoms and occasionally associated with a one of many deities maintaining exclusive reign over specific parts of the human body. The presumptive and ultimate etiology of all parasitic infestations or fungal, bacterial, and viral infections is supranatural and faith based i.e. impairments in health are the result of dissatisfied supranatural deities and recovery of good health is accomplished by calming angered deities.

Although the ultimate etiology of impaired health during the Ancient civilizations of Mesopotamia, Egypt, and surrounding areas is faith based, the Ancients offer the first beginnings of recording signs and symptoms and making empirically derived associations with earthly physical forces of nature. For example, the gods may have sent the Guinea worm to infest a patient's body (faith based system). The patient's body will respond to the infestation with the following signs and symptoms (empirically derived physical associations). The worm can be removed by a physical procedure and the patient's physical body can be expected to respond in a predictable manner (empirically derived physical associations). This exemplifies the willingness and open mindedness of the Ancient civilizations to consider a conceptual matrix, within which to understand good health and impaired health, which includes both supranatural and natural forces. Striking, how little has changed and remained the same during the past 5,000 years.

Antiquity, 500 BC - 500 AD.

The written records of Antiquity are filled with descriptive accounts of infestations by human parasites and infection by fungi, bacteria, and viruses producing impairment in health, oftentimes resulting in death.

Thucydides (460 BC-395 BC) Greek historian, eloquently describes the clinical signs and symptoms evidenced by individuals infected with the obligate intracellular bacterium, we know today as Rickettsia prowazekii, transmitted by the human body louse. Additionally, he offers detailed clinical descriptions, perhaps unmatched to date, of the Plague of Athens appearing in 431 BC- 404 BC, during which bacteria and suspected viruses (especially variola) are responsible for killing an estimated 1/3 of the entire population of Athens (1843,1910,1919/1921)[9,10,11].

The Hippocratic Collections, the majority of treaties written circa 400 BC-300 BC, collected and deposited in the Greek city of Alexandria, located in northern Egypt, reveal a familiarity with many of the parasites, fungi, bacteria, and viruses producing disease and poor health in humans from the earliest times in recorded history. Treaties within the Collection describe the epidemiology, clinical presentation of signs and symptoms, prognosis, and treatment of many of these disorders. For example, in Epidemics, Books I v, written circa 410 BC, the author (perhaps Hippocrates himself) describes the clinical presentation of individuals infected with Mycobacterium tuberculosis (TB), characterized by the classic signs and symptoms of chronic cough, blood tinged sputum, night sweats, fever, and weight loss. The author describes the condition as "…phthisis…" rather than the more familiar term used today "tuberculosis", yet the signs and symptoms are sufficiently clear to recognize the presentation as tuberculosis.

Trivia: The term "phthisis" is derived from the Greek meaning to "…dwindle or waste away…". A perhaps more familiar alternative term for TB "consumption" enters the medical literature in Book II Section 8 of Aulus Celsus' Roman encyclopedia "De Medicina" [On Medicine] circa 30 AD and commonly used until the mid-1900s. Consumption is derived from the Latin "consumptionem" referring to the appearance of the body being consumed from within as the result of disease.

Note: Medical texts of the Greeks and Romans of this period are organized differently than the medical texts of today. The Greeks and Romans organize disease and infections based upon clinical signs and symptoms, rather than the system familiar to most medical students today of organizing diseases and infections based upon the underlying etiology e.g. parasite, fungus, bacterium, or virus. This difference makes a scholarly assessment of the written records challenging, whenever attempting to identify the likely etiologies of diseases and infections across time. Many different causes of diseases and infections generated similar clinical signs and symptoms e.g. fever, nausea, rapid fatigue, weakness, delirium, and more. However, many diseases and infections produce sufficiently unique signs and symptoms to allow a reasonable comparison between the early Greek and Roman descriptions with the classification system of disease and infections based upon underlying microorganisms used today. So is the case in the interpretation of records within the Hippocratic Collections.

The Hippocratic Collections offers clinical descriptions of patients suffering infection and disease from parasites, fungi, bacteria, and viruses. Parasites (Entamoeba histolytica) reasonably account for dysentery reported in Epidemics Book I v, xv, and Book III viii, while (Plasmodium falciparum) reasonably accounts for malaria reported in Epidemics Book I ii, v, vi, xxiv, xxv and Book III xii. Bacteria (Streptococcus pyogenes) reasonably account for erysipelas described in Epidemics Book III iv; (Borrelia recurrentis) for relapsing fever described in Epidemics Book I xxi; and (Shigella) for dysentery, as an alternative to the parasite Entamoeba histolytica, in Epidemics Book I v, xv. Viruses reasonably account for mumps (mumps virus) reported in Epidemics Book I and poliomyelitis (poliovirus) described in Epidemics Book IV i (circa 410 BC/1839,1891,1923,1934,1994)[12,13,14,15,16].

The Collection, while reporting familiar endemic infections and diseases, fails to report clinical descriptions or offer case histories of smallpox, measles, bubonic plague, or syphilis. Of the 42 case histories presented in Epidemics Books I and III, 60% of the patients die. The writing of Epidemics is unique in that it offers little if any suggestions for treatments or cures. Rather, emphasis is placed upon detailing the onset, course, and resolution of clinical signs and symptoms without intervention, simply observing the body's natural response to infection and disease.

Antiquity witnesses a fundamental change in the approach as to how knowledge is acquired. The empirical-inductive methods of the Ancients are replaced by rational–deductive methods popularized by Greek mathematicians and philosophers. Careful empirical observation and inductive reasoning is replaced by careful intellectual, rational thought, and deductive reasoning followed by observation. In addition to the fundamental change in preferred methods there is also a shift in the fundamental philosophical approach and thought processes. As a whole, the Ancients' approach moves from the specific to the general, whereas the Greek natural philosophers' approach, popular during Antiquity, moves from the general to the specific.

These fundamental shifts in philosophic approaches and methods alter not only what is investigated but also how it is investigated.

Aristotle (384 BC-322 BC) Greek natural philosopher resists the prevailing change in methods, away from the empirical-inductive approach of the Ancients and towards the new rational-deductive approach characteristic of Antiquity, much to the chagrin of his teacher Plato (428 BC-348 BC). Aristotle holds fast to the old school approach of the Ancients, which emphasizes empirical observation. He is a stanch empiricist, among many now embracing the new rational-deductive investigational models.

Aristotle's contributions in general are not particularly original. However, translations of his written works reveal a detailed familiarity with parasitic infestation, especially lice, detailing their source or origin "…generated out of the flesh of animals…", their parasitic nature "…live on the juices of living flesh…", epidemiology "…boys heads are apt to be lousy but men in less degree…women are more subject to lice than men…", recognition of an association with poor health "…lice is a disease…", and their presence as a potential source of death "…men have been known to succumb to this louse disease…" (Book V, Section 31) (circa 350 BC/1910)[17].

Aristotle describes parasitic intestinal worms; proposes their classification into three species (flat-worm, round worm, and ascarid); offers his views of their origins (spontaneous generation); and provides a description of empirically derived observations which will assist physicians in making a differential diagnosis between parasitic intestinal worms. Here is an excerpt from Aristotle's writings contained in his History of Animals series; "…These intestinal worms do not in any case propagate their kind. The flat-worm, however, in an exceptional way, clings fast to the gut, and lays a thing like a melon-seed, by observing which indication the physician concludes that his patient is troubled with the worm…" (Book V, Section 19) (circa 350 BC/1910)[17].

In addition to his observations of parasitic infestations, Aristotle describes his empirical observations and familiarity with a specific viral infection. Aristotle describes rabies. He does not detail the acute brain inflammation which results from the rabies virus but rather describes the behavioral consequence of infection and a common vector of transmission; "…rabies drives the animal mad…any animal will take the disease if bitten by a dog so afflicted…the disease is fatal to the dog and any animal it may bite…" (Book VIII, Section 22) (circa 350 BC/1910)[17].

Trivia: Rabies is derived from the Greek word "lyssa" meaning "mad-frenzy". The root is preserved today in the genus classification of rabies virus, Lyssavirus.

Aristotle's writings pertaining to parasitic and viral infections offer nothing particularly new or original, yet remain relevant in the context of history in that they emphasize the natural (physical) etiology of disease and provide a written record, open for examination by other investigators.

Titus Carus (99 BC-55 BC) Roman philosopher exemplifies the shift in philosophical approaches of acquiring new knowledge, between the investigators of the Ancient civilizations (empirical-inductive) and the Greek and Roman investigators of Antiquity (rational-deductive). Adopting the rational-deductive methods and rejecting supranatural deities as reasonable explanations, Carus is among the first to record his speculations disease can be explained by invisible, although natural phenomena, which follow the fundamental laws of physics (50 BC/2008)[18]. He rejects the dogma of the supranatural in favor of physics.

Marcus Varro (116 BC-27 BC) Roman scholar extends Carus' position, infection and disease can be caused by minute, invisible entities and begins to lay the foundation of microbiology, emphasizing a natural rather than a supranatural deity model with which to explain disease. Varro warns "…Precautions must also be taken in the neighbourhood of swamps, both for the reasons given, and because there are bred certain minute creatures which cannot be seen by the eyes, which float in the air and enter the body through the mouth and nose and there cause serious diseases..." (37 BC/1934)[19].

Aulus Celsus (14 AD-37 AD) Roman encylopediaist offers his tremendously influential collection and synthesis of medical knowledge in "De Medicina" [On Medicine] (30 AD/1478,1935)[20,21]. In keeping with the format of the period, he systematically details signs and symptoms of infection and disease, provides recommendations for treatment of signs and symptoms, and conceptualizes infection and disease within the Alexandrian School's balance of humors model. Unlike medicine today, which organizes infection and disease based upon underlying microorganisms e.g. parasite, fungus, bacterium, or virus, Celsus organizes based upon clinical signs and symptoms. Both systems are effective in organizing large amounts of information and guiding behavioral, dietary, medical, and surgical treatments. Celsus' "De Medicina" (circa 30 AD/1478,1935)[20,21] provides sufficiently detailed and unique clinical descriptions to permit reasonable associations with specific parasites, fungi, bacteria, and viruses, much like the descriptions of signs and symptoms found in the Hippocratic Collections (circa 400- 300 BC/1839,1891,1923,1934,1994)[12,13,14,15,12].

Galan of Pergamum (129 AD-200 AD) a proponent of the rational-deductive methods, typical of the Greek and Roman investigators of the period, offers his views on disease, their causes, cures, and prognoses. Galen's conceptualizes infection and disease within the Doctrine of Balances models proposed by Alcmaeon 600 years earlier, Aristotle 400 years earlier, and Celsus 100 years earlier. He accepts infections and disease are the result of natural rather than supranatural forces. In his typical dogmatic, authoritarian writing style Galan offers numerous treaties listing previously reported signs and symptoms of common parasitic infestations, as well as, fungal, bacterial, and viral infections. He frequently takes credit for the work of others, claiming priority for ideas and investigative findings which are easily traceable today to their original sources. Galan is prolific in his writing efforts. His writings are accepted by most as medical dogma and remain relatively unchallenged for the next 1,700 years. Combination of the sheer volume of his writings and writing style stifle the pursuit of new knowledge as much as they offer comfort to the medical and scientific communities in their absolute dogma.

Galen describes the signs and symptoms of fevers associated with malaria and explains the fevers to be the product of imbalances in humors. For example, the quartan fever (fever cycles every three days) typical of plasmodium malaria is described based upon its periodicity and explained within the matrix of the doctrine of balances, as the result of too much black bile. Galen has no idea however that the fever is the result of a micro-organism. The micro-organism and the mosquito vector are not discovered until 1,600 years later (1880,1886)[22,23].

Galen coins the term "gonorrhea" to describe a familiar bacterial infection (circa 175 AD/1513, 1976)[24,25]. The term is derived from the Greek "gonos" meaning seed and "rhoia" meaning to run or flow. Galen's choice of term is based upon his misinterpretation of the purulent discharge characteristic of gonorrhea to be an involuntary discharge of semen. Here too, he describes a common bacterial infection without an appreciation of the micro-organism responsible for the infection. The coffee bean shaped, diplococci bacteria responsible for gonorrhea is discovered 1,600 years later (1879)[26] by German physician Albert Neisser (1855-1916).

Similarly, Galen offers clinical descriptions of tuberculosis without appreciating the micro-organism responsible. The bacteria causing tuberculosis, Mycobacterium tuberculosis is identified

1,600 years later (1882)[27] by German physician Robert Koch (1843-1910). Viral infections, including small-pox, now identified responsible for the Antonine Plague (aka Plague of Galen circa 166 AD) are reported by Galen and presented according to physical signs and symptoms. Here too he fails to appreciate the microbiology responsible for the clinical presentations of viral infections.

Galen accepts impaired physical health is due to natural, physical causes and conceptualizes infection and disease within a balance of body humors matrix. However, he dogmatically rejects alternative explanations, including "…invisible entities…natural phenomena…" proposed by a few willing to challenge the accepted medical and scientific understanding of disease (98 BC/ 1934, 50 BC/2008)[28,29]. Galen's dogmatic conceptualization of disease conditions and prolific writings on the topics actually impedes the scientific search for micro-organisms for the next 1,600 years. The mind set of Galen and his followers is basically, why look for an alternative explanation when the explanation is already known.

So true then as today is the risk of failing to understand completely when one begins to accept uncritically the knowledge passed from others, especially when the knowledge is passed in a confident, self-assured, authoritative, dogmatic style. Be willing to think for yourself as a future physician and take the risk of challenging current medical truths. The history of medicine has certainly revealed repeatedly throughout the course of time, medical truths change.

In summary, Antiquity witnesses the early development of medical microbiology as a scientific discipline. Specific and most influential records are the Hippocratic Collections, Celsus' De Medicina, and the collected works of Aristotle and Galen. Each of these collected works detail the physical consequences of infection and disease generated by parasites, fungi, bacteria and viruses and offer the treating physician guidance in diagnosis, treatment, and prognosis. Unlike the classification system of today, where infection and disease are organized based upon the microorganism responsible, the Greek and Roman system of Antiquity is based upon presentation of clinical signs and symptoms e.g. fever, diarrhea, oozing pus, skin lesions, weight loss. Writings of the period are sufficient in detail and case presentations are sufficiently unique to recognize the parasitic infestation or fungal, bacterial, or viral infections most likely responsible for the clinical presentations. Many of the same microorganisms continue to produce infections and diseases today, over 2,000 years later.

Specifically and by way of example, Thucydides eloquently details the clinical presentation of patients suffering the Plague of Athens (variola virus) unmatched by descriptions even today. The Hippocratic collection details the clinical presentation of tuberculosis (Mycobacterium tuberculosis), dysentery (Entamoena histolytica; Shigella), malaria (Plasmodium falciparum), erysipelas (Streptococcus pyogneses), mumps (mumps virus), and poliomyelitis (poliovirus). Aristotle describes lice as a disease and potential source of death. He describes intestinal worms and offers his classification into three species, flat worms, round worms and ascarids, based upon the physical properties of the parasite. He demonstrates how use of his classification system can assist treating physicians in their efforts to diagnosis, treat, and make a reliable prognostic statement regarding clinical course and likely outcome. Aristotle also describes the clinical presentation of rabies and identifies the dog as a common vector of transmission. Celsus' medical encyclopedia, "De Medicina", details most all medical knowledge assembled to date regarding infection and disease produced by parasites, fungi, bacteria, and viruses. Galan offers voluminous writings, although not particularly original, provide continuing evidence of an intimate familiarity with infestations, infections, and diseases of the period. The true source of many of these conditions, once dogmatically rejected by Galen, are known today to be microorganisms.

Medical microbiology is developing as a young science. Listing of empirically derived physical signs and symptoms accompanied by recommended treatments exemplify the written record of the period and offers guidance to the practicing physician. The preferred approach to acquiring new knowledge shifts from the empirical-inductive (specific to the general of the Ancients to the rational-deductive (general to the specific) preferred by Greek and Roman philosophers and mathematicians. Much of the western world's knowledge concerning infestation and disease is assembled and studied in the Greek City and Libraries of Alexandria. Infection and disease from microscopic organisms are conceptualized within a balance of humors matrix. Only a few challenge the dogma of the time and suggest illness may be the result of invisible, naturally occurring organisms, and which follow principles of nature and physics. Dogmatic rejection of microorganisms as possible explanations of infection or disease, especially by Galen and his unquestioning obedient followers, uniformly suppress the growth and development of medical microbiology for the next 1,600 years.

Middle Ages (Medieval Times), 500 AD - 1400 AD.

The Middle Ages witness few advances in medical microbiology.

The Middle Ages begins with the fall of the Western Roman Empire (modern-day Italy, France, Spain, Great Britain, coastal Libya, Tunisia, Algeria, and Morocco) to invading military forces. The Eastern Roman Empire (aka Byzantine Empire; modern-day Greece, Turkey, Syria, Lebanon, and Egypt) remain relatively preserved although advancement of science and medicine is greatly suppressed by military campaigns. Much of the written record of knowledge concerning science and medicine, amassed by the Roman Empire, is relocated to the Middle East for safe keeping. There, original manuscripts written in Greek and Latin are translated into Arabic. This opens the window of opportunity for access, synthesis, reflection, assessment, and reinterpretation by academics, scholars, and practicing physicians outside of the epistemological systems which originally produced this fund of knowledge. As the political, military, and economic systems stabilize in Europe, much of the materials translated into Arabic are translated once again into Latin and return to the scientific and medical communities of Europe.

Slow progress is being made in medical microbiology. For the scientific and medical communities, infectious disease resulting from microorganisms are confidently diagnoses and treated within a strict, nature based, Galenian balance of humors model. For the organized religion communities, infectious disease resulting from microorganisms are confidently explained within a strict, supranatural, faith based model, as "…the will of God…". Both positions, confident in their understandings, actively suppress further development of medical microbiology throughout the Middle Ages and beyond.

Infectious disease spreads through Europe eliminating the lives of millions and reducing the overall population by an estimated 50 percent, not once but twice. That's right, an enterobacteriaceae, Gram-negative, rod shaped bacterium, Yersinia pestis is responsible for the deaths of millions and the devastating subsequential impact upon governments, economic, and social systems across Europe. This microscopic organism, perhaps more than any other single factor, changes the course and development of Europe forever.

Two devastating epidemics are documented and attributed to this bacterium; first the Plague of Justinian in 542 AD (bubonic plague) and second the Black Death during 1347 AD-1353 AD (bubonic plague) (2010)[30]. In addition to these epidemics, micro-organisms e.g. parasites, fungi, bacteria, and viruses of the period routinely produce debilitating physical illnesses and frequent death. Yes, a simple infection we might treat medically today, as a routine part of our daily practice with little thought, would often result in the death of the patient, during the Middle Ages.

Many micro-organisms you recognize today prove to be particularly challenging to the treating physicians of the Middle Ages. Some of the most debilitating are parasites e.g. plasmodium (malaria); bacteria e.g. Mycobacterium tuberculosis (tuberculosis), Shigella (dysentery), Salmonella enteria (typhoid fever), Mycobacterium leprae (leprosy), Treponema pallidum (syphilis); and viruses e.g. morbillivirus (measles), and variola major (smallpox).

The economic, social, and political impact these micro-organism exert upon society cannot be overstated. Whenever significant numbers of the work force are eliminated due to death or disease there is a resultant consequence that changes entire economic, social, and political systems. The core foundational systems of working society are shaken. In efforts to stabilize these systems, governments and organized religions begin to introduce laws, directives, and mandates in efforts to manage the destabilizing effects infectious disease have as they spread across Europe.

Let us now take a brief look at some of the specifics events, influential people, and contributions which have impacted medical microbiology and its subsequent development, occurring during the Middle Ages.

The Middle Ages begin with its fair share of problems, least of which is the microscopic, Gram-negative, rod shaped bacterium, Yersinia pestis. The bacterium is the micro-organism most likely responsible for the deaths of millions and which reduces the population of Europe by approximately fifty percent within only a few years (circa 542 AD/1776,1788)[31,32]. This devastating epidemic is recorded in history as the Plague of Justinian or simply and more descriptive as the first bubonic plague. Medicine and science have little to offer, at the time, in explaining the underlying source or vector of transmission of this infectious and lethal bacterium.

Newly formed organized religions e.g. the Catholic Church and well established organized religions e.g. Judaism, however can and do offer an explanation. Their explanation is simple, easily understood by the masses, faith based, and supranatural. In brief, the reason people become ill and die is "…that is God's will…". Illness and death are the consequences of the person's failure to adhere to and follow Church doctrine. If you do not do as the Church instructs, you will be punished by God. The religion based matrix also provides a course of action to treat the illness. Treatments are faith based. Treatments are accomplished through prayer, appealing to a supranatural deity (God), asking a deity (God) for forgiveness. If it is "…God's will…" the person will recover from the illness. The faith based, supranatural (deity) explanation offered by organized religions stand in mark contrast to the natural (physical) based explanation offered by the Greek and Roman philosophers of Antiquity. Faith based models, to explain and guide treatment, displace natural (physical) models which have been in place for over 1,000 years.

In the absence of a demonstrable, natural (physical), scientifically sound explanation of natural phenomena, many people will readily accept an alternative faith based, supranatural (deity) explanation to understand the many causes of physical illness. In the absence of natural (physical) and effective treatments, many people engage in faith based appeals to supranatural deities (gods) to provide relief from suffering and a cure from physical illness. Oh how little human nature has changed during the past few thousand years.

OK…back to the specific events and influential people of the Middle Ages which impact the development of medical microbiology.

Paulus of Aegina (625 AD-698 AD) Greek physician systematically describes much of what is known in medicine and surgery. He presents material in the traditional format of the period by describing clinical signs and symptoms, recommending specific managements and treatments, and conceptualizing disorders within a Galenian balance of humors matrix. Visible parasites e.g. intestinal worms and Guinea worms receive dedicated discussions and are recognized as common sources of impaired physical health. Disorders recognized today as resulting from microscopic parasites, fungi, bacteria, and viruses are systematically described based upon clinical presentations. Specifically, in his major work a three volume medical encyclopedia, "De Re Medica Libir Septum" [Medical Compendium in Seven Books], he discusses malaria (Plasmodium falciform), dysentery (Entamoeba histolytica), the plague (Yersinia pestis), syphilis (Treponema pallidum), gonorrhea (Neisseria gonorrhea), tetanus (Clostridium tetani), tuberculosis (Mycobacterium tuberculosis), cholera (Vibrio cholerae), measles (Morbillivirus), and smallpox (variola major) to list only ten of over one hundred clinical descriptions (circa 675 AD/1844, 1847)[33,34]. Most of these conditions have been previously reported in a similar format by The Hippocratic Collections, Aristotle, Galen, and others.

Paulus of Aegina's "De Re Medica Libri Septum" remains unrivaled in its accuracy and completeness, serving as a major medical text throughout Europe and the Middle East for the next 1,200 years. The original work in written in Greek and is published in Venice during 1528 and translated into English in 1834. The second and third volumes, most relevant to medical microbiology, are translated into English during 1844. The text, originally written over 1,300 years ago highlights the challenges micro-organisms present to physicians, past and present, whenever diagnosing, treating, or managing potentially lethal infectious diseases.

Abu Ibn al-Razi (Latinized to Rhazes) (865 AD-925 AD) Persian scholar offers his 22 volume "Kitabu al-Hawi fi-Tibb" [The Comprehensive Book on Medicine], originally written in Arabic and subsequently translated into Latin in 1229 AD, serves as another significantly influential work with relevance to medical microbiology. The Book serves as a foundational text used in the education of physicians throughout the Middle East and Europe for over 800 years. Similar in format to previous works, detailing clinical presentations of disease through series of clinical case studies, he too emphasizes the natural, physical basis for disease. He too holds tightly to a balance of humors conceptual model whenever explaining the underlying pathologies responsible for clinical signs and symptoms and recommended course of treatment. Here too, many of the cases presented can reasonably be reorganized into the diagnostic classification systems used today, over 1,000 years later and which today places primary emphasis upon the micro-organism e.g. parasite, fungus, bacterium, or virus, responsible for producing the clinical signs and symptoms, based solely on the detailed descriptions offered in the "Kitabu'l Hawi Fi'Tabb".

Particular note with reference to medical microbiology is Al-Razi's presentation of two problematic and lethal diseases, smallpox (variola virus) and measles (paramyxovirus) (circa 900 AD/1948,1985)[35,36]. Al-Razi provides clear and succinct statements outlining the clinical signs and symptoms, clinical course, and prognostic indicators for both diseases (circa 900 AD/1948,

1985)[35,36]. His descriptions are so helpful in making a correct differential diagnosis they are used by practitioners well into the 1900s.

Ibn Sina (Latinized to Avicenna) (980 AD-1037 AD) Persian philosopher, physician, and scientist offers his "Kitab al-Qanun fil-al Tibb" [The Canon of Medicine] (1025AD,1632,1999)[37,38,39]. This text too offers essentially a restatement of European and Middle Eastern medical knowledge regarding infectious disease and the conceptual matrix within which physicians have dogmatically interpreted disease since Alcmaeon of Croton first introduces the balance doctrine (510 BC/1896, 1903/1954,1954-1964,1966)[40,41,42,43]. Nothing really new here other than a return to evidence based and experimental medicine.

Ibn Sina's "The Canon of Medicine" consists of five books. Book 1 discusses general principles of medicine, defining medicine, and identifying the subjects of medicine. Disease is conceptualized within the traditional Galenian model emphasizing balance in explaining disease, signs and symptoms, and treatments. Book 2 discusses simple medications. Book 3 discusses the physics of medicine, provides anatomical descriptions of effected body regions, and criticizes all earlier writing by others who have only presented clinical signs and symptom and associated cures, while ignoring descriptions of anatomy as an essential component of understanding disease. Book 4 is especially relevant to medical microbiology in addressing disease which effect different parts of the body, describes the periodicity of disease; common lethal viral diseases smallpox and measles, and assorted bacterial infections e.g. erysipelas and abscesses. Book 5 is essentially a pharmacopeia for Arabian practitioners.

The "Canon of Medicine" soon achieves acceptance within Arabic medicine in much the same way as Galen's writing influenced the Roman Empire. The writings become accepted as dogma and not to be challenged. Certainly the Canon influences the medical school educations of physicians and further suppresses development of medical microbiology (1507 AD/1964,1930, 1966)[44,45,46].

Organized religions are becoming powerful and influential institutions. They provide an alternative explanation of infectious disease and physical illness from that offered by the scientific and medical communities. Organized religion bases its understanding of disease and treatment within the conceptual matrix of supranatural deities (god(s)). In brief, a person who suffers disease does so as punishment from God. Recovery from disease necessitates supranatural intervention from God. The specifics as to how to satisfy an angered God e.g. prayer, confession, atonement is dependent upon the specific religion e.g. Judaism, Catholicism, or Islam.

This stands in contrast to the scientific and medical communities which base their understanding of disease and treatments upon a conceptual matrix of natural, earthly, physical forces which follow the rules of physics. In brief, a person who suffers from disease does so due to exposure to natural conditions and which produces disturbances in the normal function of the physical body. Recovery from disease necessitates natural (physical) interventions to restore the natural (physical) balances within the body. Two very different conceptual matrixes. Both establish large numbers of followers.

Organized religions of the period e.g. Judaism, Catholicism, and Islam are notable in their influence in providing guidance as to how to recognize, diagnose, treat, and manage many diseases. Leaderships within these three most popular organized religions of Europe issue orders and directives as to when, where, and how to deal with individuals suffering disease. Some orders and directives are quite humane while others much less so.

On the more humane side, the Roman Catholic Church using a monesterial system establishes monasteries throughout Europe, which provide care and comfort to people suffering disease and infection. In particular and by way of example is the monastery in southeast France, established by the Roman Catholic Church in 1095 AD, dedicated to care and suffering of individuals suffering common diseases of the Middle Ages. Specifically, the monastery specializes in the care for individuals suffering skin diseases e.g. St. Anthony's Fire (ergot poisoning) resulting from chronic ingestion of the fungus Clavicps purpurea which grow on grains, especially rye; erysipelas (red skin) resulting from an acute bacterial infection of the deep epidermis by streptococcus; and shingles (painful skin rash with blisters) resulting from viral infection of Herpes zoster-Varicella zoster. The community of monks of the monastery is known as the Hospital Brothers of Saint Anthony. Saint Anthonywithin the Catholic Church is the patron saint of infectious disease.

So successful is the monastery in providing hospital care, the St. Anthony Order quickly spreads throughout Europe and establishes hundreds of hospitals to care for individuals suffering infectious diseases. The Order further establishes its value in providing care throughout Europe during the epidemic of the second bubonic plague (Black Death) in 1347 AD-1352 AD. An estimated 25 million people, approximately 50% of the entire population of Europe at the time, die as the result of the bacterium responsible for the second bubonic plague (Yersinia pestis) (2004)[47].

Trivia: The bacterium (Yersinia pestis) responsible for two devastating epidemics effecting Europe during the Middle Ages is first identified and its vector of transmission clarified (rodent carrying fleas) by Alexandre Yersin (1863-1943) Swiss bacteriologist, while working for the Pasteur Institute (1894,1894)[48,49]. He makes the discovery while investigating the bubonic plague epidemic in Hong Kong. Yersin originally names the Gram negative, rod shaped, facultative anaerobe bacterium "Pasteurella pestis" in acknowledgement of the institute providing funding for his investigations. The name is changed to the now more familiar "Yersinia pestis" in 1967. See later in this chapter for the huge professional controversy surrounding the identification of this bacterium (Yersin-Kitasato controversy).

Tuberculosis (Mycobacterium tuberculosis) represents another bacterium which poses significant problems to the people of Europe and the physicians and clergy charged with providing medical care. Recall, tuberculosis (TB) is characterized by a chronic cough, blood tinged sputum, fever, night sweats, and weight loss. The primary mode of transmission between people is respiratory droplets. Tuberculosis is termed "phthisis" in the medical writings found within the Hippocratic Collections (Epidemics I.v.) and the writings of Aretaeus, Aristotle, and Galen. The Greek term "phthisis" when translated into Latin means "consumption" (to waste away). The term "consumption" is used well into the mid-1900s to describe the infection today we term "tuberculosis".

Tuberculosis is recognized as a communicable disease and efforts are made to control its spread. Ibn Sina's "The Canon of Medicine" (1025 AD), clearly and definitively states the disorder is contagious. This stands in contrast to the explanations offered by the Hippocratic Collections from Antiquity which state TB is an inherited condition. Ibn Sina's position is based in part upon the writings of Aretaeus (circa 100 AD/1856)[50] and Aristotle and Galen from Antiquity, who argued TB is of natural (physical) origins and spreads from person to person through the air.

An alternative and popular explanation which explains TB during the Middle Ages is based upon the supranatural (deity) models advocated by organized religions. Again in brief, these models state the origin of TB is from God; God chooses when and who are to be afflicted; the disease is sent to afflict people who fail to follow Church doctrine; and cure can only be effected thought the forgiveness of God.

Trivia: Hippocrates recognizes TB to be nearly always fatal and recommends physicians not to attempt to treat or be in the company of patients who suffer from the condition (Book 1, Epidemics) (1923)[14].

Leprosy (Mycobacterium leprae) represents another chronic disease resulting from an infectious microscopic bacterium. Leprosy, a first cousin of tuberculosis, is the most feared disease throughout most of the Middle Ages. The bacterium has devastating impact upon people physically, legally, economically, and socially. Recall, leprosy is a granulomatous disease affecting primarily the upper respiratory tract mucosa and peripheral nerves. The condition is characterized by progressive debilitating sensory loss, muscle weakness, and disfiguring skin lesions (large, discolored lumps). The bacterium is transmitted primarily by way of respiratory droplets.

Unlike many of the bacteria and viruses of the period which result in relatively quick death of a person following exposure; leprosy is a chronic condition. The long term management of leprosy falls not to physicians but rather to religious leaders, politicians, and newly developing national governments. Physicians have little to offer. Debate continues within the medical, scientific, religious, and political communities, of the times, as whether leprosy is best understood as an inherited disorder, an acquired disorder, or simply a disease "sent by an angered God". In absence of an effective cure, isolation from the general population and termination of legal civil rights is the mandated management strategy of the period.

An extensive network of small, long term care facilities are established across Europe to care for individuals identified as lepers. The facilities are typically affiliated with and funded by organized religion e.g. monasteries of The Roman Catholic Church. Most facilities care for small numbers of patients e.g. 10 or less and provide food, shelter, and religious comfort. Leprosy is widespread throughout Europe but is not particularly common.

Fear of leprosy during the Middle Ages is not based upon the physical signs and symptoms of the disorder as one might reasonably expect but rather the termination of legal rights. For example, English Common Law of the 1200s explicitly states any person identified as a leper shall no longer be permitted to own property, take possession of any inheritance, or enter into a legally binding contract (1952)[51]. A leper shall not be permitted to plead in court. The termination of civil rights are to apply equally to any son born of leper parents whether or not the son ever demonstrates any sign or symptoms of leprosy himself. The intent of the Law is clear; remove any person presenting with this bacterium from participating in society economically, socially, legally, and physically.

To me and perhaps you too, this raises many legal and ethical questions found all too frequently throughout medical history as to the role of government, legal systems, organized religion, society at large, and professional medicine. What do you think?

Leprosy witnesses a distinct dramatic decline during the late Middle Ages. It is unlikely the decline is the result of segregation or termination of legal rights of lepers and their family but rather the appearance of another bacterium, Mycobacterium tuberculosis. Recall, TB kills at a much faster rate than leprosy. As the incidence of TB increases throughout Europe, the incidence of leprosy systematically decreases. Recent reports based upon retrospective DNA analyses reveal a high incidence of co-infections, during the Middle Ages of tuberculosis and leprosy (1995, 2005)[52,53].

The increasing role of government, in its attempt to regulate microorganism based infection, is further demonstrated by the British Parliament in 1161 AD, which pass laws to control and reduce the spread of Gonorrhea (Neisseria gonorrhea). One such law explicitly states "…no stew holder (bath house/brothel operator) shall keep any woman that hath the perilous infirmity of burning…" (1161AD/1717-1719)[54].

King Louis IX of France, following a failed 1254 AD attempt to eliminate the practice of prostitution, based more on religious grounds than public health issues, revises his decree in 1256 AD in response to great public protest and permits prostitution outside of the borders (bordes) of the city walls. Houses of prostitution since have been known as "bordellos".

No discussion of the Middle Ages and microbiology would be complete without addressing the role of the bacterium Serratia marcescens. Incorrectly referred to as a fungus in early medical writings, this bacteria finds itself central to the frequent intersection of microbiology and religion (1823,1849a,1849b,1848,1850,1851a,1851b,1903,1969)[55,56,57,58,59,60,61,62].

In brief, this bacterium grows readily in damp basements and on starchy foods. It appears pink to dark red in color, which fades within a couple of days upon exposure to sun light. Religious leaders, especially from the Christian based religions, have oftentimes interpreted the growth of the bacterium on communion wafers (starchy bread) as literally "…the blood of Christ…". Consistent with the Christian Church's views on transubstantiation, the periodic appearance of the bacterium on communion bread wafers, which are used in many Christian ceremonies, provides an impressive confirmation for believers. The Pope of the Catholic Church is so impressed by the appearance of the bacteria in 1263 AD, he officially declares the "bleeding bread" to be a miracle from God. The robes, communion plates, and garments from the 1263 AD event are housed today in the Vatican Museum.

Another 560 years pass before an Italian pharmacist Bartholomeo Bizio (1791-1862) challenges the religious (supranatural) explanation, replicates the "miracle" by experimentally growing the "bleeding bread" bacterium on polenta, demonstrating a physical (natural) explanation and viewing this bacterium for the first time under a microscope (1823,1827,1924)[63,64,65].

The Middle Ages end in much the same way as they began, struggling with an epidemic spread of the microscopic bacterium Yersinia pestis. This, the second bubonic plague, also known as the Great Mortality or the Black Death, again devastates the population of Europe. Death estimates are placed around 100,000,000 (sic) in Europe alone. The epidemic peaks during 1348 AD-1350 AD.

The economic, social, cultural, religious, and political impact micro-organisms and their resultant infectious diseases cannot be overestimated. For example, as the direct result of micro-organism based diseases, much of the population of Europe is devastated, not once but twice. Image the effects of eliminating almost the entire work force of any large geographic area e.g. country or continent. Middle Age life expectancy at birth is between 20-25 years. This reflects a substantial change in expected numbers of years a person is expected to live. Prior to the Middle Ages and during Antiquity the normal life expectancy is 65-70 years (1948,1975,1994)[66,67,68]. After the Middle Ages and currently in most modern industrialized countries today, the normal life expectancy is 75-80 years.

Very few resources are committed to the early universities and medical schools of Europe to study and better understand the origins, vectors of transmission, and treatments of micro-organism based diseases. Impaired physical health is interpreted dogmatically by the scientific and medical communities within a traditional Galenian balance of humors matrix and by organized religions simply as the "…will of God…" Both positions confident in their understanding actively suppress further development of medical microbiology.

In summary, the Middle Ages witness the fall of the Western Roman Empire and separation from the Eastern Roman Empire. Centralized seats of government throughout Europe fall and are replaced by local feudal systems. Scholarship moves from Europe to the Middle East where classical Greek and Roman medical knowledge is translated, critically analyzed, reconceptualized, and modified. Europe suffers two devastating micro-organism based epidemics, the First (Plague of Justinian) and Second (Black Death) bubonic plagues. Yersinia pestis changes the face of Europe politically, economically, culturally, and socially. Natural (physical) explanations for disease are reinterpreted by popular organized religions, Judaism, Christianity, and Islam which provide supranatural (deity) based models to explain disease and illness.

Few resources are devoted to understanding microorganisms and associated disease although the microorganisms devastate the regions for centuries. Science and medical communities understand disease within dogmatic Galenian natural (physical) balance models, whereas organized religions understand disease within dogmatic faith based supranatural (deity) models. No need to understand further what is already known to be true. Right? Parasitic, fungal, bacterial, and viral diseases are common, widespread, and often result in death. Dysentery, tuberculosis, plague, and smallpox are among the most common killers.

Specifically, Paulus of Aegina systematically describes signs, symptoms, and treatments for many common micro-organism based infections in his influential encyclopedia, "Medical Compendium in Seven Books". Abu Ibn al-Razi offers his "Comprehensive Book on Medicine" and Ibn Sina offers his "Canon of Medicine", both from the Persian perspective. All three highly influential works offer little new knowledge and reflect essentially a restatement of knowledge previously reported in the Hippocratic Collections, works of Aristotle, Galen, and others. Science and medicine conceptualized disease within a natural (physical) balance model. Organized religions become influential in the practice of medicine and offer faith based, supranatural (deity) models, within which to understand disease. The Roman Catholic Church utilizes a monesterial system throughout Europe to offer care and comfort to people affected by micro-organism based disease e.g. Saint Anthony's Fire, leprosy. The same monesterial system is utilized to translate the written record of medicine into the language of the Church, Latin. Government and organized religions cooperate and become tremendously influential in the management of infectious disease, generating numerous laws, regulations, and decrees. Micro-organism based disease kill hundreds of million people and produce devastating economic, social, and political impact. The expected life expectancy plummets from 65 years during Antiquity to 25 years during the Middle Ages. Few resources are devoted to the advancement of microbiology at the newly founded universities or medical schools throughout Europe. The debate between natural (physical) and supranatural (deity) based explanations of disease is unresolved. Authoritative, dogmatic positions from both science and religion impede significant process in the advancement of medical microbiology.

The Middle Ages offer medical microbiology a rich history with few advancements.

Early Modern, 1400 AD - 1800 AD.

The Early Modern period witnesses renewed interests and associated advances in medical microbiology. Improved technologies e.g. the invention of the microscope and a growing dissatisfaction with the inadequacies of accepted theories to explain human disease and treatments, drive medical microbiology forward as a scientific discipline. New technologies provide access through direct observations to a previously "invisible" microscopic world. Scientists are now able to observe and study the "invisible" entities suspected to be responsible for disease. New conceptual matrixes are proposed to explain disease and old matrixes are revised in light of new knowledge. These are truly exciting times for medical microbiology.

Girolamo Fracastoro (1478-1553) Italian physician, scholar, and supporter of the atomist position proposes disease to be a natural (physical) condition and caused by transfer of tiny particles he terms "spores" (1546)[69]. The specifics of his theory are detailed in "De contagione et contagiosis morbis et curatione" [Contagions, contagious diseases, and treatments] published first in 1546. Fracastoro proposes contagions ("spores") are the primary cause of disease and can be transferred from person to person by three primary vectors; immediate contact (true contagion); intermediate agents such as formites; or simply through the air. He offers his theory as a plausible explanation to explain epidemic disease. The theory is noteworthy, yet not entirely original. Similar "seed" theories are proposed previously during Antiquity and the Middle Ages.

Fracastoro's conceptual matrix of "spores" as primary contributors to human disease and vector of transmission between people is developed and proposed as Germ theory, over 300 years later in 1835. As with many, his theory as an early conceptual model later to be termed Germ Theory, is not readily accepted during his lifetime and will see three hundred years before conformation by French microbiologist Louis Pasteur (1822-1895) and German bacteriologist Robert Koch (1843-1910). The more popular theories of disease at the time are Miasma theory, based upon bad air (natural) cause of disease and faith-based deity models (supranatural) causes of disease, which propose disease is the result of an angered God.

Athanasius Kircher (1601-1680) German Jesuit scholar is first to report "little worms" can be seen in vinegar and milk. Kircher views microorganisms on a screen, using a modified projection system termed a magic lantern (1646)[70]. Thirteen years later upon viewing blood of patients suffering the plague in Rome, he concludes disease can be caused by "invisible" microorganisms (1658)[71]. It is noteworthy to recognize Kircher's report appears 37 years before the more celebrated and perhaps more recognizable Antonie van Leeuwenhoek reports his microscopic observations of "invisible animals" (1676/1677)[72]. OK, given the magnification power of Kircher's instrument, Althanasius Kircher most likely sees blood cells rather than the bacteria Yersinia Pestis responsible for the plague; however his observations guide him to a correct conclusion; microscopic organisms are associated with human disease. Van Leeuwenhoek fails to make this association. An important point and one often overlooked in most histories of medicine.

Marchamont Needham (1620-1678) British pamphleteer offers the first English publication on the subject of bacteriology; provides an English translation of Kircher's Scrutinum Pestis; details Kircher's microscopic experiments which associate microorganisms with human disease; and attacks the dogmatic wisdom and authority of the (Royal) College of Physicians. He accomplishes this in his most influential work "Medela medicinae: A plea for the free profession and a renovation of the art of physicks out of the noblest and most authentick writers. Shewing the publick advantage of its liberty. The disadvantage that comes to the publick by any sort of physicians imposing upon the studies and practice of others. The alteration of diseases from their old state and condition. The causes of that alteration. The insufficiency and uselessness of mere scholastick methods and medicines, with a necessity of new. Tending to the rescue of mankind from the tyranny of diseases and of physicians themselves from the pedantism of old authors and present dictators" (sic) (1664)[73]. Now that is a book title!

Needham deplores the scientific and medical communities' reliance upon ancient authorities in medicine. He argues to move beyond the conceptual matrixes and prescribed treatments of Hippocrates, Aristotle, and Galen. He calls for new conceptual matrixes, new methods, and new medical treatments. Needham argues physicians should move towards more chemistry based treatment plans and away from the common practices of bloodletting. He believes physicians should contribute to the advancement of new knowledge through critical analyses of the existing knowledge base, utilizing thoughtful reasoning and scientific experimentation. No practicing physician should accept medical knowledge as dogma. He calls upon physicians and scientists to stop the worship of ancient medical authorities and embrace the new.

As you might reasonably expect, Needham's book and ideas meet with an immediate response from the established guard within the medical community. Robert Sprackling (1611-1670) a member of the established (Royal) College of Physicians, responds to Needham with "Medela Ignorantiae: or a just and plain vindication of Hippocrates and Galen from the groundless imputations of M. N. wherein the whole substance of his illiterate plea titled "Medela Medicinae" is occasionally considered" (1665)[74]. So begins another debate of "new school vs. old school".

Trivia: During the plague epidemics e.g. Great Plague of London (1665-1666), treating physicians often wear a "bird's beak" on their nose, containing a perfumed sponge, based upon the belief that smells (miasmas) are the cause of infectious disease.

Robert Hooke (1635-1703) English natural philosopher utilizes recently developed technologies, more specifically the microscope and revolutionizes the study of infectious disease. His major work "Micrographia" (1665)[75] is the first publication devoted entirely to microscopic observations and provides detailed descriptions of microorganisms. "Micrographia" is the first major publication of The Royal Society of London for Improving Natural Knowledge.

The Royal Society as it is more commonly referred is a learned society established for the discussion of scientific research and related topics. The Society founded in 1660 and continues today reflecting over 358 years of continuous operation. The Society acts as the UK's Academy of Sciences. The Society's motto "Nullius in verba" [Take nobody's word for it] reflects succinctly the general scientific skepticism and sentiment of its members throughout history. The Society's journal is "Philosophical Transactions" and represents the oldest and longest running scientific publication in the world. Archived publications can be found online, free of charge, dating to the first issue published in 1665 (2011)[76].

Hooke is first to report the physical structure of the fungus mold Mucor, based upon microscopic observations (chapter in "Micrographia"). He coins the now familiar term "cell" to describe the physical appearance of his microscopic observations of biological tissue. There is no evidence in his writings Hooke ever recognizes or reports the cell to be the principal organization of biological tissues, as frequently and incorrectly reported in both popular and medical literature. Recognition and report of this now fundamental statement within biology will not appear until the published works of Czech physiologist Jan Purkinje, German physiologist Theodor Schwann, German botanist Matthais Schleidnen, and French physiologist Henri Dutrochet circa 1835.

Note: Recently in January 2006, a previously unknown text written by Robert Hooke containing 650 pages of excerpts from the Royal Society's Journal Books 1661-1677 and rough minutes of the Society's meetings 1677-1691, recorded by Hooke as Society Secretary are discovered. The text and images provide new insights and perspectives into the Society's activities, research areas, topics of discussion, internal politics, and heated professional rivalries. Scanned copies of Hooke's handwritten notes, typed transcriptions, and images collectively referred to as "The Hooke Folio" are now available online (2011)[77].

No discussion of medical microbiology is complete without considering the enormous impact new technologies bring. In the case of medical microbiology, few technologies have greater importance in moving the discipline forward, during the Early Modern period, than the light microscope.

Antonie van Leeuwenhoek (1632-1721) neither a physician or scientist by education or training but rather a successful drapery business owner in Amsterdam and textile inspector offers the medical and scientific communities their first reports and microscopic descriptions of bacteria (1676/1677)[72]. He follows the initial reports with the first microscopic report of the pear-shaped protozoan parasite Giardia duodenalis (1681)[78]. Van Leeuwenhoek makes his reports through an intermediary, physician Reiner de Graaf, to the Royal Society of London. Given van Leeuwenhoek is neither a physician nor scientist he is not permitted to submit reports directly to the Royal Society. Similar restrictions prohibit direct submissions by women.

Van Leeuwenhoek's initial reports demonstrating the potential of the microscope as a new and valuable tool for medicine and science are well received by the Society (1673)[79]. However, with his submission describing single cell micro-organisms three years later quickly sours the Society's enthusiasm (1676)[72]. The report directly challenges Society dogma regarding the foundation of life. Recall, single cell organism where unknown to science and medicine at that time. Van Leeuwenhoek integrity and his work are soon questioned by the Society. An official review committee is dispatched to review his work and evaluate whether he is "…of sound mind…". The Committee confirms van Leeuwenhoek's work and mental stability, thereby beginning the necessary process of re-evaluating scientific, medical, and religious dogma regarding the core foundations of life.

Giovanni Bonomo (1663-1699) Italian physician adds another piece to the puzzle in understanding the role of parasites, fungi, bacteria, and viruses in human infectious disease. Specifically, his most significant contribution is made in letters to his professor Francesco Redi, in which he reports his "…observations concerning the flesh worms of the human body...", introducing a theory of parasitic infectious disease, describing modes of transmission, and offers drawings of the mite, which he makes from his microscopic observations. The contribution finds its importance in the history of medicine in that it unlike all previous descriptions of the mite and its well established association with itching, identifies the mite Saroptes scabies as the source of the highly contagious skin disease (1687,1703,1928)[80,81,82].

Previous reports of scabies are made by Moses, as found in the Christian Bible, Book of Leviticus, circa 1200 BC (n.d.)[83]; Aristotle's report on "...lice in the flesh...", concluding lice are born from sweat by way of spontaneous generation (circa 350 BC/1883)[84]; Roman physician Aulus Celsus whom coins the term "scabies" and describes the disease's clinical presentation and recommended treatments in a chapter devoted to the topic in "De Medicina" (circa 30 AD/1478)[20,21]; all recognize the disease, report common signs and symptoms and recommend treatments. All of these early reports fail to recognize the mites are responsible for the disease. It is not until 1687 does Bonomo report the cause of scabies. It is the scabies mite itself, rather than the mites being the resultant product of the disease, as commonly believed (1687,1928)[80,82].

Bonomo's letters and Redi's subsequent book discussing the issue quickly draws the attention of organized religion. The Pope and his medical advisers denounce Bonomo's evidence of a natural (physical) cause for the disease. Church dogma is clear as to the supranatural cause of disease. Bonomo chooses not to challenge the powerful and influential institutions of organized religion, based in part on the known consequences of doing so as clearly exemplified by the disagreement between Galileo (1564-1642) and the Church in 1615. Organized religion suppresses Bonomo's conclusions of a natural (physical) cause of disease and further delays the progress in medical microbiology. Here lies another example of organized religion's influence upon the content and process of professional science.

Trivia: The term "scabies" is derived from the Latin word "scabere" meaning "to scratch".

Carl Linnaeus (1707-1778) Swedish biologist publishes a 12 page booklet proposing a nested hierarchical structured classification system of nature; kingdoms. classes, orders, genera, species, and ranks (1735)[85]. Groupings are based upon observation of shared physical characteristics. Linnaeus' taxonomy begins with the now familiar three kingdoms; animal, plant, mineral. The original taxonomy proceeds systematically in providing finer discriminations between subgroups classes and orders. Finding the complete, formal name cumbersome, Linnaeus soon replaces the complete formal name with a more informal, binomial format, introduced in his 10th edition of "Systema Naturae" (1758)[86]. The binomial (two name) shorthand defines the species. For a modern example consider the familiar bacterium E. coli. It is found in the Kingdom: Bacteraia; Phylum: Proteobacteria; Class: Gamma Protrobacteria; Order: Enterobacteriales; Family: Enterobacteriaceae; Genus: Escherichia; Specie: Escherichia coli. Applying the informal binomial shorthand, today we refer to this bacterium simply as E. coli. The system soon gains popularity and provides the beginning of standardized nomenclature improving communication within a rapidly growing international scientific community.

The Linnaeus taxonomy has largely been displaced today by newer classification and taxonomy systems governed by international nomenclature codes e.g. International Code of Nomenclature of Bacteria (ICNB) (1992)[87], International Committee on Taxonomy of Viruses (ICTV) (2005)[88]. However, the popular binomial format of Linnaeus continues to be popular today, over 260 years after its introduction in 1758; e.g. the bacterium; Escherichia coli.

Marcus Plenciz (1705-1786) Italian physician challenges medical dogma and claims the existence of a causal relationship between microorganisms and infectious disease; the material of infectious substances are alive; infectious substances are capable of multiplying within the human body;

variability in clinical signs and symptoms accompanying infection can be explained by variability in incubation times; each microorganism is responsible for a specific disease; nothing else other than microorganisms can cause disease; and transmission of infectious disease can be accomplished through air (1762)[89]. Certainly bold statements given the current level of knowledge. Plenciz's conceptualizations are facilitated by new technologies (microscope), an openness to alternative conceptual matrixes beyond existing medical, scientific, and religious dogma, an application of the scientific-experimental method, and a refreshing willingness to bare the burden of consequence suffered by many whenever proposing innovative ideas challenging the status quo.

The Early Modern period ends making little progress in the debate between the scientific community and the organized religion community as to the etiological basis of disease and illness. The scientific community argues dogmatically the cause of disease and illness is physical, natural, and follows the laws physics. The organized religion community argues equally dogmatically the cause of disease and illness is supranatural, deity based, and follows faith based beliefs recorded in the major guiding text of each religious group e.g. Torah, Bible, and Qur'an. Both positions delay advancements in the knowledge base of medical microbiology.

In summary, the Early Modern period (1400 AD-1800 AD) witness renewed enthusiasm and excited interest in old and new models to explain human disease based upon "invisible" micro-organisms. Invention and rapid development of new technologies, including the microscope provide the necessary tools to observe the "invisible" world of microbiology unlike any before. Single cell living organisms are observed for the first time. Observed micro-organisms are quickly associated with human disease. Vectors of disease transmission begin to be understood within the matrix of microscopic pathogens. Human disease etiologies, transmission, clinical presentations, and treatments are reconceptualized by the scientific community and begin to be understood within the matrix of specific microorganisms. Medical dogma established by revered medical icons Hippocrates, Aristotle, and Galen, in place for over 1500 years, is openly challenged. The Royal Society is founded in London and the Society's journal "Philosophical Transactions" begins publication providing a new scholarly forum to discuss the rapidly developing new scientific knowledge base. Classification systems are introduced to organize the rapidly growing knowledge base of microorganisms. Standardized nomenclature is introduced to facilitate communications among investigators and medical practitioners. Philosophical battles regarding the true etiology of human disease and illness continue to be fought between the scientific community advocating a physical natural etiology and powerful, organized religion communities advocating a faith based, deity, supranatural etiology. As true throughout time, the powerful influence of organized religion and its influences upon the content and process of science further delay scientific advances. However, medical microbiology quickly establishes itself as a valued and rapidly developing scientific discipline with immediate applications for all practicing physicians.

Middle Modern, 1800 AD - 1900 AD.

The Middle Modern period witnesses tremendous growth in medical microbiology.

New and improve technologies permit observations of microbes previously unseen. The microscope and microscopic techniques are refined and result in much improved imaging. Microbe staining techniques are introduced making the identification and description of microbes easier. Microscope photography is introduced into medical microbiology offering another important format for the sharing and exchange of information between investigators.

Long held conceptual matrixes used to understand life and disease are displaced by overwhelming experimentally generated scientific data. Models of spontaneous generation (life resulting from non-living matter e.g. flies from putrid matter, mice from dirty hay, crocodiles from rotting logs) and heterogenesis (one form of life is derived from another form of life e.g. bees from flowers) are displaced by models of biogenesis (living things come from other living things). Germ theory is introduced and its basic tenant microscopic organisms can and do cause disease displaces miasma theory as primary in the physical cause of human disease. Medical diagnostic procedures and treatment interventions are modified to accommodate the new knowledge.

New professional societies and academic journals devoted specifically to microbiology and its application to human disease are founded. Rapid progress is made in understanding the interactive relationships between parasites, fungi, bacteria, viruses, and human disease. New classification systems are proposed and integrated to organize the rapidly accumulating base of new information. Medical microbiology matures from its earliest beginnings founded in general biology and establishes itself as a new and focused discipline with immediate value in understanding and treating human disease.

Fungi are studied aggressively and understood within the matrix of potential cause of human disease. The term "mycology", derived from the Greek meaning "fungus", is introduced into the scientific and medical literatures to describe a distinctly new branch of medical microbiology. Fungi are established to exist in three distinct forms; mold, spores, and yeast. Their life cycles are described and understood within the context of disease. Fungi are recognized to absorb nutrients from both living organic and non-living organics substances. This fundamental recognition, supported by new experimental data, challenges the current understanding of fungi. Fungi are associated with commonly occurring and specific medical conditions e.g. tinea (ringworm). Remember, ringworm is a fungal infection not a worm infection. Much attention is devoted to fungi and human disease especially during the early-1800s. Interests in fungi slow by the mid-1800s as a rapidly growing interest in bacteria and its association with human disease becomes the newest and latest area of discovery.

Bacteria replace fungi as the primary focus of investigation by the mid-1800s and are aggressively studied for the balance of the century. Bacteria are understood within the recently proposed matrix of Germ theory and associated with human disease. Vectors of bacteria transmission are identified. Specific bacteria are associated with specific diseases e.g. anthrax, tuberculosis, cholera, gonorrhea, and bubonic plague. Bacteria reproduction and virulence are manipulated experimentally with exposure to extreme temperatures and chemicals. Bacteria are studied in vivo and in vitro. New technologies, now familiar to every medical student, are invented to assist in the study of bacteria e.g. auger gels, Petri dish, and Gram staining. Microscope resolutions improve. The term "bacterium" is introduced into the scientific and medical literatures. Bacteria are classified into groupings based upon physical shapes and understood as a special form of life within the animal and plant kingdoms.

Viruses are discovered by the late-1800s and proposed to be causal in human diseases. Viral replication is demonstrated to be dependent upon cells and begins to be understood within the context of human disease. Viruses are identified as a new group of pathogens and different from the three more familiar established pathogens of the period, parasites, fungi, and bacteria.

Microbes are uniformly accepted within the scientific and medical communities as potential causes of human disease and poor physical health. Criteria are introduced and accepted by the scientific and medical communities which establish a causal relationship between a microbe and a disease. Microbes are also recognized by some and less uniformly by the scientific and medical communities to be equally important in maintaining good physical health.

Let us now briefly examine some of the specific events, influential people, and contributions during the 1800s which have impacted medical microbiology then and now. We will also examine a few heated professional debates regarding priority of discovery, professional rivalries, and dispel a few popular myths.

Alfred Donne (1801-1878) French bacteriologist, public health physician, and microscopist demonstrates the presence of parasite organism Trichomonas vaginalis in vaginal secretions of Parisian prostitutes (1836)[90]. Six years later he reports his discover and description of platelets in blood (1842)[91]. Perhaps much less known to many, he invents the photoelectric microscope with assistant student Leon Fourcault (1819-1869) and is among the first to apply photography to microscopic preparations (1845)[92].

Johann Schonlein (1793-1864) German naturalist is among the first to recognize the etiological role of fungi in generating infectious disease in humans. He is first to provide drawings made from microscopic observations of the fungus he recognizes to be responsible for ringworm (aka tinea) (1839)[93]. Building upon the works of the Italian farmer/lawyer Agostino Bassi (1773-1856) in which Bassi successfully identifies fungus as the microorganism responsible for an infectious disease effecting silkworms (1835)[94], Schonlein is first to demonstrate fungus to be the etiological cause of an infectious disease in humans (1839)[93]. The specific fungus identified by Schonlein is soon termed Achorion schonleinii, in his honor. The fungus is later renamed and recognized today as Trichophyton schoenleinni.

You may recognize Schonlein's name from your medical pathology course. He is perhaps most recognized today for the syndrome typically appearing in children, often following an infection (often pharyngitis), which results in a systemic inflammation of blood vessels, deposition of immune complexes in the kidneys and joints, and characterized by joint and abdominal pains and palpable small hemorrhages in the skin (purpura); Schonlein-Henoch purpura.

David Gruby (1810-1898) Hungarian microbiologist completes similar investigations into infectious disease in humans generated by fungi. He too independently identifies the fungus responsible for ringworm, recognizes it to be an infectious agent, describes its microscopic properties, and is instrumental in establishing medical mycology as a distinct branch of medicine (1841)[95]. Gruby is first to report the fungal basis of thrush in children (Candida albicans), a common and poorly understood condition of the period (1842)[96].

The works of Bassi, Schonlein, and Gruby, during the mid-1830s and early-1840s, trigger a hopeful excitement within the medical communities. There is now a clearly identifiable, natural (physical), previously invisible etiology, linked to infectious human disease. New technology (e.g. microscope) provides the technology to study the "invisible" microorganism now recognized to be causal in infectious disease. In the excitement many human diseases are immediately and oftentimes incorrectly attributed to a mycotic etiology e.g. cholera, tuberculosis. Recall, bacteria has yet to be identified and associated with specific human disease. Another 40 years will pass before Koch demonstrates convincingly cholera and tuberculosis are not produced by fungi but rather bacteria. Much attention is devoted to the study of mycology during the early-1800s with particular applications to the practice of medicine. The foundations of modern medical mycology are securely in place by the mid-1800s.

Ignaz Semmelweis (1818-1865) Hungarian obstetrician catalyzes a fundamental change in the conceptual matrix within which physicians understand disease. Semmelweis investigates disease as the product of a single and specific physical cause. His method is largely dependent upon clinical observation, logic, and statistical reasoning. Applying his method, Semmelweis identifies medical personnel and their medical instruments as primary vectors of transmission of infectious disease. Unpopular and unaccepted by the established medical community during his lifetime, Semmelweis' work provides much of the foundation for preventative medicine routinely practiced today.

For perspective, recognize Semmelweis offers his investigational work and conclusions during a period in which medical dogma clearly identifies the natural (physical), causes of disease to be understood within the matrix of two popular theories, miasma and contagions. Remember miasma theory simply states disease is caused by invisible particles suspended in "bad air" and contagion theory simply states disease is caused by direct contact with another person who suffers from the same disease. Germ theory has not been accepted by the medical community and only recently proposed by German histologist Jakob Henle (1838,1840)[97,98].

Semmelweis is struck by the inability of the two most popular and accepted theories of the period to reasonably explain his clinical observations. In brief, he observes a large number of young, healthy women dying within days to two weeks following the birth of their babies. All of the women suffer childbed fever (puerperal fever) with signs and symptom onset appearing within days of their deliveries. This in and of itself is unremarkable given many women of the period died following childbirth and often the death is associated with childbed fever. What is remarkable is Semmelweis' observation of much higher mortality rates of women when attended at the medical teaching hospital clinic compared to a non-teaching hospital clinic. This simple observation stimulates a series of investigations which will revolutionize medical microbiology.

Note: Childbed fever (puerperal fever) is derived from the Latin word "puerperal" meaning "bearing a child". The fever results from a beta hemolytic, Group A streptococcus infection, typically contracted by women within days after giving birth, characterized by infection of the placenta and uterus, and which can progress into a fatal septicemia if left untreated.

Semmelweis completes a series of studies over a period of five consecutive years (1841-1846) investigating reasonable and potential causes which might explain the differences in mortality rates between the two facilities (1847,1848,1861)[99,100,101]. He systematically evaluates such variables as delivery techniques, diet, inadequate ventilation, overcrowding, terrestrial influences, cosmic influences, weather conditions, month of the year, religious preferences, assorted psychological factors, and behavior of patients and clinic personnel. All of these variables are reasonable within the conceptual of models of disease popular during the period (1845,1849, 1857)[102,103,104].

Findings reveal an approximate two to five time higher mortality rate associated with childbed fever occurring in the teaching hospital clinic when compared to the non-teaching hospital clinic. Semmelweis identifies the single most likely cause to be attributed to the behavior of physicians and medical students within the teaching hospital clinic. Medical students are identified to be the primary vector of transmission. When in doubt, blame the medical student. Right? In this case the blame is correctly placed and justified. Medical students at the teaching hospital's clinic routinely participate in autopsies of women, whom have recently died from childbed fever. Frequently the medical students will leave the autopsy to deliver a baby in the clinic. Unaware they are transmitting the microorganism responsible for childbed fever from the autopsy suite to the clinic; they attend to the unsuspecting mother, infecting her with the bacteria which Semmelweis simply refers to as "cadaver particles". Recall, bacteria have yet to be identified as causal agents in infectious disease.

Based upon his findings, Semmelweis implements the practice of removing the "cadaver particles" by washing the hands of medical students and other clinic personal in an antibacterial mixture of chlorinated soap before attending to any expectant mother. The mortality rates associated with childbed fever now plummets in the teaching hospital clinic where the hand washing procedure is implemented. Years later he implements the procedure to include washing medical instruments in the same antibacterial mixture of chlorinated soap.

The contributions of Semmelweis while often inflammatory, unsupported during his lifetime, and seldom or never referenced subsequently by Louis Pasteur, Robert Koch, or Joseph Lister, prove significant in the early development of germ theory. Semmelweis' contributions guide the conceptual matrix of the modern understanding of disease from a simple listing of clinical signs and symptoms and associated pathological anatomical findings to the conceptual matrix of single cause - single disease model so familiar in medicine today. To be sure, Semmelweis makes significant contributions to medical microbiology. His contributions have been distorted with time; deserve recognition, and more unbiased placement within the broad context of the history of medicine.

Let us now correct some incorrect information, regarding Semmelweis' contributions, frequently appearing in the popular literature and increasingly so in the professional medical literature.

First, Semmelweis does not introduce "hand washing" to the practice of medicine, to control infectious disease. Hand washing is routinely used in medical care facilities as a component of more general efforts to improve cleanliness and hygiene decades before Semmelweis begins his landmark study series. Semmelweis is first to unequivocally demonstrate the value of combining the bactericide chlorine to the existing practice of using soap and water alone.

Second, contrary to much written in the popular literature, Semmelweis is not first to identify medical personnel as potential and frequent vectors of transmission of infectious disease. Medical personnel have long been known to be potential vectors of infectious disease transmission. For example, over fifty years before Semmelweis proposes the transmission of "cadaver particles" by medical students to their patients as causal in producing childbed fever, Alexander Gordon (1752-1799) Scottish obstetrician writes "…the cause of this disease (childbed fever) was a specific contagion, or infection, I have unquestionable proof…The disease seized such women only as were visited, or delivered by a practitioner…or nurse who has previously attended patients afflicted with the disease. It is a disagreeable declaration for me to mention that I was myself the means of carrying the infection to a great number of women..." (1795a,1795b)[105,106]. Oliver Wendell Holmes (1809-1894) American physician weighs in on the topic also before Semmelweis, publishes an essay which summarize 20 cases of childbed fever, noting "…puerperal fever is so far contagious as to be frequently carried from patient to patient by physicians and nurses…" (1843)[107].

Third, contrary to much written in the popular literature, Semmelweis is not responsible for providing early descriptions of the clinical presentation of childbed fever. The clinical signs and symptoms of childbed fever are documented in the medical literature at least as early as the Hippocratic Collections circa 400 BC. Clinical and autopsy descriptions of childbed fever and medical treatment recommendations are plentiful and readily found throughout the early-1800s. These works predate the work of Semmelweis. For example and extracted from the medical literature as written during the early and mid-1800s, case reports detail the clinical presentation and autopsy findings of women suffering childbed fever. She is "…seized with a rigor, or shivering fit, which was succeeded by a great degree of heat, often terminating in profuse perspiration, and severe pain in the abdomen. The pain had no complete intermission…the melancholy scene was usually closed in a few days…" (1815)[108]. Autopsy findings reveal "...the omentum had lost about half its substance by suppuration…there was about half a pint of pus…in the abdomen..." (1822)[109]. Recommended treatments emphasizes "…fresh air, clean linen, and avoiding tight bindings of the uterus and breasts…" (1849)[103].

Fourth, contrary to much written in the popular literature, Semmelweis does not identify the specific microorganism responsible for childbed fever. This falls to Carl Mayrhofer (1837-1882) Austrian physician, working in the same clinics as Semmelweis and approximately 13 years after Semmelweis leaves the clinic in Vienna to return to his homeland of Hungary. Mayrhofer reports his microscopic observations of "vibrions" in the uterine discharges of patients suffering childbed fever and attributes these microorganisms to be causal in the disease (1863,1865)[110,111]. Others elsewhere later identify the specific bacterium (Streptococcus pyogenes) as the beta hemolytic, Gram positive, non-motile, non-spore forming, catalase negative, opportunistic facultative anaerobe, group A streptococcus, we understand the bacterium to be today.

Trivia: Carl Mayrhofer is hired in 1862 as an assistant to Semmelweis' successor, Carl Braun (1822-1891) Austrian obstetrician, in the clinics at Vienna General Hospital. He is hired specifically to generate research in support of Carl Braun's opposition position to Semmelweis research, claiming an iatrogenic base to the spread of childbed fever. Braun is among the many incensed by the claims of Semmelweis that physicians could in any way be responsible for infecting young mothers with this potentially fatal disease (1852)[112]. Mayrhofer initially publishes several papers in support of Braun's position. Within a short period of time and by 1865 Mayrhofer reconsiders his position, agrees with Semmelweis, publishes a paper and is immediately fired (1865)[113]. So goes the consequences of publically disagreeing with those whom pay your salary.

Having attempted to bring some light on four common and frequently reported misunderstandings of Semmelweis' contributions, let me as succinctly as possible place his true contributions in historical perspective. His contributions are not to be found in specifics but rather in the much broader matrix of his methods; recognition of a problem by way of clinical observations (more women are dying at the teaching hospital than at the non-teaching hospital clinics); thoughtful conceptualization of likely casual factors based upon existing models of disease (e.g. miasmas theory: surrounding terrains and clinic ventilation), openness to alternative models of disease (recently proposed germ theory); willingness to systematically evaluate each of the most likely causal factors applying a combination of both logical and statistical reasoning (longitudinal and repeated measurement research designs with appropriate statistics; publication of his findings for peer review; and application of his finding to change well established medical procedures to improve the clinical outcome of his patients (washing of hands and instruments with bactericides).

Application of a rational approach to medicine, in the epistemological sense, and moving from a well-established system which organizes diseases based upon clinical signs and symptoms to a new system, which organizes diseases based upon universal necessary cause (microorganisms), is the value of Semmelweis' most significant contributions.

As with many throughout the history of medicine who dare challenge medical dogma and provide empirical findings in support of their position, Semmelweis is met with resistance during his lifetime. The true value of his contributions is not realized until after his death. His work proves instrumental in development of germ theory and largely unacknowledged by those most immediately associated with germ theory, during the mid and late-1800s, Louis Pasteur and Robert Koch.

By the mid-1800s experimental research provides sufficiently persuasive data that miasma and contagion based models of disease are being displaced by Germ theory. Fungi research popular during the early-1800s gives way to bacteria research. Investigations provide overwhelming data which challenge the concepts of spontaneous generation and heterogenesis and supports biogenesis. The way scientists and physicians understand the fundamentals of life are changing. The second half of the 1800s is devoted almost in its entirety to the investigation of bacteria and their associations with disease.

Casimir Davaine (1812-1882) French physician and Pierre Rayer (1793-1867) French dermatologist discover the anthrax bacillus in blood of dying animals, representing the first bacteria associated with septicemia (1850)[114]. No accident the first bacterium discovered is one of the largest.

Louis Pasteur (1822-1895) French microbiologist is perhaps most remembered by uninitiated medical students as first to propose fermentation to be a biological process (caused by microorganism) rather than a chemical process (1857)[115]; first to propose spoilage of food and beverages can be prevented by heating (pasteurization) (1865)[116]; first to propose Germ theory as a conceptual matrix to explain disease (1878,1880)[117]; and first to create vaccines to impart immunity against specific bacteria e.g. anthrax (1878)[118], cholera (1880a,1880b,1880c)[119,120,121] and viruses e.g. rabies (1885)[122]. These are among the many claims frequently reported in the popular literature. However, these claims are not supported by the published medical literature or written historical record. These and other claims made by Pasteur himself or attributed to Pasteur by others are by many reasonable accounts exaggerations and blatant misrepresentations of the factual truths (1883,1904,1912,1923,1942)[123,124,125,126,127]. Here too are found examples and great lessons in professional ethics and behavior whenever engaged in the practice of professional medicine.

Louis Pasteur certainly makes significant contributions to the advancement of medical microbiology. However, priority for which Pasteur claims discovery or for which others have assigned priority to Pasteur might more correctly be assigned to other investigators.

Priority for understanding fermentation to be a biological process mediated by microorganisms and not simply a chemical process is more correctly assigned to Theodor Schwann (1810-1882) German physiologist (1837)[128] and Antonie Bechamp (1816-1908) French biologist whom details the process at least 35 years before Pasteur's first paper on the subject.

Priority for recognizing spoilage of foods and beverages can be significantly delayed by heating (pasteurization) is more correctly assigned to Nicolas Appert (1749-1841) French chef and confectioner. Appert successfully answers the 1795 challenge of Napoleon Bonaparte, who offers 12,000 francs to anyone who can devise a technique to sterilize food and extend its time before spoilage. Appert demonstrates food and beverages spoilage times can be extended by sealing the food or beverage in a glass jar, then placing the jar in boiling water. He publishes his findings in "The Art of Preserving Animal and Vegetable Substances" (1810)[129]. Although Appert is permitted to claim the cash award, immediately he is prohibited from publishing his findings due to the strategic importance of the discovery to the ongoing military campaigns of Napoleon. Appert's book describing the process appears 55 years before Pasteur applies the process to wines and claims priority (1810,1865)[129,116].

Priority for the development of Germ theory might more correctly be assigned to Girolamo. Francastri 300 years before Pasteur (1546), Marcus Plenciz 100 years before Pasteur (1762), or Jakob Henle (1840) 22 years before Pasteur publishes his first paper on the topic (1862). Priority for early vaccines against cholera, anthrax, and rabies might more correctly be assigned to Emile Roux (1853-1933) French immunologist and close colleague of Pasteur rather than Pasteur himself.

To be sure, assignment of priority for any major scientific discovery to only one person is difficult. The process of discovery is in and of itself is a group process. The final assignments is often based upon intra and inter institutional politics, effective self and institution assisted promotion, and decisions made within governing professional societies, rather than the individual efforts of any single person. So true is the case with many of Pasteur's discoveries. He devotes as much energy to self-promotion as to investigational research. As with others before him, for example Hippocrates and Galen, if you publish a lot, claim priority for discoveries whether justified or not, with time those who actually make the discoveries will be lost in the memories of time. Only the well published and promoted will be most remembered. So is the history of medicine.

Ferdinand Cohn (1828-1898) German biologist brings order and a popular classification system to bacteria. He organizes bacteria into four primary groupings based upon shape: Sphaero-bacteria (spherical or rounded), Micro-bacteria (short rods or cylinders), Desmo-bacteria (long rods or threads), and Spiro-bacteria (spirals or screws). He publishes the system in his landmark three volume treaties "Researches on Bacteria" (1875)[130]. Systems which classify bacteria based upon shape continue to be used today. At the time of Cohn's research, bacteria are considered by many to be animals, based upon their apparent voluntary movements and activity, while others consider bacteria to be plants. His research proves instrumental in establishing bacteria as a separate group of living organisms, different from plants and animals (1872a,1872b/1881)[131,132]. Cohn is not particularly interested in the study of bacteria associated diseases as are Pasteur and Koch. However he does complete seminal research demonstrating most bacteria can be destroyed with heat, while a small number remain insensitive to heat and can survive following high heat exposure. Hummm....who do you think quickly claims priority for this discovery?

Robert Koch (1843-1910) German bacteriologist and past student of Henle describes bacteria responsible for several devastating diseases of the period e.g. Bacillus anthrax (1876)[133], Tuberculosis bacillus (1882)[134], and Vibrio cholera (1884)[135]. He modifies original criteria used to identify specific microbes as causal in producing a specific disease, proposed 44 years earlier by his major professor Jakob Henle (1884)[136]. These four modified criteria will become known simply as Koch's postulates and continue to be used for the next 125 years with minimal modifications. In brief and in essence the 1884 criteria are as follows: If a specific microorganism is to be identified as responsible for causing a specific disease it should: 1) be found in abundance in each case of the disease; 2) not be found in other diseases; 3) when inoculated into a healthy animal the animal should reveal the specific disease; and 4) be recovered from the inoculated animal and re-grown in pure culture. Robert Koch further develops and extends the use of microscopic medical photography as part of his investigations into microbes responsible for disease (1877)[137]

Koch and Pasteur are contemporaries and both provide research in support of Germ theory models of disease, Pasteur representing the French academic institutions' positions and Koch representing the German academic institutions' positions. Pasteur and Koch are extremely competitive investigators. My personal review of the literature reveals Pasteur to be more of a self-promoter while Koch a more careful scientific investigator. Koch too is not beyond self-promotion or claiming priority for discoveries made by others. On balance with Pasteur, he appears to be a more careful scientist, more sophisticated in the politics of professional science, and less brazen in claiming priority for discoveries made by others. Koch is awarded the Nobel Prize in Physiology or Medicine "...for his investigational discoveries in relation to tuberculosis..." (1906)[138].

Trivia: Before Robert Koch describes the bacillus Vibrio cholera in 1884, the bacillus has already been identified and described in detail by Italian anatomist Filippo Pacini (1812-1883), 30 years earlier (1854)[139]. Perhaps you might recognize Pacini from your medical school's neuroscience course. Pacini discovers the small sensory organs at the end of peripheral nerves, which detect vibration and pressure sensations from the skin. These sensory receptor organs are the Pacinian corpuscles (1835,1840)[140,141]. The term "Pacini's corpuscle" is coined not by Pacini, but rather Jakob Henle (1844)[142]. Recall, Jakob Henle proposes the criteria, which will later be known as the Koch's postulates, 44 years before being proposed by Koch. Are these additional examples, in the history of medicine, of misassigned priority for significant professional contributions? You decide.

Charles Sedillot (1848-1892) French surgeon brings uniformity to the terminology of recently identified and rapidly growing list of pathogenic microorganisms. During the 1870s and 1880s microorganisms are being described by different investigators, using a wide range of terms to describe the same microorganism. The variability in terms, as in any new and developing discipline is characteristic of a maturing discipline, leads to unnecessary confusion in communication between investigators from different academic institutions, different countries, and different theoretical models. The terms microzoaria, microphyta, microgerms, germs, vibrios, protista, and infusoria are all used to refer to pathogenic microorganisms.

The term "microbes" is suggested by Sedillot and proposed during a lively discussion between advocates of the terms microzoaria and microphyta at the 1878 annual meeting of the Paris Academy of Sciences. The term is free from implications as to whether the small living beings are plants or animals (topic under discussion), soon gains acceptance among French investigators and helps to standardize communication (1878)[143]. German and English investigators are less accepting initially of the term and the term does not find its way into these literatures on a regular basis for another five years. The term "microbe" is derived from the Greek "micro" meaning small. The term is still used today.

Albert Neisser (1855-1916) German bacteriologist identifies the microbe responsible for gonorrhea (1879)[144]. This Gram negative, coffee bean shaped, diplococci bacteria, Neisseria gonorrhea, recall is transmitted by sexual contact. Perhaps unknown to many medical students, Neisser plays an instrumental role in identification of the bacterium responsible for leprosy. The same year he publishes his work identifying the bacterium responsible for gonorrhea he travels to Norway and collects samples from 100 patients suffering leprosy. He returns with the samples to Germany where he identifies the bacilli and publishes his findings (1880)[145]. The paper immediately generates a heated dispute regarding priority between Neisser and Norwegian bacteriologist Gerhard Hansen (1841-1912).

You might recall from your pathology course the term Hansen disease as an alternative name for the chronic infectious disease caused by Mycobacterium leprae and characterized by granulomatous lesions of the skin, mucous membranes, bones, and peripheral nerves (1874)[146]. The professional debate between Neisser and Hansen regarding priority for discovery consumes much of both men's remaining careers (1880,1881)[147,148]. Today, following a retrospective analysis of available information, many agree, Hansen is first to identify the leprosy bacillus (Mycobacterium leprae), while Neisser is first to identify it as the causal agent of the disease leprosy (1955)[149]. Another valuable lesson here in professional ethics and behavior.

Trivia: Gonorrhea today is informally referred to as "the clap". The informal term is derived from the French word "clapoir", a term referring to a sexual sore and "clapier" a "brothel" where one is likely to acquire the clapoir.

Investigators refine existing technologies in efforts to move medical microbiology forward. Three notable refinements occur during the early-1880s and are recognizable to all medical students today. Agar gels replace liquid solutions as media for growing bacteria. The Petri dish is introduced and becomes the preferred glass vessel for growing bacteria. Ziehl-Neelsen and Gram stains are introduced, permitting improved microscopic inspection and new classification of bacteria.

Walther Hess (1846-1911) German pathologist, with much assistance from his wife and while working in the laboratory of Robert Koch in Germany, discovers the value of adding agar to the gels of media used to grow bacteria cultures. The techniques eliminates the need to use liquid solutions, offers a medium not easily degraded by microorganisms, and provides a more flexible medium upon which to grow cultured strains of bacteria (circa 1881). Agar gels provide a stable medium upon which to grow bacteria and change microbiology forever.

Julius Petri (1852-1921) German bacteriologist invents the Petri dish while working as an assistant to Robert Koch soon after the laboratory begins using the agar gels discovered by another Koch assistant Walther Hess (circa 1887). The "Petri Plate", a glass dish containing culture media with a slightly larger glass lid to cover the bottom dish, proves to be simpler and more reliable than the bell jar system used before Petri introduces his dish.

Hans Christian Gram (1853-1938) Danish scientist develops the staining technique still used today which differentiates bacteria into two large groups, Gram positive and Gram negative, based upon properties of the bacterium's cell wall (1884)[150].

Franz Ziehl (1859-1926) German neurologist and Friedrich Neelsen (1854-1898) German pathologist introduce their special stains for acid-fast microorganisms. Recall, acid fast microorganisms are resistant to Gram and standard hematoxylin and eosin (H+E) staining (1882)[151]. The Ziehl-Neelsen proves particularly important in medical microbiology in that it is responsible for identifying the acid fast fungus Mycobacterium tuberculosis responsible for the disease tuberculosis (1882,1883a,1883b)[151,152,153] and the acid fast bacteria Mycobacterium leprae responsible for leprosy.

Trivia: The compound term "Ziehl-Neelsen" stain first appears in the literature in the fourth edition of Edgar Crookshank's textbook on bacteriology, while both Ziehl and Neelsen have published independently their acid fast staining methods for more than ten years prior to the term "Ziehl-Neelsen" entering the literature (1896)[154].

Richard Pfeiffer (1858-1945) German bacteriologist recognizes a heat stable toxin bound to the membrane of the bacterium Vibrio cholerae and which is only released after the cell walls are disintegrated. He terms this new material "endotoxin" to distinguish it from toxic materials released from healthy bacteria (1894)[155]. His discovery provides another important piece to the puzzle in understanding bacteria and their potential to produce illness and disease.

Alexandre Yersin (1863-1943) Swiss bacteriologist, long time investigator at Louis Pasteur's research laboratories and close collaborator with French immunologist Emile Roux, identifies rod-shaped, Gram positive, bacterium responsible for the bubonic plague and the bacterium's primary vector of transmission, fleas carried by rats (1894)[156]. Yersin originally refers to the bacterium simply as "…bacille de la peste…". The bacterium is assigned different names during the next 100 years e.g. "Pasteurlla pestis" in recognition of Pasteur Laboratories. The bacterium today is known simply as "Yersinia pestis" in recognition of Yersin's many contributions to the discipline of bacteriology (1944)[157].

Prior to the identification of the bacterium responsible for the plague, Yersin contributes to the development of the anti-rabies serum, completed at the Pasteur Laboratories, during the mid-1880s; investigates tuberculosis, during the late-1880s; studies briefly with Robert Koch in Germany, and returns to the Pasteur Institute in Paris, where he and Emile Roux report their discovery of an antitoxin, capable of neutralizing the toxic poisons released by the bacterium responsible for diphtheria (Corynebacterium diptheriae) in 1889.

Subsequent to Yersin's identification of the "…bacilli de la peste…", Yersin leaves France for Vietnam to manufacture and dispense one of the first anti-plague scrums. He remains in Vietnam until his death and is instrumental in the founding of the Medical School of Hanoi.

Yersin's discovery of the "bacilli de la peste" is not without controversy.

In brief, Shibasaburo Kitasato (1853-1931) Japanese bacteriologist also claims priority for the discovery of the bacterium responsible for the bubonic plague and identification of its primary vector of transmission, while investigating the plague epidemic in Hong Kong, during the same time as Yersin (1894). Kitasato represents the German schools of investigation having studied with Robert Koch and Emil von Behring and contributing substantially to the development of an understanding of the medical microbiology of tetanus, diphtheria, anthrax, and tuberculosis, during the late-1800s. Alexandre Yersin represents the French schools of investigation having studied with Emile Roux and Albert Calmette (BCG vaccine fame) at the Pasteur Institute and contributing substantially to the development of an understanding of medical microbiology of rabies, diphtheria, and tuberculosis, during the late-1800s. Both investigators are dispatched by their respective institutions, during the summer of 1894, to Hong Kong for the purpose of investigating the current plague epidemic sweeping across the region of southern China. Both investigators within days of arriving in Hong Kong summit papers for publication claiming identification and description the bacterium found in blood of plague victims and causal for bubonic plague (1894a,1894b,1884a,1884b)[158,159,160,161].

My own personal translation and review of both original papers reveals sufficient evidence to reasonably assign priority of discovery to Yersin. Both investigators do observe the bacterium responsible for producing the plague at approximately the same time, while Yersin is more successful in isolating the bacterium from others. Yersin applies more careful methods and is more cautious with his findings. More importantly than retrospective analysis of priority for discovery, demonstration of fierce competition between research institutes and investigators, or national pride, is the identification of the microbe responsible for the deaths of millions.

Throughout the mid to late-1800s there is great competition between the French and German bacteriologists. The French are most represented by Louis Pasteur and his followers while the German are most represented by Robert Koch and his followers. Both groups are tenacious in their scientific methods, brutal in their professional science politics, and make substantial contributions which significantly advance the field of medical microbiology at an unprecedented rate.

Before the end of the 1800s a new microscopic pathogen is discovered and opens new lines of investigations to complement ongoing investigations of parasites, fungi, and bacteria causal in producing human disease. The virus.

Martinus Beijerinck (1851-1931) Dutch microbiologist recognizes a new infectious agent smaller than a bacterium and terms the new pathogen "virus" (1898)[162]. He is unable to culture the agent, however observes the agent can replicate and multiply in living tissues and produce disease. Beijernick opens doors for new areas of investigation with his discovery of the new infectious agent. Medical microbiology no longer limits itself to the investigation of parasites, fungi, and bacteria. Medical microbiology is never again the same.

Trivia: Beijernick use of the term "virus" is actually a reintroduction of the term with a new meaning. The term is derived from the Latin "virus" meaning "poison" and usually associated with the poisonous sap of plants. The term along with its original meaning of poison and other noxious substances is first introduced into English circa 1392 AD (2011)[163]. The term as we use it today, a distinct pathogen, can reasonably be attributed to Beijernick

As the 1800s come to a close, professional academic organizations and associated academic journals are founded, reflecting the growing interests in medical microbiology and maturation of the discipline. The first meeting of the Society of American Bacteriologists is held at Yale, December 27, 1899 and publishes its first abstracts in "Science" (1900)[164]. Here is a sampling of topics discussed at the first meeting; "Generic nomenclature of bacteria" by Erwin Smith; "Natural varieties of bacteria" by H.W. Conn; "Methods employed in the teaching of bacteriology" by H.C. Ernst; and "A new pathogenic fungus - the sporothrix of Schenck" by L. Hektoen. The Society's objectives are stated simply "...the promotion of the science of bacteriology, bringing together of American bacteriologists, the demonstration and discussion of bacteriological methods and the consideration of subjects of common interest..." (1899)[165]. The Society soon establishes and begins publication of its official journal in 1916, the "Journal of Bacteriology". The Journal remains the official journal of the Society and continues publication today, over 100 years later. In keeping with the broad interests of its members and to more accurately reflect its membership, the Society is renamed the American Society of Microbiology in December of 1960. Starting with an initial membership of 60, the Society today maintains over 43,000 members, representing true international collections of scientists and ideas from around the world. No longer restricted to bacteria the Society represents much more diverse areas of interests of medical microbiology.

In sum, the Middle Modern period (1800-1900) witness tremendous advances in medical microbiology as a scientific discipline. Fungi are aggressively investigated and associated with specific human diseases. Mycology establishes itself as a respected sub-discipline within medical microbiology. Fundamental shifts in the conceptual matrix within which the very basic origin of life is understood appear during the early-1800s, in the presence of extensive scientific generated data. Models of spontaneous generation and heterogenic origins of new life give way to models built upon biogenesis. Similarly, long held models of disease, miasma theory and contagion theory give way to the newly proposed models of germ theory. By the mid-1800s bacteria displace fungi as the primary focus of investigations. Bacteria are quickly identified and associated with specific human disease and illnesses. Classification of bacteria based upon physical characteristics e.g. cocci, rods and staining properties e.g. Gram positive, Gram negative, acid fast, provide a new system within which to understand human disease. Previously, human diseases are frequently organized according to clinical signs and systems. With the recognition of specific bacteria producing specific disease, human disease is now organized according to the underlying microorganism producing the disease e.g. Gram positive cocci. The new classification system additionally provides guidance for specific pharmacological treatments directed toward the destruction of the specific disease causing bacteria. By the late-1800s a new pathogen is identified which in addition to parasites, fungi, and bacteria cause disease in humans, the virus.

Medical microbiology matures as a scientific academic discipline with clinical relevant and immediate applications of methodologies, technologies, and content knowledge to the practicing physician. New professional societies and academic journals appear devoted specifically to the understanding and promoting the advancement of scientific knowledge pertaining to microorganisms responsible for human disease. Standardization of vocabulary appears within the discipline and facilitates communication between investigators and practicing physicians. New training programs and modifications in medical school curriculum are introduced to provide investigators and future practicing physicians the necessary knowledge to better understand, diagnose, and successfully treat human disease and illness.

Specifically, ringworm is recognized to result from a fungus; microscopic parasites are observed in vaginal secretions of Parisian prostitutes by the same investigator first to discover and describe blood platelets; photography is introduced into microbiology; thrush appearing in children is recognized to result from a fungus; tuberculosis and cholera believed to result from fungi are recognized to result from bacteria; childbed fever triggers a series of landmark hospital based investigations which utilize novel integrated research methodologies and provide a model for hospital based investigations still used today over 150 years later; medical personnel are recognized as potential vectors of transmission of disease causing microbes; the first bacteria producing septicemia are identified; Germ theory is proposed and soon displaces miasmas and contagion theories as most responsible for human disease; fermentation is identified as a biological rather than chemical process; pasteurization as a process of heating foods and beverages to delay spoilage is introduced and demonstrated over 65 years before Louis Pasteur claims priority for its discovery; it is recognized most bacteria can be destroyed by heat; specific criteria are established which must be uniformly satisfied before a specific microorganism is recognized as causing a specific human disease; the term "microbe" is introduced into the scientific literature avoiding the hotly debated issue of the period as to whether microorganisms are best understood and classified as plants or animals; the bacterium responsible for gonorrhea is identified by the same investigator instrumental in the identification of the bacterium responsible for leprosy; agar gels replace liquid solutions as media for growing bacteria; the Petri dish is introduced and becomes an essential laboratory glass wear of all who investigate bacteria; Ziehl-Neelsen and Gram introduce their stains and provide a new method to identify and classify disease causing bacteria; endotoxins are recognized; the bacterium responsible and vector of transmission are identified for the bubonic plague; a new microscopic pathogen is first identified and termed virus; and heated professional battles regarding claims of priority of discovery often overshadow the value of the discoveries themselves.

Medical microbiology is now well established as a valued academic professional discipline with clinical relevance to the practicing physician and medical patient.

Late Modern, 1900 AD - 2000 AD.

The Late Modern period witnesses the continued development and maturation of medical microbiology as a professional discipline.

The first half of the 1900s continues with investigations of bacteria and the recently discovered virus as causal pathogens of human disease. Vectors of transmissions are discovered and described; interactions between bacteria and viruses are detailed for the first time; virology is defined as a distinct area of scientific investigation; the electron microscope is invented; and the first prototypical antibiotics are released by medical pharmaceutical companies.

The first decade 1900-1910 focuses attention upon understanding insect vectors and their roles in transmitting disease. Particular attention is directed to the mosquito's transmission of the virus responsible for yellow fever, the tick's transmission of the bacterium responsible for Rocky Mountain spotted fever, the louse's transmission of the bacterium responsible for typhus fever (not to be confused with typhoid fever) and the reduviid (kissing) bug's transmission of the parasitic protozoa responsible for Chagas disease.

The second decade 1910-1920 further expands investigations of viruses and attempts to better understand their roles as pathogens of human disease. Particular attention is directed to understanding the roles of viruses in cancers. Viruses are recognized to invade bacteria and the role of the bacteria is understood within the matrix of viral sustainability and replication. The bacteriophage is discovered, described, and understood within the matrix of human disease. By the end of the decade the world is engulfed in a worldwide viral epidemic. The virus underlying the epidemic effects only humans and results in the estimated deaths of millions worldwide.

The next three decades 1920-1950 witness the establishment of virology as a separate area of study distinct from bacteriology; the life cycle of a virus is described; the electron microscope is invented; electron microscopy produces images of bacteria and viruses at 200,000 - 300,000x magnification available by light microscopy; aggressive programmatic investigations of chemotherapies are completed which focus upon the identification and development of medications capable of destroying numerous microscopic pathogens; medical pharmaceutical companies aggressively compete for market shares; and two prototypical antibiotics are introduced to the market, penicillin effective against Gram positive bacteria and streptomycin effective against Gram negative bacteria.

The second half of the 1900s is devoted largely to the investigations of disease causing parasites, fungi, bacteria, and viruses, at the molecular level. Attention is focused upon understanding genetic material and its role in human disease. By the end of the 1900s human genetic material is manipulated and often with the assistance of viruses. Specific human diseases are understood within the matrix of retroviruses both as causal e.g. AIDS and therapeutic e.g. SCIDS. Advances in technology e.g. polymerase chain reaction (PCR) and other molecular based procedures open the doors for rapid expansion of medical microbiology laboratories providing essential, timely, and cost effective information to practicing physicians regarding the nature of the underlying causes of a patient's medical condition. Prions are identified as a new and previously unrecognized pathogen. Rapid diagnostic testing technologies become more sophisticated, less expensive, and more available to the practicing physician.

Let us now briefly examine some of the specific events, influential people, and contributions, during the 1900s which have impacted medical microbiology.

Walter Reed (1851-1902) American military physician and bacteriologist is perhaps most recognized by medical students from the military hospital in Washington, D.C. which bears his name, Walter Reed Army Medical Center. His contributions to medical microbiology are perhaps less known and come at the end of his life when he is assigned to administratively head a military board, charged with the investigation of tropical diseases in Cuba. Prior to Reed's investigations of tropical diseases, he spends most of his military career stationed on U.S. Army outposts in the American western frontier. His reassignment is initiated as the result of thousands of United States military personnel stationed in Cuba contracting yellow fever. The infection of military personnel devastates U.S. military forces, during the Spanish-American War (April 21,1898 - August 13, 1898).

Recall, the U.S.S. Maine mysteriously explodes in Havana harbor on February 15, 1898 and kills 266 sailors. This event occurs during Cuba's War of Independence from Spain. In response, U.S. president William McKinley concedes to popular opinion pressures and declares war on Spain in retaliation and in support of Cuba. The United States direct military involvement in the Cuban War of Independence lasts approximately 10 weeks (Spanish-American War). The U.S. military occupying force in Cuba are quickly devastated by yellow fever and necessitates their withdrawal. More U.S. military die from yellow fever during this period than from combat.

Walter Reed and members of the U.S. Army Yellow Fever Commission in Cuba under his administrative direction quickly identify the mosquito as the vector of transmission of yellow fever. Prior to the Commission's celebrated findings, medical dogma considers yellow fever to be transmitted from person to person by contagions via formites e.g. contaminated beddings and clothing. Reed receives much credit for the discovery of the mosquito vector, not because he or the Commission actually identify the vector, but as the product of a very effective political-military information campaign which assigns discovery to Reed and the Commission (1900,1901)[166,167].

Carlos Finlay (1833-1915) Cuban medical investigator is first to identify the mosquito as the vector of transmission for yellow fever. Finlay and his research group identify, describe, detail, and report the mosquito vector over 20 years before Reed is ever assigned to investigate the issue (1881a,1881b)[168,169]. Finlay and his group, in addition to identifying the mosquito as the vector of yellow fever, identify the specific mosquito (Aedes aegypti) responsible for transmission of the "fever", and recognize the spread of yellow fever can be controlled by simply controlling the mosquito vector (1881a,1881b,1901)[168,169,170]. Yes, the U.S. Army Yellow Fever Commission in

Cuba, aka the Reed Commission, discovers in 1900 that which is already discovered, 20 years earlier in Cuba; yellow fever is transmitted by a mosquito vector and the disease can be controlled by controlling the vector.

Trivia: Yellow fever is an acute viral hemorrhagic disease resulting from an enveloped RNA virus (Flaviviridae) transmitted my female mosquitoes. The "flavus" is derived from the Latin meaning "yellow". The term "yellow fever" is descriptive of the clinical sign of jaundice, characteristic of the disease.

Howard Ricketts (1871-1910) American bacteriologist is instrumental in identifying the microorganism and vector of transmission of Rocky Mountain spotted fever (a form of typhus fever). Ricketts, as a young professor is funded by the McCormick Memorial Institute and the State of Montana to investigate the etiology of a relatively low base rate disease, Rocky Mountain fever. The disease at the time of funding is responsible for only a dozen deaths a year in the United States (1902). However, the mortality rate for the disease is close to 90%. At the time of funding there is a cluster of high incidence of the disease appearing in a wealthy and influential community in the Bitter Root Valley of Hamilton, Montana. Well-funded, Howard Ricketts and Josiah Moore (1886-1964) biology undergraduate student at Montana State University soon identify the microorganism responsible for producing the disease (later termed Rickettsia rickettsii) and the vector of transmission, the wood tick (Dermacentor occidentalis) (1906,1909)[171,172]. A year later, Ricketts identifies the microorganism and vector of transmission responsible for typhus fever while investigating the typhus epidemic in Mexico City (1910a,1910b)[173,174].

The genus Rickettsia, characterized by the non-motile, Gram negative, non-spore forming, highly pleomorphic bacteria responsible for Rocky Mountain spotted fever and typhus is named in honor of Ricketts' significant contributions towards understanding the microorganism and after his death (1916)[175]. Remember, Howard Ricketts and Rickettsias have nothing to do with rickets, the softening of bones in children due to a vitamin D deficiency.

Note: Rocky Mountain spotted fever (RMSF) is the most lethal and most frequently reported rickettsial infection in the USA. The name is misleading. Rocky Mountain spotted fever occurs throughout many other regions of the United States, Canada, Mexico, Central America, and South America.

Carlos Chagas (1879-1934) Brazilian bacteriologist discovers Chagas disease (aka American trypanosomiasis). Recall from your pathology course, Chagas disease is a tropical disease caused by the parasitic flagellate protozoan Trypanosoma cruzi and transmitted most commonly by the "kissing bug" (insect vector). Chagas details the new infectious disease, its pathogen, its vector of transmission, clinical signs and symptoms, and epidemiology (1909a,1909b,1910)[176,177,178]. This is no trivial accomplishment. He sequences the disease from vector to clinical presentation. The insect vector-disease paradigm is still used today over 100 years later. Chagas names the parasite "Trypanosoma cruzi". The terms "trypano" and "soma" are derived from the Greek meaning "borer" and "body" and describe the corkscrew movement of the protozoa observed by Chagas. The additional term "cruzi" completes the name and is coined by Chagas in honor of his friend and colleague Brazilian bacteriologist Oswaldo Cruz (1872-1917), founder of the Oswald Cruz Biomedical Research Institute located in Rio de Janeiro and where Chagas is employed.

The works of Finlay, Reed, Ricketts, and Chagas represent a distinct line of investigations in medical microbiology. All four investigate protozoa or other complex microorganism which require an intermediary host to complete their life cycle and require a vector of transmission different from the mechanical vectors of transmission of bacteria or viruses. Similar works completed by Charles Laveran (1845-1922) French physician identification of the malaria Plasmodium parasites (1880a,1880b)[179,180]; Ronald Ross (1857-1932) British physician identification of the malaria mosquito vector (1899)[181]; William Leishman (1865-1926) Scottish pathologist and Charles Donovan (1863-1951) Indian-Irish physician identification of the protozoan parasite transmitted through the bite of female sand fleas (1903,1903,1903)[182,183,184]; Charles Nicole (1866-1936) French bacteriologist identification of human body lice as vector of transmission of epidemic typhus (aka jail fever, ship fever, camp fever) (1909)[185]; and Piraja da Silva (1873-1961) Brazilian parasitologist and Robert Leiper (1881-1969) British helminthologist identification of the life cycle of parasitic fluke Schistosoma (1908,1915,1916)[186,187,188], represent additional investigations occurring at approximately the same time and significantly contribute to this line of investigation.

Trivia: The word "mosquito" is derived from the Latin meaning "little gnat". The term "Schistosoma" is derived from the Greek meaning "split body" reflecting the physical appearance of this fluke.

To put this body of work into perspective, the insect vector-disease model provides the necessary scientific data to understand and thereby control an entire category of devastating human diseases. Control of these diseases is essential in completing major infrastructure building projects in various regions of the world. Building the Panama Canal is only possible after yellow fever and malaria are controlled (1904-1914). Recall, construction of the Panama Canal is initiated by the French (1881-1889) following their success with the construction of the Suez Canal. The Panama Canal, although only half the length of the Suez Canal is abandoned following debilitating high numbers of deaths and illness associated with insect vector diseases e.g. malaria. Estimates of approximately 22,000 workers die during the initial French construction. The Canal's successful construction led by the United States resumes in 1904 and only after the microbiology underlying insect-vector diseases is understood. Arguably, without an understanding of insect-disease vectors, this and other infrastructure constructions may never have been completed. Consequently, the knowledge and understanding of insect-vector disease plays an important role in geo-economical and geopolitical landscape of the modern world.

The importance of these collective works into insect vectors and disease is quickly recognized by the scientific community. Several of the principle investigators are nominated for or are awarded the newly established Nobel Prize in Physiology or Medicine. Specifically, Ronald Ross is awarded the Nobel Prize in Physiology or Medicine " …for his work on malaria, by which he has shown how it enters the organism and thereby has laid the foundation for successful research on this disease and methods of combating it…" (1902)[189]; Charles Laveran is awarded the Nobel Prize in Physiology or Medicine "…in recognition of his work on the role played by protozoa in causing disease…" (1907)[190]; and Charles Nicole is awarded the Nobel Prize in Physiology or Medicine "…for his work on typhus…" (1928)[191]. Carlos Finlay is nominated seven times (1905, 1906, 1907, 1912, 1913, 1914, and 1915) and Carlos Chagas is nominated two times (1913,1921) yet neither ever receive the Nobel Prize (2011)[192]. Do you have any ideas why? Politics within the communities of professional science and medicine? Nationality biases? Ruthless competitiveness from rival investigators? You decide.

Francois Rous (1879-1970) American virologist is first to recognize and report the role of viruses in the transmission of cancer (1911)[193]. Forty year later he is awarded the Nobel Prize in Physiology or Medicine "…for his discovery of tumour-inducing viruses…" (1966) [194].

Many investigators are focusing on the identification and description of specific microbes responsible for specific diseases, while others focus their attention instead upon identification and development of effective treatments against these newly described microbes.

Paul Ehrlich (1854-1915) German immunologist recognizes specific microbial pathogens bind specific chemical structures. Ehrlich proposes pharmacological treatments can be delivered and targeted to specific microbial pathogens, utilizing the pathogens' inherent affinity to specific chemical structures (1898,1900)[195,196]. Schachiro Hata (1873-1938) Japanese bacteriologist, while working in the laboratory of Paul Ehrlich, successfully demonstrates the effectiveness of the delivery approach and produces an effective treatment against the spirochete responsible for syphilis (1910,1913)[197,198]. The compound is an organoaresenic compound, also known by the trade name Salvarsan or by its original compound number "606" assigned in Ehrlich's lab.

Salvarsan offers the first new and effective treatment against the bacteria responsible for syphilis in 70 years. The compound is expensive, difficult to prepare, difficult to distribute, difficult to administer (usually injected), required weekly administrations over the course of a year or more, and produces many toxic side effects e.g. rashes, liver damage, and reactions requiring limb amputations (1915)[199].

Medical treatments prior to the introduction Salvarsan are limited. Although syphilis has affected patients for thousands of years the medical dogma of the time is to treat the sexually transmitted infection with either mercury or potassium iodide (1915,1918)[199,200]. Both are administered topically, orally, rectally, or by injection. The mercury treatments prove much more effective than potassium iodide, however it produces many more serious and oftentimes life threatening side effects. The often repeated adage, "…spend one night with Venus and then spend the rest of your life with Mercury…", has its roots in the medical treatment of syphilis.

Salvarsan is slow to be accepted by the medical community yet it and its second generation modified compound Neo-salvarsan prove to be the standard treatment until both are displaced by penicillin approximately 35 years later.

Salvarsan's place in the history of medicine is not so much in its effectiveness in treating syphilis but rather in that it represents one of the first synthetic compounds derived from an understanding of biochemistry and a clear conceptual matrix which successfully guides the delivery of a specific chemical to a specific pathogen, resulting in the destruction of the pathogen, while permitting the host to survive. Notice this is a distinctively different approach towards infectious disease. This approach does not use the body's immune system to effect a therapeutic result as in immunization; rather it introduces a synthetic compound of chemicals, which in effect poison the pathogen.

Paul Ehrlich's successful approach applied to the treatment of bacteria stimulates a flurry of investigations during the next 40 years which focus upon the discovery of the next chemical compound effective in destroying other disease producing bacteria. Welcome the discovery of the corporate scientist. Academic investigators are quickly introduced to the large financial rewards available in commercial medicine, particularly in the area of synthetic pharmaceuticals. Paul

Ehrlich's scientific knowledge coupled with his business acumen provides an impressive model for the aspiring commercial scientist.

Trivia: Paul Ehrlich coins the term "chemotherapy" during his address at the opening of the George Speyer Haus Biomedical Research Institute, Frankfurt, Germany. He first offers the term within the context of a mission statement for the Research Institute; "…curing organisms infected by certain parasites in such a way that the parasites are exterminated within the living organism… not by the use of protective substances produced by the organism itself through a process of immunization, but by substances which have had their origin in the chemist's retort…" (1906)[201].

As Ehrlich and others aggressively pursue investigations and commercialization of therapies based upon immunizations capitalizing upon the normal response of a patient's own immune system (aka serum theories) and chemotherapies capitalizing upon the chemical affinities of specific chemicals to specific pathogens, during the early-1900s, an innovative alternative treatment approach emerges. The use of bacteria and viruses to treat bacterial and viral diseases.

Frederick Twort (1877-1950) English bacteriologist and Felix d'Herelle (1873-1949) Canadian microbiologist discover the "bacteriophage" (1915,1917)[202,203]. Recall, bacteriophages are viruses which infect and can destroy bacteria. The discovery is embroiled in heated disputes of priority for many years and frequent topic of debate at professional meetings for decades (1921,1921)[204, 205]. The issue for some remains unresolved today, over 95 years later. Independent of the dispute for priority of discovery, the discovery itself offers medical microbiology an essential component in understanding infectious disease and an innovative approach to treatment.

Medical microbiology is tested by nature once again in 1918. The world experiences an influenza pandemic, which results in an estimated death toll between 50 and 100 million people. Most affected are young healthy adults rather than the elderly, children, or immunocompromised. The pandemic is defined by the 2.5 year period June 1918 to December 1920. The viral infections abruptly stop, perhaps as the result of a mutation of the virus to a less lethal strain. The 1918 virus pandemic has tremendous economic, social, political, and religious impact. The impact is similar major bacterial and viral epidemics of the past e.g. Plague of Athens (431 BC-404 BC; Rickettsia prowazekii, Yersinia pestis, variola), Plague of Justinian (541-542 AD; Yersinia pestis); bubonic plague (1347 AD-1353 AD, Yersinia pestis). As with past epidemics and pandemics, medicine has little to offer beyond palliative care and symptom relief.

Thomas Rivers (1888-1962) American bacteriologist and virologist challenges scientific dogma in the same address in which he reports his observations and defines the fundamental nature of all viruses. Eloquently stated, before the newly founded Society of American Bacteriologists, "…In all fields of work, times come when one must stop and take thought. New facts, new ideas, and new suggestions alter lines of endeavor in every field of research. We are here today for the purpose of taking thought…". Thomas continues the address and reports his observations which revolutionize the way in viruses are conceptualized. He states "…Viruses appear to be obligate parasites in the sense that their reproduction is dependent upon living cells…" (1926,1927)[206,207].

Prior to Rivers' bold statement, viruses are simply understood as a filterable agent. Stated differently, prior to Rivers' statement, a virus is defined and understood as an infectious agent which passes through a fine porcelain filter, which holds back bacteria. Rivers' observations are challenged by many established investigators of the period, including Simon Flexner (1863-1946), director of the powerful Rockefeller Institute. Flexner recently claims to have isolated and cultured the polio virus in a cell-free medium. Rivers stands firm and is later proven correct.

Thomas Rivers provides medical microbiology with the critical observations which opens the door to a new and specialized area of scientific investigations, virology, as a distinct and independent area of investigation from bacteriology (1928)[208] .

You might be thinking…hummm…Flexner….didn't he produce the famous Flexner Report which radically reformed medical education in the United States and Canada (1910)[209] ? Close. The Flexner Report is written by Simon Flexner's younger brother, Abraham Flexner (1866-1959) a non-physician, public educator, and ardent critic of the American medical education system.

The investigation of viruses attracts much attention during the early-1900s. The unique characteristics of the virus which distinguishes it from bacteria are detailed. The virus is understood within the matrix of a potential disease producing pathogen and a potential treatment agent. As virology established itself as a new and valued sub-discipline of medical microbiology, investigations of bacteria continue.

Albert Calmette (1863-1933) and Camille Guerin (1872-1961) French bacteriologists, working in the Pasteur Institute in Lillie, introduce a living non-virulent strain of tuberculosis sufficiently safe to be used in the immunization of humans against the disease, the bacillus Calmette-Guerin (BCG) vaccine (1920,1921,1957)[210,211,212]. This is one of the first relatively safe and effective prophylactic interventions against tuberculosis. The vaccine is slow to be accepted by the medical community. Today, over 98 years since its introduction, the BCG vaccine continues to be used in many countries throughout the world.

Notice the difference in the fundamental approach of Calmette and Guerin which utilize the body's innate immune system to generate antibodies against tuberculosis bacteria (vaccination) and the alternative approach popularized by Paul Ehrlich and others which utilize antibiotic pharmaceuticals to attack bacteria directly. Both approaches prove effective in the management of bacterial infections and provide the foundational base for investigations throughout the balance of the 1900s.

Alexander Fleming (1881-1955) Scottish biologist and perhaps most recognized by medical students from childhood stories identifying him as the man whom discovers penicillin from mold growing on an old slice of bread. Actually, he never discovers penicillin. That's right. Alexander Fleming does not discover penicillin nor is he first to recognize the bactericidal properties of molds. Fleming also is frequently credited with the discovery of the enzyme lysozyme. Fleming does not discover lysozyme either. Here lies another case of priority assigned incorrectly and perpetuated by popular myths. As future physicians, you are entitled to an alternative truth supported by historical records.

First, the issue of the lysozyme. Recall, a lysozyme is simply a particular enzyme that catalyzes a biochemical reaction (hydrolysis), in the mesh like layer outside the plasma membrane of bacteria cell walls (peptidoglycans), resulting in destabilization and ultimately lysis of the bacteria's cell wall. Don't confuse lysozyme with lysosomes, which are the membrane bound organelles found inside of many cells. Lysozymes are enzymes, found in abundance in body secretions such as tears, saliva, and mucus. Before Fleming coins the term "lysozyme", demonstrates its presence in nasal mucus, or claims priority of discovery many less familiar investigators have already identified, described, and detailed the enzyme as well as its bactericidal properties (1907,1919, 1922,1922)[213,214,215,216].

Second, the issue of penicillin. The name Alexander Fleming will always be linked to the discovery of penicillin. However, there is more to the story. Fleming more correctly "rediscovers" penicillin (1929)[217]. Thirty-five years before Fleming's first paper on the topic, Ernest Duchesne (1874-1912) a 23 year old, French medical student, becomes fascinated by molds which kill bacteria. Unconfirmed medical history lore tells of Duchesne first observing stable boys keeping saddles in a darkened moist area of the stables, in order to grow mold on the saddles. The mold provides a natural treatment against infections generated by saddles rubbing against the horses. Independent of any confirmation of the authenticity of this frequently repeated story, Duchesne does complete a series of carefully designed and executed experiments investigating the relationship between molds and their potential use to kill bacteria. The experiment series and his rational are detailed in his medical school thesis titled "Contribution à l'étude de la concurrence vitale chez les micro-organismes: antagonisme entre les moisissures et les microbes" [Contribution to the study of vital competition in micro-organisms: antagonism between fungi and microbes] (1897)[218].

Specifically, Duchesne's thesis can be reduced to two fundamental questions. Is the competition for survival recognized among man, animals, and plants present among micro-organisms? Can micro-organisms or substances produced by micro-organisms used to insure their natural survival be used as potential treatments against other disease producing micro-organisms? More specifically, Duchesne investigates the response of the bacteria Escherichia coli and Salmonella typhi to the exposure of the fungus Penicillum glaucum. Duchesne investigations generate a wealth of new information. He scientifically demonstrates the bactericidal properties of fungus and additionally demonstrates the systemic bactericidal effects when a penicillum compound is injected into animals (1897)[218]. Duchese reports his findings over three decades before Fleming's begins his first investigations and claims priority of discovery of penicillin.

Alexander Fleming, while often failing to recognize contributions of others, readily accepting priority for discoveries made by others, and never missing an opportunity to perpetuate the penicillin myth, he does contribute to the advancement of medical microbiology. Fleming offers many investigations and discussions of antiseptics and their potential for use in clinical medicine.

Recall, antiseptics are antimicrobial agents used for topical use only, usually due to high toxicity. While Alexander Fleming does not discover the lysozyme, he does make contributions which advance the scientific understanding of the lysozyme. His publications and other document records reveal he is a keen observer and a financially successful corporate scientist. Alexander Fleming establishes and maintains a financially lucrative agreement with Park, Davis, and Company (pharmaceutical company), supplying prepared vaccines, serums, and antitoxins, for over 30 years.

Returning briefly to the issue of penicillin, all available written information e.g. publications, letters, notes, and correspondences, indicate Fleming initially fails to appreciate the significance of his observations regarding Penicillum's antibacterial properties. His studies investigate the mold only within the matrix of a topical antiseptic agent. Fleming abandons his work of Penicillum by the early-1940s assured, it is too toxic to be used systemically; it cannot survive long enough inside the human body to effectively kill disease producing bacteria; and cannot be produced commercially in sufficiently large quantities to ever be useful in the clinical treatment of infections.

Ernst Chain (1906-1979) German biochemist and Howard Florey (1898-1968) Australian pathologists are most responsible for moving forward the simple observation Penicillium inhibits the growth of Staphylococcus on plated cultured medium. They develop the observation into a useful medical treatment against Gram positive bacteria and change medical microbiology forever. Alexander Fleming, Ernst Chain and Howard Florey are jointly awarded the Nobel Prize in Physiology or Medicine "...for the discovery of penicillin and its curative effect in various infectious disease..." (1945)[219].

So goes another example in the history of medicine of a medical student, in this case Ernest Duchesne, who actually makes original and seminal observations, designs and completes meticulous experimental studies substantiating his/her observations, completes additional studies which moves basic science findings into the arena of potentially revolutionary medical treatments only to be ignored by the established scientific and medical communities with rewards of scientific discovery priority and finances gains misdirected to more senior and better marketed investigators. Oh, the world of professional science and medicine. How little people, professional science, and professional medicine have changed over time.

Helmut Ruska (1908-1973) German biologist offers the first electron microscopic images of bacteria, viruses, and bacteriophages (1940a,1940b)[220,221]. The electron microscope offers images unseen previously by traditional light microscopy. The new technology quickly proves essential in the study of pathogenic microorganisms and soon allows imaging at magnification greater than 1,000,000x. Helmut Ruska's elder brother Ernst Ruska (1906-1988) German physicist is instrumental in the invention and development of the first electron microscopes. Ernst Ruska is awarded the Nobel Prize in Physics "...for his fundamental work in electron optics, and for the design of the first electron microscope..." (1986)[222].

Albert Schatz (1922-2005) American microbiologist, Elizabeth Bugie-Gregory (1921-2001) American biochemist, and Selman Waksman (1888-1973) American biochemist offer another blow to disease producing bacteria with their discovery of streptomycin (1944,1945)[223,224]. Streptomycin proves to be the first antibiotic effective against Mycobacterium tuberculosis and several Gram negative bacteria unaffected by penicillin. Beyond the tremendous impact this discovery brings to medicine as a new and effective pharmaceutical it too brings another example of misguided claims and rewards of priority for discovery. Selman Walkman is awarded the Nobel Prize in Physiology or Medicine "...for his discovery of streptomycin, the first antibiotic effective against tuberculosis..." (1952)[225].

However, it is Albert Schatz, working as a graduate student at Rutgers University who actually formulates the conceptual matrix designed to find a cure for tuberculosis and Gram negative disease producing bacteria, completes the necessary experiments, and makes the discovery of streptomycin. The story of another misguided claim of priority is all too familiar.

In brief, Schatz does the science and Waksman claims credit, since the science is completed in Waksman's laboratory space at Rutgers. Waksman receives worldwide recognition in the form of the Nobel Prize for discoveries made by Albert Schatz. Waksman and Rutgers University receive millions of dollars in royalties collected from the U.S. priority patents on streptomycin (1948)[226]. Schatz's contributions are minimized or neglected completely by Waksman, the University, and the Nobel Awards Committee. Only after successful litigation against the University and Waksman is Albert Schatz compensated financially for his work and more correctly recognized as the investigator responsible for completing the science, culminating in discovery of streptomycin, the antibacterial agent which successfully treats tuberculosis and many Gram negative bacteria causing disease (1950,1993)[227,228].

The first half of the 1900s devotes much effort to the investigation of bacteria and development of antibiotics designed to kill disease producing bacteria. The second half of the 1900s devotes much more effort to the investigation of disease producing viruses, understanding bacteria, viruses, fungi, and parasites at the molecular level, developing new and more effective immunizations, and developing clinical microbiology laboratory services for use by the practicing physician.

Jonas Salk (1914-1995) American virologist develops a safe and effective vaccine against poliomyelitis (polio) while working with the University of Pittsburg, School of Medicine (1953)[229]. Salk's vaccine consists of three inactivated polioviruses. The vaccine's effectiveness, as with other vaccines, is based upon stimulation of the person's own immune system. The fundamental principle upon which this active immunization is based is that once a person is exposed to a pathogen via immunization the body's immune system is primed to response effectively in the event the person is ever exposed to the pathogen again. Salk's injected vaccine confers IgG mediated immunity in the bloodstream and thereby offers protection against viremia, eliminating the risk of paralysis upon subsequent exposure to the polio virus.

Salk's vaccine is field tested in the United States in one of the largest medical experiments in history. Field testing is directed by the University of Michigan's Thomas Francis (1900-1969) American virologist and epidemiologist. The testing involves approximately 1.8 million children, in school grades 1-3, approximately 6 to 8 years of age, distributed across 44 of 48 states in the U.S.A., as well as Canada and Finland. Approximately 420,000 children receive injection of the vaccine, approximately 200,000 receive injection of a harmless placebo, and approximately 1.2 million children receive no vaccination and serve as a control group (1955,1955)[230,231]. The massive field testing of the Salk inactivated polio vaccine (IPV) is conducted 1954-1955. Field testing findings are interpreted as demonstrating the vaccine's effectiveness and safety in light of appropriate concerns regarding research design and statistical methodologies (1955,1957)[230,232]. Immediately a nationwide immunization campaign is launched, promoted by the National Foundation for Infantile Paralysis (aka March of Dimes). The incidence of polio in the United States plummets.

Jonas Salk refuses to patent the vaccine, making it available to all.

Alick Isaacs (1921-1967) Scottish virologist and Jean Lindenmann (1924-2015) Swiss virologists discover interferon (INF), an antiviral protein produced by the body to fight viral infections (1957,1957)[233,234]. Their experiments demonstrate a cell when infected by virus will release interferon. The interferon protein blocks the growth of another virus when another virus attempts to infect the same cell. The interferon protein is the factor responsible for the "inference phenomenon" in which the cell once infected interferes with any other viruses which attempts to infect the same cell. The interference phenomenon has been known to virology and reported for at least 20 years before Isaacs and Lindenmann discover the specific protein responsible (1937,1942,1950)[235,236,237]. Today, it is recognized interferon is made within hours of a viral infection of a cell and is specie specific. That is, interferon produced by human cells is protective only for other human cells. Interferon while having many other biological effects, its primary function is antiviral defense.

Albert Sabin (1906-1993) Polish pathologist reports development of an oral polio vaccine. He offers an attenuated oral vaccine, attenuated sufficiently not to produce the disease yet still imparting immunity to the person. It blocks the polio virus from entering the bloodstream at the level of the intestines. Sabin identifies the intestines as the location where polio multiplies and first attacks the body.

Initial testing of the Sabin vaccine is completed in the Chillicothe Ohio reformatory during 1954. Recall, Salk tested his vaccine in an orphanage. Sabin's vaccine is soon dispensed to approximately 100 million people, residing in the USSR, Mexico, the Netherlands, and Eastern Europe, during 1955-1961, and before beginning large scale clinical trials in the USA, during 1960. The first large scale USA clinical trial is conducted on 180,000 Cincinnati, Ohio school children. Based upon clinical trials, the new Sabin attenuated oral polio vaccine (OPV) is determined to be effective. The Sabin OPV meets with much resistance from supporters of the successful Salk vaccine and is actively opposed by the March of Dimes organization. In light of stiff opposition, the Sabin vaccine is licensed for production and U.S. distribution in 1962. Sabin, an ardent, vocal critic of the Salk's inactivated polio vaccine, unsuccessfully attempts to block the use of the Salk vaccine.

Trivia: Albert Sabin is not his birth name. Sabin changes his name in 1930 when he becomes a naturalized citizen of the United States. His original family name is Saperstein.

Clinical microbiology and the clinical microbiology laboratory becomes an integrated part of clinical medicine during the second half of the 1900s. Adaptation of microbiology techniques perfected in basic science laboratories are made available to practicing clinicians. Large centrally located clinical microbiology laboratories process delivered samples and generate clinically valuable information regarding specific, infectious bacteria, fungi, viruses, and parasites. The information guides clinical treatment and management decisions made by practicing physicians.

Direct fluorescent antibody testing is introduced and uses chemically labeled antibodies as reagents for the detection of antigenic materials (1944)[238]. Radioimmunoassay (RIA) testing is introduced to assess concentrations of antibody or antigen in a sample material by radioactively labeling antigen or antibody then detecting the radioactivity signal intensity. RIA is first described by Rosalyn Yalow (1921-2011) American physicist and Solomon Berson (1918-1972) American internal medicine physician (1960)[239]. RIA is soon applied to measurement of specific hormones in the human body e.g. hormones of thyroid function T3, T4, TBG, TRH (1975)[240].

Rosalyn Yalow is awarded the Nobel Prize in Physiology or Medicine "…for the development of radioimmunoassay of peptide hormones…" (1977)[241]. She is the second woman to be awarded the Nobel Prize in Physiology or Medicine, the first is Gerty Cori in 1947. Gerty Cori shares the 1947 Prize with her husband Carl Corti. You might remember them from your biochemistry course. Remember the pathway for the catalytic conversion of glycogen?

The single standardized antibiotic disk is introduced and offers a quick and easy test of antibiotic susceptibility (1966)[242]. Recall from your biochemistry/microbiology lab in medical school, when you place the disk on a cultured medium in a Petri dish, bacteria susceptible to the antibiotic contained within the disk will fail to grow in the area of the disk while growing readily on other parts of the medium. Low tech in retrospect but useful at the time in guiding antibiotic selection.

Given concerns of potential risks associated with radioactivity inherent in the RIA, a new enzyme linked immunosorbent assay (ELISA) is introduced and displaces RIA (1971,1971)[243,244]. The direct and indirect ELISA tests capitalize upon the introduction and economical production of monoclonal antibodies (MAbs) (1975)[245]. Recall, monoclonal antibodies are derived from a single clone cell and have the same specificity. This provides a tremendous advantage over naturally occurring antibodies. The ELISA tests allows for the rapid detection of both a pathogenic antigen (direct ELISA) and antibody produced by the body against a pathogenic antigen (indirect ELISA). The ELISA tests provide a very sensitive and simple test. ELISA testing is often used to screen for the presence of antibodies, for example HIV proteins in a person's blood sample.

Immuno-blotting tests e.g. Western blot are introduced and provide a test capable of identifying proteins in complex biochemical mixtures (1981)[246]. The blotting tests use gel electrophoresis to separate specific proteins. The Western blot test is often performed to detect individual antibodies to HIV proteins in serum samples to complement and confirm a HIV positive result identified by an ELISA test (1986)[247]. The tests in combination improve accuracy of diagnosis.

As medical microbiology focuses upon developing newer, faster, and more economical diagnostic tests, developing more effective pharmacological treatments against, bacteria, viruses, fungi, and parasites, exploring the new opportunities offered by the production of monoclonal antibodies, and exploring the molecular basis of disease causing micro pathogens, advancements are being made in the clinical application of the rapidly developing microbiology knowledge base.

By the late-1970s the world proclaims smallpox to be successfully eradicated globally (1979)[248]. The viral infection (variola major and variola minor viruses), carried and transmitted only by humans, which results in a distinctive maculopapular rash followed by disfiguring raised fluid filled blisters, viremia, and frequent fatalities, is certified by the World Health Organization (WHO) to be officially eradicated worldwide. The successful eradication is attributed in large part to the result of focused and aggressive immunization efforts worldwide. Smallpox is the first infectious disease to be successfully eradicated, as the result of immunization.

Trivia The term "variola" is derived from the Latin word meaning "spotted".

The United States Supreme Court injects itself into medical microbiology in 1980. The Court issues a landmark decision in the case Diamond vs. Chakrabarty (1980)[249]. The decision in brief states life forms which naturally occur in nature and which until now have fallen outside the scope of U.S. patent law can now be patented, if the life form is genetically modified to produce a life form which does not naturally appear in nature. Specifically, the Diamond vs. Chakrabarty case deals with a genetically modified bacterium designed to dissolve oil. However, the decision has much greater implications given the recent and rapidly developing sophistication in molecular biology. The Court decision stimulates a frenzy of patent applications and U.S. patent awards to investigators and corporations for DNA sequences with both known and unknown functions. Science once again is altered by attorneys, government, and commercial corporate capitalism. So goes another example of modifying influences which mold and direct scientific knowledge.

The 1980s and 1990s witness the discovery of a new infectious pathogen which is neither parasite, fungus, bacteria, nor virus. The primary infectious agent responsible for the devastating poorly understood and recently recognized acquired immunodeficiency syndrome (AIDS) is identified to be a retrovirus. The human immunodeficiency virus (HIV) kills more than 12 million people worldwide, reaching pandemic proportions. Tremendous efforts are made to increase social awareness of AIDS / HIV. Tremendous financial and scientific resources are devoted to understanding, controlling, and treating HIV and associated disorders. Medical dogma continues to be challenged. Stomach ulcers are no longer believed to result from eating spicy foods and emotional stress and now understood to result from the bacterium Helicobacter pylori. Recently discovered bacteria which can survive in extreme environmental conditions are utilized in the development of innovative molecular biology techniques necessary to the identification, replication, and manipulation of genetic materials. Rapid diagnostic testing becomes more widely available. Complete genomes of bacteria are sequenced. Clinical medical microbiology laboratories become integrated into the daily and routine practice of medicine. Medical microbiology embraces molecular biology. Medical school curriculum require medical students to demonstrate a fundamental command of new molecular biology technologies with application to the practice of medicine.

Stanley Prusiner (1942-) American neurologist identifies a new and previously unknown infectious protein he terms "prions" (1982)[250]. This new group of self-reproducing pathogens is unique in that the protein's misfolded configuration is associated with its infectious characteristics. Prions are soon identified to be causal in the invariably fatal degenerative neurological condition Creutzfeldt-Jakob disease and other transmissible spongiform encephalopathies. Prusiner is awarded the Nobel Prize in Physiology or Medicine "…for his discovery of Prions - a new biological principle of infection…" (1997)[251].

Luc Montagnier (1932-) French virologist and Robert Gallo (1937-) American biochemist, leading independent research groups announce discovery of the human immunodeficiency virus (HIV), a retrovirus to be the cause of acquired immunodeficiency syndrome (AIDS) (1983,1984, 1984)[252,253,254]. Montagnier and his colleague French virologist Francoise Barre-Sinoussi (1947-) are awarded the Nobel Prize in Physiology or Medicine for "…discovery of human immunodeficiency virus…" (2008)[255].

John Warren (1937-) Australian pathologist and Barry Marshall (1951-) Australian microbiologist challenge and displace medical dogma regarding the source of stomach ulcers. Prior to Warren and Marshall it is universally believed by the established medical community peptic ulcers are caused by stress, spicy foods, and too much stomach acid. Warren and Marshall correctly identify the cause to be a bacterium. They correctly identify the bacterium to be Campylobacter pylori (later called Helicobacter pylori) revolutionizing the understanding of peptic ulcers and their treatments (1983)[256]. Warren and Marshall are recognized for their contributions and awarded the Nobel Prize in Physiology or Medicine "…for their discovery of bacterium Helicobacter pylori and its role in gastritis and peptic ulcer disease…" (2005)[257].

Kary Mullis (1944-2019) American biochemist uses Thermophilus aquaticus (Taq), a heat insensitive bacterium found in hot springs to develop the polymerase chain reaction (PCR) method of duplicating segments of DNA (1986)[258]. Recall, the PCR process requires repeated cycles of heating and cooling. The extreme heat permits separation of DNA strains necessary for replication and the DNA polymerase (Taq enzyme) provides the necessary heat-stable enzyme necessary for the enzymatic replication of strains. The replicated copies of DNA provide the necessary material to conduct a wide number of molecular based diagnostic tests. The improvement in PCR methods by Mullis and his group makes the amplification of selected segments of DNA affordable and subject to automation. Medical microbiology moves quickly to providing clinical microbiology diagnostic services to the practicing physician, utilizing automatic molecular biology techniques e.g. PCR. Kary Mullis is awarded the Nobel Prize in Chemistry "…for his invention of the polymerase chain reaction (PCR) method…" (1993)[259].

Rapid diagnostic testing becomes popular during the 1990s and offers an alternative to lengthy and expensive microbiology laboratory testing. Rapid diagnostic testing during the 1990s is directed to providing a fast, usually less than 20 minutes, inexpensive, accurate result, generated at the point of service e.g. the physician's office or clinic rather than a large central clinical microbiology laboratory and provides information as to which specific bacteria is responsible for an infection. The information is then used to guide clinical treatment decisions e.g. selection of an appropriate antibiotic.

By the late-1990s the genomes of several bacteria are sequenced, opening new doors to guide identification of bacteria, using molecular technologies, and a greater understanding of the molecular basis responsible for the mechanisms of actions of common disease producing bacteria. By the end of the 1990s the following bacteria genomes are sequenced in full: Haemopilius influenza (1995)[260] (the first complete genome sequence from a free living organism); Escherichia coli (1997)[261]; Helicobacter pylori (1997)[262]; Chlamydia trachomatis (1998)[263]; and Mycobacterium tuberculosis (1998)[264].

In summary, the first half of the 1900s witness medical microbiology's continued, rapid develop, and maturation as a scientific based discipline with applied applications to clinical medicine. Early in the 1900s insects are recognized to be intermediate hosts for numerous bacteria, viruses, and parasites, providing the essential knowledge necessary to effectively control an entire category of devastating human diseases. Much attention is devoted to the investigation of bacteria. Particular attention is focused upon better understanding the vectors of bacteria transmission, role of intermediate hosts, development of pharmacological treatment agents specifically designed to chemically bind and destroy disease producing bacteria, and utilization of attenuated bacteria strains in producing immunization against devastating disease producing bacteria. Chemotherapy is introduced as a complementary approach to immunization. Salvarsan is introduced as one of the first effective chemotherapy treatments, synthesized and based upon an understanding of the biochemistry responsible for directing a pharmacological agents to a specific disease producing pathogen, resulting in this case with the destruction of the bacteria responsible for syphilis, while permitting the host to survive. Bactericidal properties of molds are recognized and quickly extended resulting in the introduction of penicillin as an effective treatment against Gram positive bacteria. Streptomycin is subsequently introduced as the first antibiotic effective against Mycobacterium tuberculosis and other Gram negative bacteria. The BCG vaccine is introduced. The BCG vaccine offers a conceptual model and intervention strategy distinctly different from the chemotherapy models and strategies for controlling bacteria responsible for tuberculosis.

The virus, the recently discovered new human pathogen, is aggressively investigated. The virus is understood within the matrix of replication, vectors of disease transmission, and specific human diseases. Viruses are recognized to be obligate parasites with survival dependent upon living cells. Virology is recognized as a distinct scientific discipline. Virus and bacterium interactions begin to be understood. The bacteriophage is identified and begins to be understood within the matrix of human disease, both as cause and potential vehicle for effective treatments. Advances in technology such as invention of the electron-microscope provide imaging resolutions of fungi, parasites, bacteria, and viruses unmatched in history. Professional battles between academic institutions and between investigators, often surrounding claims of priority of discovery and the rich financial rewards associated with priority of discovery punctuate the early-1900s. Opportunities for tremendous amounts of money to be earned are quickly recognized by academics and capitalists alike as the basic science knowledge base of microbiology finds its place in clinical applications for the practicing physician.

The second half of the 1900s witness a shift from interests in bacteria producing disease and their destruction by pharmacological agents to much greater interests in understanding viruses and their role in human disease. Viruses are more completely understood both as disease producing pathogens as well as their roles in providing effective immunization against disease and providing new, innovative treatments for many human diseases. Jonas Salk and Albert Sabin introduce their polio vaccines and complete clinical trials which include millions of children. Interferon is discovered and applied to the treatment of viral infections. The retrovirus responsible for acquired immune deficiency syndrome (AIDS) is identified. The World Health Organization declares smallpox globally eradicated, as the result of effective worldwide immunization efforts. The long held belief and medical dogma, stomach ulcers are the result of psychological stress or eating spicy foods is recognized to be false and replaced upon the discovery of the bacterium Helicobacter pylori as the true etiological agent producing these common and debilitating ulcers. The prion is discovered and aggressively investigated. Innovative advances in technology moves medical microbiology further into molecular levels of analysis. Parasites, fungi, bacteria, and viruses producing human disease are more completely understood at the molecular level. Radioimmunoassay (RIA) provides technology permitting the analysis of antibody and antigen concentrations. Additionally, RIA provides early quantitative laboratory based measurements of specific hormones levels in any specific patient and offers the practicing physician another tool from the medical microbiology laboratory to better diagnose and treat clinical patients.

The antibiotic disk is introduced and widely used as a rapid diagnostic tool in identifying specific bacteria. Enzyme linked immunosorbent assay (ELISA) soon displaces RIA. Rapid and economical production of monoclonal antibodies (MAbs) opens new doors for the medical microbiology laboratory and rapid diagnostic testing services. Rapid diagnostic testing moves from the large shared medical microbiology laboratories to the practicing physician's office. Diagnostic testing times are reduced from weeks to minutes. Rapid diagnostic testing becomes affordable and available to physicians providing health care services in the world's most remote areas. Discovery of the heat insensitive bacterium Thermophilus aquaticus (Taq) provides an essential component necessary for the successful duplication of DNA segments within the laboratory via the polymerase chain reaction (PCR) method. Much of medical microbiology moves to a DNA level of analysis. Many bacteria genomes are sequenced and human disease begins to be understood and conceptualized within the matrix of genetic materials. Medical microbiology goes molecular.

Current Modern, 2000 AD - 2019 AD.

Medical microbiology continues to grow as a respected scientific discipline and one which provides essential clinical diagnostic service to the practicing physician. The discipline is recognized as a leader in both basic and applied medical sciences, routinely applying the latest interdisciplinary molecular technologies to better understand the fundamental basis of disease causing microorganisms and offering the practicing physician with timely information used to make more informed clinical diagnostic and treatment decisions. Recent advances are offering new ways to understand old problems. Medical microbiology no longer restricts itself to understanding microorganisms as cause of disease. Greater attention is being directed to understanding microorganisms within the matrix of good health and normal bodily functions. Recently developed molecular technologies coupled with new and innovative thinking utilize microorganisms to treat disease.

The American Society for Microbiology is now over 100 years in existence and claims over 43,000 members throughout the world. Most modern developed countries contribute to the advancement of medical microbiology through the free exchange of scientific information. The development of the World Wide Web internet offers immediate communication between investigators, clinical service laboratories, and the practicing physician. The Canadian Association for Microbiology and Infectious Disease, the Society for General Microbiology located in the United Kingdom, and other respected professional societies continue to offer training, education, and platforms for the exchange of ideas, technologies, and science throughout the world for students, clinical practitioners, investigators, and yes, even old, gray haired, tenured medical school professors (2011,2011,2011)[265,266,267]. Medical microbiology is alive and well in the world today.

Bacteria are becoming resistant to antibiotic treatments. Specifically, strains of Staphylococcus aureus are becoming resistant to the antibiotic vancomycin (VRSA). This is particularly disturbing given vancomycin has been in use for more than 30 years, without emergence of marked resistance, and is the preferred treatment of choice for methicillin resistant Staphylococcus aureus (MRSA) and oxycillin resistant Staphylococcus aureus (ORSA) (2001)[268]. Enterococcus bacteria are also demonstrating resistance to vancomycin (VRE) (2000)[269]. Bacteria are mutating their genetic materials in an adaptive defense against antibiotics.

New viruses are identified and create worldwide pandemics e.g. SARS coronavirus (SARS-CoV), a positive strained, enveloped, RNA virus. This virus is responsible for the Severe Acute Respiratory Syndrome (SARS), a respiratory disease in humans, infecting thousands, in over 37 different countries, and producing death in many infected by the virus (2003)[270].

Molecular diagnostic testing becomes more readily available with highly automated nucleic acid-based testing. Real time PCR combines nucleic acid amplification with fluorescent detection within the same closed system (2004,2004)[271,272].

Rapid diagnostic testing is becoming more available, fast, and less expensive. New technologies offer identification of wide range of pathogens, including all known bacteria, all major pathogenic fungi, and major families of viruses along with detection of virulence factors and antibiotic resistance markers (2008)[273]. Routine HIV screening can be completed in less than 60 seconds (2010)[274]. Tuberculosis screening and assessment of rifampin resistance can be completed in less than 2 hours (2010)[275]. Other rapid diagnostic tests available identify MRSA, malaria, helicobacter, gonorrhea, chlamydia, and hundreds more. The rapid diagnostic test have not yet replaced the clinical microbiology laboratory, which still maintains typically better sensitivity and specificity than the rapid point of service tests. Rapid diagnostic tests are proving especially useful in the public health area identifying infectious pathogens in patients who may not return for follow up or must travel great distances to receive health care services.

Pharmaceutical companies are recognizing the financial benefit of investigating new medications which will be taken long term by patients. Very few new antibiotics are being introduced or investigated. The reasons include a much lower financial return- investment cost ratio, bacteria's increasing resistance, and the explosion of much more profitable pharmaceuticals which require long term use rather than the 2-3 week episodic use typical of antibiotics. Pharmaceutical used in treatment and management of cardiovascular diseases or neurological diseases prove much more profitable. Similarly, consider the financial profits generated from sildenafil (Viagra) to that which might be recovered from introduction of a new antibiotic. Yes, Virginia, there is no Santa Claus.

Medical school Basic Sciences program curricula (first two years of medical school) in the United States and Canada combine microbiology, genetics, and immunology into an integrated single course. Few medical schools continue to teach separate courses in these three critically important disciplines, emphasizing the growing overlap in topic materials and technologies.

Molecular analyses of bacteria continue. The complete genome of the bacterium responsible for the Black Death plague, which swept through Europe between 1347 AD-1351 AD and killed approximately 30 to 50 percent of the entire population of Europe, is successfully sequenced (2011)[276].

The future of medical microbiology is molecular.

In sum, the first twenty years of the 2000s demonstrates medical microbiology to be alive and well. Worldwide membership in professional societies devoted to microbiology as both as a basic science and an applied medical science have never been higher. Sharing of new information between investigators and practicing physicians has never been greater. Information is shared at high speed, no longer requiring communications to be completed at societal meetings, publication in hard copy journals, or personal correspondence through traditional mail systems. Information is shared electronically and instantaneously. Medical microbiology more than ever before continues to make meaningful contributions to the new scientific knowledge base, embracing intra and inter disciplinary collaborations and sharing new innovative technologies. Rapid diagnostic testing is more available, faster, and less expensive. Molecular diagnostic testing is now highly automated and much more available. Bacteria are becoming resistant to antibiotic treatments and are accomplishing the resistance by mutating their genetic materials. New viruses are continuing to be identified. Some have recently created worldwide pandemics not too different from similar worldwide pandemics over 90 years ago. Medical microbiology continues to lead in finding effective solutions to these new problems. Medical school curriculums are responding to these and other changes by combining basic science program course work into more integrated courses which now include microbiology, genetics, and immunology rather than teaching them as traditionally independent discipline based courses. Medical microbiology is well positioned to make continued substantial contributions in both the basic and applied medical sciences.

Yes, the future of medical microbiology certainly should be exciting.

References.

[1] Dirckx, J. (1997). Stedman's concise medical dictionary for the health professional. 3rd edition. Baltimore: William and Wilkins.

[2] Griffith, F. (circa 1800 BC/1898 AD). The Petrie papyri: Hieratic papyri from Kahun and Gurob. London: Bernard Quaritch. Retrieved September 2011 from http://www.archive.org/stream/hieraticpapyrifr00grifuoft#page/n7/mode/2up

[3] Ebers Papyrus (circa 1550 BC). Compendium of the whole Egyptian medicine (Georg Ebers), Columns 1-2. University of Leipzig Library, Special Collections. Leipzig, Germany.

[4] Edwin Smith Surgical Papyrus (circa 1500 BC). [Online English translation]. Retrieved September 2011 from http://www.touregypt.net/edwinsmithsurgical.htm.

[5] Thompson, R. (1923). Assyrian medical texts from the originals in the British Museum. London: H. Milford. Oxford University Press.

[6] Zink, A., Sola, C., Reischl, U., Grabner, W., Rastogi, N., Wolf, H., and Nerlich, A. (2003). Characterization of Mycobacterium tuberculosis complex DNAs from Egyptian mummies by spoligotyping. Journal of Clinical Microbiology, 41(1):359–67.

[7] Scurlock, J. and Anderson, B. (2005). Diagnoses in Assyrian and Babylonian medicine: Ancient sources, translations, and modern medical analyses. Chicago: University of Illinois Press.

[8] Labat, R. (circa 800 BC/1951). Treate akkadien de diagnostics et pronostics medcicaux [Treaties of Medical Diagnoses and Prognoses]. Leiden. Brill.

[9] Thucydides (1843). The Peloponnesian War. Translator Thomas Hobbes. Perseus Digital Library, Tufts University. Retrieved September 2011 http://www.perseus.tufts.edu/hopper/text?doc=Perseus:text:1999.01.0200.

[10] Thucydides. (1910). The Peloponnesian War. Translation by Richard Crawley. London, J. M. Dent; New York, E. P. Dutton.

[11] Thucydides. (1919,1921). History of the Peloponnesian Wars; Books Vol I: Books 1-2; Vol II: Books 3-4; Vol III: Books 5-6. Translation by C.F. Smith. Loeb Library Collection. Retrieved August 81, 2011 from http://www.hup.harvard.edu/collection.php?cpk=1031

[12] Hippocrates and Littre, E. (1839). Oeuvres complétes d'Hippocrate, traduction nouvelle avec le texte Grec en regard, collationn sur les manuscrits et toutes les éditions: accompagnée d'une introduction, de commentaires médicaux, de variantes et de notes phiologiques. Paris: J. B. Bailliere.

[13] Adams, F. (1891). The Genuine works of Hippocrates. New York: William Wood and Company. Retrieved from http://classics.mit.edu/Hippocrates/epidemics.1.i.html

[14] Hippocrates and Jones, W. (1923). Hippocrates Volume 1: Ancient Medicine. Airs, Waters, Places. Epidemics 1 and 3. The Oath. Precepts. Nutriment. Loeb Classical Library 147, Harvard University Press.

[15] Goodall, E. (1934). On infectious diseases and epidemiology in the Hippocratic Collection. Section of the History of Medicine. Proceedings of the Royal Society of Medicine, March 27(5):525-534.

[16] Hippocrates and Smith, W. (1994). Hippocrates Volume VII, Epidemics 2, 4-7. Edited and translated by Wesley D. Smith. Loeb Classical Library 477.

[17] Aristotle and Thompson, D. (350 BC/1910). Aristotle's history of animals. Book V, Section 31. Translated by D'Arcy Wentworth Thompson. Adelaide: eBooks@Adelaide. Retrieved August 17, 2011 from http://ebooks.adelaide.edu.au/a/aristotle/history/

[18] Carus, T. (circa 50 BC). On the Nature of Things. The Project Gutenberg EBook #785. Translated by William Leonard. (July 31, 2008). Volume 1-6. Retrieved January 2012 from http://www.gutenberg.org/files/785/785-h/785-h.htm

[19] Varro, M. (circa 37 BC). De Re Rustica, Loeb Classical Library, 1934. Marcus Teretius Varro on Agriculture Book I, Sec 12, 2. Lacus Curtis. Retrieved September 2011 from http://penelope.uchicago.edu/Thayer/E/Roman/Texts/Varro/de_Re_Rustica/1*.html#12.2

[20] Celsus, A. (circa 30 AD). De Medicina [On Medicine]. First printed 1478. Florence Nicolaus Laurentii. Rare Book Collection, Countway Medical Library, Boston.

[21] Celsus, A. (circa 30 AD). De Medicina [On Medicine]. Online English translation by W. Spencer (1935) Loeb Classical Library Edition. Retrieved November 2009 from http://penelope.uchicago.edu/Thayer/E/Roman/Texts/celsus/home.html

[22] Laveran, A. (1880). Note sur un nouveau parasite trouvè dans le sang de plusieurs malades atteints de fièvre palustre. Bull. Acad. Med., 9:1235-1236.

[23] Golgi, C. (1886). Malarial infection. Arch. Sci. Med., 10:109-135.

[24] Galien, C. (1513). De affectorum locorum notitia: libri sex. Guilielmo Copo Basileiensi interprete. Paris: Henrici Stephani. Bibliotheque nationale de France. Retrieved January 2012 from http://gallica.bnf.fr/ark:/12148/bpt6k543808

[25] Galen. (circa 175 AD). De Locis Affectis, Book VI. Translated by Rudolph Siegel. Galen on the affected parts: translation from the Greek text with explanatory notes (1976). Basel, Switzerland: S. Karger.

[26] Neisser, A. (1879). Über eine der Gonorrhoe eigenthümliche Micrococcusform. Ctrbl f med Wiss., 17:497-500. Trans in Med Life, 1932, 39:507-10.

[27] Koch, R. (1882). Die aetiologie der tuberculose. Berliner Klinische Wochenschrift, 19:221-30.

[28] Varro, M. (1934). De Re Rustica. On Agriculture Book I, Sec 12, 2. Translated by W. Hooper and H. Ash. Edited by Bill Thayer. Loeb Classical Library. Retrieved September 2011. http://penelope.uchicago.edu/Thayer/E/Roman/Texts/Varro/de_Re_Rustica/1*.html#12.2.

[29] Carus, T. (circa 50 BC). On the Nature of Things. Volume 1-6. Translated by William Leonard. (July 31, 2008). The Project Gutenberg EBook #785.

[30] Morelli, G., Song, Y., Mazzoni, C., Eppinger, M., Roumagnac, P., Wagner, D., Feldkamp. M., Kusecek, B., Volger, A., Li, Y., Cui, Y., Thomson, N., et al (2010). Yersinia pestis genome sequencing identifies patterns of global phylogenetic diversity. Nature Genetics, 42(12):1140–3.

[31] Gibbon, E. (1776-1788). The History of the Decline and Fall of the Roman Empire, 6 Volumes. Volume 4: 327-331. London: W. Strahan and T. Cadell in the Strand.

[32] Procopius. (1914). History of the Wars, 7 Volumes, translated by H. B. Dewing, Loeb Library of the Greek and Roman Classics, Cambridge, Mass.: Harvard University Press. Volume. I, 451-473.Retrieved January 2012 from http://www.fordham.edu/halsall/source/542procopius-plague.asp

[33] Aenineta, P. (1844.) The seven books of Paulus Aegineta. Translated from the Greek with a commentary embracing a complete view of the knowledge possessed by the Greeks, Romans, and Arabian, all subjects connected with medicine and surgery. Translated by Francis Adams in three volumes. Printed for the Sydenham Society: London. Retrieved online from the Open Library.org
http://www.archive.org/stream/sevenbooksofpaul01pauluoft#page/n1/mode/2up

[34] Aegineta, P. (1847). The seven books of Paulus Aegineta: Translated from the Greek with a commentary embracing a complete view of knowledge possesses by the Greeks, Romans, and Arabians on all subjects connected with medicine and surgery. Translated by Francis Adams. London: Sydenham Society. C. and J. Adlard.

[35] Rhazes. (1848). A Treatise on the Small-Pox and Measles, English translation by W.A. Greenhill. London: Sydenham Society.

[36] Rhazes. (1985). Rhazes' Liber Continens. [An encyclopedia of Medicine] by Abu Bakr Muhammand B. Zakariyya Ar-Razi, Part XVII on Smallpox, Measles and Plagues. Edited and collated with Escuriall MSS. Nos 817 & 856 and the MS of Hakeem Ashufta preserved in the Da'iratus'l-Ma'arif-il-Osmania. Hyderabad, India: Osmania Oriental Publications Bureau, Osmania University.

[37] Abu Ali al Husayn ibn Abd Allah Ibn Sina (aka Avicenna). (1025 AD). Kitab al-Qanun fi al-tibb (The Canon of Medicine. MS A 53, Islamic Medical Manuscripts at the National Library of Medicine.

[38] Ibn Sina (Avicenna). (1025 AD). Kitab al-Qanun fi al-tibb (Canon on Medicine). London Welcome Library for the History and Understanding of Medicine, MS Arab. 155, copied in 1632 (1042 H).

[39] Avicenna (1999). Canon of Medicine. (English.) Chicago: Kazi Publications.

[40] Wachtler, J. (1896). De Alcmaeone Crotoniata. Leipzig: Teubner. (The only full-scale commentary devoted to Alcmaeon. Greek texts of the fragments and testimonia with commentary in Latin).

[41] Diels, H. and Kranz, W. (1952). Die Fragmente der Vorsokratiker (in three volumes), 6th edition, Dublin and Zürich: Weidmann, Volume 1, Chapter 24, 210-216. Greek texts of the fragments and testimonia with translations in German. (Originally published 1903).

[42] Timpanaro-Cardini, M. (1958-64). Pitagorici, Testimonianze e frammenti, 3 vols., Firenze: La Nuova Italia, Vol. 1, 124-153 (Greek texts of the fragments and testimonia with translations and commentary in Italian).

[43] Freeman, K. (1983). Ancilla to the Pre-Socratic Philosophers. Cambridge: Harvard University Press. (reprint edition). This book is a complete English translation of the 'B' passages–the so-called 'fragments'–from Die Fragmente der Vorsokratiker.

[44] Avicenne. (1507). Liber Canonis Avicennae. Venice, Apud Simonem Papiensem. Facsimile by George Olms, Hildesheim (1964).

[45] Avicenna and Gruner, R. (1930). A treatise on the Canon of Medicine incorporating a translation of the First Book. London.

[46] Avicenna. (1966). The general principles of Avicenna's Canon of Medicine. English translation by Mazhar Shah. Karachi. (Book 1 with summaries of Books 2-5).

[47] Smallman-Raynor, M. and Cliff. A. (2004). War Epidemics. Oxford University Press.

[48] Yersin, A. (1894). La peste bubonique a Hong Kong. Comptes Rendus de l'Academie des Sciences, 119:356.

[49] Yersin, A. (1894). La peste bubonique a Hong Kong. Ann. Inst. Pasteur., 8:662-667.

[50] Aretaeus (circa 100 AD). De causis et signis diuturnorum morborum. [On the causes and symptoms of chronic disease]. The exact works of Aretaeus. The Cappadocian. Book 1. Edited and translated into English by Francis Adams. Boston Milford House Inc. (1972)). Republication of the 1856 edition. Retrieved online 9-22-2011. Digital Hippocrates - A collection of Ancient Medical Texts. http://www.chlt.org/sandbox/dh/aretaeusEnglish/index.html.

[51] Pollock, F. and Maitland, F. (1952). The History of English Law before the time of Edward I. Cambridge: Cambridge University Press.

[52] Roberts, C. and Manchester, K. (1995). The archaeology of disease. Ithaca, New York: Cornell University Press.

[53] Donoghue, H., Marcsik, A., Matheson, C., Vernon, K., Nuorala, E., Molto, J., Greenblatt, C., Spigelman, M. (2005). Co-infection of Mychobacterium tuberculosis and Lycobacterium leprae in human archaeological samples: A possible explanation for the historical decline of leprosy. Proc Royal Society B., 272:389-394.

[54] Beckett, W. (1717-1719). An attempt to prove the antiquity of the venereal disease, long before the discovery of the West Indies; in a letter from Mr. William Beckett, Surgeon to Dr. James Douglas, M.D. and R. Soc. Soc. and by him communicated to the Royal Society. Philosophical Transactions 1717-1719, 30(351-363):839-47.

[55] Bizio, B. (1823). Lettera di Bartholomeo Bizio sopra il fenomeno della polenta porporina. Biblioteca Italiana ossia Giornale di Letteratura Scienze ed Arti. 30:275-295. Retrieved January 2012 http://emeroteca.braidense.it/eva/sfoglia_articolo.php?IDTestata=110&CodScheda=207&CodVolume=2449&CodFascicolo=15991&CodArticolo=301633

[56] Ehrenberg, C. (1849a). Observations on the so-called bleeding bread caused by Monas prodigiosa. Bericht u. d. z. Bekanntmachung geeigneten Verhandlungen d. Kgl. preuss. Acad. d. Wissenschaften, October 26, 1848, 349-353.

[57] Ehrenberg, C. (1849b) Fortsetzung der Beobactung des sogenannten Blutes im Brode als Monas prodigiosa. [Continuation on the observations on the so-called bleeding bread caused by Monas prodigiosa] An appendix to the previous article prepared after the first paper was read before the Academy of Science. Bericht u. d. z. Bekanntmachung geeigneten Verhandlungen d. Kgl. press. Acad. d. Wissenschaften, October 26, 1848, p.354-362.

[58] Ehrenberg, C. (1850). Fernere Mittheilungen uber Monas prodigiosa oder die Purpurmonade. Bericht u. d. z. Bekanntmachung geeigneten Verhandlungen d. Kgl. press. Acad. d. Wissenschaften. March 15, 1849, p.101-116.

[59] Ehrenberg, C. (1851a). Hochst wahrscheinlicher Grund d. Verbotes d.Bohnengenusses bei. d. Pythagoraern. Bericht u. d. z. Bekanntmachung geeigneten Verhandlungen d. Kgl. press. Acad. d. Wissenschaften. January 17, 1850, p.5-9.

[60] Ehrenberg, C. (1851b). Eine Centurie historischer Nachtrage zu den blutfarbigen Meteoren und sogenannten Prodigien. Bericht u. d. z. Bekanntmachung geeigneten Verhandlungen d. Kgl. press. Acad. d. Wissenschaften. June 27, 1850, p.215-246.

[61] Hefferan, M. (1903). A comparative and experimental study of bacilli producing red pigment. Centralbl. f. Bakt., Abt. II, 11, 311-317, 397-404, 456-475, 520-540.

[62] Gaughran, E. (1969). From superstition to science: the history of a bacterium. Trans. N.Y. Acad. Sci., 31:3-24.

[63] Bizio, B, (1823). Lettera di Bartolomeo Bizio al chiarissimo canonico Angelo Bellani sopra il fenomeno della polenta porporina. Biblioteca Italiano o sia Giornale di Letteratura, Scienze e Arti. Appendice Tomo 30, Anno 8, Aprile, Maffio, e Giugno, 275-295. [Batolomeo Bizio's letter to the most eminent priest, Angelo Bellani, concerning the phenomenon of the red-colored polenta]. Translated from the Italian by C. Merlino. J. Bacteriology, Nov, 1924, 9:527-543. Retrieved August 17, 2011 http://jb.asm.org/cgi/reprint/9/6/527

[64] Bizio, B. (1827). Del fenomemo della polenta porporina. [The phenomenon of red corn meal mush]. Opuscoli Chimicofisici, Tomo 1, Parte 2, Richerche e spiegazioni di alcuni fenomeni, Articolo 1, 261-298, Venezia, Giuseppe Antonelli.

[65] Merlino, C. (1924). Bartolomeo. Bizo's letter to the most eminent priest, Angelo Bellani, concerning the phenomenon of the red colored polenta. Journal of Bacteriology, 9:527-543.

[66] Russell, J. (1948). British medieval populations. Albuquerque: University of New Mexico Press.

[67] Hollingsworth, T. (1975). A Note on Mediaeval Longevity of the Secular Peerage, 1350-1500. Population Studies, 29(1):155-159.

[68] Montague. J. (1994). Length of life in the ancient world: a controlled study. Journal of the Royal Society of Medicine, Vol. 87. Jan., 25-26.

[69] Fracastoro, G. (1546). De contagione et contagiosis morbis et curatione. Venetis: L. Iuntae.

[70] Kircher, A. (1646). Ars Magna Lucis et Umbrae. [The Great Art of Light and Shadow]. Rome. (British Library, London: 536. I. 25).

[71] Kircher, A. (1658). Scrutinium Physico-Medicum contagiosae Luis, quae Pestis dicitur quo'origo, causae,signa, prognostica Pestis, nec non involentes malignantis Naturae effectus, qui statis temporibus, caelestium influxuum, virtute et efficacea, tum in elementis; tum in epidemiishominum animantiumque morbis elucescunt, una cum appropriatis remediorum Antidotis nova doctrina in lucem eruuntur. Dedicated to Pope Alexander VII. Rome.

[72] Leeuwenhoeck, A. (1676/1677). Observations, communicated to the publisher by Mr. Antony van Leeuwenhoeck, in a Dutch letter of the 9th Octob. 1676. Here English'd: concerning little animals by him observed in rain-well-sea-and snow water; as also in water wherin pepper had lain infused. Philisolical Transactions, 12(133):821-831. doi:10.1098/rstb.2014.0344.

[73] Needham, M. (1665). Medela medicinae: A plea for the free profession and a renovation of the art of physicks out of the noblest and most authentick writers. Shewing the publick advantage of its liberty. The disadvantage that comes to the publick by any sort of physicians imposing upon the studies and practice of others. The alteration of diseases from their old state and condition. The causes of that alteration. The insufficiency and uselessness of mere scholastick methods and medicines, with a necessity of new. Tending to the rescue of mankind from the tyranny of diseases and of physicians themselves from the pedantism of old authors and present dictators. Printed for Richard Lowndes at White Lion in St. Pauls Church Yard, near the Little North door.

[74] Sprackling, R. (1665). Medela Ignorantiae: Or a just and plain vindication of Hippocratres and Galen from the groundless imputations of M. N. wherein the whole substance of his illiterate plea, entitled "Medela Medicinae" is

occasionally considered. London: Printed by W.G. for Robert Crofts at the Crown in Chancery lane under Serjeants Inn.

[75] Hooke, R. (1665). Micrographia: Or some physiological descriptions of minute bodies made by magnifying glasses with observations and inquires thereupon. London: Jo Martyn and Jason Allestry.

[76] Royal Society (2011). Serial Archive listing for the Philosophical Transaction of the Royal Society of London. Retrieved October 2011. http://onlinebooks.library.upenn.edu/webbin/serial?id=philtransactions

[77] Royal Society (2011). The Hooke Folio Online. Retrieved October 2011. http://webapps.qmul.ac.uk/cell/Hooke/Hooke.html

[78] Leeuwenhoek, A. (1681). Ontdeckte onsightbaarhede. Leiden. [The original description is in a letter in Dutch, dated November 4, 1681. It was read, translated into English at a meeting of the Royal Society, London, November 9, 1681].

[79] Leeuwenhoek, A. (1673). Letter 1 to Henry Oldenburg, Secretary of England's Royal Society and editor of the Society's journal Philosophical Transactions, dated April 28, 1673, appearing in Philosophical Transactions May 19, 1673, no. 94. Attached figure drawing appear in Philosophical Transactions, no. 97, October 6, 1673.

[80] Redi, F. (1687). Osservazioni intorno a pellicelli del corpo umano fatte dal Dottor Gio: Cosimo Bonomo e da lui com altre osservazioni scritte in una lettera all'illustriss. Sig. Francesco Redi. Florence: Piero Matini.

[81] Mead, R. (1703). Translation of part of Bonomo's letter to Redi, 1687. Philosophical Trans., 23:1296-9.

[82] Lane, J. (1928). Bonomo's letter to Redi - an important document in the history of scabies. Arch. Dermatol. Syphilogr., 18:1-25.

[83] Leviticus 15: verse 2-11, Holy Bible (King James Version).

[84] Aristotle (circa 350 BC). Aristotle's history of animals in ten books. Translated by Richard Cresswell, St John's College, Oxford (1883). London: George Bell and Sons, York Street, Covent Garden.

[85] Linnaeus, C. (1735). Systema naturæ, sive regna tria naturæ systematice proposita per classes, ordines, genera, & species. [1–12]. Lugduni Batavorum. (Haak).

[86] Linnaeus, C. (1758). Systema naturae per regna tria naturae: secundum classes, ordines, genera, species, cum characteribus, differentiis, synonymis, locis (10th edition ed.). Stockholm: Laurentius Salvius. Retrieved January 2012 http://www.biodiversitylibrary.org/bibliography/542

[87] Lapage, S., Sneath, P., Lessel, E., Skerman, V., Seeliger, H., Clark, W. (1992). International code of nomenclature of bacteria: 1990 revision. Washington DC: American Society for Microbiology Press.

[88] Fauquet C., Mayo, M, Maniloff, J., Desselberger, U., Ball, L. (2005). Virus taxonomy VIIIth report of the International Committee on taxonomy of viruses. San Diego: Elsevier Academic Press.

[89] Plenciz, M. (1762). Opera medico-physica: De contagio, Volume 1. Vindobona. Vienna: Joannis Trattner.

[90] Donne, A. (1836). Animalcules observés dans les matières purulentes at le produit des sécretions des organes génitaux de l'homme et de la femme. Comptes Rendus de l'Académie des Sciences, Paris, 3:385-186.

[91] Donne, A. (1842). De l'origine des globules du sang de leur mode de formation et leur fin. Comptes Rendus de l'Académie des Sciences, 14:366-368.

[92] Donne, A. and Foucault, J. (1845). Atlas du cours de microscopie exécuté d'après nature au microscope-daguerréotype. Paris: J. B. Bailliere.

[93] Schonlein, J. (1839). Zur Pathogenie der Impetigines. Auszug aus einer brieflichen Mitteilung an den Herausgeber. [Müller's] Archiv für Anatomie, Physiologie und Wissenschaftliche Medicin, 82.

[94] Bassi, A. (1835). Del mal del segno calcinaccio o moscardino. Submitted to Faculty University of Pavia.

[95] Gruby, D. (1841). Mémoire sur une vegétation qui constitue la vraie teigne. Comptes rendus hebdomadaire des séances de l'Académie des Sciences, Paris, 13:72-75.

[96] Gruby, D. (1842). Recherches anatomiques sun une plante cryptogame qui constitue le vrai muguet des enfants. Comptes rendus hebdomadaire des séances de l'Académie des Sciences, Paris, 14:634-636.

[97] Henle, J. (1838). On Miasmata and Contagie. English translation by George Rosen. Baltimore: Johns Hopkins Press.

[98] Henle, J. (1840). Pathologische Untersuchungen. [Pathological studies]. Berlin: Verlag von August Hirschwald.

[99] Hebra, F. (1847). Höchst wichtige Erfahrungen über die Aetiologie der an Gebäranstalten epidemischen Puerperalfieber. Zeitschrift der k.k. Gesellschaft der Ärzte zu Wien., 4(1):242–244.

[100] Hebra, F. (1848). Fortsetzung der Erfahrungen über die Aetiologie der in Gebäranstalten epidemischen Puerperalfieber, Zeitschrift der k.k. Gesellschaft der Ärzte zu Wien., 5: 64f.

[101] Semmelweis, I. (1861). Die aetiologie, der begriff und die Prophylaxis des Kindbettfiebers. [The etiology, concept and prophylaxis of childbed fever]. C.A. Hartleben Verlag in Pest, Vienna, and Leipzig. Translated into English by Kay Codell Carter (1983), Madison: University of Wisconsin Press.

[102] Lumpe, E. (1845). Die Leistungen der neuesten Zeit in der Gynaekologie. [The achievements of modern times in Gynaecology] Zt. k. k. Ges. Aerzte zu Wien., 1(34):1-371.

[103] Churchill, F. (1849). Essays on the Puerperal Fever. London: The Sydenham Society.

[104] Braun. C. (1857). Lehrbuch der Geburtshilfe mit Berücksichtigung der Puerperalprocesse und der Operationstechnik. [Textbook of obstetrics concerning the puerperal process and surgical technique]. Wein.

[105] Gordon, A. (1795aa). A treatise on the epidemic puerperal fever of Aberdeen. Chapter IV Cause of Disease. In: F. Churchill editor (1849). Essays on the puerperal fever and other diseases selected from the writings of British authors previous to the close of the eighteenth century. London: Sydenham Society, 445-500.

[106] Gordon, A. (1795b). A treatise on the epidemic puerperal fever of Aberdeen, London, printed for G. G. and J. Robinson, 5–13.

[107] Holmes, O. (1843). The contagiousness of puerperal fever. New England Quart. J. Med. Surg., 1:503-530.

[108] Hey, W. (1815). A Treatise on the Puerperal Fever. London: Longman, Hurst, Rees, Orme and Brown, 21-25, 44.

[109] Mackintosh, J. (1822). A treatise on the disease termed puerperal fever. Edinburgh: William Blackwood. 197.

[110] Mayrhofer, C. (1863). Untersuchungen uiber Aetiologie der Puerperalprocesse, Z. k. k. Ges. Aertze. Wien., 19:28-42.

[111] Mayrhofer, C. (1865). 0'Zur Frage nach der Aetiologie der Puerperalprocesse', Mschr. Geburtsk. Frauenkr., 25: 112-134.

[112] Hodge, H. (1852). On the non-contagious character of puerperal fever. An introductory lecture. Delivered Monday, October 11, 1852. Philadelphia: T.K. and P.G. Collins, Printers.

[113] Mayrhofer, C. (1865). Zur Frage nach der Aetiologie der Puerperalprocesse', Mschr. Geburtsk. Frauenkr., 25:112-134.

[114] Rayer, P. (1850). Inoculation du sang de rate. Comptes Rendus de l'Académie des Sciences Soc. Biol., 11:141-144.

[115] Pasteur, L. (1857). Mémoire sur la fermentation appelée lactique. Comptes Rendus, 45:913–916.

[116] Pasteur, L. (1865). Procédé pratique de conservation et d'amélioration des vins. Comptes Rendus, May 1, 60:899-901.

[117] Pasteur, L. (1880). Extension of the Germ Theory to the etiology of certain common disease. Paper presented to the French Academy of Sciences, May 3, 1880. Published in Comptes rendus de l'Academie des Sciences, XC, 1033-44.

[118] Pasteur, L. (1878). Germ Theory and its applications to medicine and surgery. Paper presented to the French Academy of Sciences, April 29th. Published in Comptes Rendus de l'Academie des Sciences, LXXXVI:1037-43

[119] Pasteur, L. (1880a). Sur le Cholkra des poules estudes des conditions de la non-recidive de la maladie et de quelques autres de ses caracteres. Comptes Rendus de l'Acadmie des Sciences, 90:954.

[120] Pasteur, L. (1880b). Sur les maladies virulentes, et en particulier sur la maladie appelee vulgairement cholkra des poules. Comptes Rendus de l'Acadkmie des Sciences, 90:242.

[121] Pasteur, L. (1880c). Experiences tendant de demontrer que les poules vaccinees pour le cholera sont refractaires au charbon, Comptes Rendus de l'Académie des Sciences, 91:315.

[122] Pasteur, L. (1885). Methode pour preventir la rage après morsure. Comptes Rendus Acad Sci., 101:765-844.

[123] Béchamp, A. (1883). Les Microzymas: L'hétérogénie, l'histogenie, la physiologie et la pathologie. Librairie J. B. Baillière, Paris.

[124] Béchamp, A. (1903). Louis Pasteur: ses plagiats chimicophysiologiques et medicaux. Chez l'auteur, Paris.

[125] Bechamp, A. (1912). The blood and its third anatomical element. Translated from French into English by Montague Leverson. London: John Ouseley Limited.

[126] Hume, E. (1923). Béchamp or Pasteur? A lost chapter in the history of biology. Chicago: Covici-McGee.

[127] Pearson, R. (1942). Pasteur, plagiarist, imposter!: The germ theory exploded. Reprinted by Health Research Books. Washington: Pomeroy. Retrieved from http://books.google.com/books?id=KfehqKQWwNIC&printsec=frontcover&source=gbs_ge_summary_r&cad=0#v=onepage&q&f=false

[128] Schwann, T. (1837). Ann. Phys. Chem. (Poggendorff), 41:184-193.

[129] Appert, N. (1810). Le livre de tous les manges, ou l'art de conserver, pendant plsieurs années, toutes les substances animales et vegetales. Paris: Chez Patris er Cie, Imprimeurs-Libraires, quai Napoleon, au coin de la'rue de la colombre, no. 4.

[130] Cohn, F., 1875. Untersuchungen ueber bakterien. Beitraege zur biologie der planzen [Investigations about bacteria. Contributions to the biology of the plants] 1:127-222.

[131] Cohn, F. (1872a). Ueber Bakterien, die kleinsten lebenden Wesen. Lüedritz'sche Verlagsbuchhandlung [About bacteria, the smallest living beings], Berlin: Carl Habel.

[132] Cohn, F. (1872b). Bacteria: The smallest living organisms. Translated by Charles S. Dolley (1881). Rochester, New York: Frank D. Phinney.

[133] Koch, R. (1876). Untersuchungen ueber bakterien v. die aetiologie der Milzbrand-Krankheit, begruendent auf die entwicklungsgeschichte des bacillus anthracis. Beitr. z. Biol. D. Pflanzen., 2:277-310.

[134] Koch, R. (1882). Die Aetiologie der Tuberculose. Berliner Klinische Wochenschrift, 19:221-230.

[135] Koch, R. (1884). Cholera-Berichte aus Egypten und Indien. Deutsche Vierteljahrsschrift für öffentliche Gesundheitspflege, 16:493-515.

[136] Koch, R., Gaffky, G., Loeffler, F. (1884). Experimentelle studien über die künstliche Abschwächung der Milzbrandbazillen und Milzbraninfection dürch Fütterung. Mittheilungen aus dem Kaiserlichen Gesundheitsamte, 2:147-181.

[137] Koch, R. (1877). Verfahrungen zur Untersuchung, zum Conserviren und Photographiren der Bacterien. Beiträge zur Biologie der Pflanzen., 2(3):300-434.

[138] Nobel Prize in Physiology or Medicine 1905. Nobelprize.org Retrieved 11-16-2011.

[139] Pacini, F. (1854). Osservationi microscopiche e deduzioni pathologiche sul cholera asiatico. [Microscopical observations and pathological deductions on cholera]. Comptes Rendus Academy Sciences, Paris, 40, 30.

[140] Pacini, F. (1835). Sopra un particulare genere di piccoli corpi globulari scoperti nel corpo umano da Filippo Pacini. Archivio delle scienze medico-fisiche toscana, 8.

[141] Pacini, F. (1840). Nuovi organi scoperti nel corpo umano. Pistoia: Cino.

[142] Henle, J. and Killiker, A. (1844). Ueber die Pacini'schen Körperchen. Zurich.

143 Sedillot, C. (1878). Paris Academy of Sciences Meeting March 11, 1878, From Trouessart, E. L. Microbes, Ferments and Moulds (1892). International Scientific Series, Vol. 57. New York: D. Appleton.

[144] Neisser, A. (1879). Ueber eine der Gonorrhoe eigenthumliche micrococcusform. [A form of micrococcus peculiar to gonorrhea].Vorlaufige Mitteilung. Cbl. F. d. Med. Wiss., 28:497-500.

[145] Neisser, A. (1880). Ueber die Aetiologie des Aussatzes. Jahresberichte der schlesischen. Gesellschaft für Vaterländische Cultur, Breslau, 57:65-72.

[146] Hansen, G. (1874). Undersøgelser angaende spedalskhedens arsager [Investigations concerning the etiology of leprosy]. Norsk Mag. Laegervidenskaben, 4:1-88.

[147] Hansen, G. (1880). Bacillus leprae. Quarterly Journal of the Microscopical Science, 20:92-102.

[148] Neisser, A. (1881). Weitere Beiträge zur Aetiologie der Lepra. Virchows Archiv für pathologische Anatomie und Physiologie und für Klinische Medicin., Berlin, 84:514-542.

[149] Fite, G. and Wade, H. (1955). The contribution of Neisser to the establishment of the Hansen bacillus as the aetiologic agent of leprosy and the so-called Hansen-Neisser controversy. International Journal of Leprosy, 23:418-27.

[150] Gram, H. (1884). Uber die isolierte Färbung der Schizomyceten in Schnitt- und Trockenpräparaten. Fortschritte der Medizin., 2:185–9.

[151] Ziehl, F. (1882). Zur farbung des tuberkelbaclilus. Deutsche Medizinische Wochenschrift, 8:451.

[152] Ziehl, F. (1883a). Uber die farbung des tuberkelbacillus. [On staining of tubercle bacilli]. Deutsche Medizinische Wochenschrift, 9:247.

[153] Neelsen, F. (1883b). Ein casuistischer beitrag zur lehre von der tuberkulose. [A causistic note on the theory of tuberculosis]. Centralblatt fur die medicinischen Wissenschaften, 28:497.

[154] Crookshank, E. (1896). A textbook of bacteriology: Including the etiology and prevention of infective diseases and a short account of yeasts and moulds, haematozoa, and psorosperms. 4th edition.London: H.K. Lewis.

[155] Pfeiffer, R. (1894). Weitere Untersuchungen ueber das Wesen der Choleraimmunitat und ueber specifisch baktericide Processe. Ztschr. f. Hyg. u. Infektionskrankh. XVIII, 1-16.

[156] Treille, G. and Yersin, A, (1894). La Peste Bubonique A Hong-Kong. Paper presented at the VIII Congress International d'Hygiene et de Demographie de Budapest du 1 August - 9 September. Budapest, Hungary. Subsequently published in the Annales de l'Institut Pasteur., 8:662-667.

[157] Loghem, J. (1944). The classification of the plague bacillus. Antonie van Leeuwenhoek, 10(1):15-16.

[158] Yersin, A. (1894a). La peste bubonique a Hong-Kong. Ann. Inst. Pasteur Paris, 8:662-667. Retrieved December 2011 http://www.archive.org/stream/journaldemicrob01frangoog#page/n748/mode/2up

[159] Yersin, A. (1894b). La peste bubonique a Hong-Kong. C. R. Acad. Sci., 119:356. Paper presented to the Academy of Sciences July 30, 1894 by Emil Duclaux on behalf of A. Yersin.

[160] Kitasato, S. (1894a). The bacillus of bubonic plague. Lancet, 2:428-430.

[161] Kitasato, S. (1894b). Preliminary notice of the bacillus of bubonic plague. Practitioner, 53:311.

[162] Beijerinck, M. (1898). Uber ein contagium vivum fluidum als ursache der fleckenkrankheit der tabaksblatter. [Over a contagion vivum fluidum as the cause of the tobacco leaf spot disease.]. Verhandelingen der Koninklyke akademie van Wettenschappen te Amsterdam, 65:1-22.

[163] Online Etymology Dictionary (2011). Virus. Retrieved October 2011 http://www.etymonline.com/index.php?term=virus

[164] Society of American Bacteriologists (1899). First meeting December 27, 28, 29, at Yale University. New Haven: Abstracts published by H.W. Conn (1900) in Science N.S. Vol XI, March; No. 273; 455-463.

[165] Society of American Bacteriologists (1899). Constitution of the Society of American Bacteriologist, Draft. First meeting December 27-29 at Yale University, New Haven, Connecticut.

[166] Reed, W., Carroll, J., Agramonte, A., Lazear, J. (1900). The etiology of Yellow Fever - A preliminary note. Reprinted from the Proceedings of the Twenty-eighth Annual Meeting of the American Public Health Association in Indianapolis, October 22-26, 1900.

[167] Reed, W., Carroll, J., Agramonte, A. (1901). The etiology of Yellow Fever: An additional note. Reprinted from the Proceedings of the Pan-Am. Medical Congress in Havana, February 4-7, 1901.

[168] Finlay, C. (1881a). The mosquito hypothetically considered as an agent in the transmission of yellow fever poison. Paper presented at the Medical, Physical, and Natural Sciences of Habana, August 14, 1881.

[169] Finlay, C. (1881b). El mosquito hipoteticomente considerado como agente transmisor de la fiebre amarilla. Anales de la Academia de Ciencias, 27:147-169.

[170] Finlay, C. (1901). Advances made during the XIX century on the Yellow fever propagation. Paper presented at the Third Pan-American Medical Convention, February 4-7 1901, Habana, Cuba.

[171] Ricketts, H. (1906).The transmission of Rocky Mountain spotted fever by the bite of the wood-tick (Dermacentor occidentalis).The Journal of the American Medical Association, Chicago, 47:358.

[172] Ricketts, H. (1909). A micro-organism which apparently has a specific relationship to Rocky Mountain spotted fever. A preliminary report. The Journal of the American Medical Association, 52:379-380.

[173] Ricketts, H. and Wilder, R. (1910a). The relation of typhus fever (tabardillo) to Rocky Mountain spotted fever. Archives of Internal Medicine, Chicago, 5:361-370.

[174] Ricketts, H. and Wilder, R. (1910b). The etiology of the typhus fever (tabardillo) of Mexico City. A further preliminary report. The Journal of the American Medical Association, 54:1373-1375.

[175] Rocha-Lima, H. (1916). Zur Aetiologie des Fleckfiebers. [The etiology of typhus] Berliner klinische Wochenschrift., 53:567-569.

[176] Chagas, C. (1909a). Nouvelle espèce de Trypanosomiase humaine. Bulletin de la Société de pathologie exotique, 2: 304-307.

[177] Chagas, C. (1909b). Nova trypanozomiaze humana. Estudos sobre a morfolojia e cíclo evolutivo do Schizotripanum cruzi n. gen. n. sp., ajente etiolòjico de nova entidade morbida do homem. Memòrias di Instituto Oswaldo Cruz, Rio de Janeiro, 1(2):159-218, ests 9-13.

[178] Chagas, C. (1910). Nova entidade morbida do homem. Brazil Médico, 43: 423-428; 44, 433-437; 45, 443-447.

[179] Laveran, A. (1880a). New parasite found in the blood of several patients suffering from marsh fever. Two notes to the Academy of Medicine in Paris, November and December 1880.

[180] Laveran, A. (1880b). A new parasite found in the blood of malarial patients. Parasitic origin of malarial attacks. Bull. Mem. Soc. Med. Hosp. Paris. 17:158-164.

[181] Ross, R. (1899). Mosquitoes and malaria. Brit. Med. J., 432-433.

[182] Leishman, W. (1903). On the possibility of the occurrence of trypanosomiasis in India. Br. Med. J., 1:1252-1254.

[183] Donovan, C. (1903). On the possibility of the occurrence of trypanosomiasis in India. Br. Med. J., 2:79.

[184] Ross, R. (1903). Further notes on Leishman's bodies. British Medical Journal, 2, 1401.

[185] Nicolle, C., Comte, C., Conseil, L. (1909). Transmission expérimentale du typhus exanthématique par le pou du corps. Comptes Rendus Hebdo-Madaires des Seeances de l'Académie des Sciences, 149:486–9.

[186] Silva, P. (1908). Contribuicaso para o estudo da schistosomiase na Bahia. Brasil Med., 22:281-283.

[187] Leiper, R. (1915). Report on the results of the bilharzia mission in Egypt, Part I. Transmission. Journal Royal Army Med. Corps, 24:1-48; 25:1-55.

[188] Leiper, R. (1916). Observations on the mode of spread and prevention of vesical and intestinal Bilharziosis in Egypt with addition to August 1916. Proc. R. Soc. Med., 9 (Gen Rep), 145-172.

[189] The Nobel Prize in Physiology or Medicine 1902. Nobelprize.org. 25 Nov 2011 http://www.nobelprize.org/nobel_prizes/medicine/laureates/1902/

[190] The Nobel Prize in Physiology or Medicine 1907. Nobelprize.org. 25 Nov 2011 http://www.nobelprize.org/nobel_prizes/medicine/laureates/1907/

[191] The Nobel Prize in Physiology or Medicine 1928. Nobelprize.org. 25 Nov 2011 http://www.nobelprize.org/nobel_prizes/medicine/laureates/1928/

[192] Nomination Database - Physiology or Medicine. Nobelprize.org. 25 Nov 2011 http://www.nobelprize.org/nobel_prizes/medicine/nomination/nomination.php?

[193] Rous, P. (1911). Transmission of a malignant new growth by means of a cell-free filtrate. J. Am. Med. Assoc., 56:198.

[194] The Nobel Prize in Physiology or Medicine 1966. Nobelprize.org. 25 Nov 2011 http://www.nobelprize.org/nobel_prizes/medicine/laureates/1966/

[195] Ehrlich, P. (1900). Cellularbiologische Betrachtungen über Immunität. [Cellular biological observations on immunity.]. Bericht der Senckenbergischen Naturforschenden Gesellschaft in Frankfurt am Main., 147-150

[196] Ehrlich, P. (1898). Ueber den Zusammenhang von chemischer Constitution und Wirkung. [On the relation of chemical constitution and effect.]. Münchener Medizinische Wochenschrift, 51:1654-1655.

[197] Ehrlich, P. (1910). Diskussionsbemerkungen zum vortrag von wechselmann: Chemotherapie der syphilis. [Discussion comments on the presentation chemotherapy of syphilis.]. Bericht ueber die Tagung der Freien Vereinigung fuer Mikrobiologie, 47:223-224.

[198] Ehrlich, P. (1913). Uber chemotherapie: Die behandlung der syphilis mit Salvarsan und verwandten stoffen. [About chemotherapy: The treatment of syphilis with Salvarsan and related materials]. Paper presented to the Seventeenth International Congress of Medicine, Section 13, London.

[199] McDonough, J. (1915). Practitioner's Encyclopedia of Medical Treatment. Oxford Medical Publications.

[200] Thibierge, G. (1918). Syphilis and the Army. Edited by C. Marshall. London: University of London Press.

[201] Ehrlich, P. (1906). Address delivered at the dedication and opening of the George-Speyer Haus Biomedical Research Institute. Collected papers, extracted from Vol 3, 53-63.

[202] Twort, F. (1915). An investigation on the nature of ultra-microscopic viruses Lancet, 2:1241-1243.

[203] d'Herelle, F. (1917). Sur un microbe invisible antagonistic des bacilles dysenterique. Comptes Rendus de l'Académie des Sciences Paris, 165:373-375.

[204] Bordet, J. and Ciuca, M. (1921). Remarques sur l'historique des recherches concernant la lyse microbienne transmissible. Comptes Rendus de l'Académie des Sciences Biol. Paris, 84:745-747.

[205] d'Herelle, F. (1921). Sur l'historique du bacteriophage. Comptes Rendus de l'Académie des Sciences Biol. Paris, 84:863-864.

[206] Rivers, T. (1926). Filterable viruses: A critical review. Paper presented to the XXVIII annual meeting of the Society of American Bacteriologists, Philadelphia, Pennsylvania, December 29, 1926.

[207] Rivers, T. (1927). Filterable Viruses: A critical review. J. Bacteriol., 14:217-258.

[208] Rivers, T. (1928). Filterable Viruses. Baltimore: Williams and Wilkins.

[209] Flexner A. (1910). Medical Education in the United States and Canada: A Report to the Carnegie Foundation for the Advancement of Teaching. Bulletin No. 4. Boston, Mass: Updyke.

[210] Calmette, L. (1920). L'infection bacillaire et la tuberculose chez l'homme et chez les animaux. [The tuberculosis infection in humans and animals,] Paris: Masson.

[211] Calmette, L. (1921). Preventive vaccination against tuberculosis with BCG. Proceedings of the Royal Society of Medicine, 24:85–94.

[212] Guerin, C. and Rosenthal, S. (1957). Early history of BCG. London: Little Brown.

[213] Nicolle, M. (1907). Ann. Inst. Pasteur., 21:613-621.

[214] Bloomfield, A. (1919). Bull John Hopkins Hospital, 30:317-322.

[215] Fleming, A. (1922). Proc. R. Soc. London, Ser B, 93:306-317.

[216] Fleming, A. and Allison, V. (1922). Br. J. Exper. Pathology, 3:252-260.

[217] Fleming, A. (1929). On the antibacterial action of cultures of a Penicillium, with a special reference to their use in the isolation of B. influenza. Brit. J. Exp. Path., 10:226-236.

[218] Duchesne, E. (1897). Contribution a l'etude de la concurrence vitale chez les microorganisms antagonisme entre les moisissures et les microbes. [Contribution to the study of the struggle for life in microorganisms: antagonism between fungi and microbes] Thesis presented to the Faculty of Medicine and Pharmacy, Lyon to obtain the degree of Doctor of Medicine. Publicly defended December 17, 1897. School of Military Health Sciences, Lyon, France.

[219] The Nobel Prize in Physiology or Medicine 1945. Nobelprize.org. 15 Nov 2011

[220] Ruska H, von Borries B, and Ruska E. (1940). Die Bedeutung der Übermikroskopie für die Virusforschung. Arch ges Virusforsch [The significance of electron microscopy for virus research], 1:155-69.

[221] Ruska, H. (1940). Die Sichtbarmachung der bakteriophagen lyse im ubermikroskop. Naturwissenschaften. [The visualization of the bacteriophage lysis by electron microscopy, Natural Sciences], 28:45-6.

[222] Press Release: The 1986 Nobel Prize in Physics. Nobelprize.org. 21 Nov 2011 http://www.nobelprize.org/nobel_prizes/physics/laureates/1986/press.html

[223] Schata, A., Bugie, E., and Waksman, S. (1944). Streptomycin, a substance exhibiting antibiotic activity against gram-positive and gram-negative bacteria. Proc. Soc. Exp. Biol. Med., 55:66-69.

[224] Schatz, A. (1945). Streptomycin, an antibiotic produced by Actinomyces griseus. Ph.D. Dissertation. Rutgers University.

[225] Nobel Prize in Physiology or Medicine 1952. Nobelprize.org Retrieved 11-16-2011.

[226] Anonymous (1948). U.S. Patent Office File Wrapper and Contents. Improvement in Streptomycin and Processes of Preparation. No. 2,449,866. Granted Sept. 21, 1948, to S.A. Waksman and A. Schatz.

[227] Anonymous (1950). Civil Action Judgment. Albert Schatz, Plaintiff, versus Selman A. Waksman and Rutgers Research and Endowment Foundation, a corporation of New Jersey. Superior Court of New Jersey, Chancery Division, Middlesex County. Docket No. C-1261-49. December 29.

[228] Schatz, A. (1993). The true story of the discovery of streptomycin. Actinomycetes, 4(2):27-39.

[229] Salk, J. (1953). Studies in human subjects on active immunization against poliomyelitis. A preliminary report of experiments in progress. JAMA, 151:1801.

[230] Francis, T., Korns, R., Voight, R., Boisen, M., Hemphill, F., Napier, J, et al. (1955). An evaluation of the 1954 poliomyelitis vaccine trials: summary report. Am. J. Public Health, 45(suppl): 1–50 with 63 page supplement.

[231] Brownlee, K. (1955). Statistics of the 1954 Polio Vaccine Trials. Journal of the American Statistical Association, 50:1005-1013.

[232] Meier, P. (1957). Safety of the Poliomyelitis Vaccine. Science, 125:1067-1071.

[233] Isaacs, A. and Lindenmann, J. (1957). Virus interference; I. The interferon. Proc. Roy. Soc. Series B, 147:258-267.

[234] Isaacs, A., Lindenmann, J., Valentine, R. (1957). Virus interference: II. Some properties of interferon. Proc. R. Soc., 147:268-73.

[235] Findlay, G. and MacCallum, F. (1937). An interference phenomenon in relation to yellow fever and other viruses. The J. of Path. and Bac., 44 (2):405-424.

[236] Andrewes, C. (1942). Interference by one virus with the growth of another in tissue-culture. Br. J. Exp. Path., 23:214-220.

[237] Henle, W. (1950). Interference phenomena between animal viruses: A review. J. Immunol., 64, 203-236.

[238] Coon, A., Creech, H., Jones, R., Berlinger, E. (1944). The demonstration of pneumococcal antigen in tissues by the use of fluorescent antibody. J. Immunolog,. 45:159-70.

[239] Yalow, R. and Berson, S. (1960). Immunoassay of endogenous plasma insulin in man. J. Clin. Invest., 39(7): 1157–75.

[240] Stahl, T. (1975). Radioimmunoassay and the hormones of thyroid function. Semin. Nucl. Med., Jul 5(3):221-46.

[241] The Nobel Prize in Physiology or Medicine 1977. Nobelprize.org. 29 Nov 2011.

[242] Bauer, A. Kirby, W., Sherris, J., Turk, M. (1966). Antibiotic susceptibility testing by a standardized single disk method. The Am. J. Clinic. Path., 45(4):493-496.

[243] Engvall, E. and Perlman, P. (1971). Enzyme-linked immunosorbent assay (ELISA). Quantitative assay of immunoglobulin G., Immunochemistry, 8(9):871–4.

[244] Van Weemen, B. and Schuurs, A. (1971). Immunoassay using antigen-enzyme conjugates. FEBS Letters 15(3): 232–236.

[245] Kohler, G. and Milstein, C. (1975). Continuous cultures of fused cells secreting antibody of predefined specificity. Nature, 256:495-497.

[246] Burnette, W. (1981). Western blotting: electrophoretic transfer of proteins from sodium dodecyl sulfate-polyacrylamide gels to unmodified nitrocellulose and radiographic detection with antibody and radioiodinated protein A. Anal.Biochem., 112:195-203.

[247] Gallo, D., Diggs, J., Shell, G., Dailey, P., Hoffman, M., and Riggs, J. (1986). Comparison of detection of antibody to the acquired immune deficiency syndrome virus by enzyme immunoassay, inmmunofluorescence, and Western blot methods. J. Clinical Microbiology, June, 23, (6):1049-1051.

[248] World Health Organization (1979). Resolution WHA33.3 Formal declaration of the global eradication of Smallpox, based upon the report of the Global Commission to the Director General of WHO, as adopted unanimously by the Thirty-third World Health Assembly on 8 May 1980.

[249] U.S. Supreme Court (1980). Diamond, Commissioner of Patents and Trademarks v. Chakrabarty, 447 U.S. 303 (1980). Retrieved 11-30-2011 from http://caselaw.lp.findlaw.com/cgibin/getcase.pl?navby=case&court=us&vol=447&invol=303

[250] Pruiner, S. (1982). Novel proteinaceaous particles cause scrapies. Science, 216:136-144.

[251] The Nobel Prize in Physiology or Medicine 1997. Nobelprize.org. 18 Nov 2011 http://www.nobelprize.org/nobel_prizes/medicine/laureates/1997/

[252] Gallo, R., Sarin, P., Gelmann, E., Robert-Guroff, M., Richardson, E., Kalyanaraman, V., Mann, D., Sidhu, G., Stahl, R. (1983). Isolation of human T-cell leukemia virus in acquired immune deficiency syndrome (AIDS). Science, 220:865-867.

[253] Popovic, M., Sarngadharan, M., Read, E., Gallo, R. (1984). Detection, isolation, and continuous production of cytopathic retroviruses (HTLV-III) from patients with AIDS and pre-AIDS. Science, 224 (4648):497–500.

[254] Montaigner, L., Duquet, L., Axler, C., Chamaret, S., Gruest, J., Nugeyre, M., Rey, F., Barne-Sinoussi, F., Chermann, J. (1984). A new type of retrovirus isolated form the patients presenting with lymphadenopathy and acquired immune deficiency syndrome: structural and antigenic relatedness with equine infectious anemia virus. Ann Virol., 135:119-134.

[255] The Nobel Prize in Physiology or Medicine 2008. Nobelprize.org. 29 Nov 2011.

[256] Warren, J. and Marshall, B. (1983). Unidentified curved bacilli on gastric epithelium in active chronic gastritis. Lancet, 1: 1273.

[257] The Nobel Prize in Physiology or Medicine 2005. Nobelprize.org. 29 Nov 2011. http://nobelprize.org/nobel_prizes/medicine/laureates/2005/illpres/. Retrieved 11-18-2011.

[258] Mullis, K., Faloona, F., Scharf, S., Saiki, R., Horn, G., Erlilch, H. (1986). Specific enzymatic amplification of DNA in vitro: the polymerase chain reaction. Cold Spring Harbor Symp. Quant. Biol., 51:263-73.

[259] The Nobel Prize in Chemistry 1993. Nobelprize.org. 29 Nov 2011. http://www.nobelprize.org/nobel_prizes/chemistry/laureates/1993/

[260] Fleischmann, R., Adams, M., White, O., Clayton, R., Kirkness, E., Kerlavage, A., Bult, C., Tomb, J., Dougherty, B., Merrick, J., et al. (1995). Whole genome random sequencing and assembly of Haemophilus influenza Rd. Science, Jul 28, 269(5223):496-512.

[261] Blattner, F., Plunkett, G., Bloch, C., Perna, N., Burland, V., Riley, M., Collado-Vides, J., et al. (1997). The complete genome sequence of Escherichia coli K-12. Science, 277:1453-74.

[262] Tomb, J., White, O., Kerlavage, A., Clayton, R., Sutton, G., Fleischmann, R., Ketchum, K., Klenk, H., Gill, S., Dougherty, B., Nelson, K., et al (1997). The complete genome sequence of the gastric pathogen Helicobacter pylori. Nature, Aug 7; 388(6642):539-47.

[263] Stephens, R., Kalman, S., Lammel, C., Fan, J., Marathe, R., Travind, L., Mitchell, W., Olinger, L., Tatusove, R., Zhao, Q., Koonin, E., Davis, R. (1998). Genome sequence of an obligate intracellular pathogen of humans: Chlamydia tracomatis. Science, Oct, 32, 282(5389):754-9.

[264] Cole, S., Brosch, R., Parkhill, J., Garnier, T., Churcher, C., Harris, D., Gordon, S., et al. (1998). Deciphering the biology of Mycobacterium tuberculosis from the complete genome sequence. Nature, 393:537-44.

[265] American Society for Microbiology. Official website retrieved 11-22-2011 from http;//www.asm.org/

[266] Canadian Association for Clinical Microbiology and Infectious Disease. Official website retrieved 11-22-2011from http://www.cacmid.ca/

[267] Society for General Microbiology. Official website retrieved 11-22-2011 from http://www.sgm.ac.uk

[268] Hiramatsu, K. (2001). Vancomycin resistant Stapylococcus aureus: a new model of antibiotic resistance. The Lancet-Infectious Disease, 1(3):147-155.

[269] Cetinkaya, Y., Falk, P., Mayhall, C. (2000). Vancomycin resistant Enteroccoci. Clin. Microbiol. Rev., Oct 13(4), 686-707.

[270] World Health Organization (2003). Summary tables of SARS cases by country, 1 November 2002-7 August 2003. Retrieved WHO website 11-22-2011.

[271] Bankowski, M. and Anderson, S. (2004). Real-time nucleic acid amplification in clinical microbiology. Clin. Microbiol. Newsl., 26:9-15.

[272] Boivin, G., Cote, S., Dery, P., DeSerres, F., Bergeron, M. (2004). Multiplex real-time PCR assay for detection of influenza and human respiratory syncytial viruses. J. Clin. Microbiol., 42:45-51.

[273] Ecker, D., Sampath, R., Massire, C., Blyn, L., Hall, T., Eshoo, M., Hofstadler, S. (2008). Ibis T5000: a universal biosensor approach to microbiology. Nature Reviews Microbiology, 6:553-558.

[274] Haukoos, J., Hopkins, E., Conroy, A., et al. (2010). Routine opt-out rapid HIV screening and detection of HIV infection in emergency department patients. JAMA, 304:284-292.

[275] Boehme, C., Nabeta, P., Hillemann, D., Nichol, M., Shenai, S., Krapp, F., Allen, J., et al. (2010). Rapid molecular detection of tuberculosis and rifampin resistance. N. Eng. J .Med., 363:1005-1015.

[276] Bos, K., Schuenemann, V., Golding, G., Burbano, H., Waglechner, N., Coombes, B., McPhee, J., DeWitte, S., Meyer, M., Schmedes, S., Wood, J., Earn, D., Herring, D., Bauer, P., Poinar, H., Krause, J. (2011). A draft genome of Yersinia pestis from victims of the Black Death. Nature, 478(7370):506-10.

Chapter 7

Medical Immunology

Definition.

Immunology is "…a science that deals with the immune system and the cell mediated and humoral aspects of immunity and immune responses…" (2018)[1]. The word immunology is a compound word derived from the Latin "immunis" meaning exempt and "logos" from the Greek meaning the study of a subject. Medical immunology is the study of "…all aspects of the immune system, including structure and function, disorders of the immune system, blood banking, immunization, and organ transplantation…" (2018)[2]

Classical immunology deals with the molecular and cellular components of the immune systems, their functions, and interactions. Medical immunology expands the definition, emphasizes the study and understanding of the many disorders and diseases of the systems with application of the knowledge to the treatment and management of human disease.

Traditionally, the immune system is divided into the innate immune system and the acquired immune system. Recall, the innate immune system is concerned primarily with barriers to primary infections e.g. bacteria, viruses, fungi, the process of phagocytosis, the complement system, and inflammatory mediators. The acquired immune system in contrast is primarily concerned with self vs non-self identifications, antigen recognition molecules, clonal selection, and memory (2017)[3].

In classical immunology, innate and acquired systems are further divided into their humoral and cellular components. Recall, humoral components include the soluble molecules, for example the antibodies produced by B cells, complement, interferons, collectins, and C reactive proteins. Cellular components of the system include numerous cells with specific functions, for example neutrophils, macrophages, B cells, T cells, and dendritic cells.

Clinical medical immunology is primarily concerned with the study of diseases caused by disorders of the immune system and strategies of using the immune systems to provide treatment and management of human disease conditions. Developmental immunology investigates the changes in the immune system across the lifespan. Diagnostic immunology utilize antibodies specific to specific antigens to label and subsequently detect specific antigens, typically associated with a disease process. Remember, an antigen is anything, yes anything that will generate an immune response. Collectively classical, clinical, developmental, and diagnostic immunology will form the cornerstones for the discussion of the history of medical immunology presented in this chapter.

Introduction.

Immunology has always been important to the science and clinical practice of medicine. From the time of the earliest written records, which appear on ancient clay tablets inscribed over 5,000 years ago in Mesopotamia, to the world wide electronic postings on the internet today, immunology has always been with us. Immunology, as a modern science, however is relatively new. Its roots are firmly planted in the discipline of microbiology. During the immediate past 100 years, immunology has developed, matured, and successfully established itself as an independent, much respected scientific discipline. The scientific contributions made by immunology throughout the 1900s and early-2000s are unmatched by any other time in history. The discipline, like all other scientific disciplines throughout history has capitalized upon technological advancements and applied these new technologies to advancing the knowledge base. Immunology is continually changing its conceptual matrixes and research approaches to better understand the mechanisms of actions used by the human body to defend and repair itself from infection and disease.

This chapter outlines the development of Immunology as a scientific discipline throughout time with special emphasis placed upon relevance for the medical student who is attempting to understand the history of a discipline, which so greatly impacts the routine practice of clinical medicine today.

This chapter is organized chronologically for consistency with other chapters and to provide you an opportunity to easily follow major developments, significant milestones, and the most influential people who have guided the development of immunology over time. Additionally, the chapter considers factors oftentimes neglected, political, social, economic, religious, and professional which have influenced the content, direction, and speed in which advances have been made or impeded.

Upon completion of this chapter you will have had an opportunity to develop a fundamental understanding of the history of medical immunology as it relates to the modern practice of medicine today. Perhaps too, you will begin to acknowledge the dangers inherent in the sirens' call for unquestioned acceptance of medical dogma and the comfort, security, and self-confidence medical dogma brings to so many.

History.

Early Records, 3500 BC - 500 BC.

There is very little known today of systematic or scientific study of immunology prior to 500 BC. The ancient civilizations of Mesopotamia (Mesopotamia literally means between two rivers; the Euphrates and Tigris) and ancient Egypt have however left many clues, in the form of cuneiform inscribed clay tablets and hieroglyphics. These written and pictorial inscriptions, from over 5,000 years ago, are only today beginning to reveal the content, level, and application of immunological knowledge, during the time of the Ancient civilizations of Sumeria circa 3500 BC, Egypt circa 3200 BC, and Babylonia circa 2000 BC. Much of the record is found on the thousands of clay tablets discovered during 1849 AD- 1852 AD, at two principle sites, the Royal Library of King Sennacherib (705 BC- 681 BC) and the Royal Palace/ Libraries of King Assurbanipal (668 BC- 627 BC), located in northern Mesopotamia (present day Iraq). The tablets discovered at these sites represent collected tablets from all regions of the Neo-Assyrian Empire (934 BC- 608 BC). Assyria is arguably one of the most powerful nations on earth and located primarily in northern

Mesopotamia. The rival nation of Babylonia controls the southern regions of Mesopotamia. These clay tablets contain knowledge reflecting the period during which they were inscribed and the history of knowledge accumulated over the previous thousands of years. Today, most of the tablets are housed in the British Museum. Recent translations from these and similar ancient civilization tablets are beginning to reveal an understanding of fundamental immunology previously unrecognized (2005)[4].

It is now clear. Ancient civilizations possessed not only an understanding of basic fundamental immunological principles e.g. an understanding of infectious communicable disease, innate immunity, and acquired immunity; they organized their knowledge into conceptual matrixes which guided observations, diagnosis, prognosis, and treatment.

In addition to the clay tablets from northern Mesopotamia, tablets from southern Mesopotamia region, dating to the First Babylonian Dynasty (1830 BC-1530 BC) provide supportive written evidence of the ancient civilizations understanding and application of fundamental immunological principles. Arguably, the most extensive medical text written during the period is the "Babylonian Diagnostic Handbook". The Handbook is contained in forty clay tablets, dates to approximately 1050 BC, and offers much insight into the conceptual matrixes used by the ancients to report and organize their knowledge in regard to disease and how the body responds (2005,2000,1976,1964, 1951)[4,5,6,7,8,9].

Early translations and interpretations of these and other tablets, during the late-1800s AD and 1900s AD, result in mischaracterizations of much of the knowledge known to these ancient civilizations. Often the knowledge is misrepresented as poorly organized, unsophisticated, based upon unscientific principles, and infused with magic and sorcery. These initial interpretations are today quickly being recognized to be incorrect. In fact, current translations and interpretations suggest just the opposite. The ancient civilization indeed maintained a rather sophisticated understanding of basic immunological principles and applied their knowledge to the diagnosis, treatment, and management of several disease processes. The epistemological approach applied by these Ancient civilizations is logical, rational, and based heavily upon empiricism.

True enough, the overriding conceptual matrix of the ancient civilizations often assigns the cause of diseases to the actions of angered deities and treatments are indeed steeped in mysticism. Upon reflection, similar interpretations can be made today regarding modern disease and treatments. It is easy enough to recall someone you have met during your lifetime who is equally prepared to argue the reason some individuals are afflicted by disease and suffering is simply due to punishment by God. The punishment is imposed upon the individual for deviating from the teachings and beliefs of any of the many organized religions of today and the result of a deviant lifestyle. Common examples I have heard during my lifetime, attributing illness, disease, and suffering to be punishments sent from God, are applied to homosexuals now suffering AIDS and IV drug users now suffering hepatitis.

Similarly, medical treatments offered by physicians today can be easily conceptualized as a constellation of arcane medical procedures and arcane recommendations to patients to ingest assorted pills and potions, many of which the scientific and medical communities do not understand exactly how they work or why they are effective. For those of you who have been in any hospital, how many of the hospitals have professional members of organized religions e.g. priest, rabbi, minister or places of worship within the hospital, available to the patient, family, and friends to appeal to their god for comfort or cure?

There are many similarities between the conceptual matrixes and healing practices applied by the Ancient civilizations with the conceptual matrixes and common healing practices of the modern-day practicing physician. Take a little time now and think about the similarities and differences. You will never have more free time than you do now for the remainder of your professional career. Think about it.

OK…back to ancient Mesopotamia and their approach to understanding disease and the immune systems. The written records reveal the ancient civilizations of Mesopotamia and neighboring Egypt developed and recorded empirically derived lists of observations, symptoms, and associated effective treatments. These empirically and experientially derived associations, accumulated over thousands of years, provided the empirical knowledge base from which diagnosis, treatment, management, and prognosis were based. Many of these detailed and accurate descriptions inscribed upon clay tablets closely parallel descriptions of signs and symptoms listed today in modern-day medical textbooks. The tablets reveal an understanding of infectious disease, transmission vectors, the body's immunological response to infection, and offer a comprehensive, integrated conceptual matrix from which to organize knowledge and generate effective medical treatments.

The methods of the ancient Mesopotamians and neighboring Egyptians are not that different from methods used today in the primary care setting. The concepts of collecting a history from a patient, associating information with known diseases, consulting a well-established empirical database as to what treatments and potions are most effective, prescribing a treatment program, following the patient for changes in their condition, and providing palliative care when no effective treatment is known is the same over 5000 years ago as it is today. Indeed many of the same diseases assessed and treated 5000 years ago are still assessed and treated today, often using similar diagnostic procedures and treatments. More on this later.

In summary, immunology and the medical interests in the immune response by the body has a long history. The immune response is detailed in the earliest written records. The immune response is identified as a normal process in the recovery of the body following disease or injury. Treatments designed to facilitate or regulate the immune response have also been detailed from the earliest history. Recovered and recently translated records from both ancient civilizations of Mesopotamia and neighboring Egypt reveal an impressive awareness of and interest in recording immunological knowledge. A foundational understanding of innate and acquired immunity is evident in the earliest written records. Yes, the specifics as to what generates an immune response and the mechanisms of actions responsible for maintaining and terminating the response have become more clear during the past 5000 years, however, the foundations of immunology remain firmly placed in ancient history. Only recently have we recognized and begun to reinterpret our misunderstandings, entrenched in academic and medical dogma. Immunology maintains an ancient history too often neglected and provides the foundation upon which many new and exciting advances in immunology stand today.

Antiquity, 500 BC - 500 AD.

Immunology witness many advancements during Antiquity. Greek pre-Socratic natural philosophers of the period explore natural, physical based models of disease and immunity, as an alternative to the supranatural, deity based models. Both natural and supranatural models account for and readily explain the source, presence, course, and resolution of disease. Both models provide predictions as to who are at risk for contracting a disease (natural immunity) and who are at reduced risk for recontracting the disease following an initial exposure (acquired immunity). Both models provide guidance to practitioners attempting to treat and comfort individuals suffering disease.

The polarizing effect of the two dominant models of the period, natural (physical) and supranatural (deity), soon lead proponents of each model to extreme positions. The two models follow separate courses of development and maturation with each establishing its own dogma.

The supranatural (deity) model of disease and immunity is embraced by organized religions. Written records reflecting the history and beliefs of three popular religions, Judaism, Christianity, and Catholicism of this period reveal a shared belief, as it relates to disease and immunity. In brief, disease is sent by an angered "God" to punish an individual, often due to the individual's failure to adhere to the fundamental teachings, beliefs, and behaviors approved by organized religion. The severity of a disease is dependent upon the degree of deviation from the guidelines or established rank ordering of specific thoughts and behaviors, specified by the respective religions. For example, a person committing homicide is more likely to suffer a severe disease and associated severe clinical course than a person who commits a theft. Recovery from the disease is based upon forgiveness from "God".

Specific examples are readily available in the early written records and teachings of each organized religion. Below are a few examples from taken from the Christian Bible, Jewish Torah, and Islamic Quran.

The Christian Bible for example, written over the course of perhaps 1500 years, during the period of 1000 BC through 500 BC, is filled with specifics e.g. Deuteronomy 7:15 "…and the Lord will take from thee all sickness and will put none of the evil diseases of Egypt which thou knowest upon thee; but will lay them upon them that hate thee…"; Deuteronomy 28:22 "…the Lord will smite thee with a consumption (old term for tuberculosis) and with fever and with an inflammation….until thou perish…"; Numbers 11:33 "…the Lord smote the people with a very great plague…"; Job 2:7 "…So went Satan forth from the presence of the Lord and smote Job with sore boils from the sole of his foot unto his crown…."; Leviticus 13:3-4 "…a plague of leprosy: and the priest shall look on him and pronounce him unclean…then the priest shall shut up him that hath (isolate) seven days…"; Samuel 5:6 "…the Lord's hand was heavy upon the people…he brought devastation upon them and afflicted them with tumors (for stealing the Ark of the Convenient)…" (circa 500 BC/2011)[10].

The Jewish Torah shares the books of Genesis, Exodus, Leviticus, Numbers, and Deuteronomy with the Christian Bible (circa 1300 BC/2011)[11]. Judaism and Christianity emphasize the role of the supranatural in understanding the source of disease and a person's response to disease.

Trivia: Moses, born in Egypt circa 1300 BC-1000 BC, is frequently credited throughout history with "writing" the first five books of the Bible; Genesis, Exodus, Leviticus, Numbers, and Deuteronomy.

The Islamic Quran, believed to have been written circa 610 AD- 632 AD, takes a slightly different approach than the Christian Bible. Disease and illness are not sent from God as punishment, rather they are sent to test an individual's commitment to Islam. Treatments for specific disease conditions appear throughout the Quran and most typically contain repeating specific phrases from the Quran, supplication, and performing symbolic, ritualistic behaviors (circa 632AD/1998)[12].

The second dominant belief system of the period emphasizes the role of the natural (physical) forces when attempting to understanding sources of disease and the human body's response to the disease. This belief system is advocated not by organized religions, rather by the pre-Socratic Greek natural (physical) philosophers.

Alcmaeon of Croton (557 BC-491 BC) pre-Socratic Greek, natural philosopher provides many of the earliest known writings, describing human body functions within the matrix of physical processes and openly challenges deity models, popular during this period. He offers a "natural" model, based upon physical process occurring within the body. The new physical process model receives much support and is aggressively investigated at the new medical school, founded by Alcmaeon at Croton, located in southern Italy. A rational-empirical approach, free from magic and religious elements is applied to acquiring new knowledge and understanding how the body works. The natural model is embraced by the faculty and medical students studying at Croton.

It is Alcmaeon who is first to propose the doctrine of balanced physical forces, rather than Hippocrates, as oftentimes popularly reported. Alcmaeon's model emphasizes a balance between the physical and naturally occurring qualities of wet, dry, cold, hot, bitter, and sweet. Alcmaeon's balance model emphasizes and describes normal and abnormal functioning of the body, including immune responses, within a model which emphasizes physical (natural), observable, and qualitatively measureable events and processes. This conceptualization stands in mark contrast to the supranatural (deity) based models of the ancient civilizations and organized religion.

Medical students at Croton are exposed to another influential and notable contemporary of Alcmaeon, Pythagoras of Samos, the Greek philosopher, mathematician, and founder of a mystic religious movement, subsequently termed Pythagoreanism.

Pythagoras of Samos (570 BC-495 BC) blends philosophy, mathematics, mysticism, and religion into his teachings. Of interest here is his emphasis upon proportions. Building upon Alcmaeon's matrix balance between qualities i.e. hot, cold, wet, dry, bitter, and sweet, Pythagoras introduces mathematical formulations and numerical quantifications into the matrix, allowing qualitative and quantitative measurements of change in the balances of these specific qualities held important in normal bodily functions. It is the change in proportions which is central to Pythagoras in understanding good health and disease.

By 500 BC the dogma of supranatural forces as being solely responsible for disease and the body's response to disease or infection is beginning to be questioned by a few willing to question authority. Alternative, natural (physical) based explanations are beginning to be explored and accepted. Mathematical relationships of proportions begin to be relevant in the practice of medicine. Given Alcmaeon's conceptualization of balanced physical qualities as necessary for good physical health and imbalance of these qualities result in illness, Pythagoras suggest proportional change in qualities should be assessed and can be associated with specific illnesses and diseases.

Hippocrates (460 BC-370 BC) Greek, itinerant practitioner of medicine, personally contributes little if at all to the development or advancement of immunology. The Hippocratic Collection, assembled circa 300 BC in the Libraries of Alexandria, however include a listing of commonly occurring diseases, their associated signs, symptoms, and recommended treatments. The Collection reflects the emphasis upon natural (physical) causes and natural (physical) body reactions rather than the supranatural (deity) models held by others. For example, tetanus

(Epidemics), tuberculosis (Afflictions), bubonic plague (Afflictions), malaria (Afflictions), and other commonly occurring diseases and infectious are extensively described and attributed to natural (physical) rather than supranatural causes (circa 300 BC/1525 AD-1595 AD)[13].

Thucydides (460 BC-395 BC) the much respected Greek historian, details vividly the gruesome signs and symptoms revealed by those afflicted by the Plague of Athens, circa 431 BC. His writings clearly state any person who contracts the illness and recovers will not contract the illness for a second time and can treat the sick without fear of a second illness (acquired immunity) (431BC/1934AD,2004AD)[14,15].

The Plague of Athens, caused by the obligate intracellular bacterium we know today as Rickettsia prowazekii and transmitted by the human body louse, results in the death of one of every three citizens of Athens. Within the course of two years, the entire population of the region is reduced by approximately thirty three percent (33%). The Plague has devastating political, social, religious, and economic effects upon the region.

During the Plague of Athens, four important observations are made and applied to the understanding of disease and the body's natural (physical) reactions to infection. First, disease and infection are the result of natural (physical) processes and not the result of displeased super-natural deities. Second, disease and infections can be transmitted between individuals following contact and not the result of spontaneous generation. Third, individuals who contract the disease follow a relatively common clinical course, characterized by predictable and time linked signs and symptoms. Fourth, individuals exposed to disease often develop an "acquired immunity" resulting in much reduced signs and symptoms in the event the individual is ever exposed to the disease for a second time. Certainly if the individuals contract the disease for a second time, the second episode rarely if ever will result in death.

During Antiquity, efforts are made by world leaders, led by the recently self-proclaimed King of Egypt (King Ptolemy I), to collect, consolidate, and organize records of human knowledge, including medical knowledge. Much of the Western world's written records of knowledge are brought to the Greek city of Alexandria, located on the western end of the Nile delta, in northern Egypt. The City is recognized as one of major cities in the world and center for scholarship, knowledge, and new learning. The City and Libraries flourish from its founding circa 323 BC until its initial decline circa 47 BC when the City and Libraries are unintentionally burned by invading Roman military forces led by Julius Cesar. The City and much of the deposited knowledge in the Libraries are intentionally destroyed in 392 AD, under order of the Roman Empire to destroy all non-Christian temples and non-Christian contents within.

The multi-authored Hippocratic Collections, reflects medical knowledge of the period and is assembled in the Libraries of Alexandria circa 300 BC. The Collection sheds much light on the understanding of disease and immunology of early-Antiquity. Inspection of the Collection reveals organized collections of written materials devoted specifically to epidemics and disease. Consistent with the usual and customary style of writing of the period, epidemics and diseases are recorded primarily as a listing of signs and symptoms. This stands in contrast to today in that most epidemics and diseases are recorded not by a constellation of signs and symptoms but rather the organism or infectious agent responsible for the disease. Many of the diseases recorded in the Collection can be easily identified today based upon their detailed descriptions. Yes, many of the diseases treated over 2000 years ago and described in the Hippocratic Collections are diagnosed and treated by physicians today.

Aristotle (384 BC-322 BC) Greek philosopher-scientist, stanch empiricist, proponent of the balance of humors doctrines, and committed exponent of the Miasma theory of disease, influences the direction of immunology for the next two thousand years. In brief and in regard to immunology, Aristotle's contributions are not particularly original. However, they do provide a point in history to introduce a then commonly held belief within the scientific and medical communities regarding the natural (physical) cause of disease, which is held as dogma well into the late-1800s, Miasma theory of disease.

Miasma theory of disease states, disease is caused by noxious, foul smelling vapors, generated from decomposing organic materials. Mists filled with particles of decomposed materials are the source of disease. The vapors coming from the ground (miasmata) are most common in low lying grounds such as swamps. Miasmatic theory provides a reasonable explanation, based upon the knowledge of the period. When a rational or empirical approach is applied to test the theory, end results are similar and supportive of the theoretical matrix. For example, consider the mosquito-borne infectious disease malaria. Think about it. Where are cases of malaria most prevalent? Who is most likely to suffer from malaria? The very term "malaria" is based upon miasmatic theory of disease and is derived from the Italian meaning "bad air" (mal= bad, aria = air). Miasmic theory of disease is very much a part of medical and scientific dogma well into the 1800s, at which time it is displaced by Germ theory. More on Germ theory later.

Aristotle is an avid proponent of the balance of humor doctrines, which provides a conceptual matrix within which to understand the body's physical immunological reaction to disease. Diseases, whether the result of natural (physical) spontaneous generation, miasmas, or transmission between infected people as purported by Aristotle or the result of supranatural forces as purported by organized religions, generates an observable, natural (physical) reaction from the body. According to Aristotle, disease is simply the antecedent cause, which produces a disturbance in the natural proportion of humors within the body and it is the disturbance in the balance of proportioned humors which is most responsible for the natural (physical) response from the body. He offers little else in regard to specifics.

Following Aristotle's logic, treatment for any disease therefore is simple; restore the balance of humors within the body and the body will return to a state of good health. There is nothing original here. Aristotle simply restates a minimally modified version of Alcmaeon's doctrine of balances, proposed and taught to medical students studying at the medical school founded by Alcmaeon, in Croton, a Greek city located in southern Italy, over 150 years before Aristotle.

Original contributions leading to a more complete understanding of disease and the immune response will soon come with the work of Herophilus and Erasistratus, co-founders of the medical school in Alexandria, Egypt.

Herophilus (325 BC-280 BC) and Erasistratus (304 BC-250 BC) Greek natural philosophers and experimentalists, working in arguably one of the world's most academic and scholastic cities, Alexandria, offer new and original insights into the area of medicine later to be termed immunology. These two men are most recognized for their application of a systematic, experimental approach into anatomy and physiology. Their investigations result in many of the foundational observations and conceptual thoughts which guide medical research for the next two thousand years. They are among the first to systematically investigate and document results of their empirical observations regarding the body's immunological response. Records reveal an awareness of bodily changes associated with infection, disease, and trauma. The immune reaction is outlined based upon empirical observations, including events necessary to trigger an immune response, the time dependent nature of the response, and probable outcome. While the physiology underlying the mechanisms of actions of the immune response are not reported and will not be well understood for another two thousand years, the point here is the immune response and its systematic study has a much older and richer history than many today recognize.

By the middle of Antiquity, philosophical, scientific, and religious forces are well established in influencing the content and direction of immunology. Government based political leaders soon too find opportunities to influence advances in immunology.

Mithridates VI, King of Pontus (Turkey) (120 BC-63 BC) issues royal directives to systematically investigate the prophylactic effect of repeated exposure of injecting increasingly small dosages of assorted poisons and snake venoms. The directives are issued in an effort to obtain the necessary knowledge to protect the King from potential poisonings from others. Remaining true to a common practice evident throughout the history of medicine and still practiced in several countries in the world today; testing is completed on State criminals. The royal directives from Mithridates VI perhaps represents the first documented, State funded investigation, specifically focusing upon the development of a greater understanding of the immune system and more specifically acquired immunity (200 AD/1914-1927)[16].

OK…as we transition from BC to AD time periods, it seems logical to briefly summarize here what we know today, in regard to the history of immunology, and perhaps correct a few popular misconceptions too.

First the popular and oftentimes reported belief, immunology has a short and only recent history is simply false. The common practice of introducing the history of immunology with its beginnings couched in the work of Edward Jenner in the late-1700s is misleading at best and minimizes the full and lengthy history of medicine.

Second, the belief early immunology is entrenched in mysticism, sorcery, an unorganized collection of random associations, and reliance upon supranatural deities to explain disease, infection, and treatments is true only in part and is extremely misleading. Most practices of the healing arts historically are couched in conceptual matrixes which rely upon the supranatural in order to explain that which we don't understand. It should not be surprising, this is also the case with the immune systems. If it cannot be understood within the matrix of current knowledge and technologies, it must be explained by the supranatural. This is only part of the story. Written records from the ancient civilizations of Mesopotamia circa 3500 BC reveal evidence both natural and supranatural conceptual matrixes are used to understand immune responses. Both models reveal a written history of organized and thoughtful observations. By 500 BC the natural (physical) models displaces most supranatural models. By 300 BC immunology is studied in a systematic, experimental, natural (physical) matrix by faculty and medical students at the medical school and Libraries in Alexandria.

Third, the fundamental concepts of innate and acquired immunity are recognized even among the lay public. True enough, the physiological and molecular basis responsible for innate and acquired immunity have yet to be established, yet the fundamental concepts are described from an empirical observational perspective. A person who is injured by cutting of the skin will invariably react with signs and symptoms of inflammation, characterized by localized swelling, redness, warmth, and pain (innate immunity). A person who suffers an initial exposure to the plague and survives is more likely to suffer a less intense clinical course upon a subsequent exposure (acquired immunity). The concepts of innate and acquired immunity at this point in time are not the primary result of careful, systematic, experimental, scientific-method based investigations (though some do exist) but rather emerge from a collective awareness among people of the millions of people who have cut their skin and suffered plagues throughout history.

Fourth, the fundamental concept of infectious disease, reservoirs, and vectors of disease transmission are recognized. It is known animals and insects can carry diseases (e.g. rabies, bubonic plague, smallpox); drinking stagnant water or eating spoiled foods can produce violent immune gastrointestinal reactions (e.g. dysentery, food poisoning); living close to a swamp oftentimes produces recurring fevers (e.g. malaria); a person infected by a disease can transmit the disease to a non-infected person by physical or close contact (e.g. syphilis, leprosy, tuberculosis (aka consumption), plague). While this knowledge is perhaps better classified as epidemiological rather than immunological, most people of the period make an empirical-experiential association with specific environmental conditions and a predictable immune response.

Fifth, it is recognized the body's innate immune system and consequently the body's recovery from infection can be supported through the application of therapeutic plasters (e.g. honey's antibacterial effect), ingestion of specific and empirically derived potions, cleaning and drainage of wounds, establishing good personal hygiene, modifying diet, and engaging in moderate exercise. All of these simple supports of the immune system are known and have been practiced for thousands of years. Today, throughout most of the world in most every medical center, these simple guidelines to support a patient's immune systems are still recommended by most treating physicians. The modern idea that many of these are new and relatively recent discoveries simply challenge the written records of medical history.

Sixth, mithridazation, the practice of intentionally self-administering progressively larger and larger non-lethal amounts of poisons or snake venom, for the purpose of developing immunity to the poison or venom is known and practiced by a select few during the early years of Antiquity. Mithridazation is still practiced today, in limited settings, especially by individuals working routinely with venomous snakes or insects in medical research settings. See Bill Hasst (1910-2011) notable and founding director of the Miami Serpertarium Laboratories. While limited then and today, recent and renewed interests in the role of venoms e.g. bee venom, is currently being investigated as to its role in stimulating and manipulating the immune response for therapeutic purposes. The point here is there is a written history documenting recognition and investigation of poisons and venoms roles in manipulation of the body's immune systems, over 2000 years old and modern investigations currently being conducted today, in laboratories around the world, continue to investigate the relationship between poisons, venoms, and the immune systems' response.

Seventh, hypersensitivity immune reactions, especially type I e.g. food allergies, occupational rhinitis, asthma, hay fever, bee sting anaphylaxis are recognized and described from an experiential, observational matrix thousands of years ago. The conditions necessary to trigger reactions are described along with resultant signs and symptoms and empirically derived effective courses of treatment. Although the molecular bases we use today to describe and understand the mechanisms responsible for these reactions are not revealed for another 1,800 to 2,000 years, the scientific, medical, and religious communities of the period all provide written records documenting their understanding and their proposed mechanisms of actions responsible for the hypersensitivity reactions.

Eighth, immune systems and immune responses have been systematically studied and findings recorded in the written record since the time of the Ancient civilizations. Familiar medical documents such as the Edwin Smith papyrus dated approximately 1550 BC for example describe specific immune reactions e.g. asthmas and allergies, along with effective treatments. More recently, during Antiquity, systematic, scientific based, experimental investigations conducted and recorded at the medical school and Libraries of Alexandria circa 300 BC-1 BC have been discovered and translated.

Ninth, two broad conceptual matrixes prove most prominent in organizing knowledge of immune systems and immune responses by 1 BC, the supranatural (deity) models preferred by organized religions and the natural (physical) models preferred by natural philosophers and natural medical scientists. Both models provide the organization and structure to permit diagnosis, guide treatments, and predict clinical outcomes. By 1 BC the natural (physical) model is the more favored model among medical investigators, although both affect the progress in efforts to better understand immune systems and their manipulation for therapeutic purposes.

In summary, by 1 BC immunology has established a rather lengthy written history; two competing conceptual matrixes organize immunological knowledge, the supranatural (deity) and the natural (physical) models; the basic concepts of innate and acquired immunity are recognized; the basic concepts of infectious disease, disease reservoirs and disease vectors are recognized; specific therapies which can augment immune system function and speed body healing are recognized; repetitive exposure of small, non-lethal doses of specific antigens bolsters tolerance for the antigen; hypersensitivity reactions are recognized and systematically studied; the immune system and immune responses are systematically studied in the world's major medical centers and medical schools; and both competing conceptual matrixes which organize immunological knowledge of the period provide the structure to guide diagnosis, treatment, and predict clinical outcome.

Let us consider now the history of immunology as it moves through the balance of Antiquity.

Aulus Celsus (14 AD-37 AD) Roman encylopediaist offers his tremendously influential treaties "De Medicina", circa 30 AD, which describes in part the state of medical knowledge of the period. Celsus describes good health, infectious disease, physical trauma and the body's immune reactions within the contemporary conceptual matrix of the Alexandrian School's balance of humors models. Good health is maintained by good hygiene, diet, and exercise. Poor health is the result of imbalance within and between body humors. Treatment is directed to restoring balance within and between body humors.

Perhaps more importantly, Celsus in "De Medicina" distills much of the Alexandrian School's observations of the immune response into the four cardinal signs of inflammation, with which we are most familiar today; calor (warmth), dolor (pain), tumor (swelling), and rubor (redness) (circa 30 AD/1478,1935)[17,18]. That's right. Celsus succinctly summaries the clinical signs of the immune response over 2,000 years ago. These four cardinal signs of inflammation (actually 3 signs and 1 symptom) are still taught to medical students, in medical schools around the world today.

Much of the popular and the professional medical literature of today blindly and incorrectly assign credit to Galen of Pergamum for adding a fifth sign, "impaired function" (function laesa) to Celsus' original four clinical signs of inflammation. Recent and extensive examinations of the original written records fail to support the recurring claim Galen ever made this observation

(1971)[19]. True in the history of medicine and true in professional medicine today, credit for specific contributions are often assigned to an individual based upon the combined efforts of many or simply as the result of repeated, blind reporting of secondary referenced sources from the professional medical literature. The earliest known written evidence of the addition of "impaired function" to Celsus' original tetrad first appears approximately 150 years ago, in a handbook of general pathology (p441), printed in Germany (1864)[20].

Galen of Pergamum (129 AD-200 AD) born in the Greek city of Pergamum, located in Turkey (sic) and then part of the Roman Empire, offers numerous treaties describing the immune response. In brief, Galen's conceptualizes the body's immune response to infectious disease and trauma within the matrix of a balance of humors model. The immune response is a normal, beneficial, adaptive response, and essential to the healing process. The immune response, independent of the source of the antigen, is simply a natural response by the body in its efforts to restore balance within and between body humors.

Several of Galen's treaties focus upon a product of the immune response, the viscous fluid containing leukocytes and debris of dead cells, "pus". Within Galen's conceptual matrix, "pus" is to be encouraged to form and represents materials to be eliminated by the body in its effort to restore balance between body humors. Given Galen's tremendous authoritarian influence, dogmatic confidence, and prolific medical writings, result in acceptance within the medical community of his conceptualization of pus. Simply stated: "pus" is good and the absence of "pus" is bad. It takes another 1,700 years for the medical community to modify and subsequently displace Galen's dogma with a reinterpretation of the source of "pus" and its role in the immune response.

Antiquity ends with the last emperor of the combined Western and Eastern Roman Empires Flavius Theodosius I (347 AD-395 AD), upon the recommendation of a Christian Bishop of Alexandria, orders the destruction of Libraries and Temples of Alexandria and "…destruction of all non-Christian knowledge within…". So goes another example in history of organized religions in cooperation with state government deciding what knowledge is and is not acceptable for science, medicine, and the masses.

In summary, the second half of Antiquity develop established empirical observations characterizing antecedent conditions which routinely and reliably trigger immune responses and the immune responses themselves; Celsus offers "De Medicina" and the four cardinal signs of inflammation; immune responses are recognized as normal, adaptive responses essential for healing; Galen writes extensively about "pus" and its role in the immune response; organized religion influences government leaders resulting in the intentional destruction of recorded knowledge housed in the Libraries and Temples of Alexandria, one of the world's largest centers and depository of scientific and medical knowledge. And so it goes….

Middle Ages (Medieval Times), 500 AD - 1400 AD.

The Middle Ages begin with the fall of the Western Roman Empire (modern-day Italy, France, Spain, Great Britain, coastal Libya, Tunisia, Algeria, and Morocco) to military invading forces. The Eastern Roman Empire (aka Byzantine Empire; modern-day Greece, Turkey, Syria, Lebanon, and Egypt) remains relatively preserved, although advancement of science and medicine is greatly suppressed by military campaigns between governments seeking to control lands, people, culture, and commerce. Scientists and philosophers are greatly restricted by government and religious influences and many exodus to Persia (modern-day Iraq and Iran).

Much of the written scientific and medical knowledge of the Roman Empire is relocated to the Middle East and translated from the original writing in Greek and Latin into Arabic by an outcast Christian sect known as the Nestorians. This sect is devoted to scholarship and learning and translates many of the original manuscripts written by Aristotle and Galen into Arabic. Very few advances in science or medicine are made during the Middle Ages in Europe. Scholarship in Europe is restricted largely to translation of Greek records of knowledge into Latin, the official language of the Church. During translation, much of the information is modified from its original form to better conform to the teachings and dogma of the Church. The Church is gaining tremendous influence and powers and provides much of the funding for scholarship throughout Europe. Most original scholarship is occurring in the Middle East rather than Europe. Later, as scientists return to Europe from the Middle East, they bring with them the new knowledge and integrate the information into the Western European medical and scientific knowledge bases.

Procopius (500 AD-565 AD) notable Byzantine historian provides insight into and reiterates the fundamental understanding of the period, in regard to infectious disease and the body's immune response. Procopius describes in detail the immune response associated with infection of the first known bubonic plague (Plague of Justinian) circa 541 AD, and notes the well-established empirically derived fact, individuals once infected by the plague and if survive will upon exposure to the plague a second time will experience a much less severe clinical course and most certainly are much less likely to die as the result of the second exposure (acquired immunity) (1914)[21].

Estimates of 25% to 50% of the region's entire population is lost to the first known bubonic plague epidemic in Europe (Plague of Justinian). In light of the hundreds of thousands deaths which result from this plague, few advances are made in understanding the body's immune response within the matrix of the natural (physical) science model, popular at the time. In fact, the natural (physical) models are challenged by the religion based supranatural, religion favored (deity) based models. In the absence of science's ability to explain natural (physical) events (including disease), historically supranatural models are quickly substituted as an alternative. So too during the first half of the Middle Ages in regard to understanding immunology. Supranatural (deity) based models compete once again in providing an understanding of disease and immune reactions.

Islam, a new and popular organized religion first appears circa 600 AD. The religion advocates a supranatural bases for disease and immune reactions, similar to other popular organized religions of the period Judaism, Christianity, and Catholicism. The fundamental belief of Islam in regard to disease and the body's immune responses is best understood within a modified and integrated super-natural and natural matrix model. In brief, disease, infection, and immune responses are the result of natural (physical) events. Disease and infection are provided by God (Allah), as well as their cures, to "test" the sincerity of one's belief in the religion of Islam. The clinical course of a disease and the associated physical immune response, provide the follower the necessary time to reflect upon their commitment to their religious beliefs. According to the Islamic belief system, if one survives the "test" they are rewarded with earthly and non-earthly rewards.

Abu Ibn al-Razi (Latinized to Rhazes) (865 AD-925 AD) Persian scholar provides the first meaningful synthesis of immunological knowledge since Galen. Building upon the foundations of the natural (physical) model of infectious disease and immune response, Razi applies a rational investigational approach, makes original, clinical observations, develops an integrated conceptual matrix which accommodates past knowledge, clinical observations and systematically guides diagnosis, treatment, and prognosis. He holds firmly to the balance of humors models whenever discussing his conceptual matrix of disease and immune responses.

Perhaps one of Abu Ibn al-Razi's most substantial contribution is found in his treaties complied in his 22 volume "Kitabu al-Hawi Fi'Tibb" [The Comprehensive Book on Medicine] (1094 AD)[22]. The "Comprehensive Book on Medicine" is a collection of case histories of various diseases, supplemented by extracts from earlier authors' discussions of disease and therapies. The book, written originally in Arabic is first translated into Latin in 1297 AD, by Farai ben Salim, and later into French, Italian, and Greek. The book serves as a major resource for medical education throughout the Middle East and Europe through the 1700s. Of particular interest is volume 17 which discusses the similarities and differences of two problematic diseases of the period smallpox (variola virus) and measles (paramyxo virus) (1094 AD/1848,1297 AD/1985)[23,24]. Al-Razi provides clear and succinct statements outlining the clinical presentation of signs and symptoms, clinical course, and prognostic indicators for both diseases (1848)[23.] His descriptions prove so helpful in making a correct differential diagnosis between smallpox and measles, they are used by practitioners well into the 1900s.

Al-Razi's conceptual model of smallpox and measles provide a matrix to organize clinical signs and symptoms, explain changes in signs and symptoms across the clinical course, and make accurate prognostic statements regarding probabilities of recovery. The matrix additionally provides a conceptual frameworks within which to explain why children are at greater risk for contracting the disease than the elderly; why individuals once exposed and who have recovered suffer much less severe clinical course if at all, upon subsequent exposure; why individuals once exposed maintain lifelong immunity; identifies blood to be essential in understanding these two infectious diseases; emphasizes the role of person to person transmission; emphasizes sanitation to be an important risk factor in contracting the disease and in the recovery from the disease; recognizes the advantages and disadvantages of segregating infected individuals from noninfected individuals; recognizes fever to be a necessary part of the immune response; and fever is the result of the body's defense against the disease rather than a disease itself.

Al-Razi offers one of the first scientific treaties which discuss allergies and associated immune reactions. He addresses the subject in multiple treaties. The "Kitab-al-Hawi" reports and describes 33 clinical cases on the topic. Case 29 addresses specifically "hay fever" (1094AD/1955-1971)[25]. Al-Razi further addresses the topic of seasonal rhinitis in "The Sense of Smell" (1094AD,1094AD /2000)[26,27]. This article additionally appears under the title of "An article on the reason why Abou Zayd Balkhi suffers from rhinitis when smelling roses in spring", in the collected bibliography of Razi numerous works, compiled approximately 50 years after his death (1048AD/1987)[28]. The Sense of Smell provides recognition seasonal and environmental factors contribute to the initiation of what we describe today as a Type I hypersensitivity immune reaction and offers a lengthy listing of prophylactic measures to reduce the onset of the reaction and specific measures to be taken to effectively treat and manage the reaction once triggered.

Trivia: The term "hay fever" is first introduced into the medical literature by John Macculloch (1773-1835) Scottish physician and noted geologist (sic) (1828)[29]. Subsequently that year, John Bostock (1773-1846) British physician recommends the continued use of the term "hay fever" in a series of articles in which he address the topic of seasonal allergies. Although Bostock had published an article ten years before Macculloch, offering clinical descriptions of seasonal allergic rhinitis, Bostock never used the term "hay fever", until after reading Maccolloch's papers describing seasonal allergies (1819, 1828)[30,31].

Ibn Maymoun (Latinized to Moses Maimonides) (1135 AD-1204 AD) Spanish philosopher, religious scholar, and physician, approximately three hundred years after Razi, publishes "Maqala fi al rabw" [Treatise on Asthma]. "Treaties on Asthma" emphasize the modifying and beneficial effects of diet, climate, clean air, exercise, rest, sleep, and sexual intercourse in regard to chronic disease and health in general (1190 AD/2001)[32]. "Treaties on Asthma" is certainly not an organized treatment of asthma as the title might suggest. The document is important in its role in communicating Greek and Arabic medicine to medieval Europe rather than any original work by Maimonides or insights into the immunology of asthma. The Treatise is best understood as an aphoristic guide to good health and healthy living.

World health is challenged in 1348 AD by one of the most devastating pandemics in human history, the Great Plague of London, renamed approximately 500 years later as The Black Death (1832)[33]. This bubonic plague (derived from the Greek word bubo meaning "swollen gland") is caused by the bacterium Yesinia pestis, which is most often transmitted to humans from infected fleas living on rats and other small rodents. When the flea bites the skin the bacteria is transmitted through the lymphatics and results in painful swollen lymph nodes, high fever, and chills, as the body mounts an immune response to the infection. Without treatment, this plague kills two out of three people within six days. The Great Plague sweeps through Europe, at approximately six kilometers a day, during the mid-1300s and in the course of approximately two years had killed an estimated 75 million people (sic), reducing the entire European population by approximately 50% (2005)[34].

Trivia: In response to the Great Plague of 1348 AD, the city of Venice begins requiring ships arriving from infected ports to sit at anchor for 40 days before coming ashore. This 40 day restriction was known as "quarantena" and became the familiar term "quarantine" used to describe the isolation of an infected individual.

The Middle Ages witness resurgent interests in organized religion. Organized religions, as always, provide an explanation for disease and direction for those affected by illness. In absence of any persuasive natural (physical) explanations for disease and suffering, such as that brought on by the Great Plague, religious (supranatural) models quickly displace natural models. Recall, the model of disease promoted by the Christian and Catholic Church is as follows: you do not get sick if you have not sinned (natural immunity); you become sick because you have sinned, you do not become sick again if you have repented for your sins (acquired immunity); if you sin a little you become a little sick, if you sin a lot you become very sick. Christianity, Catholicism, Islam, Judaism, and other popular organized religions of Europe all provide supranatural based guidance to individuals to insure good health, explain illness and disease, and offer specific recommendations as to how one can mitigate illness and disease once present. Religion and deity based models provide comfort and reassurance to justifiably frightened people in ways natural (physical) based models of science and medicine are unable to offer, given the knowledge of the period. Religion, once again is substituted for science and becomes the preferred model among the masses, from which to understand sickness and immune responses.

In summary, the Middle Ages witness the fall of the Western Roman Empire; much of the written scientific and medical knowledge of Western Europe is relocated to the Middle East where original Greek and Latin medical writings are translated into Arabic; the immune response is described in detail by Procopius circa 541 AD; natural (physical) models of disease are displaced by supranatural, deity models when science and medicine cannot explain the plagues, which repeatedly spread rapidly across Europe, taking the lives of millions, devastating families, communities, workforces, and commerce; Abu Ibn al-Razi provides the first truly original, reevaluation and detailed description of the immune response, within a natural (physical) conceptual matrix since Galen; Abu Ibn al-Razi offers his "Comprehensive Book on Medicine" and eloquently describes the similarities and differences between smallpox and measles, describes their clinical course, person to person transmission, importance of good sanitation, explains why individuals once exposed to not suffer the extreme clinical sign and symptom upon a second exposure, discusses the value of segregating the infected from the uninfected, and recognizes fever to be a part of a necessary immune response and not a disease itself; Abu Ibn al-Razi offers the first scientific treaties on allergies and describes their triggers and immune responses; Ibn-Maymoun builds upon Ibn al-Razi's description of allergies and offers recommended guidelines to avoid allergies and live a healthy life; organized religions' faith based, supranatural, deity models of disease displace natural models, which once again slows the advancement of understanding immune systems and immune responses from the scientific perspective.

Early Modern, 1400 AD - 1800 AD.

The European Renaissance period enjoys resurgence in the interests in original scientific thought and investigation. Organized religions remain tremendously influential in guiding scholarly activities. Much of the new knowledge and methodologies acquired in the Middle East during the Middle Ages moves into Europe and is integrated into scientific and medical knowledge bases. Many of the original ancient Greek and Roman medical and scientific writings translated into Arabic in the Middle East during the Middle Ages are translated again, now into Latin by academics funded by the major organized religions of Europe, especially the Christian and Catholic Churches. Many of the translations are modified to better conform to religious dogma. Simultaneously however, there is movement away from supranatural explanations of life in nature, including vitalism and towards natural (physical) base explanations, which rely upon the laws of physics. Original, innovative thought and investigation is encouraged and rewarded. Early in this period Copernicus, Galileo, Newton, and Descartes are vocal proponents of the new "scientific method" as the favored process in acquiring scientific knowledge. Empiricism rather than rationalism is the favored epistemology (1637)[35]. Scientific, medical, and religious dogma, in place for thousands of years, is challenged by new discoveries.

Technological advances contribute to the forward movement of medical knowledge with the invention of the printing press, during the 1400s and subsequent mass printing, allowing mass circulation of new knowledge and ideas and in effect establishing a more integrated community of scientists. The printing press also makes scientific and medical knowledge much more available to the general public. The printing press provides the ability to print materials in local languages rather remaining restricted to language of scholars, Latin. The microscope is invented during the 1500s and offers the necessary technology permitting investigation of cell based models of inflammation. During the 1600s the microscope is refined. The cell is seen through the microscope for the first time. Microorganisms previously speculated to exist and associated with disease and resultant immune responses are seen for the first time. The 1700s witness the wide spread use of variolation throughout Europe and the New England colonies of North America. Epidemiological methodologies and associated statistical probabilities are applied to the scientific study of infectious disease and associated immune responses. By the end of the 1700s vaccination replaces variolation as the preferred method of establishing acquired immunity for immunological protection against smallpox.

Modern immunology owes much to the foundational contributions made by investigators of the Early Modern period. It is during the Early Modern period (1400s-1800s), that many of the anatomical structures of the immune systems are identified, described, and integrated into a functional system matrix which displaces much of the scientific and medical dogma firmly enriched for over two thousand years. Emphasis during the Early Modern period is directed to the investigations of the immune systems, at the level of gross anatomical structure. These structures are then integrated into functional, physiological organ systems. Efforts are made to understand immune systems and the body's physical reaction to infection, disease, and trauma, within the popular mechanical models of the period. That is, efforts are made to understand the body in the same way one can understand a machine. Identify and describe all of the "parts" (anatomy); identify and describe what each part does do (functional anatomy); and finally describe how all of the "parts" work together with all the other "parts" (physiology).

Bone marrow, thymus, spleen, lymph nodes, lymphatic vessels, mucosa associated lymphoid tissues (MALT) e.g. tonsils, adenoids, Peyer's patches, are recognized and aggressively investigated as important structures essential to a healthy, competent, immune system.

Marco Aurelius Severino (1580-1656) Italian anatomist identifies and describes an elongated thickening of intestinal epithelium of a few centimeters in length, located in the lowest portion of the small intestine ileum in humans. This is the first published description of the aggregated lymphoid tissue (1645)[36], later to be termed "Peyer patches" by Swiss anatomist Johann Peyer (1653-1712) (1677)[37]. These and other lymphoid tissues are independently detailed by Danish anatomist Niels Stensen (1638-1686), the same person who first describes the ducts which carries saliva from the parotid gland to the mouth (Stensen ducts) (1662)[38]. The Peyer patches are of particular interests, during this time period, in that they are a common site of intestinal ulceration, hemorrhage, and perforation, in patients suffering typhoid fever.

Recall, typhoid fever (enteric fever) is a bacterial infection characterized by fever, abdominal pain, diarrhea, and occasionally a "rose spots" rash on the chest and belly. Most commonly caused by Salmonella typhi. The bacteria is spread through contaminated food, drink, or water. Once a person eats or drinks something which is contaminated, the bacteria travels through the intestines and into the bloodstream, inflaming the Peyer's patches, lymph nodes, liver, spleen and other immune organs. Some people become carriers of the bacteria and continue to release the bacteria in their stool for years, spreading the disease (2011)[39].

Perhaps the most familiar carrier in United States' history is Mary Mallon (1869-1938), aka Typhoid Mary. Mary Mallon, an Irish immigrant, working many years as a cook in New York City, during the early-1900s, is suspected of transmitting the bacterium Salmonella typhi, as the result of failing to routinely wash her hands before preparing foods. She is quarantined and involuntarily confined, by order of the New York City Department of Health, for years, as a significant and potentially lethal health risk to the general public. She remains in involuntary confinement, until her death in 1938. Do you see any ethical issues here? Professional issues?

Olof Rudbeck (1630-1702) Swedish, Professor of Medicine is among the first to clearly describe the anatomy and outline the multiple functions of the lymphatic systems. Until this time, the lymphatic system is viewed within a Galenian matrix and responsible only for the distribution of food derived nutrients from the GI system to the liver for additional processing. Rudbeck identifies and reports a previously unrecognized clear fluid (lymphatic fluid) and its associated vessels (lymphatic vessels). He suggest, for the first time, the clear fluid and vessel system are essential in maintaining body immunity against infection and are instrumental in mounting a healthy immune response (1653)[40].

Thomas Bartholin (1616-1680) Danish anatomist is also among the first to publish full descriptions of the lymphatic systems in humans. He correctly describes the thoracic duct and explains how lymphatic fluid is moved into blood without moving through the liver (1653,1654)[41,42]. He too explores the additional roles of the lymphatic system beyond the traditional role of moving nutrients from the small intestines to other body organs. Bartholin, like Rudbeck soon begins to explore the role of the lymphatic system structures in maintaining body immunity against disease.

Olof Rudbeck and Thomas Bartholin soon enter one of the most public and hotly disputed debates over professional priority for discovery. The debate is fueled not by Rudbeck or Bartholin but rather individuals working within their research groups in Sweden and Denmark. In brief, one of Rudbeck's medical students publically accuses Bartholin of plagiarizing Rudbeck's recent work on the lymphatic system. In response, one of Bartholin's medical students, Martin Bogdan, publically attacks Rudbeck's work accusing him of plagiarizing Bartholin's recent work on the lymphatic system. In a series of publications, the debate attracts much attention within the professional community (1654,1654,1654,1657)[43,44,45,46]. This very public debate raises once again the age old question of how priority for significant discoveries should be best assigned. Are we any closer to answering the question today?

Frederik Ruysch (1638-1731) Dutch anatomist adds another bit of information which helps to better understand the immune systems. He established the existence of valves in the lymphatic vessels and establishes the mechanism of action which explains unidirectional flow of lymphatic fluids (1665)[47].

Very little attention is devoted to the study of lymphatics and their role in immunology during the next 120 years. Attention is directed instead to the study and practice of variolation. Efforts are focused upon understanding the scientific and medical basis of innate and acquired immunity, with particular interest in applying this knowledge to the management of smallpox.

Variolation, the practice of intentionally infecting noninfected individuals with a virus, in an effort to impart immunity, by way of scratching the noninfected person's skin with a sharp object contaminated by the virus from pustules of an infected individual or inhaling dried scabs harvested from an infected patient, has been practiced for thousands of years, yet the basic science as to how and why it works are first investigated during the 1600s. Most documented written records identify its common use in the Far East, Africa, and India. Variolation is introduced into Turkey from the Far East circa 1670 and subsequently introduced into Western Europe during the early-1700s (1913)[48].

The procedure is typically performed by non-medical personal e.g. elderly woman. By the time the procedure is introduced into Turkey and Western Europe it has an established, demonstrated history of providing acquired, natural, active immunity. The procedure goes by many names, in Western Europe, most often referred to by 1700s investigators as variolation, inoculation, insertion, engrafting, or transplantation. Variolation is most often used to impart immunity to the variola virus, the virus responsible for the highly infectious disease smallpox.

Smallpox, a serious, oftentimes fatal, infectious disease, unique to humans, characterized by high fever and an extensive rash, is one of several life threatening infections capable of quickly eliminating substantial numbers of individuals from any given population and is especially feared by most communities. The virus is transmitted between people upon direct, prolonged face to face contact or direct contact with contaminated objects such as clothing and bedding.

The clinical presentation is characterized by an approximate 14 day incubation period, following initial exposure to the virus, during which the patient is asymptomatic; a prodromal period of approximately 2-4 days, characterized by first symptom onset which includes fever, malaise, head and body aches sufficient to interfere with normal daily activities; an early rash period lasting approximately 4 days, during which small red spots appear on the tongue and mouth and which develop into sores that eventually break open and spread the virus into the mouth and throat, making the patient highly contagious; at the time the sores in the mouth break, a rash on the skin of the face develops and quickly spreads within 24 hours to the arms, legs, hands, and feet; at about day 3 the rash changes into small bumps and fill with opaque fluid, often with a characteristic "smallpox" indentation in the center of the bump; the bumps soon become pustules; a pustular rash period follows lasting approximately 5 days and characterized by raised pustules, firm to the touch and reportedly feel a lot like BB pellets embedded in the skin; a scabbing period follows, of an approximate 5 days duration, during which the pustules form a crusty scabs; this is followed by a period of resolution of approximate 5 days, during which the scabs begin to fall off, leaving the characteristics marks on the skin, which eventually scar; after the scab falls off, the patient is no longer contagious (2011)[49].

Variola (smallpox virus), the large, biscuit shaped, double stranded DNA virus, which codes for 200 proteins, is derived from the Latin words "varius" meaning pimpled or perhaps "varus" meaning spotted or mark on the skin. Although the disease is known for thousands of years the term "variola" is first introduced in Europe by Bishop Marius of Avenches (Switzerland) circa 570 AD, in referring to the disease, later to be known as smallpox (1815)[50]. The term "variolation" is first reported in the medical literature by Heinrich Vollgnad (1634-1682) in his publication "Globus Vitulinus" (1671)[51]. The term "smallpox" first appears in Europe during the 1400s and used to distinguish the condition from the "great pox" (syphilis). The term "pox" refers to a disease which results in pockmarks, the permanent residual pitting scars of the skin evident following infection of a pox disease.

Emanuele Timoni (1670-1718) Greek physician and Giacomo Pylarino (1659-1718) Italian physician introduce the practice of variolation, as it is successfully practiced in Constantinople, to the Royal Society of London in 1713. They report success in preventing severe outbreaks of disease, specifically smallpox, in other countries of the world and its protective benefits of imparting acquired, natural, active immunity to an individual (1714,1715,1715)[52,53,54]. Timoni and Pylarino's reports are met with much skepticism by the English medical community and considered by many too dangerous and controversial to be taken seriously as a line of investigation or clinical application. It will take the unrelenting work and influence of a London socialite, Mary Montague, to persuade and move the English medical community into action.

Mary Montague (1689-1762) English aristocrat and champion of variolation in England, perhaps more than any physician or medical society is instrumental in bringing the practice of variolation to the people of England. She learns of the practice and witnesses its effectiveness against smallpox while living two years in Turkey (1717-1718), as her husband serves as the English ambassador to Turkey. She writes of the procedure and describes graphically both the process and effectiveness in a series of now historically significant letters referred to today as simply the "Turkish Embassy Letters" (1717,1718)[55,56]. Convinced of the protective value of variolation, she soon has herself and immediate family members inoculated. Upon her return to England, Lady Mary Montague calls upon her many political and social relationships in relentless efforts to champion the value of variolation. Against much resistance from the established medical community she succeeds in 1721-1722 in having the English medical community investigate the effectiveness of variolation, to impart immunity against smallpox, utilizing a simple, small sample, and clinical trial research design.

The initial clinical trials investigate the safety and effectiveness of variolation and are conducted by English physician Charles Maitland, in England. The trials are completed with the support of the Royal family and are soon to be known collectively and simply as the Royal Experiment of 1721-1722 (1722)[57].

In brief, Maitland inoculates seven condemned prisoners housed at Newgate prison in London and follows their clinical course. The prisoners volunteer for the investigative study in exchange for potential immunity from smallpox and their freedom, in the event they survive. The investigation is successful. The study is soon repeated on orphaned children residing in a local London orphanage. Again the findings are favorable. So impressed by the findings members of the Royal family are soon inoculated and variolation quickly becomes popular throughout England, while many within the established medical community remain actively opposed to the practice.

Variolation is soon widely practiced throughout England. The procedure is performed by both non-medical and medical personnel and remains central to the prevention of smallpox for the next 130 years. The procedure is declared illegal in England in 1840. Variolation is replaced by the vaccination procedures popularized by Edward Jenner during the late-1700s and early-1800s. Vaccination is made compulsory by the English Parliament for all subjects of the English Crown in 1853.

Throughout the 1700s, the clinical benefits of variolation are well documented. James Jurin (1684-1750) an English scientist is among the first to publish a series of epidemiological articles reporting empirically derived base rates for smallpox and comparing non-inoculated and inoculated persons. His serial investigations conducted in England, primarily during the period 1722-1727, reveal approximately 1:6 deaths occur following infection of smallpox without prior variolation; whereas 1:60 deaths occur following infection of smallpox with prior variolation (1722)[58].

Similar findings are being reported from the New England colonies of North America, where smallpox outbreaks are common. Cotton Mather (1633-1728) a non-physician publishes his epidemiological findings from Boston, demonstrating the safety and clinical value of the practice of variolation (1722)[59]. Zabdiel Boylston (1679-1766) a Boston physician inoculates over 200 people in Boston, during an outbreak of smallpox in 1721. His inoculations provide immunity to many. He reports the result of his inoculations in his book on the subject titled "Historical account of the smallpox inoculated in New-England, upon all sorts of persons, whites, blacks, and of all ages and constitutions: with some account of the nature of the infection in the natural and inoculated way, and their different effects on human bodies: with some short directions to the unexperienced in this method of practice" (1726)[60]. The four year delay in reporting his results is due to the adamant outrage from Boston's organized religious groups opposing the practice of variolation. Boylston is arrested in Boston for engaging in the practice of variolation. He publishes his findings only upon his release and return to England. Here is another example in the history of medicine as to how organized religion can and does impede the quest for new knowledge, whenever the quest or new knowledge is at odds with religions' theological dogma.

Opposition to variolation, in the new American colonies, is not restricted to organized religions. Members of the medical community are equally and quite emotionally opposed to the practice of variolation. Several publications by William Douglass (1691-1752) Scottish physician and longtime resident of Boston details his opposition and encourages all others to join him in his opposition to the practice (1722)[61]. Douglass argues against variolation based upon his assessment the practice is unproven to be effective in preventing smallpox and that the procedure actually increases the incidence of smallpox; "…I shall forever exclaim against, especially that detestable wickedness of spreading infection…" (1722)[62].

Variolation, as a procedure for imparting acquired immunity against smallpox is debated within medical, political, religious circles, as well as the lay community for much of the 1700s. Refinements in the procedure are proposed and implemented in England. Statistical studies in England and the new American colonies consistently reveal its prophylactic value (1721,1722, 1726,1754,1754,1759,1762,1978)[63,58,60,69,64,65,66,67].

In light of the demonstrated effectiveness, variolation is opposed in England by many within the established medical community (1748)[68]. Additionally, the powerful and influential Protestant and Catholic Churches oppose the practice. However, in the mist of the oftentimes heated debate, the London Small-Pox and Inoculation Hospital is established in 1746. Together with the Foundling Hospital of London, these two institutions offer variolation against smallpox for free.

Note: The Foundling Hospital is not a medical hospital as we think of a hospital today, but rather a children's home, established for the education and daily care of deserted children. The term "hospital" refers to the more general use of the term than we use today and refers to the "hospitality" offered to those less fortunate.

In France and Italy, the Catholic Church presses its influential opposition to variolation upon the medical communities and as a consequence is slow to recognize or embrace the procedure's demonstrated effectiveness in imparting acquired immunity. Not until French explorer-scientist Charles-Marie de La Condamine (1701-1774) addresses the Royal Academy of Sciences in Paris on the effectiveness of inoculation observed during his explorations of South America (1754)[69], Italian physician Giovanni Targioni Tozzetti (1712-1783) reports his experiments on children of the Ospedale degli Innocenti (Hospital of the Innocents) a children's orphanage in Florence (1757)[70], and Italian physician Angelo Gatti (1724-1798) publishes his critical review of inoculation practices and effectiveness (1764)[71] does France and Italy begin to accept the value of variolation for the prophylaxis of smallpox.

In the new colonies of America, variolation is recognized and accepted by the late-1700s. Benjamin Franklin is a vocal proponent of the procedure and publishes his own statistical based studies in support of his position (1759)[66]. General George Washington recognizes the military advantages of having troops inoculated against smallpox and orders mandatory inoculation of all persons enlisting in the Continental Army (1777)[72]. By the end of the 1700s, variolation is widely accepted throughout the new American colonies and Western Europe as an effective prophylactic against smallpox, yet little is known as to exactly how or why variolation is effective.

Church dogma remains explanatory in religious circles. Simply stated in brief, people who contract smallpox do so because they have sinned and are being punished by God. Individuals who might survive smallpox do so at the mercy of a forgiving God. Man should not interfere with God's will by offering immunity. In contrast, the medical and scientific communities recognize the clinical value of variolation, yet fail to understand the physical mechanisms responsible in producing the immunity beyond "…people who have smallpox must have something remaining in their body which overcomes subsequent contagious infection…" (1738)[73] or something was depleted from the blood during the initial exposure or resulting from variolation, resulting in immunity as the result of "…its seeds were sown in an exhausted soil…" (1764)[71]. The answers as to how and why become more clear during the 1800s.

Attention shifts during the mid to late-1700s from variolation to vaccination. Vaccination, although similar to variolation, utilizes the cowpox virus, a complex, double stranded DNA virus which codes for approximately 200 proteins rather than the variola virus used in variolation to impart immunity to smallpox. Vaccination utilizes the less lethal cowpox virus compared to the smallpox variola virus. The advantages and demonstrated clinical equality in providing immunity against smallpox using the cowpox virus is well recognized in rural England by 1776.

The term "vaccination" is derived from the Latin word "vaccinus", meaning "of or from cows". The term is introduced by Edward Jenner in 1798 in reference to the procedures used to confer immunity against smallpox (1798a)[74]. Over eighty years later, Louis Pasteur extends the use of the term and generalizes it to include preventive inoculations of all kinds of infectious agents (1881)[75]. The term is still in use today.

John Fewster (1738-1824) English surgeon is among the first medical professionals to discuss the immunological properties of cowpox in its ability to confer immunity against smallpox. He articulates his position in a paper titled "Cowpox and its ability to prevent smallpox" he reads to the London Medical Society (1765)[76]. He concludes infections by the cowpox, like infection by smallpox, provides a prophylactic immunity upon subsequent exposures. However, he fails to offer a conceptual model or offer any hypothesis as to why. The paper simply makes the conclusion based upon anecdotal reports and casual observations made by dairy farmers throughout England and surrounding countries. Fewster never publishes his own observations. He does however discuss his observation with his friend, English scientist Edward Jenner and encourages local medical practitioners to establish a house where all can come to receive inoculation by medical practitioners.

Fewster's efforts are met with much resistance from the medical community (challenges medical dogma), the Church (interfering with God's work); the government (potential spread of infectious disease) and the general public (concerns regarding mixing human and animal bloods and possible consequence of the human subsequently taking on animal characteristics e.g. growing horns). In light of considerable resistance, the immunological advantages and potential risks of cowpox inoculations, as a new procedure for reducing the devastating consequences of smallpox infection, continues to be explored.

Benjamin Jesty (1737-1816) a dairy farmer located in southern English and aware of the prophylactic benefits cowpox offers dairy maids against smallpox, is among the first to vaccinate his own family with the cowpox virus in 1774. While his family enjoys the immunological benefits of the inoculation he and his family are subject to much criticism from those around them, similar to John Fewster described above. With time, the value of Jesty's contribution is recognized by others. England's House of Commons officially recognizes Jesty's contribution with a financial award in 1803, noting his valuable contributions and preceding by over 25 years the works of Edward Jenner, whom most often receives the lion's share of recognition, whenever discussing vaccination.

Edward Jenner (1749-1823) English surgeon and perhaps most recognized by medical students as the single person responsible for the discovery of vaccination, in fact did not discover vaccination at all. Vaccination is a well-known procedure, long before Jenner publishes his first papers on the topic. His primary contributions are found in his application of the scientific method to investigate vaccination; its applications to the protection against smallpox; offering a hypothetical model to explain the protective effects against smallpox, as the result of vaccination; and his unrelenting efforts to popularize the procedure throughout England, Western Europe, and the United States of America.

Jenner completes his first inoculation experiment in 1796, approximately 30 years after first learning of the procedure from his friend John Fewster. Jenner submits the findings from the experiment to the influential Royal Society of Medicine in 1797 and the paper is quickly rejected and never published. Undaunted by the Society's rejection, Jenner adds a few more cases to his initial experiment and self-publishes the now historically significant 64 page booklet titled "An inquiry into the causes and effects of the variolae vaccinae, a disease discovered in some of the western counties of England, particularly Gloucestershire and known by the name of cow pox" (1798a,1798b)[74,77].

The booklet can be organized into three general sections. First; Jenner describes the suspected source of the cow pox, its mode of transmission from horse to cow to humans, and describes the typical signs, symptoms, and clinical course of a cow pox infection. In his own words, the following describes the suspected source of the cow pox virus. "…There is a disease to which the horse, from his state of domestication, is frequently subject. The farriers have called it "the grease". It is an inflammation and swelling in the heel, from which issues matter possessing properties of a very peculiar kind, which seems capable of generating a disease in the human body, after it has undergone the modification which I shall presently speak of, which bears so strong a resemblance to the smallpox that I think it highly probable it may be the source of the disease…." (1798)[774].

The second section of the booklet presents 23 clinical cases ranging in age from young children to the elderly. He offers his cases in support of his proposed "horse origination hypothesis" and as demonstration of the effectiveness of surgeon Robert Sutton's method of inoculation. In brief, Sutton's method is first developed in England during the mid and late-1700s; utilizes the clear lymphatic fluid from a developing pox lesion as the source material for the inoculant rather than that the matured pus filled pustule; and eliminates the need to extract the necessary inoculant material from cows, using humans instead. The method has a demonstrated history of effectiveness, spanning approximately 50 years before Jenner's paper is published. The Sutton family establishes an extremely lucrative business spanning several generations during the mid and late-1700s, providing inoculations (variolation) for a fee. The Sutton's advertise the availability of the procedure, easy availability, costs, and benefits in local newspapers, pay for endorsements from local church officials, and create an extremely successful business model based upon providing a simple, routine procedure to thousands of people (1798)[78].

The third section of Jenner's booklet offers assorted general observations e.g. cowpox provides immunity against smallpox in humans; the problems associated with conducting experiments; the problems in controlling experimentally extraneous and potentially confounding variables; the recognition of the infectious properties of the lymph fluid from lesions is active before it is secreted as pus; seasonal variability in the presence of the disease (spring and early summer highest); the suspected likelihood of multiple and variable forms of the smallpox virus; his observation of limited transmission of the cowpox or smallpox virus through sexual intercourse; the strengths and weaknesses of various inoculation procedures; lack of fatalities following cowpox inoculations in comparison to smallpox variolation; and the lack of viral transmission by way of physical contact with intact skin.

Jenner quickly follows his original publication with three subsequent papers in which he extends his original observations, interpretations, and details the history of the discovery and development of vaccination (1799,1800,1801)[79,80,81]. Jenner's publications are met initially with mixed reviews by the medical community. Vaccination, however is soon recognized as a much safer alternative to variolation and quickly spreads throughout Western Europe. Vaccination soon becomes the preferred means of imparting prophylactic immunity against smallpox. Variolation is soon thereafter outlawed by the British government.

Trivia: Edward Jenner, in light of his substantial contributions, is never admitted into the Royal Society of Medicine.

William Woodville (1752-1805) and George Pearson (1751-1828) English hospital based physicians conduct several large scale clinical trials, in efforts to assess the comparative value of variolation and vaccination (1799,1803)[82,83]. Their findings support a rapidly growing body of scientific publications of the period, reporting the clinical effectiveness and advantages of vaccination in imparting immunity against smallpox (1896)[84].

By the end of the 1700s and early-1800s, inoculation is well established as an effective procedure in the prophylactic management of smallpox. Vaccination is preferred over variolation. Napoleon Bonaparte mandates the compulsory vaccination of his military troops in 1805. The Catholic Church announces endorsement of immunization by the Pope in 1814. Several Western European governments e.g. Bavaria (SE Germany) (1807), Denmark (1810), Norway (1811), Sweden (1816), and Hanover (NW Germany) (1821), legislatively mandate immediate and compulsory vaccination of all of its citizens. England follows with similar mandates requiring compulsory vaccinations in 1853.

Advancements in immunological knowledge, specifically variolation and vaccination, trigger a storm of social, philosophical, legal, ethical, and religious issues.

Governmental mandates requiring immediate and compulsory vaccination raise questions among many within governmental, religious, medical, and scientific leaderships, and the public at large. Who is responsible for determining who and when a person is to be subjected to an involuntary medical procedure? Who determines costs? How will the costs be paid? Who determines qualifications required to safely execute the harvesting, storage, and distribution of the infectious materials? Who is qualified to administer the procedure? Is it the role of government to provide compulsory medical care to its citizenry? What is to be done when the governmental imposed mandate is at odds with a person's religious belief? Is the procedure safe? Who is responsible and what are the remedies when the procedure results in an unexpected or undesirable outcome e.g. death. Does potential protection of a large population group, achieved through compulsory submission to a medical procedure mandated by government officials, outweigh an individual's choice to participate or not participate in a medical procedure?

These are among the questions asked and struggled with by many, both then and now.

As the 1700s come to a close, Western Europe is aware acquired immunity against specific viral infections e.g. smallpox, is possible by variolation or vaccination. Knowledge is limited and based largely upon observation; if you do this, then this will happen and this is a good outcome; if you do that, then that will happen and that is a bad outcome. Little is known as to how the immunity is actually generated within the body. Immunology becomes an area of much interest during the next 100 years and produces many milestone advances. The mechanisms of actions within the body producing immunological responses and acquire immunity become more clear.

In summary, the Early Modern Period 1400-1800, includes the scientific and cultural revolution of Western Europe, the Renaissance, and witnesses resurgence in original scientific thought and investigation. Invention of the printing press allows for mass sharing of information and scientific knowledge. Anatomical studies identify major organ systems and associated structures of the immune systems. Cells are seen through the microscope for the first time. Microscopic investigation of the immune systems is now available and opens new lines of investigations. Epidemiological studies demonstrate repeatedly the advantages of acquired immunity. Medical dogma entrenched for over two thousand years is displaced. Advances made early in this period in understanding the basic sciences of the immune systems are soon integrated into immediate clinically oriented application of immunological principles. Variolation is recognized in Western Europe as an effective procedure in providing prophylactic immunity against the fatal variola virus (smallpox). The procedure is refined and demonstrated effective in imparting acquired immunity. Variolation is replaced by vaccination by the end of the period, as the most desired procedure to stimulate the immune systems and provide acquired immunity against the variola virus. The study and practice of providing protection against variola in the clinical setting dwarfs all investigations directed towards understanding the basic sciences underlying and responsible for producing acquired immunity. The immediate rewards of clinical service delivery are embraced at the expense of basic research. Manipulation of immune systems is demonstrated and clinical value well proven. However, an understanding of the mechanisms of actions and the basic science responsible for the clinical effects will have to wait until the 1800s to be elucidated. Advances in clinical immunology, between 1400-1800, raise numerous political, social, philosophical, professional, economical, legal, ethical, and religious questions. Many of these questions remain relevant today and continue to have no unanimously agreed best answer.

Middle Modern, 1800 AD - 1900 AD.

The 1800s witness continuing interests and growth in immunology. Technological advances in microscopy open new windows of investigation into the body's defense systems and infectious disease. A new theory, Cell theory, challenges medical and religious dogma and proposes cells are the basic unit of structure of all living things and should be the primary unit of study. Cells, important in normal body defense systems are viewed for the first time and their role in establishing and maintaining body immunity are described. Dendritic cells, mast cells, basophils, eosinophils, neutrophils are first identified. Identification of the specific functions of these fundamental immune system cells however will not be realized until the late-1900s. Processes of phagocytosis and diapedesis are observed and detailed for the first time. The cell becomes central to understanding the body's normal defense against infection and disease.

Non-cellular, soluble substances found in blood and other body fluids continue to be studied. New humoral substances are identified e.g. complement and antibodies. Chemistry of the immune system is aggressively investigated. A passionate scientific debate between cellularists and humoralists, as to which component of the immune system is primary and which is secondary, dominate much of the scientific literature. The debate is slow to resolve, yet by the end of the 1800s most agree. To understand the human immune system one must recognize the dynamic interaction between cellular and humoral components of the systems. However, rigid division remain within the medical and scientific communities regarding which component, cells or humors, is most important. As the 1800s come to a close and the 1900s begin, the discovery of antibodies and complement move non-cellular soluble substances in blood to the forefront of immunological investigations and move cellular investigations into the background.

Germ theory is introduced and proposes many diseases can be produced by microscopic organisms and each microscopic organism produces a specific disease. The dogma of spontaneous generation of disease is replaced with recognition that many disease causing microorganisms reproduce themselves in a reliable and predictable manner. Reproduction of these disease producing microorganisms is accomplished by biogenesis and cell division and not by spontaneous generation. Germ theory is met with predictable initial resistance by many; however the theory stands the test of scientific scrutiny and is soon accepted by the scientific and medical communities.

Equipped with new technologies and new conceptual matrixes, investigators of the 1800s soon lay the foundation upon which much present day knowledge of the immune systems will build.

The early-1800s focus upon description and structure of cells of the immune systems, whereas the second half of the 1800s focus upon the systems' chemistry.

Let us now take a look at some of the specific, notable people and their contributions to immunology during the 1800s, which have relevance to you as a future physician.

Theodor Schwann (1810-1882) German physiologist and Matthias Schleiden (1804-1881) German botanist revolutionize biology with their proposal of Cell Theory (1830,1839,1847)[85,86,87]. In brief, Cell theory states the cell is the basic unit of structure of all living things and new cells are produced from preexisting cells. The theory changes the unit of study and directly challenges the dogma of vitalism and spontaneous generation. Truly a revolutionary idea of the time and one that will influence the course of immunology for the next 188 years.

Recall, Vitalism states living organisms are the result of vital principles (life forces) distinct from biochemical reactions; the processes of life are not explicable by laws of physics and chemistry alone; and life is in some part self-determined. Spontaneous generation theory, in brief states life originates from inanimate, non-living matter, and not from reproduction. Schwann and Schleiden's Cell theory directly challenges both traditional belief systems.

The year after Schwann and Schleiden introduce Cell theory, another well recognized investigator introduces a model to explain the probable source of disease.

Jakob Henle (1809-1895) German histologist is among the first to propose the fundamental tenants which will later become known as Germ theory (1838,1840)[88,89]. Germ theory simply states, disease is caused by microorganisms. Henle's theory directly challenges the dogma of two popular theories used to conceptualize the causal factors of disease for centuries, miasma and contagions.

Recall, Miasma theory in brief states disease is caused by the presence of "miasma" in air, a poisonous vapor containing suspended particles of decaying matter and which characteristically produces a foul smell. Contagion theory in brief states disease is caused by direct contact with a person suffering from a disease.

Germ theory as proposed by Henle, later modified by his student Robert Koch (1843-1910), and developed by Louis Pasteur (1822-1895), is soon accepted by the medical and scientific communities and provides an alternative to the dogma of miasma and contagion theories of disease.

Trivia: Henle, perhaps most recognized for his "loops" in the kidneys is additionally instrumental in modifying medical dogma concerning polio. The same year Henle publishes his paper proposing Germ theory, he publishes a series of 29 case studies demonstrating polio to be a specific clinical disorder and not simply another form of paralysis (1840)[90]. Certainly a busy year for Henle. What have you done this year?

Rudolf Virchow (1821-1902) Polish pathologist extends Cell theory, to explain disease. Simply stated; disease is the result of abnormal cells (1858)[91]. This is a non-trivial statement for the time. Recall, medical dogma until the mid-1800s states disease is the result of an imbalance of non-cellular humors. Virchow's cell model of disease is revolutionary for its time. As are many new ideas, the cell model of disease is slow to be accepted by some and simply rejected by many others in the scientific and medical communities. Many scientists and medical practitioners of the time are still struggling with the acceptance of Germ theory, introduced a mere 18 years earlier and which challenged medical dogma, well entrenched for thousands of years.

The events offer another excellent lesson to be learned and remembered. Scientific and medical truths change. As you are preparing to enter the medical profession, try to remain open to new ideas and alternative explanations when presented, even when the new and alternative ideas challenge what you have been taught, have learned, or believe to be true. An open mind is a valuable and essential resource if medical knowledge is to advance beyond its present state. Will you be among the few who will contribute?

By the mid-1800s, investigators of the immune systems are poised to make substantial advances. Fundamental components of the healthy immune systems are identified, described, and major functions detailed. Immunology as a discipline expands its investigations of normal structures and body defense systems to include changes in immunological defense systems which generate new, previously unrecognized diseases. Well established disease are reexamined within the context of the immune systems.

Gabriel Andral (1797-1876) French, Professor of Medicine and William Addison (1802-1881) English country physician simultaneously first describe leukocytes and note a change in these cells in the presence of disease (1843,1843)[92,93]. Do not confuse William Addison with British contemporary physician Thomas Addison (1793-1860) who describes pernicious anemia (1849)[94] and Addison's disease (1855)[95]. William Addison is among the first to report the movement of leukocytes from blood circulation into inflamed and diseased tissues (1843)[93]. The description of diapedesis provides another piece in the puzzle of understanding processes of the innate immune response. Diapedesis further reinforces recognition of the importance the cell and its role in the body's defenses against infection and disease.

Recall, leukocytes are simply white blood cells and are found throughout the blood and lymphatic systems. The word "leukocyte" is derived from the Greek "leuko" meaning "white" and "kytos" meaning cell. These cells are involved primarily in defending the body against infectious disease. They can be classified based upon the presence of granules (granulocytes) e.g. polymorphonuclear leukocytes (PMN) neutrophils, basophils, and eosinophils or the absence of granules (agranulocytes) e.g. mononuclear leukocytes, lymphocytes e.g. B-cells, T-cells, natural killer cells, monocytes, and macrophages.

Recall too, the main targets and functions of each leukocyte are as follows: neutrophils defend primarily against bacteria and fungi; eosinophils defend primarily against large parasites and modulate allergic inflammatory responses; basophils primarily release histamine as part of the inflammatory response; B-cells mature into plasma cells which release antibodies and assist in the activation of T-cells; T-helper cells primarily activate and regulate T-cells and B-cells; CD8 cytotoxic T-cells defend primarily against virus infected cells and tumor cells; regulatory (suppressor) T-cells protect against misidentifying "self from nonself"; natural killer cells defend primarily against virus infected cells and tumor cells; monocytes move out of the blood and into tissues where they differentiate into tissue specific macrophages e.g. microglia cells in brain, Kupffer cells in liver, alveolar macrophages in lung, or dendritic cells aka Langerhan cells in skin. In general, macrophages are responsible for detecting, engulfing, and destroying pathogens and apoptotic cells.

Ernst Haeckel (1834-1919) German marine biologist is among the first to report leukocytes physically ingest foreign particles. He describes his finding and the process of phagocytosis based upon his studies of mollusks (1862)[96]. The following year, Max Schultze (1825-1874), German biologist and Friedrich von Recklinghausen (1833-1910), German pathologist, independently report similar findings and descriptions of phagocytosis in mammals (1863,1863)[97,98]. Yes, this is the same von Recklinghausen who 18 years later writes his now classical article on neurofibromatosis, aka von Recklinghausen's disease (1882)[99].

Paul Langerhans (1847-1888) German pathologist, medical student of Ernst Haeckel and perhaps most recognized by medical students as the person who first describes the histology of the insulin producing cells of the pancreas as an "…island of clear cells throughout the gland, staining differently than the surrounding tissue…" and initially mistakenly believes them to be lymph nodes (1869)[100]. Today these islands of cells are simply referred to by the term introduced by French pathologist Edouard Laguesse (1861-1927), the Islets of Langerhans (1893)[101]. Twenty years after Langerhans identifies these cells, Oscar Minkowski (1858-1931) Lithuanian medical investigator and Josef von Mering (1849-1908) German medical investigator working at the University of Strasbourg, identity the hormone "insulin", its source the pancreas, and make the first connections with diabetes (1889,1890)[102,103]. Another 22 years will pass before medical research physiologist Frederick Banting and research assistant Charles Best, at the University of Toronto, termed this pancreatic extract "insulin" in 1922.

Langerhans' contribution to immunology is found in his paper he publishes while in medical school, in which he first describes the histology of the dendritic cells of the skin (1868)[104]. Using a gold chloride staining technique, developed by his teacher Julius Cohnheim and while investigating the neural innervation of the skin, Langerhans details the histology of the dendritic cells and mistakenly believes them to be part of the nervous system. He has no idea of their role in the immune system as a bone marrow derived macrophage, antigen presenting cell, or its many other roles in cell mediated immunity. The functions of these dendritic cells and their role in the immune system will have to wait another 100 years before they are recognized.

Julius Cohnheim (1839-1884) German pathologist offers two notable contributions to immunology. First, he offers his observations and conclusions on the source of pus. He correctly recognizes pus to be comprised of protein rich fluids and dead leukocytes, which have moved into the intercellular space of infected tissues (1867)[105]. Secondly, he reports his microscopic observations of the movement of leukocytes and chemical analyses of humoral substances from systemic blood circulation into inflamed tissues (1873)[106].

It is Cohnheim who is among the first to scientifically study the body's response to infectious agents producing inflammatory responses and provides a synthesis of cellular and humoral components contributing to the inflammatory reaction. Although the concept of inflammation has been known since the Ancient civilizations and the term appears in the earliest medical documents e.g. Smith's Papyrus, and Cornelius Celsus gives us the familiar definition "…rubor et tumor cum calore et dolare…" (redness, swelling, heat, pain) circa 30 AD, Julius Cohnheim provides in vivo studies demonstrating a reliable sequence of vascular dilation, increased blood flow to the area, plasma leakage, leukocyte margination, and leukocyte diapedesis (1873)[106].

Paul Ehrlich (1854-1915) German immunologist is fascinated with the new cell staining dyes and techniques made popular during the 1800s. In 1878 he publishes his medical school dissertation in which he identifies the mast cell, a large, basophilic granulated cell, he names "mastzellen". Mastzellen is from the German word "mast" meaning "food" and reflects Ehrlich's initial thoughts as to the function of the cell (1878)[107]. He believes the cell's function is to provide nourishment to surrounding tissues. Only later the mast cell is recognized to play critical roles in the inflammatory process e.g. degranulation producing capillary dilation, localized edema, and irritation of local nerve endings, resulting in itching or pain. Recall, today we know mast cells originate in bone marrow, from the myeloid cell line and mature in connective and mucosal tissues. Mast cells are essential to the innate immune system and release a variety of substances e.g. histamine, serotonin, heparin, serine proteases, and most associated with allergic, Type I hypersensitivity reactions (immediate hypersensitivity) such as hay fever, food allergies, bee sting anaphylaxis, asthma, atopic eczema, and dermatitis.

Paul Ehrlich's contributions to immunology are numerous. His interests in staining leads to a new classification of cells based upon the cell's response to three distinctly different dyes he classifies as basic, acidic, or neutral (1879)[108]. In this 1879 paper he first offers his classification of polymorphonuclear leukocytes (PMN), basophils, eosinophils, and neutrophils, based upon staining characteristics. Yes, Paul Ehrlich is responsible for the classification of leukocytes, basophils, eosinophils, and neutrophils you learned in your histology course, during your first year of medical school.

Three years later he introduces a method for staining tubercle bacillus bacteria, which proves to be the foundation upon which the now familiar Gram stain is based (1882,1883)[109,110]. Based upon his staining studies, Ehrlich quickly recognizes specific pathogens bind with specific chemical structures. Expanding his thinking, he then proposes and provides experimental data in support of his conceptualization that specific pathogens can be targeted by specific medications, based upon their chemical structure that will allow them to bind to each other. This offers a new method for matching pathogens with specific medications and delivery of pharmacological treatments. Ehrlich terms these specific pathogen-medication matchings, based upon the chemical structure of the medication binding with specific pathogens, "magic bullets" (1898,1903)[111,112]. He demonstrates the effectiveness of his "magic bullet" model in his research group's discovery of a successful and effective treatment of the spirochete responsible for syphilis (1910,1913)[113,114].

His investigations into the interaction of cells and humors lead him to additionally propose another novel idea; cells have surface receptors which bind specific toxins and the binding of the two trigger antibody production (1885,1897)[115,116]. This idea is developed into a theory and later comes to be known simply as the side chain theory for antibody and antigen interaction (1900,1902)[117,118]. Paul Ehrlich shares the 1908 Nobel Prize in Physiology or Medicine with Ilya Mechnikov "…in recognition of their work on immunity…" (1908)[119].

Recall, antibodies are simply Y-shaped proteins, produced by plasma cells (differentiated B cells), and occur in two physical forms, soluble and non-soluble. The soluble forms are secreted from plasma cells and circulate in blood and other body fluids. The non-soluble forms are membrane bound and attach to the surface of B cells and function as a B-cell receptor. Both forms are used by the immune system to identify antigens such as bacteria and viruses. Antibodies are a main component of the humoral immune system.

Trivia: The term "antibody" first appears in the medical literature in an article written in German by Paul Ehrlich, titled "Experimental Studies on Immunity" (1891)[120]. The term is not immediately accepted by the medical or scientific communities.

Trivia: The term "antigen" is introduced into the scientific literature by Ladislas Deutsch (1874-1939) Hungarian microbiologist (1899). Antigen recall is anything, yes anything, when introduced into the body triggers the production of antibody. The term is derived from the combination of two words "antibody" and "generation".

Ilya Mechnikov (1845-1916) Ukrainian biologist builds upon the research of others earlier in the 1800s and extends the concept of phagocytosis to better understand the biological mechanisms most responsible for inflammation. Mechnikov is often and incorrectly credited with the discovery of phagocytosis. Phagocytosis is well known before Mechnikov begins his investigations on the topic. His contribution is not with the discovery but with a reconceptualization of the role of phagocytosis within the immune systems. The dogma of the period is phagocytosis of bacteria is a bad thing, in that it is one mechanism which distributes bacteria from a sight of inflammation throughout the entire body. Mechnikov argues phagocytosis is a good thing, in that it does not redistribute harmful bacteria throughout the body but rather eliminates it.

A frequently recited anecdote, often by Mechnikov himself, describes Mechnikov inserting a splinter into a large transparent starfish (Bipinnaria) and observing the migration and accumulation of cells around the splinter. The event occurs during the summer of 1883, while briefly living on the Italian island of Sicily and is often credited with stimulating Mechnikov's interests in the inflammation response. Mechnikov throughout his career maintains an unwavering commitment to the cell, as the primary element responsible for generating the immune response (1883)[121].

Mechnikov is one of the most vocal advocates of the cellularist position. He makes the observation PMN leukocytes (which he terms microphages (sic)) are most active when in the presence of bacteria, while monocytes and other macrophages are most active in the absence of bacteria. Mechnikov additionally observes PMNs leukocytes are eventually phagocytized by macrophages. He completes his work on phagocytosis and the immune response with his opus magnum summarizing his work and the current state of immunology in "L'Immunitl dans les Maladies Infectieuses" (1901)[122].

He now focuses his efforts on developing a phagocytosis based model to explain normal aging. Mechnikov suggests aging is the result of an autoimmune based macrophage phagocytosis of altered cells in tissue (1903)[123]. Although the phagocytosis model of aging never finds the necessary experimental support, Ilya Mechnikov is credited with coining the term "gerontology" (1907,1908,1908/2004)[124,125,126]. The term "gerontology" is derived from the Greek "geron" meaning "old man" and "ology" meaning the "study of". Mechnikov shares the 1908 Nobel Prize for Physiology or Medicine with Paul Ehrlich "…in recognition of their work on immunity…" (1908)[127].

Trivia: The term "phagocytosis" is coined by Carl Claus (1835-1899) Austrian marine biologist. Claus recommends the term to Mechnikov in 1882 as an alternative to the currently used German term "fresszellen" the "eating cell". The term "phagocytosis" is derived from the Greek "phago" to eat + "cyte" cell + "osis" action.

Robert Koch (1843-1910) German microbiologist and student of German histologist Jakob Henle, is among the first to provide experimentally derived data demonstrating an association between specific bacteria and specific disease. He provides experimental data which confirm the propositions set in Germ theory and proposed over 30 years earlier by Henle. Specifically, Koch demonstrates the association of anthrax with the bacterium Bacillus antracis (1876)[128], tuberculosis with Tuberculosis bacillus (1882)[129], and cholera with Vibiro cholera (1884)[130]. All three bacteria are sources of disease resulting in frequent mortality. Remember, antibiotic treatments have yet to be discovered.

Trivia: Thirty years before Robert Koch makes his report of an association of the bacterium Vibiro cholera with the frequently fatal infectious disease of the small intestines, typically sourced from contaminated water and characterized by severe vomiting and diarrhea i.e. cholera, Filippo Pacini of Florence, Italian anatomist publishes "Microscopical observations and pathological deductions on cholera" (1854)[131]; a paper in which Pacini describes the association and reports the same conclusions Robert Koch will report 30 years later. Humm…coincident or not? You decide.

Pacini's innovative work describing the relationship between Vibro cholera pacini (formal nomenclature for the bacterium) and cholera is initially rejected and ignored by the medical and scientific communities in Italy, given the dogma of the period attributes cholera to miasma.

Perhaps you recognize Pacini from your medical neuroscience course. He describes the Pacinian corpuscle. The specialized, encapsulated, sensory, mechanoreceptor found at the beginning of peripheral nerves, located in glabrous (hairless) skin, and especially sensitive to vibrations.

Robert Koch is instrumental in developing new techniques, allowing bacteria to be grown, stained, examined, and photographed in the laboratory (1877)[132]. He is first to describe the complete life cycle of bacteria. Koch's investigations into tuberculosis results in the identification of the

Tuberculosis bacillus bacteria as the primary underlying etiology and supplants the popular medical dogma of the time that tuberculosis is the result of a nutritional deficit (1882)[129]. He is responsible for first describing the delayed hypersensitivity reaction associated with TB, resulting in granuloma formations, and the induration associated with now familiar purified protein derivative (PPD) skin test for TB exposure. He publishes the Henle-Koch postulates which outline four criteria necessary to establish a causal relationship between a microbe and a disease (1890)[133]. These criteria are still used today. Robert Koch receives the 1905 Nobel Prize in Physiology or Medicine "…for his investigations and discoveries in relation to tuberculosis…" (1905)[134].

Koch's contributions to microbiology are clear. Perhaps, less clear are his contributions to immunology. To reiterate in brief, his work is instrumental in supplanting medical dogma regarding the fundamental cause of disease e.g. miasma and contagion theories, with Germ theory. Acceptance of Germ theory opens new lines of investigations and offers a conceptual matrix within which to accommodate the explosion of new information of the immune system during the 1800s.

Trivia: Robert Koch's assistant Julius Petri (1852-1921) German bacteriologist, invents the "Petri dish", the shallow, lid covered, glass dish used for the purpose of growing bacteria and other cells in the laboratory (1887)[135]. The Petri dish continues to be used today and is familiar to every modern medical student.

Emil von Behring (1854-1917) German physiologist and student of Robert Koch, further advances immunology with his investigations into passive immunity. He and his colleague Shibasaburo Kitasato (1853-1931) Japanese bacteriologist, also a student of Robert Koch, recognize certain bacteria produce toxins. It is the toxins released by the bacteria that are responsible for the clinical signs and symptoms associated with certain bacterial infections. Normally, in response to the presence of toxins, the body responds by releasing chemicals into blood which neutralize the toxins, making them harmless. Von Behring and Kitasato term these chemicals "antitoxins". Antitoxins will later be renamed "antibodies".

Studying bacteria responsible for diphtheria and tetanus, von Behring and Kitasato soon realize animals immunized with a weakened forms of the bacteria still produce the antitoxins and without the associated clinical signs and symptoms (1890)[136]. Two years later von Behring in collaboration with Erich Wernicke (not to be confused with Karl Wernicke of cortical language area fame) demonstrate transferring the antitoxin produced in one animal into another animal offers protection to the second animal against the bacterial toxins, introducing "passive immunity" (1892)[137]. Von Behring in collaboration with Paul Ehrlich soon demonstrate large amounts of antitoxin can be produced from horses and provide a large sustainable source of antitoxin for use in wide scale immunization. Emil von Behring is awarded the 1901 Nobel Prize in Physiology or Medicine "…for his work on serum therapy, especially its application against diphtheria, by which he has opened a new road in the domain of medical sciences and thereby placed in the hands of the physician a victorious weapon against illness and deaths…" (1901)[138].

Richard Pfeiffer (1858-1945) German bacteriologist, builds upon von Behring's findings working with diphtheria and tetanus bacteria, demonstrates similar finding using Vibrio cholera pacini bacteria (1894)[139]. Pfeiffer successfully demonstrates when blood plasma is extracted from an animal, previously immunized with the cholera bacteria and combined with the live bacteria in vitro, the bacteria will lyse and die. The same year he demonstrates live cholera bacteria injected into a previously immunized animal will not experience the debilitating clinical signs and symptoms evidenced by a non-immunized animal. Pfeiffer and von Behring provide the classic foundations for what we know today as passive immunity.

Pfeiffer makes additional contributions to immunology. Perhaps one of the most relevant is his recognition certain bacteria only release their toxins when the bacteria cell wall is lysed. Pfeiffer terms these toxins "endotoxins" to differentiate them from other toxins released by bacteria, without the necessity of membrane wall lysis. His observations have significant explanatory powers in understanding why a patient who is suffering a specific bacterial infection oftentimes can become more ill with antibiotic treatments which lyse bacteria cell walls e.g. penicillin.

Jules Bordet (1870-1961) Belgian immunologist discovers the lysis of bacteria in vivo can be significantly enhanced in the presence of specific, innate, cell bound and soluble proteins. Bordet is first to recognize and describe two distinct humoral components of blood serum, which work together to lyse bacteria, a heat stable component (antibodies) and a heat sensitive, fragile, labile component (alexins). The term antibody, coined by German immunologist and contemporary of Bordet, Paul Ehrlich, is still used today. The original term "alexins", proposed by Bordet to describe the heat sensitive, fragile, component of blood serum, which contributes to the lysis of bacteria is derived from the Greek meaning "…to ward off…to keep protected". The term alexins is soon changed by Paul Ehrlich to the more familiar term we use today "complement". Recall, complement "completes" the killing of bacteria coated with specific antibody.

Bordet recognizes and describes the interaction of antibodies and complement, not only in the lysis of bacteria but also in the lysis of the red blood cell (RBC). Emphasizing the humoral elements of the immune system, Bordet offers a scientific foundation of core knowledge which predicts and explains the risks and benefits associated with the exchange of blood, especially blood serum, between animals. His investigations prove instrumental in the formulation of procedures which allow manipulation of antibody production in animals as an alternative to injecting bacteria (1898)[140]. Twenty years later Jules Bordet is awarded the 1919 Nobel Prize in Physiology or Medicine "…for his discoveries relating to immunity…" (1919)[141].

Trivia: The taxonomic classification of the Gram-negative aerobic coccobacilli bacteria Bordetella, the pathogen responsible for the respiratory disease pertussis (whooping cough) is named in recognition of Bordet and his efforts in isolating the pathogen (1906)[142].

Throughout much of the 1800s, polarization within the scientific and medical communities between cellularists and humoralists is evident in the professional literature. These polarized scientific positions soon take on institutional and national boundaries. The cellularists' position, championed by Ukrainian biologist Ilya Mechnikov and others working in France, especially at the Pasteur Institute in Paris, advocate recognition of the importance and primacy of the cell e.g. polymorphonuclear leukocytes (PMN), macrophages, and the process of phagocytosis as most responsible for the body's defense against pathogens. The humoralists' position, championed by German microbiologist Robert Koch and others working in Germany, especially at the Koch Institute in Berlin, advocate recognition of the importance and primacy of non-cellular, soluble substances in blood e.g. antibodies and complement, as most responsible for the body's defense against pathogens.

By the end of the 1800s, following almost 100 years of debate, immunological investigations return to and once again emphasize the importance of humoral components of the human immune system. Research efforts led primarily by the German humoralists are fueled by demonstrated dramatic clinical rewards of successfully and effectively managing and treating common deadly bacterial infections e.g. diphtheria, tetanus, and cholera, utilizing passive immunity principles and procedures. Mortality rates plummet.

In summary, the 1800s witness tremendous activity in the discovery of new knowledge in immunology. These 100 years establish the foundation upon which most modern immunology is based. Primary components of the immune systems are identified, mechanism of actions detailed, and newly discovered basic science knowledge is quickly and successfully integrated into clinical medical practice.

Specifically, the cell is introduced as the basic unit of life and investigated extensively. The dogma of vitalism and spontaneous generation are rejected and replaced with models emphasizing laws of physics and chemistry. Leukocytes are identified as essential to the body's normal immune response and classified into the now familiar sub-types neutrophils, basophils, eosinophils, monocytes, and macrophages we still use today. Phagocytosis is observed for the first time and recognized as a fundamental process in maintaining normal body functions and to be an essential process within the immune systems. Diapedesis is observed for the first time. Movement and chemical analyses of non-cellular humoral substances from systemic blood into inflamed tissues is detailed. The mechanisms of actions responsible for the four cardinal signs and symptoms of inflammation, redness, swelling, heat, and pain are made clear for the first time, based upon microscopic observations and chemical analyses of the process. Mast cells are identified and their role in allergic reactions detailed. Antibodies and complement are recognized as soluble substances, moved by systemic blood and essential in the normal immune response to bacterial infections. The conceptual model of antigen-antibody interaction is introduced. Old models as to the source of disease e.g. Miasma theory and Contagion theory, are replaced by Germ theory. Bacteria are aggressively investigated which result in a new understanding of their potential source for disease and an essential understanding of their mechanisms of action. Endotoxins and exotoxins are identified. The combined study of specific bacteria e.g. Corynebacterium diphtheriae, Vibiro cholerae, Clostridium tetani, Bordetella pertussis, Mycobacterium tuberculosis, and the human immune system's response provides the necessary basic science knowledge which soon leads to an understanding of passive immunity and its application to clinical medicine. Infectious disease mortality rates plummet worldwide, as the principles and procedures of basic science immunological investigations of the 1800s are integrated into the daily practice of clinical medicine.

Yes, the 1800s prove to be an exciting and productive period in the discovery and understanding of the human immune system. These 100 years offer the solid foundation upon which much of our current knowledge of the immune system is based and reveals only the tip of the iceberg of things to come during the next 118 years.

Late Modern, 1900 AD - 2000 AD.

The 1900s quickly build upon the foundation laid during the 1800s and rapidly advance the understanding of individual biological components which make up the immune system; the genetic origins of these components; how the components function both individually and interactively to form a dynamic biological system; and how the immune system is involved in maintaining good physical health and its role in injury and disease.

The first half of the 1900s remain focused upon understanding more completely the humors of the immune system. Very little attention is focused upon investigations or study of the cell as important to body immunity. Most within the scientific and practicing clinical medical communities are content with the dogma of circulating antibodies as knowledge sufficient in explaining the basic sciences underlying the human immune system and guiding proven and effective clinical treatments.

From a professional development perspective, the first half of the 1900s witness the founding of professional societies and journals devoted specifically to the advancement of immunology as a separate scientific discipline. Universities and medical schools establish departments of immunology. Basic research findings are quickly reinterpreted within a medical clinical service delivery system matrix and integrated into routine medical care and treatments.

The first half of the 1900s witness the introduction of the now familiar ABO classification of blood types, which is based upon the recognition of antibody-antigen interactions. Hypersensitivity reactions are described and mechanisms of actions detailed. The American Association of Immunologists is founded and the "Journal of Immunology" begins publication. Antibodies are investigated in detail and recognized to be both cell bound and soluble serum proteins. The shape of antibodies is recognized to be more important than chemistry when interacting with antigens. The functions and process of opsinization are introduced and detailed. Rh factor is identified on RBCs and leads to the development of a blood group classification system based upon the presence of the newly discovered RBC antigens. Rh factor is understood within the matrix of blood transfusions and its cause of hemolytic disease of the newborn. The B-cell is identified as the source of antibody production. Electrophoresis is perfected and serum antibodies identified. Clinical blood tests are introduced to quickly assess the presence of specific antibodies in blood serum. New knowledge discovered and developed during the first half of the 1900s, concerning the humoral components of the immune system provide critical information and upon which much of immunology is still based today.

Let us take a look at some of the specific, notable people and their contributions to immunology during the first half of the 1900s, which have immediate relevance to you as a future physician.

Karl Landsteiner (1868-1943) Austrian biologist introduces the now familiar ABO classification of main blood groups, based upon identification of agglutinins in blood. Specifically, he observes RBCs clump together when RBCs are mixed with antibodies incompatible with the glycoprotein antigen expressed on the RBC (1900)[143]. For example, when type A blood (type A antigen expressed on RBCs) is mixed with serum from type B blood (contains antibodies which bind type A antigen) the RBCs within the type A blood will begin to clump together. The clumping of RBC is termed "hemagglutination", derived from the Latin word "agglutinare" meaning "to glue". This fact is the basis for typing blood before transfusions to ensure hemagglutination does not occur in your patient receiving the transfusion. Landsteiner is awarded the 1930 Nobel Prize in Physiology or Medicine in recognition "…for his discovery of human blood groups…" (1930)[144].

Alfred von Descastello (1872-1960) and Adriano Sturli (1873-1964) recognize some RBCs express both A and B surface antigens. They designate this distinct blood type as AB (1902)[145].

Trivia: Landsteiner in his original paper refers to ABC blood groups and not the ABO groups we recognize today. Since the ABC system (later the same year 1900 is renamed the ABO system) is based upon which antigen A, B, or neither is expressed on the RBC. Landsteiner replaces the "C" blood group, which expresses neither the A or the B antigen, with "O". The "O" term is derived from the German word "ohne", meaning "without" and to emphasize the absence of A or B antigen on the RBC.

Remember, the ABO blood groupings are based upon the presence or absence of the inherited antigen(s) on the RBC. The groupings are not based upon the presence or absences of antibodies to the antigens. This is a common source of error among many medical students. Don't forget it. The classifications are based upon antigen(s) not the antibodies.

Patients with type AB blood, A and B antigens present on their RBCs, do not produce A or B antibodies. Therefore, your AB patients can receive blood from any group; AB (preferred), A, B, or O. However, they can only donate blood to another AB patient. We often refer to these patients as universal blood recipients. In contrast, patients with type O blood, no A or B antigens present on their RBCs, do produce A and B antibodies. Therefore, your type O patients can receive blood only from another type O person. However, your type O patients can donate blood to any blood group; A, B, AB, or O. We often refer to these patients as universal blood donors. Be careful; there is more to the story. Your type O patients can donate blood to patients in any blood group, A, B, AB, or O, if and this is a big if, if the O type blood to be donated is O-Rh negative.

Landsteiner introduces the Rhesus factor: (Rh), approximately 40 years after introducing the familiar ABO blood groups, to describe an additional antigen, which may or may not be present (Rh + or Rh -) on any specific individual patient's RBCs. This now extends the ABO classification system to include the presence or absence of the Rh factor e.g. AB+ or AB- (1941)[146]. The Rh factor's role in the immune response is soon associated with blood transfusions and identified as a common and potential lethal cause of hemolytic disease of the newborn (1939,1940)[147,148]. The discovery of blood groups, based upon antigen-antibody interactions, explains the mechanisms of actions responsible for many disorders of blood and the variability in success whenever transfusing blood from one person to another.

Trivia: The original term "Rh", assigned by Karl Landsteiner and Alexander Wiener (1907-1976), indicate the source of RBCs injected into their research rabbits, taken from their research Rhesus monkeys.

Perhaps unknown to most medical students, Landsteiner in collaboration with Austrian physician Erwin Popper (1879-1955) identifies the polio virus as the causative agent responsible for poliomyelitis, six years after introducing the ABO blood groups and thirty three years before introducing the Rh factor (1908)[149].

Recall, polio is an acute viral infection which typically spreads from person to person via the fecal-oral route. The virus can enter the central nervous system, where it preferentially attacks neuronal cell bodies located in the gray matter of the anterior horns of the spinal cord or occasionally motor nuclei of cranial nerve systems located in the brain stem. The infection produces muscle weakness and paralysis.

The term "polio" is derived from the Greek word "polios" meaning gray, "myelos" from the Ancient Greek referring to the spinal cord, and the suffix "itis" from the Ancient Greek meaning inflammation.

Martinus Beijerinck (1851-1913) Dutch microbiologist is first to publish the discovery of a new, disease causing agent, smaller than a bacterium (1898)[150]. He terms this new agent "virus", a reintroduction of an English word from the late-1300s and early-1400s, then used to refer simply to poisonous substances. While Beijerinck is rightfully credited with the first published account of a virus, Russian biologist Dimitri Ivanovsky (1864-1920) actually discovers the "virus" six years earlier, while investigating a disease affecting tobacco leaves. He never publishes his findings. Instead, he presents his findings at a meeting of the St. Petersburg Academy of Imperial Sciences (1892)[151].

Here lies another good lesson for you the medical student. If you present a paper at a local, national, or international professional society meeting, complete the professional process. Rewrite your paper putting it in the necessary journal format and submit it for publication. Do not be satisfied with an abstract published in the society's summary of papers presented at the meeting. Journals are always looking for new ideas and well conducted research projects. If you need assistance in completing the process, seek out one of your faculty members who might share an interest in your project. They can help.

At the time Ivanovsky and Beijernick first introduce their findings identifying a new infectious agent the "virus", most research investigators are focusing efforts upon bacteria. Ivanovsky's and Beijernick's work receives little recognition or attention from the scientific and medical communities of the period. Their work later proves to be the foundations for all modern viral immunology.

Here too lies another valuable lesson for the medical student. Often the most valuable contributions are made in areas where few investigators are working. Don't be afraid to be creative and spend at least some of your time thinking in original, innovative, and different ways from all others. Question the dogma you learn in medical school. If you choose to contribute to the profession through academic research as part of your professional practice don't restrict yourself solely to the pursuit of Normal Science, to use a term coined by Thomas Kuhn (1922-1996)[152]. Don't be satisfied with adding simply another brick to the massive building of scientific knowledge; consider the role of architect instead.

OK…back to history.

Wilhelm Ellerman (1871-1924) Danish physician and Oluf Bang (1881-1937) Danish veterinarian are among the very few willing to devote resources to investigating this new infectious agent, the virus. Ellerman and Bang are first to report a virus containing cell free filtrate, can cause leukemia (1908)[153]. They are first to report a virus can and do cause certain cancers. Today, we simply refer to these cancer causing viruses as oncoviruses. Holding to the time honored tradition in medicine, not to quickly reject established medical dogma, their work is largely ignored by the professional and medical communities.

Francois Rous (1879-1970) American pathologist extends the work of Ellerman and Bang to solid tumors. Rous is first to demonstrate tumors can be transmitted from one animal to another by injecting small pieces of a tumor into a healthy animal (1910)[154]. The following year he demonstrates tumors can be transmitted from animal to animal without cells and simply injecting virus containing filtrate (1911)[155]. His work too is not widely accepted. Late in life and four years before his death, his contributions are recognized. He is awarded the Nobel Prize in Physiology or

Medicine in recognition of his work "…for his discovery of tumour-inducing viruses…" (1966)[156]. Sometimes a good idea takes a little time to catch on.

Only a small number of researchers worldwide are interested in investigating the recently identified new infectious agent, the virus. Fewer still are interested in investigating the virus within the matrix of the immune system. Many of the technologies necessary to study viruses are yet to be invented. Most investigators during the early-1900s who do investigate the immune system, limit their investigations to immune reactions triggered by common immunogens e.g. allergens and contagious bacteria. The investigators use conventional chemical analytic techniques. Few investigate viruses.

Charles Richet (1850-1935) French physiologist and Paul Portier (1866-1962) French marine physiologist report findings of their initial investigations leading to their discovery of the severe immune reaction, termed anaphylaxis (1902)[157]. The initial experiments are conducted aboard the yacht Princess Alice II, owned by Prince Albert of Monaco, which set sail in the summer of 1901 from Toulon France for the West African coast, near the Cape Verde Islands. Aboard are Richet, Portier, and Prince Albert's son Albert Grimaldi whom is an avowed oceanographer. Upon the recommendation of Prince Albert the three are encouraged to study the toxin of the Portuguese man-o-war (Physalia) during the voyage. Upon injecting the toxin into one of the ships dogs, they observe the now classic reactions. A single injection produces no apparent ill effects whereas a second injections weeks later produces a severe, violent reaction resulting in death. Richet is awarded the Nobel Prize in Physiology or Medicine in 1913 "…in recognition of his work on anaphylaxis…" (1913)[158].

Nicolas Arthus (1862-1945) French immunologist is among the first investigators of the early-1900s to systematically study the body's severe, acute, multi-system, immune responses. Building upon the foundational study recently reported by Richet and Portier, Arthus correctly describes the mechanisms of action underlying anaphylaxis. He correctly describes the binding of antigen with antibody bound to mast cells; describes the subsequent degranulation of the mast cell; correctly observes the reaction occurs only after a second exposure to a specific type of antigen; correctly observes the immune reaction is severe, immediate, and involves the whole body; and correctly observes the reaction to be potentially life threatening (1903,1921)[159,160].

The anaphylaxis reaction and the underlying mechanisms responsible is not the reaction most medical students associate with Nicolas Arthus. Most medical students associate Nicolas Arthus with the "Arthus reaction", also known as the "Arthus phenomenon" (1903)[159]. The Arthus reaction, in contrast to the generalized anaphylaxis reaction, is a local, immune complex mediated, type III hypersensitivity reaction, characterized by deposition of antigen-antibody complexes in the vascular walls, pleura, pericardium, synovium, and renal glomeruli.

Almroth Wright (1861-1947) British academic immunologist and Stewart Douglas (1871-1936) discover serum fluids which prepare bacteria for phagocytosis (1903)[161]. They term these serum fluids "opsonin". The term "opsonin" is derived from the Greek meaning "to prepare for a meal", reflecting their identified function. The serum fluids which coat bacteria and prepare it for phagocytosis, described by Wright and Douglas, later prove to be antibody and complement.

Clemens von Pirquet (1874-1929) Austrian pediatrician and Bela Schick (1877-1967) Hungarian pediatrician observe patients who have received smallpox vaccinations or injections of antibodies from horse serum, oftentimes develop severe immune reactions when given a second injection.

They coin the term "allergy", derived from the Greek "allos: meaning "other" and "ergon" meaning "function". The term is used to describe the clinical presentation of an immune hypersensitivity reaction "…the other function…" which occasionally occurs in response to immunization, in addition to the "…primary function…" of immunization to provide protection against specific viruses or bacteria (1906)[162]. The immune reaction they describe is simply a Type I immune-complex hypersensitivity reaction and familiar to most practicing physicians as an occasional reaction to penicillin injections.

Von Pirquet soon extends his work to investigate tuberculin generated from the bacteria which produces tuberculosis and its role in producing a hypersensitivity reaction similar to that produced by smallpox vaccinations or antibodies from horse serum reported earlier. He develops a quick procedure to assess if a patient has ever been exposed to a tuberculosis infection. The procedure consists of scratching a drop of tuberculin into the surface of a small area of skin and examining the site the next day for development of redness, hardness, and other signs of localized immune response (1908)[163].

Charles Mantoux (1877-1947) French physician builds upon Pirquet's original work and develops the Mantoux test, in which tuberculin is injected into the skin and is used as a diagnostic test for tuberculosis (1907)[164].

Bela Schick later develops his test for detecting susceptibility to diphtheria, based upon a simple, clinical procedure of injecting a small amount of diluted diphtheria toxin into the skin and observing redness and swelling at the injection site, as clinical indicators of an immune response (Schick test). If the patient's immune system is adequate, there is no evidence of redness or swelling at the injection site. If the immune system is compromised, the patient will reveal redness and swelling at the injection site (1910)[165]. This represents one of many clinical diagnostic tests soon to be developed and widely used in clinical medicine, based directly upon an understanding of the mechanism of actions of the immune systems.

As investigators during the early-1900s focus upon hypersensitivity reactions, providing clinical descriptions, postulating mechanisms of actions, and developing quick clinical diagnostic procedures based upon an understanding of the immune systems, the discipline of immunology matures, as a recognized and respected discipline, separate from microbiology. Immunology establishes its own professional societies and journals devoted specifically to the advancement of immunology as a professional discipline. The American Association of Immunologists (AAI) is founded June 19, 1913, on the campus of the University of Minnesota (2013)[166]. The "Journal of Immunology" begins publication in 1916 (1916)[167]. Today, over 100 years later, both the AAI and Journal are active, highly respected and continue to make innovative contributions, moving the discipline of immunology forward, as a much respected scientific discipline with knowledge immediately applicable to the practice of high quality clinical medicine.

Linus Pauling (1901-1994) American molecular biologist, biochemist, and two time Nobel Prize recipient proposes the shape of antibodies and antigen are primary in determining their interaction within the immune systems rather than their chemistry (1940)[168]. His proposal challenges conventional thinking and medical dogma of the time, antibodies and antigen bind via chemical interactions. Over the course of approximately 10 years during the 1940s, Pauling establishes a detailed model of the binding of antibody and antigen, at the molecular level (1943,1945)[169,170]. The model is very similar in concept to the "lock and key" model proposed by Emil Fischer 46 years earlier to describe high specificity of enzymes to substrates (1894)[171].

Linus Pauling makes numerous and substantial contributions throughout his career and proves to be one of the most influential scientists in the areas of quantum chemistry and molecular biology, during the twentieth century. Pauling is awarded the 1954 Nobel Prize in Chemistry "…for his research into the nature of the chemical bond and its application to the elucidation of the structure of complex substances…" (1954)[172]. He is awarded the 1962 Nobel Prize for Peace "…for his opposition to weapons of mass destruction…" (1962)[173]. The same year Francis Crick, James Watson, and Maurice Wilkins are awarded the Nobel Prize for Physiology or Medicine "…for their discoveries concerning the molecular structure of nucleic acids and its significance for information transfer in living material…" (1962)[174].

Astrid Fagraeus (1913-1997) Swedish immunologist experimentally confirms differentiated B-cells i.e. plasma cells, to be the source of antibody production. She presents the idea as part of her doctoral dissertation (1948)[175] extending the works of Jens Bing who first identifies the relationship between plasma cells and antibody production 10 years earlier (1937,1943, 1946) [176,177,178].

Arne Tiselius (1902-1972) Swedish chemist and Elvin Kabat (1914-2000) American quantitative immunochemist perfect the electrophoresis technique and classify gamma globulins, with the most significant gamma globulin being immunoglobulins (Igs), also known as antibodies (1938)[179]. Tiselius is awarded the Nobel Prize in chemistry "…for his research on electrophoresis and adsorption analysis, especially for his discoveries concerning the complex nature of the serum proteins…" (1948)[180].

Frank Burnet (1899-1985) Australian immunologist and Peter Medawar (1915-1987) British transplant biologist identify elements of the immune system responsible for organ transplant rejection and offer theories of self tolerance and clonal selection. Burnet's monograph "The Production of Antibody" introduces the now familiar concept of "self vs non-self" and moves immunology from a pursuit in chemistry to one of biology (1949)[181].

Peter Medawar extends the work of Frank Burnet and investigates the role of the immune system as it impacts the success of skin graphing procedures offered to individuals suffering burns received during World War II. Medawar's investigations provide the necessary insights and experimental data which demonstrate an advantage in suppressing a patient's healthy immune system immediately before and immediately following tissue transplant. This manipulation significantly improves the probability of the recipient's body not rejecting donor tissues. Peter Madawar and Frank Burnet are awarded the Nobel Prize in Physiology or Medicine "…for discovery of acquired immunological tolerance…" (1960)[182].

The first half of the 1900s closes, having made significant advances in the understanding of the humoral components of the immune system e.g. antibodies, complement, and opsins. The ABO blood group classification is introduced with an understanding as to why blood transfusions between people can result in lethal outcomes. The Rh factor is discovered and understood, reducing hemolytic disease of the newborn. Viruses are recognized and understood as potential disease causing non-cellular pathogens. Leukemia is recognized as one condition which can be caused by cell free filtrate containing virus. Immune reactions are better understood. Anaphylaxis is detailed and understood within the matrix of an immune system response. Allergies are understood as immune reactions. Rapid skin tests are introduced to evaluate a person's prior exposure to tuberculosis or diphtheria. The interactions of antibodies with antigen within the immune systems is recognized to be accomplished primarily by physical shape characteristics rather than chemical reactions. Immune systems are studied at the molecular level. Production of antibodies from plasma cells, differentiated B-cells, is discovered and confirmed by experimental investigations. Electrophoresis is introduced and used to separate serum proteins e.g. immunoglobulins (antibodies). Tissue transplant begins to be better understood and introduces the concept of "self" vs "non-self". Suppression of the immune system is recognized to be beneficial, reducing tissue transplant rejection and in the management of select disease conditions. Professional societies e.g. the American Association of Immunologists and professional journals e.g. The "Journal of Immunology" are founded for the specific purpose of exchanging information and advancing immunology as a scientific discipline.

The second half of the 1900s opens by expanding investigations into the humoral components of immune systems and placing more focus upon understanding cellular components and their roles in the body's defenses.

Humors continue to be investigated and provide much new information regarding their sources, structures, mechanisms of actions, and roles in cell to cell signaling. New antibodies are discovered and classified into the now familiar five classes: IgA, IgD, IgE, IgG, and IgM. Antibody structures are detailed, revealing the Fc and Fab components of these proteins. Interferons (IFNs) are first identified and their roles in activating immune cells are detailed. Interleukins (ILs) and other secreted protein signaling molecules are first identified. Interleukins are recognized to be released by leukocytes and to be important in promoting normal T-cells and B-cells development.

Cells soon become the focus of most immunological investigations during the second half of the 1900s. T-cells are discovered and their importance as fundamental components of the immune system recognized and aggressively studied. The thymus is recognized as essential for normal T-cell development. Dendritic cells are identified as primary antigen presenting cells. Natural killer cells are identified and their role in the immune system described. Much attention is directed to systematic investigation of cell receptors. Specifically, B-cell receptors, T-cell receptors, and HLA (human leukocyte antigen) receptors are identified for the first time. Their structures and physiology detailed, co-receptor complexes identified, and roles in signal transduction detailed. The CD (cluster of differentiation) system is introduced to describe the chemical molecule which coats cell surfaces, useful in cell identification, receptor binding, and cell signaling of leukocytes (white blood cells). The MHC (major histocompatibility complex) are identified on all cells and subclassified into the now familiar MHC Class I and MHC Class II classification system. The MHC complex's role in both cell to cell signaling and antigen presentation within the immune system are detailed.

Let us now take a look at some of the specific, notable people and their contributions to immunology during the second half of the 1900s, which have relevance to you as a future physician.

Alick Isaacs (1921-1967) British virologist and Jean Lindenmann (1924-2015) Yugoslavian microbiologist discover and coin the term "interferons" (INFs), the proteins made and released by host cells in response to presence of viruses, bacteria, parasites, tumor cells and other pathogens (1957)[183]. Recall, interferons are a subclass of cell signaling molecules which interfere with viral replication within host cells, activate natural killer cells and macrophages, and up regulate antigen presentation to T-cells.

The discovery of interferons during the late-1950s signals a milestone and the emphasis placed upon understanding cell to cell signaling. Immunology devotes considerable resources to understanding cell to cell communication at the molecular level, for the next 50 years.

Jean Daussett (1916-2009) French investigator discovers the human leukocyte antigen (HLA). This leukocyte antigen in humans is simply termed the major histocompatibility complex (MHC) and encodes cell surface antigen presentation proteins. Recall, the body's immune system uses a person's HLAs to differentiate self-cells from non-self cells. Daussett makes his discovery of the MHC while searching to understand the basis of histocompatibility between tissues transplanted from a graph donor to a graph recipient (1958)[184]. Daussett shares the Nobel Prize in Physiology or Medicine with Baruji Benacerraf (1920-2011) Venezuelan immunologist and George Snell (1903-1996) American transplant immunologist "...for their discoveries concerning genetically determined structures on the cell surface that regulate immunological reactions..." (1980)[185].

James Gowans (1924-2020) British researcher and E. Julie Knight (unknown-) British researcher demonstrate lymphocytes recirculate from lymph back into blood via lymphatic sinuses located primarily in lymph nodes. This data requires a radical change in the way lymphocytes are understood within the immune system (1964)[186]. They additionally establish once lymphocytes re-enter blood circulation, they rapidly migrate to specific tissues e.g. lymph nodes, the white pulp of the spleen, Peyer's Patches of the intestines, but not thymus or bone marrow (1964)[186]. Gowan and Knight further demonstrate cell to cell signaling of lymphocytes in their 1964 paper, however another twenty years will pass before the surface molecules on lymphocytes are identified responsible for organ specific homing and lymphocyte trafficking (1983)[187].

At the time Gowans and Knight make their seminal 1964 contribution, most in immunology are studying humoral components of the immune system with little interests in cellular components. For perspective on the level of knowledge of the cells' roles in the immune system, during the mid-1960s, dogma at the time Gowans and Knight publish is as follows; given lymphocytes are loaded with DNA, have very little cytoplasm, and circulate widely throughout the body, their primary function must be to deliver DNA to cells throughout the body, "...like mobile filling stations delivering DNA to cells in need of a fill up..." (2006)[188].

Rodney Porter (1917-1985) British biochemist mixes papain, an enzyme from papaya juice, with IgG and successfully breaks the 1,300 amino acid IgG molecule into smaller pieces which he subjects to additional analysis (1948)[189]. He soon identifies the Fc (fraction crystallizable) one third portion of the IgG molecule and demonstrates the Fc portion is constant between all IgG antibodies, does not bind antigen, and fixes complement. He quickly observes the antigen-binding portion of the IgG molecule is found on the other two thirds of the molecule and is variable between IgG molecules. He terms this section the Fab portion (fragment antigen-binding) (1958)[190].

Gerald Edelman (1929-2014) American biologist identifies the heavy and light chain protein subunits of the antibody molecule, their disulfide bonds, and their variable and constant domains (1969)[191]. Collectively, Porter and Edelman detail the basic structure of the antibody. Rodney Porter and Gerald Edelman share the 1972 Noble Prize in Physiology or Medicine "...for their discoveries concerning the chemical structure of antibodies..." (1972)[192].

Henry Kunkel (1916-1983) American immunologist and Jacques Oudin (1908-1985) French immunologist independently provide additional research on antibody structure and classify antibodies according to idiotypes (1963,1963)[193,194].

Recall, an idiotype is simply the unique sequence of amino acids located on the variable region of the Fab fragment of an antibody or T-cell receptor, which determines the antigen specificity to the receptor. Don't confuse idiotype with isotype. This is a common mistake among medical students. Recall, an isotype defines an antibody, based upon its constant regions of the heavy and light chains and provides the basis for the classification of antibodies into the five familiar groupings: IgA, IgD, IgE, IgG, and IgM. Don't forget it.

Jacques Miller (1931-) French research scientist identifies two major subsets of lymphocytes, the T-cell and the B-cell and describes their functional significance (1961,1964)[195,196]. Miller discovers the thymus is necessary to the normal development and education of lymphocytes. He is first to recognize and demonstrate the thymus is the location where removal of auto-reactive T-cells occurs and is accomplished before T-cells are released into systemic circulation (1967)[197]. Miller and his research group subsequently provide the necessary data which demonstrates an interaction of T and B cells is necessary for normal antibody production (1971)[198].

Robert Good (1922-2003) American immunologist and Jacques Miller (1931-) are among the first to emphasize the importance of the thymus and document the important role of the palatine tonsils in the developing immune system. Their work move the tonsils from the widely accepted category of useless, unnecessary, and dispensable tissue to one essential in normal immune system development and function (1962,1966)[199,200].

Robert Good is a member of the transplant team completing the first successful bone marrow transplant. The successful transplant is completed on a child suffering from X-SCID (X-linked severe combined immunodeficiency) (1968)[201].

Successful bone marrow transplants are routinely completed in children with immune deficiency diseases. Can you reason why? Correct. Given their T-cell deficiency, these children do not require the cyto-ablation and post-graph immunosuppression necessary in patients presenting with an intact immune system.

This provides an example in medical research where thoughtful analysis and a conceptual model permits one to take advantage of naturally occurring pathologies to study, better understand, and contribute to the advancement of knowledge of both normal and pathological process, occurring in biological systems. Recognition that it is the immune system which is primarily responsible for tissue transplant rejection opens new avenues of scientific investigations and leads to rapid advances in the success of tissue transplants and transplant immunology during the second half of the 1900s.

Philip Gell (1914-2001) and Robert Coombs (1921-2006) British immunologists publish their classification system of four clinically distinguishable hypersensitivity reactions (1963)[202]. Their classification system is familiar to all in medical school today. The classification organizes hypersensitivity responses into four basic groups, differentiated upon clinical responses and independent whether the trigger is environmental, infectious, or self antigens: Type I immediate hypersensitivity reactions e.g. hay-fever, food allergies; Type II antibody mediated cell-bound antigen hypersensitivity reaction e.g. penicillin induced immune hemolytic anemia, hemolytic disease of the newborn, Graves disease; Type III immune antigen-antibody complex hypersensitivity reactions e.g. post streptococcal glomerulonephritis, systemic lupus erythematosus; and Type IV delayed hypersensitivity reactions e.g. contact dermatitis, rheumatoid arthritis, multiple sclerosis.

Hypersensitivity reactions have been known for thousands of years and studied extensively during the late-1800s and early-1900s. Gell and Coombs' contribution is in the organization of the literature, classification of the most common forms of hypersensitivity reactions into four major categories based upon clinical presentation, and offering a conceptual matrix within which to organize, synthesize, and understand fundamental mechanisms of action responsible for each major category.

As immunology moves into the early-1970s, subtypes of T- lymphocytes are discovered and their specialized functions detailed. Natural killer cells are first discovered. The functional roles of the dendritic cell are finally made clear, approximately 100 years after the cell is first identified by Paul Langerhans.

Nicholas Mitchison (1928-) British immunologist is among the first to describe a subset of T-lymphocytes demonstrating helper activity (1971)[203]. Helper T-cells have no phagocytic or cytotoxic capabilities by themselves. They are essential in directing and coordinating the phagocytic and cytotoxic activities of other immune cells. Helper T-cells are essential in determining B-cell antibody class switching, maximizing phagocytic actions of macrophages, and activating cytotoxic CD-8 T-cells.

Richard Gershon (1932-1983) and Kazunari Kondo (unknown-) are among the first to demonstrate the role of the suppressor T-cell, a subpopulation of lymphocytes that suppresses antibody formation by B-cells and down regulates the ability of T-cells to mount a cellular response (1971)[204].

Rolf Kiessling (unknown -) Swedish researcher identifies a subpopulation of lymphocytes which appear to lyse tumor cells and cells infected by viruses. He names these special cells "Natural killer" cells based upon initial beliefs during the early-1970s these cells kill any cell missing the major histocompatibility complex (MHC-I) which identifies the cell as "self" and that the killing is "natural", that is occurring without activation which is required of all other known lymphocytes (1975)[205]. Today, natural killer cells are recognized as important cytotoxic lymphocytes essential in the innate immune system response; however they are now known to require activation via interleukins, macrophage cytokines, or antibody. Additionally, natural killer cells are recognized today not to lyse cells as originally suspected but rather accomplish their killing via apoptosis; an important distinction.

Ralph Steinman (1943-2011) and Aanvil Cohn (1926-1993) American immunologists recognize the "dendritic cell" to be the primary antigen presenting cells of the immune system (1973)[206]. Recall, dendritic cells are immune cells present in tissue in contact with the external environment, such as the skin (Langerhans cells), nose, lungs, stomach, and intestines. Once activated they migrate to lymph nodes and interact with T-cells and B-cells to help guide the initial adaptive immune response. While Paul Langerhans first describes this cell in 1868 it is not until 1973 their functional role within the adaptive immune system is identified (1973)[206].

Peter Doherty (1940-) Australian veterinarian immunologist and Rolf Zinkernagel (1944-) Swiss immunologist are among the first to report how the body's immune system protects against viruses, at the cellular level.

Peter Doherty and Rolf Zinkernagle propose, when a virus infects a host cell, the virus molecule alters the host's marker protein, which identifies the cell as belonging to the host. The alteration of the host's marker self protein provides the necessary signal which informs T-lymphocytes the cell is now infected and marks the cell for destruction by the immune system. Building upon the work by Jean Daussett from the 1950s with the major histocompatibility (MHC) antigens and recognizing it is the MHC that is altered by the virus that opens the doors to understanding for the first time the concepts of MHC restriction and cell mediated dual recognition, involved in the body's normal immune response to viral infections (1974)[207]. T-cells do not recognize a virus directly, but only in conjunction with MHC molecules. The immune system needs to recognize both self and foreign molecules in order to initiate an effective response to viral infections. Doherty and Zinkernagle share the Nobel Prize in Physiology or Medicine "...for their discoveries concerning the specificity of the cell mediated immune defense..." (1996)[208].

Kendall Smith (unknown -) and Steve Gills (unknown -) first describe interleukin IL-2 and advances the understanding of cell to cell signaling used within the immune system to regulate and coordinated system activities (1977)[209]. The term interleukin is selected to emphasize the function of this protein, cell secreted signaling molecule, to carry messages between leukocytes. Two years later, Lymphocyte Activating Factor (LAF), the term used by investigators to describe the substance which make T-cells proliferate, is changed to the new nomenclature, IL-1. The change is made during a meeting in France to establish new and uniform nomenclature within the field of immunology (1979)[210]. Additional investigations soon clarify more completely the roles of IL-2 and mechanisms of action, which establishes IL-1 as a distinct cytokine from IL-2 (1980)[211]. IL-1 is named and detailed two years after IL-2, making IL-2 the first interleukin identified, detailed and purified (1980)[212]. The IL-2 receptor is described one year later (1981)[213].

By the early-1980s significant and rapid advances are being made in the field of immunology. The 1980s witness the discovery of new cell signaling molecules e.g. additional interleukins; a new infectious agent prions; a group of viruses with affinity for cells of the human immune system e.g. the human immunodeficiency virus (HIV); discovery of T-cell receptor complexes; introduction of the cluster of differentiation (CD) classification system of leukocytes; and an understanding of the production of antibodies sufficient to produce large amounts of specific monoclonal antibodies.

Stanley Prusiner (1942-) American neurologist and biochemist, working with the University of California San Francisco discovers a new class of infectious, self-reproducing pathogens, comprised primarily of proteins in a misfolded form. He terms these new infectious agents "prions", derived from the words "protein" and "infection" (1982)[214]. He is awarded the Nobel Prize in Physiology or Medicine "...for the discovery of prions as a new biological principle of infection..." (1997)[215]. The award immediately generates much controversy within the discipline of immunology and remains unresolved today, twenty years after the award is made. The controversy centers around Stanley Prusiner's claim of discovery and the Nobel Prize Committee's recognition prions are "... a new biological principle of infection...", joining the list of bacteria, viruses, and fungi. Many question the capability of prions to induce disease given they contain no genetic material. What do you think?

Francoise Barre-Sinoussi (1947-) and Luc Montagnier (1932-) French virologists are first to correctly identify and report the science which explains the immunological basis of a new and devastating medical condition, which rapidly spreads worldwide and first identified in the early-1980s, acquired immunodeficiency syndrome (AIDS) (1893) [216]. They are awarded the Nobel Prize in Physiology or Medicine in recognition "…for their discovery of human immunodeficiency virus…" (2008)[217].

Ellis Reinherz (unknown-), Philppa Marrack (1945-), John Kappler (1943-), James Allison (unknown -) describe the T-cell antigen receptor (TCR) (1983)[218]. The TCR recognizes and engage antigen bound to MCH molecules on cells in conjunction with CD4 and CD8 surface molecules (1983)[219]. The TCR complex is soon defined, including both the TCR and co-receptor molecules. The CD-4 molecule is recognized as a co-receptor and maintains selectivity for cells presenting antigen in combination with MHC class II molecules. The CD-8 molecule is recognized as a co-receptor and maintains selectivity for cells presenting antigen in combination with MHC class I molecules. Activation of the TCR complex is necessary to generate the normal T-cell immune response.

The cluster of differentiation (CD) classification system of leukocytes is introduced as a protocol for the identification of cell surface molecules on leukocytes (1982)[220]. Specific CD molecules act as receptor or ligands, are important in cell signaling, and play important roles in cell adhesion. All leukocytes e.g. neutrophils, basophils, eosinophils, monocytes, T-helper cells, T-suppressor cells, cytotoxic T-cells, B-cells, platelets, and natural killer cells, all express CD molecules. Identification of CD molecules and combination of multiple CD molecules appearing on specific leukocytes provide molecular markers for rapid sorting of leukocytes and an understanding of how leukocytes recognize, respond to, and interact with antigens. Today, more than 370 unique clusters of differentiation have been identified in the human.

Trivia: The term "cluster of differentiation" (CD) is derived from the statistical method used to identify statistical "clusters of antibodies" with very similar patterns of binding to leukocytes at various stages of development "differentiation". Hence the term "clusters of differentiation".

During the early-1980s, immunologists are generating large numbers of monoclonal antibodies reactive to leukocyte cell markers. In an attempt to standardize the nomenclature, the profession holds a workshop to resolve the rapidly growing problem of unstandardized nomenclature. The first International Workshop and Conference on Human Leukocyte Differentiation Antigens (HLDA) is held in Paris in 1982. Standardization of nomenclature is a sign of maturation within a developing scientific professional community. Efforts continue today to standardize nomenclature within immunology.

Niels Jerne (1911-1994) British immunologist, George, Kohler (1946-1995) German immunologist, and Cesar Milstein (1927-2002) Argentine biochemist share the Nobel Prize in Physiology or Medicine "…for theories concerning the specificity in development and control of the immune system and the discovery of the principle for production of monoclonal antibodies…" (1984)[221].

Recall, each B-cell in your patient's body is capable of synthesizing only one kind of antibody. There are billions of B-cells in the body. Therefore there are billions of possible variations in the antibodies produced in any single patient (antibody diversity). The antibody produced by B-cells in any one patient is dependent upon the antigens to which the patient has been exposed.

Antibodies are typically used by the body to identify antigens and mark the antigens for destruction by phagocytosis. Once the mechanisms of action are identify as to how antibodies identify and bind to the short sequences of antigens comprising the antigen epitope, it is soon recognized antibodies can also be used to function as marker molecules of any short sequence of amino acids occurring on the surface of specific cells. This opens the door for the identification of specific cell subtypes, cell receptors, bacteria, and most anything expressing a short sequence of amino acids on its surface.

The technological problem of culturing a large population of B cells, to produce a large amount of a single antibody, is solved by Niels Jerne, George Kohler, and Cesar Milstein by the early-1980s. The process of culturing a large population of B-cells from a single ancestral B-cell permits the harvesting of a single kind of antibody which then can be used to mark other cells. The population of the cultured B-cells is termed "monoclonal" and the antibody produced from the B-cells is termed "monoclonal antibodies" (MAbs). Jerne, Kohler, and Milstein are awarded the 1984 Nobel Prize in Medicine or Physiology "…for theories concerning the specificity in development and control of the immune system and the discovery of the principle for production of monoclonal antibodies…" (1984)[221].

Monoclonal antibodies are successfully used in immunology and numerous other areas of medicine for the balance of the 1900s. Monoclonal antibodies are soon used in ELISA (1971)[222], useful in the diagnosis of HIV during the 1980s and 1990s. Today, monoclonal antibodies continue to be used as essential components in numerous diagnostic tests, effective treatments, and provide investigators with another powerful tool to better understand the human immune system.

As immunology moves into the 1990s, the field witnesses much research devoted to the understanding of the immune systems within the matrix of its underlying genetic material. Genetics are introduced to explain the molecular basis of antibody diversity, selected mechanisms of immune system activation, the molecular basis of several inter and intra cellular signaling systems, and the molecular basis of many well-known inherited disorders, which result in impaired immune system function.

Susumu Tonegawa (1939-) Japanese immunologist introduces the genetic principle, to explain antibody diversity. Given B-cells can potentially manufacture billions of different antibodies and a B-cell carries only about 100,000 genes on its chromosomes, a mechanism of action and conceptual matrix is required to explain the tremendous diversity available to B cells in producing antibody specific to antigens. The answer, at least for now, is offered by Tonegawa and his research group. They demonstrate the genes coding for antibody are shuffled at random, so in the mature cell a cluster of functional genes is formed which is unique to that specific cell. Each individual mature cell therefore produces its own specific antibody. This diversity is further amplified given each antibody molecule is comprised of four protein chains, all with highly variable terminal regions. Tonegawa is awarded the Nobel Prize in Physiology or Medicine "…for his discovery of the genetic principle for generation of antibody diversity…" (1987)[223].

Charles Janeway (1943-2003), Paula Preston-Hurlburt (unknown-), and Ruslan Medzhitov (1966-) working with the recently discovered Toll receptor, demonstrate when a Toll like receptor (TLR) is bound by antibody, the interaction triggers activation of genes necessary for initiating an adaptive immune response, characterized by activation of naive T-cells (1997)[224]. This research group and others e.g. Susumu Tonegawa, begin to provide the necessary and essential knowledge required to understand the human immune system within a new conceptual matrix of function and genetic material.

Recall, Toll like receptors (TLR) are a class of membrane bound proteins which recognize shared patterns within molecules of pathogens, distinct from host molecules. They receive their name from their similarity to the protein, coded by the Toll gene found in the fruit fly (Drosophila melanogaster) and which play a significant role in the fly's immunity to fungal infections.

Trivia: The term "Toll" is derived from the German word "toll", which when translated into English means "great".

Gunter Blobel (1936-2018) German molecular biologist identifies and details the molecular processes used by newly synthesized proteins to direct proteins to specific locations inside of the cell. He formulates and provides experimental evidence in support of a "signal hypothesis" for guiding transport of proteins to specific targets within a cell. The molecular mechanism described is similar to the mechanisms described by Romanian cell biologist and Nobel Prize recipient George Palade (1912-2008) over 25 years earlier and used to direct proteins to specific targets outside of the cell. Gunter Blobel is awarded the 1999 Nobel Prize in Physiology or Medicine "…for discoveries concerning signal transduction…" (1999)[225], further emphasizing the importance immunology, as a discipline, places upon molecular communications as the 1900s come to a close.

In summary, during the first half of the 1900s, immunology witnesses rapid growth in content knowledge and matures as a scientific discipline. Blood is sub-typed into the ABO classification system based upon antigens expressed on the surface of RBCs and antibody reactions to these cell bound antigens. Anaphylaxis and other hypersensitivity reactions are described and their mechanisms of actions detailed. The concept of opsonization is introduced and understood within the matrix of phagocytosis. Several quick clinical diagnostic tests are introduced which rapidly identify previous exposure to specific bacterial infections e.g. tuberculosis, diphtheria, based upon the patient's observed immune response. These tests are quickly integrated into clinical medicine. The American Immunological Society is founded and its "Journal of Immunology" begins publication. The structure of antibodies are identified and recognized to be essential in the binding of antibody to antigen. Differentiated B-cells (plasma cells) are recognized to be the source of antibody production. Electrophoresis helps identify and classify serum proteins, including antibodies.

During the second half of the 1900s immunology continues its rapid growth and maturation as a discipline. Interferons are identified. The concept of "self vs. non-self", based upon theories of self tolerance and clonal selection in antibody formation, is introduced and moves immunology from a pursuit in chemistry to one of biology. HLA is discovered and recognized important in antigen presentation and essential in discrimination of "self from non-self" cells. Lymphocytes are recognized to recirculate and their mechanism of actions identified. Antibody Fc and Fab fragments are identified and functions detailed. Antibody idiotypes are identified and examined at the molecular level. Antibody isotypes are identified and classified into the five major classes, IgA, IgD, IgE, IgG, and IgM. T-cells are discovered. The interaction between B-cells and T-cells become more clear. Thymus is recognized to be essential in T-cell development. Palatine tonsils are recognized to be important in immune system development and no longer regarded as unnecessary and dispensable. Subtypes of T cells are identified and organized according to suspected functions e.g. T-helper and T-suppressor cells. Type I, Type II, Type III, and Type IV hypersensitivity reactions classification system is introduced, based upon clinical presentation. MHC complexes are understood within the matrix of viral infections. A new conceptual matrix is introduced to understand how the immune system deals with viral infections, augmenting immune system knowledge built upon an understanding of bacterial infections. Natural killer cells e.g. dendritic cells are identified and their function detailed. Antigen presenting cells are recognized and their mechanisms of action detailed. Interleukins are discovered, stimulating investigations into cell to cell signaling, within the immune systems. Prions are introduced as a new biological principle of infection. The HIV virus responsible for AIDS is identified. B-cell, T-cell, and HLA receptor complexes are identified and described in detail. Receptor complexes are described at the molecular level and understood within the conceptual matrix of a receptor complex containing co-receptors, series of biochemical enzymatic reactions, and production of genetic transcription factors. The cluster of differentiation (CD) system is introduced. CD-8 and CD-4 cells are described. MHC-I and MHC-II are identified and their roles in cell to cell signaling and antigen presentation detailed. Monoclonal antibodies are produced and immediately incorporated into clinical immunology, forming the basis of many new immunological test procedures e.g. ELISA which are used in the rapid diagnosis of immune system disorders. The genetic basis accounting for antibody diversity is introduced and detailed.

Yes, the 1900s prove to be an exciting time in immunology.

Current Modern, 2000 AD - 2019 AD.

Immunology is very much alive and well as we step into the early-2000s. Currently the field is making rapid advances in understanding the immune systems at the molecular level. Attention is being focused upon genetic materials and their roles in determining structure, mechanisms of action, and variability between individuals. Many research immunologists today are filing patents to protect their professional and financial interests. Discoveries are quickly integrated into clinical commercial medicine. Staggering profit margins are being enjoyed by large pharmaceutical corporations, as pharmacological management of the immune systems becomes a routine part of clinical practice of medicine. Many of the innovative research advances being made in medical immunology are now funded by private, for profit, startup companies.

Rodcrick Nairn (1951-) American biochemist and Matthew Helbert (unknown-) British clinical immunologist make a significant contribution to the field of immunology and perhaps more than any other has immediate relevance for all currently enrolled medical students. In 2002 they release their first edition of "Immunology for Medical Students" (2002)[226]. This book masterfully integrates the massive and rapidly changing knowledge of immunology into an easily readable, understandable, and relevant text for the first or second year student. The text is elegant in its ability to identify major topic areas, convey essential content information, and provides a matrix within which to understand material with clear relevance to the practice of medicine. The book is now in its third and updated edition (2017)[3].

Harald zur Hausen (1936-) German virologist is awarded the Nobel Prize in Physiology or Medicine 2008 "…for his discovery of human papilloma viruses causing cervical cancer…" (2008)[227]. His work is based upon the knowledge cell growth, division, and death are regulated by a cell's genes. When the genes of healthy cervical cells are altered by the human papilloma virus (HPV type 16 and 18, wart viruses) cervical cancer results. At the time Harold zur Hausen makes his discovery, cervical cancer is the second most common tumor in women worldwide and is killing over 260,000 women annually. Given the new understanding as to how these viruses invade cells and alter cell DNA, a vaccine, 100% effective against the HPV type 16 and 18 is soon produced and approved by the US Food and Drug Administration (2006)[228]. The vaccine today continues to be safe and effective, and its benefits continue to outweigh its risks (2018)[229].

Francoise Barre-Sinoussi (1947-) and Luc Montagnier (1932-) French virologists share the Nobel Prize in Physiology or Medicine 2008 with Harold zur Hausen "…for their discovery of the human immunodeficiency virus…", responsible for autoimmune deficiency syndrome (AIDS) (2008)[230]. The notable works of Francoise Barre-Sinoussi and Luc Montagnier focus on their discovery of the retrovirus responsible for invading the DNA of CD 4 T-helper cell lymphocytes, which incorporate the RNA of the virus into the lymphocyte's DNA and produce the devastating condition, AIDS.

Three years later American immunologist Bruce Beutler (1957-) and French biologist Jules Hoffmann (1941-) are awarded the Nobel Prize in Physiology or Medicine 2011 "…for their discoveries concerning the activation of innate immunity…" (2011)[231]. Bruce Beutler's research team discovers a Toll-like receptor (TLR), which when it binds the bacterial product lipopolysaccharide (LPS), signals are activated that cause inflammation and when in excess septic shock (1998)[232]. Jules Hoffmann's team discover the product of the Toll gene is necessary in recognizing pathogenic microorganisms and activation of the innate immune system response (1996)[233].

The same year Ralph Steinman (1943-2011) Canadian physician and medical researcher shares the Nobel Prize in Physiology or Medicine 2011 "…for his discovery of the dendritic cell and its role in adaptive immunity…" (2011)[231]. Ralph Steinman discovers a new cell type, he terms the dendritic cell (1973)[234]. He demonstrates the dendritic cell can activate T-cells, which play essential roles in adaptive immune system response (1978)[235].

Today, new, exciting, and substantive contributions are being made to the immunology knowledge base. Current areas of research are reflected in seven general areas of investigation now being completed at the National Institutes of Health (NIH), in over 200 NIH labs. These seven representative areas are: immune cell signaling and cell biology; developmental immunology; allergy, autoimmunity and immunoregulation; structural/molecular immunology and immunogenetics; tumor immunology, infectious diseases and vaccines; mucosal and innate immunity; and adaptive immunity and lymphocyte biology (2011)[236].

From a medical education perspective, all medical schools in the United States, Canada, and Europe require medical school training and a demonstrated competency in understanding of the fundamentals of medical immunology of all future physicians.

In summary, the early-2000s are witnessing much interest in immunology. New and rapid advances in molecular technologies are now allowing levels of investigation previously barely imaginable. Many of the brightest medical and graduate students have accepted the challenge of contributing to the existing knowledge base of medical immunology. They are now actively acquiring the skill sets necessary and collectively offer an exciting future for medical immunology. The complete history of immunology of the 2000s is yet to be known or written; however it is most certainly going to be an exciting time for medical immunology.

References.

[1] Merriam-Webster's Medical Dictionary. (2018). Immunology. Retrieved 7-10-2018 from https://www.merriam-webster.com/dictionary/immunology

[2] MedicineNet. (2018). Definition of Immunology. MedicineNet.com. Retrieved 7-10-2018 from https://www.medicinenet.com/script/main/art.asp?articlekey=3941

[3] Helbert, M. (2017). Immunology for medical students. 3rd edition. New York: Elsevier.

[4] Scurlock, J. and Anderson, B. (2005). Diagnoses in Assyrian and Babylonian medicine: Ancient sources, translation, and modern medical analyses. Chicago: University of Illinois Press.

[5] Heessel, N. (2000). Babylonisch-assyrische Diagnostik, Alter Orient und Altes Testament, Band 43. [Babylonian-Assyrian diagnosis, Ancient Orient and Old Testament, Volume 43]. Munster:Ugarit-Verlag.

[6] Hunger, H. (1976). Spaet babylonische text aus uruk. Vol 1. Berlin: Mann.

[7] Kocher, F. (1964). Die babylonisch-assyrische medizin in testen und untersuchungen . Vols 1-6. Berlin: Walter de Gruyter.

[8] Labat. R. (1951). Traite akkadien de diagnostics et prognostics medicaux. Collection des travaux de l'Academie internationale d'histoire des sciences. Vol 7. Academie Internationale d'histoire des sciences. Wiesbaden: Franz Steiner Verlag.

[9] Thompson, R. (1923). Assyrian medical texts from the originals in the British Museum. London: H. Milford, Oxford University Press.

[10] The Official King James Bible Online. Retrieved 3-11-2011 from http://www.kingjamesbibleonline.org/1611-Bible/

[11] Torah. (circa 1300 BC). An online searchable version. Retrieved 3-11-2011 from http://www.templesanjose.org/JudaismInfo/Torah/Torah.htm.

[12] Ali, A. (circa 310-332 AD/1998). The Qur'an: Text, translation, and commentary. The meaning of the Holy Qur'an. English translation, complete online text. Retrieved 7-10-2018 from http://www.wright-house.com/religions/islam/Quran.html

[13] Hippocratic Collection. (circa 300 BC).[Digitized copies of the first printed editions (1525-1595) housed at the Biblioteque Interuniversitiarire de medicine of Paris]. Retrieved November 2009 from http://www.bium.univ-paris5.fr/histmed/medica/hipp_va.html

[14] Thucydides. (circa 431 BC/ 1934). Thucydides: The Peloponnesian War. Richard Crawley translation. New York: Modern Library.

[15] Thucydides. (circa 431 BC/2004). The History of the Peloponnesian War. The Second Book, Chapter VI. Translated by Richard Crawley. Whitefish, Montana: Kessinger Publishing. Retrieved 2-2-2011 from http://classics.mit.edu/Thucydides/pelopwar.2. second.html

[16] Dio, C. (circa 200 AD). Roman History: The Text of Cassius Dio on Lacus Curtius. Volumes 1-80. Loeb Classical Library. Harvard University Press, 1914-1927. Translation by Earnest Cary. Retrieved January 2011 from http://pcnelope.uchicago.edu/Thayer/E/Roman/Texts/Cassius_Dio/home.html

[17] Celsus, A. (circa 30 AD). De Medicina [On Medicine]. First printed 1478. Florence Nicolaus Laurentii. Rare Book Collection, Countway Medical Library, Boston.

[18] Celsus, A. (circa 30 AD). De Medicina [On Medicine]. Online English translation by W. Spencer (1935) Loeb Classical Library Edition. Retrieved November 2009 from http://penelope.uchicago.edu/Thayer/E/Roman/Texts/celsus/home.html

[19] Rather, L. (1971). Disturbance of function (functio laesa): The legendary fifth cardinal sign of inflammation, added by Galen to the four cardinal signs of Celsus. Bull. N. Y. Acad. Med., 47(3).

[20] Uhle, P. and Wagner, E. (1864). Handbuch der allgemeinen Pathologie. Lepzig: Otto Wigand.

[21] Procopius. (1914). Procopius; with English translation by H. B. Dewing in six volumes. History of the Wars, Books I and II. London: Macmillan and Company. Retrieved 2-2-2011 from http://www.archive.org/details/procopiuswitheng01procuoft

[22] Razi, A. (1094 AD). Al-Kitab al-hawi fi al-tibb [The Comprehensive Book on Medicine]. New York University, Institute for the Study of the Ancient World. MS A 17 OV1. Retrieved from http://isaw.nyu.edu/exhibitions/romance-reason/rrobjects/comprehensive-medicine-purgatives

[23] Razi, A. (1094/1848). Kitab fi-al Jadari wa-al-Hasbah. Treatise on the Small-Pox and Measles, English translation by W.A. Greenhill. London: Sydenham Society.

[24] Rhazes, A. (1094/1297/1985). Liber Continens [An encyclopedia of Medicine] Part XVII on Smallpox, Measles and Plagues. Edited and collated with Escuriall MSS. Number 817 & 856 and the MS of Hakeem Ashufta preserved in the Da'iratus'l-Ma'arif-il-Osmania. Hyderabad, India: Osmania Oriental Publications Bureau, Osmania University.

[25] Razi, M. (1094/1955-1971). Al Hawi fi al Teb (Continent, Continenes). Edited by Muhammad Abd al Moid Khan, 22 volumes. Dekan, India: Encyclopedia Press of Ossmania.

[26] Razi, M. (1094). The Sense of Smell: An article on the reason why Abu Zayd Balkhi suffers from rhinitis when smelling roses in spring. MS no. 4573, Malek National Library, Tehran; also MS no. 461, Bodleian Library, Oxford.

[27] Razi, M. (1094/2000). The Sense of Smell: An article on the reason why Abu Zayd Balkhi suffers from rhinitis when smelling roses in spring. English translation in Tadjbakhsh, H. (2000). The life of Muhammad Ibn Zakariya Razi and the discovery of allergic asthma. Iranian Journal of Allergy, Asthma and Immunology, 1(1):3-9.

[28] Birouni, A. (1048/1987). Fi Fehrest al Kotob al Razi [Bibliography of Razi's Books]. Edited by Mehdi Mohaghegh. Tehran University Press.

[29] Macculloch, J. (1828). An essay on the remittent and. intermittent diseases, including, generically marsh fever and neuralgia. Comprising, under the former various anomalies, obscurities, and consequences, and under a new systematic view of the latter, treating tic douloureux, sciatica, headache, ophthalmia, toothache, palsy, and many other modes and consequences of this generic disease, in two volumes. Vol 1, 394-397. London: Longman, Rees, Orme, Brown, and Green.

[30] Bostock, J. (1819). Case of a periodical affection of the eyes and chest. Medico-Chirurgical Transactions, 10:161.

[31] Bostick, J. (1828). On the catarrhus aestivus or summer catarrh. Medico-Chirurgical Transactions, 14:437-46.

[32] Maimonides, M. and Bos, G. (2001). On asthma: A parallel Arabic-English text edited, translated, and annotated by Gerrit Bos. Volume 1 of the complete medical works of Moses Maimonides. Provo, Utah: Brigham Young University Press.

[33] Hecker, J. (1832). Der schwarze Tod im vierzehnten Jahrhundert: Nach den Quellen für Ärzte und gebildete Nichtärzte bearbeitet. [The Black Death in the 14th century: from the sources by physicians and non-physicians]. Berlin: Herbig.

[34] Christakos, G., Olea, R., Serre, M., Yu, H., Wang, L, (2005). Interdisciplinary public health reasoning and epidemic modeling: the case of Black Death. Berlin: Springer.

[35] Descartes, R. (1637). Discourse on the Method. Translated by John Veitch (2008). New York: Cosimo.

[36] Severion, M. (1645). Zootomia Democritus: Id est Anatome generalis totius animatum opificii quinque linbris distincta. [Zootomy: General anatomy of animals divided into five separate books]. Nuremberg: Endterius.

[37] Peyeri, J. (1677). Exercitatio anatomico-medica de glandulis intestinorum earumque usu et affectionibus. Cui subjungitur anatome ventriculi Gallinacei; in Parerga anatomica et medica septem. Ratione ac experientia parentibus concepta et edita (1682). Amsterdam: Hemricus Westentius.

[38] Stensen, N. (1662). Observtiones anatomicae, quinus caria oris, oculorum & narium vas describuntur novique salivae, lacrymarum & muci fonts detefuntur. Lugduni Batacorum: J. Chouet.

[39] National Institute of Health. (2011). Typhoid fever. Pub Med Health: Retrieved 3-10-2011 from http://www.ncbi.nlm.nih.gov/pubmedhealth/PMH0002308/

[40] Rudbeck, O. (1653). Nova Exercitatio Anatomica, exhibens ductus hepaticos aquosos et vasa glanularum serosa, nunc primum in venta, aeneisque figures delineate. Vesteras: E. Lauringer.

[41] Bartholin, T. (1652). De lacteis thoracis in homine brutisque nuperrime observatis: historia anatomica. Hafniae (Copenhagen): M. Martzan.

[42] Bartholin, T. (1654). Vasa lymphatica in homine nuper inventa. Haffniae (Copenhagen): M. Martzan.

[43] Hemsterhuis, S. (1654). Messis aurea triennalis, exhibens; anatomica: novissima et utilissima experimenta. Edited by Siboldus Hemsterhuis. Leyden: Adriaan Wyngaerden.

[44] Bogdan, M. (1654). Apologia pro vasis lymphaticis. Thomas Bartholini. Hafniae: Georgii Lamprechti.

[45] Rudbeck, O. (1654). Insidiae structae Olai Rubeckii Sueci ductibus hepaticis aquosis, et vasis glandularum serosis contra Bogdani libellum scriptum. Lugdunum Batavorum (Leyden).

[46] Rudbeck, O. (1657). Ad Thomam Bartholinum danum epistola, qua sibi primam inventionem vasorum serosorum hepatis asserit. Ubsalice.

[47] Ruysch, F. (1665). Dilucidatio valvularum in vasis lymphaticis etlacteis. Hagae: Harmani Gael.

[48] Klebs, A. (1913). The historic evolution of variolation. Bulletin of the Johns Hopkins Hospital, 24:69-83.

[49] Center for Disease Control and Prevention (2018). Smallpox. (2018). Atlanta Georgia. Retrieved 7-22-2018 from https://www.cdc.gov/smallpox/index.html

[50] Moore J. (1815). The History of the Smallpox. London, Longman, Hurst, Rees, Orme & Brown.

[51] Voognad, H. (1671). Globus vitulinus. Miscellanea Curiosa, sive Ephemiridum Naturae Curiosorum 2, Dec. 1, Jena.

[52] Timoni(us) E. (1714). An account, or history, of the procuring of the smallpox by incision or inoculation, as it has for some time been practised at Constantinople. Philosophical Transactions of the Royal Society, 1714-1716; 29:72-82.

[53] Pylarino G. (1714). Nova et tuta variolas excitandi per transplantationem methodus, nuper inventa et in usum tracta. Philosophical Transactions of the Royal Society, 1714-1716; 29:393-9.

[54] Pylarino, G. (1715). Nova Et Tuta Variolas Excitandi per Transplantationem Methodus: Nuper inventa & in usum tracta: Qua ritè peracta, immunia in posterum praeservantur ab hujusmodi contagio corpora. Venetiis: Jo. Gabrielem Hertz.

[55] Montague, M. (1717). Letter from M. Montague to Sarah Chiswell dated April 1, 1717 discussing the process and benefits of variolation. Retrieved 3-9-2011 from UCLA Louise M. Darling Biomedical Library. Retrieved from http://unitproj.library.ucla.edu/biomed/his/smallpox/inoculation.html

[56] Montague, M. (1718). Letters of the right Honorable Lady Mary Wortley Montague: Written during her travels in Europe, Asia and Africa to persons of distinction, men of letters and in different parts of Europe, which contain, among other curious relations, accounts of the policy and manners of the Turks; drawn from the sources that have been inaccessible to other travelers. Letter 31 to Sarah Chiswell, dated April 1, 1718. Vol 2, 41-47. London: Printed for T. Becket and P. A. De Hondt, in the Strand.

[57] Maitland, C. (1722). Mr. Maitland's account of inoculating the smallpox. London: J Downing.

[58] Jurin, J. (1722). A letter to the learned Dr. Caleb Cotesworth containing a comparison between the danger of the natural smallpox, and of that given by inoculation. Philosophical Transactions of the Royal Society, 32:213-7.

[59] Mather, C., Dummer, J., Tumain, W. (1722). An Account of the Method and Success of Inoculating the Small-Pox in Boston in New England. London: J Peele.

[60] Boylston, Z. (1726). Historical account of the smallpox inoculated in New-England, upon all sorts of persons, whites, blacks, and of all ages and constitutions: with some account of the nature of the infection in the natural and inoculated way, and their different effects on human bodies: with some short directions to the unexperienced in this method of practice. Humbly dedicated to her Royal Highness The Princess of Wales, 2nd ed. London: Printed for S. Chandler, at the Cross-Keys in the Poultry.

[61] Douglass, W., Stuart, A., and Franklin, J. (1722). The abuses and scandals of some late pamphlets in favour of inoculation of the smallpox, modestly obviated, and inoculation further considered in a letter to A-S-M.D. & F.R.S. in London. Boston: Printed and sold by J. Franklin, at his printing house in Queen-Street, over against Mr. Sheaf's school.

[62] Douglas, W. (1722). The abuses and scandals of some late pamphlets in favour of inoculation of the smallpox, modestly obviated, and inoculation further considered in a letter to A.S. M.D. and F.R.S. in London. Boston.

[63] Mather, C. (1721). Some account of what is said of inoculating or transplanting the smallpox. By the learned Dr. Emannuel Timonius and Jacobus Pylarinus with some remarks thereon, to which are added a few queries in answer to the scruples of many about the lawfulness of this method. Boston: Zabdiel Boylston. Sold by S. Gerrish at his shop in Corn-Hill.

[64] Kirkpatrick, J. (1754). The analysis of inoculation: Compromising the history, theory, and practice of it: with an occasional consideration of the most remarkable appearances in the Smallpoxs. 2nd edition (1761), London: Printed for J. Buckland in Pater-Noster-Row and R. Griffiths opposite Somerset-House in the Strand.

[65] Sutton, R. (1762). Ipswich Journal, 25 September.

[66] Franklin, B. (1759). Some account of the success of inoculation for the smallpox. London: W. Strahan.

[67] Zwanenberg, D. (1978). The Suttons and the business of inoculation. Medical History, 22:71-82.

[68] Mead, R. (1748). A discourse on the smallpox and measles, by Richard Mead to which is annexed a treaties of the same diseases by the celebrated Arabian physician Abu-Beker Rhazes; the whole translated into English under the authors inspection by Thomas Stack. London. John Brindley, New Bond Street.

[69] La Condamine, C. (1754). A discourse on inoculation, Paper presented to the Royal Academy of Sciences in Paris, April 24, 1754. Translated into English by M. Maty. Printed for Vaillant 1755.

[70] Tozzetti, G. (1757). Relazion d'innesti de vaiuolo fatti in Firenze nell'autunno 1756. [Relations of grafts from variolation made in Florence in autumn 1756]. Andrea Bonducci.

[71] Gatti, A. (1764). Ré'flexions sur les pré'juge's qui s'opposent aux progre`s et a` la perfection de l'inoculation, [Thoughts on the prejudices that oppose progress and to the perfection of inoculation,] Bruxelles: Musier.

[72] Beebe, L. (1776). Journal of Lewis Beebe: A Physician on the campaign against Canada, 1776. Edited by Frederick Kirkland (1935). Philadelphia: Historical Society of Pennsylvania.

[73] Boerhaave, H. (1738). Praxis Medica: sive commentarium in aphorismos. Vol. V, London: Sumtibus Societatis.

[74] Jenner, E. (1798a). An inquiry into the cause and effects of the variolae vaccinae, a disease, discovered in the western counties of England, particularly Gloucestershire and known by the name of cow pox London: Sampson Low, Berwick Street, Soho.

[75] Pasteur, L., Chamberland C., Roux E. (1881). De l'attenuation des virus et de leur retore a la virulence. C. R. Seances Acad. Sci., 92:430–435.

[76] Fewster J. (1765). Cowpox and its ability to prevent smallpox. Unpublished paper read to the Medical Society of London, 1765.

[77] Jenner, E. (1798b). An inquiry into the causes and effects of the variolae vaccine, or cowpox, 1798. The Three Original Publications on Vaccination Against Smallpox, The Harvard Classics. http://bartleby.com/38/4/1.html

[78] Van Zwanenberg, D. (1798). The Suttons and the Business of inoculation. Medical History, 22:71-82.

[79] Jenner, E. (1799). II. Further Observations on the Variolae Vaccine, or Cow-Pox.1799. Harvard Classics. The three original publications on vaccination against smallpox. http://barthleny.com/38/4/2.html

[80] Jenner, E. (1800). III. A Continuation of facts and observations relative to the variolæ vaccine, or cowpox. Harvard Classics. The three original publications on vaccination against smallpox. Retrieved from http://barthleny.com/38/4/3.html

[81] Jenner, E. (1801). The origin of the vaccine inoculation. London: Printed by D. N. Shury, Berwick Street, Soho.

[82] Woodville, W. (1799). Reports of a series of inoculations for the variolae vaccine or cow-pox. London.

[83] Pearson, G. (1802). Report on the cow-pock inoculation during the years 1800, 1801, and 1802. London.

[84] McVail. J. (1896). Cow-pox and small-pox: Jenner, Woodville, and Pearson. The British Medical Journal, May 12, 1271-1276.

[85] Schwann, T. (1839). Mikroskopische Untersuchungen uber die Ubereinstimmung in der Struktur un dem Wachstum der Thiere and Pflanzen. [Microscopic studies of the agreement in the structure of the growth of animals and plants]. Berlin: Verlag der Sanderischen Buchhandlung, G. E. Reimer.

[86] Schawann, T. and Schleyden, M. (1839). Microscopic investigations on the accordance in the structure and growth of plants and animals. Berlin. English translation by the Sydenham Society, 1847, London.

[87] Schwann, T. (1847). Microscopical researches on the similarities and the growth of animals and plants. Translated from the German (1839) by Henry Smith. London: Printed for the Sydenham Society; C. and J. Aslard printers.

[88] Henle, J. (1838). On Miasmata and Contagie. English translation by George Rosen. Baltimore: Johns Hopkins Press.

[89] Henle, J. (1840). Pathologische Untersuchungen. [Pathological studies]. Berlin: Verlag von August Hirschwald.

[90] Heine, J. (1840). Beobachtungen uber Lahmungszustande der untern Extremitaten und deren Behandlung. [Report Concerning a Laming-illness of the Lower Extremities and Its Management]. Monograph of 29 cases. Stuttgart: F.H. Kohler.

[91] Virchow, R. (1858). Die Cellularpatholgie in ihrer Begrundung auf physiologische und pathologische Gewebelehre. Berlin: A. Hirschwald.

[92] Andral, G. (1843). Essai d'Hematologie Pathologique. Paris: Fortin, Masson & Co.

[93] Addison, W. (1843). Experimental and practical researches on inflammation and on the origin and nature of tubercles of the lung. London: J. Churchill.

[94] Addison, T. (1849). Anaemia-disease of the suprarenal capsules. Medical Gazette. 43:517-518.

[95] Addison, T. (1855). On the constitutional and local effects of disease of the supra-renal capsules. London: Samuel Highley.

[96] Haeckel, E. (1862). Die Radiolaren. 1:135-140. Leipzig: Karl Riemer.

[97] Schultze, M. (1863). Das Protoplasma der Rhizopoden und der Pflanzenzellen. Leipzig: Verlag Wilhelm Englelman.

[98] Recklinghausen, F. (1863). Uber Eiter und Bindegewebskorperchen. (Virchows) Archiv fur Pathologische Anatomie und Physiologie, und fur. Klinische. Medicin., 28:157-197.

[99] Reckinhausen, F. (1882). Uber die multiplen Fibrome der Haut der ihre Beziehung zu den multiplen Neuromen. Festschrift fur Rudolf Virchow. Berlin.

[100] Langerhans, P. (1869). Beitrage zur mikroscopischen anatomie der bauchspeichel druse. [Contributions to the microscopic anatomy of the pancreas]. Dissertation. Berlin: Gustav Lange.

[101] Laguesse, E. (1893). Sur la formation des ilots de Langerhans dans le pancreas. Comptes. Rend. Soc. Biol., 5 (Series 9):819-20.

[102] Mering, J. and Minkowski, O. (1889). Diabetes mellitus nach Pankreasextirpation. Centralblatt für klinische Medicin, Leipzig, 10(23):393-394.

[103] Mering, J. and Minkowski, O. (1890). Archiv für experimentelle Patholgie und Pharmakologie, Leipzig, 26:37.

[104] Langerhans, P. (1868). Ueber die nerven der menschlichen. [On the nerves of the human skin] Haut. Virchows Arch.[B] 44:325-37.

[105] Cohnheim, J. (1867). Ueber Entzundung und Eiterung. Archiv fur Pathologische Anatomie und Physiologie und fur Klinische. Medizin., 40:1-79.

[106] Cohnheim, J. (1873). Neue Untersuchungen uber die Entzundung. Berlin: A. Hirschwald.

[107] Ehrlich, P. (1878). Beiträge zur Theorie und Praxis der histologischen Farbung. Test (Hrsg.), I. Teil: Die chemische Auffassung der Farbung. II. Teil: Die Anilinfarben in chemischer, technologischer und histologischer Beziehung. 65 S. [Ehrlich, P: contributions to the theory and practice of histological staining. Test (eds), Part I: The chemical view of the staining. Part II: The aniline dyes in a chemical, technological and histological relationship.] Dissertation. Leipzig.

[108] Ehrlich, P. (1879). Ueber die specifischen Granulationen des Blutes. [About the specific granulations of blood.] Archiv fuer Anatomie und Physiologie: Physiologische Abteilung, 571-579.

[109] Ehrlich, P. (1882). Über die Färbung der Tuberkelbazillen. [The staining of tubercle bacilli.] Deutsche Medizinische Wochenschrift, 269-270.

[110] Ehrlich, P. (1883). Über eine neue Methode der Färbung von Tuberkelbacillen. [On a new method of staining tubercle bacilli]. Berliner Klinische Wochenschrift, 20:13.

[111] Ehrlich, P. (1898). Ueber den Zusammenhang von chemischer Constitution und Wirkung. [On the relation of chemical constitution and effect]. Münchener medizinische Wochenschrift, 1654-1655.

[112] Ehrlich, P. (1900). Cellularbiologische Betrachtungen über Immunität. [Cellular biological observations on immunity.]. Bericht der Senckenbergischen Naturforschenden Gesellschaft in Frankfurt am Main, 147-150.

[113] Ehrlich, P. (1910). Diskussionsbemerkungen zum Vortrag von Wechselmann (Chemotherapie der Syphilis). [Discussion comments on the presentation by von Wechselmann- chemotherapy of syphilis]. Bericht ueber die Tagung der Freien Vereinigung fuer Mikrobiologie, 47:223-224.

[114] Ehrlich, P. (1913). Uber Chemotherapie: Die Behandlung der Syphilis mit Salvarsan und verwandten Stoffen. [About chemotherapy: The treatment of syphilis with salvarsan and related materials]. Münchener medizinische Wochenschrift.

[115] Ehrlich, P. (1885). Das Sauerstoff-Bedürfniss des Organismus: eine farbenanalytische Studie. [The oxygen needs of the organism: a color-analytic study]. Berlin: Hirsch Forest.

[116] Ehrlich, P. (1897). Zur Kenntnis der Antitoxinwirkung. [On the knowledge of the anti-toxin effect]. Fortschritte der Medizin, 15:41-43.

[117] Ehrlich, P. (1900). On immunity with special reference to cell life. Proceedings of the Royal Society of London, Series B: Biological Sciences, 66:424-448.

[118] Ehrlich, P. and Morgenroth, J. (1902). Die Seitenkettentheorie der Immunität. [The side-chain theory of immunity]. Anleitung zu hygienischen Untersuchungen: nach den im Hygienischen Institut der königl. Ludwig-Maximilians-Universität zu München üblichen Methoden zusammengestellt 3. Aufl: 381-394. [Guidance to health investigations: in accordance with the Royal Hygiene Institute. Ludwig-Maximillians University in Munich, conventional methods compiled 3rd Edition: 381-394].

[119] Nobel Prize in Physiology or Medicine 1908. Nobelprize.org. Retrieved 7-22-2018 from https://www.nobelprize.org/nobel_prizes/medicine/laureates/1908/.

[120] Ehrlich, P. (1891). Experimentelle Untersuchungen über Immunität. [Experiemntal studies on immunity]. I. Ueber Ricin. II. Ueber Abrin. Deutsche medicinische Wochenschrift, Berlin, 17:976-979, 1218-1219

[121] Metchnikoff, E. (1883). Untersuchungen uber die intracellulare Verdauung bei wirbellosen Tieren, Arb. zool. Inst. Univ. Wien, 5:141-168.

[122] Metchnikoff, E. (1905). Immunity in infective diseases. English translation by F. G. Binnie. Cambridge: Cambridge University Press.

[123] Metchnikoff, E. (1903). The Nature of Man: Studies in Optimistic Philosophy. London: G. Putnam and Sons.

[124] Metchnikoff, E. (1907). Essais optimists. Paris. [Optimistic Studies]. Translated and edited by P. Chalmers Mitchell. London: Hainemann.

[125] Mechnikoff, E. and Mitchell, P. (1908). The prolongation of life: Optimistic studies. New York: Putman.

[126] Mechnikoff, E. and Mitchell, P. (1908/2004). The prolongation of life: Optimistic studies. Classics in Longevity and Aging. New York: Springer Publishing Company.

[127] The Nobel Prize in Physiology or Medicine 1908. Nobelprize.org. Retrieved 7-22-2018 from https://www.nobelprize.org/nobel_prizes/medicine/laureates/1908/

[128] Koch, R. (1876). Die Aetiologie der Milzbrand-Krankheit, begründet auf die Entwicklungsgeschichte des Bacillus anthracis. [The etiology of anthrax disease, based on the history of Bacillus anthracis.]. Beiträge zur Biologie der Pflanzen, 2:277-310.

[129] Koch, R. (1882). Die Aetiologie der Tuberculose. [The etiology of tuberculosis].Berliner Klinische Wochenschrift, 19:221-230.

[130] Koch, R. (1884). Sechster Bericht der deutschen Wissenschaftlichen Commission zur Enforschung der Cholera, Geh Regierungsraths Dr Koch. Dtsch. Med. Wochenschr., 10:191-2.

[131] Pacini F. (1854). Osservazioni microscopiche e deduzioni patologiche sul cholera asiatico. Firenze: Bencini.

[132] Koch, R. (1877).Verfahren zur Untersuchung, zum Conservieren und Photographieren der Bakterien. [Methods for studying, preserving, and photographing bacteria.]Beiträge zur Biologie der Pflanzen, 2:399-434.

[133] Koch, R. (1890). Ueber bakteriologische Forschung. Verhandlungen des X. internationalen medizinische Kongresses. [An Address on Bacteriological Research]. Berlin,1:35-47; British Medical Journal, 2:380-383.

[134] The Nobel Prize in Physiology or Medicine 1905. Nobelprize.org 26 April 2011.

[135] Petri, R. (1887). Eine kleine modification des Koch'schen plattenverfahrems. [A small modification of Koc's plating method] Centralblatt fur Bacteriologie und Parasitenkunde, 1:279.

[136] Behring, E., and Kitasato, S. (1890). The Mechanism of Immunity in Animals to Diphtheria and Tetanus. Deutsch. Med.Wochenschr., 16:1113.

[137] Behring, E. and Wernicke, E. (1892). Z. Hyg. 12:10-45.

[138] The Nobel Prize in Physiology or Medicine 1901. Nobelprize.org. Apr 26, 2011.

[139] Pfeiffer, R. (1894). Ueber die specifische Bedeutung der Choleraimmunität (Bakteriolyse). Zeitschrift für Hygiene und Infektionskrankheiten, 17:355-400; 1895;18:1-16.

[140] Bordet, J. (1898). Sur l'agglutination et la dissolution des globules rouges par le serum d'animaux injectes de sang defibrine. Ann. De l'Inst. Pasteur., 12:688-695.

[141] The Nobel Prize in Physiology or Medicine 1919. Nobel Prize.org. May 10, 2011.

[142] Bordet J. and Gengou U. (1906). Le microbe de la coqueluche. Ann Inst Pasteur., 20:731.

[143] Landsteiner, K. (1900). Zur Kenntnis der antifermentativen, lytischen und agglutinierenden Wirkungen des Blutserums und der Lymphe. Zentralblatt Bakteriologie, 27:357–62.

[144] The Nobel Prize in Physiology or Medicine 1930. Nobel Foundation. Retrieved 5-30-2011.

[145] von Decastello, A. and Sturli, A. (1902). Ueber die Isoagglutinine im Serum gesunder und kranker Menschen. Mfinch. Med. Wschr.,, 49:1090–5.

[146] Landsteiner, K. and Wiener, A. (1941). Studies on an agglutinogen (Rh) in human blood reacting with anti-rhesus sera and with human isoantibodies. Journal Experimental Medicine, 74(4):309–320.

[147] Levine, P. and Stetson R. (1939). An unusual case of intragroup agglutination. JAMA, 113:126–7.

[148] Landsteiner, K. and Wiener, A. (1940). An agglutinable factor in human blood recognized by immune sera for rhesus blood. Proc. Soc. Exp. Biol. Med., 43:223–4.

[149] Landsteiner, K. und Popper, E. (1909). Übertragung der Poliomyelitis acuta auf Affen in Zeitschrift für Immunitätsforschung und experimentelle Therapie, 2:377-390.

[150] Beierinck, M. (1898). Concerning a contagium vivum fluidum as a cause of the spot-disease of tobacco leaves. Verh. Akad. Wet. Amsterdam II, 6:3-21.

[151] Ivanovsky, D. (1882). Concerning the mosaic disease of the tobacco plant. Saint Petersburg Acad. Imperial Sci. Bul., 35:67-70.

[152] Kuhn, T. (1970). The Structure of Scientific Revolution. 2nd edition. Chicago: Chicago University Press.

[153] Ellerman, C., and O. Bang. (1908). Experimentelle Leukämie bei Hühnern. Zentralblatt fur Bakteriologie. 46:595–609.

[154] Rous, P. (1910). Transmissible avian neoplasm [Sarcoma of the common fowl]. Exp. Med., 12:696–705.

[155] Rous, P. (1911). Transmission of a malignant new growth by means of a cell-free filtrate Exp. Med., 13:397–411.

[156] The Nobel Prize in Physiology or Medicine 1966". Nobelprize.org. 22 Jun 2011.

[157] Portier, P. and Richet, C. (1902). De l'action anaphylactique de certains venins. C. R. Seances Soc. Biol., 54:170.

[158] The Nobel Foundation. Nobel Lectures, Physiology or Medicine 1901-1921. The Nobel Prize for Physiology or Medicine, 1913.

[159] Arthus, M. (1903). Injections répétées de serum du cheval zhez le lapin. Comptes Rendus des Séances de la Societe de Biologie., 55:817.

[160] Arthus, M. (1921). De l'anaphylaxie à l'immunité; anaphylaxie, protéotoxies, evenimations, anaphylaxie-immunité, sérums antivenimeux. [Of anaphylaxis to immunity, anaphylaxis, proteotoxic, evenimations, anaphylaxis-immunity, antivenoms.]. Paris: Masson.

[161] Wright, A. and Douglas, S. (1903). An experimental investigation of the role of the body fluids in connection with phagocytosis. Proc. R. Soc. London, 72:357-370.

[162] Pirquet, C. (1906). Allergie. Münch. Med. Wochenschr., 53:1457-1458.

[163] Pirquet, C. (1908). The frequency of tuberculosis in childhood. Transaction of the Sixth International Congress on Tuberculosis, Washington, D.C., Sept 28 to Oct. 12, 1908.

[164] Mantoux, C. (1908). Intradermo-reaction de la tuberculine. Comptes rendus de l'Académie des sciences. Paris. 147:355-357.

[165] Schick, B. (1913). Die Diphtherictoxin-Hautreaktion del Menschen als Vorprobe der prophylaktischen Diphtherie-heilseruminjection. Münchener medizinische Wochenschrift 60:2608–2610.

[166] American Association of Immunologist. (2013). American Association of Immunologist, About Us, History, History of Immunology and Science. Retrieved 7-18-2018 from http://www.aai.org/timeline/

[167] The Journal of Immunology. (February 1916). The Journal of Immunology, 1(1):1-128. Retrieved 7-18-2018 from http://www.jimmunol.org/content/1/1

[168] Pauling, L. (1940). A theory of the structure and process of formation of antibodies. J. Am. Chem. Soc., 62:2643-57.

[169] Pauling, L., Campbell, D., Pressman, D. (1943). The nature of the forces between antigen and antibody and the precipitation reaction. Physiological Reviews, 22(3).

[170] Pauling, L. (1945). Molecular Structure and Intermolecular Forces. Part VIII in The Specificity of Serological Reactions. Edited by Karl Landsteiner. Cambridge, MA: Harvard University Press.

[171] Fischer, E. (1894). Berichte der deutschen chemischen Gesellschaft., 27:2985-2993.

[172] The Nobel Foundation. Nobel Prize in Chemistry 1954. Nobelprize.org. 2 Jun 2011.

[173] The Nobel Peace Prize 1962. Nobelprize.org. Nobel Media AB 2014. Retrieved 7-18-2018 from http://www.nobelprize.org/nobel_prizes/peace/laureates/1962/

[174] The Nobel Foundation. Nobel Peace Prize 1962. Nobelprize.org. 2 Jun 2011.

[175] Fagraeus, A. (1948). Antibody production in relation to the development of plasma cells: In vivo and vitro experiment. Stockholm: Ph.D. dissertation.

[176] Bing, J. and Plum, P. (1937). Serum proteins in leucopenia: Contribution on the question about the place of formation of the serum proteins. Acta. Medica. Scandinavia, Vol XCII fasc IV-V.

[177] Bing, J. and Christensen, N. (1943). The connection between plasma cells and the occurrence of hyperglobinemia in horses and cattle. Acta. Medica. Scandinavia, Vol CXVI, fasc III-IV 1944.

[178] Bing, J. (1946). Histological changes after intraperitoneal injection of proteins and proteinhydrolysates. Acta Pathologica, Microbiologicia et Immunologica Scandinavica., 23(6):540-548.

[179] Tiselius, A. and Kabat, E. (1938). Electrophoresis of immune serum. Science. May 6; 87:416-417.

[180] The Nobel Prize in Chemistry 1948. Nobelprize.org. 2 Jun 2011.

[181] Burnet, F. and Fenner, F. (1941). The Production of Antibodies. Melbourne: Macmillan.

[182] The Nobel Prize in Physiology or Medicine 1960. Nobelprize.org. 3 Jun 2011

[183] Isaacs, A. and Lindenmann, J. (1957). Virus interference. I. The interferon. Proc. R. Soc. Lond. Biol. Sci., 147(927):258–67.

[184] Dausset, J. (1958). Iso-leuco-anticorps. Acta. Haematol., 20:156-166.

[185] The Nobel Prize in Physiology or Medicine 1980". Nobelprize.org. 3 Jun 2011.

[186] Gowans, J. and Knight, J. (1964). The route of recirculation of lymphocytes in the rat. Proc. Royal Soc. (London); Series B, 159:257-259.

[187] Gallatin, W., Weissman, I., Butcher, E. (1983). Nature, 304:30.

[188] Lynch, R. (2006). Lymphocyte Traffic. American Society for Investigative Pathology Bulletin, 9:2.

[189] Porter, R. (1948). Doctoral dissertation. Cambridge, Department of Biochemistry.

[190] Porter, R. (1958). Separation and isolation of fractions of rabbit gamma-globulin containing the antibody and antigenic combing sites. Nature, Sept. 6, 182(4636):670-1.

[191] Edelman, G., Cunningham, B., Gall, W., Gottlieb, P., Rutishauser, U., Waxsal, M. (1969). The covalent structure of an entire G immunoglobulin molecule. Proceeding of the National Academy of Sciences of the United States of America. (63)1:78-85.

[192] The Nobel Prize in Physiology or Medicine 1972. Nobelprize.org. 3 Jun 2011.

[193] Kunkel, H., Mannik, M., and Williams, R. (1963). Individual antigenic specificity of isolated antibodies. Science, 140:1218-1219.

[194] Oudin, J. and Michel, M. (1963). Une nouvelle forme d'allotypie des gloulines gamma du serum de lapin, apparemment liee a la fonction eta la specificite anticorps. C.R. Hebd. Seances Acad. Sci., 257:805.

[195] Miller, J. (1961). Immunological function of the thymus. Lancet. Sep 30, 2:748-9.

[196] Miller, J. (1964). The thymus and the development of immunologic responsiveness. Science, Jun 26, 144:1544-51.

[197] Miller, J. and Mitchell, G. (1967). The thymus and the precursors of antigen reactive cells. Nature. Nov 18, 216(5116):659-663.

[198] Miller, J. and Sprent, J. (1971), Cell-to-cell interaction in the immune response. VI. Contribution of thymus-derived cells and antibody-forming cell precursors to immunological memory. J. Exp. Med. ,Jul 1; 134(1):66-82.

[199] Good, R, Dalmasso, A., Martinez, C., Archer, O., Pierce, J. and Papermaster, B. (1962). The role of the thymus in development of immunological capacity in rabbits and mice. The Journal of Cell Biology, 116(5):773-796.

[200] Good, R., Cooper, M., Peterson, R., Kellum, M., Sutherland, D., Gabrielsen, A. (1966). The role of the thymus in immune process. Annals of the New York Academy of Science, 135:451-478.

[201] Gatti, R, Meuwissen, H., Aleen, H, Hong, R., Good, R. (1968). Immunological reconstruction of sex-linked lymphopenic immunological deficiency. Lancet. Dec 28, 2(7583):1366-9.

[202] Gell, P. and Coombs, R. (1963). Clinical Aspects of Immunology. Oxford, England: Blackwell.

[203] Mitchison, N. (1971). Carrier effect in the secondary response to hatpin-protein conjugates II. Cellular cooperation, European Journal of Immunology, 1(1):18-27.

[204] Gershon, R. and Kondo, K. (1971). Antigenic competition between heterologous erythrocytes: I Thymic dependency. J. Immunol., 106:1524-1531.

[205] Kiessling, R., Klein, E., Wigzell, H. (1975a). Natural killer cells in the mouse. I. Cytotoxic cells with specificity for mouse Moloney leukemia cells. Specificity and distribution according to genotype. European Journal of Immunology, Feb 5 (2):113-7.

[206] Steinman, R. and Cohn, Z. (1973). Identification of a novel cell type in peripheral lymphoid organs of mice. I. Morphology, quantitation, tissue distribution. J. Exp. Med., 137(5):1142–62.

[207] Zinkernagel, R. and Doherty, P. (1974). Immunological surveillance against altered self components by sensitized T lymphocytes in lymphocytes choriomeningitis. Nature, 251(5475):547-548.

[208] The Nobel Prize in Physiology or Medicine 1996. Nobelprize.org. 6 Jun 2011.

[209] Gillis, S. and Smith K. (1977). Long term culture of tumor-specific cytotoxic T cells. [Letter] Nature. 268:154-156.

[210] Proceedings of the 2nd International Lymphokine Workshop. (1979), Lake Constance - Ermatingen, Switzerland. May 27-31.

[211] Smith, K., Gilbride, K., Favata, M. (1980). Lymphocyte Activating Factor Promotes T-cell Growth Factor Production by Cloned Murine Lymphoma Cells. Nature. Oct. 30; 287(5785):853-855.

[212] Smith, K., Lachman, L., Oppenheim, J., Favata, M. (1980). The functional relationship of the interleukins. J. Exp. Med., June 1, 151:1551-1556.

[213] Robb, R., Munck, A., Smith, K. (1981). T cell growth factor receptors. Quantitation, specificity, and biological relevance. J. Exp. Med., Nov 1, 154(5):1455-1474.

[214] Prusiner, S. (1982). Novel proteinaceous infectious particles cause scrapies. Science. April 9: 216 (4542):136-144.

[215] The Nobel Prize in Physiology or Medicine 1997. Nobelprize.org. 6 Jun 2011.

[216] Barré-Sinoussi, F., Chermann, J., Rey, F., Nugeyre, M., Chamaret, S., Gruest, J., Dauguet, C., Axler-Blin, C., Vezinet-Brun, F., Rouzioux, C., Rozenbaum, W., Montagnier, L. (1983). Isolation of a T- lymphotropic retrovirus from a patient at risk for acquired immune deficiency syndrome (AIDS). Science, 220(4599):868–71.

[217] The Nobel Prize in Physiology or Medicine 2008. Nobelprize.org. 28 Jun 2011.

[218] Reinherz, E., Meuer, S., Schlossman, S. (1983). The human T-cell receptor: Analysis with cytotoxic T-cell clones. Immunol. Rev., Sept. 74:83-112.

[219] Swain, S. (1983. T cell subsets and the recognition of MHC class. Immunol. Rev., 74: 129-142.

[220] First International Workshop and Conference on Human Leukocyte Differentiation Antigens (HLDA). (1982). Paris.

[221] The Nobel Prize in Physiology or Medicine 1984. Nobelprize.org. 6 Jun 2011.

[222] Engvall, E. and Perlman, P. (1971). Enzyme-linked immunosorbent assay (ELISA). Quantitative assay of immunoglobulin G. Immunochemistry, 8(9):871-4.

[223] The Nobel Prize in Physiology or Medicine 1987. Nobelprize.org. 6 Jun 2011.

[224] Medzhitov, R., Preston-Hurlburt, P., Janeway, C. (1997). A human homologue of the Drosophila Toll protein signals activation of adaptive immunity. Nature, 388 (6640): 394–7.

[225] The Nobel Prize in Physiology or Medicine 1999. Nobelprize.org. 6 Jun 2011.

[226] Nairn, R. and Helbert, M. (2002). Immunology for Medical Students. New York: Mosby.

[227] The Nobel Prize in Physiology or Medicine 2008. Nobelprize.org. Retrieved 7-21-2018 from https://www.nobelprize.org/nobel_prizes/medicine/laureates/2008/

[228] U.S. Food and Drug Administration. (2006). June 8, 2006 Approval Letter – Human Papillomavirus Quadrivalent (Types 6, 11, 16, 18) Vaccine, Recombinant. Retrieved 7-21-2018 from https://wayback.archive-it.org/7993/20170722145339/https://www.fda.gov/BiologicsBloodVaccines/Vaccines/ApprovedProducts/ucm111283.htm

[229] U.S. Food and Drug Administration. (2080. Gardasil Vaccine Safety. Information from FDA and CDC on the safety of Gardasil Vaccine. Retrieved 7-2-2018 from https://www.fda.gov/biologicsbloodvaccines/safetyavailability/vaccinesafety/ucm179549.htm

[230] The Nobel Prize in Physiology or Medicine 2008. Nobelprize.org. Retrieved 7-21-2018 from https://www.nobelprize.org/nobel_prizes/medicine/laureates/2008/

[231] The Nobel Prize in Physiology or Medicine 2011. Nobelprize.org. Retrieved 7-21-2018 from https://www.nobelprize.org/nobel_prizes/medicine/laureates/2011/

[232] Poltorak, A., He, X., Smirnova, I., Liu, M., Van Huffel, C,, Du, X., Birdwell, D., Alejos, E., Silva, M., Galanos, C., Freudenberg, M., Ricciardi-Castagnoli, P,, Layton, B., Beutler, B. (1998). Defective LPS signaling in C3H/HeJ and C57BL/10ScCr mice: Mutations in Tlr4 gene. Science, 282:2085-2088.

[233] Lemaitre, B., Nicolas, E., Michaut, L., Reichhart, J., Hoffmann, J. (1996). The dorsoventral regulatory gene cassette spätzle/Toll/cactus controls the potent antifungal response in drosophila adults. Cell, 86:973-983.

[234] Steinman, R. and Cohn, Z. (1973). Identification of a novel cell type in peripheral lymphoid organs of mice. I. Morphology, quantitation, tissue distribution. J. Exp. Med., 137:1142–1162.

[235] Steinman, R. and Witmer, M. (1978). Lymphoid dendritic cells are potent stimulators of the primary mixed leukocyte reaction in mice. Proc. Natl. Acad. Sci., 75:5132–5136.

[236] Immunology@NIH. (2011). Immunology. Our research. U.S. Department of Health and Human Services – National Institute of Health. Retrieved 7-27-2011.

Chapter 8

Medical Neurosciences

Definition.

Neuroscience is "…a branch of science that deals with the anatomy, physiology, biochemistry, or molecular biology of nerves and nervous tissues." (2016)[1]. Others define neuroscience as "…the study of the brain and nervous system, including molecular neuroscience, cellular neuroscience, cognitive neuroscience, psychophysics, computer modeling and diseases of the nervous system…" (2016)[2]. Clinical neuroscience "…is a branch of neuroscience that focuses on the fundamental mechanisms that underlie diseases and disorders of the brain and central nervous system… (2016)[3].

The medical neurosciences are a collection of neuroscience sub-specialties, committed to the study and understanding of the nervous systems, with particular emphasis placed upon the clinical application of the knowledge base to the diagnosis, treatment, and management of patients presenting with impaired neurological functions. Specific sub-specialties contributing to the broadly defined discipline of medical neurosciences are medical genetics, molecular biology, neurobiology, neuroanatomy, neurophysiology, neurochemistry, neuroradiology, neurosurgery, and neurology.

Introduction.

This chapter explores the historical development of the medical neurosciences from their earliest beginnings, as practiced by the ancient civilizations of Mesopotamia, Egypt, and Greece to its current state, as practiced by modern Western medicine. Emphasis is placed upon developing a fundamental understanding of the course of medical neurosciences across time. Attention is focused on providing you, the medical student, an opportunity to understand what, when, where, and how the past has guided and shaped our current understanding of the medical neurosciences. Medical dogma is explored across time, as are the reasons it is embraced, modified, rejected, and displaced. Influential people and their contributions are highlighted. People, terms, and concepts introduced to you, during your medical neuroscience course, are placed into a historical context and explored. Knowing how the medical neurosciences have developed through time will provide you with a greater understanding of the neurosciences of the past, present, and future.

Let's begin.

History.

Early Records, 3500 BC - 500 BC.

The earliest history of the medical neurosciences is just now beginning to be revealed. Ancient civilization of Mesopotamia, Egypt, and Greece have a rich history and interests in the medical neurosciences. Each civilization offers recorded evidence of their interests. Recent works by Professor JoAnn Scurlock (1953-), Professor Burton Andersen (1932-), and their students are contributing much to unlocking the history of the medical neurosciences of the ancient civilizations of Mesopotamia (2005)[4]. Based largely on their recent translation of sections of forty, cuneiform inscribed medical clay tablets, dated circa 3500 BC to 1600 BC, we know the ancient people of Mesopotamia (modern-day Iraq) are keenly aware of changes in body functions and patient behavior, whenever the nervous system is altered by disease or trauma.

Clinical presentations of patients impaired by neurological disease or trauma are systematically documented. Records reveal clinical presentations are organized accordingly: a brief listing of presenting signs and symptoms, clinical diagnosis, prognosis, recommended treatment(s), and clinical outcome. The collection of recorded clinical presentations is impressive, detailing many of the conditions seen today by practicing physicians, over 5,000 years later and since their initial documentation e.g. head traumas, seizure disorders, stroke syndromes, paralysis, sensory loss, pain syndromes, cranial nerve disorders, movement disorders, spinal cord injuries, and coma (circa 3,500 BC/2005)[4].

Ancient Mesopotamia conceptualizes disease and impaired neurological function, as intervention from supranatural gods and demons. Clinical signs and symptoms result from impairment of physical body functions, which have their source of origins in the supranatural. Treatments are characterized by medical, mechanical, and environmental interventions e.g. eat this plant, rub this on it, drink this herb tea, wash your hands, clean the house, eat more healthily. All improvements in an individual's condition following treatment, are interpreted to be treatment interventions pleasing to the god(s) or demon(s). Empirical records are maintained as to what and which treatments please the god(s) and demon(s) and which treatments further anger these supranatural entities and thereby exacerbate the clinical condition.

Ancient Egypt recognizes the importance of neurological disorders and too systematically record the clinical presentation of signs and symptoms, offers diagnoses, and recommend specific treatments based upon diagnosis. Prognostic statements are associated with each diagnoses. Like the Ancients of Mesopotamia, the ancient Egyptian knowledge base, clinical observations, diagnoses, and treatments are rationally formulated and empirically derived.

Two historically important papyri, the Edwin Smith Papyrus and the Georg Ebers Papyrus, provide much of the preserved, written historical record of the conceptual models and the medical and surgical practices of ancient Egypt, known to us today (1700BC/1930,1500BC/1987)[5,6].

The Edwin Smith Papyrus, written circa 1700 BC, in essence is a surgical papyrus and reports 48 cases. The first 27 cases describe head injuries. The balance of cases describe 6 cases of throat and neck injuries (cases #28-33), 2 cases describing clavicle injuries (cases #34-35), 3 cases describing arm injuries (cases #36-38), 8 cases describing sternum injuries (cases #39-46), 1 case describing a shoulder injury (case #47), and 1 case describing a spine injury (case #48). Each case is presented in a rational, systematic manner. First a title with a brief description of the injury is presented; followed by instruction as to how the injury should be examined e.g. sensory testing, probing of the wound, moving various body parts; followed by a diagnosis; followed by three choices for possible intervention "…An ailment which I will treat… An ailment which I will contend… An ailment not to be treated…"; followed by the treatment e.g. cauterization of the wound, smearing grease or honey into the wound; and then followed by additional explanatory notes as necessary (1700BC/1930,2016)[5,7]. The Edwin Smith Papyrus cases are among the first to systematically describe the clinical presentation, examination, diagnosis, prognosis, and treatment interventions of many familiar conditions affecting the nervous systems seen today, over 5,000 years since they were described by the ancient Egyptians e.g. paralysis, aphasia, meningitis, epilepsy, cerebral edema, and spinal edema (1700BC/1930,2016)[5,7].

The Ebers Papyrus, written circa 1500 BC, is essentially the pharmacopeia of ancient Egypt. The Papyrus contains approximately 850 recommended medicinal and topical remedies, directed to the treatment of a wide range of conditions. Specific formulations are offered for the treatment of migraine headaches, body pains, and cognitive impairment associated with organ failure. The Ebers Papyrus offers one of the first descriptions of vascular dementia, "…as to perishing of the mind and forgetfulness…the mind becomes confused…drying up of the mind…his mind passes away…" (1500BC/1937)[8]. All of these cognitive impairments are attributed to disturbances of the heart, resulting in disturbances in normal blood flow to the brain and the consequential impairments in normal cognitive functions (1500BC/1937)[8].

The Ebers Papyrus is written within the contextual matrix and dogma of the period. The medical dogma of ancient Egypt states the brain and its surface blood vessels serve essential and necessary functions. They cool blood. The brain's function is much like that of a car radiator. It cools fluids. When the normal cooling function of the brain is disrupted, impaired cognitive functioning results.

Note: The ancient Egyptians held the heart to be the organ responsible for cognition and mood. The brain simply serves to cool the fluids of the heart and other body organs. It will be another 1,200 years before the brain begins to displace the heart as the organ responsible for human thoughts, cognitions, and emotions (circa 500BC,1903,1948)[9,10,11].

Unlike the Edwin Smith Papyrus which focuses on surgical treatments, the Ebers Papyrus focuses on medical treatments. When these two papyri are examined in combination with other notable ancient Egyptian medical papyri e.g. Hearst (2000 BC), Berlin (1800 BC), Kahun (1800 BC), London (1300 BC), and Beatty (1200 BC), they offer insight into the conceptual matrix within which neurological and other organ system disorders are understood and treated.

Given retrospective analyses of these papyri, a few general observations can be made. First, the papyri reveal the ancient Egyptians to be keen and accurate observers. Second, they recognize the value of recording observations for diagnostic, treatment, prognostic, and training purposes. Third, practitioners of the period are conducting systematic medical assessments. Fourth, they are making and evaluating the value of diagnosis. Fifth, they are making and evaluating the value of prognosis. Finally, they are compiling an empirically generated and recorded knowledge base, as to which diagnoses, prognoses, treatments, and management strategies are proving most effective (1935)[12].

Ancient civilizations of Mesopotamia and Egypt recognize neurological impairments and systematically record clinical presentations, examination procedures, diagnosis, treatment interventions, and prognosis of numerous neurological conditions. The records are descriptive and empirically derived. Disease, injury, and clinical outcomes are determined by supranatural entities e.g. god(s) and demon(s). Physical (natural) intervention e.g. medical or surgical, in combination with an appeal to supranatural forces, result in effective treatment interventions. The system and conceptual matrix is rational, empirically derived, based upon repeated observation over time, and establishes a reliable and stable knowledge base.

The primary points to be made here are neurological impairments have been recognized since the beginning of recorded history, the conditions occur with sufficient frequency to warrant recording the constellation of presenting signs and symptoms, recording empirically demonstrated effective and ineffective treatments, recording empirically derived prognoses, and developing a rational conceptual matrix to understand the presenting signs and symptoms sent by an unseen, angry, supranatural god(s) or demon(s), and to guide effective treatments which satisfy the god(s) or demon(s).

The Ancient civilization of Greece introduces a new approach to conceptualizing neurological impairments and stands in contrast to the ancient civilizations of Mesopotamia and Egypt. The ancient Greeks propose all neurological impairment can be explained by natural (physical) forces, which are knowable, observable, and follow the same physical properties observed throughout all of nature.

Two individuals exemplify the new approach to conceptualizing, understanding, and treating neurological impairments, Pythagoras of Samos and Alcmaeon of Croton.

Pythagoras of Samos (582 BC-510 BC) exemplifies the pre-Socratic philosophers and conceptualizes nature within the matrix of dynamic balances of opposing natural (physical) forces. He conceptualizes the entire universe to be ordered and bound by knowable physical properties. He is among the first to offer a rational conceptual matrix which attributes disturbances in body functions to be the result of imbalances in natural (physical) forces.

Note: Samos is a Greek island located in the eastern Aegean Sea between Greece and Turkey and located approximately one mile off the coast of Turkey.

The Pythagorean model offers guidance as to how to prevent illness, by manipulating natural (physical) forces, operating within the human body. Specifics treatments are recommended to restore and maximize normal balance. For example, modifying one's lifestyle to incorporate a vegetarian diet, daily meditation, daily physical exercise, organized and structured daily routines, residence in a healthy climate, and maintaining belief systems which provide a positive attitude towards life. Sound familiar? These recommendations are made today, every day, by practicing physicians around the world, over 2,100 years after Pythagoras first offers his recommendations.

Pythagoras emphasizes natural (physical) causes for impaired body functions and seeks to identify the mathematical relationships between normal balanced physical forces and imbalances of physical forces associated with impaired physical bodily functions. He quantifies the ratio of bodily fluids necessary for good physical health and applies number theory to medicine whenever possible e.g. periodicity of fevers. He is tremendously influential in guiding the philosophical perspective on medicine, as taught in the medical school at Croton, located in southern coastal Italy.

Alcmaeon of Croton (557 BC-491 BC) is among the first to propose the brain, rather than the heart, to be the organ responsible for sensation and cognition. This proposal challenges medical dogma. Alcmaeon declares all senses are connected to the brain. The connection between the source of sensations i.e. the outside world, is carried through channel tubes within the body to the brain. Alcmaeon proposes channels for all special sensory systems; seeing, hearing, smelling, and tasting. He identifies two channels which he places much emphasis. The two channels originate from the back of the eye and carry visual information to the brain; yes cranial nerves II (circa 500 BC/1871)[13].

Note: Croton is located on the sole of the boot of coastal, southern Italy and is a medical metropolis during ancient Greece. Croton is home to Pythagoras of Samos, circa 530 BC.

Alcmaeon embraces empirical observation as essential to understanding the physical (natural) world and the physical (natural) processes upon impaired neurological function result. He embraces a rational conceptual matrix and one which explains the natural (physical) causes of normal and abnormal neurological functions. The matrix guides rationally derived treatments and interventions, in efforts to restore balances among internal, natural, physical, body forces. He advocates the position all disturbances in body functions are the result of natural (physical) events, which are knowable and follow the same physical laws of nature as do all other natural phenomena. He rejects dogma attributing neurological impairment to supranatural causes. For Alcmaeon, all body illnesses, disease, and trauma can be and should be explained within a conceptual matrix which emphasizes the physical properties of dynamic physical forces operating within the physical human body. Treatments are directed to restoring balance between disordered internal physical forces.

As with most investigators who make meaningful contributions to the advancement of medical and scientific knowledge, he makes a few mistakes along the way. For example, Alcmaeon proposes one of the first rational theories for sleep, proposing sleep occurs when blood drains from the body and fills the vessels in the brain. The awake state and consciousness occurs when brain blood vessels empty, returning blood to the rest of the body. His vascular model for sleep is based in part on the observation of the period, apoplexy (strokes syndrome) is associated with decreased levels of conscious e.g. stupor. The vascular model proposed by Alcmaeon ultimately proves to be incorrect with time; however it persists in varying forms and permutations for the next 2,000 years.

The point here is two-fold. First, if you are thinking for yourself and choose not to follow the conventional dogma of the time, you are at risk and very likely to make a few mistakes in your thinking along the way. Second, if you never think for yourself or never challenge the prevailing dogma and if the prevailing dogma is indeed correct, you will never make a mistake. However, if the dogma is incorrect and you fail to challenge it, you will always be in error and never in a position to advance knowledge or offer a more innovative, more effective, or more correct care to your patients. Something to think about.

In summary, the history of the medical neurosciences has a rich and well documented past. The earliest known civilizations evidence interests and commit valued resources to attempting to understand neurological conditions, their etiologies, and effective treatment interventions. The ancient civilizations of Mesopotamia and Egypt offer written records of systematic observations of many neurological conditions familiar to most practicing physicians today. The Ancients conceptualize neurological impairments to be the result of unseen, supranatural origins, and can be modified only by executing the proper treatment intervention, empirically proven to be pleasing to the supranatural forces e.g. god(s) or demon(s) responsible for the impairment(s). Non-pleasing interventions, which anger the god(s) or demon(s), result in a worsening of the patient's condition are documented with the same care as interventions which please the god(s). Treatments utilize a multidimensional approach, attending to medical, mechanical, and environmental factors. Treatments are empirically based and rational. Ancient Egyptians formalize the recording of observations, introducing the now familiar process of observing the patient, documenting presenting signs and symptoms, conducting a physical examination, generating a diagnosis based upon the observations, history, and physical findings, generating a prognosis based upon a diagnosis, and instituting a rational treatment based upon the conceptual matrix of the period and demonstrated success with other patients presenting with similar conditions.

Ancient Greece builds upon the knowledge of the ancient civilizations of Mesopotamia and Egypt. Ancient Greece introduce the new idea, neurological conditions can be understood and explained by natural (physical) forces, rather than supranatural forces. Two individuals, Pythagoras and Alcmaeon, prove especially influential and advocate rejection of period dogma, proposing replacement of supranatural explanatory models with new models based upon natural (physical) forces. Particular attention is directed to quantifying these physical forces and noting changes, as a function of healthy or impaired body function. Effective treatments of neurological conditions are directed to restoring balance of body natural (physical) forces.

The ancient civilizations of Mesopotamia, Egypt, and Greece lay the foundation upon which all future developments in the medical neurosciences will build.

Antiquity, 500 BC - 500 AD.

Antiquity witnesses radical changes in the conceptual matrix used to understand neurological conditions.

Early-Antiquity builds upon the empirical knowledge base established by the Ancient civilizations of Mesopotamia, Egypt, and Greece. Emphasis continues to be placed upon observation, examination, and understanding of the physical (natural) basis of impaired bodily function and rejects supranatural explanations. By late-Antiquity, physical models are displaced by supranatural (deity) models. The two models are diametrically opposed, based upon their suppositional foundations, however they do share several commonalities. Both models offer a rational conceptual matrix within which to understand neurological impairment. Both models explain the origins of neurological impairments; how and why the conditions are manifested; how the conditions should best be treated; and under what conditions the patient's condition can be expected to improve.

Let us examine a few of the most influential factors contributing to the changes in conceptual models across Antiquity. What factors influence the change in the conceptual models? Do similar factors influence conceptual models today? Let us also review a few of the most influential people, making significant contributions, during Antiquity and how their contributions influence the early development and future direction of the medical neurosciences.

Empedocles of Agrigento (495 BC-435 BC) Greek pre-Socratic natural philosopher builds upon the Pythagorean and Alcmaeonean models, emphasizing an essential and necessary balance among four natural (physical) and opposing forces within the human body, Earth, Wind, Fire, and Water.

Similar to Pythagoras, Empedocles emphasizes the ratios between these forces, rather than their absolute quantity, quality, or anatomical location, to explain impaired physical health. Empedocles embraces a cardio-centric model, placing the anatomical location for all cognitive processes, sensations, and movement in the heart. Blood is conceptualized as the essential medium for all thought. A person's degree of intelligence depends upon the composition of their blood. Neurological impairments are understood as disordered ratios of the four naturally opposing fundamental forces within the human body. Treatment interventions are all directed to restoring disordered ratios to normal.

Note: The city of Agrigento is located on the southern coast of Sicily and is one of the great centers of Greek medicine.

Diogenes of Apollo (460 BC-390 BC) born in the Greek settlement of Apollonia, located on the Mediterranean Sea coast of modern-day Bulgaria, influentially proposes the conceptual model which emphasizes the flow of "pneuma" (a vital life giving force) through body channels (blood vessels), as essential and necessary for normal brain function and good physical health. Diogenes is one of the influential pre-Socratic natural (physical) philosophers, emphasizing the physical nature of the world. He explains the physical world within the matrix of elemental physical constituents, which in varying combinations make up all physical matter, including the human body. According to Diogenes' conceptual matrix and in regard to the nervous system, normal perceptions and cognitions occur when "pneuma", carrying sensory information from the external environment, is inhaled into the body by inspiration, mixes with blood, flows through the body via the blood vessel systems, ultimately reaching the brain. It is the brain and not the heart, in which sensory perception and cognition take place. Movement results when "pneuma" flows through blood vessels to the limbs. Neurological disorders, sensory, motor, or cognitive, result when the normal flow of "pneuma" through blood vessel channels is obstructed. Treatments of neurological impairments are directed to restoring the normal flow of "pneuma" through the body.

Diogenes of Apollo systematically details the gross anatomy of blood vessel systems of the human body. The observations and descriptions of the "pneuma" carrying channels (blood vessels) are extensive, accurate, and provide the foundation upon which all future descriptions of major blood vessels will be based (On Nature, DK 64 B 6/1887,1948,1966,2006)[14,15,16,17]. In combination, his model of "pneuma" and associated anatomical channels within which it flows, offers a rational, conceptual matrix, firmly planted in the natural (physical) world and offers a model within which to rationally understand clinical presentations of neurological impairments and guide treatment interventions.

As a medical student today, over 2,400 years after Diogenes first proposes his model, consider now the many neurological conditions you have learned in medical school, which result when there is disruption in blood flow to your patient's brain, or when oxygen levels in blood are reduced, as the result of poor respiratory ventilation.

Hippocrates (460 BC-377 BC) of Cos extends the developing conceptual matrix of four humors. Hippocrates embraces natural (physical) rather than supranatural origins of impaired body function. Pathologies develop when humors appear in excess or insufficient amounts. Treatment interventions are directed to restoring balance among natural bodily humors, especially blood (heart), phlegm (brain), yellow bile (liver), and black bile (spleen). Hippocrates clearly states the brain is responsible for sensation, movement, and cognition.

Note: Cos is one of the many Greek islands found in the south Aegean Sea, located between Greece and Turkey, and the site of an early Greek medical school (Coan School), devoted to the training of future physicians, emphasizing the physical (natural) rather than the supranatural (deity) bases of disease and illness.

Hippocrates describes two common neurological conditions; epilepsies and stroke syndromes (apoplexy). Both conditions are familiar to practicing physicians today, over 2,400 years after Hippocrates describes the conditions. Hippocrates describes both conditions within the matrix of natural origins and natural (physical) body pathologies e.g. disordered balance of body humors. He specifically rejects medical dogma of the period which state these conditions originate from supernatural origins (deities). He describes common clinical signs and symptoms of each condition and associates these with environmental factors e.g. climate, time of day, season of the year, and living conditions and moderator variables such as age, family history, and diet.

Hippocrates descriptions of the epilepsies are discussed in the Medical Psychology chapter and will not be reiterated here.

Hippocrates description of stroke syndromes (apoplexy) emphasizes presentation of sudden paralysis or sudden death. Here too the condition is interpreted within the matrix of humors imbalances, with congestion of cold and moist phlegm or cold and dry black bile in the head, as explanatory physical causes of apoplexy. As with epilepsies, Hippocrates associates subject variables with apoplexy, noting older individuals are much more likely to experience an episode of apoplexy than younger individuals (Aphorism III:31) and more specifically "...persons are most subject to apoplexy between the age of forty and sixty..." (Aphorism VI:57)[18,19]. Old individuals experiencing an episode of apoplexy are much more likely to die suddenly, than a younger individual experiencing an episode of apoplexy. Environmental factors are associated with the onset of apoplexy, noting the apoplexy is most likely to occur during the winter months and less likely in the summer months (Aphorism III:23)[18,19]. From a diagnostic perspective, Hippocrates distinguishes two sub-types of apoplexy "...strong and weak...". The classification system is based upon the severity of signs and symptoms evident at first presentation for diagnosis and treatment. Hippocrates reports prognosis is poor "...for a strong attack of apoplexy...and not easy to remove for a weak attack..." (Aphorisms II:47) (400BC/1849)[18,19].

In addition to the epilepsies and stroke syndromes, Hippocrates describes many other familiar neurological conditions, including speech and language disorders, sensory and motor impairments resulting from spinal cord lesions, and cerebral palsies. All syndromes are conceptualized within the balance of humors, natural (physical) models and offer rational treatments, based upon the conceptual framework which explain the underlying pathologies responsible i.e. imbalance of humors.

Hippocrates' commitment to the natural (physical) explanation of neurological conditions is exemplified in his self-assured and adamant comments regarding seizure disorders; "...those who first called this disease sacred...we now call quacks and charlatans...by invoking a divine element...and call this a sacred malady is to conceal their ignorance of nature..." (400 BC/ 1950)[20].

Aristotle (384 BC-322 BC) born in the region of Chalcidice, Greece, located on the large, three finger peninsula of north-central Greece, stretching into the northwestern Aegean Sea, relocates to

Athens and joins Plato's Academy, at the age of 18 years. He resides in Athens for most of his adult life, only to be forced from the city during his last year of life by political pressures.

Aristotle actively investigates and writes prolifically in the area of zoology for most of his very productive life. He offers an alternative conceptual matrix within which to understand the function of the brain and other parts of the nervous system. His alternative model directly challenges the rapid developing brain models proposed by Alcmaeon and Hippocrates. Aristotle, while embracing the physical (natural) rather than supranatural (deity) models shared by Alcmaeon and Hippocrates, rejects the brain as being primary to sensations and movement. He dogmatically insist the heart, rather than the brain, to be central to all sensation and movement. Aristotle confidently and without reservation emphatically states "…of course, the brain is not responsible for any sensation at all. The correct view (is) that the seat and source of sensation is the region of the heart…the (e)motions of pleasure and pain, and generally all sensations plainly have their source in the heart…" (350 BC/1955,1995)[21,22].

Aristotle throughout history is often misunderstood in regard to his position on the centrality of the heart and its role in neurological functions. Most writers simply report Aristotle rejects the brain and substitutes the heart. This is an over simplification. Aristotle indeed places the heart at the center of a "heart-brain" system, however; he does not reject or deny the importance of the brain in mediating normal sensations, cognition, memory, or movement. He simply assigns the brain a secondary, albeit an important and necessary role, in all sensations, perceptions, cognitions, and movement.

The brain's secondary assignment is based upon Aristotle's rational conceptual model. The heart is naturally a "hot organ" and requires cooling. The brain and lungs are naturally "cool organs" and provide the necessary cooling required for normal heart functioning and by extension normal sensation, perception, cognition, and movement. In the absence of sufficient cooling, as the result of old age, injury, or brain disease, the heart will fail, thereby producing the observed clinical syndromes.

Aristotle assigns blood cooling functions to the brain, based upon the premise the brain is a "cool organ", blood vessels of the brain are thin, thereby allowing for evaporation and cooling of blood, as it flows through the "cool and moist" brain. Neurological impairments result when the brain fails in its ability to cool blood or the brain's ability to produce phlegm. Phlegm is a natural body humor, produced in the brain, when "hot vapors" generated in the heart reach the brain and mix with blood. Phlegm is essential for good health. Failure to produce phlegm results whenever normal blood flow through the brain is obstructed or when the brain becomes hard and dry. Aristotle notes old age is associated with an overly dry and hard brain, thereby increasing the probabilities of observing neurological impairments in older patients.

Treatment interventions are directed to restoring balance among the four normal body humors (blood, phlegm, yellow bile, black bile), restoring flow of the humors through the body, and restoring organs to their usual natural quality state. For example, returning the brain to its natural healthy state of "moist and cool". Common procedures used to achieve treatment objectives are purging and bleeding and application of the Principle of Opposites. Purging and bleeding are used to eliminate excess body fluids and restore the quantity and balance of body humors. The Principle of Opposites states "…if it is hot then cool it, if it is cool then warm it, if it is dry then moisten it, and if it is moist then dry it…". The Principle of Opposites is used to restore the physical body, especially organs to their natural, healthy, quality state of hot, cool, moist, or dry.

Aristotle further encourages manipulation of the patient's physical environment, habits, and activities of daily living e.g. altering the climate and or living conditions of patient's place of residence, maintaining good physical hygiene, following a vegetarian diet, and engaging in regular moderate exercise. Treatment interventions are all directed to restoring balance and harmony in the patient's physical body and immediate physical surrounding environment.

Sound familiar? These are recommendations made every day, by practicing physicians around the world today, over 2,300 years after Aristotle makes the recommendations to patients in his care.

Moving now from the Greek cities and settlements of Italy (Croton and Agrigento), modern-day Bulgaria (Apollonia), Turkey (Cnidus), and Greece (Samos, Cos and Athens), to the Greek City of Alexandria, Egypt (sic), medical neurosciences take a historically significant turn in development. The investigative paradigm shifts from the philosophical approach of the natural philosophers, which rely upon thoughts to generate new ideas and evaluate conceptual models, to the physical observations of the empiricists, which rely upon sensory experiences to acquire and evaluate new knowledge. This notable shift in the approach to the study of the brain and brain functions is most evident in the City of Alexandria, approximately 50 years after the death of Hippocrates. This new approach introduces human dissection as an essential and acceptable investigational tool. Advances are quickly made in the areas of gross anatomy, physiology, and in particular gross human neuroanatomy.

Herophilus (335 BC-280 BC) an empirical neuroanatomist, working in the City of Alexandria, makes significant contributions. He differentiates sensory from motor nerves, more than 2,100 years before Scottish surgeon Charles Bell (1774-1842) and French physiologist Francois Magendie (1783-1855) claim credit for this discovery, based upon their own investigations. Herophilus reports damage to motor nerves cause paralysis. He names the meninges, names the cerebral ventricles, describes CN II, CN III, CN V, CN VII, CN VIII, and XII, and describes the gross anatomical differences and functional significance between the cerebral hemispheres and cerebellar hemispheres. Herophilus challenges and uniformly rejects Aristotle's conceptual model, which attributes the primary function of brain to cooling of blood. Herophilus localizes intelligence and reasoning to the brain, based upon empirical evidence collected by way of systematic, experimental investigations, conducted in Alexandria.

Erasistratus (310 BC-250 BC) an empirical neuroanatomist, working in the City of Alexandria, and colleague of the more senior Herophilus, makes significant contributions, which advance the methods used in the discovery of new knowledge, the assessment of existing knowledge, and challenge medical dogma. He describes the cerebral ventricular system, choroid plexus, and describes the gross anatomy of sensory and motor nerves as they enter and exit the brain and spinal cord. Erasistratus embraces experimentation as primary to the discovery of new knowledge and assessment of old knowledge. He is among the first to describe and detail anatomical changes associated with stroke syndromes.

Many advances are made in understanding the anatomical and physiological basis of the human nervous system, during the brief 30 to 40 year period human dissection is conducted in the City of Alexandria, primarily by Herophilus and Erasistratus, before governmental sanctions specifically prohibit all human dissections or human eviscerations. Human dissection is explicitly prohibited by government and organized religions, for the next 1,800 years. Legal and Church approved human dissection reappears only in the mid-1500s (1543)[23]. Rapid advancements being made through the investigational use of human dissection, quickly stall.

At approximately the same time human dissection is first prohibited by government sanctions, in the City of Alexandria, external forces e.g. introduction of organized religion, war, and changes in ruling governments contribute significantly to the absence of meaningful progress being made in the medical neurosciences. City-States of Greece give way to a rapidly expanding Roman Empire. Rome quickly controls Italy, Greece, and most all of the eastern Mediterranean City-States, and North Africa.

In the absence of the generation of new knowledge, efforts are soon directed to organizing and summarizing existing knowledge.

Aulus Celsus (25 BC-50 AD) Roman encyclopedist offers his eight book encyclopedia, "De Medicina" [On Medicine]. "De Medicina" is written circa 50 AD and summarizes with much editorial license, the medical knowledge of ancient Greek and Alexandrian medicine (50AD/1498)[24]. As characteristic of the Romans of the period, the Romans identify selected elements of culture and knowledge of civilizations they conquer and simply claim them to be their own. So too is the case with medical knowledge during this period of rapid expansion of the Roman Empire, circa 200 BC-200 AD.

Galen of Pergamum (129 AD-200 AD) is arguably one of the most prolific writers in medical history, writing over 600 treatises. His writings are largely restatements of existing knowledge. He is born in Pergamum and soon travels to the city of Alexandria to study anatomy. He returns to Pergamum in his late 20s and works briefly as a surgeon to the gladiators. He travels extensively throughout the Mediterranean and spends most of his adult life in Rome, writing and providing medical services to successive Roman emperors.

Note: Pergamum is an ancient Greek city, located close to the modern-day city of Bergama, Turkey, approximately 16 miles inland from the Aegean Sea.

Galen writes extensively on the nervous systems and approaches these systems primarily from an anatomical perspective. His writings are authoritative and dogmatic. For example, Galen rejects Aristotle's proposition the brain serves as a cooling system for the heart, emphatically stating "…the supposition that the encephalon was formed for the sake of the heat of the heart, to cool it and bring it to a moderate temperature, is utterly absurd…"(circa 173AD/1968)[25]. He argues instead vital spirits produced in the left ventricle of the heart are carried to the brain via the carotid arteries and then transformed into psychic pneuma (animal spirits), in the anatomical structure "rete mirabile", located at the base of the brain.

The "rete mirabile" does not exist in humans. Perhaps Galen is describing what latter will be termed the Circle of Willis and its penetrating arteries into the hypothalamus. According to Galen, psychic pneuma (animal spirits) are stored in brain ventricles and when needed, move through hollow nerves. Movement of psychic pneuma through hollow nerves, allows movement of sensory information from a person's external environment to the brain, resulting in the perception of sensations. Movement of psychic pneuma through hollow nerves, from brain ventricles to skeletal muscles, initiates and maintains movement. Galen argues all memories, imaginations, intellectual resources, and cognitions are located within the cerebral spinal fluid filled brain ventricles.

Galen identifies, describes, illustrates, and assigns function to many neuroanatomical structures familiar to you as a medical student; for example, the corpus callosum, fornix, superior and inferior colliculi, sympathetic chain ganglia, optic chiasm, brachial plexus, and pineal gland (circa 173AD/1968,177AD/1956,1962,2010)[25,26,27].

Galen contributes meaningfully to the foundation of our understanding of the spinal cord and the consequential results when the spinal cord is lesioned. In a series of experiments, conducted circa 177 AD, he systematically and methodically, surgically introduces lesions into the spinal cord at differing spinal segments and reports the consequential results. He describes changes in sensory and motor functions, based upon the spinal cord segment level lesioned. Here is a brief excerpt from the translation of Galen's notes.

> "...If you sever it completely between the third and fourth vertebrae, the animal at once ceased to breathe. Not only does the thorax become motionless, but also the whole body below the section... If beyond the sixth vertebra, all muscles of the thorax become motionless immediately and the animal breathes in only by the means of the diaphragm...". (Galen, 117 AD/1956, Book VIII, Chapter 9, Transverse section of spinal cord, Section 696, p221)[28].

Galen reports any transection lesion of the spinal cord will always produce loss of sensory and motor functions below the level of the lesion. Lesions made in the high cervical segments result in disruption of respiration. Lesions of the lower cervical segments result in preserved respiration with paralysis and somatosensory loss of the upper extremities. When lesions are made to the lower spinal cord segments, only the lower extremities evidence paralysis and impaired sensory functions and the upper extremities remain unaffected. He additionally describes the consequence of hemi-section of the spinal cord; noting only one half of the body, below the level of the hemi-section is affected (circa 177AD/1956,2010)[29].

Much of Galen's writings, summaries, and conceptualizations of the nervous systems go unchallenged, for the next 1,500 years.

Newly organized religions e.g. Judaism, Christianity, Catholicism, and Islam begin to greatly affect the development of the medical neurosciences. Empirical science is displaced by faith based belief systems. The emphasis once placed upon the natural (physical) bases of normal and disordered neurological function, shifts once again to the supranatural (deity) based models. According to most organized religions the cause of neurological impairment is an angered god. Conceptualization of the nervous system and associated functions are understood within the matrix of faith based belief systems of organized religions.

Treatment interventions are guided by the accepted models of organized religion. For example, conditions such as epilepsies are considered to be the consequence of an angry God, who has sent the condition as punishment upon an individual, whom has failed to accept the teachings and practices of the organized religion. The treatment of epilepsies, therefore is best accomplished through spiritual healing, accomplished by prayer, acknowledgment to others of one's spiritual transgressions, and engaging in ritualistic behaviors guided by the leaders of organized religions rather than physicians, in hopes these actions will appease the angry God, and the God will return the person's neurological condition to normal by removing the God sent punishment.

Some individuals within organized religion, attempt to reconcile the long established history and conceptual models attributing neurological function and neurological impairments to physical causes with the beliefs of the newly organized religions, which emphasize the supranatural (deity) based models of neurological function and neurological impairments. One influential individual attempting to reconcile physical models with faith based models is Nemesius.

Nemesius (circa 390 AD) Catholic bishop of Emesa (modern-day Homs, Syria) attempts to reconcile the natural (physical) models established by the Greeks and summarized by Galen, with the faith based supranatural (deity) models embraced by organized religions, and combination models such as Plato's tripartite model of the soul. Certainly an ambitious effort. For the purpose of this writing, Nemesius' most important contribution to the development of the medical neurosciences is his manuscript outlining his doctrine of ventricular localization of mental functions (circa 415AD/1955, 2008)[30,31].

In brief, Nemesius asserts sensory perception and imagination are mediated by the anterior ventricles (two lateral ventricles), intellectual abilities the middle ventricle (third ventricle), and memory the posterior ventricle (fourth ventricle). He bases his anatomical location of function upon the summary writings of Galen, who implicated the ventricles as the anatomical location of sensory, motor, and cognitive functions, over two hundred years earlier.

Specifically, Nemesius points to the observations, lesions of the brain in and around the ventricles result in different clinical presentations e.g. lesions of the anterior ventricles (lateral ventricles) impair sensations, perception, and movement, while intellect and cognition remains unaffected; lesions of the middle ventricle (third ventricle) impair intellect and cognition; lesions of the posterior ventricle (fourth ventricle) affects memory, while sensation, perception, and movement remain unaffected.

He expands upon Plato's tripartite model of the soul and Aristotle's model of the soul (life-force) to incorporate both natural and supranatural dimensions to explain healthy and impaired neurological conditions. Nemesius conceptualizes the soul as an indestructible, spiritual substance, distinctly separate from the physical body, yet linked allowing the physical body to perceive, think, and remember experiences.

Ventricle models, which localize sensory, motor, and cognitive functions to brain ventricles, are largely unchallenged until the mid-1600s. The ventricle doctrine of localized mental functions is taught to medical students, as medical dogma, at all major medical centers throughout the Mediterranean and Western Europe for nearly 1,200 years. Renaissance artist Leonardo da Vinci pours casts, illustrates, describes, and documents in detail, the ventricles along with their assigned functions, sensation, movement, and cognition (1504-1507/1935,1970)[32,33]. Andreas Vesalius influential Belgium anatomist, discusses and reinforces the ventricular doctrines in his major work "De Humani Copris Fabrica" [On the fabrics of the human body] (1543,1543/1555,2015)[34,35]. Thomas Willis (circle of Willis fame) is first to reject this long-standing medical dogma that brain ventricles are the locations of sensory perception, cognition, and memory. He attributes these functions instead to the cerebral cortex (1664,1672)[36,37].

In summary during Antiquity medical neurosciences undergoes a radical shift in paradigms within which neurological conditions are understood, investigated, diagnosed, managed, and treated. Early in Antiquity the conceptual matrix used to understand neurological impairments is strongly rooted in the natural (physical) world. Neurological disorders follow the same physical principles of nature as the physical universe. Neurological conditions have physical origins; can be investigated like all other physical events; and can be understood, treated, and managed by applying fundamental principles of physics. This conceptual matrix is displaced midway through

Antiquity with the introduction of organized religion. Faith based, supranatural (deity) models replace natural (physical) models, within which to understand neurological conditions. Faith based models attribute neurological impairments to an angered, supranatural deity (God) who sends neurological impairments as punishments to those whom refuse or fail to adhere to the faith based beliefs and practices of organized religions. Treatments focus on appeasing the angered, supranatural deity, though prayer, confession of transgressions and sins, performing penance, and embracing the teachings, practices, and belief systems of organized religions.

In early-Antiquity Empedocles offers his model of four, natural, physical, and opposing forces, operating within the body Earth, Wind, Fire, and Water. In order for a person to maintain good physical health, the proper ratio between these forces must be maintained. In the event the ratios are disordered impairment in body function will result. Treatment is directed to restoring normal ratios between the four forces.

Diogenes proposes the flow of "pneuma" model, emphasizing normal sensory perception, cognition, and movement occurs when pneuma is inhaled, mixes with blood, flowing through the body by way of blood vessel channels, bringing sensory information from the environment to the brain, where perception and cognition takes place, and to the limbs to produce movement. Disturbances in the flow of pneuma results in impaired functioning. Treatments are directed to restoring normal flow.

Hippocrates develops the four natural humors model, assigning production of each humor to a specific organ. Neurological impairments result when there is too much or too little humor or when the balance between humors is disordered. Treatment is directed to restoring the quantity in and balance between humors. Hippocrates describes several familiar neurological disorders, two in detail, epilepsies and strokes. He introduces the importance of moderator variables e.g. age, family history, diet, living conditions, climate, and season of the year, to understanding any disease condition.

Aristotle introduces the heart-brain system, emphasizing each organ is equally important for maintaining normal neurological function. In the event the system is disordered impaired neurological function results. The brain is assigned the function of cooling the "hot vapors" produced in the heart. Blood circulates the "vapors" between the heart, brain, and distant body parts. In addition to disorders of brain and its cooling function, disorders of the blood circulation contribute to impairments in sensory perception, cognition, memory, and movement. Treatments are directed to restoring the cooling function of the brain and restoring normal blood circulation in brain and throughout the whole body.

Herophilus details much neuroanatomy and associated functions, during his work in the City of Alexandrea, and relies heavily upon human dissection as an essential investigative tool. He differentiates sensory and motor nerves, reports damage to motor nerves produce paralysis, names the meninges and cerebral ventricles, describes cranial nerves, and describes the anatomical and functional differences between the cerebral and cerebellar hemispheres. He localizes intelligence and cognition to the brain, based upon empirical evidence collected through systematic, experimental investigations.

Erasistratus also details much human anatomy and associated functions, during his work in the City of Alexandria and also relies heavily upon human dissection. He describes cranial and spinal nerves, along with their associated sensory and motor functions, as they enter and exit the brain and spinal cord. He describes the choroid plexus, located inside of the ventricles and identifies its primary function, production of cerebral spinal fluid. He is among the first to describe in detail the anatomical changes in brain associated with stroke syndromes.

By mid-Antiquity organize religions and governments in response to the presses of organized religion prohibit human dissection. Advancement of new knowledge stalls. Medical knowledge is for all intent and purposes simply summarized and modified to better align with the beliefs of the Roman Empire and organized religions.

Aulus Celsus summaries and modifies existing scientific and medical knowledge from ancient Greece and Alexandria medicine, in his influential, historically important, landmark encyclopedia "De Medicina".

Galen offers his summary of existing medical neuroscience knowledge; introduces a modified version of Diogenes' "pneuma" model, identifies, names, and assigns function to numerous neuroanatomical structures e.g. corpus collosum, fornix, sympathetic chain ganglia, optic chiasm, brachial plexus, and the pituitary gland. He offers original contributions in understanding spinal cord lesions, reporting different sensory and motor outcomes, based upon the location of a lesion within the spinal cord and emphasized the importance of spinal cord level. Galen's extensions and summaries, in all areas of medical knowledge, are soon accepted as medical dogma and remain effectively unchallenged for the next 1,500 years.

Nemesius attempts to integrate the natural models of early-Antiquity with the supranatural, faith based models of mid and late-Antiquity, in a less than successful effort to accommodate everyone, including organized religion. He introduces the concept of brain localization of function e.g. sensory perception, intellect, thought, memory, and movement to the four brain ventricles. The model is taught to medical students as dogma for the next 1,200 years.

By the end of Antiquity organized religions have displaced scientific investigations with faith based belief systems embracing supranatural deity models within which to understand neurological impairments and to guide treatments. Progress in the advancement of scientific knowledge in the medical neurosciences stalls.

Middle Ages (Medieval Times), 500 AD - 1400 AD.

The Middle Ages witness the fall of the Western Roman Empire circa 500 AD. There is a fundamental restructuring of the geographic, political, economic, and social dimensions of Europe. Intellectual interests in the medical neurosciences become secondary in importance and priority. Europe is reorganizing at every level. Organized religions continue to be tremendously influential in determining the reorganization of Western Europe and what and how new knowledge will be generated. Many scholars flee Europe to the Middle East, especially Iran, to escape academic, geopolitical, and economical persecution. Middle East scholars soon begin to summarize the medical writings of the Greeks and Romans into encyclopedia form. Original medical writings of the Greeks and Romans, carried to the Middle East by fleeing scholars, are translated into Syric and Arabic. The Nestorian Christian Sect are responsible for many of the translations during the 600s-900s AD, in the Middle East. Scholars whom remain in Europe translate original Greek and Roman medical documents, with liberal editorial license to modify the translations to be more in line with the beliefs of organized religions, into the preferred language of the Christian Protestant and Catholic Church, Latin.

Medical school education and training is formalized. New medical schools are founded in Italy and affiliate with established universities. Governments regulate the practice of medicine, requiring formal training in medicine and formal examination by medical school faculty before an individual is permitted to practice medicine.

King Ruggiero (1095 AD-1154 AD) King of Sicily, aka King Roger II, proclaims by royal decree "…whoever from this time forth desires to practice medicine must present himself before our officials and judges, and be subject to their decision…Anyone audacious enough to neglect this shall be punished by imprisonment and confiscation of goods. This decree has for its object the protection of subjects of our kingdom from the dangers arising from the ignorance of practitioners…" (1140AD/1904-1905)[38].

The prevailing conceptual matrix within which to understand neurological impairment and disease is squarely centered in organized religions' dogma. Rejecting physical (natural) models, well established within Greek and Alexandrian medicine and embracing supranatural (deity) faith-based models established by relatively new organized religions reframes the content and process of medical and scientific investigations leading to new knowledge. Investigative studies, exploring the physical basis of the nervous systems and neurological impairment are severely restricted by organized religion. Only at the end of the Middle Ages, does the pendulum swing and return once again to conceptualizing neurological conditions within a physical matrix and without supranatural intervention.

Human dissection returns to university affiliated medical schools and becomes an important component of the new medical school curriculum. Illustrations of neuroanatomical structures are introduced to accompany neuroanatomical text and facilitate learning. Most major contributions are coming from the medical schools and universities of Italy. Neuroanatomy returns as an important area of investigation and contributes significantly to the advancement of the medical neurosciences. Human dissection performed within the medical schools correct many errors in Galenian medical dogma.

Before moving forward too quickly, let us place in context major events, contributions, and people who significantly influence the advancement and development of the medical neurosciences through the Middle Ages.

Ibn-San (aka Avicenna) (980 AD-1037 AD) Persian (Iranian) polymath and encyclopedist summarizes Greek and Roman medical writings, which have recently been translated into Syric and Arabic. Ibn-San offers his major and tremendously influential work, "al-Qanun fi-al-Tibb" [The Canon of Medicine], circa 1025 AD. The "al-Qanun fi-al-Tibb" is a five volume, medical encyclopedia, heavily influenced by the work and summaries of Galen. The encyclopedia is primarily a summary and reiteration of Greek and Roman medical writings. The "al-Qanun fi-al-Tibb" serves as the primary source of medical information, for the next five hundred years, throughout the Middle East and Europe. The encyclopedia contains descriptions of numerous and familiar neurological conditions. For example epilepsies, dementias, stroke syndromes, movement disorders, inflammation of the meninges, disorders characterized by impairments in the form and content of thought (possible schizophrenia), severe and debilitating impairments in mood, and hallucinations. The encyclopedia embraces a modified version of the balanced four natural humors model, within which to conceptualize and understand physical health. This stands in contrast to the rapidly developing bias evident in Europe and the Middle East, which rejects physical (natural) cause models in favor of supranatural, faith-based models, offered by relatively new, organized religions e.g. Christianity and Islam.

In Europe, as the Western Roman Empire falls and as part of the restructuring process, new organized religions e.g. Christianity, Catholicism, and Islam have increasing influence in guiding the conceptual matrix within which to understand the human body, disease, and neurological impairment. Organized religions guide not only the conceptual matrix, they greatly influence the investigative methodologies and procedures used to investigate, study, and understand neurological impairments. Scholasticism, an intellectual approach to acquiring new knowledge through the process of joining faith and reason, through the process of dialectical reasoning and resolution of contradictions, gains popularity and is applied to understanding neurological function and neurological disorders. Scholasticism stands in marked contrast to the practical empiricism applied by the ancient civilizations of Mesopotamia, Egypt, Greece or the Libraries of Alexandria.

Thomas Aquinas (1225 AD-1274 AD) Italian, Dominican friar, Catholic priest, and influential Catholic theologian embraces the Doctrine of ventricular localization of mental functions.

Without offering an extended discussion of Thomas Aquinas' philosophical and theological views, let it suffice to say, from a historical perspective of the medical neurosciences, Thomas Aquinas embraces the natural (physical) explanation of disease. As a Catholic theologian he equally embraces the concept of a non-physical soul, which too can become diseased and disordered. In its most simple form, Thomas Aquinas argues when a person sins (transgressions against organized religions values or teachings) the soul is disordered. When the soul is disordered, the disorder is manifested as an illness of the physical body. Treatment interventions required to restore the physical body to good health are achieved through healing the soul. When the soul is healed, the body heals.

Thomas Aquinas' hybrid model, in efforts to reconcile natural and faith-based models, incorporates the doctrine of ventricular localization of mental functions, originally proposed by Catholic bishop Nemesius over 800 years earlier. Thomas Aquinas argues human sensation and perception are localized to the anterior (two lateral ventricles), memories to the middle (third ventricle), and movement to the posterior (fourth ventricle). In combination, Thomas Aquinas acknowledges the brain to be the organ of primary importance when considering perception, cognition, memory, and movement. However, it is the condition and health of the soul which determines the condition and health of the body.

The ventricular model of localization of mental functions (aka Cell doctrine; not to be confused with Cell theory) remains medical dogma well into the mid-1500s, when it is challenged by Renaissance period Belgium anatomist Andreas Vesalius (1514-1564). Andreas Vesalius offers anatomical evidence based upon his observations, the ventricles observed in the human brain are very similar to the ventricles observed in many animal brains. Given the anatomical similarities and assumption animals cannot house a human soul, it follows therefore the ventricles cannot possibly house the human soul and all of its associated mental processes (1543)[34,35]. Later and more convincingly, English neuroanatomist Thomas Willis (1621-1675) challenges the ventricular model of localization of mental functions, based upon evidence from patients presenting with acquired brain injuries, congenital brain abnormalities, and personally conducted brain dissections (1664)[39]. Thomas Willis offers an alternative explanation, localizing specific mental functions to the cerebral cortex rather than the ventricles. As with most challenges to medical dogma, Willis' localization of cognitive functions to the cerebral cortex is not immediately accepted by the professional or medical communities.

Return now with me to the late-1200s AD, soon after Thomas Aquinas proposes his modified version of Diogenes' ventricular model, localizing sensory, motor, and higher order brain functions to the cerebral spinal fluid filled cerebral ventricles. Advancements continue to be made in the area of human gross anatomy and in particular human neuroanatomy. Manuscripts detailing and illustrating human brain anatomy are being collected, reproduced, made available, and circulated among medical school faculty and medical students. While the printing press will not be invented for another 200 years, during the mid-1400s and only later developed sufficiently during the early-1500s to the point mass printing and distribution of manuscripts are made available to medical schools and universities, important work is completed during the early-1300s AD, advancing the understanding of neuroanatomical structure and function.

Mondino de Luzzi (1270 AD-1326 AD) Italian anatomist, working at the University of Bologna located in north-central Italy, prepares and distributes "Anathomia Corporis", an instructional dissection manual of the human body prepared specifically for medical students (1316AD)[40]. This dissection manual remains the standard until Andreas Vesalius publishes "De Human Corporis Fabrica" (1543,1555/2015)[34,35]. The efforts of Mondino de Luzzi and other investigators working in newly founded Italian universities and associated medical schools reintroduce the systematic teaching of anatomy into the medical school curriculum.

Guido da Vigevano (1280 AD-1349 AD) Italian physician, student of Mondino de Luzzi, while attending medical school at the University of Bologna and noted inventor, offers an important manuscript in the development of medical neuroanatomy, "Anathomia Designate per Figures" (1345AD,1926)[41,42]. Here he offers for the first time, illustrations of brain, spinal cord, and spinal nerves as a complement to anatomical descriptions. This is a significant change and greatly influences how neuroanatomy is introduced and taught to medical students for the next 670 years.

"Anathomia Designate per Figures" contains six illustrated plates which offer systematic anatomical drawings of dura and pia mater (XI), cerebral convolutions (XII,XIII,XV,XVI), ventricles (XV), spinal cord and the origin of spinal nerves (XVI). Viewing these plates, one immediately recognizes a marked and distinctive lack of perspective in the drawings. Recall, introduction of perspective into drawings appears later, in Italy at the beginning of the Italian Renaissance, circa 1413.

Prior to the neuroanatomical contributions of Mondino de Luzzi and Guido da Vigevano, most gross anatomy and specifically neuroanatomy knowledge taught to medical students is presented without the aid of human dissection or illustrations of internal body structures and based upon the summary writings of Galen 200 years earlier. Imagine for a moment, trying to learn human anatomy without the aid of a human cadaver (real or virtual) or anatomical photographs or illustrations. You are now sitting in class, listening to your anatomy professor read aloud from text written by Galen 200 years earlier. This should put into perspective any challenges you might be having today in your modern medical school's gross anatomy or neuroanatomy course.

Much time and energies during the Middle Ages are committed to reconciling differences between the natural (physical) models used to understand neurological function, embraced by the Greeks and Romans during early-Antiquity with the supranatural (deity, faith-based) models proposed by organized religions during mid and late-Antiquity. Proponents of both models are equally self-assured, their position is absolutely correct and the opposing position is absolutely wrong. Recall, the Greeks and Romans traditionally approach discovery by means of an empirical process, accumulating and amassing a practical compendium of information from which to understand normal and impaired health. This stands in contrast to the new alternative which emphasizes faith based belief in a supranatural deity. Both conceptual matrixes assign primary cause for neurological disease and impaired neurological function (natural vs supranatural), define fundamental approaches to discovery (empirical observation vs faith), and offer a rational approach to understand, diagnose, treat, and manage individuals suffering neurological disease or impairment (physics vs faith).

By the end of the Middle Ages, several new medical schools are founded throughout Europe. The first and most prestigious are founded in Italy and France. Each medical school quickly formalizes its medical school curriculum, affiliates with a university, and adopts preferred philosophical principles which guide their medical education program content, process, training, and methods applied to generate new knowledge.

By way of example, consider the Salerno School of Medicine, founded during the early-800s AD, on the coast of southeastern Italy, approximately 38 miles southeast of Naples.

The Salerno School of Medicine is the first modern medical school established in Europe. The School has its origins as a Benedictine monastery dispensary and hospital. Formalized education and training of future physicians is established by the late-800s AD. The medical curriculum and training is based upon the writings of Hippocrates and Galen. The School offers a liberal atmosphere, which embraces diversity and opportunity for many and encourages original thought. The School admits students without regard to national origin, religion, cultural background, or financial resources. Women are admitted, a practice quite unusual for the period. Cultural and intellectual diversity is embraced, resulting in a medical school and medical center reaching the height of its prestige around 1100 AD and rivaling the medical center of Alexandria, Egypt, at the height of its prestige circa 300 BC.

Trivia: The first medical school founded in the United States (USA) is founded in 1765 and associated with the University of Pennsylvania. The first medical school in Canada is founded in 1824 and associated with the Montreal Medical Institute, which later becomes the Faculty of Medicine at McGill University.

In summary, the Middle Ages witness the fall of the Western Roman Empire and significant geopolitical, economic, and social change. Many of the original Greek and Roman manuscripts, tablets, and papyri, containing the record of past and current medical knowledge are carried to the Middle East by scholars fleeing persecution in Europe. The medical record is translated into languages of the Middle East, North Africa, and Latin. Ibn-Sin (aka Avicenna) offers his influential five volume, encyclopedia of medical knowledge "al-Qanun fi-al-Tibb" [The Canon of Medicine]. Europe and the Middle East are greatly influenced by organized religions, Judaism, Christianity, Catholicism, and Islam. Organized religions significantly influence the direction, methods, and conceptual matrix applied to understand neurological conditions. Emphasis moves from the natural (physical) models of the Greeks and Romans to faith based, supranatural (deity) models. Advancement of new neuroscience knowledge stalls, as organized religions exert their powers on governments and impose restrictions on investigations which reveal findings inconsistent with the teachings of the organized religions. Human dissections is prohibited.

Investigators funded by organized religions are encouraged to insure all new medical knowledge is consistent with the beliefs and teachings of organized religion.

Historic medical knowledge of the ancient civilizations of Mesopotamia, Egypt, Greece, and the collected world medical knowledge archived in the Libraries of Alexandria is reinterpreted and translated to better agree with faith-based conceptual matrixes of new organized religions. Scholasticism is introduced as an acceptable and preferred approach to acquiring new knowledge. The ventricular theory of localization of mental function is reintroduced by Thomas Aquinas, in efforts to reconcile the opposing conceptual matrixes of the natural philosophers of Greece and Roman with the supranatural, faith-based conceptual matrix of organized religion. Governments place restrictions on the practice of medicine, in efforts to insure practitioners receive proper formal training and supervision before offering services to the community. New medical schools are founded in Europe and associate with universities. The Medical School at Salerno is the first established in Europe and offers a liberal atmosphere, embracing student and faculty diversity, open mindedness, and commitment to excellence in clinical practice and research. The medical school in Salerno soon establishes itself as a world class center, much in the same fashion as Alexandria 1,400 years earlier. Mondino de Luzzi offers his human dissection manual, prepared specifically for medical students. Guido da Vigevano offers the first illustrated manuscript of the brain, spinal cord, and spinal nerves to accompany anatomy text and specifically prepared to facilitate learning by medical students.

Medical neuroscience stands on the threshold of radical changes to come, during the Italian and European Renaissances of the Early Modern Age.

Early Modern, 1400 AD - 1800 AD.

The Early Modern Age witnesses rapid advancements in the medical neurosciences. Functions are associated with newly discovered neuroanatomical structures. Galenian dogma is challenged and corrected. Ventricle models used to understand mental functions, such as cognition, memory, and imagination are replaced by models localizing these functions to the cerebral cortex. Books devoted specifically to the description of neurological disease and recommended treatments are printed and widely distributed throughout Europe. Many neuroanatomical structures and cerebral vessels are described, detailed, illustrated, and formally named e.g. hippocampus, substantia nigra, and the Circle of Willis. Stroke syndromes are understood to result from occlusion or hemorrhage of cerebral blood vessels. Models of neural transmission, emphasizing movement of "animal spirits" or "fine particles" through hollow tubes (nerves), are displaced by new models emphasizing bioelectricity as the primary means of neural transmission. Neurological diseases are organized into taxonomies, based upon observation of clinical presentations of signs and symptoms and similar to the new taxonomies applied to plants and animals e.g. kingdom, class, order, genus, and species. New vocabulary is introduced to describe new discoveries and facilitate communication between investigators. Advancements in technology e.g. the introduction of the microscope, offers opportunities to study the nervous systems at the microscopic level and reveals structures never observed before e.g. cross section of nerve fibers and the neuromuscular junction.

Medical neurosciences are once again making forward movements, rethinking, revising, challenging, and displacing medical dogma. New technologies and procedures are introduced and applied resulting in many new discoveries. The medical neurosciences return to the empirical, observational, experiential methodologies and establishes itself as a valued, contributing, scientific discipline.

Let us briefly review a few of the most influential people making significant contributions during the Early Modern Period and begin to understand how and why their contributions have influenced the development of modern medical neurosciences.

Leonardo da Vinci (1452-1519) Italian Renaissance polymath makes wax casts of the human cerebral ventricles and quickly recognizes the casts do not match anatomical drawings of the cerebral ventricles (1490-1492,1490,1490,1504-1507/1952)[43,44,45,46]. Rather than challenging medical dogma and the very popular ventricle theory (Cell doctrine) of localization of mental functions, he offers anatomically correct illustrations of the human cerebral ventricles and accommodatingly assigns the traditional functions memory, cognition, and imagination to each ventricle. Leonardo da Vinci contributes meaningfully to the advancement of medical neurosciences, offering for the first time anatomically correct illustrations of the human nervous systems. He leaves the debate as to the purpose and function of the cerebral ventricles to others.

Italian Renaissance artists contribute much to the understanding of human anatomy, perhaps more than the medical schools of the period. In the artists' efforts to embrace Naturalism, as an artistic painting style, artists observe with great detail the human form. Leonardo da Vinci alone is believed to have participated in the dissection of no less than 300 cadavers and generates approximately 1,500 anatomical drawings, associated with these dissections. Many errors in understanding of human anatomy are exposed by the artists. Remember, human dissection has been prohibited by the Church and government for the proceeding 1,300 years. Only with the open-minded advancements now being achieved in Italy, during the mid-1300s to late-1500s, are long held medical dogma challenged by new information.

Niccolo Massa (1488-1569) Italian anatomist offers one of the first clear account and complete description of cerebral spinal fluid (CSF) and its presence within the cerebral ventricles (1536)[47]. He identifies the liquid state of CSF and its location deep within the cerebral hemispheres' ventricles. Niccolo Massa's paper proves influential in understanding the physical causes of hydrocephalus and changes treatment interventions directed to the treatment and management of hydrocephalic conditions.

At the time Niccolo Massa offers his CSF paper, the scientific and medical communities continue to embrace Galenian dogma. Galen describes the content of the ventricles to be vapors of purified "animal spirit" (aka "psychic pneuma") produced by the "rcte mirabile". The vaporous "animal spirts" are stored in the cerebral ventricles and when needed move through hollow nerves to move sensory information from a person's external environment to the brain for sensations or from the ventricles through hollow nerves to skeletal muscle to initiate and maintain movement. The "animal spirit" stored in the cerebral ventricles additionally carry waste products from the brain through the pituitary gland, for discharge from the body, through the nose as "pituita" (173AD/ 1968,177AD/1956)[25,26].

Trivia: The term "pituitary" originates from the Latin word "pituita", when translated means "phlegm" (2016)[48].

Prior to Niccolo Massa's description of the contents of the cerebral ventricles in 1536, investigators speculate as to their contents, air, vacuum, vapors, or water. Speculation is required, in the absence of the opportunity for physical inspection, given the restrictive sanctions against human dissection imposed by governments and organized religion during the preceding 1,200 years.

Niccolo Massa emphatically rejects all models attributing sensation, perception, cognition, memory, or body movement to the brain ventricles. So begins the challenge to Galenian dogma and ventricle models (Cell doctrine) of localization of perception, cognition, and memory to the cerebral ventricles (1536)[47].

Andreas Vesalius (1514-1564) Belgium anatomist, offers his landmark publication "De Humani Corporis Fabrica" [On the fabric of the human body], working as a Professor of Anatomy at the University of Padua, located in northern Italy, approximately 25 miles west of Venice (1543)[49]. This publication is based largely upon human dissections conducted at the University of Padua. Andreas Vesalius unapologetically proclaims numerous errors in descriptions and illustrations of the human brain and nervous systems, which have been held as medical dogma since the time of Galen, spanning 1500 years. Vesalius claims to have identified no less than 200 anatomical errors in Galen writings (1952,2001)[50,51]. Among the many errors actually discovered or claimed to be discovered by Vesalius, perhaps the one most frequently and popularly attributed to Vesalius is his self-proclaimed observation, the "rete mirabile" does not exist in man. In fact, Vesalius is not first to make this observation. Jacopo da Carpi (1460-1530) Italian anatomist is first to report the absence of "rete mirabile" in humans, thirteen years earlier and before Andreas Vesalius makes his claim of first discovery (1530)[52]. And so it goes…

Recall, the "rete mirabile", an anatomical structure identified and described by Galen, is a structure complex of arteries and veins found in numerous vertebrates, which according to Galen permits the mixing of "animal spirits" with life giving and life sustaining "vital spirits". Today, approximately 2000 years later, the "rete mirabile" is recognized to functions as a metabolic heat exchanger. For example, in ducks, the legs and webbed feet have a "rete mirabile" which allows transfer of heat from arterial blood to the cooler incoming venous blood, providing a useful heat exchanger, allowing the ducks feet and legs to remain close to ambient temperature, thereby reducing heat loss.

Andreas Vesalius, as a student attending medical school at the University of Paris, challenges his major anatomy professor Jacques Dubois (aka Jacobus Sylvius) (1478-1555). Vesalius brashly rejects conventional ideas and the dogmatic beliefs of the established academic medical community of Paris. As a consequence of his open and brash challenges, the faculty first attempt to have him conform and accept the well-established medical dogma taught at the medical school. When he refuses to conform and abandon his unconventional ideas, he is ostracized by the faculty and fellow students. Soon he transfers to the more open-minded University of Padua in Italy and completes his medical education. He is soon offered a faculty position in the Department of Anatomy at the University of Padua.

The point here is Vesalius' experience offers another example in the history of the medical neurosciences of the resistance by established authorities to change when dogma is challenged and the potential consequences to anyone who dares to challenge the established facts of the day. Are you willing to challenge medical dogma? Are you willing to suffer the potential consequences for doing so?

Jacques Dubois is adamant and vocal in his discontentment with his student (Vesalius) "…I urge you to pay no attention to a certain ridiculous madman, one utterly lacking in talent who curses and inveighs impiously against his teacher …Let no one give heed to that very ignorant and arrogant man, who, through his ignorance, ingratitude, impudence, and impiety denies everything his deranged or feeble vision cannot locate…" (1551,1964)[53,54]. Vesalius counters with the bold statement he was never better able to see more clearly than when he removed himself from the blinding Galenian indoctrination he received while in Paris. He states if he had not rejected the indoctrination in Paris he would have never discovered the truths of the inter-workings of the human body.

If you as a medical student, resident, or young faculty member choose to challenge established medical dogma, be prepared to bear the criticism and slings and arrows from those who find comfort and ease in their acceptance of medical dogma, as you pioneer newer truths.

Note: Jacques Dubois (aka Jacobus Sylvius) (1478-1555) French, Professor of Anatomy at the University of Paris is not Franz de la Boe (aka Franciscus Sylvius) (1614-1672) German/Dutch, Professor of Anatomy at Leiden University. Both men are anatomist. Jacques Dubois (Jacobus Sylvius) is born about 100 years before Franz de la Boe (Franciscus Sylvius). Both make meaningful contributions to the field of anatomy.

Jacques Dubois is responsible for naming many of the familiar muscles you memorized in your gross anatomy course e.g. biceps, triceps, serrati, and naming many of the blood vessels e.g. femoral, popliteal, jugular, subclavian, renal, spermatic, superior and inferior mesenteric. Before assigning names to specific muscles, muscles were simply numbered by anatomists. Jacques Dubois encourages medical students to learn anatomy by way of dissection and physical examination of anatomical structures, rather than reading about anatomical structures in textbooks or hearing about the structures in a medical school lecture hall (1555)[55]. He offers at least one manuscript outlining the suggested daily routine for all medical students, in order to remain healthy and maximize their opportunities for learning, while in medical school (1530,1962)[56,57]. Many of the same recommendations might well be offered to you by your own medical school faculty today.

Jason Pratensis (1486-1558) Dutch physician, offers the first printed book devoted specifically to neurological disease, "De Cerebi Morbis" (1549)[58]. Thirty-three chapters discuss symptom complexes of tremors, epilepsies, vertigo, tetanus, memory loss, headaches, and more. This book is largely a review of Greek, Roman, and Arabic approaches to understanding neurological diseases through observation of clinical signs and patient reported symptoms. The book offers little new information. The book emphasizes the important role of the brain in all sensory and motor functions and disruption of brain effects sensory and motor functions. The book reflects a return to the natural (physical) models used to understand the nervous systems offered by the Greeks and Romans of Antiquity, rather than the supranatural (faith-based, deity) models popularized by organized religions, during the early-Middle Ages.

Medical neuroscience continues to develop and establish itself as a specialized branch of medicine and scientific investigations, requiring specialized knowledge and training. New terminology is required and introduced into the professional and scientific literatures. Specialized journals devoted specifically to the scientific investigation and clinical practice of the medical neurosciences begin to appear.

Giulio Aranzi (1530-1589) Italian anatomist of Bologna, describes and coins the now familiar term "hippocampus" to describe bilateral nuclei located deep inside the temporal lobes of the cerebral hemispheres. The term "hippocampus" is derived from the Greek "hippo" meaning "horse" and "kampos" meaning "sea monster". He first uses the term in his book of anatomical observations "Observationes anatomicae libre" (1579)[59] and subsequently in his book on his observations of the human fetus "Observationes Anatomicicae: De humano foetu liber" (1587)[60].

A brief reading of Giulio Aranzi's original description quickly leaves one wondering what he is actually trying to describe. How does this structure resemble a sea-horse? At least one professor of anatomy has unapologetically commented, this is perhaps the worst anatomical description ever (1923)[61]. If you or your neuroscience professor cannot see the "sea-horse" you are not alone. Throughout history, many have expressed frustration in their inability to see the "sea horse". The fact is, the structure does not look like a "sea-horse", unless you dissect the brain in a very specific and somewhat unique manner, as did Swedish neuroanatomist Gustav Retzius (see Plate XLVI) (1896)[62,63]. Now and only now can you begin to see what Aranzi saw over 440 years ago.

Rene Descartes (1596-1650) French mathematician and philosopher describes the pineal gland as the control center of body and where thoughts are formed (1649,1664)[64,65]. Recall, today we recognize the pineal gland as a single midline structure, located in the back of the midbrain, behind the third ventricle, and functions as an endocrine gland, releasing primarily melatonin. The primary functional result is regulation of sleep-awake cycles and seasonal and circadian rhythms (2013)[66].

Descartes offers a rational model, built around the location and presumed function of the pineal gland to explain body sensations, movement, and human emotions. The model conceptualizes the physical body as a mechanical apparatus and therefore all of the natural laws of physics apply. The model explains sensation, movement, emotions, and sleep-wakefulness.

The model in brief states the pineal gland is mechanically stimulated by sensory systems, causing the gland to vibrate. The vibration of the pineal gland gives rise to somato-sensations, movement, and emotions. Somato-sensations e.g. hot, cold, pain, vibration, touch result when materials inside of neural tubes (peripheral nerves) resonate in response to sensory stimulation. These resonating materials are responsible for the mechanical transmission of sensory signals to the brain. At the brain, resonating signals are transduced into conscious sensory experiences e.g. pain or movement. Movement results when resonating sensory transmissions received by the brain open valves located in the walls of the cerebral ventricles and allow movement of cerebral spinal fluid (CSF) from the cerebral ventricles into neural tubes (peripheral nerves). Vibrations of the pineal gland generates vibrations of materials inside of neural tubes, which mechanically transmit vibrations to peripheral muscles, resulting in movement. Graduated movements are dependent upon the frequencies of resonation (1649,1664)[64,65].

Similarly, human emotions result when resonating material contained within sensory neural tubes reach the brain and stimulate the brain. Resonations at different frequencies generate different emotions. Resonating vibrations within the brain are then transmitted through neural tubes to the body's extremities, resulting in physical movement and observable reactions to internal human emotions (1649,1664)[64,65].

Rene Descartes offers an additional model, also dependent upon the pineal gland, within which to understand sleep and wakefulness. Briefly, when one is awake, "animal spirits" flow through the brain causing the brain to distend. When one is asleep, less "animal spirits" flow through the brain, thereby reducing brain volume. The pineal gland by its nature of location exerts regulation and control of "animal spirits" (1649,1664)[64,65].

The mid-1600s witness continuing advancements in the identification and description of normal neuroanatomical structures. Interests increase in applying this new knowledge to better understand clinical presentations of abnormal neurological functions associated with neurological disease and trauma.

Franz de la Boe (aka Franciscus Sylvius) (1614-1672) German/Dutch anatomist is most recognized for his descriptions and naming of neuroanatomical structures e.g. the septum pellucidum (septum between the two lateral cerebral ventricles), dural venous sinus (sinuses between layers of dura mater which channel venous blood and CSF away from the brain), lateral cerebral fissures (cerebral fissures separating the cerebral temporal lobe from the frontal and parietal lobes) (1641)[67]. He additionally introduces the term "aqueduct of Sylvius" to label the channel located in the posterior brainstem, allowing movement of CSF from the third cerebral ventricle down into the fourth ventricle, although this structure and its associated function had been well known, at the time Sylvius introduces the term "aqueduct of Sylvius". For example, Niccolo Massa (1536)[47] describes the structure and function over 100 years before Sylvius names the structure after himself.

Johannes Wepfer (1620-1695) Swiss pathologist describes all major cerebral arteries in detail. He identifies the two internal carotid arteries and the two vertebral arteries as the primary arterial blood supplies to the brain. He is first to attribute and document post-mortem, pathologies of cerebral blood vessels result in stroke syndromes (1658,1658/1704)[68,69]. In his book, "Observationes Anatomicae", he describes a series of four patients presenting with clinical stroke syndromes and upon post-mortem examination of the brains, reveal evidence of brain cerebral blood vessel hemorrhage and vessel occlusions. He correctly associates these two general vascular pathologies to the stroke syndromes and explains the stroke syndrome signs and symptoms within the matrix of the current understanding of neuroanatomical structures and associated function (1658,1658/1704)[68,69].

Thomas Willis (1621-1675) English, Professor of Natural Philosophy at Oxford University is perhaps most remembered by medical students as the person describing and illustrating the network of arterial blood vessels located as the base of the brain, termed the Circle of Willis. Thomas Willis does not discovered the "Circle", is not the first person to describe it, nor does he assign his name to the "Circle". The "Circle of Willis" is known for over 1,500 years before Thomas Willis offers his description. Galen identifies this network of cerebral vessels and assigns function. These are the cerebral blood vessels Galen refers to when discussing the "rete mirabile" (173 AD)[70]. Many others before Willis also describe and illustrate this network of blood vessels and attribute varying functions. For example, Guilio Casserus (1552-1616) Italian anatomist offers a clear illustration of the "Circle of Willis" in his influential human anatomical atlas, Plate X, published post humously (1627)[71]. Johannes Wepfer describes the "Circle of Willis" six years before Thomas Willis publishes his description and includes English architect, astronomer, and medical student Christopher Wren's drawing of the "Circle of Willis (1658,1658/1704,1664, 1681)[68,69,72,73]. The term "Circle of Willis" is coined 110 years later by Swiss anatomist Albrecht von Haller (1708-1777) (1774)[74].

Thomas Willis offers more meaningful and influential contributions to medical neurosciences. He directly challenges the medical dogma of the doctrine of ventricular localization of mental and cognitive functions. He offers instead a new model localizing cognitive processes to the cerebral cortex and intellectual resources e.g. memories to cortical gray and subcortical white matter structures (1664,1672/1683)[72,75]. Willis views the cerebral ventricles as nothing more than the catchment structure for waste products produced by the brain. He localizes the primary anatomical structures responsible for voluntary movement to be the basal nuclei and cortex of the cerebral hemispheres. He localizes involuntary movements to the cerebellar hemispheres. Thomas Willis offers a conceptual model which emphasizes association of function with each anatomical structure and organizing cognitive processes and behaviors into an ordered hierarchical system.

Thomas Willis embraces new technologies and new procedures to advance the study of the human brain and nervous systems. He is among the first to routinely inject dyes into anatomical structures and follow the dye as it is forced through anatomical structures e.g. blood vessels, cerebral ventricles. He uses microscopy and determines nerves are not hollow and instead filled with fine string like material running the entire length of the nerve.

New and developing disciplines require new terms and vocabulary to describe new discoveries, new concepts, and to facilitate communications between professionals. So too is the case with the medical neurosciences. Thomas Willis contributes several new and now familiar terms. For example, he introduces terms for the large paired basal nuclei structure (corpus striatum), as well as cerebral hemispheres, and cerebellar hemispheres. Perhaps the most noted new term introduced by Thomas Willis is that of "neurologie", the term originally introduced to describe the study of nerves and distinguishing this study from the study and investigation of central nervous system structures brain, brainstem, cerebellum, and spinal cord (1664)[72]. This term is translated into English as "neurology" 17 years later, as it appears in Samuel Pordage's English translation of Thomas Willis' book "Cerebi Anatome" (1664,1681)[72,73]. By the end of the 1700s the term's original restriction to the study of nerves is abandoned and the term soon includes the study of all elements of the nervous systems. The term is subsequently adopted to describe the medical sub-discipline committed to the assessment, diagnosis, and treatment of neurological conditions.

Thomas Willis offers several early descriptions of now familiar neurological conditions, for example myasthenia gravis (1667,1672/1683)[76,77]. Recall, myasthenia gravis today, over 345 years since first described by Willis is known to be a chronic autoimmune disorder in which the patient's immune system attacks cholinergic receptors located on skeletal muscles. The characteristic and consequential result is weakness experienced by the patient. The weakness increases with activity and improves following periods of rest. The term "myasthenia gravis" is derived from the Greek meaning "grave muscle weakness".

Below is an expert from Thomas Willis book, published in 1672, describing one of his patients, whom is most likely suffering from the condition "myasthenia gravis".

> "…There is another kind of this disease depending on the scarcity and fewness of the spirits, in which the motion fails wholly in no part or member, yet it is performed weakly only, or depravedly by any; those who be in trouble with a scarcity of spirits, are able at first rising in the morning to walk, move their arms this way and that, or to lift up a weight with strength; but before noon, the stores of spirits which influenced the muscles being almost spent, they are scarce able to move hand or foot. I have now a prudent and honest woman in cure, who for many years has been obnoxious to this kind of bastard palsy not only in the limbs, but likewise in her tongue; this person for some time speaks freely and readily enough, but after long, hasty, or laborious speaking, she becomes mute as a fish and cannot bring forth a word, nay, and does not recover the use of her voice till after an hour or two…" (1672/1683)[77].

Thomas Sydenham (1624-1689) English physician, perhaps most remembered by medical students today as the person who first describes an acute, self-limiting, choreiform movement disorder, most often evident in children between 5-15 years of age, appearing three time more often in females than males, associated with rheumatic fever, often appearing following strep throat infection (Group A beta hemolytic streptococci bacteria), and typically resulting in complete recovery from abnormal movements within one to two months after onset of the abnormal choreiform movements.

Thomas Sydenham originally describes the condition:

> "…There is a kind of convulsion, which attacks boys and girls from the tenth year to the time of puberty. It first shows itself by limping or unsteadiness in one of the legs, which the patient drags. The hand cannot be steady for a moment. It passes from one position to another by a convulsive movement, however much the patient may strive to the contrary. Before he can raise a cup to his lips, he does make as many gesticulations as a mountebank; since he does not move it in a straight line, but has his hand drawn aside by the spasms, until by some good fortune he brings it at last to his mouth. He then gulps it off at once, so suddenly and so greedily as to look as if he were trying to amuse the lookers-on…" (1686)[78].

Today, approximately 330 years after Thomas Sydenham first describes the condition, which he terms "chorea minor"(1686)[78], we understand the movement disorder to result from an antibody cross-reaction to the neuronal cell wall membranes of basal nuclei structures (molecular mimicry). The body's immune system disrupts the normal function of the child's basal nuclei, inhibiting movements at rest, thereby resulting in the characteristic movement disorder. Thomas Sydenham refers to the abnormal movement disorder as "chorea minor" and "Saint Vitus dance". It is not until the late-1800s, almost 200 years after his death, is the condition increasingly referred to as the "chorea of Sydenham" (1878)[79].

Trivia: The term "chorea" originates from the Ancient Greek word "choreia" meaning "to dance". The term "Saint Vitus" dance originates from the traditional, medieval practice of dancing in front of statues of the Roman Catholic patron Saint Vitus, in annual celebration of his ultimate battle against Roman, anti-Christian government rule, circa 300 AD. According to the Catholic faith, Saint Vitus is the patron Saint of epileptics, children suffering Saint Vitus dance (Sydenham's chorea), dancers, actors, and the protector against storms.

While Sydenham is most associated with the movement disorder which now bears his name, he really is not interested in movement disorders. Sydenham's primary professional interests are found in fevers, gout, and nosology. He publishes three major works addressing each primary area of interest (1666,1676,1683)[80,81,82].

Sydenham approaches the diagnosis and treatment of neurological conditions from a common sense approach. He uniformly rejects traditional humor models and Galenian dogma. He rejects the use of invasive pathological procedures such as human dissection and equally rejects the use of new technologies e.g. microscopy, due to firmly held religious beliefs. He embraces instead the ideals of Hippocrates and argues in favor of the physician providing support and comfort to patients, allowing nature to take its course and heal the patient. He encourages bedside examination and careful observation as primary tools of the practicing physician. Thomas

Sydenham offers one of the early classification systems of disease, based upon observation of clinical signs and patient report of symptoms (1676)[81].

Domenico Mistichelli (1625-1715) Italian physician embraces traditional doctrines of humors models and Galenian dogma when he reports his observations, in his treaties on apoplexy (stroke syndromes), proclaiming when a lesion occurs in one cerebral hemisphere, the patient will reveal motor impairment on the side of the body opposite to the side of the lesion (1709)[83]. He observes and reports fibers responsible for controlling movement decusate at the level of the medulla and can be observed by visual inspection on the front of the medulla. Here is an excerpt from the English translation from the original Italian text;

> "…if on the right side of the …cerebral hemisphere of the cerebrum, or the extension of the medulla oblongata, through oppressive humors, or through convulsions, strangulation, or some other defect, the transit of the animal liquid (vital spirit) through very interstices is impeded, it will soon happen the arm or leg or other left part, with which those nerve filaments are in agreement, will remain either convulsed or paralyzed, or deprived of sensation and motion, because the nerves of those parts do not receive the necessary supply of spirit from the opposed part that has been injured…" (1709,1996)[83,84].

The observation that a lesion of the cerebral hemisphere often results in contralateral loss of sensory and/or motor function is nothing new. These observations are made during Antiquity and documented by Greek/Roman anatomists Cassius (circa 150AD/1841)[85] and Aretaeus (circa 150AD/1856)[86], approximately 1,600 years before Mistichelle offers his observations (1709)[83].

What is important here is not so much Domenico Mistichelli's description of the decussation of the motor pathways, which are believed to be tubes, allowing for the movement of "vital spirits" through the body, resulting in mechanical body movement. Rather, what is important is the adherence to Galenian dogma and the doctrine of humors model to explain clinical presentation of neurological impairments. Balance of humors and mechanical models continue to be used well into the mid-1600s to explain neurological conditions and their associated impairments in sensation, movement, and cognition.

Alexander Monro (secundus) (1733-1817) Scottish anatomist describes the anatomical channels connecting the left and right lateral cerebral ventricles to the single midline third ventricle, allowing flow of cerebral spinal fluid down through the ventricular system. He offers his observations in a paper he reads to the Philosophical Society of Edinburgh, describing the blockage of these channels, in a case of a three year old boy suffering hydrocephalus (1764)[87]. The boy is examined at autopsy by Monro's elder brother, physician Donald Monro (1728-1802) and Robert Whytt (1714-1766). Autopsy findings reveal blockage of CSF flow through the ventricular system, resulting in the condition, non-communicating hydrocephalus. Alexander Monro offers a more complete description of this important neuroanatomical condition and associated clinical presentation nineteen years later, in his atlas of human and comparative neurology titled, "Observations on the structure and function of the nervous system" (1783)[88]. The inter-ventricular channels, connecting the two lateral channels with the single mid-line third ventricle, are known as the foramina of Monro, in recognition of Monro's anatomical descriptions of the foramina and the pathologies which result when the foramina are obstructed.

Trivia: Scottish physician family Alexander Monro (primus) (1697-1767), Alexander Monro (secundus) (1733-1817), and Alexander Monro (tertius) (1773-1859) collectively hold the Chair of

Anatomy at the University of Edinburgh for three consecutive generations, spanning 126 years (2012)[89].

Medical neurosciences are continuing to develop and mature as a specialized discipline. Advancements and refinements in technologies now permit examination of the nervous systems at levels previously impossible. Improvements in lens technologies and microscope technologies contribute significantly to the movement of medical neurosciences into the exciting and new world of the microscopic examination and study of the human nervous systems.

Antony van Leeuwenhoek (1632-1723) Dutch, non-physician, non-scientist, and textile retailer, offers the necessary development in lens technologies which permit movement of the medical neurosciences into the microscopic world. He offers to the Royal Society one of the first descriptions of a nerve fiber, in cross-section, viewed under the lens of a microscope (1675)[90].

Herman Boerhaave (1668-1738) Dutch, Professor of Medicine at Leiden University provides medical neurosciences its first illustration of the neuromuscular junction (1735)[91]. Boerhaave proposes muscle contract when fluid, within nerve fibers, moves from the nerve into the muscle. The transfer of fluid occurs at the neuromuscular junction. The increase of fluid inside of the muscle shortens the muscle and thereby results in movement (1735)[91].

Dutch microscopist Jan Swammerdam (1637-1680) completes a series of physiology experiments, published posthumously, which unequivocally demonstrate muscles do not contract as the result of an influx of fluid from connecting nerve fibers or any other fluid source (1738)[92]. The whole hydraulic - mechanical model of movement as offered by Galen, Rene Descartes, and Herman Boerhaave, embraced as medical dogma for over 1,500 years is now brought back into question. Could Galen, Descartes, Boerhaave and others possibly be wrong?

New conceptual models begin to appear and are rigorously tested, in efforts to understand the biological mechanisms responsible for movement. Fifty years of additional investigations, major development and refinements in essential technologies, and an intellectual willingness by some investigators to boldly question medical dogma, begins to answer fundamental questions regarding movement. The answer, bioelectricity (1791)[93]. This discovery opens new doorways of investigation and establishes the foundation upon which the modern conceptualization of neural transmission will build for the next 225 years.

Advancements continue to be made in neuroanatomy during the late-1700s. Advancements are being made at both the gross and microscopic levels. Cranial nerves (CN) are organized into the now familiar 12 pair CN system; nuclei deep inside of the brain and brainstem are identified and detailed e.g. locus ceruleus, substantia nigra, caudate, putamen, and globus pallidus; the cerebral cortex is recognized to be heterogeneous in its cytoarchitectural structure; channels connecting cerebral ventricles are identified; and peripheral nerve fibers are described at 700x magnification power, detailing the inside of neural fibers unlike at any other time in history.

Samuel von Sommerring (1755-1830) German anatomist restructures and modifies existing cranial nerves (CN) organizational systems. He proposes a 12 pairs CN classification system. The CN classification system proposed by von Sommerring, as a 23 year old medical student in his doctoral dissertation while studying at the University of Gottingen (Germany), over 240 years ago is the system still used today (1778)[94].

As with most classifications systems, the CN systems have been revised multiple times, through the course of time. For example years before von Sommerring, Galen and Andreas Vesalius offer their CN classification system based upon only 7 pairs of CNs (1543)[95]; Gabriel Fallopius proposes a system based upon 8 pairs of CNs (1561)[96]; Thomas Willis proposes a system based upon 9 pairs of CNs (1664)[72]; and Bartolomeo Eustachi offers his classification system of CN based on 10 pairs of CN (1552,1714)[97,98].

Trivia: Samuel von Sommerring publishes a popular and influential paper titled "On the injurious effect of tight lacing of the corset" (1793)[99]. The paper identifies the health hazards of compressing ribs and internal organs, for the sole purpose of achieving the highly fashionable, female hour glass silhouette of the period. The paper is quickly translated into several languages, becomes a best seller, and impacts women's fashion throughout Europe. You can view online images of the illustrations published in this paper and made available by the National Library of Medicine (2002)[100].

Felix Vicq d'Azyr (1748-1794) French anatomist organizes the cerebral hemispheres according to lobes, gyri and fissures; he describes the heterogeneity in cerebral cortex cytoarchitectural structure; differentiates white matter into three primary fiber bundle types (commissures, association, and projection fibers), and identifies major paired basal nuclei structures (caudate, putamen, globus pallidus) (1786)[101]. Two years earlier he identifies the locus ceruleus ("the blue spot") and substantia nigra ("the black substance") nuclei (1784)[102]. Felix Vicq d' Azyr advocates a functional approach to investigating anatomy, proposing a suspected or demonstrated primary function should be identified and associated with each anatomical structure. The functional-anatomical approach guides medical neuroanatomical investigations for the next 200 years.

Felice Fontani (1730-1805) Italian anatomist describes the anatomy of the direct and consensual pupillary light reflexes (1765)[103]. Two years later he describes the small trabecular meshwork located at the iris-cornea angle, which drains aqueous humor form the anterior chamber of the eye into the venous sinus of the sclera (spaces of Fontani; aka canal of Schlemm) (1767a)[104].

Felice Fontana utilizes recent advancements in microscope technologies and describes the gross and microscopic anatomy of peripheral nerves and central nervous system white matter tracts, noting their similar characteristics and functions.

> "…The basic structure of nerves is as follows: a nerve is formed of a large number of transparent, uniform, and simple cylinders. These cylinders seem to be fashioned like a very thin, uniform wall of tunic which is filled, as far as one can see, with transparent, gelatinous fluid insoluble in water. Each of these cylinders receives a cover in the form of an outer sheath…Several of these nerves together for the larger nerves…I am fully convenience by my own observations, which I repeated many times with the same result, that the cylinders I have described are the simple and first organic elements of nerves, for I never succeeded in dividing them further, no matter what investigation I carried out with the help of the sharpest and finest needles…" (1781)[105].

Using a single lens microscope capable of 700 x magnification, he correctly describes structures and substances within the neuron and the myelin producing cells surrounding neurons. His observations lead him to reject popular models of neural transmission e.g. vibrations models proposed by Herman Boerhaave and Alexander Monro which state sensory information is carried mechanically through the vibration of substances contained within the nerve, from peripheral sensory receptors to the brain, and traditional Cartesian models proposed by Descartes and others which state fine particles originating from animal spirits contained in blood, physically move through the nerve and are exuded from the nerve, resulting in a mechanical hydraulic effect on the brain (sensory system) or muscle (motor system) (1767b,1781)[106,105].

Given the evidence presented by Felice Fantana, an alternative model is needed to explain neural transmission. Ten years later, Italian anatomist Luigi Galvani provides a reasonable alternative model and conceptual matrix within which to understand neural transmission. Bioelectricity (1791)[93].

Luigi Aloysii Galvani (1737-1798) Italian anatomist offers experimental data and changes the conceptual model within which to understand neuronal transmission of information. He rejects medical dogma of 1,500 years and introduces data which revolutionize the way in which neural transmission is understood. Galvani states simply, transmission of information along nerve fibers is accomplished by bioelectricity (1791)[107]. "Animal spirits" and "fine particles" become bioelectricity. Technologies to measure small bioelectrical currents in tissues develop over the next fifty years. Experimental investigations into "animal electricity", the term used by Galvani, soon develop into the foundational studies upon which modern electrophysiology will build.

Trivia: Luigi Galvani and Antonio Scarpa (1752-1832) Italian anatomist and colleagues (yes, the same Scarpa you remember from your gross anatomy course as Scarpa's fascia) engage in one of the many passionate and heated professional debates regarding priority of discovery and failure to acknowledge others. Available records strongly suggest Antonio Scarpa claims priory of discovery for many discoveries reported by Luigi Galvani. Specifics claims focus primarily upon structures of the inner ear (1772,1783)[108,109]. The debate is never resolved during the two men's lifetime and remain open today, over 245 years later. So goes another example, in the history of medicine, of brilliant investigators committing much time, energies, and professional resources to managing claims for priority of discovery.

In summary, the Early Modern period is a period of tremendous growth and development for the medical neurosciences. Many new and now familiar anatomical structures are identified and associated with function e.g. the hippocampus (memory) and substantia nigra (muscle tone and inhibition of movement). Galenian dogma is challenged, corrected, and many times simply replaced. The cerebral cortex is clearly identified as the primary anatomical location for neural activities resulting in sensations, perceptions, movement, and higher order functions, language, memory, and cognition. Old models which have explained neural transmission of information for over 1,800 years are displaced by new models emphasizing neural transmission by way of bioelectricity. Neurological disorders are organized into a systematized taxonomy. Tools and technologies are significantly improved e.g. microscope. New vocabulary is introduced and facilitates communication between investigators and clinical practitioners. Medical neurosciences return to the physical (natural) origins to understand and explain impaired neurological functioning. Progress once again is being made in advancing the medical and scientific knowledge base of the medical neurosciences.

Of particular note and in summary, eighteen individuals and their contributions exemplify progress throughout the Early Modern Period, 1400 AD -1800 AD.

During the 1400s and 1500s, Leonardo da Vinci offers anatomically correct illustrations of the human nervous systems. Niccolo Massa describes CSF, cerebral ventricles, and offers a new understanding as to the origins and treatment of hydrocephalus. Andreas Vesalius offers his "De Humani Corpus Fabrica" based on human dissection, identifies no less than 200 anatomical errors revealed by dissection of the human body, and ostracized by established medical school faculty for challenging medical dogma. Jacques Dubois (Jacobus Sylvius) describes and names many now familiar muscle groups and blood vessels e.g. biceps, triceps, femoral, popliteal muscles; subclavian arteries, jugular veins, and proclaims human dissection to be essential for all medical students when learning anatomy. Franz de la Boe (Francious Sylvius) describes and name now familiar neuroanatomical structures e.g. septum pallucidum, dural sinuses, aqueduct of Sylvius, and lateral cerebral fissures (Sylvian fissures). Jason Pratensis offers the first printed book devoted specifically to neurological diseases, devoting chapters to tremors, epilepsies, vertigo, memory loss, headaches and other commonly occurring neurological disorders. Giulio Aranzi describes and coins the term hippocampus.

During the 1600s, Rene Descartes details the pituitary gland and places it at the center of his new model to explain normal and abnormal neurological functions. Johannes Wepfer details cerebral blood vessels and associates specific vessels with specific stroke syndromes. Thomas Willis challenges the ventricular model of localization of cerebral function and proposes an alternative emphasizing the roles of the cerebral cortex, basal nuclei, and cerebellum. Thomas Willis details several neurological disorders e.g. myasthenia gravis and introduces the term "neurologie" into the professional literature. Thomas Sydenham describes his chorea, details conditions associated with fevers, extensively investigates gout, and offers original insights into a new diagnostic nosology, built upon careful clinical observation of patient signs and symptoms.

During the 1700s, Domenico Mistichelli reiterates findings first reported over 1,600 years earlier that cerebral vascular disorders effecting a single cerebral hemisphere will result in contralateral deficits. Domenico Mistichelli perpetuates traditional Galenian dogma explaining all normal and abnormal neurological functions within a matrix of a mechanical - balance of humors model. Antony van Leeuwenhoek offers greatly improved lens for use in microscopes, revolutionizing the study of the nervous systems. Herman Boerhaave illustrates the neuromuscular junction. Jan Swammerdam successfully challenges the 1,500 year dogma of Galen and Descartes, demonstrating experimentally, movement is not the result of hydraulic-mechanical processes, rather it is bioelectrical signaling which is responsible for the contraction of muscle groups and consequential movements. Samuel von Sommerring proposes the 12 pair organization of cranial nerves and draws attention to the dramatic, non-healthy, physical consequences of wearing high fashion clothing. Felix Vicq d'Azyr organizes the brain into the now familiar lobes, gyri, and fissures, differentiates three types of white matter tracts, the commissures, projection fibers, and association fibers, describes the cytoarchitectural structure of the cerebral cortex, identifies important paired nuclei e.g. substantia nigra and locus ceruleus, describes microscopic structures inside of neurons, and details the microscopic anatomy of peripheral nerves. Luigi Galvani revolutionizes the understanding of neural transmission by introducing and demonstrating bioelectricity as primary in transmission of sensory and motor information traveling through neurons.

Yes, the Early Modern Period, 1400 AD-1800 AD witness many important advancements in the medical neurosciences and prepares the discipline for many more advancements to be made during the Middle Modern Period. Hold on; things are about to get very interesting.

Middle Modern, 1800 AD - 1900 AD.

The 1800s embrace a rapidly growing interest in the medical neurosciences. The spinal cord is organized into functional systems e.g. motor systems are positioned primarily in the front of the spinal cord while sensory systems are positioned primarily in the back of the spinal cord. The anatomy of the cerebral ventricular system is developed and the channels responsible for flow of CSF from the ventricles into the subarachnoid space are identified. Pathologies associated with blockage of these channels, the midline foramen of Magendie or the two lateral foramina of Luschka, are explained within the matrix of impaired CSF flow through these channels. The source of CSF is correctly identified to be the choroid plexus.

The nervous systems are investigated at the microscopic level. The six cell layers of the cerebral cortex and three cell layers of the cerebellum are identified. Myelinated and unmyelinated neural fibers are identified and differentiated. Anterograde and retrograde degeneration of neural fibers following injury is explained. Organelles inside of the neuron are identified e.g. Nissl substance. Innovative cell staining techniques, development of the microtome, and improvements in microscope technologies greatly improved investigations of the nervous systems at the cellular and subcellular levels. Embryological and fetal developments of the nervous systems are investigated, resulting in the identification of neural crest cells and the tremendously important process of gastrulation.

The nervous system is now understood to be composed of interconnected cells. Two principal models of brain functioning are introduced and debated; the equipotentiality model which argues the brain functions as an indivisible whole and the localizationist model which argues the brain and brain functions can be localized to specific anatomical areas of the brain. Clinical pathologies are interpreted within the conceptual matrix of both models. Electrophysiology and innovative recording techniques are introduced and provide a new technology which allows for the study of neural systems in real time. Study of the nervous system is no longer restricted to anatomy and clinical observations.

Clinical observations however continue to be tremendously important in understanding brain-behavior relationships. Disorders and conditions familiar to all medical students today are described and systematically investigated e.g. Bell's palsy, Parkinson's disease, Huntington's disease, phantom limb phenomena, aphasia, multiple sclerosis (MS), and amyotrophic lateral sclerosis (ALS).

New instruments and clinical procedures are invented, developed, and refined allowing for improved bedside examination of the nervous systems. For example, the ophthalmoscope, tuning forks, and reflex hammer are introduced into the clinical examination of the nervous systems. Deep tendon reflex (DTR) testing is introduced, the neuroanatomy underlying the reflex arch explained, and the clinical value of DTR testing appreciated. The Romberg test is introduced for bedside examination of proprioceptive systems. Weber and Rinne tests are introduced to clinically assess hearing systems. Clinical signs are associated with specific underlying neuropathologies e.g. Babinski sign and Gower's sign.

New vocabulary is introduced to facilitate communication between investigators and define newly discovered structures, instruments, procedures, and findings. For example, the terms neuron, axon, dendrite, synapse, autonomic nervous system, action potential, electroencephalogram (EEG), reflex hammer, ophthalmoscope, deep tendon reflex (DTR), Bell's palsy, Broca's aphasia,

Wernicke's aphasia, and Babinski sign are all introduced into the professional literature during the 1800s.

New professional societies and associated professional journals committed to the advancement of medical neurosciences are founded. For example, in France the Societe de Neurologie de Paris and its journal "Le Revue Neurologie" and in Great Britain the Neurological Society of London and its journal "Brain" are two of the earliest professional organizations and journals committed specifically to the advancement of the medical neurosciences in Europe. Professional societies and associated journals in the USA and Canada will be founded later, in the 1900s.

"…Times are a changing…" for medical neurosciences. Let's take a brief look at some of the specific individuals and events which greatly influence the development of this rapidly developing specialty area within medicine.

Charles Bell (1774-1842) Scottish anatomist extends localization of brain functions to the spinal cord. He is particularly interested, as many before him, in the seemingly marked differences in functions evidenced by the cerebral hemispheres compared to the functions of the cerebellar hemispheres. Can these observed functional differences be extended into the spinal cord? He presents his early ideas in a small, self-published, limited edition pamphlet (approximately 100 copies) and distributes the pamphlet to friends and close colleagues (1811)[110].

In this pamphlet he organizes the spinal cord into two primary divisions. The anterior half of the spinal cord to which he attributes the functions of voluntary movement and somato-sensations (sic), noting these to be cerebral hemisphere functions and the posterior half of the spinal cord to which he attributes involuntary, reflexive, and visceral functions, noting these to be cerebellar hemisphere functions. While recognizing the anterior half of the spinal cord is essential to normal motor function, he fails to recognize the posterior half of the spinal cord is essential to normal somato-sensory functions. He reports stimulation of the anterior rootlets of the spinal cord produce convulsions, whereas stimulation of the posterior spinal rootlets produce no visible signs (1811)[110].

Given a retrospective review of Charles Bell's reported experiments and claims to priority of discovery that the anterior spinal rootlets carry neural signals essential for voluntary movement and the posterior spinal rootlets carry neural signals essential for somato-sensations, appear to me to be unjustified. Yes, Charles Bell is among the first to demonstrate the anterior half of the spinal cord is essential for normal voluntary movement and fails to recognize or demonstrate the essential somato-sensory functions of the posterior half of the spinal cord (1810,1811)[111,110].

Ten years later, French physiologist Francois Magendie of Bordeaux (1783-1855) publishes the definitive paper, differentiating the posterior rootlets into primary somato-sensory functions and the anterior rootlets into primary somato-motor functions (1822)[112]. Charles Bell quickly reinterprets his own findings and claims priority of discovery for identifying the motor function of the anterior spinal rootlets and the sensory functions of the posterior rootlets. An arguably significant modification from Bell's original interpretation reported in his 1811 pamphlet. Bell's claim of priory of discovery triggers a heated professional debate, which continues well past the death of both men and persist today in the halls of many medical schools.

Trivia: Charles Bell publishes a collection of essays on the anatomy of facial expressions, which he prepares not for physicians but rather for artists (1806)[113].

Charles Bell is most remembered by medical students for his description of the unilateral facial paralysis resulting from the disruption of normal CN VII function, later termed Bell's palsy (1821,1829-1830)[114,115].

Charles Bell's original description of Bell's palsy, which results from a unilateral lesion of CN VII, is first described by Bell in a presentation to the Royal Society of London, July 12, 1821. The facial paralysis is originally observed following an induced unilateral lesion of CN VII of a donkey (sic). Bell in his original paper repeatedly refers to CN VII as the "respiratory nerve of the face". He additionally offers experimental studies using assorted animals and clinical case reports of humans in support of the reliable observation of facial paralysis, whenever CN VII is lesioned.

Below is a brief expert from the 1821 paper, in which Bell recounts one case history, in his own words, after removing

> "… a tumor from before the ear of a coachman: a branch of the nerve which goes to the angle of the mouth was divided. Sometime after he returned to thank me for ridding him of a formidable disease, but complained that he could not whistle to his horses…" (July 12, 1821)[114].

As a medical student, do you recognize why the patient is no longer able to whistle? While the surgery is successful, has the successful treatment also resulted in a functional impairment? Is the functional impairment occupationally debilitating?

Here is another brief excerpt, eight years later, taken from a 1829 letter from Charles Bell to an attending physician, regarding a patient examined by Bell as a consultation and describing in Charles Bell's own words the left sided facial palsy, known today simply as Bell's palsy.

> "…The face is twisted to the right side. The left nostril does not move in respiration. The eye-lids of the left side are not closed when he winks, although, when he attempts it, the eye-ball is turned up, the cheek is relaxed, and the forehead on the left side unruffled…" (1829-1830)[115].

Charles Bell brings attention to the functional organization of the spinal cord and offers his landmark observations of facial paralysis caused by a lesion of CN VII and independent of lesions located in the cerebral hemispheres. Recall lesions of the cerebral hemispheres, located in the primary somato-motor strip or descending white mater tracts from the cortex to brain stem CN VII nuclei can also produce facial weakness; however the paralysis of these lesions can be readily differentiated upon visual inspection and clinical assessment of the face. As a medical student do you remember why? Hint: remember the bilateral intervention of CN nuclei from the cerebral cortex. A unilateral upper motor neuron lesion will produce a contralateral facial paresis most evident in the lower quadrant of the face with the upper quadrant less affected. A lesion of the lower motor neuron (CNVII) produces an ipsilateral paralysis of both upper and lower quadrants of the face. Bell's palsy by definition is produced with a lesion of the lower motor neurons (CN VII) only.

James Parkinson (1755-1824) English apothecary offers his landmark essay on the Shaking Palsy (1817)[116]. Fifty-five years later, French neurologist Jean Charcot (1825-1893) of the Salpetriere Hospital in Paris renames the condition Parkinson's disease, in acknowledgement of James Parkinson's original contribution to describing the disorder (1872)[117]. Jean Charcot additionally introduces bradykinesia and rigidity to the original constellation of signs and symptoms reported by James Parkinson and noting two primary sub-types, with tremor and without tremor with rigidity (1872)[117].

James Parkinson describes the condition, which today we simply term Parkinson's disease, as an

> "…involuntary tremulous motion, with lessened muscular power, in parts not in action and even when supported, with a propensity to bend the trunk forward, and to pass from walking to a running pace, the essence of intellect being uninjured…So slight and nearly imperceptible are the first inroads of this malady, and so extremely slow its progress, that it rarely happens, that the patient can form any recollection of the precise period of its commencement. The first symptoms perceived are, a slight sense of weakness, with a proneness to trembling in some particular part, sometimes the hands and arms. These symptoms gradually increase in the part first affected; and at an uncertain period, but seldom in less than twelve months or more, the morbid influence is felt in some other part…and becomes similarly affected…" (1817)[116].

James Parkinson prefaces his now landmark paper in neurology with a few words of caution; reminding the reader the following report is based upon clinical observations and without support of experimental study or anatomical examination. He openly admits to having no answers as to the cause of the condition or how to effectively treat it. Rather he offers his observations of a condition which does not fit into any current diagnostic taxonomy and for the purpose of bringing attention to the condition, perhaps having it entered into a current diagnostic taxonomy and "…having excited the attention of those, who may point out the most appropriate means of relieving a tedious and most distressing malady…" (1817)[116].

James Parkinson reports his clinical observations of the Shaking Palsy, based upon observation of three of his own patients and three additional individuals appearing in the local streets, that he observes and appear to be suffering the condition. While prefacing his paper with a cautionary note, he speculates as to possible causes, recommended treatments, and suggestions to assist in differential diagnosis (1817)[116]. Another seventy-eight years will pass before the anatomical location responsible for producing the syndrome of Parkinson's disease is identified to be the substantia nigra nuclei of the mid-brain (1895)[118].

Marie Flourens (1794-1867) French experimental physiologist challenges the rapidly growing popularity of the localizationist's model of brain function. In his efforts to systemically and objectively investigate the localizationist model, he conducts a series of experiments which introduce specific brain lesions to different regions of the brain and observes the changes, if any in behavior or demonstrated cognitive functions (1824)[119]. Flourens' findings are unexpected to him and reveal specific brain functions can be localized to specific areas of the brain and brain stem e.g. cognitive functions to the cerebral cortex, motor coordination to the cerebellum, and respiratory controls to the medulla. Unwilling to accept a pure localizationist position he offers an alternative explanation. Flourens interprets the findings to indicate brain functions can only be localized to specific lobes of the cerebral hemispheres, cerebellar hemispheres, or regions of the brainstem. No more detailed localization of function is possible. He argues once function is localized to a general area of the brain e.g. lobe of the cerebral hemisphere or "vital node" of the medulla, any further detailed localization is simply impossible. Any observed impairment in function and the degree of impaired function is determined by the amount of brain tissue ablated and not by any narrow localization of the tissue ablated. Flourens confidently argues against the localizationist model of brain functions and argues brain functions are the result of the brain working as an integrated whole, supporting the equipotential model of brain functions.

Perhaps Marie Flourens' own words will further clarify his position;

> "...a large section of the cerebral lobes can be removed without loss of function. As more is removed, all functions weaken and gradually disappear. Thus the cerebral lobes operate in unison for the full exercise of their functions ... The cerebral cortex functioned as an indivisible whole ... an essentially single faculty of perception, judgement and will ..." (1824)[119].

So begins the debate between investigators arguing in favor of the localizationist model of brain functions and investigators arguing in favor of the equipotential model of brain functions. This debate remains unsettled throughout the 1800s.

Independent of Marie Flourens' position as to the localization or lack of localization of brain functions, he makes a significant contribution to the advancement of new knowledge through his application of the scientific method and systematic experimental investigations designed to answer specific questions e.g. are brain functions localized to specific and definable areas of the brain? His experimental approach to the study of the nervous systems complements and extends the clinical observation and descriptive approaches embraced by clinicians and which characterizes many investigations during the 1800s, for example investigations conducted by James Parkinson.

Marie Flourens applies his experimental methodologies to the investigation of the vestibular system and offers seminal papers identifying the system's importance for maintaining normal balance and posture (1830a,1830b)[120,121].

Jean-Baptiste Bouillaud (1796-1881) French internist is among the first to identify and report impairments in the frontal lobes of the cerebral hemispheres can and do result in impairments in speech and language (1825,1825,1827)[122,123,124]. These are among the first documented cases of localized higher cortical functions specially addressing areas of brain essential for normal and abnormal speech and language. Jean- Baptiste Bouillaud precedes more recognizable investigators of this subject Paul Broca and Carl Wernicke by more than 36 and 49 years respectively.

Robert Remak (1815-1865) Polish neurologist and microscopist describes myelinated and unmyelinated neuronal fibers (doctoral dissertation) (1836,1838)[125,126]; offers microscopic descriptions of the nervous system, describing the absence of myelin covering autonomic system fibers; reports fibers from motor neurons in the spinal cord continue uninterrupted through the anterior roots of the spinal cord and into peripheral muscles (1836,1838)[125,126]; offers microscopic evidence nerves are not empty or filled with fluid, rather they contain small fibrils encased in a cylinder and connected to a cell body (1843)[127]; and describes the six neuronal cell layers of the cerebral cortex (1844)[128].

In addition to his influential contributions to better understanding the nervous system structure at the microscopic level, Robert Remak offers additional insights into the embryological development. He builds upon the work of German embryologist Heinz Pander (1794-1865) whom identifies embryonic germ cell layers and the process of gastrulation (1817)[129] and refines the germ cell layer model (1843,1855)[130,131].

Note: The now familiar terms, identifying the three germ cell layers which result from the process of gastrulation during week three of embryological development, endoderm and ectoderm are introduced into the professional literature by Irish naturalist George Allman (1812-1898) of Trinity College - Dublin (1853)[132] and mesoderm by British biologist Thomas Huxley (1825-1895) (1871)[133] .

Johannes Purkinje (1787-1869) Czech experimental physiologist embraces microscope technologies and describes the cells of the cerebellum (1837)[134]. Early in his professional career, Johannes Purkinje conducts studies into sensory physiology focusing on vision, equilibrium, and vertigo (1819,1825)[135,136]. He additionally recognizes human fingerprints can be used as a reliable form of identification and introduces a nine group classification system for fingerprints which continues to be employed, in a modified form today, over 195 years after first introducing the classification system (1823)[137]. After acquiring a compound microscope in 1832, he and Adolph Wendt, a medical student working in Purkinje's laboratory, discover and describe the sweat glands of the human skin (1833)[138]. Five years later Purkinje describes the pair shaped cells of the cerebellar cortex which bear his name today, the Purkinje cells (1837)[139]. Purkinje along with Bogislaus Palicki, a medical student working in Purkinje's laboratory, describe the specialized fibers which conduct electricity from the atrioventricular (AV) node of the heart, through the inner walls of the ventricles in order synchronize heart contractions and maintain a consistent heart rhythm (1839,1839)[140,141]. These are the same fibers you studied in your physiology course and known today simply as Purkinje fibers.

The development of the compound microscope and microtome, significantly improve investigations being conducted at the cellular and subcellular levels and offer new opportunities to study the nervous systems unlike ever before.

Trivia: Purkinje introduces the term "protoplasm" into the scientific vocabulary, while studying animal embryos (1839)[142].

Theodor Schwann (1810-1882) German physiologist is perhaps most remembered by medical students as the person who first describes the myelin forming Schwann cells of the peripheral nervous systems (PNS) (1838,1839,1860)[143,144,145]. Perhaps more importantly and less often recognized is his contributions to the introduction and development of the Cell theory (not to be confused with the ventricular cell doctrine which localizes mental functions to cerebral ventricles). Cell theory states the cell is the basic unit of structure for all living things; all living things are composed of cells; and all new cells are produced from pre-existing cells (1839)[144]. This builds on the work of German botanist Matthias Schleiden (1804-1881) who originally proposes the idea of Cell theory (1838)[146]. Schwann openly challenges the dogma of spontaneous generation and provides a series of microscopic observations in support of his position all new cells arise from preexisting cells. Schwann challenges his major professor, German physiologist Johannes Muller (1801-1858) and breaks with scientific and religious dogma and the doctrine of vitalism. Challenging scientific and medical dogma is always a risky choice and one with potentially great scientific reward or disastrous professional consequences. Theodor Schwann accepts the risks. Will you?

Recall, Vitalism states the functions of living organism are the result of vital principles distinct from biochemical reactions; the processes of life are not explicable by laws of physics and chemistry alone; and that all life is in some part self-determined. Prior to Schwann's challenge, many neurological conditions are conceptualized within the matrix of an imbalance in the vital energies, whether the vital forces are defined as four humors (Hippocrates), four temperaments (Galen), qi and prana (Eastern religion), or the soul (Christian religion). Today and consistent with Schwann's early conceptualizations, disease and illness are conceptualized within the matrix of physical and biochemical disturbances in otherwise healthy tissues.

The neurosciences are slow to embrace the Cell theory due to technical difficulties with the microscope's resolution and inherent structure of neural tissues. However, by the end of the 1800s improvements in the microscope and technology allows neuroscience to join in the support of the Cell theory model and to better understand the fundamental organizational structure of the nervous systems, at the level of the basic structural unit, the cell.

Trivia: Thomas Schwann is interested in and investigates physical properties of skeletal muscles, establishing the first tension-length diagrams (1837)[147]. He actively investigates the physiology of the digestive systems and is first to discover and isolate the enzyme primarily responsible for digestion in the stomach. He names the substance pepsin (1836)[148]. Thomas Schwann coins the term "metabolism" to describe the chemical changes which occur in animal tissues (1839)[149].

Marshal Hall (1790-1857) English physiologist introduces a new term into the scientific vocabulary, the "reflex arc" (1833)[150]. The term describes the neural pathway that controls reflexive actions and is composed of a primary sensory input from a peripheral receptor to the central nervous system and a primary motor output from the central nervous system to a muscle group. Marshal Hall describes the reflex arc and offers sneezing, coughing, and vomiting as examples. Charles Bell reports his own observations of a "nervous circle" seven years before Marshal Hall publishes his paper which introduces the term "reflex arc" to the scientific and medical communities. Charles Bell reports "…Between the brain and the muscles there is a circle of nerves; one nerve conveys the influence from the brain to the muscle, another gives the sense of the condition of the muscle to the brain…" (1826, p170)[151]. It will be another 42 years before the value of routine, clinical assessment of deep tendon reflexes is acknowledged (1875)[152].

Marshal Hall offers the important observation, under conditions of darkness, many patients experience severe impairment in proprioception and consequently impaired posture control. He soon recognizes, vison plays an important role in regulation of normal posture and can partially compensate for impaired proprioception (1836)[153]. His observations and conceptualization of how sensory systems influence motor control required for normal posture and balance lay the foundation for what will soon become a routinely administered component of the modern neurological examination, the Romberg test.

Mortiz von Romberg (1795-1873) German neurologist builds upon Marshal Hall's original work and observes patients with tabes dorsalis, a condition associated with late stage syphilis infection and characterized by unsteady gait, shooting pains, and urinary incontinence, noting these patients often loose postural control when in darkness or whenever they close their eyes. Here in his own words, he describes his observations of patents suffering tabes dorsalis.

> "…If the patient is told to shut his eyes while in the erect posture, he immediately begins to move from side to side, and the oscillations soon attain such a pitch that unless supported he falls to the ground . . . The eyes of such patients are their regulators, or feelers; consequently in the dark, and when amaurosis supervenes, as is not unfrequently the case, their helplessness is extreme..." (1853, p226-227)[154].

"…The feet feel numbed in standing, walking, or lying down, and the patient has the sensation as if they were covered with a fur . . . The gait begins to be insecure, and the patient attempts to improve it by making a greater effort of the will; as he does not feel the tread to be firm, he puts down his heels with greater force. From the commencement of the disease the individual keeps his eyes on his feet to prevent his movements from becoming still more unsteady. If he is ordered to close his eyes while in the erect posture, he at once commences to totter and swing from side to side; the insecurity of his gait also exhibits itself more in the dark. It is now ten years since I pointed out this pathognomonic sign…" (1840, p395-396)[155].

Mortiz von Romberg devises a quick bed-side procedure, specifically designed to evaluate the integrity of conscious proprioceptive systems (1846)[156]. This bedside assessment today (2018) is simply termed the Romberg test and is a routine part of the modern neurological examination.

Note: Tabes dorsalis when translated from its modern Latin origin means "wasting of the back". Recall, it is the posterior columns of the spinal cord, which carry conscious proprioceptive information, necessary for knowing where the patient's body is in space, that are most effected by the syphilitic condition.

Emil Du Bois-Reymond (1818-1896) German physiologist extends the works of Luigi Galvani, reconciles Alessandro Volta (1745-1827) criticisms of Galvani's work, discovers and explains the neuron's action potential, and establishes the field of experimental electrophysiology. Most of his influential work is completed between 1841 and 1843 (1841,1843)[157,158]. Later he summaries much of his work in his book titled "Untersuchungen uber thierische elektricitat" [Research on Animal Electricity] (1848-84)[159]. His works describe electricity generated by both neural and muscle tissues. Emil Du Bois-Reymond provides medical neurosciences with a new methodology and associated technology which allows investigations into the nervous systems unlike any before, electrophysiology. The new methodology will greatly influence the direction and future investigation of the nervous systems for the next 175 years and most likely beyond.

Charles Brown-Sequard (1818)-1894) French physiologist reports changes in movement and somato-sensations, upon hemi-sectioning of the spinal cord (1846,1851,1855)[160,161,162]. The constellation of signs and symptoms characterized by same side paralysis, same side loss of sensation for vibration, two-point discrimination, conscious proprioception, and opposite side loss of sensation for pain and temperature, all occurring at or below the level of the spinal cord lesion, is the Brown-Sequard syndrome. Perhaps Brown-Sequard's own words, as they appear in a 1869 issue of The Lancet best describe his syndrome;

"…a lesion in one of the lateral halves of the spinal cord produces: 1st, paralysis of voluntary movements in the same side; 2nd, anesthesia to touch, tickling, painful impressions, and changes of temperature in the opposite side; 3rd, paralysis of the muscular sense in the same side…" (1869)[163].

The Brown-Sequard syndrome is familiar (or should be) to every modern medical student today.

Trivia: The Brown-Sequard syndrome is named in recognition of the single individual (Brown-Sequard) who describes the condition during the mid-1800s. Often medical students are under the misunderstanding the condition is named in recognition of two individuals, Brown and Sequard.

Hermann von Helmholtz (1821-1894) German, Professor of Physics and Physiology introduces an instrument which changes how the nervous system is clinically examined, the ophthalmoscope (1851)[164]. In his original 1851 publication, he refers to his new instrument as an augenspiegel (eye mirror), describes the optic disc, and the central arteries, and veins of the retina (1851)[164]. This new instrument is quickly embraced by investigators and reports quickly begin to appear in medical and professional journals describing pathologies, for example a detached retina (1854)[165], the cupped optic disc of glaucoma (1854,1857)[166,167], central artery retinal embolism (1859)[168], and the neurological significance of papilledema (swelling of the optic disc due to increased intracranial pressure) (1860,1870,1871)[169,170,171].

Practicing physicians are slow to accept the new technology. As improvements and modifications are made to Hermann von Helmholtz original instrument e.g. in 1851 introducing two rotating discs containing a series of correcting convex lens, correcting for refraction errors of patient and examiner, the instruments is made more user friendly. The instrument slowly gains acceptance by practicing physicians and is integrated into the routine, clinical assessment of patients, as its value is repeatedly demonstrated in the medical literature and books begin to appear which discuss the use of the instrument and how the instrument can be used to identify specific pathologies effecting the eye directly and other medical conditions indirectly e.g. kidney impairments (1855,1871, 1879)[172,173,174].

Clinical description of neurological syndromes is popular during the 1800s and reinforces the functional application of discoveries being made by the academic anatomists and pathologists at the gross anatomical and microscopic levels and the experimental physiologists at the electrophysiological level. The basic sciences underlying the normal and abnormal function of the human nervous systems are more completely understood and applied to the clinical practice of medicine.

Augustus V. Waller (1816-1870) English physiologist, not to be confused with his son Augustus D. Waller (1856-1922), describes the degeneration of neural fibers as viewed with the microscope "...after their continuity with the brain has been interrupted by section..." (1850)[175]. Recall, Wallerian degeneration is the result of degeneration of the distal segment of a neural fiber once it has been severed from the nutritive centers of the cell body (1852,1857)[176,177].

Francois Magendie (1783-1855) French physiologist describes the Foremen of Magendie (1842)[178]. Recall, the Foremen of Magendie is the single median channel which allows for the flow of CSF from the fourth ventricle into the subarachnoid space. This channel is one of three channels which move CSF into the subarachnoid space. The other two channels are the two lateral Foramina of Luschka, which will be described thirteen years later (1855)[179].

Perhaps unknown to many medical students, Francois Magendie triggers a heated professional debate with Scottish anatomist Charles Bell, as to priority for discovery of the sensory and motor functions of the spinal rootlets, as they enter and exit the spinal cord (1822)[180,181]. Both men claim priority, although differentiation between the posterior sensory rootlets and the anterior motor rootles are first reported by Erasistratus, in the City of Alexandria over 2,000 years before Magendie or Bell publish their first papers on the topic. The debate, accusations, and denials, as to who did what and when, continue well past the death of Bell in 1842 and Magendie in 1855 (1868,1868,1869)[182,183,184]. The debate continues today, in many hallways and lounges of medical schools throughout Europe, USA, and Canada. What do you think? Which man, if either has a legitimate claim to the priority of discovery?

Hubert von Luschka (1820-1875) German anatomist, correctly describes the source of the production of CSF to be the choroid plexus, located within the brain ventricles; correctly describes the directional flow of CSF through the ventricular system; identifies two lateral channels which allow for the movement of CSF from the ventricular system into the subarachnoid space, at the level of the pons and which he terms the lateral Foramina of Luschka (1855)[179]. In this same paper, Hubert von Luschka openly rejects Francois Magendie's earlier claims, pia mater produce CSF (1825,1855)[185,179].

By the mid-1800s, the basic functional organization of the spinal cord is known, somato-sensory systems are principally located in the posterior half of the spinal cord and somato-motor systems are principally located in the anterior half of the spinal cord; the anatomy of the ventricle system is understood along with the production and flow of CSF through the system; the microscope proves to be an essential tool and assist in detailing the cellular organization of the nervous systems; microscopic findings provide support in favor of the Cell theory (the cell is the basic structural unit of all living things, all living things are composed of cells, and all new cells are produced from pre-existing cells); the six cell layers of the cerebral cortex and the three cell layers of the cerebellar cortex are detailed; myelinated and unmyelinated fibers are identified and associated with the speed in which information is transmitted through neural fibers; the nervous system is understood to be composed of interconnecting cells; humor balance models of brain function are displaced by models of localization and equipotentiality; systematic clinical observations and descriptions of now familiar neurological conditions are reported and re-interpreted within the new models of brain functions e.g. Parkinson's disease, Brown-Sequard syndrome, and aphasias; new clinical bedside diagnostic procedures are introduced e.g. assessment of deep tendon reflexes (reflex arch); Romberg test (proprioception), Rinne and Weber tests (hearing); new clinical diagnostic instruments are introduced and become a part of the practicing physicians tool box e.g. tuning forks and ophthalmoscope.

The second half of the 1800s witness many new advancements and continuing developments. Paul Broca and Carl Wernicke describe their aphasias; Jean-Marie Charcot describes multiple sclerosis, amyotrophic lateral sclerosis, and provides explanations as to the underlying neuropathologies responsible for each condition; Johann Horner describes the Horner's syndrome; George Huntington describes Huntington's disease; George Giles de la Tourette describes assorted movement disorders, Richard Caton records electricity generated by brain tissues and introduces the electroencephalogram (EEG); Louis Ranvier describes the nodes of Ranvier; Franz Nissl discovers Nissl substance; Camillo Golgi describes the Golgi tendon organ and introduces the silver nitrate method for staining neurons; Wilhelm Erb and Karl Westphal introduce and explain the clinical value of deep tendon reflex (DTR) assessment e.g. patellar reflex; Jason Taylor introduces the familiar Taylor reflex hammer; Joseph Babinski introduces his clinical procedure for assessing neuronal inhibition of lower motor neuron systems (Babinski sign); new terms and vocabulary are introduced to define new concepts and discoveries e.g. the terms neuron, dendrite, axon, synapse, and autonomic nervous system; new professional societies and associated journals are founded and committed to the advancement of the medical neurosciences.

Let's take a brief look now of a few of the specific people and their contributions which significantly impact the direction and development of medical neurosciences during the second half of the 1800s.

Paul Broca (1824-1880) French anatomist is perhaps best remembered by medical students and most physicians as the person who describes impairments in speech and language, whenever a patient suffers a lesion localized to the posterior aspect of the left inferior frontal gyrus of the cerebral cortex of the brain (Broca's area). He reports the clinical and autopsy findings of his 51 year old patient "Tan" to the Societe d'Antrohpolige in Paris, noting the importance of the condition and assigns the term "aphemie" to the condition, characterized by impairment in speech and language with comprehension of langue remaining intact and terms the cortical area affected " the convolution du language" (1861b,1861c,1861d)[186,187,188].

Three years later French internist Armand Trousseau (1801-1867) renames the condition "aphasia" in his provocative paper titled "De l'aphasia, maladie decrite recemment sous le nom improper d'aphemia" [On aphasia, a sickness formerly wrongly referred to as aphemia] (1864)[189]. Armand Trousseau points out the term chosen by Broca "aphemia" is derived from the Greek, meaning "without speech" whereas the newly proposed term "aphasia", also derived from the Greek, meaning "without language" better describes this important condition(1864)[189].

Twelve years after Paul Broca first reports "the convolution du language", Scottish neurologist David Ferrier (1843-1928) most remembered for his seminal work in the application of faradic stimulation of brain cortex and providing one of the earliest maps of cortical brain functions, renames the area "Broca's convolution" (Broca's area) (1873)[190].

Perhaps less known are some of Paul Broca's numerous additional contributions. He writes more than 500 scientific papers and books, each offering his unique insights. For example in brief, he describes the microscopic changes associated with muscular dystrophies (1851)[191], osteoarthritis (1850)[192], and rickets noting the bone impairments characteristic of rickets interfere with ossification and can be attributed to a single factor, poor nutrition (1852)[193]. He applies microscope technologies to investigate cancer and describes how cancer is carried from one part of the body to another through the blood (1850,1852)[194,195]. He is first to recognize and describes the high prevalence of breast cancer occurring within families, noting breast cancer can be inherited (1866-1869)[196].

Jean-Marie Charcot (1825-1893) French neurologist and Professor of Pathological Anatomy at the University of Paris makes tremendous contributions to the advancement of medical neurosciences, while working as a scientist-practitioner and administrator, at the celebrated large public Salpetriere Hospital, located in Paris. He maximizes his opportunities to observe a wide range of patients presenting with neurological signs and symptoms and identifies many of the conditions familiar to medical students today. For example, he is first to describe the clinical presentation and underlying neuropathological changes of multiple sclerosis (the condition he terms "la sclerose en plaques") (1868)[197]; describes amyotrophic lateral sclerosis (ALS, Lou Gehrig's disease) (1869)[198]; and describes Charcot-Marie-Tooth disease, importantly noting the pathology is a neuropathy rather than a myopathy (1886)[199].

Jean-Marie Charcot is an influential mentor to many students who will make their own substantial contributions to the advancement of medical neurosciences e.g. Joseph Babinski and George Gilles de la Tourette. In addition to training students, conducting research, writing scientific papers, teaching, and providing clinical services, he is largely responsible for establishing the Salpetriere Hospital as a world class center for neurology. Jean Marie Charcot is a passionate advocate for making extensive, careful, systematic observations and recording signs and symptoms of clinical patients, then correlating these observations and signs and symptoms with microscopic and gross anatomical pathologies observed at autopsy. He provides a striking example of an individual who excels within the Scientist-Practitioner model.

While rapid progress is being made in the observation and description of clinical neurological syndromes, progress is too being made at the microscopic level of investigations.

Wilhelm His, Sr. (1831-1904) Swiss embryologist develops the microtome, allowing for the preparation of extremely thin layers of tissue for observation under the light microscope (1870)[200]. He applies microscopic technologies to investigate embryological development of the nervous systems. He identifies the migration and positioning of embryonic cells, which later form the spinal and cranial nerve ganglia. Wilhelm His, Sr. terms these cells "Zwischenstrang" (1868)[201]. You recognize them by their English terms "neural ridge" or "neural crest cells" (1878)[202].

Camillo Golgi (1843-1926) Italian pathologist, Professor of Histology at University of Pavia, and Nobel Prize Laureate in Physiology or Medicine (1906)[203] "…in recognition of their work on the structure of the nervous system…" uses the microscope to describe the Golgi tendon organ (1878)[204] and the intracellular Golgi apparatus complex (1886)[205]. He introduces an innovative silver staining technique which he initially terms "la reasione near" (black reaction). The revolutionary staining technique, soon renamed the Golgi stain, allows for the visualization of individual cell structures when viewed under the light microscope (1873)[206]. The staining technique allows investigators to follow and visualize in fine detail the entire length of the neuron and visualize connections between neurons.

Observations made using Golgi's new staining method contribute significantly to data supporting the Neuron doctrine. The Neuron doctrine is one of two competing conceptual models passionately debated and used to explain the organization of the nervous system, at the cellular level, during the second half of the 1800s. Proponents of the Neuron doctrine argue the nervous system is composed of distinct, identifiable, separate elements i.e. neurons, which are interconnected by a network of neural branching. The second conceptual model of this period is the nervous system is composed of a reticulum, a continuous network of a single tissue consisting of fused neuronal dendrites and axons. The Neuron doctrine proves to be the conceptual matrix upon which future neuroscience builds.

Johann Horner (1831-1886) Swiss, Professor of Ophthalmology, while working with the University of Zurich, describes the sympathetic nervous system disorder syndrome with which most medical students are familiar, Horner's syndrome (1869)[207]. He offers his findings of a 40 year old female presenting with the now classic signs of Horner's syndrome. In his own words he describes the syndrome;

> "…slight drooping of the right upper eyelid…the upper lid covers the right cornea to the upper edge of the pupil, the lid is not loose or wrinkled…The pupil of the right eye is considerably more constricted than that of the left, but reacts to light…the right side of her face became red and warm, the color and heat increasing in intensity under our observation, while the left side remained pale and cool…the patient thereupon told us that the right side never perspired…" (1869). (English translation by J. F. Fulton, appearing in Arch Neurology, 1968, Vol 19 (5) Nov., p541-542)[208].

Silas Mitchell (1829-1914) American neurologist with an army hospital based practice in Philadelphia, Pennsylvania during the American civil war, focuses on the treatment and management of soldiers with nerve injuries. He discovers and describes two particularly important pain syndromes. First is complex regional pain syndrome (CRPS), aka reflex neurovascular dystrophy, characterized by chronic, severe pain, swelling, and changes in the skin. The second is phantom pain syndrome, characterized by intense pain or other sensations e.g. tingling, cramping, hot, and cold, seemingly originating in a part of the body which has been traumatically amputated. Silas Mitchell describes both conditions in his book "Injuries of Nerves and their Consequences" (1872)[209]. Wars and their resulting injuries to the human body offer unique opportunities to investigate the effects of trauma on the human nervous systems.

George Huntington (1850-1916) American physician from New York, describes the autosomal dominant form of an inherited chorea, which he terms the "heredity chorea" (1872a,1872b)[210,211]. Later the "hereditary chorea" described by Huntington will be termed Huntington's chorea and recognized to be the result of the neuropathological changes which characterize Huntington's disease e.g. bilateral degeneration of the head of the caudate nuclei, located deep inside of the brain cerebral hemispheres. The neuropathological changes result from a mutation of a gene located on chromosome 4 (4p16.3) which codes for the cytoplasmic protein huntingtin (HTT). The mutation is characterized by CAG tri-nucleotide repeats greater than 35. The condition today is recognized to evidence genetic anticipation (signs and symptoms of the disorder have earlier onset with increased severity of signs and symptoms with successive generations) and almost complete penetrance.

Charles Waters (1816-1892) upstate New York physician, reports the same signs and symptoms of the "hereditary chorea", as reported by George Huntington. However, Charles Waters does it thirty-one years before George Huntington. He describes and details the condition's clinical presentation in Dutch settlers, its characteristic chorea, adult onset, strong pattern of heredity, progressive nature of the clinical signs and symptoms, irreversibility or resolution of signs and symptoms once they appear, and emphasizes this chorea is different from other movement disorders evidencing chorea as a prominent sign (1841/1848)[212]. Yet, George Huntington is awarded professional recognition and priority of discovery. George Huntington authors only two journal papers in his professional career, both recounting his observations of the "hereditary chorea" (1872b,1910)[211,213]. Has the history of medicine made an error in awarding him priority for discovery? What do you think?

Carl Wernicke (1848-1905) German neuropathologist, at age 26 years, publishes his landmark paper describing a specific type of language disorder he terms "sensory aphasia" (1874)[214]. The impairment typically results from a cerebrovascular lesion located in the cerebral cortex of the posterior aspect of the left superior temporal gyrus. This aphasia is characterized by the loss of comprehension of the spoken word, loss of the ability to read silently and understand what has been read, and loss of the ability write, while retaining memory for words and with primary sensory and motor functions remaining intact (1874)[214]. You might recognize this aphasia by its alternative name used commonly today, "Wernicke's aphasia". Carl Wernicke's observation and description of sensory aphasia provides additional support in favor of the localizationists' position, specific functions can be localized to specific areas of the cerebral cortex. Wernicke's aphasia complements the "motor aphasia" described by Paul Broca (1861)[186].

Three years later Carl Wernicke describes his findings of a 20 year old seamstress suffering sulphuric acid poisoning and recognizes cranial nerve (CN) motor nuclei of the brainstem have properties similar to the motor nuclei of the anterior horns of the spinal cord, in that they can be uniquely affected by disease processes in much the same way as poliomyelitis affects the lower motor neurons of the spinal cord (1877,1881)[215]. He describes specifically the impact of the toxic exposure upon the CN motor nuclei principally responsible for eye movements (CN III, CN VI), disrupting normal conjugate eye movements. He emphasizes the selective impairment in the patient's lateral gaze, noting the left and right eyes fail to move laterally, suggesting selective impairment of the CN VI nuclei, bilaterally or perhaps the parapontine reticular nuclei formation and their associated medial longitudinal fasciculi, bilaterally. He offers different terms for the observed impairment of lateral conjugate gaze e.g. lateral nystagmus, ataxia, and the syndrome of acute hemorrhagic superior polio encephalitis (1881,1881/1968)[216,217]. Today, almost 140 years after Carl Wernicke first reports his observations, we associate the syndrome with the condition we simply term Wernicke's encephalopathy. Today, Wernicke's encephalopathy is well recognized and most typically associated with a nutritional deficiency of vitamin B1 (thiamine).

Carl Wernicke in his early thirties offers his three volume book "Lehrbuch der Gehirnkrankheiten fur Aerzte und Studirende" [Textbook of Brain Disorders: For physicians and students] (1881-1883)[215]. The book attempts to comprehensively account for all brain diseases within the conceptual matrix of cerebral localization. He reviews the anatomic-physiologic works of Theodore Meynert, offers a classification of brain diseases, and discusses the pathology of focal cerebral lesions. The book is embraced by the Localizationists of the period and offers guidance to understanding brain disorders from the Localizationist position, for the next 100 years.

New investigative tools are introduced during the late-1800s which open new lines of investigation into the nervous systems, moving beyond simple descriptions of gross anatomy, gross anatomical pathologies, and their association with clinical syndromes. Measurement of electrical brain potentials is introduced and developed, leading to a new understanding of brain cell and tissue physiology.

Richard Caton (1842-1926) English, pioneer of brain electrophysiology, measures electrical activity generated by brain and recognizes "…the electrical currents of the grey matter appear to have a relation to its function…" (1875a,1875b)[218,219]. His seminal experiments and pioneering applications of new technology allow for the direct measurement of electrical activity generated by the brain. He successfully demonstrates increased electrical activity in specific regions of the cerebral cortex associated with specific functions e.g. visual cortex when light is shined into the eyes. Richard Canton offers additional data in support of period models which conceptualize the localization of specific functions to specific brain regions. He follows his initial experiments with a series of repeated experiments with a larger number of animals and confirms his initial findings; electrical activity is generated from brain tissues; this electrical activity can be measured and recorded; and electrical brain activity varies dependent upon the location of the recording and the type of sensory stimulation presented to the animal (1877,1887)[220,221].

Richard Canton provides the foundation, upon which Hans Berger will build and allow Hans Berger to record electrical activity from humans, using non-invasive recording procedures (1929)[222]. Neuro-electrophysiology will prove to be tremendously influential in moving the medical neurosciences forward during the next 140 years. The capability to record and measure electrical bran activity provides both a new technology for investigating the normal basic science physiology of the nervous systems, it provides clinically useful tools to assist in the measurement of abnormal electrical brain activity associated with brain pathologies e.g. electroencephalogram (EEG) for epilepsies, visual evoked potentials (VEP) for multiple sclerosis, brainstem auditory evoked potentials (BAEP) for neurosensory hearing loss.

The microscope continues to be an essential investigative tool during the late-1800s. When coupled with innovative staining techniques, improvement in lens resolutions, and improved specimen preparation techniques, the microscope contributes to many of the advancements in medical neurosciences often taken for granted today.

Louis Ranvier (1835-1922) French histologist using the microscope discovers and describes the periodic, regularly spaced, gaps in the insulating myelin sheath surrounding myelinated neurons and correctly deduces their important role in conduction of signals through neurons (1871,1872, 1874,1878)[223,224,225,226]. These microscopic anatomical structures Ranvier termed "etranglements annulaires" for the nodes and "segments interannularies" for the internodes, are known today simply as the "nodes of Ranvier". The term "Ranvierschen Schnurringe" [nodes of Ranvier] is offered by Rudolf Albert von Kolliker (1817-1905) Swiss histologist (1896)[227]. Many of the leading French anatomists of the period simply reject the use of the microscope, in part to their lack of acceptance and open rejection of Cell theory. Ranvier pushes against the established authorities and finds value in the microscope as an essential tool to better understanding neuropathologies.

Franz Nissl (1860-1919) German neuropathologist introduces the Nissl stain. The stain and staining techniques allows for the first time visualization of components of neurons previously unknown. He introduces the stain while a medical student (1884)[228]. Ten years later, Franz Nissl discovers and reports the presence of rough endoplasmic reticulum inside of neurons and terms this intracellular structure Nissl substance (1894)[229].

Trivia: Franz Nissl is great friends with Alois Alzheimer and serves as Best Man in Alois Alzheimer's wedding in April 1894.

Investigators identify new clinical syndromes and develop new clinical procedures to assess the nervous systems at bedside. Many of the procedure continue to be used today, over 100 years since they are first introduced.

Wilhelm Erb (1840-1921) German neurologist offers significant contributions to the identification, classification, and treatment of muscular dystrophies. Perhaps you remember him from your first semester gross anatomy course when you learned about Erb's palsy, a paralysis of the arm caused by an injury of the neuronal fibers innervating the upper limb and trunk (e.g. C4-C6) as they pass through the brachial plexus, typically resulting from a dislocation of the shoulder, during the birthing process, and characterized by a flaccid paralysis of the shoulder and arm, with no loss of sensation (1874)[230].

Wilhelm Erb is instrumental in describing the clinical value of the deep tendon reflex (DTR) and offers instruction as to how to properly elicit the DTR, using only the examiner's fingers or "reflex" hammer (1875)[152]. Wilhelm Erb recognizes the great clinical diagnostic value of routinely evaluating DTRs and reports the first examination of a DTR which he terms the "patellarshnenreflex" (patellar tendon reflex). Evaluation and interpretation of DTRs are now a routine part of every neurological examination conducted by physicians today, over 140 years since Wilhelm Erb first introduces the procedure and reports the importance and clinical value.

Wilhelm Erb offers additional contributions in the area of electro-diagnostics in neurology. He authors an influential book outlining the potential and demonstrated value of applying electricity to the diagnosis and treatment of neurological disorders, titled "Handbuch der Elektrotherapie" [Handbook of electrotherapy] (1882)[231]. He is instrumental in founding one of the earliest journals committed to the advancement of medical neurosciences, the" Deutsche Zeitschrift fur

Nervenheilkunde" [German Journal of Neurology] (1891)[232]. Erb contributes to the Journal's first issue with articles discussing assorted nerve pathologies and a survey of the muscular dystrophies (1891a,1891b)[233,234].

Karl Westphal (1833-1890) German neurologist describes the spinal reflex, the same year as Wilhelm Erb (1875)[235]. Karl Westphal terms the reflex response "unterschenkelphanomen" (lower leg phenomenon). This reflex response is exactly the same DTR Wilhelm Erb describes and terms "patellar tendon reflex". Karl Westphal publishes his paper after reading Erb's paper and while serving as the editor of the "Archive fur Psychiarie und Nervenkrankheitern" [Archives for Psychiatric and Mental Illnesses]. However, Westphal offers an alternative explanation to account for the observed sign. He interprets the DTR phenomena not as a reflex, but as a local muscle contraction, induced by sudden tension and resulting from a physical blow to the tendon (1875)[235]. Westphal's interpretation proves to be incorrect. Wilhelm Erb's original interpretation of the DTR, with sensory input into the spinal cord and motor output from the spinal, proves to be correct.

Perhaps you recognize Karl Westphal from the parasympathetic nuclei, which bear his name. Recall these nuclei, the parasympathetic nuclei of CN III or alternatively the Edinger-Westphal nuclei, are located in the back of the midbrain and responsible for the constriction of the pupils (1885,1887)[236,237]. Whenever you assess a patient's pupillary light reflex, direct or consensual, you are assessing these nuclei described by German anatomist Ludwig Edinger (1855-1819) first in the human fetus brain (1885)[236] and two years later by Karl Westphal in the adult human brain over 130 years ago (1887)[237].

Georges Giles de la Tourette (1857-1904) French neurologist and student of Jean-Marie Charcot, describes nine patients presenting with repetitive, stereotyped, involuntary movements, echolalia, coprolalia, and tic vocalizations, which he identifies as a special subtype of movement disorder from chorea and terms the condition "maladie des tics" (1884,1885)[238,239]. As an investigator and clinical practitioner at the large public Salpetriere Hospital in Paris, Giles de la Tourette applies the recommended investigative strategies of his mentor Jean-Marie Charcot; careful, systematic observations and correlation with patient history and autopsy findings. Giles de la Tourette recognizes and reports the movement disorder appears primarily in males, onset of signs and symptoms typically occur during childhood or adolescences, patients oftentimes report a family history of other members evidencing similar movement disorders, and patients often tend to live in the same general area of the city. Jean-Marie Charcot, at the time Giles de la Tourette first describes this unique movement disorder, is constructing and developing a new classification system for neurological disorders. He accepts his student's assessment of the identification of a new and unique movement disorder and it is Charcot who proudly assigns the eponym "Giles de la Tourette syndrome" to the clinical presentation of this movement disorder.

Trivia: Georges Giles de la Tourette is shot in his head by one of his patients, a paranoid schizophrenic, claiming she had been hypnotized against her will and involuntarily hospitalized by Giles de la Tourette, at the Salpetriere Hospital in Paris (1893)[240]. Authorities subsequently find the patient's charges to be unfounded. Giles de la Tourette survives the gunshot wound.

William Gowers (1845-1915) British neurologist, Professor of Medicine University College London, and scientist-practitioner at the National Hospital for the Paralyzed and Epileptics, located in Queen's Square, London, offers his two volume, tremendously influential, "Manual of Diseases of the Nervous System" (1886,1893)[241,242]. Volume I addresses diseases of the nerves and spinal cord and volume II addresses issues of the brain, its structure and functional organization, disease of the cranial nerves, localization of cerebral disease, diseases of the meninges, organic brain diseases, degenerative diseases of the brain, all followed by discussion of specific conditions e.g. epilepsy, paralysis agitans (Parkinson's disease), tetanus, chorea, alcoholism, and headaches. Each condition is organized according to its etiology, presenting symptoms, varieties, pathological anatomy, pathology, diagnosis, and treatment. He offers illustrations and photographs to accompany text descriptions e.g. brain anatomy, spastic paralysis, cranial nerve palsies, dystonias, flexed posture of Parkinson's disease, wrist drop associated with lead poisoning, and the now familiar Gowers' sign (vol.I, fig.150, p511). The inclusion of illustrations and photographs greatly facilitate understanding by the reader.

William Gowers' Manual offers a comprehensive text of neurological conditions unmatched by all others to date. It serves as the primary resource for applied medical neurosciences well into the early-1900s. Simply, an impressive contribution to the medical neurosciences.

William Gowers embraces the scientist-practitioner model, making careful, systematic observations, maintaining extensive records of patients, compiling the information, identifying commonalities shared among the clinical presentations, then searching for a common etiology and an effective treatment. He contributes at least a dozen books within his thirty year career, summarizing, clarifying, and advancing the medical and scientific knowledge base, Specific conditions and procedures are noted in medical ophthalmology (1879)[243], paralytic disorders (1879)[244], epilepsy and chronic convulsive disorders (1881)[245], diseases of the nerves, spinal cord, brain, and meninges (1886,1893)[246], as well as migraines, sleep disorders, and conditions producing vertigo (1907)[247].

Trivia: William Gowers invents the first practical and useful hemoglobin meter (1879)[248]. Assessment of hemoglobin is among the first diagnostic blood tests available to clinicians and today, over 139 years later, is one of the most frequently requested blood test ordered by practicing physicians.

As the 1800s come to a close, new instruments are invented and become a familiar addition to every physician's tool box used during the bedside examination. Pathognomonic signs are discovered and applied to clinical practice and assist in the diagnosis of neurological disorders.

John Taylor (1855-1931) American pediatrician, designs the now familiar, triangle shaped head, "reflex hammer", thirteen years after Wilhelm Erb introduces the "patella tendon reflex". Very little has changed from its original design introduced at the annual meeting of the Philadelphia Neurological Society (1888)[249].

Joseph Babinski (1857-1932) French neurologist and one of many who investigate neurological disorders at the Salpetriere Hospital in Paris, under the guidance of Jean-Marie Charcot. He offers his original papers on the Babinski sign and details its clinical significance (1896,1896, 1898)[250,251,252]. The original paper describing the abnormal reflex characterized by dorsiflexion of the toes, upon stimulation of the sole of the foot, and associated with lesions affecting the inhibitory pathways running with the lateral cortico-spinal motor tracts (Babinski sign), is first presented in a brief, 26 line presentation at the 1896 meeting of the Societe de Biologie. Later Joseph Babinski includes fanning of the toes in addition to the dorsiflexion of the toes (1903)[253]. The Babinski sign continues to be used today, as a clinical indicator of upper motor neuron impairment of inhibitory motor systems.

Joseph Babinski maintains an interest in photography and incorporates his interest into the documentation of the toe movements of the "Babinski sign" through photographs. He joins an increasing number of investigators during the 1800s who recognize the value of medical photography. For example, French neurologist Guillaume Duchenne (1806 -1875) also working at the Salpetriere Hospital in Paris, offers several books and atlases using photography to document neurological conditions (1862)[254]. Yes, this is the same Duchenne responsible for the identification of Duchenne's muscular dystrophies. Jean-Marie Charcot embraces medical photography as valuable for both education and patient care, at the Salpetriere Hospital in Paris and establishes a medical photography unit at the Hospital in 1878. Medical photography quickly becomes a routine part of the practice of neurology at the Salpetriere (1888,1893)[255,256].

The late-1800s witness the founding of several professional societies and journals devoted to the advancement of the medical neurosciences. Distribution and sharing of new information increases. The first issue of "Brain" is published in 1878 and serves as the official Journal of the new Neurological Society of London, founded by Hughlings Jackson (1878)[257]. Jean-Marie Charcot and French neurologist Desire Bourneville (1840-1909) found the "Archives of Neurologie" (1880). Wilhelm Erb is instrumental in founding "Deutsche Zeitschrift fur Nervenheilkunde", later renamed "Zeitschrift fur Neurologie", which finally became the "Journal of Neurology" (1891). Erb contributes to the first issue with a survey of muscular dystrophies (1891)[258]. The "Le Revue Neurologie" begins publication and serves as the official Journal of the newly established Societie de Neurologie de Paris (1893). Much progress is being made in Europe which advances the medical neurosciences.

In addition to the establishment of new professional societies and associated journals, another indicator of a maturing discipline becomes evident. New vocabulary is introduced to define new, previously unknown structures, and to facilitate communication between investigators and practitioners. Fundamental medical neuroscience terms are coined and introduced into the professional literature. Wilhelm His, Sr. introduces the term "dendrite" (1889)[259]; Wilhelm von Waldeyer-Hartz introduces the term "neuron" (1891)[260]; Albert von Kolliker coins the term "axon" (1896)[261]; Charles Sherrington introduces the term "synapse" (1897)[262]; and Cambridge physiologist John Langley (1852-1925) introduces the term "autonomic nervous system" (1898)[263].

Medical neurosciences continue to develop and make substantial contributions to the medical and scientific knowledge base. The foundation is laid, upon which the next 100 years of new information builds. The 1800s have been good to the development of the medical neurosciences and the discipline matures.

In summary the Middle Modern Period, 1800-1900, witness many important advancements in the medical neurosciences. The spinal cord is organized into functional systems e.g. motor and sensory; CSF production, movement, and removal is described from its source the choroid plexus, through the ventricles, through the subarachnoid space, and into the superior sagittal sinus; underlying mechanisms responsible for hydrocephalus are described; the six cell layer structure of the cerebral cortex is identified; myelinated and unmyelinated fibers are differentiated; new staining procedures are introduced e.g. Nissl and Golgi stains; the microtome is developed allowing for greatly improved microscopic inspection of the nervous system; embryological and fetal development of the nervous systems are described; new conceptual models from which to understand brain function are introduced e.g. equipotentiality and localizationist; electroencephalography is introduced allowing for the real time recording of electrical brain activity generate by brain; the ophthalmoscope becomes a popular tool for the practicing physician; clinical syndromes are described e.g. Bell's palsy, Erb's palsy, Parkinson's disease, Huntington's disease, aphasias, multiple sclerosis, amyotrophic lateral sclerosis (ALS), Brown-Sequard, syndrome, Horner syndrome, Giles de la Tourette syndrome, and phantom limb syndrome; deep tendon reflexes are described and recognized as important systems lending themselves to bedside examination and offering much information about a patient's sensory and motor systems; clinically useful diagnostic signs evidenced during clinical examination are identified e.g. Romberg, Babinski, Gower; new professional societies and associated journals committed to the advancement of neurosciences are founded e.g. "Brain", "Journal of Neurology"; and new vocabulary is introduced to facilitate communication among investigators and describe newly discovered structures and functions e.g. axon, dendrite, neuron, synapse, nodes of Ranvier, Wallerian degeneration, and autonomic nervous system.

The 1800s are very good to the medical neurosciences.

Late Modern, 1900 AD - 2000 AD.

The 1900s witness refinement in microscopic techniques which lead to a clear proclamation the nervous system is comprised of separate, individual cells, which communicate primarily by way of release of chemical substances, across a synapse, which binds to the next cell in series and propagates transmission of information through the nervous systems' fibers by way of bioelectricity. Neuropathological changes observed at the microscopic level are associated with clinical syndromes e.g. Alzheimer's disease, Parkinson's disease.

Neuro-electrophysiology develops quickly and offers new insights into neural transmission at the cellular level. The principles of "all or none firing of neurons" and "reciprocal inhibition" underlying reflexes and coordinated movement is understood. At the clinical level, electrical brain wave activity is recorded noninvasively from scalp electrodes, described, and specific changes in electrical brain activity are associated with brain pathologies e.g. epilepsies, tumors, encephalitis.

Dermatome maps are introduced. Sensory systems are aggressively investigated and better understood. Somato-sensory system neuropathologies are explained e.g. pain syndromes, shingles.

The autonomic nervous systems are aggressively investigated and better understood from an anatomical, neurochemical, and clinic-pathological perspectives.

Investigations of normal and abnormal brain functions become integrated components of neurosurgical procedures. Localization of brain functions identified through use of neurosurgical procedures are more frequently reported in professional journals.

Importance of early brain stimulation by the environment is recognized as essential for normal early brain development.

New brain models are offered to explain normal and abnormal brain functions e.g. Alexandria Luria's model of hierarchical organization of functional brain systems, and models emphasizing cerebral dominance and lateralization of specific higher order cortical functions to left and right cerebral hemispheres.

New commercial neuro-pharmaceuticals are introduced and improve clinical conditions e.g. Sinemet for Parkinson's disease, Dilantin for epilepsies.

Governments establish specialized research, training, and treatment centers committed to excellence and advancements of medical neurosciences e.g. Montreal Neurological Institute, National Institute of Neurological Diseases and Blindness.

Neuroimaging procedures are introduced, developed, and become routine in the assessment of patients presenting with impaired neurological functions. Specific notable procedures introduced are pneumoencephalograghy, cerebral angiography, computerized axial tomography (CAT), magnetic resonance imaging (MRI), single photon emission computerized tomography (SPECT), positron emission tomography (PET), functional magnetic resonance imaging (fMRI), and magnetic resonance angiography (MRA).

Let's take a look now at a few specifics.

Alois Alzheimer (1864-1915) German neuropathologist, working closely together with Franz Nissl (1860-1919) German neurologist and Gaerano Perusini (1879-1915) Italian neuropathologist, describe the microscopic, neuropathological changes associated with early onset dementia (1906a.1906b)[264,265]. Alzheimer describes patient AD, a 56 year old female with a clinical presentation of impaired orientation, impaired memory, and difficulties with language functions, especially reading, writing, and speaking (1906a,1906b)[264,265]. Neuropathological changes evidenced upon autopsy of patient AD, reveal thinning of the cerebral cortex, presence of senile plaques (inter-cellular inclusions) and neurofibrillary tangles (intra-cellular tangles) (1906a,1906b)[264,265]. Alois Alzheimer and Gaerano Perusini, working closely together, identify and report additional patients evidencing similar clinical presentations and neuropathological findings (1907,1909)[266,267].

Complementing their clinical descriptions and autopsy findings, Alzheimer and Perusini prepare detailed drawings of the neuropathological changes, including drawings from patient AD (1909-1910,1911)[268,269]. Alzheimer and Perusini prepare their detailed drawings, using a projection camera attached to a microscope, allowing detailed tracings of images they view under the microscope. The drawings clearly reveal and document the observed changes appearing in the cerebral cortex of patients presenting with dementia and provide additional evidence of the use and value of the microscope, in the hands of thoughtful investigators.

Emil Kraepelin (1826-1926) German psychiatrist reviews the presentations and papers offered by Alois Alzheimer and Gaerano Perusini, determines the condition is sufficiently distinct and requires its on diagnostic designation, and chooses to term this condition Alzheimer-Perusini disease (1910)[270]. Today, over 110 years since the condition and neuropathology are offered by Alois Alzheimer and Gaerano Perusini, the neuropathological changes are simply termed Alzheimer's disease and the clinical presentation, until recently known as dementia of the Alzheimer's type (2000)[271]. The new and most recent term for this clinical presentation is Major Neurocognitive Disorder due to probable Alzheimer's disease (2013)[272].

Camillo Golgi (1843-1926) Italian histologist shares the 1906 Nobel Prize in Physiology or Medicine with Spanish histologist Santiago Ramon y Cajal (1852-1934) "…in recognition of their work on the structure of the nervous system…" (1906)[273]. The recognition is made in large part as the result of the innovative staining method developed by Golgi, by impregnating neurons with silver nitrate, allowing for the structure of the cell to be clearly visualized with the light microscope. This contribution opens a new branch of investigation of the nervous system, at the microscopic level, unlike anything before. Camillo Golgi, applies his new staining procedure, "la reazione nera" (the black reaction) (1873)[274] with improved microscope technology to identify new microscopic structures e.g. Golgi tendon organ (aka neurotendonous spindles, a proprioceptive sensory nerve ending embedded into tendons) (1880a)[275]; describes the anatomy of brain and spinal cord multipolar motor and sensory neurons, organizing them into Golgi type I (long axon processes) and type II (short axonal processes) (1880b)[276]; the intracellular Golgi complex (Golgi terms the "internal reticular apparatus" and is essential for packaging synthesized proteins into membrane bound vesicles for transport) (1886,1898)[277,278]; and describes the developmental cycle of Plasmodium (parasite responsible for malaria) in red blood cells and associates recurrent fevers and chills with the release of the parasite into blood (1886,1889)[279,280].

Santiago Ramon y Cajal applies Golgi's new staining technique and describes in much detail the cell structure of the neuron. He is first to demonstrate each neuron is an independent structure and neural information is transferred by neural impulse form one cell to another. Santiago Ramon y Cajal's works prove monumental in helping to resolve the passionate debate, during the 1800s as to whether the central nervous systems is comprised of a single net of neural fibers, as argued by Camillo Golgi, or as a collection of individual cells communicating with each other in a coordinated manner, as argued by Santiago Raymon y Cajal (1899,1904)[281]. Assisted by Golgi's staining method, Santiago Raymon y Cajal's position proves to be correct and provides the foundation upon which the human nervous systems will be understood, during the next 120 years.

Trivia: Although the 1906 Nobel Prize in Physiology or Medicine is shared by Camillo Golgi and Santiago Raymon y Cajal, the Nobel Prize Committee debates whether the Prize should be awarded to Golgi alone, given the work of Santiago Ramon y Cajal is so heavily dependent upon the contributions made by Golgi (1999)[282]. What do you think?

Korbinian Brodmann (1868-1918) German neurologist describes fifty- two distinct cortical areas, based upon microscopic examination of cerebral cortex cytoarchitectural structure and using the Nissl staining technique (1909)[283]. Perhaps you recognize a few of the more common cortical regions e.g. Brodmann's areas 44, 45 (Broca's area), Brodmann's area 22 (Wernicke's area), Brodmann's area 4 (primary somato- motor strip), Brodmann's areas 1, 3, 2 (primary somato-sensory strip) and Brodmann's area 8 (frontal eye fields). Other investigators propose similar brain maps and numbering systems, many with more areas (several hundreds) and other with less areas, however, the fifty-two areas defined by Brodmann continue to serve as the gold standard today, over 109 years after he first introduces his organizational system.

Friedrich Lewy (1885-1950) German neuropathologist first describes intracytoplasmic inclusion bodies, later to be termed Lewy bodies, in neurons located in the parasympathetic nuclei of CN X (dorsal vagal nuclei) of the medulla, Nucleus of Meynert (substania innominate) located in the basal forebrain below and anterior to the thalamus, and basal nuclei putamen and globus pallidus located deep inside the cerebral hemispheres (1912,1913)[284,285].

The same intracytoplasmic inclusions are identified six years later, in the substantia nigra nuclei, located in the anterior midbrain, in patients presenting with clinical signs and symptoms of paralysis agitans (Parkinson's disease). This seminal observation is made by Russian neuropathologist Konstantin Tretiakoff (1892-1958) while conducting research, in fulfillment of his medical school doctoral thesis requirement, at the University of Paris (1919)[286].

Konstantin Tretiakoff studies 54 brains, 9 having clinically evidenced paralysis agitans (Parkinson's disease). He observes 6 of 9 patients have a distinct loss of pigmentation in the substantia nigra nuclei and the remaining cells are swollen. It is in the swollen cells he observes the inclusion bodies and notes these inclusions are invariably associated with impaired mental functions. He terms these intracellular aggregate protein inclusions "…corps de Lewy…" [Lewy bodies] and importantly notes these inclusions do not occur only in patients with paralysis agitans (Parkinson's disease). Lewy bodies are observed in brains of patients clinically presenting with a wide range of movement disorders e.g. chorea and cervical dystonia (1919)[286].

Neurohistology is instrumental in the rapid development of the medical neurosciences during the 1800s. Neurohistology offers a methodology providing unique and essential new information, which guides medical neuroscience research for the next 100 years.

Georges Guillain (1876-1961) French neurologist, Jean Barre (1880-1967) French neurologist, and Andre Strol (1887-1977) French physiologist describe the syndrome affecting primarily young adults characterized by ascending progressive muscle weakness of the extremities, which can result in paralysis, termed simply Guillain-Barre-Strol syndrome (1916)[287].

Note: Most Americans pronounce Guillain's name incorrectly and most often when referring to the Guillain-Barre syndrome. The correct pronunciation of Guillain's name, according to his extern training with him in 1939, is "… "ghee-lain", with the final ain nasalized…" (1977)[288].

Henry Head (1861-1940) English neurologist pioneers work in the somato-sensory systems, offering highly influential theoretical conceptual models and empirically derived experimental observations, which establish the foundation upon which much modern clinical neurosciences builds. His commitment to understanding the workings of the human nervous systems and applying new information to the diagnosis, treatment, and management of neurologically impaired patients is exceptional. Perhaps no better example of his commitment is demonstrated when he enlist medical colleagues and friends William Rivers (1864-1922) and James Sherren (1872-1945) to sever and suture all cutaneous branches of Henry Head's left radial nerve, in order to determine how long it takes to regrow the nerve, the time it takes sensations to return, and in which order do sensations return following nerve injuries (1908)[289]. For those of you are curious, access the 1908 paper and see what part of Henry Head's body is used by William Rivers as a control. If you do, you will better understand Henry Head's complete and total commitment to understanding the somato-sensory systems (1908,2009)[289,290]. Would you be willing to use this part of your body in replicating their original experiment?

Henry Head offers one of the first dermatome maps of the human body and explains the characteristic restricted rash distribution and pain associated with shingles (herpes zoster virus) (1900,1920a,1920b)[291,293,294]. Henry Head originally refers to sensory dermatomes, in his original publications, simply as "pain spots". Henry Head is first to offer a systematic description of the function of specific thalamic nuclei and their connections to the cerebral cortex (1911)[292].

Henry Head offers his extremely influential two volume series, "Studies in Neurology", which is based on over eighteen years of clinical observation and research (1920a,1920b)[293,294]. Volume I presents instructions and methods for examining somatosensory systems e.g. vibration sense, two-point discrimination, conscious proprioception, sharp and dull pain, hot-cold; identifies lesion locations within the peripheral and central nervous systems which effect normal sensations; details consequences of injury to peripheral nerves and provides evidence based research on recovery of nerves and function following injury (1920a)[293]. Volume II presents information on the afferent impulses within the spinal cord and associated consequences of lesions to the spinal cord; autonomic disorders resulting from spinal cord lesions; sensory disturbances resulting from lesions of white matter tracts of the brainstem and cerebral hemispheres; and sensory disturbances associated with lesions of the cerebral cortex (1920b)[294]. No publication to date details and summarize the neurosciences underlying human sensation with applications to clinical practice more than "Studies in Neurology". William Rivers and James Sherren join Henry Head, eight years after severing his radial nerve, as contributing authors to "Studies of Neurology".

Henry Head, while focusing on clinical observations and investigations into the nervous systems he develops passionately held opinions regarding the proper training of medical students and medical residents. He argues individuals who choose to teach medical students should first be academics, well trained in the basic sciences and devoted to the continued advancement of the medical and scientific knowledge through thoughtful basic or applied research and only secondarily practice occasionally as a clinician.

Henry Head briefly summarizes his concerns on this topic:

> "…Medical education in England suffers from the fact that the great hospitals are manned by practitioners of medicine who sometimes teach, instead of professors of science who occasionally practice…" (1902 p15)[295].

Recall, around 1900 in Europe and in the United States of America (USA) many physicians are educated and trained in free standing, poorly regulated, privately owned and operated schools of medicine and not exposed to or trained to contribute to the research process, which allows the clinical practice of medicine to move forward. This concern is shared by many in the USA and Canada at the time, resulting in the now well recognized Flexner Report, which changes medical education in the USA and Canada for the next 100 years, requiring medical schools to associate with universities (1910)[296].

As any new professional discipline develops, advances in new and innovative technologies are required to move the scientific and clinical knowledge bases forward. So too is the case with the medical neurosciences. During the early-1900s, developmental advances in the recording of electrical brain activity, originally demonstrated by neuroelectrophysiology pioneers Richard Caton (1842-1926) Liverpool physician and Adolf Beck (1863-1942) Polish, Professor of Physiology, using invasive procedures on animals are evidenced and the technique modified and applied to humans. Neuroelectrophysiology is soon to become an integrated component of the assessment of the human nervous system and proves especially valuable in the assessment and understanding of seizure disorders.

Hans Berger (1873-1941) German psychiatrist, records electrical signals generated from the human brain in 1924, using non-invasive techniques and recording signals from scalp electrodes. Five years later he publishes the first paper describing his procedures and is first to record, electrical brain signals from the human brain (1929)[297]. In the long held tradition and practice of many researchers, Hans Berger uses his children as early test subjects to help develop and refine the recording procedures and equipment. Recording of human brain electrical activity, as proposed by Hans Berger, is replicated in independent laboratories throughout Europe and soon acknowledged as a truly new and innovative procedure. Hans Berger terms the recording and procedure the electroencephalogram.

Recording electrical brain activity by non-invasive procedures open many new avenues of investigations into the medical neurosciences. The procedure quickly reveals its value in the investigations of seizure disorders. The electroencephalogram (EEG) soon becomes a mainstay procedure for the assessment and monitoring of neurological impairment. The procedure continues to be used today, over 95 years since first introduced and continues to provide essential information regarding electrical brain activity to assist in diagnosis and to guide clinical treatments.

Charles Sherrington (1857-1952) and Edgar Adrian (1889-1977) English neurophysiologists are awarded the 1932 Nobel Prize in Physiology or Medicine "…for their discoveries regarding the functions of neurons…" (1932)[298]. Charles Sherrington discovers and demonstrates the principle of reciprocal intervention of muscles and displaces medical dogma regarding reflex muscle movements. Reflexive movements are not the result of a simple reflex arch as previously understood, rather reflexes result from unconscious neural integration and coordination which produce contraction of an agonist muscle group and reciprocal inhibition of the antagonist muscle group (1906)[299]. The same principle explains the underlying neuronal mechanism responsible for coordinated movement. Many disorders of movement can now be understood within this conceptual matrix.

Edgar Adrian (1889-1977) English neuro-electrophysiologist and colleague Swedish neuro-electrophysiologist Yngve Zotterman (1898-1982) discover and demonstrate the now fundamental principle of the " all or none law of nerve firing". Intensity of a sensory stimulus does not result in a stronger or weaker neural signal, rather the signals are sent either more often or less often and through more or less numbers of nerve fibers. Muscles respond to neural stimulation independent of the strength of the neural input. Edgar Adrian and Yngve Zotterman achieve their discovery by applying new neuro-electrophysiology recording techniques which allow for the recording of a single afferent neuron firing, which allows for the study and description of neuron firing properties, as a function of varying stimuli intensities (1926)[300].

Henry Dale (1875-1968) English pharmacologist and Otto Loewi (1873-1961) German neurophysiologist share the 1936 Nobel Prize in Physiology or Medicine "…for their discoveries relating to chemical transmission of nerve impulses…" (1936)[301]. Henry Dale is first to identify and describe acetylcholine (ACh) and demonstrate its role in chemical synaptic transmission between neurons and at the neuromuscular junction (1914)[302]. He discovers acetylcholine to be the primary neurotransmitter used in the parasympathetic nervous system and is released onto heart muscles to regulate and dampen heart rate (1914)[302]. He demonstrates it is the primary neurochemical substance used at the autonomic ganglia of both the parasympathetic and sympathetic nervous systems. He demonstrates the role of ACh in constricting the pupil of the eyes. He is instrumental in resolving the debate as whether neural transmission occurs electrically or chemically at the synapse.

Before Dale's contributions it is widely recognized neurons and muscle use electricity. In order to explain the speed of neural transmission, it makes sense to explain neural transmission via electricity jumping across, "sparking", from cell to cell. However, Dale challenges this dogma and offers the alternative, chemical transmission model to explain neural transmission. The debate continues well in to the late-1930s (1939,1039)[303,304] and exemplified in the passionate exchanges between himself and future 1963 Nobel Prize in Physiology or Medicine recipient Austrian neurophysiologist John Eccles (1903-1997). John Eccles discovers inhibitory and excitatory post synaptic potentials (IPSP and EPSP) and is an unyielding proponent of electrical transmission model of neural transmission.

Henry Dale is responsible for the separation of acetylcholine and their receptors into the nicotinic and muscarinic subtypes (1914)[302]. He identifies acetylcholine to be a naturally occurring substance in the human body (1929)[305]. Prior to his contribution, only adrenaline is known to exist in animals and acetylcholine is unknown to exist in animals and only to exist as a plant extract.

It is Henry Dale whom first proposes classifying neurons based upon the principle neurotransmitter released, specifically cholinergic and adrenergic neurons (1933)[306]. The same year, two of Henry Dale's students identify acetylcholine to be present in the ganglia of sympathetic nervous systems (1933)[307]. Henry Dale further advances the understanding of the autonomic nervous systems and demonstrates some components of the sympathetic nervous system e.g. sweat gland, actually release acetylcholine rather than epinephrine as commonly believed at the time (1934)[308]. Finally, it is Henry Dale who definitively demonstrates, it is acetylcholine released by neurons which stimulated nicotinic receptors on skeletal muscles, producing skeletal muscle contraction and the resultant movement of the body (1953)[309].

Otto Loewi extends the original work of British pharmacologist Walter Dixon (1871-1931) and in effect replicates Walter Dixon's 1907 experiment, in which he demonstrates the inhibitory effect of cranial nerve X on the heart and proposes it is the result of the release of a chemical substance from a neuron that is responsible (1907)[310]. It is the seeming replication of Walter Dixon's experiment for which Otto Loewi is frequently remembered by medical students and contributes to sharing the 1936 Nobel Prize in Physiology or Medicine with Henry Dale.

Otto Loewi does offer a series of influential papers; specifically investigating the role of the neurochemical substance he initially terms "vagustoff", which is later identified to be acetylcholine (1921)[311]. Otto Loewi confirms Walter Dixon's original hypothesis, CN X (vagus nerves) have an inhibitory effect on heart rate and use "vagustoff", released from the neurons to effect the inhibition on heart rate. His more original contributions are found in providing additional experimental evidence demonstrating neural transmission is chemical rather than electrical, as popularly believed at this time. Arguably more importantly, he offers original and influential insights into the underlying chemical mechanisms responsible for the metabolism of acetylcholine and how its metabolism is inhibited (1926)[312]. From a pharmacological perspective and working primarily with the cholinergic systems, he is instrumental in clarifying two mechanisms responsible for many medical treatments, the blockade or augmentation of neuronal systems and associated functions by use of medications which target specific neurotransmitter systems.

Wilder Penfield (1891-1976) American, Professor of Neurology and Neurosurgery at McGill University, Montreal, Quebec, Canada revolutionizes the understanding of the brain with introduction of the "Montreal Procedure". In brief, the Procedure introduces brief bursts of electrical current, applied by a probe, to a focused and localized area of brain, while the patient is awake, in order to report what the patient experiences whenever the electrical current is applied e.g. sensation, hallucinations, illusions, mood, déjà vu, jamais vu, memories (1952,1954)[313,314]. The Procedure proves revolutionary in helping to understand the functional localization in brain, especially the cerebral cortex. The Procedure produces the now familiar sensory and motor homunculi (1937,1954)[315,314]. Wilder Penfield is primary in establishing the Montreal Neurological Institute. He founds the Institute with an initial endowment of approximately 1.25

million dollars from the Rockefeller Foundation for the committed "… investigation of the brain and mind as a way to human betterment…" (1934)[316].

Today, the Montreal Neurological Institute is a world leader for brain research and advanced patient care. It offers world-class training opportunities for both clinicians and researchers. The Institute offers a seemingly seamless integration of research, patient care, and training. Today, the Institute offers the largest neuroscience graduate program in North America and has provided advanced education and training to professionals from over 60 countries throughout the world (2016)[317].

Brenda Milner (1918-) Canadian neuropsychologist and Professor of Psychology at the Montreal Neurological Institute exemplifies one of the many exceptional investigators working today at the Institute and making substantial contributions to the advancement of the medical neurosciences. Perhaps most recognized for her extensive evaluation of patient H.M., between 1957-2008, she offers new and thoughtful insights into changes in higher order cortical functions, such as memory, language, cognition, as the consequence of lesions of the cerebral hemispheres. Recall, patient HM (1926-2008), at 31 years of age undergoes a bilateral medial temporal lobotomy resecting the anterior two thirds of the temporal lobes and removing most of the hippocampi nuclei and associated white matter tracts bilaterally (1957,1958)[318,319]. Subsequent to the surgery, he evidences significant impairments in memory. Brenda Milner details the patient's condition and meticulously assesses change across time. She offers much to our understanding of memory and other higher order cortical functions and how these functions change as the result of brain lesions.

Trivia: Patient H.M. donates his brain to the University of California, San Diego, where it is sliced into histological sections December 4, 2009, digitized, and made available to investigators around the world, via the internet (2009,2010,2014)[320,321,322].

The United States government creates a new Institute committed to the advancement of neuroscience knowledge and offers high quality training opportunities for future researchers and clinicians interested in the basic and applied medical neurosciences. The National Institute of Neurological Diseases and Blindness (NINDB) is created by the United States Congress, Public Law 81-692, signed by US President Harry S. Trumann, August 15, 1950 "…for research on neurological diseases (including epilepsy, cerebral palsy, and multiple sclerosis) and blindness…" (1950)[323]. The mission of the Institute has always been "…to reduce the burden of neurological disease - a burden borne by every age group, every segment of society, and people all over the world…" and to accomplish this mission "… supports and conducts basic, translational, and clinical research on the healthy and diseased nervous system; fosters the training of investigators in the basic and clinical neurosciences; and seeks better understanding, diagnosis, treatment, and prevention of neurological disorders…" (1950,2016)[323,324].

The Institute has undergone four names during its 70 years in existence, The Institute is originally named the National Institute of Neurological Disease and Blindness (NINDB) in 1950, changes its name in 1968 to the National Institute of Neurological Diseases and Stroke (NINDS), changes its name in 1975 to the National Institute of Neurological and Communicative Disorders and Stroke (NINCDS), and again changes its name in 1988 to its present name, the National Institute of Neurological Disorders and Stroke (NINDS) (2016)[324].

The United States joins a long lists of governments throughout the history of medicine, in recognizing the need to support research and training of individuals committed to understanding, treating, and managing impairments in neurological functions, as a responsibility government has to society and the people it governs.

Ulf von Euler (1905-1983) Swedish neurophysiologist and Julius Axelrod (1912-2004) American neurophysiologist, both working at the National Institute of Neurological Disease and Stroke, share the 1970 Nobel Prize in Physiology or Medicine with German neurophysiologist Bernard Katz (1911-2003) for "…their discoveries concerning the humoral transmitters in the nerve terminals and the mechanism for their storage, release and inactivation…" (1970)[325].

Ulf von Euler discovers norepinephrine, details its role in producing the fight or flight responses, details how norepinephrine is formed, stored, and packaged, and describes how neurotransmitters pass between cells via synapses for neural transmission and stimulation of target tissues (1946a,1946b,1948)[326,327,328]. Julius Axelrod studies and reports seminal works regarding norepinephrine and its role during aggression and danger responses. He details how norepinephrine is released from neurons and returned to and stored in the presynaptic neuron (1957)[329]. Bernard Katz further develops and details the release of acetylcholine into the synapse of the neuromuscular junctions and how the neurotransmitter initiates muscle contractions, complementing the work of contemporary Henry Dale (1952,1954)[330,331].

Increased understanding of the underlying mechanisms of neural transmission and neurotransmitter substances leads to increased interests in developing pharmaceuticals capable of modifying the naturally occurring processes with the intent to produce medications capable of modifying these systems, in order to produce meaningful improvement in patients presenting with impaired neurological functions.

One of the first pharmaceuticals, demonstrating early promise in the treatment of neurological impairments is suggested by Swedish pharmacologists Avid Carlsson (1923-2018) and Nils-Ake Hillarp (1916-1965). Capitalizing on their recent technological advancements in their ability to quantify small amounts of catecholamines in biological tissue, they propose L-dopa, as a potential pharmacological agent which should improve the debilitating impairments in movement, characteristic of Parkinson's disease (1958)[332]. The proposal is rational, based upon the current understanding of brain chemistries, identified brain regions deficient in a specific neurotransmitter substance (basal nuclei; dopamine), and preliminary animal studies demonstrating improvement in impaired motor function when brain dopamine levels are increased (1957,1958)[333,332].

Levodopa (L-dopa) is introduced for the treatment of Parkinson's disease and evidences promising results (1961,1968,1969)[334,335,336]. Addition of an inhibitor of dopa decarboxylase further reduces the necessary amounts of L-dopa required to be administered and reduces side effects. The compounded pharmaceutical, L-dopa + a decarboxylase inhibitor (carbidopa) is marketed by Merck Pharmaceuticals as Sinemet and proves to be more beneficial than L-dopa alone (1973,1973)[337,338]. Sinemet continues to be one of the most prescribed drugs for the treatment and management of Parkinson's disease today (2016)[339].

The introduction and development of pharmaceuticals designed to alleviate signs and symptoms of neurological impairment play an important role in the development of the medical neurosciences. New and effective treatments attract young clinicians and investigators to the medical neurosciences, open new lines of investigation, and offer another important tool to be used in investigations to better understand the complexities of the human nervous systems.

Note: Avid Carlsson shares the 2000 Nobel Prize in Physiology or Medicine with Eric Kandel (1929-) Austrian neurophysiologist and Paul Greengard (1925-2019) American neurophysiologist "…for their discoveries concerning signal transduction in the nervous system…" (2000)[340].

New conceptual models of brain organization are offered and applied to understanding neurological impairments.

Roger Sperry (1913-1994) American neurophysiologist and Michael Gazzaniga (1939-) American neuropsychologist offer a model of functional brain organization which gains much popularity during the 1960s and 1970s. Based largely on their work with patients suffering refractory epilepsy and the neurosurgical procedure of cutting the corpus callosum to prevent abnormal electrical brain activity responsible for seizures, from spreading from one cerebral hemisphere to the other, they offer the conceptual model of cerebral lateralization of brain functions.

In brief, the model states the left cerebral hemisphere is more specialized for processing verbal information, syntactic and semantic aspects of language, and analytic thought. The right cerebral hemisphere is more specialized for processing non-verbal components of language e.g. prosody, visual spatial tasks, music, and holistic thought. The model generates an oversimplified understanding of lateralization of cognitive processes by many and contributes to the popular misunderstanding the left hemisphere is dominant for processing verbal information and the right hemisphere is dominant for processing non-verbal information. While the oversimplified model of lateralization of cognitive brain functions continues to be perpetuated in the popular literature, from a scientific perspective, the over-simplified understanding of left brain right brain dichotomy of cerebral lateralization of cognitive function is simply wrong (1978,1982,1985)[341,342,343].

Roger Sperry shares the 1981 Nobel Prize in Physiology or Medicine "…for his discoveries concerning the functional specialization of the cerebral hemispheres…" (1981)[344]. David Hubel (1926-2013) Canadian neurophysiologist and Torsten Wiesel (1924 -) Swedish neurophysiologist shares the Prize with Roger Sperry "…for their discoveries concerning information processing of the visual system…" (1981)[345]. David Hubel and Torsten Wiesel detail how the eye captures light, how light waves are converted into bioelectrical signals at the level of the retina, how visual signals are sent to the visual cerebral cortex, and how specialized cells interpret contrast, patterns, and movement (1959,1962)[346,347].

David Hubel and Torsten Wiesel additionally offer their seminal works detailing the importance of early sensory and motor stimulation of animals to ensure normal brain development and offer innovative insights into brain plasticity (1963a,1963b,1965)[348,349,350]. An animal's environment has a demonstrable effect on the normal development of brain tissue. Poor environmental conditions result in poor brain development.

Alexander Luria (1902-1977) Russian neuropsychologist offers his conceptual model within which to understand normal and disordered brain functions, with particular attention to higher order cortical functions (1973)[351]. The model is conceptually simple and provides a conceptual matrix within which to understand both normal and abnormal neurological function. In brief, Alexander Luria's model sates the human brain processes information in a systematic and predictable fashion. Impairment in function can result from impairment anywhere along the way from initial sensory stimulation, flow through neural pathways, nuclei, and cortex, or the cortical processing of information. Similarly for motor systems, impairment in function can result anywhere along the way from the initial thought to engage in volitional movement, to the preprocessing of the movement at the level of the cerebral cortex before being transmitter to the neural pathways which will transmit the processed signal through the brain, brainstem, spinal cord, and peripheral nerve to stimulate muscle fibers, initiating contraction of the muscle and producing movement. Particular attention within the model is directed to the processing or preprocessing of information at the cortical level. For example, he introduces the concept of primary, secondary, and tertiary cortex.

For somatosensory information, once a signal has passed from the peripheral sensory receptor, through a peripheral or cranial nerve to the spinal cord or brain stem, then on to the thalamic nuclei, and on to the cerebral cortex, the signal is initially received and processed in the primary somatosensory cortex. At this point a person perceives sensation and without attributing meaning to the sensation. The signals move from primary sensory cortex to secondary and tertiary association cortex where the signal is further processed and meaning is associated with the signal. This basic model holds true for all sensory systems.

Similarly, the conceptual model is applied to the motor system. Thoughts of movement generate brain bioelectric signals which are transmitted from basal nuclei to the cerebral cortex, initially processed at the cortical level in the tertiary and secondary pre-motor cortex before moving to the primary somato-motor cortex. From the somato-motor cortex of the precentral gyrus, the signal is sent away from the cerebral cortex, through neural pathways cursing through the cerebral hemispheres, brain stem, spinal cord, and peripheral or cranial nerves on to muscles.

Simply an elegant conceptual model. Neurological impairment can be interpreted within the model and signs and symptoms explained and predicted by understanding where in the system a lesion exist. Understanding of any functional impairment necessitates an understanding where the flow of information through the neural system is first disrupted and how that will effect transmission and processing further along in the system.

For example, in the somatosensory system, a lesion of the primary somatosensory cortex will result in a primary loss of somato-sensation. However, if the primary somatosensory cortex remains intact and the lesion occurs in the secondary or tertiary association cortex, the patient will maintain perception of sensation, however will be unable to associate meaning to the sensation, resulting in an agnosia, a higher order cortical impairment.

Luria advocates flexibility in the diagnostic assessment process, adjusting clinical examination procedures to accommodate or stress specific functional systems, in an effort to identify the neurological basis for impaired function. Alexander Luria's conceptual model of functional systems remains a mainstay in the medical neurosciences throughout the balance of the late-1900s.

New technologies open new lines of investigations in the medical neurosciences during the 1900s. The most significant advances are made in the area of neuroimaging.

In brief, early in the 1900s neuroimaging is restricted to two primary procedures, pneumoencephalography (PEG) introduced by American neurosurgeon Walter Dandy (1886-1946) and cerebral angiography introduced and developed by Portuguese neurologist and future Nobel Prize Laurette in Physiology or Medicine Egas Moniz (1874-1955). Both procedures utilize the recently discovered X-ray technology and offer images of brain structures previously unseen without opening the skull.

Pneumoencephalography extends Walter Dandy's earlier and less successful work in brain imaging with ventriculography. Pneumoencephalography requires draining CSF from the subdural space by spinal tab, injecting air into the subarachnoid space, and by mechanical manipulation of the patient's head working the air into the cerebral ventricles. Once the air is positioned inside of the ventricles, conventional X-ray images are made of the head and brain. Given air absorbs no x-ray, images of the ventricles and any ventricular displacement by space occupying lesions can be imaged. Although with its own risk of mortality associated with the procedure and painful to patients, it offers one of the first neuroimaging procedures used in medicine (1919)[352]. Yes, this is the same Dandy who describes the Dandy-Walker malformation and syndrome (1921)[353].

Cerebral angiography is pioneered by Portuguese neurologist and Nobel Prize Laurette Egas Moniz as a safer and more exact method than Walter Dandy's pneumoencephalography, to identify space occupying brain lesions, specifically brain tumors (1927)[354]. The procedure requires injection of a contrast agent containing iodine into the carotid artery. Once injected the contrast material fills the arteries of the brain, which then can be imaged using conventional X-ray technology of the period to reveal displacement of the arteries from their usual positons. Displacement of the arteries suggests a space occupying brain lesion, such as tumors, while absence of filling of arteries suggest cerebral arterial blockage.

Trivia: Egas Moniz is awarded the 1949 Nobel Prize in Physiology or Medicine for "… his discovery of the therapeutic value of leucotomy in certain psychoses…". Years later, Egas Moniz is shot in his office by a delusional and paranoid patient. The injuries suffered, confine him to a wheel chair for the balance of his life.

Pneumoencephalgraphy and cerebral angiography remain mainstay procedures for imaging brain for the next 50 years, when they begin to be displaced by computerized axial tomography (CAT scans), magnetic resonance imaging (MRI), and magnetic resonance angiography (MRA).

Computerized axial tomography is introduced for medical purposes by Godfrey Hounsfield (1919-2004) British electrical engineer working with EMI Laboratories and Alan Cormack (1924-1998) South African physicist working with Tufts University. The procedure uses X-ray technologies to generate brain images, based upon calculations using X-ray absorption coefficients to reconstruct images of brain. Tissues absorb different amounts of X-ray based upon their density e.g. bone absorbs a lot of X-ray, brain tissue a moderate amount, and CSF in the ventricles very little. The initial images generated for medical purposes during the early-1970s are restricted to the axial plane, resulting in the procedure's initial name, CAT scan (computerized axial tomography). CAT scanners are widely available by the 1980s and non-invasive brain imaging is made readily available to the practicing physician. With development over the next 25 years, the procedure is capable of producing images in additional planes e.g. coronal plane, radiation exposure is reduced, scanning times and therefore radiation exposure reduced, image resolution greatly improved, and cost of imaging reduced. Today, the procedure is simply termed CT and continues to be an essential tool available to professionals charged with the diagnosis, treatment, and management of individuals suffering impaired neurological functions due to structural lesions of the nervous systems.

Godfrey Hounsfield and Alan Cormack share the 1979 Nobel Prize in Physiology or Medicine "…for the development of computer assisted tomography…" (1979)[355]. In the true spirit and conventional practice of numerous researchers throughout the history of medicine, Godfrey Hounsfield tests the CAT procedure on himself before using it to successfully image a cerebral cyst in a patient at Atkinson Morley Hospital located in London, October 1, 1971, the first human documented to be scanned for medical purposes.

Trivia: The Company which supports the early development of the CT scanner is EMI (Electric and Musical Industries). This is the same EMI responsible for producing the 1960s pop band, the Beatles. Profits generated by the music division of EMI contribute importantly to the early development of the CT scanner, then known simply as the EMI scanner.

Magnetic resonance imaging (MRI) is introduced during the early-1970s and begins to become available for medical use, at large medical centers during the mid-1980s. The procedure utilizes magnetic field technologies rather than X-ray technologies to non-invasively generate high resolution images of brain and spinal cord structures. The MRI provides an attractive alternative to the CT procedure and images by not requiring the use of ionizing radiation to generate images, providing high resolution brain stem images, and greater differentiation between white matter and gray matter structures.

Magnetic resonance imaging results from the combined efforts of numerous investigators contributing to its development beginning during the early-1950s (1950,1952,1952)[356,357,358]. Three individuals working during the early-1970s conventionally receive most credit for developing the procedure for medical purposes, American chemist Paul Lauterbur (1929-2007) working at the State University of New York (SUNY) Stoney Brook, English physicist, Peter Mansfield (1933-2017) working at the Max-Plank Institute for Medical Research, and Raymond Damadian (1936-) American physician-scientist working at the State University of New York (SUNY) Downstate Medical Center in Brooklyn.

Application of MRI during the early-1970s reliably differentiates normal brain tissues from brain tumors. Given cerebral tumors contain more water than normal brain tissues and the magnetic properties of the tissues differ when placed in a strong magnetic field and an external resonating frequency applied to the magnetic field, begins to establish the MRI as a new procedure for non-invasively revealing brain structure, useful in the practice of medicine and surgery (1971, 1973)[359,360]. By the mid-1980s MRI is proving to be especially useful in imaging assorted neuropathologies e.g. multiple sclerosis (1981)[361], acoustic neuromas (1983)[362], cerebral infarctions (1983)[363], brainstem tumors (1985)[364], and brain cancers (1985)[365].

Paul Lauterbur and Peter Mansfield are awarded the 2003 Nobel Prize in Physiology or Medicine "….for their discoveries concerning magnetic resonance imaging…" (2003)[366]. Raymond Damadian is not included in the award and ignites a professional debate, as to the possible reasons why. The debate continues today with most knowledgeable professionals within the medical neurosciences maintaining a clear position and opinion. So goes the politics within professional science and medicine.

The next step in development of medical neuroimaging is the introduction of procedures, during the 1970s through 1990s, which use radioactive emission tomography technologies and which allow for assessment of metabolically active brain tissues and imaging of regional cerebral blood flow.

Single photon emission computerized tomography (SPECT), using gamma-ray emission technologies, allows for a direct assessment of cerebral blood flow and an indirect measurement of metabolic brain activity. The procedure requires inhalation or injection of a radioactive isotope into the bloodstream, which is then carried to the brain areas with increased metabolic demand. The gamma radiation released is collected by gamma cameras surrounding the head and signals are then converted to brain images, revealing brain areas of increased or decreased metabolic activity. Spatial resolution of tissues is approximately one centimeter. The first SPECT scanners developed for medical use are introduced during the early-1970s. The procedure continues to be used today and offers a relative inexpensive procedure to evaluate cerebral blood flow and generate functional images of brain activity. The procedure is frequently used today in the assessment of several neurocognitive disorders e.g. Major Neurocognitive disorders (dementia) resulting from Alzheimer's disease, Parkinson's disease, brain trauma, toxin exposure, and cerebral vascular disease processes.

Positron emission tomography (PET), also using emission tomography technologies is introduced for medical neuroimaging (1973)[367]. Similar to SPECT, the PET scan uses emission technologies. Positron-emitting radionuclides are introduced into the body via the bloodstream, on a biologically active molecule. In the case of the PET, the positron emitting radionuclide molecule most often used is fluorine-18 (F-18) and is tagged most commonly to fludeoxyglucose (FDG) an analogue of glucose (FDG-PET). Brain areas with high metabolic demand and high demand for glucose e.g. brain areas in which rapid cell division is occurring (rapidly growing tumors), will localize the greatest concentration of the radioactively tagged molecule, allowing for external detection of the materials' radioactive decay and construction of brain images based upon the radioactive decay information. Spatial resolution of PET images are much higher than SPECT images. Temporal resolution for both procedures is poor.

Functional magnetic resonance imaging (fMRI) is introduced during the early-1990s and offers a relatively easy, non-invasive procedure to assess cerebral blood flow which is not dependent upon radioactive tracers or emission technology (1991,1991,1992)[368,369,370]. The procedure is unique in that it does not require the use of ionizing radiation. The most common fMRI protocol used during the 1990s is termed blood-oxygen-level-dependency (BOLD). The protocol allows computer generated brain images based upon differential changes in brain tissue utilization of oxygen. Temporal and spatial resolutions are poor.

Magnetic resonance angiography (MRA) is applied to cerebral vessels and offers a new, minimally invasive, and relatively safe procedure to assess cerebral blood vessels (1992, 1992)[371,372]. MRA offers an attractive alternative to conventional brain angiography. The procedure uses magnetic field technologies, rather than x-ray or emission technologies, to generate computer images of brain blood vessels. Intravenous injection of contrast material, most commonly gadolinium, allows imaging of cerebral and brainstem arteries and veins, with relatively good resolution.

In summary, the 1900s witness tremendous advancements in the medical neurosciences. Microscopic investigations identify and associate changes in the nervous systems with specific clinical syndromes. Alois Alzheimer describes the thinning of the cerebral cortex, presence of extracellular senile plaques, and intracellular neurofibrillary tangles to be associated with dementia. Medical student Konstantin Tretiakoff identifies the presence of Lewy bodies in patients presenting with Parkinson's disease. New histological staining procedures prove especially useful in the investigation of the nervous systems. Camillo Golgi and Santiago Cajal are awarded Nobel Prizes for their discovery and application of innovative staining techniques. Korbinian Brodmann describes the cytoarchitectural structure of the cerebral cortex, offering his fifty- two distinct areas.

Neural transmission is understood within the matrix of bioelectricity and excitatory and inhibitory neurotransmitter systems. Chemical neurotransmission, at the synapse is understood. Production, storage, release, metabolism, reuptake, and elimination of neurotransmitters are understood. Acetylcholine is identified as a naturally occurring neurotransmitter substance in animals and humans, its role in muscle contraction and importance in autonomic nervous systems functions are detailed.

Somatosensory systems are aggressively investigated and better understood. Dermatome mapping is introduced. Pain syndromes are identified and interpreted within a conceptual matrix recognizing not all pain is the same and is differentially generated dependent upon which neural systems are affected.

Motor systems and associated disorders are detailed. New clinical syndromes are identified e.g. Guillain-Barre syndrome. Basal nuclei systems are recognized to be essential for normal movement and when disordered result in abnormal movement syndromes characterized by increased muscle tone (rigidity) and abnormal movements at rest (tremors, chorea). Basal nuclei disorders are differentiated from cerebellar and cortico-spinal motor system disorders.

Commercial neuropharmaceuticals are introduced and prove effective in the treatment and management of neurological conditions e.g. Sinemet (carbidopa-levodopa) for Parkinson's disease and Dilantin (phenytoin) for seizure disorders.

Neuroelectrophysiology is developed and contributes meaningfully to the study of the nervous systems, at the cellular level. Recording of electrical brain activity becomes a much valued clinically useful procedure for evaluating brain electrical activity in real time and proves especially useful in the diagnosis and assessment of seizure disorders. Computer technologies allow for the introduction and development of evoked potentials and too prove useful in the assessment of normal and impaired neurological systems.

Brain surgical procedures e.g. the Montreal Procedure and Split Brain, contribute to a rapidly developing dogma of localization of cortically mediated brain functions, such as language, memory, and cognitive processes.

New conceptual models are introduced and displace conventional medical dogma. Alexandrea Luria introduces his model based upon systematic, hierarchical organization and ordered information processing.

Governments of Canada and the USA establish research, training, and treatment centers dedicated to the advancement of medical neuroscience knowledge e.g. the Montreal Neurological Institute and National Institute of Neurological Disease and Blindness.

Neuroimaging is responsible for astonishing advancements. The following procedures are all introduced, developed, refined, and revolutionize the way we assess the nervous system: pneumoencephalography (PEG), cerebral angiography (CA), computerized axial tomography (CT), magnetic resonance imaging (MRI), single photon emission computerized tomography (SPECT), positron emission tomography (PET), functional magnetic resonance imaging (fMRI), and magnetic resonance angiography (MRA).

Investigations of brain and associated impairment in function are high priorities and well-funded during the 1900s. Many new and innovative advancements are made and new lines of investigation opened. Professional journals enjoy a surge in articles addressing brain and brain functions. International collaborative networks are established and permits rapid sharing of information among investigators. The general public is educated on neurological diseases, especially Alzheimer's disease, Parkinson's disease, multiple sclerosis, amyotrophic lateral sclerosis, and epilepsies. Medical neurosciences attract many of the brightest and innovative minds graduating from graduate and medical schools throughout the world. Medical neuroscience establishes itself as a mature and clinically valuable professional discipline.

Current Modern, 2000 AD - 2019 AD.

Medical neurosciences continue to pioneer the search for new knowledge and "…boldly go where no man has gone before…". Innovative technologies and ideas continue to play critical roles in advancing the medical neurosciences. The human nervous systems and all of its complexities continue to challenge the brightest of minds. Much emphasis in medical neuroscience research today is being placed upon better understanding of genetic materials and their roles in the origins, amelioration, and potential treatments of neurological diseases and conditions. Medical school education and training in the medical neurosciences is highly emphasized and fundamental to every modern medical student's knowledge base, whether choosing academia or clinical service delivery. Continued, rapid, and significant advancements are reasonably expected in the next few years.

Advancements in imaging technologies continue. For example, one impressive imaging tool benefiting from recent developments is Diffusion Tensor Imaging (DTI) and a second is CLARITY.

Diffusion tensor imaging (DTI) uses MRI technologies to map and characterize the three dimensional diffusion of water, as a function of spatial localization in brain. Images generated reveal estimates of white matter connectivity patterns, termed tractographs (1999,2001, 2007)[373,374,375]. The procedure is being applied to the imaging of assorted brain pathologies such as brain ischemia associated with stroke syndromes (1999)[376], multiple sclerosis (1999, 2003)[377,378], cerebral tumors (2002)[379], vascular malformation (2006)[380], and children with autism (2007)[381]. More recently the procedure has been applied to the investigation of brain trauma (2008,2012,2016)[382,383,384], psychiatric disorders e.g. schizophrenia, bipolar disorder, major depression (2009,2011,2013)[385,386,387], mild cognitive impairments associated with suspected Alzheimer's disease (2011)[388], amyotrophic lateral sclerosis (2012)[389], and Parkinson syndromes (2013)[390].

Karl Deisseroth (1971-) Professor of Bioengineering, Psychiatry and Behavioral Sciences at Stanford University and Kwanghun Chung (unknown-) Assistant Professor of Medical Engineering and Sciences introduce a new technology which allows for making brain tissues transparent and labeling of specific proteins within tissues. They term the new technique CLARITY (2013,2013)[391,392].

CLARITY places tissues within a transparent scaffolding and lipid components are then removed. What remains are proteins and nucleic acids. Contrast agents are introduced such as antibodies, DNA or RNA labels, or fluorescent molecule tags, which bind to special target substances. Using specialized microscopy, a high resolution, three dimensional image can be observed (2013)[393]. An equally exciting element of this new procedure is that it is possible to remove antibodies and reapply new ones, enabling the tissue sample to be targeted with more than one group of antibodies, targeting different proteins, and generating new images from the same original tissue (2013)[394]. When applied to brain tissue, the procedure allows for imaging of local neural circuits and tracing of specific neurotransmitter systems previously unseen. CLARITY has been applied to the examination of brain tissues sampled from animals demonstrating autistic like behaviors and reveals an unusual and characteristic "ladder" pattern where neurons connect back to themselves and other local neurons (2013)[395]

Advancements continue in our understanding as to how the brain processes information. Neuronal firing patterns are now being better understood within specific sensory modalities and related to brain information processing.

John O'Keef (1939-) American physiologist, May-Britt Moser (1963-) Norwegian neurophysiologist, Edward Moser (1962 -) Norwegian neurophysiologist share the 2014 Nobel Prize in Physiology or Medicine "… for their discoveries of cells that constitute a positioning system in the brain…" (2014)[396]. Data indicate specific cell types located close to the hippocampus nuclei are differentially activated as an animal moves through their environment. The activation pattern of the specialized cell appears to form a kind of coordinate systems essential for normal navigation.

Personalized medicine also known as precision medicine is a model receiving increased attention and with potential application to the medical neurosciences. The model allows for medical decisions to be based upon individual biological characteristics e.g. genetic material profiles, to guide treatment interventions. The fundamental idea is to design treatment interventions based upon identified patient characteristics which best responds to specific treatment interventions rather than recommending general treatment interventions which have proven effective for most patients presenting with any given neurological condition. There is much optimism today that genetic materials hold the next key which will unlock the answers to allow advancement to the next level of understanding of the human nervous system and provide solutions for individuals experiencing nervous system dysfunction and impairment.

New and exciting opportunities are now available to graduate and medical students choosing to pursue careers or additional training in the medical neurosciences. The future of medical neurosciences is filled with opportunity. Are you interested? Will you be the next person to make a meaningful contribution to the medical neurosciences?

References.

[1] Neuroscience. (2016). Merriam-Webster. Medical definition of neuroscience. Retrieved 1-22-2016 from http://www.merriam-webster.com/medical/neuroscience
[2] Neuroscience. (2016). MedicineNet.com. Retrieved 1-22-2016 from http://www.medicinenet.com/script/main/art.asp?articlekey=25656
[3] Clinical Neuroscience. (2016). Clinical neuroscience. University College of London. Retrieved 1-22-2016.
[4] Scurlock, J. and Andersen, B. (2005). Diagnoses in Assyrian and Babylonian medicine: Ancient sources, translation, and modern medical analyses. Chicago: University of Illinois Press. Retrieved 1-25-2106 from https://books.google.com.ai/books?id=alBmzfP3cpoC&printsec=frontcover&dq=scurlock+andersen+diagnosis&hl=en&sa=X&redir_esc=y#v=onepage&q=scurlock%20andersen%20diagnosis&f=false
[5] Breasted, J. (1700BC/1930). The Edwin Smith Surgical Papyrus. Chicago: University of Chicago Press.
[6] Ghalioungui, P. (1500BC/1987). The Ebers Papyrus. A new English translation, commentaries and glossary. Cairo: Academy of Scientific Research and Technology.

[7] U.S. National Library of Medicine. (1700BC/2016). Edwin Smith Papyrus. Retrieved 1-26-2016 from https://ceb.nlm.nih.gov/proj/ttp/flash/smith/smith.html

[8] Ebbell, B. (1500BC/1937). The Papyrus Ebers. The greatest Egyptian medical document. Copenhagen: Levin and Munksgaard.

[9] Plato (circa 360 BC). Timaeus. Translated by Benjamin Jowett. The Internet Classic Archives. Retrieved 1-27-2016 from http://classics.mit.edu/Plato/timaeus.html

[10] Diels, H. (1903). Die fragmente der Vorsokratiker griechissch und deutch. Berlin: Widenmannsche Buchhandlung.

[11] Freeman, K. (1948). Ancilla to the Pre-Socratic Philosophers: A complete translation of the Fragments in Diel's Fragmente der Vorokratiker. Cambridge: Harvard University Press.

[12] Grapow, H. (1935). Die Agyptischen medizinischen papyri und was sie enthalen [The Egyptian medical papyri and what they include]. Munch Med Worchenschr. 82:958-962; 1002-1005.

[13] Theophrastus (circa 500 BC/1871). H. Diels, Doxographi Graeci. Berlin: De Gruyter, (1879) p. 497-527, Fragment on Sensation, DK 24 A5.; Also Alcmaeon peripheral sense organs connect channels to central organ (DK 24 A5,cf A11).

[14] Diels, H. (1887). Leukippos und Diogenes von Apollonia. RM 42:1-14.

[15] Freeman, K. (1948). Ancilla to the Pre-Socratic Philosophers: A complete translation of the Fragments in Diels, Franmente der Vorsokratiker. Reprint edition 1983. Harvard University Press. Retrieved 2-25-2016 .http://www.sacred-texts.com/cla/app/index.html

[16] Diels, H. and Kranz, W. (1966). Die Fragmente der Vorsokratiker [Fragments of the pre-Socratic philosophers]. Berlin: Weidmann Verlag.

[17] Crivellato, E., Mallardi, F., Ribatti, D. (2006). Diogenes of Apollonia: A pioneer in vascular anatomy. The Anatomical Record (Part B: New Anat.), 289B:116-120.

[18] Hippocrates (circa 400 BC/1849). The genuine works of Hippocrates. Translated and edited by Francis Adams. London: Sydenham Society.

[19] Hippocrates. (circa 400 BC). Aphorisms. Retrieved from http://classics.mit.edu/Hippocrates/aphorisms.html

[20] Hippocrates. (circa 400BC/1950). On the sacred disease. In Chadwick, J. and Mann, W. translation of The Medical Works of Hippocrates. p179-189. Oxford: Blackwell.

[21] Aristotle (350BC/1955). Parts of Animals. Movement of Animals. Progression of Animals. Translation by A. L. Peck and E. S. Forster. Loeb Classical Library. 656a, 666a. Cambridge, MA: Harvard University Press.

[22] Gross, C. (350BC/1995). Aristotle on the Brain. The Neuroscientist, 1(4):245-250.

[23] Vesalius A. (1543). De humani corporis fabrica, libri septum. Basel: Ioannis Oporini. Retrieved 3-7- 2016. https://ceb.nlm.nih.gov/proj/ttp/flash/vesalius/vesalius.html.

[24] Celsus, A. (circa 50AD/1478). De Medicina. Retrieved 3-8-2016. See especially Book V and Book VIII. http://penelope.uchicago.edu/Thayer/E/Roman/Texts/Celsus/home.html

[25] Galen. (circa 173AD/1968). De usu partium. [On the usefulness of the parts of the body]. Translated from the Greek with an introduction and commentary by M. May. Two volumes. Ithaca, NY: Cornell University Press.

[26] Galen and Singer, C. (circa 177AD/1956). Galen on anatomical procedures. De Anatomicis Administrarionibus. New York: Oxford University Press. Retrieved 3-10-2016. https://archive.org/details/b20457194

[27] Galen (circa 177AD), Duckworth, W. (1962/2010). Galen on anatomical procedures. Edited by M. Lyons and B. Towers. Book IX, On the brain. New York: Cambridge University Press. Retrieved 3-10-2016. https://books.google.com.ai/books?id=OvJgbFMv1oYC&pg=PA266&dq=galen+173+177&hl=en&sa=X&redir_esc=y#v=onepage&q=galen%20173%20177&f=false

[28] Galen. (circa 177AD/1956). Galen on Anatomical Procedures. Translation of the surviving books with introduction and notes by Charles Singer. Book VIII, Chapter 9, Section 696, p221. London: Oxford University Press. Retrieved 3-22-2016. https://archive.org/stream/b20457194#page/n7/mode/2up

[29] Galen, Duckworth, W., Lyons, M., Towers, B. (2010). Galen on Anatomical Procedures: The later books. Cambridge: Cambridge University Press.

[30] Telfer, W. (1955). Cyril of Jerusalem and Nemesius of Emesa. Volume 4 of the Library of Christian Classics. London: SCM Press.

[31] Nemesius, Van der Eijk, P., Sharples, R. (circa 414 AD/2008). Nemesius: On the nature of man. Translated for historians. Translated by P. Van der Eijk and R. Sharples. Liverpool: University Press.

[32] Clark, K. (1935). A catalogue of the drawings of Leonardo da Vinci at Windsor Castle. Cambridge: Cambridge University Press.

[33] Richter, J. (1970). The notebooks of Leonardo da Vinci, compiled and edited from the original manuscripts. Dover: New York.

[34] Vesalius, A. (1543). Humani corporis fabrica. National Library of Medicine. Retrieved 3-23-2016 from https://ceb.nlm.nih.gov/proj/ttp/flash/vesalius/vesalius.html

[35] Vesalius, A., Garrison, D., Hast, M. (1543,1555/2015). The fabric of the human body: An annotated translation of the 1543 and 1555 editions of De humani corporis fabrica libri septem. Basel: A. G. Karger.

[36] Willis, T. (1664). Cerebri anatome: cul accessit nervorum description et usus. Londini: Typis Flesher, Impernsis Martyn & Allestry.

[37] Willis, T. (1672). De anima brutorum quae hominis vitalis ac sensitiva est, excertitationes duae; prior physiologica ejusdem naturam, partes, potentias et affectiones tradit; altera pathologicca morbos qui ipsam, et sedem ejus primarium, nempe cerebrum et nervosum genus atticiunt, explicat, eorumque therapeias insituit. Oxford: R. Davis. English translation by Samuel Pordage (1683). London.

[38] Stirling, W. (1904-5). Salerno. The oldest school of medicine in Medieval Europe. In The Medical Chronicle, E. M. Brockbank editor, Whole series, vol. XLI; Fourth series, vol. XIII, p. 85. Manchester: University Press.

[39] Willis, T. (1664,1670). Cerebri anatome: cui accessit nervorum descriptio et usus.[The Anatomy of the brain and nerves]. Londini, typ. J. Flesher, imp. J. Martyn & J. Allestry; Amsterdam 1664, 1665/1666, 1667, 1676, 1683. English translation by S. Pordage (1681). London.

[40] Luzzi, M (1316 AD). Anathomia corporis humani. Padua: Petrus Maufer.

[41] Vigevano, G. (1345 AD). MS Library at Chantilly, Conde Museum MS 569.

[42] Vigevano, G., de Luzzi, M, Wickersheimer, E. (1926). Ernest Wickersheimer. Anatomies de Mondiono dei Luzzi et de Guido de Vigenvano. Paris: E. Droz.

[43] Da Vinci, L. (1490-92). Recto: The layers of the scalp, and the cerebral ventricles. Verso: Studies of the head. RCIN 912603. Royal Collection Trust.

[44] Da Vinvi, L. (1490). An early drawing of the eye and cerebral ventricles of the brain. Royal Library in Windsor Castle, W12603r.

[45] Da Vinci, L. (1490).The ventricles based on wax injection and the rete mirable. Royal Library in Windsor Castle, W19127r.

[46] Da Vinci, L. (1504-1507/1952). The ventricles based on wax injection and (lower) the rete mirable, W19127r. In Charles O'Malley and J. Saunders (eds.), Leonardo da Vinci on the human body: The anatomical and embryological drawings of Leonardo da Vinci with translations, emendations and a biographical introduction. Retrieved from https://www.princeton.edu/~cggross/BVM_ch2.pdf

[47] Massa, N. (1536). Liber introductorius anatomiae, sive dissectionis corporis humani, nunc primum ab ipso auctore in lucem aeditus. Venice: Birdonus and Pasinus.

[48] Online Etymology Dictionary (2016). Pituitary. Retrieved 3-1-2016. http://www.etymonline.com/index.php?term=pituitary

[49] Vesalius, A., Garrison, D., and Hast, M. (1543, 2015). The fabric of the human body: An annotated translation of the 1543 and 1555 editions of De humani corporis fabric libri septem. Basel: S. Krager AG.

[50] Vesalius, A. (1543/1952). Vesalius on the human brain. Translation by Charles Singer. Wellcome Historical Medical Museum (Book 4). Oxford University Press.

[51] Finger, S. (2001). Origins of Neuroscience: A history of explorations into brain function. Oxford University Press.

[52] Da Capri, J. (1530). Isagogae breues et exactissimae in anatomia humani corporis. Henricus Sybold. Retrieved 3-23-2016 from https://books.google.com.ai/books?id=fgamMN9j69EC&pg=PT6&dq=Jacopo+Berengario+da+Carpi&source=gbs_toc_r&cad=4#v=onepage&q–Jacopo%20Bcrcngario%20da%20Carpi&f=false

[53] Sylvius, J. (1551). Vaesani cuiusdam calumniarum in Hippocratis Galenique rem anatomicam depulsio. [A refutation of the slanders of a madman against the anatomy of Hippocrates and Galen]. Paris: Jacopo Gazell.

[54] O'Malley, C. (1964). Andreas Vesalius of Brussels, 1514-1564. p239. California: University of Californian Press: Berkley and Los Angeles. Retrieved 3-23-2016 from https://books.google.com.ai/books?id=HCA6wGaU8PUC&printsec–frontcover&dq–O%27Malley+1964&hl=en&sa=X&ved=0ahUKEwivqoCin9fLAhVjsIMKHRkvDYMQ6AEIGzAA#v=onepage&q=O'Malley%201964&f=false

[55] Sylvius, J. (1555). Introduction sur l'anatomique partie de la phisiologie d'Hippocras and Galien, faite par Jaques Sylvius …and distribuee en tris livres. [The introduction to the anatomy and physiology of Hippocrates and Galen] Paris: John Hulpeau. A guide to French books before 1601 on 35 mm microfilm Reels 1-530. Reel 386. New York: Norman Ross Publishing Inc.

[56] Sylvius, J. (1540). Victus ratio, scholasticis pauperibus partu facilis and slubris. [A regimen for poor scholars, readily observed and wholesome]. Parisisiis: Iacobum Gasellum. Original manuscript located at the Yale History of Medicine Library, New Haven, Connecticut, USA.

[57] O'Malley, C. (1962). Jacob Sylvius' advice for poor medical students. Journal of the History of Medicine and Allied Sciences, 17(1) (January), p 141-151. Retrieved from https://www.jstor.org/stable/24620863?read-now=1&refreqid=excelsior%3A93445c344adbd40ba8c93dacfa8190cc&seq=1#metadata_info_tab_contents

[58] Pratensis, J. (1549). De cerebri morbis. Basel: Per Henrichum Petri. Retrieved 3-23-2016 from https://books.google.com.ai/books?id=FGgI2Th8zYwC&printsec=frontcover#v=onepage&q&f=false

[59] Arantius, J. (1579b). Observationes anatomicae. Basileae.

[60] Aranzi, G. (1587). De humano foetu liber tertio editus, ac recognitus: Ejusdem anatomicarum observationum liber ac de tumoribus secundum locus affectos liber nunc primum editi. Venetiis: Jacobum Brechtanum.

[61] Lewis, F. (1923). The significance of the term hippocampus. J. Comp. Neurol., 35:213-230.

[62] Retzius, G. (1896). Das Menschenhirn - Studien in der makroskopischen Morphologie. Text und Atlas. Stockholm: Königliche Buchdruckerei P. A. Norstedt & Soner.

[63] Judas, M. and Pletikos, M. (2010). A note on the seahorse in the human brain. Translational Neuroscience, 1(4) 335-337. See Figure 1.

[64] Descartes, R. (1649). Les passions de l'ame, Amsterdam: Lodewijk Elsevier. (In French.) Reprinted in AT, vol. XI. Electronic text available online. English translation in CSM, vol. I.

[65] Descartes, R. (1664). L'Homme, Paris: Charles Angot. (In French). Reprinted in Adam and Tannery vol. XI. Partial English translation in CSM, vol. I. Complete English translation in Hall 1972.

[66] Axelrod, J., Fraschini, F., and Velo, G. (2013). The pineal gland and its endocrine role. NATO Advanced Science Institute Series, Series A: Life Sciences, vol. 65. Plenum Publishing Corporation.

[67] Bartholini, C. (1641).Thomas Bartholini, ed. Institutiones anatomicae, novis recentiorum opinionibus and observationibus quarum innumerae hactenus editae non sunt, figurisque auctae ab auctoris filio Thoma Bartholino (in Latin). Lugdunum Batavorum: Apud Franciscum Hackium.

[68] Wepfer, J. (1658). Obserationes anatomicae, ex cadaveribus eorum quos sustulit apoplexia, um exerciatione de eius loco affecto. Shaffhuasen: Sutur.

[69] Wepfer, J. (1658). Historiae apoplecticorum. English translation from Bagvili Practice of Physik, London 1704.

[70] Galen. (173AD/1968). De usu partium corporis humani. [Galen on the usefulness of the parts of the body]. Translated from the Greek with introduction and commentary by Margaret Tallmadge May (1968), 2 vols, Ithaca: Cornell University Press.

[71] Casserius, J. (1627). Tabulae anatomicae. See Plate X. Venetiis: Apud E. Deuchinum,

[72] Willis, T. (1664). Cerebri Anatome, cui accessit nervorum descriptio et usus. [Anatomy of the brain, with a description of the nerves and their function]. London: type. J. Flesher, imp. J. Martyn, and J. Allestry.

[73] Willis T. (1681). The remaining medical works of that famous and renowned physician Dr. Thomas Willis. English translation by S. Pordage. London: Dring, Harper, Leigh & Martyn.

[74] Haller, von A. (1774). Bibliotheca anatomica. Tiguri (Zurich): Orell, Gessner, & Fuessli.

[75] Willis, T. (1672/1683). De Anima brutorum quæ hominis vitalis ac sensitiva est, excercitationes duæ; prior physiologica ejusdem naturam, partes, potentias et affectiones tradit; altera pathologica morbos qui ipsam, et sedem ejus primarium, nempe ceerebrum et nervosum genus atticiunt, explicat, eorumque therapeias instituit. Oxford (UK): Oxonii Theatro Sheldoniano. English translation by Samuel Pordage 1683, London

[76] Willis, T. (1667). Pathologiae Cerebri et Nervosi Generis Specimen [An Essay of the Pathology of the brain and nervous stock in which convulsive diseases are treated]. English translation by Samuel Pordage, 1681. London: T. Dring.

[77] Willis, T. (1672). De Anima brutorum quæ hominis vitalis ac sensitiva est, excercitationes duæ; prior physiologica ejusdem naturam, partes, potentias et affectiones tradit; altera pathologica morbos qui ipsam, et sedem ejus primarium, nempe ceerebrum et nervosum genus atticiunt, explicat, eorumque therapeias instituit. Oxford (UK): Oxonii Theatro Sheldoniano. pp. 404-407. English translation by Samuel Pordage, 1683, London.

[78] Sydenham, T. (1686). Schedula monitoria de novae febris ingressu. Londini, Kettilby, p. 25-28.

[79] Charcot, J. (1878). A lecture on rhythmical hysterical chorea. The British Medical Journal. Feb. 16.

[80] Sydenham, T. (1666). Methodus curandi febres. [A method for curing fever, based upon my own observations] 1666, 1668. Amsterdam.

[81] Sydenham, T. (1676). Observationes medicae circa morborum acutorum historiam et curationem. London.

[82] Sydenham, T. (1683). Tractatus de podagra et hydrope.Londini, G. Kettilby.

[83] Mistichelli, D. (1709). Trattato dell'Apoplessia. Rome: Rossi.

[84] Clarke, E. and O'Malley, C. (1996). The human brain and spinal cord: A historical study illustrated by writings from antiquity to the twentieth century. Norman Publishing.

[85] Cassius (circa 150AD/1841). Physici et medici Graeci minors, Problems 41, editor Iulius Ideler, Berolini: G. Reimeri.

[86] Aretaeus (circa 150AD/1856). The Exant works of Aretaeus, The Cappadocian. Edited and translated by Francis Adams. On the cause and symptoms of chronic disease. Book I. Boston: Milford House, Inc. Reproduction of the 1856 edition, London: printed for the Sydenham Society, 1972. Retrieved from National Library of Medicine, History of Medicine Division, Digital Hippocrates 6-30-2016. http://www.chlt.org/sandbox/dh/aretaeusEnglish/page.60.a.php?size=240x320

[87] Monro, A. (1764). On the communication of the ventricles of the brain with each other. Paper read to the Edinburgh Philosophical Society, December 13, 1764. Unpublished.

[88] Monro, A. (1783). Observations on structure and functions of the nervous system. Edinburgh, UK: Creech and Johnson.

[89] Wu, O., Manjila, S., Malakooti, N., Cohen, A. (2012). The remarkable medical lineage of the Monro family: Contributions of Alexander primus, secondus, and tertius. Journal of Neurosurgery, 116:1337-1346.

[90] Leeuwenhoek, A. (1674). Microscopic observations of Mr. Leeuwenhoek concerning the optic nerve. Philosophical Transactions of the Royal Society of London, 10:377-380, fig. 117.

[91] Boerhaave, H. (1735). Institiones medicae, in usus annuae exertationis domesticos digestae ab Hermann Boerhaave. Leyden.

[92] Swammerdam, J. (1738). Biblia Naturae [The Book of Nature]. Experiments on the particular motion of the muscles of the frog; which may be also, in general, applied to all the motions of the muscles in men and brutes. Published posthumously by Hermann Boerhaave. English translation by Thomas Floyd (1958). Revised and improved by John Hill London: C. G. Seyffert.

[93] Galvani, L. (1791). De viribus electricitatis in motu musculari commentariu. Bologna: Accademia delle Scienze.

[94] Soemmering, S. (1778). Dissertatio de basi encephali et originibus nervorum cranio egredientium libri quinque. Goettingae: Vandenhoeck Viduam.

[95] Vesalius, A. (1543). De humani corporis fabrica libri septem [On the fabric of the human body in seven books]. Basel: Johannes Oporinus.

[96] Fallopius, G. (1561). Observationes Anatomicae. Venice: Marcus Antonius Ulmus.

[97] Eustachius, B. (1552). Tabulae anatomicae. Rome: Lancisi.

[98] Eustachius, B. (1714). Tabulae anatomicae Bartholomaei Eustachii quas e tenebris tandem vindicatas præfatione notisque illustravit, ac ipso suæ bibliothecæ dedicationis die publici juris fecit Jo. Maria Lancisus. Rome: Francesco Gonzaga, Folio.

[99] Sommerring S. (1793). Uber die Wirkungen der Schnürbrüste. Berlin: Neue Auflage.

[100] Sommerring. S. (1793/2002). The effects of the corset. Images of health. National Library of Medicine Newsletter Jan-June, 57 (1,2):17. Retrieved 8-31-2016 from https://www.nlm.nih.gov/archive/20120906/pubs/nlmnews/janjun02/57n1-2Newsline.pdf

[101] Vicq d'Azyr, F. (1786). Traite d'anatomie et de physiologie. Paris: Didot.

[102] Vicq d'Azyr, F. (1784). Recherche sur la structure du cerveau. Mémoires de l'Académie Royale des Sciences de Paris, p.495-622.

[103] Fontana, F. (1765). Richerche de motu dell'iride. Lucca: J. Giusta.

[104] Fontana, F. (1767a). Ricerhche fisiche sopra il veleno della vipera. Lucca: J. Giusti. English translation 2 volumes, 1787, London.

[105] Fontana, F. (1781). Observations sur la structure des nerfs faites a Londres en 1779. In Traite sur le venin de la viper. Florence, 1781, 2:187-208, 207-208

[106] Fontana, F. (1767b). De irritabilitatis legibus, nunc primum sancitis, et de spirituum animalium in movendis musculis inefficacis. Lucca: J. Giusta.

[107] Galvani, A. (1791). De Viribus electricitatis in motu musculari commentarius. [Commentary on the Effect of Electricity on Muscular Motion]. De Bononiensi Scientiarum et Artium Instituto atque Academia Commentarii. 7: 363-419. Bologna: Lelio della Volpe.

[108] Scarpa, A. (1772). De structura fenestrae rotunda auris et de tympano secundario, anatomicae observations. [The structure of the round window of the ear and the ear drum, anatomical observations]. Sociertatem Typographicam – Superiorum facultate, Mutiane.

[109] Galvani, L. (1783). De volatilium aure. De Bononiensi Scientiarum et Artium Instituto atque Academis Commentarii, 6:90-91

[110] Bell, C. (1811). Idea of a New Anatomy of the Brain – submitted for the observations of his friends. London: Strahan and Preston; 1811. Reprint retrieved 7-21-2016 from www.ncbi.nlm.nih.gov/pmc/articles/.../pdf/janatphys00211-0151.pdf

[111] Bell, C. (1810). Letter from Charles Bell to elder brother George Joseph Bell, dated March 12, 1810. In Letters of Sir Charles Bell. London: John Murray (1870). Retrieved 7-21-2016 fromhttps://archive.org/stream/letterssircharl00bellgoog#page/n12/mode/2up

[112] Magendie F. (1822). Note sur le siège du mouvement et du sentiment dans la moelle épinière. J. Physiol. Exper. Path., 2:366–371.

[113] Bell, C. (1806). Essays on the anatomy of expression in painting. London.

[114] Bell, C. (1821). On the nerves: Giving an account of some experiments on their structure and functions, which lead to a new arrangement of the system. Paper presented to the Royal Society, July 12, 1821. Philosophical Transactions of the Royal Society of London, 111:398-424; p 416-417. Retrieved 7-20-2016 from http://rstl.royalsocietypublishing.org/content/111/398.full.pdf+html

[115] Bell, C. (1829-1830). The Nervous System of the Human Body, embracing the papers delivered to the Royal Society on the subject of the nerves, (with) Appendix, containing cases and letters of consultation on nervous diseases, submitted to the author since the publication of his papers on the function of the nerves, in the Transactions of the Royal Society, and illustrative of the facts in the preceding pages. Longman, London

[116] Parkinson, J. (1817). An essay on the shaking palsy. London: Whittingham and Rowland.

[117] Charcot, J. (1872. De la paralysie agitante. In Oeuvres Complètes (t 1) Leçons sur les maladies du systeme nerveux, p.155–188, Paris: A Delahaye. [English trans. by G. Sigerson, On Parkinson's disease. In Lectures on diseases of the nervous system delivered at the Salpêtrière, p.129–156. New Sydenham Society, London.

[118] Brissaud, E. (1895).Lecons sur les maladies nerveuses.p.469–501. Paris: Masson.

[119] Flourens, M. (1824). Recherches expérimentales sur les proprietes et les fonctions du système nerveux, dans les animaux vertebres (ed 1), vol 26, p 20. Paris: Chez Crevot. Retrieved 8-24-2016 from http://books.google.co.uk/books?id=b-NiqvJXS4UC&ots=GEVKSH7mTO&dq=flourens+%22Recherches+exp%C3%A9rimenta.

[120] Flourens, M. (1830a). Experiences sur les canaux semicirculaires de l'oreille chez les oiseaux et chez les mammiferrer. Mem. Acad. Roy. Sci. Paris, 9:455–475.

[121] Flourens, P. (1830b). Experiences sur les canaux semicirculaires de l'oreille dans les mammifères. Mem. Acad. Roy. Sci. Paris, 9:467–477.

[122] Baptiste-Bouillaud, J. (1825). Traite clinique et physiologique de l'encephalite, ou inflammation du cerveau.Paris.

[123] Baptiste-Bouillaud, J. (1825). Recherches cliniques propres à démontrer que la perte de la parole correspond a la lesion des lobules antérieures du cerveau. Archives Generales de Medecine, Paris, 8:25-45.

[124] Bouillaud, J. (1827). Recherches experimentales tendant à prouver que le cervelet préside aux actes de la station det de la progression, et non a l'instinct de la propagation. Archives Generales de Medecine, Paris, 15:64-91, 225-247.

[125] Remak, R. (1836). Observationes anatomicae et microscopicae de systematis nervosi structura: dissertatio inauguralis Berolini: Formis Reimerianis. Originally published in Latin.

[126] Remak, R. (1838). Observationes anatomicae et microscopicae de systematis nervosi structura: dissertatio inauguralis Berolini: Formis Reimerianis.

[127] Remak, R. (1843). Uber den Inhalt der Nervenprimitivrohren. Müller's Archiv., 8:197–201.

[128] Remak R. (1844). Neurologische Erläuterungen. Arch. Anat. Physiol. Wiss. Med., 12:463–472.

[129] Pander, H. (1817). Beiträge zur Entwicklungsgeschichte des Huhnchens im Eye. Wurzburg.

[130] Remack, R. (1843). Ueber die Entwicklung des Hühnchens im Ei. [Müller's] Archiv. für Anatomie, Physiologie und Wissenschaftliche Medicin. Berlin.

[131] Remak, R. (1855). Untersuchungen über die Entwickelung der Wirbelthiere. Berlin: G. Reimer.

[132] Allman, G. (1853). On the anatomy and physiology of cordylophora, a contribution to our knowledge of the tubularian zoophytes.Philosophical Transactions of the Royal Society of London.143:367–384. Retrieved 8-15-2016 from http://rstl.royalsocietypublishing.org/content/143/367.full.pdf+html (Accessed November 30, 2013).

[133] Huxley, T. (1871). A Manual of the anatomy of vertebrated animals. New York: D. Appleton and Company. Retrieved 10-2013 from http://dx.doi.org/10.5962/bhl.title.49320

[134] Purkinje, J. (1837). Neueste Untersuchungen aus der Nerven- und Hirnanatomie. (Uber die gangliöse Natur bestimmter Hirnteile). In: Bericht über die Versammlung deutscher Naturforscher und Aerzte in Prag im September [Recent studies from the nerve and brain anatomy [About the ganglionic nature of certain parts of the brain].In Report of the meeting of German naturalists and physicians in Prague, September] p.177-180. Prague. 6:235-237.

[135] Purkinje, J. (1817). Beiträge zur Kenntniss des Sehens in subjectiver Hinsicht. [Contributions to the knowledge of vision from a subjective perspective]. Doctoral dissertation, University of Prague, 1819.

[136] Purkinje, J. (1825). Beobachtungen und Versuche zur Physiologie der Sinne.2 volumes. Berlin. (Observations and experiments investigating the physiology of senses). The first volume is a re-publishing of his dissertation (1823). Second volume with subtitle: Neue Beiträge zur Kenntnis des Sehens in subjectiver Hinsicht (New Subjective Reports about Vision) (1825).

[137] Purkinje, J. (1823). Commentatio de examine physiologico organi visus et systematis cutanei. Breslau, Prussia: University of Breslau Press.

[138] Wendt, A. (1833). De Epidermide Humana [Human Epidemics]. Dissertation thesis. University of Breslau, Breslau.

[139] Purkinje, J. (1837). Nueste untersuchungen aus der nerven und hirn-anatomie. [New analysis of the nerves and brain anatomy].Amtlicher Bericht uber die Versammlung Deutscher Naturforscher und Arzte, Sept., 177-80.

[140] Palicki, B. (1839). De Musculari Cordis Structura [The Muscle Structure of the Heart]. Dissertation thesis. Breslau, Breslau.

[141] Purkinje, J. (1839). Nowe spostrzezenia i badania przedmiocie Fizyologii i drobnowidzowéj Anatomii udzielone przez naszego Czlonka korrespondenta Dr. J. E. Purkiniego. Rocznik wydzialu lekarskiego w uniwersytecie Jagiellonskim. Krakow. Tom II, p.44-67.

[142] Purkinje, J. (1839). Paper presented to the Silesian Society for National Culture, January.

[143] Schwann, T. (1838). Mikroskopische untersuchungen iiber die struktur der tiere und pflanzen [Microscopic analysis via the structure of animals and plants]. Neue. Notizen. aus dem Gebiete. der Natur. und Heilkunde., 5:228.

[144] Schwann, T. (1839). Mikroskopische untersuchungen uber die ubereinstimmung in der struktur und dem wachsthum der thiere und pflanzen [Microscopical researches into the accordance in the structure and growths of Animals and Plants]. Berlin: G.E. Reimer.

[145] Schwann, T. (1847). Microscopical researches into the accordance in the structure and growth of animals and plants. London: The Sydenham Society.

[146] Schleiden, M. (1838). Beitrage zur Phytogenesis. Müller's Archiv für Anatomie, Physiologie und Wissenschaftliche Medicin, 137-176. French translation in Annales des Sciences Naturelles. Botanique, (1839), 11:242-252, 362-370. English translation in Scientific Memoirs, (1841) 2:281-312.

[147] Schwann, T. (1837c). Auszug seiner untersuchungen uber die gesetze der muskelkraft [Investigation into the law of muscle power]. (Versammlung der naturforscher und aertze zu Jena am 18 September 1836), [Paper presented to a meeting of naturalists and medical practitioners]. Isis von Oken, 5-7:523-524.

[148] Schwann, T. (1836). Uber das Wesen des Verdauungsprocesses.Muller's Archiv für Anatomie, Physiologie und Wissenschaftliche Medicine, Berlin. 90-119.

[149] Schwann, T. (1839). Mikroskopische untersuchungen uber die ubereinstimmung in der struktur und dem wachstum der thiere und pflanzen. [Microscopic studies on the match in the structure and growth of animals and plants]. See Chapter "Theory on cells" Section III. Berlin, Sander, 1839. English translation by the Sydenham Society, 1847, p.193.

[150] Hall, M. (1833). On the reflex function of the medulla oblongata and medulla spinalis. Phil. Trans. R. Soc., 123:635-665.

[151] Bell, C. (1826). On the nervous circle which connects the voluntary muscles with the brain. Phil. Trans. R. Soc., 116(ii):163-173.

[152] Erb, W. (1875). Uber sehnenreflexe bei gesunden und bei ruckenmarkskranken. Arch Psychiat. Nerv Krankh., 5:792-802.

[153] Hall, M. (1836). Lectures on the Nervous System and Its Diseases. 27. London: Sherwood, Gilbert, and Pyer.

[154] Romberg, M. (1853). In Sieveking, E. ed., trans. Lehrbuch der Nervenkrankheiten des Menschen [A Manual of the Nervous Diseases of Man]. London: Sydenham Society, 226-227, 395-401.

[155] Romberg, M. (1840). Lehrbuch der nervenkrankheiten des menschen, [Textbook of nervous diseases in man] vols 1-2. Duncker.

[156] Romberg, M. (1846). Tabes dorsalis. Lehrbuch der Nervenkrankheiten des Menschen.,1:795. Berlin: Duncker.

[157] Du Bois-Reymond, E. (1841). Untersuchungen uber thierische electrical. Vol 1. Berlin: Georg Reimer.

[158] Du Bois-Reymond, E. (1843).Vorlaufiger Abriss einer Untersuchung uber den sigenannten Froschstrom und umber die elektromotorischen Fische. Annl. Phys., 58:1–30.

[159] Du Bois-Reymond, E. (1848-84). Untersuchungen über thierische Elektricität [Reserach on Animal Electricity]. Vol 2. Berlin: Georg Reimer.

[160] Brown-Sequard, C. (1846). Recherches et experiences sur la physiologie de la moëlle epiniere.These de Paris. Doctoral thesis.

[161] Brown-Sequard, C. (1851). De la transmission croisée des impressions sensitives par la moelle épinière [Of cross-transmission of sensory impressions through the spinal cord].Comptes Rendus de la Société de Biologie, 2:33-44.

[162] Brown-Sequard, C. (1855). Experimental and clinical researches on the physiology and pathology of the spinal cord and some other parts of the nervous centers. Richmond: Cloin and Nowland.

[163] Brown-Sequard, C. (1869). Lectures on the physiology and pathology of the nervous system and on the treatment of organic nervous affections: Lecture II, part 1. Lancet, 1:1–3.

[164] Helmholtz, H. (1851).Beschreibung eines augen-spiegels zur untersuchung der netzhaut im lebendem auge.[Description of an eye - for the examination of the retina in the living eye] Berlin: A Förstner'sche Verlagsbuchhandlung. Retrieved 8-2-2016 from https://books.google.com.ai/books?id=839dAAAAcAAJ&pg=PA1&dq=von+Helmholtz,+H.+(1851).++Beschreibung +eines+augen-spiegels+zur+untersuchung+der+netzhaut+im+lebendem+auge.+Berlin:+A+F%C3%B6rstner%27sche +Verlagsbuchhandlung&hl=en&sa=X&redir_esc=y#v=onepage&q=von%20Helmholtz%2C%20H.%20(1851).%20% 20Beschreibung%20eines%20augen-spiegels%20zur%20untersuchung%20der%20netzhaut%20im%20 lebendem%20auge.%20Berlin%3A%20A%20F%C3%B6rstner'sche%20Verlagsbuchhandlung&f=false

[165] Graefe, A. (1854). Notiz uber die ablosungen der netzhaut von der chorioidea. [Note on the detachment of the retina form the choroid]. In A. Grefe Archiv fur Ophthamologie, p.362- 371. Berlin: Verlag von P. Jeanrenau.

[166] Graefe, A. (1854-1855). Vorlaufige notiz uber das wesen de glaucoms [Preliminary note on the nature of glaucoma]. Archives of Ophthalmology, 1(1):371-382.

[167] Graefe, A. (1857). Concerning iridectomy in glaucoma and concerning the glaucomatous process. Arch. of Ophth., 456-560.

[168] Gaefe, A. (1859). Uber emnolie der arteria centralis retinae [About retinal embolism of the central artery]. Arch. of Ophthalmology, 5:136.

[169] Graefe, A. (1860). Ueber complication von sehnervenentzundung mit gehirnkrankheiten [About complication of optic neuritis with brain diseases]. Archiv fur Opthalmologie, 7(2):58-71.

[170] Allbutt, C. (1870). Cases of intra-cranial disease with ophthalmoscopic observations. Lancet, 96, (2463):670-671.

[171] Broadbent, W. (1871). On the causation and significance of the chocked disc in intra-cranial diseases. The British Medical Journal, June 15, 1872, p 633-635.

[172] Jones, T. (1855). The principles and practice of ophthalmic medicine and surgery. London: John Churchill.

[173] Allbutt, T. (1871). On the use of the ophthalmoscope in diseases of the nervous system and of the kidneys; also in certain other general disorders. London and New York: Macmillan

[174] Gowers, W. (1879). A manual and atlas of medical ophthalmoscopy. London: Churchill.

[175] Waller, A. (1850). Experiments on the section of the glossopharyngeal and hypoglossal nerves of the frog, and observations of the alterations produced thereby in the structure of their primitive fibers. Philosophical Transactions of the Royal Society of London, 140:423-429.

[176] Waller, A. (1852). Observations sur les effects de la section ds raciness spinales et du nerf pneumogastrique au dessus de son ganglion inferieur chez les mammiferes. Comptes Rendus Hebdomadaires des Seances de l'Academie des Sciences, Paris 34:582-587.

[177] Waller, A. (1857). Experience sur les sections des nerfs et les alterantions. Comptes Rendus de la Societe de Biologie, Paris, 2(3):6.

[178] Magendie, F. (1842). Recherches physiologogiques et cliniques sur le liquid cephalo-rachidien ou cerebro-spinal. 1 volume and atlas. Paris: Mequignon-Marvis.

[179] Lushka, H. (1855). Die Adergeflechte der menschlichen gehirnes. Eine Monographie. Berlin: G. Reimer.

[180] Magendie, F. (1822). Experiences sur les fonctions des raciness des nerfs rachidiens. Journal de Physiologie Experiemntale et Pathologie, 2:276-279.

[181] Magendie, F. (1822). Experiences sur les fonctions des raciness des nerfs qui naissent de la moelle epiniere. Journal de Physiologie Experiemnetale et de Pathologie, 2:366-371.

[182] Shaw, A. (1868). Magendie and Bell. Correspondence, British Medical Journal, August 15, p 179.

[183] McDonnell, R. (1868). Magendie and Bell correspondences, British Medical Journal, 2:319.

[184] Hawkins, C. (1869). Sir Charles Bell and Francios Magendie on the functions of the spinal nerves. British Journal of Medicine, 1:21.

[185] Magendie, F. (1825). Memoire sure un liqide qui se trouve dans le crane et le canal vertebral de l'homme et des animaux mammifieres. [Memory on a liquid found in the skull and vertebral canal of man and animal mammals]. Journal de Physiolgie Experimentale et Pathologie, Paris 5:27-37.

[186] Broca, P. (1861b). Perte de la parole, ramollissement chronique et destruction partielle du lobe antérieur gauche. [Sur le siege de la faculte du langage.]. Bulletin de la Societe d'Anthropologie, 2:235-238.

[187] Broca, P. (1861c). Remarques sur le siege de la faculté du langage articule, suivies d'une observation d'aphémie. Bulletin de la Société Anatomique, 1861c, 36:330-357. English translation retrieved 8-6-2016 from http://psychclassics.yorku.ca/Broca/aphemie-e.htm

[188] Broca, P. (1861d). Nouvelle observation d'aphémie produite par une lésion de la moitié postérieure des deuxième et troisième circonvolution frontales gauches. Bulletin de la Societe Anatomique, 6:398-407.

[189] Trausseau, M. (1864). De l'aphasia, maladie decrite recemment sous le nom improper d'aphemia. [On aphasia, a sickness formerly wrongly referred to as aphemia].Gazette des Hopitaux Civils et Militaires. No. 4; Mardi 12, Janvier.

[190] Ferrier, D. (1873). Experimental researches in cerebral physiology and pathology. Journal Anat. Physiol., 8(pt1): 152-155.

[191] Broca, P (1851). Description de la dystropie muscularie. Bulletin de la Société Anatomique de Paris, 26:50-64.

[192] Broca, P. (1850). Rescherches sur l'arhrite sech et les corps etrangers articullaires. Bull. Soc. Anatomy, 435-455.

[193] Broca, P. (1852). Recherches sur quelques points de l'anatomie pathologique du rachitisme [Research on some points on the pathological anatomy of rickets]. Moquet.

[194] Broca, P. (1850). Cancer dans les veines. Revue d'Anthrolologie, 2nd edition serie. T III.

[195] Broca, P. (1852). Bulletin de la Société Anatomique de Paris, 27:141 et seq., 542 et seq.

[196] Broca, P. (1866-1869). Traite des tumeurs. 2 volumes. Paris: P. Asselin.

[197] Charcot, J. (1868). Histologie de la sclerose en plaques. Gazette des Hopitaux, Paris; 41:554-5.

[198] Charcot, J. and Joffroy, A. (1869). Deux cas d'atrophie musculaire progressive avec lesions de la substance grise et des faiseaux antérolateraux de la moelle epiniere. Archives de Physiologie Normale et Pathologique, Paris, 2:354-367, 629-649, 744-760.

[199] Charcot, J. and Marie, P. (1886). Sur une forme particulière d'atrophie musculaire progressive, souvent familiale débutant par les pieds et les jambes et atteignant plus tard les mains. Revue Medicale, Paris, 6:97-138.

[200] His, W. (1870). Beschreibung eines Mikrotoms.Archiv für Mikroskopische Anatomie, Bonn, 6:229-232.

[201] His, W. (1868). Untersuchungen uber die erste anlage des wirbeltierleibes: Die erste entwicklung des huhnchens im ei. [Investigations of the first system of the vertebrate body: The first development of the bird egg]. Leipzig: Vogel.

[202] Marshall, M. (1878). The Development of the Cranial Nerves in the Chick. Journal of Cell Science, s2-18:10-40.

[203] Golgi, C. (1906). Camillo Golgi - Biographical.Nobelprize.org.Nobel Media AB 2014. Retrieved 8-8-2016 from http://www.nobelprize.org/nobel_prizes/medicine/laureates/1906/golgi-bio.html

[204] Golgi, C. (1878). Intorno alla distribuzione e terminazione dei nervi nei tendini dell'uomo e di altri vertebrati Rend. R. Ist Lomb. Sci. Lett. B11 445–53 (Reproduced in Golgi, C. (1903). Opera Omnia, 1:133–42. Milano: Hoepli).

[205] Golgi, C. (1886). Studii sulla fina anatomia degli organi centrali del sistema nervoso. Milano: Ulrico Hoepli.

[206] Golgi, C. (1873). On the structure of the brain grey matter. Gazzetta Medica Italiana, 6:244-246.

[207] Horner, J. (1869). Ueber eine form von ptosis. Klinische Mnatsblatter fur Augenbeilkunde, 7:193-198.

[208] Horner, J. (1869/1968). Ueber eine form von ptosis. Klinische Mnatsblatter fur Augenbeilkunde, 7:193-198. English translation by J.F. Fulton (1968). On a form of ptosis. Archives of Neurology, 19(5):541-542.

[209] Mitchell, S. (1872). Injuries of nerves and their consequences. Philadelphia: J.B. Lippincott and Company.

[210] Huntington, G. (1872a). On chorea. Paper presented to the Meigs and Mason Academy of Medicine. February 15, Middleport, Ohio.

[211] Huntington, G. (1872b). On chorea. The Medical and Surgical Review: A Weekly Journal, April 26, 15:317-321.

[212] Waters, C. (1841,1848). Letter to Professor R. Dunglison from Charles Waters, dated May 5, 1841, Franklin, New York, appearing in Dunglison, R. (1848). The Practice of Medicine: A treatise on special pathology and therapeutics, 3rd edition, 2 volumes, p. 216-218. Philadelphia: Lea and Blanchard. Retrieved 8-9-2016 from https://archive.org/stream/practiceofmedici248dung#page/n5/mode/2up

[213] Huntington, G. (1910). Recollections of Huntington's Chorea, as I saw it at East Hampton, Long Island, during my boyhood, by George Huntington, M.D., Journal of Nervous and Mental Diseases, April, 37:553.

[214] Wernicke, C. (1874). Der aphasische symptomencomplex. Eine Psychologische Studie auf Anatomischer Basis. Breslau.

[215] Wernicke, C. (1881-1883). Lehrbuch der gehirnkrankheiten für aerzte und studirende.[Textbook of brain diseases: For physicians and students]. 3 volumes, Kassel und Berlin: Fischer.

[216] Wernicke, C. (1881). Die acute, hamorrhagische polioencephalitis superior. In his book Lehrbuch der Gehirnkrankheiten [Textbook of brain diseases: For physicians and students]; 2:229-242. Kassel und Berlin: Fischer.

[217] Wernicke, C. (1881/1968). Acute hemorrhagic superior polioencephalities. English translation by Brody and Wilkins, Arch. Neurology, 19:229.

[218] Canton, R. (1875a). The electrical currents of the brain. Abstract presented to the 43rd Annual Meeting of the British Medical Association meeting, Edinburgh, August 4th, Section F. - Physiology.

[219] Caton, R. (1875b). The electric currents of the brain, British Medical Journal, 2:278.

[220] Caton, R. (1877). Interim report on investigations of the electric currents of the brain. British Medical Journal, 1:62–65.

[221] Caton, R. (1887). Researchcs on electrical phenomena of cerebral gray matter. Paper presented to the 9th International Medical Congress, Washington, D.C., IX International Congress. Med., 3:246.

[222] Berger, H. (1929). Uber das Elektrenkephalogramm des Menschen. [On the electroencephalogram of humans].Archiv. fur Psychiatrie und Nervenkrankheiten., 87:527–570.

[223] Ranvier, L. (1871). Sur la distribution des entanglements annulaires des tubes nerveux. Compte. Revue. Soc. Biol. (Paris).

[224] Ranvier, L. (1872). Recherches sur l'histologie et la physiologie des nerfs. Archives de Physiologie Normale et Pathologique.

[225] Ranvier, L. (1874). De quelque faits relatifs a l'histologie eta la physiologie des muscl stiles. Arch. Physiol. Norm. Path., 2 Ser. 1:5-15.

[226] Ranvier, L. (1878). Lecons sur l'histologie du systeme nerveux, par M. L. Ranvier et recueillies par M. Ed Weber.2 volumes. Paris, Libraire F. Savy. Retrieved 9-7-2016 from https://archive.org/stream/b21922494_0001#page/n7/mode/2up.

[227] Koelliker, A. (1896). Handbuch der Gewebelehre. [Handbook of histology]. Leipzeg: Engelmann.

[228] Nissil, F. (1884). Resultate und erfahrungen bei der untersuchung der pathologischen Veränderungen der Nervenzellen in der Grosshirnrinde. Doctoral dissertation (unpublished).

[229] Nissil, F. (1894). Uber die sogenannten granula der nervenzellen. Neurologisches Centralblatt, Leipzig, 13:676-685, 781-789, 810-814.

230 Erb, W. (1874). Ueber eine eigenthümliche localisation von lähmungen im plexus brachialis. Verhandlungen des naturhistorisch-medicinischen vereins zu Heidelberg, Neue Folge, 1:130-137.

231 Erb, W. (1882). Handbuch der Elektrotherapie. Leipzig: Verlag von F.C.W. Vogel.

232 Deutsche Zeitschrift fur Nervenheilkunde (1891). First issue of the German Journal of Neurology, April 30, 1(1-2). Retrieved 8-13-2016 from http://link.springer.com/journal/415/1/1/page/1

233 Erb, W. (1891a). Uber die nachsten augaben der nervenpathologie. Deutsche Zeitschrift fur Nervenheilkunde. April 30, 1(1):1-12.

234 Erb, W. (1891b). Dsytrophia musularis progressive: Klinische und pathologisch-anatomische studien. Deutsche Zeitschrift fur Nervenheilkunde, April 30, 1(1):13-94.

235 Westphal, K. (1875). Uber einige bewegungs-erscheinungen an gelahmten gliedern. Arch Psychiat. Nerv Krankh., 5:803-834.

236 Edinger L. (1885). Uber den Verlauf der centralen hirnnervenbahnen mit demonstrationen von praparaten. Arch. Psychiatr. Nervenkrankheiten., 16:858–859.

237 Westphal, K. (1887). Ueber einen fall von chronischer progressiver lahmung der augenmuskeln (ophthalmoplegia externa) nebst beschreibung von ganglienzellengruppen im bereiche des oculomotoriuskerns.Arch. Psychiat. und Nervenkrankheiten., 18:846–871.

238 Giles de la Tourette, G. (1884). Jumping, latah, myriachit. Archives de Neurologie, Paris, 8:68-74.

239 Giles de la Tourette, G. (1885). Etude sur une affection nerveuse caracterisee par l'incoordination motrice, accompagnee d'echolalie et de coprolalie. Archives de Neurologie, Paris, 9:19-42, 158-200.

240 Guinon, G. (1893). Attentat contre le Dr. Gilles de la Tourette [Attack against Dr. Tourette]. Le Progress Medical. 9 December, 21(19):466. Retrieved 8-11-2016 from http://www.baillement.com/lettres/tourette_attentat.html

241 Gowers, W. (1886). Manual of the nervous system. Volume II. Brain: General and functional diseases. London: Churchill. Retrieved 8-15-2016 from https://archive.org/stream/manualofdiseases02goweuoft#page/n3/mode/2up

242 Gowers, W. (1893). Manual of the nervous systems, Volume I, Diseases of the nerves and spinal cord with one hundred and eighty illustrations including three hundred and seventy figures. Philadelphia: Blakiston, Son, and Company. Retrieved 8-15-2016 from https://archive.org/stream/manualofdiseases01gowe#page/n7/mode/2up

243 Gowers, W. (1879). A manual and atlas of medical ophthalmoscopy. London: J. and A. Churchill.

244 Gowers, W. (1879). Pseudo-hypertrophic muscular paralysis. London: J. and A. Churchill.

245 Gowers, W. (1881). Epilepsy and other Chronic Convulsive Disorders, their Causes, Symptoms and Treatment, London: J. and A. Churchill.

246 Gowers, W. (1886,1888). A manual of diseases of the nervous system, Vol 1-2. London: J. and A. Churchill.

247 Gowers, W. (1907). The borderland of epilepsy: Faints, vagal attacks, vertigo, migraine, sleep symptoms, and their treatment. London: J. and A. Churchill.

248 Gowers, W. (1879). An apparatus for the clinical estimation of haemoglobin. Transactions of the Clinical Society of London, 12: 64-67.

249 Taylor, J. (1888). New form of percussion hammer. Journal of Nervous and Mental Disease, 15:253.

250 Babinski, J. (1896). Sur le reflexe cutane plantaire dans certaines affections organiques du systeme nerveus central. Paper presented to the Societe de Biologie in Paris, Feb 22.

251 Babinski, J. (1896). Sur le reflexe cuntane plantaire dans certaines affetions organiques du systems nerveux central. Societe de Biologie, Seance du 22 Fevrier, 3:207-208.

252 Babinski, J. (1898). Du phenomene des orteils et de sa valuer semiologique. Sem Med., 18:321-322.

253 Babinski, J. (1903). De l'abduction des orteils. Rev. Neurol., 11:728-729.

254 Duchenne, G. (1962). Album de photographies pathologiques, complementaire du livre insitule de l'electrisalation localisee. Paris: J. B. Bailliere et Fils.

255 Charcot, J. (1888). Nouvelle iconographie de la Salpetriere. [Photos to show clinical case presentations at Salpetriere].

256 Londe, A. (1893). La photographie medicale, application aux sciences medicales et physiologiques. Paris: Gauthier-Villars et Fils. Retrieved 9-7-2016 from http://cnum.cnam.fr/PDF/cnum_8KE360.pdf

257 Brain (1878). The official Journal of the Neurological Society of London. http://brain.oxfordjournals.org/content/1/1

258 Erb, W. (1891). Dystrophia muscularis progressive. Klinishee und pathologisch-anatomische studien. Dtsch. Z .Nervenheilkd., 1:173-261.

259 His, W. (1889). Die neuroblasten und deren entstehung im embryonalen mark. Abhandlungen der mathematisch-physischen classe der Koniglich Sachsischen Gesellschaft der Wissenschaften, 15:133-372.

260 Waldeyer, W. (1891). Uber einige neuere forschungen im gegiete der anatomie des central nerven systems. Deutsch Med. Wschr., 17:1352-1356.

261 Kolliker, A. (1896). Handbuch der gewebelehre des menschen, 6th ed., Zweiter Band: Nervensytem des menschen und der thiere. Leipzig: Engelmann.

[262] Foster, M. (1897). A textbook of physiology. London: Macmillan and Company.

[263] Langley, J. (1898). On the union of cranial autonomic (visceral) fibers with the nerve cells of the superior cervical ganglion. Journal of Physiology, July, (23):240-270.

[264] Alzheimer, A. (1906a). Paper presented to the 37th annual meeting of the South –West German Psychiatrist meeting, Tubigen.

[265] Alzheimer, A. (1906b). Uber einen eigenartigen schweren Krankheitsprozess der Hirnrinde. [About a peculiar severe disease process of the brain cortex].Zentralblatt für Nervenkrankheiten, 25:1134.

[266] Alzheimer A. (1907). Uber eine eigenartige Erkrankung der Hirnrinde. [About a rare disease of the cerebral cortex]. Allg. Zschr. Psychiatr. Psych. Gerichtl. Med., 64:146-148.

[267] Perusini G. (1909). Uber klinisch und histologisch eigenartige psychische Erkrankungen des späteren Lebensalters. In: Nissl F, Alzheimer, A., eds. Histologische und histopathologische Arbeiten über die Gehirnrinde, Vol III, 297–351. Jena, Germany: Fischer.

[268] Perusini, G. (1909-1910). Uber klinisch und histologisch eigenartige psychische Erkrankungen des späteren Lebensalter. In Histologische und histopathologische Arbeiten über die Großhirnrinde mit besonderer Berücksichtigung der pathologischen Anatomie des Geisteskranken, p.297-358, Plates XVII-XXIII. Jena: G. Fischer.

[269] Alzheimer, A. (1911). Uber eigenartige krankheitsfälle des späteren alters (On certain peculiar diseases of old age with 10 text figures and 2 plates.

[270] Kraepelin, E. (1909/1910). Psychiatrie, 8th ed. Vol I: Allgemeine Psychiatrie; Vol II: Klinische Psychiatrie. Leipzig, Germany: Barth.

[271] American Psychiatric Association. (2000). Diagnostic and Statistical Manual Text Revision, DSM-IV-TR. American Psychiatric Association.

[272] American Psychiatric Association. (2013). Diagnostic and Statistical Manual of Mental Disorders, DSM-5, fifth edition. Arlington, VA, American Psychiatric Association.

[273] The Nobel Prize in Physiology or Medicine 1906. Nobelprize.org.Nobel Media AB 2014. Web. 16 Aug 2016. Retrieved from http://www.nobelprize.org/nobel_prizes/medicine/laureates/1906/.

[274] Golgi, C. (1873). On the structure of the brain gray matter. Gazzetta Mdica Italiana Lombardo, 6:244-246.

[275] Golgi, C. (1880a). Sui nervi dei tendini dell'uomo e di altri vertebrati e di un nuovo organo nervosa terminale musculo-tendrineo. Mem. R. Accad. Sci. Torino, 32:359-385.

[276] Golgi, C. (1880b). Sulla struttura della fibre nervosa midollate periefriche e centrali. Archivio per le Scienze Mediche, Torino, 4:221-246.

[277] Golgi, C. (1886). Studii sulla fina anatomia degli organi centrali del sistema nervoso. Milano.

[278] Golgi, C. (1898). Intorno alla struttura delle cellule nervose. Bollettino della Societa Medico-Chirurgica di Pavia, 13(1):316.

[279] Golgi, C. (1886). Sull' infezione malarica. Archivio Per le Scienze Mediche, Torino, 10:109-135.

[280] Golgi, C. (1889). Sul ciclo evolutivo dei parassiti malarici nella febbre terzana diagnosi differenziale tra i parassiti endoglobulari malarici della terzana e quelli della quartana. [On the cycle of development of malarial parasites in tertian fever: differential diagnosis between the intracellular parasites of tertian and quartant fever]. Archivio per le Scienza Mediche., 13:173–196.

[281] Raymon y Cajal, S. (1899,1904). Textura del system nervioso del hombre y de los vertebrados. Madrid: Moya.

[282] Grant, G. (1999). How Golgi shared the 1906 Nobel Prize win Physiology or Medicine with Cajal. Retrieved 8-17-2016 from https://www.nobelprize.org/nobel_prizes/medicine/laureates/1906/article.html

[283] Brodmann, K. (1909). Vergleichende Lokalisationslehre der Grosshirnrinde in ihren Principien, dargestellt auf grund des Zellenbaues. Leipzig, Johann Ambrosius Barth Verlag.

[284] Lewy, F (1912). Paralysis agitans: pathologische anatomie. Handbuch der Neurologie, 3:920-33. Springer: Berlin.

[285] Lewy, F. (1913). Zur pathologischen anatomie der paralysis agitans. Deutsche Zeitschrift Nervenheilkunde, 50: 50-55.

[286] Tretiakoff, C. (1919). Contribution a l'etude de l'anatomie du locus niger de Soemmering avec quelques deductions relatives a la pathologenie des troubles du tonus muscularie et de la Maladie de Parkinson [A Study of the pathological anatomy of the locus niger of Soemerring and its relevance to the pathogenesis of changes in muscular tone in Parkinson's disease]. Doctoral dissertation, The University of Paris.

[287] Guillain, G., Barre, A., Strohl, A. (1916). Sur un syndrome de radiculonévrite avec hyperalbuminose du liquide céphalo-rachidien sans réaction cellulaire. Remarques sur les caractères cliniques et graphiques des réflexes tendineux. Bulletins et Mémoires de la Societé des Medecins des Hôpitaux de Paris, 40:1462-1470.

[288] Rogoff, J. (1977). Pronunciation of Dr. Georges Guillain's name. JAMA, 237(23):2470.

[289] Rivers, W. and Head, H. (1908). A human experiment in nerve division. Brain, November, 31(3):323-450.

[290] Compston, A. (2009). A human experiment in nerve division by W.H.R. Rivers MD FRS, Fellow of St Johns's College, Cambridge and Henry Head MD FRS, Physician to the London Hospital, Brain (1908), 31;323-450. Published online 27 October 2009. Retrieved 8-19-2016 from http://brain.oxfordjournals.org/content/132/11/2903.

[291] Head, H. and Campbell, A. (1900). The pathology of herpes zoster and its bearing on sensory localization. Brain, Part III, 23:353-529.

[292] Head, H. and Holmes, G. (1911). Sensory disturbances from cerebral lesions. Brain, 34:102-254.

[293] Head, H., Rivers, W., Sherren, J., Holmes, G., Thompson, T., Riddoch, G. (1920a). Studies in Neurology. Volume I, 333-839. London: Henry Frowde, Oxford University Press. Retrieved 8-18-2016 from https://archive.org/stream/studiesinneurolo01headiala#page/n7/mode/2up

[294] Head, H., Rivers, W., Sherren, J., Holmes, G., Thompson, T., Riddoch, G. (1920b). Studies in Neurology. Volume II, 1-327. London: Henry Frowde, Oxford Unvieristy Press. Retrieved 8-18-2016 from https://archive.org/stream/studiesinneurolo02headiala#page/viii/mode/2up

[295] Head, H. (1902). London –October 29. Rag Book, Volume 1 A, October 1901- July 1902, p.15.

[296] Flexner, A. (1910). Medical Education in the United States and Canada: A report to the Carnegie Foundation for the advancement of teaching. The Carnegie Foundation, Bulletin Number Four. New York City, New York.

[297] Berger H. (1929). Uber das Elektrenkephalogramm des Menschen. [On the electroencephalogram of humans]. Archiv. fur Psychiatrie und Nervenkrankheiten, 87:527–570.

[298] The Nobel Prize in Physiology or Medicine 1932. Nobelprize.org. Nobel Media AB 2014. Web. Retrieved 8-25-2016 from http://www.nobelprize.org/nobel_prizes/medicine/laureates/1932/

[299] Sherrington, C. (1906). The integrative action of the nervous system. New Haven Connecticut: Yale University Press.

[300] Adrian, E. and Zotterman, Y, (1926). The impulses produced by sensory nerve endings. Part 2. The response of a single end-organ. The Journal of Physiology, 61(2). Retrieved 8-16-2016 from http://onlinelibrary.wiley.com/doi/10.1113/jphysiol.1926.sp002281/pdf

[301] The Nobel Prize in Physiology or Medicine 1936. Nobelprize.org. Nobel Media AB 2014. Web. Retrieved 8-25-2016 from http://www.nobelprize.org/nobel_prizes/medicine/laureates/1936/.

[302] Dale, H. (1914). The action of certain esters and ethers of choline and their relation to muscarine. J. Pharmacol. Exp. Ther., 6:147-190.

[303] Erlangcr, J. (1939). The initiation of impulses in axons. J. Neurophysiol., 2:370-379.

[304] Loreintc, R. (1939). Transmission of impulses through cranial motor nuclei. J. Neurophysiol. 2:402-464.

[305] Dale, H. (1929). Some chemical factors in the control of the circulation. Lancet, 1179-1183; 1233-1237; 1285-1290.

[306] Dale, H. (1933). Nomenclature of fibers in the autonomic system and their effects. J. Physiol., 80:0-11.

[307] . Chang, H. and Gaddum, J. (1933). Choline esters in tissue extracts. J. Physiol., 79:255-285.

[308] Dale, H. and Feldberg, A. (1934). The chemical transmission of secretory impulses to the sweat glands of the cat. J. Physiol., 82:121-128.

[309] Dale, H. (1953). Adventures in Physiology, Pergamoni: Lonidoni.

[310] Dixon, W. (1907). On the mode of action of drugs. Med. Megaz., 16:454–457.

[311] Loewi, O. (1924). Uber humorale Ubertragbarkeit der Herznervenwirkung. Pflügers Archiv für die Gesamte Physiologie des Menschen und der Tiere., 204:629–640

[312] Loewi, O. and Navratil, E. (1926). Uber humorale Ubertragbarkeit der Herznervenwirkung. XI Mitteilung. Uber den mechanismus der vaguswirkung von physostigmin und erotamin. Pflugers Archiv fur die gesamte Physiologie des Menschen und der Tiere, 214:689-96.

[313] Penfield, W. (1952). Memory Mechanisms. AMA Archives of Neurology and Psychiatry, 67:178-198.

[314] Penfield, W and Jasper, H. (1954). Epilepsy and the functional anatomy of the human brain. Boston: Little, Brown & Co.

[315] Penfield, W. and Boldfrey, E. (1937). Somatic motor and sensory representation in the cerebral cortex of man as studied by electrical stimulation. Brain, 60(4):389-443.

[316] Penfield, W. (1934). The significance of the Montreal Neurological Institute. In Neurological Biographies and Addresses; Foundation Volume. Published for the Staff, to Commemorate the Opening of the Montreal Neurological Institute of McGill University (on 27th September, 1934), p.37-54. London: Oxford University Press.

[317] Montreal Neurological Institute and Hospital (2016). About McGill University - Montreal Neurological Institute and Hospital. Retrieved 8-19-2016 from http://www.mcgill.ca/neuro/about

[318] Scoville, W. and Milner, B. (1957). Loss of recent memory after bilateral hippocampal lesions.Journal of Neurology, Neurosurgery & Psychiatry, 20(1):11–2.

[319] Penfield, W. and Milner, B. (1958). Memory deficit produced by bilateral lesions in the hippocampal zone. Archives of Neurology and Psychiatry, 79:475-497.

[320] Buchen, L. (2009). Famous brain set to go under the knife. Nature, 462:403.

[321] Annese, J. (2010). Deconstructing Henry: the neuroanatomy and neuro-informatics of the brain of the amnesic patient H.M. Program No. 397.18. 2010 Neuroscience Meeting Planner. San Diego, CA: Society for Neuroscience, 2010.

[322] Annese, J., Schenker-Ahmed, N., Bartsch, H., Maechler, P., Shen, C., Thomas, N., Kayano, J., Ghatan, A., Bresler, N., Rosch, M., Klaming, R. and Corkin, S. (2014). Postmortem examination of patient HM's brain based on histological sectioning and digital 3D reconstruction. Nature Communications, 5, no. 3122, January 28, 2014.

[323] United States Congress (1950).Title IV-National Research Institutes. Establishment of Additional Institutes. Public Laws, chapter 714, August 15, 1950, 58 Stat. 707,42 U.S.C. 281-286;Sup. III, 281 et seq.; Sec, 431.

[324] NIND (2016). About NIH; The NIH Almanac. Retrieved 8-17-2016 from https://www.nih.gov/about-nih/what-we-do/nih-almanac/national-institute-neurological-disorders-stroke-ninds

[325] The Nobel Prize in Physiology or Medicine 1970. Nobelprize.org. Nobel Media AB 2014. Retrieved 8-12-2016 from http://www.nobelprize.org/nobel_prizes/medicine/laureates/1970/

[326] Euler, U. (1946a). A specific sympathomimetic ergone in adrenergic nerve fibers (sympathin) and its relation to adrenaline and noradrenaline. Acta Physiol. Scand., 12:73-97.

[327] Euler, U. (1946b). Sympathin in adrenergic nerve fibers. J. Physiology, Sept 18, 105:26.

[328] Euler, U. (1948). Synpathin E and noradrenaline. Science, 107(2782) April, p. 22.

[329] Axelrod, J. (1957). O-Methylation of epinephrine and other catechols in vitro and in vivo. Science, 126:400–401

[330] Fatt, P. and Katz, B. (1952). Spontaneous subthreshold activity at motor nerve endings. J Physiol.,117:109–128.

[331] del Castillo, J. and Katz, B. (1954). Quantal components of the end-plate potential. J. Physiology, June 28, 124(3):560-573.

[332] Carlsson A, Lindquist M, Magnusson T, Waldeck .B. (1958). On the presence of 3 hydroxytyramine in brain. Science, 127:471-472.

[333] Carlsson, A., Linquist, M., Magnusson, A., Waldeck, B. (1957). 3-4-dihydroxyphenylalamine and 5-hydroxytryptophan as reserpine antagonist. Nature, 180:1200.

[334] Birkmayer, W. and Hornykiewicz, O. (1961). The L-3,4-dioxyphenylalanine (DOPA)-effect in Parkinson-akinesia.Wien. Klin. Wochenschr., 73:787–8.

[335] Cotzias, G. (1968). L-dopa for Parkinsonism. New England Journal of Medicine, 278: 630.

[336] Cotzias, G., Papavasiliou, P., Gellene, R. (1969). Modification of Parkinsonism-chronic treatment with L-dopa. New England Journal of Medicine, 280:337-345.

[337] Marden, C., Parkes, J., Rees, J. (1973). A year's comparison of treatment of patients with Parkinson's disease with levodopa combined with carbidopa versus treatment with levodopa alone. Lancet, 2:1459.

[338] Hunter, K., Laurence, D., Shaw, K., Stern, G. (1973). Sustained levodopa therapy in Parkinsonism. Lancet, 2:929-931.

[339] Parkinson's Disease Foundation. (2016). Understanding Parkinson's disease: Medications and treatments. Retrieved 8-23-2016 from http://www.pdf.org/parkinson_prescription_meds

[340] The Nobel Prize in Physiology or Medicine 2000. Nobelprize.org. Nobel Media AB 2014. Web. Retrieved 8-24-2016. http://www.nobelprize.org/nobel_prizes/medicine/laureates/2000/.

[341] Keller, W. (1978). Hemispheric asymmetries: A tachistoscopic investigation into verbal and spatial encoding strategies. Master thesis. Ball State University.

[342] Keller, W. (1982). Personal communication Roger Sperry.

[343] Keller, W. (1985). Forty hertz EEG activity in the elderly: dementia, depression, and normal aging. Doctoral dissertation. University of Houston.

[344] The Nobel Prize in Physiology or Medicine 1981. NobelPrize.org. Retrieved from https://www.nobelprize.org/prizes/medicine/1981/summary/ ry, R. (1981)

[345] The Nobel Prize in Physiology or Medicine 1981. NobelPrize.org. Retrieved from https://www.nobelprize.org/prizes/medicine/1981/summary/ ry, R. (1981)

[346] Hubel, D. and Wiesel, T. (1959). Receptive fields of single neurons in the cat's striate cortex. J. Physiol., 48:574–591.

[347] Hubel, D. and Wiesel, T. (1962). Receptive fields, binocular interaction and functional architecture in the cat's visual cortex. J. Physiol., 160:106–154.

[348] Hubel, D. and Wiesel, T. (1963a). Shape and arrangement of columns in cat's striate cortex. J. Physiol., 165:559–568.

[349] Hubel, D. and Wiesel, T. (1963b). Receptive fields of cells in striate cortex of very young, visually inexperienced kittens. J. Neurophysiol., 26:994–1002.

[350] Hubel, D. and Wiesel, T. (1965). Binocular interaction in striate cortex of kittens reared with artificial squint. J. Neurophysiol., 28:1041-1059.

[351] Luria, A. (1973). The Working Brain: An introduction to neuropsychology. Translated by Basil Haigh. Basic Books.

352 Dandy, W. (1919). Röntgenography of the brain after the injection of air into the spinal canal. Annals of Surgery, Philadelphia, 70:397-403.

353 Dandy, W. (1921). The diagnosis and treatment of hydrocephalus due to occlusion of the foramina of Magendie and Luschka. Surgery, Gynecology and Obstetrics, Chicago, 32:112-124.

354 Moniz, E. (1927). L'encephalographie arterielle, son importance dans la localisation des tumeurs cérébrales. Revue Neurologique, Paris, 2:72-90.

355 The Nobel Prize in Physiology or Medicine 1979. Retrieved from https://www.nobelprize.org/prizes/medicine/1979/summary/

356 Hahn, E. (1950). Spin echoes. Physical Review, 80:80–594.

357 Carr, H. (1952). Free precession techniques in nuclear magnetic resonance (PhD thesis). Cambridge, MA: Harvard University.

358 The Nobel Prize in Physics 1952. Nobelprize.org. Retrieved 8-24-2016 from http://www.nobelprize.org/nobel_prizes/physics/laureates/1952

359 Damadian, R. (1971). Tumor detection by nuclear magnetic resonance. Science, March 19, 171:1151–1153.

360 Lauterbur, P. (1973). Image formation by induced local interactions: Examples employing nuclear magnetic resonance. Nature, March 16, 242:190-191.

361 Young I, Hall A, Pallis C, Legg, N., Bydder, G., Steiner, R. (1981). Nuclear magnetic resonance imaging of the brain in multiple sclerosis. Lancet, 2:1063-6.

362 Young, I, Bydder, G, Hall, A, Steiner, R., Worthington, B., Hawkes, R, Holland, G. Moore, W. (1983). The role of NMR imaging in the diagnosis and management of acoustic neuroma. Am. J. Neuroadiol., May/June, 4:223-4.

363 Sipponen, J., Kaste, M., Ketonen, L., Sepponen, R., Katevuo, K., Sivula, A. (1983). Serial nuclear magnetic resonance (NMR) imaging in patients with cerebral infarction. J. Comput. Assist. Tomography, 7:585-9.

364 Peterman, S., Steiner, R., Bydder, G., Thomas, D., Tobias, J., Young, I. (1985). Nuclear magnetic resonance imaging (NMR), (MRI), of brain stem tumors. Neuroradiolog., 27:202-7.

365 Lauterbur, P. (1986). Cancer detection by nuclear magnetic resonance zeugmatographic imaging. Accomplishments in Cancer Research, 1985 Prize Year, General Motors Cancer Research Foundation, Philadelphia: J. B. Lippincott Co.

366 The Nobel Prize in Physiology or Medicine 2003. NobelPrie.org. Retrieved from https://www.nobelprize.org/prizes/medicine/2003/summary/

367 Ter-Pogossian. M., Phelps, M., Hoffman, E., Mullani, N. (1975). A positron-emission transaxial tomograph for nuclear imaging (PET). Radiology, 114(1):89–98.

368 Belliveau, J., Kennedy, D., McKinstry, R., Buchbinder, B., Weisskoff, R., Cohen, M., Vevea, J., Brady, T., Rosen, B. (1991). Functional mapping of the human visual cortex by magnetic resonance imaging. Science, 254(3032):716-719.

369 Kwong, K, Hopkins, A., Belliveau, J., Chesler, D., Porkka, L.; McKinstry, R., Finelli, D., Hunter, G., Moore, J. et al. (1991). Proton NMR imaging of cerebral blood flow using (H2O)-O17. Magnetic Resonance in Medicine, 22(1):154–158.

370 Kwong, K., Belliveau, J., Chesler, D., Goldberg, I., Weisskoff, R., Poncelet, B., Kennedy, D., Hoppel, B., Cohen, M., Turner, R., Cheng, H., Brady, T., Rosen, B. (1992). Dynamic magnetic resonance imaging of human brain activity during primary sensory stimulation. PNAS., 89(12):5951–55.

371 Mattle, H. and Edelman, R. (1992). Cerebral magnetic resonance angiography. Neurological Research, 14(2 suppl):118-121.

372 Nussel, F, Wegmuller, H., Huber, P. (1992). Comparison of magnetic resonance angiography, magnetic resonance imaging and conventional angiography in cerebral arteriovenous malformation. Neuroradiology, January, 3 (1):56-61.

373 Conturo, T., Lori, N., Cull, T., Akbudak, E., Snyder, A., Shimony, J., McKinstry, R., Burton, H. Raichle, M. (1999). Tracking neuronal fiber pathways in the living human brain. Proc. Natl. Acad. Sci. USA, August 31, 96 (18):10422–10427.

374 Stieltjes, B., Kaufmann, W., van Zijl, P., Fredericksen, K., Pearlson, G., Soaiyappan, M. Mori, S. (2001). Diffusion tensor imaging and axonal tracking in the human brain. Neuroimage., 14:723–735.

375 Alexander, A., Lee, J., Lazar, M., Field, A. (2007). Diffusion tensor imaging of the brain. Neurotherapeutics, July 4(3):316-329.

376 Sorensen, A., Wu, O., Copen. W., Davis, T., Gonzalez, R., Koroshetz, W., Reese, T., Rosen, B., Wedeen, V., Weisskoff, R. (1999). Human acute cerebral ischemia: detection of changes in water diffusion anisotropy by using MR imaging. Radiology, 212:785-792.

377 Werring, D., Clark, C., Barker, G., Thompson, A., Miller, D. (1999). Diffusion tensor imaging of lesions and normal-appearing white matter in multiple sclerosis. Neurology, 52:1626-1632.

378 Henry, R., Oh, J., Nelson, S., Pelletier, D. (2003). Directional diffusion in relapsing-remitting multiple sclerosis: a possible in vivo signature of Wallerian degeneration. J. Magn. Reson. Imaging, 18:420-426.

[379] Witwer, B., Moftakhar, R., Hasan, K., Deshmukh, P., Haughton, V., Field, A., Arfanakis, K., Noyes, J., Moritz, C., Meyerand, M., Rowley, H., Alexander, A., Badie, B. (2002). Diffusion-tensor imaging of white matter tracts in patients with cerebral neoplasm. J. Neurosurg., 97:568–575.

[380] Lazar, M., Alexander, A., Thottakara, P., Badie, B., Field, A. (2006). White matter reorganization after surgical resection of brain tumors and vascular malformations. Am. J. Neuroradiology, 27:1258-1271.

[381] Alexander, A., Lee, J., Lazar, M., Boudos, R., DuBray, M., Oakes, T., Miller, J., Miller, J., Lu, J., Jeong, E., McMahon, W., Bigler, E., Lainhart, J. (2007). Diffusion tensor imaging of the corpus callosum in autism, Neuroimage., Jan 1;34(1):61–73.

[382] Wilde, E., McCauley, S., Hunter, J., Bigler, E., Chu, Z., Wang, Z., Hanten, G., Troyanskaya, M., Yallampalli, R., Li, X., Chia, J., Levin, H. (2008). Diffusion tensor imaging of acute traumatic brain injury in adolescents. Neurology, 70(12):948-955.

[383] Aoki, Y., Inokuchi, R., Gunshin, M., Yahagi, N. (2012). Diffusion tensor imaging studies of mild traumatic brain injury: A meta-analysis. Journal of Neurology, Neurosurgery, and Psychiatry, 83:870-876.

[384] Sener, S., Parizel, P., Maas, A. (2016). Diffusion tensor imaging in traumatic brain injury. In diffusion tensor imaging: A practical handbook. (Eds.) Wi Van Hecke, Louise Emsell, Stefan Sunaert. p. 373-380, Springer

[385] Ellison-Wright, I. and Bullmore, E. (2009). Meta- analysis of diffusion tensor imaging studies in schizophrenia, Schizophrenia Research, 108(1-3):3-10.

[386] Vederine, F., Wessa, M., Leboyer, M., Houenou, J. (2011). A meta-analysis of whole brain diffusion tensor imaging studies in bipolar disorder. Progress in Neuro-Psychopharmacology and Biological Psychiatry, 35:1820-1826.

[387] Liao, Y., Huang, X., Wu, Q., Yang, C., Kuang, W., Du, M., Lui, S., Yue, Q., Chan, R., Kemp, G., Gong, Q. (2013). Is depresssion a disconnection syndrome? Meta- analysis of diffusion tensor imaging studies in patients with MDD. Journal of Psychiatry & Neuroscience, 38(1) 49-56.

[388] Sexton, C., Kalu, U., Filippini, N., Mackay, C., Ebmeier, K. (2011). A meta-analysis of diffusion tensor imaging in mild cognitive impairment and Alzheimer's disease. Neurobiology of Aging, 32(12): 2322.35-2322.e18.

[389] Foerster, B., Dwamena, B., Petrou, M., Carlos, R., Callaghan, B., Pomper, M. (2012). Diagnostic accuracy using diffusion tensor imaging in the diagnosis of ALS: A Meta-analysis. Academic Radiology, 19(9):1075-1086.

[390] Cochrane, C. and Ebmeier, K. (2013). Diffusion tensor imaging in Parkinsonian syndromes: A systematic review and meta- analysis. Neurology, 80(9):857-864.

[391] Chung, K., Wallace, J., Kim, S., Kalyanasundaram, S., Andalman, A., Davidson, T., Mirzabekov, J., Zalocusky, K., Mattis, J., Denisin, A., Pak, S., Bernstein, H., Ramakrishnan, C., Grosenick, L., Gradinaru, V., Deisseroth, K. (2013). Structural and molecular interrogation of intact biological systems. Nature, 497(7449):332–337.

[392] Underwood, E. (2013). Tissue imaging method makes everything clear. Science, 340(6129):131–132.

[393] Geaghan-Breiner, C. (2013). CLARITY brain imaging. Stanford University.

[394] Shen, H. (2013).See-through brains clarify connections.Nature News, April 10.

[395] Deisseroth, K. (2013). See through brains. Nature Video. Retrieved 8-25-2016 fromchttps://www.youtube.com/watch?v=c-NMfp13Uug&feature=youtu.be

[396] The Nobel Prize in Physiology or Medicine 2014. Nobelprize.org.Nobel Media AB 2014. Retrieved 8-25-2016 from http://www.nobelprize.org/nobel_prizes/medicine/laureates/2014/

Chapter 9

Medical Pharmacology

Definition.

Pharmacology is "…the science concerned with drugs, their sources, appearance, chemistry, actions, and uses…" (1997)[1]. The term is derived from the Greek word "pharmaco" meaning drugs and poisons plus the familiar suffix "logy", meaning the study of a subject (2018)[2]. More specifically, medical pharmacology is the study of chemical substances and their effect on biological systems with an ultimate goal to understand these relationships and apply the knowledge to the diagnosis, prevention, management, or treatment of human disease and suffering.

Introduction.

This chapter traces the history of medical pharmacology from its earliest beginnings, as practiced by the ancient civilizations of Mesopotamia, Samaria, Babylonia, and Egypt to its current state today, as practiced by modern Western medicine. Emphasis is placed upon the development of medical pharmacology as a scientific discipline. Particular attention is devoted to developing an appreciation and understanding of the most influential people who shaped the discipline throughout history, milestone discoveries, and recognition of changes in conceptual matrixes which have led to our current knowledge of medical pharmacology today.

The chapter is organized chronologically for consistency with other chapters and for quick, easy reference.

Upon completion of this chapter you will understand and appreciate the foundation upon which the practice of modern medical pharmacology stands. You will be better prepared as future physicians to contribute to the advancement of new knowledge and apply current knowledge to the treatment of patients seeking your care. You will recognize that facts and truths change with new information. You will recognize our knowledge base of medical pharmacology is much more than an ordered accumulation of information over time. It develops as a function of multiple dynamic external and internal forces which influence content and process. You will recognize your responsibility as future physicians to continue to challenge medical dogma when necessary, remain open to new and innovative ideas, and embrace opportunities to learn from those who have gone before you. One day you will be expected to pass your knowledge on to others.

History.

Early Records, 3500 BC - 500 BC.

The written records of the ancient civilizations of Mesopotamia and ancient Egypt have recently enjoyed a resurgence in scholarly interests and are continuing to reveal a more complete history of the early beginnings of medical pharmacology (2010,2005,1923,1898,1500BC,1550BC)[3,4,5,6,7,8,9].

The most recent advances in understanding the historical foundations of medical pharmacology are being made today as more focus is being placed upon the translation and analyses of the written records from ancient Mesopotamia. Largely previously ignored by scholars, in favor of Egyptian artifacts and written medical papyri, the written records of the older ancient civilizations of Mesopotamia, Sumer, Babylon, and Assyria are now beginning to reveal their rich wealth of medical pharmacological knowledge. The new information provides an exciting complement to the more recognized and studied knowledge mined from the records of nearby ancient Egypt and offers a more complete understanding of the ancient foundations of medical pharmacology.

If you are an American or Canadian medical student your knowledge of ancient world geography is probably as poor as mine. If you are the exception and are indeed familiar with the geography and cultures of ancient Mesopotamia and Egypt, enjoy the next three paragraphs as a brief review.

Most of us know where Egypt is located. Right? North coast of Africa, the Mediterranean Sea to the north, the Red Sea to the east, Sudan to the south, and Libya to the west. Many of us however, are clueless as to the location of Mesopotamia. In brief, this ancient region of the world today is called Iraq. The term Mesopotamia literally means "between the rivers". The rivers are the Tigris and Euphrates. More completely, Mesopotamia includes not only the land between the rivers but also the surrounding plains on either side of the rivers. The region is bound to the north and east by mountain ranges. To the south is the Persian Gulf and to the west is Syria. To the southwest are the massive deserts of Syria and Saudi Arabia.

Most of us educated in North America have some familiarity with Egypt by way of its geographical landmarks e.g. the Nile River and Sahara Desert, the ancient structures e.g. the pyramids of Gaza and the Great Sphinx, the ruins of ancient cities e.g. Memphis and Thebes, the Valley of the Kings, as well as vivid images of ancient artifacts, mummified remains, sarcophagi, hieroglyphics, and medical papyri. All contribute to an accurate impression of a well-organized, sophisticated, knowledgeable, vibrant, ancient civilization.

In contrast, few of us have an equal familiarity with the geographic location of Mesopotamia and its many contributions to medicine. The mere introduction of the topic for discussion to most medical students is typically met by blank or oftentimes dazed stares, as of a deer caught in one's automobile headlights. Massive sympathetic nervous system activation is readily apparent, characterized by dilated pupils, accelerated heart rates, and profuse sweating. No need for concern any longer. The ancient civilizations of Mesopotamia can be divided into three geographical regions. Sumer, is the oldest of the three regions and is located in the southern most part of Mesopotamia (southern Iraq). Babylon, the second oldest of the three regions is located in the middle region of Mesopotamia. Assyria the youngest of the three regions, is located to the north.

Ancient records from all three Mesopotamia regions reveal a progressive, organized, culture with interests in documenting observations of the natural world e.g. movement of celestial bodies, changes in plants and animals as a function of the celestial body movement, and the amount of time before recovery or death of a medical patient when presenting with specific clinical signs and symptoms of disease, illness, or trauma. Characteristically, the observations of natural events are recorded in the form of lists and without an apparently clear conceptual matrix to organize the observations.

The Sumerian oral language provides the basis for the development of one of the world's earliest written languages, cuneiform script. The written language and all of its modified permutations over time provide the necessary and essential tool for record keeping. The written language originally develops from a need to maintain records of the thousands of trade transactions made throughout the commercially vibrant, international seaport in Sumer, record laws and regulations which govern the societal organization of the ancient civilizations, and record observations of the natural world.

The written language is recorded onto numerous and varied writing surfaces, including erasable wax tablets, sheets of papyrus, and the much more durable and permanent, clay tablets or stone.

Most of the surviving written records from the ancient civilizations of Mesopotamia and in particular the medical pharmacological treatment recipes are written in cuneiform script and on clay tablets. The Sumerian language and cuneiform script become the language of science and remain the preferred language of science, until the first century AD, at which time it begins to be displaced by the preferred language of the Roman Empire, Latin.

Written records from the ancient civilizations of Mesopotamia and Egypt document well the many efforts to relieve pain and suffering associated with illness, disease, or trauma. Most efforts are directed to drinking, eating, inserting, inhaling, or rubbing substances on or into the human body. The specific substances, process of substance selection, route of administration, and conceptual matrix which guide the use of one or a combination of substances for any particular sign or symptom vary. However, the ultimate goal and objectives remain the same; relieve human pain and suffering by use of medicinal substances.

Ancient Mesopotamian clay tablets reveal an empirical-inductive epistemological approach is applied to understanding relationships between physical signs and symptoms and the therapeutic values of plants, minerals, and animal products. The observed relationships are recorded and passed from generation to generation. Emphasis is placed upon collection of individual experiences e.g. I had a fever, I ate this root, and my fever disappeared; he had a fever, he ate this root, and his fever disappeared; she had a fever, she ate this root, and her fever disappeared. The collection of individual experiences is generalized to produce a general statement about the relationship between fever, the root, and the therapeutic clinical outcome. The process over time results in a rather stable base of information and when applied, produces a reasonably reliable predictable outcome.

Clay tablets recovered and translated from the ancient civilizations typically reveal a characteristic listings of a clinical sign or symptom, along with a simple or compound mixture of plant, mineral, or animal substance, designated as therapeutic in the treatment or management of the particular sign or symptom. The listing of signs, symptoms, and recommended therapies are among the earliest surviving written records, documenting relationships between impaired physical health and a medical approach, rather than a surgical approach to treatment. The written records recovered from Mesopotamia clearly reveal a favored medical (pharmacological) approach to treatment, whereas the written records recovered from Egypt reveal a favored surgical approach.

In addition to listing of signs or symptom and accompanying therapeutic plant, mineral, or animal substance to be used in their treatment, the recovered clay tablets frequently include and list an accompanying incantation, to be recited as a complement to the administration of the plant, mineral, or animal substance.

Early translations of the tablets, frequently interpret these accompanying incantations as simply magical spells and of little value in understanding the foundation of ancient medical pharmacology, beyond the implication ancient medical pharmacology is based heavily upon sorcery, and magical spells.

However, recent modern translations and thoughtful analyses of the ancient clay tablets suggest an alternative explanation for the accompanying incantations. The incantations complement the pharmacological treatment not as sorcery, as easily mistaken by early translations, but rather serve as an essential component of the therapeutic process. Much more than a placebo effect, the incantation or perhaps today a brief prayer, provides reassurance to the patient that she or he has officially begun treatment and can now reasonably expect an improvement in their medical condition.

Yes, the pharmacologically active agent contained in the plant, mineral, or animal substance is most responsible for modifying the body's physiology and producing the physiological improvements in the patient's condition, yet the impact of enlisting a patient's belief system e.g. religious, cultural, societal, geographically regional, or economical cannot be overestimated in facilitating a positive therapeutic outcome. The practice of administering pharmacologically active agents in combination with authoritative reassurance from a practitioner whom instills confidence to their patient by working within the patient's belief system continues today, five thousand years after it is documented in the clay tablets of ancient Mesopotamia.

Cultural belief systems of ancient Mesopotamian emphasize the role of gods, ghosts, and spirits in every aspect of life, including healing. Records from the period suggest there may have been many as 3000 identifiable gods, ghosts, and spirits. Typically a god, ghost or spirit is responsible for a specific function. For example, in reference to the disease of the body, one god is responsible for the stomach, another for the eye, another for the bowels. Specific gods, ghosts, or spirits are considered causal in symptom development. Placating the god, ghost, or spirit results in symptom relief and return to normal bodily function. Given the cultural belief system, it makes sense to include appeasement of the god, ghost, or spirit, be it through reciting incantations or other ritualistic behaviors. To ignore this component of a treatment program makes no sense if the ultimate objective is to improve the patient's physical condition. Similarly, to offer treatment based entirely upon incantations and in the absence of empirically derived effective chemical based treatments extracted from plants, minerals, and animal substances also would make no sense. It is the combination of both approaches which produce the effective medicinal treatments, provided by the astute medical practitioners of ancient Mesopotamia.

The written records of ancient Mesopotamia reveal a rich, cumulative, and empirically derived medical pharmacopeia. Of specific note are the approximate 1600 plus medical clay tablets recovered and translated by modern-day scholars, especially French Assyriologist Rene Labat (1904-1974) (1951)[10], British Assyriologist Campbell Thompson (1876-1941) (1923,1924,

1949)[11,12,13], German Assyriologist Franz Kocher (1916-2002) (1955,1963-1980)[14,15], and JoAnn Scurlock (1953-) and Burton Andersen (1932-) (2005)[16].

The medical tablets emphasize the role of botanicals, animal substances, and minerals in descending order of use. The tablets further reveal the ancient civilizations of Mesopotamia possess at least a fundamental working knowledge of organic chemistry (1959,1973,2010)[17,18,19]. Aromatics and oil extracts are frequently used as therapeutic remedies. Beer and wine are referenced repeatedly and frequently used in combination with other pharmacological active ingredients. Cultivation and harvesting of the opium poppy for medicinal use is recorded and appears to be used liberally in treating a wide range of illnesses.

The ancient written records of neighboring Egypt similarly reveal a documented history and familiarity with the fundamentals of medical pharmacology. Similar to the ancient Mesopotamians the ancient Egyptians recognize the use of botanicals, animal substances, and minerals. The ancient Egyptians also emphasize the roles of gods and spirits as essential to understanding and successfully treating disease and illness. A combination of equal attention to both pharmacologically active substances and the patient's culturally structured belief system is recognized as necessary to effect a clinically positive therapeutic outcome. Identified, effective pharmacological treatments are passed from generation to generation through written language, inscribed on clay tablets, stone, or papyri.

In contrast to the ancient Mesopotamians' empirical-inductive epistemology, ancient Egyptians apply a rational-deductive epistemology in acquiring new knowledge. This approach is applied to the relationships between therapeutic substances and good physical health. The Egyptians reveal a much greater familiarity with human anatomy when compared with the Mesopotamians and are more likely to apply surgical therapeutic interventions. The Egyptians organize their written records of pharmacological and surgical treatments based upon anatomy, while the Mesopotamians organize their written records based upon clinical signs and symptoms. Egyptian medical care and clinical service delivery emphasize a specialist model in contrast to the generalist model applied in Mesopotamia.

Much of what we know today of the ancient Egyptian medical pharmacology is based heavily upon modern translations, during the past 125 years of multiple ancient Egyptian papyri. The most studied and recognizable of these papyri, dated to approximately 2000 BC-1500 BC are the Hearst, Kahun, and Ebers papyri. Each papyrus provides a written record of prescribed pharmacological treatments recommended in the treatment of specific and general medical conditions of the period. Given the importance of these papyri in the history of medicine, let's take a very quick look at each papyrus.

The Hearst Papyrus, dated to approximately 2000 BC is named after the American publishing mogul William Randolph Hearst (1905)[20]. The Hearst family funds the expedition, through the University of California, which leads to the discovery of the papyrus, during the spring of 1901. This papyrus offers approximately 18 pages of prescriptions which focus upon pharmacological treatments of specific anatomical systems e.g. urinary, pulmonary, gastrointestinal, and cerebro-vascular. The original, 1905 translation of the papyrus, is housed today in the University of California - Berkley Bancroft Library.

The Kahun papyrus, dated to approximately 1800 BC is named after the name of the ancient worker's village in which the papyrus is discovered (1931)[21]. The worker's village is located close to and housed the workers whom constructed the ancient Pyramid of Lahun (aka pyramid of Senusret), located in northeast Egypt. The papyrus is also known as the Petrie papyrus, in recognition of Flinders Petrie (1853-1942) British Egyptologist whom discovers the papyrus in 1889. The papyrus is first translated in 1893 (1893)[22]. The Kahun papyrus offers non-surgical pharmacological prescriptions, which focus upon women heath issues and emanating from disturbances of the anatomical uterus. Specifics prescriptions are offered for fertility, contraception, and pregnancy. The papyrus is also known and frequently referenced as the Kahun gynecological papyrus. The original papyrus is housed today in the Petrie Museum of Egyptian Archaeology of the University of London.

The Ebers papyrus, dated to approximately 1500 BC is named for Georg Ebers, German Egyptologist, who purchases the papyrus in the ancient city of Thebes, Egypt (modern-day Luxor) in 1872 (1890)[23]. The papyrus is believed to have been recovered from a necropolis (cemetery) of the ancient city of Thebes (1904)[24]. It is first translated in 1890, by Heinrich Joachim (1890)[23]. Approximately 110 pages in length, the papyrus offers pharmacological prescriptions which focus on specific anatomical systems e.g. head and neck (face, ear, nose throat, eye, and teeth), reproductive, urinary, cardiac, skin, gastrointestinal, pulmonary, abdomen, chest, female genitals, rectum, and more. Over 700 different substances, from plants, animals, and minerals, act as stimulants, sedatives, analgesics, antispasmodics, astringents, antipyretics, diuretics, hypnotics, diaphoretics, expectorants, emetics, antiemetics, and purgatives are presented.

The Ebers papyrus is largely organized by organ systems. This papyrus also introduces treatments for mental disorders e.g. depression and dementia, suggesting the ancient Egyptians make no distinction or separation between physical and psychological illness, offering pharmacological treatments for both. Treatments are administered by way of injection, inhalation, ingestion, suppositories, and topical applications. Therapeutic substances are prepared in the form of pills, tablets, capsules, powders, gases, smoke, lotions, ointments, and plasters. The Ebers papyrus is housed today in the Library of the University of Leipzig. An English translation is now available online (1937)[25].

All three representative ancient Egyptian papyri presented and the ancient Mesopotamia clay tablets presented earlier share numerous similarities in content of knowledge. Specific plants, animal substances, and minerals are found in both written records and are applied to the treatment of similar medical conditions. Many of these early recognized associations are utilized today in modified form. For example, the papyri and clay tablets frequently reference opium extracted from the poppy plant as a recommended treatment for pain, coughs, and diarrhea. Honey is frequently recommended for its antiseptic properties. Willow and myrtle plants, rich in salicylate (active ingredient in aspirin), are recommended for their anti-pyretic, analgesic, and anti-inflammatory properties. Castor and olive oils are recommended laxatives. Wine and beer are frequently recommended for their sedative and analgesic effects. Aloe is recommended for the treatments of burns.

Written records of ancient Mesopotamia and ancient Egypt contain additional treatment recommendations, using seemingly odd and usual selections of single or combinations of plants, animal substances, and minerals, which challenge the limits of understanding when analyzed within the matrix of modern-day pharmacology. Perhaps the treatment contains no active pharmacological agent at all or perhaps it does and we just don't know enough today to correctly identify it, given the limitations of our knowledge. This offers you the medical student, an opportunity to piece together further the chemical basis of the now seemly odd and unusual combinations of medical pharmacological substances preserved in the written records of these two great ancient civilizations.

In summary, the cuneiform inscribed written clay tablets of ancient Mesopotamia, in combination with the cursive hieroglyphic and hieratic writings of ancient Egypt recorded in ink on papyri, document the rich and dynamic early history of medical pharmacology. The written record reveals both civilizations emphasize the healing and palliative powers of plants, animal substances, and minerals. All pharmacological treatments are administered within the contextual matrix of cultural and religious belief systems of each civilization. Whether the desired treatment and management results are the product of pharmacologically active ingredients, administration of ingredients within a culturally defined belief system, or an interaction of multiple variables, the written historical records reveal pharmacological treatments are effective. Efforts to understand the factors responsible for effective treatments and to preserve the knowledge, for future generations, is evident from the earliest of known ancient civilizations. These same efforts continue today, over five thousand years after first being documented in the written historical records.

Antiquity, 500 BC - 500 AD.

Medical pharmacology of Antiquity builds upon the foundations laid by the ancient civilizations of Mesopotamia, Egypt, and Greece. The knowledge base is expanded and refined. Pharmacological treatments continue to rely almost exclusively on the three previously established primary sources; plants, animals, and minerals. Pharmacological ingredients continue to be administered to patients in single or compounded mixtures based upon empirically derived demonstration of effectiveness. The practice of simply listing pharmacological ingredients, followed by clinical signs and symptoms of illness or disease for which administration of the pharmacological ingredient have demonstrated effectiveness continues.

Ancient civilizations of Mesopotamia, Egypt, and Greece are integrated geographically into a rapidly expanding Roman Empire. The Roman Empire soon controls most all coastal regions of the Mediterranean Sea, including southern Europe, the Middle East, and northern Africa. Pharmacological knowledge of Mesopotamia, Egypt, and Greece is soon combined and claimed by the Roman Empire to be its own.

Cuneiform tablets, hieratic papyri, and other sources of written knowledge are translated from their original languages of Sumerian, Egyptian, and Greek into the preferred language of the Roman Empire, Latin. Pharmacological knowledge, traditionally passed from generation to generation by the oral tradition is committed to the written record. The world's knowledge under control of the Roman Empire is collected and assembled in central locations e.g. the Libraries of Alexandria. Collection and organization of these materials generate impressive collections of knowledge known to the period, including but not limited to the multi-authored Hippocratic Collections (400 BC). Materials are studied, translated, reproduced, and oftentimes modified in style and content.

Beyond the Hippocratic Collections (400 BC), six notable medical pharmacology texts of Antiquity reflect typical content, format organization, and methodologies representative of this period; "Historia Plantarum" [Inquiry into Plants- 300 BC]; "De mediciona octo libri" [The Eights Books of Medicine- 45 AD]; "Compositiones Medicamentorium" [Compounds of Medicines- 45 AD]; "De Materia Medica" [Concerning Medical Substances- 65 AD]; "Naturalis Historia"

[Natural History- 75 AD]; and "De Simplicium Medicamentorum Temperamentis et Facultatibus" [On the mixtures and properties of simple medications- 170 AD].

The earliest of these influential texts summarize knowledge established by the ancient civilizations and reflect empirical (experiential) models of epistemology. The later texts attempt to move pharmacology from experiential models to rational models. A shift from the empirical paradigm to a rational paradigm defines Antiquity.

The Ancient civilizations recall, embraced the empirical approach i.e. these particular plants, animal substances, and minerals have a demonstrated history of being effective in treating these signs and symptoms; so let us continue to use them. Perhaps in the future we will discover additional plants, animal substances, and minerals which will prove to be effective too. When this occurs we will record the associations and incorporate them into our current treatment regimens. The Roman Empire on the other hand embraces a rational approach i.e. this is the way we know the body works; so if we use these particular plants, animal substances, and minerals, it make sense they should be effective in treating these signs and symptoms. The shift in paradigm represents an important change in the way medical pharmacology knowledge is created, organized, and applied.

The paradigmatic shift during Antiquity incorporates movement away from a deity (supranatural) conceptual matrix, within which to understand human disease and illness, to a physical (natural) conceptual matrix. Pharmacological treatment effectiveness e.g. relieving patient pain and suffering and facilitating recovery of good health, now begins to be understood within the matrix of physics, chemistry, and physical laws of nature, rather than supranatural intervention.

Let us consider a few specifics.

Hippocratic Collection (circa 400 BC), the now familiar, multi-authored collection of approximately 60 assorted ancient Greek medical treaties, notes, and lectures provide insights into the early beginnings of medical pharmacology. The Collection evidences an endorsement of an introduction of pharmacologically active ingredients into the treatment process only to the degree the ingredients facilitate the natural recovery processes of body healing. The therapeutic approach most reflected within the Collection is based upon the healing powers of nature. More specifically, weather, location, season of the year, and the human body's innate physical processes are considered more important than pharmacological ingredients, in effecting a successful therapeutic outcome. Pharmacologically active ingredients are used as an adjunct in treatment to help restore and facilitate the body's natural physical recovery process.

Pharmacological ingredients in the Collection can be organized according to their source; plants, animal substances, or minerals. This reflects the Collection's simple reiterations of pharmacological ingredients and medical applications established during the ancient civilizations of Greece, Egypt, and Mesopotamian. Few if any new ingredients are introduced by the Collection. The usual, garden varietal assortment of plants, animal fats, honeys, and beers/wines comprise the majority of pharmacological recipes.

The Hippocratic Collection contains approximately 3,100 formulated pharmaceutical recipes. A total of 380 plants can be identified which are used in the formulas. Approximately half of the formulas (approximately 1,500) are made with only 45 plants. A third of the formulas (approximately 1,100) are made with 80 different plants. The remaining 500 formulas are made with 255 plants (400BC,1843,1923,2004)[26,27,28,29].

The medicinal plants most mentioned in the Hippocratic Collection are hellebore, garlic, French mercury, parsley, and leek (400BC/1998)[30]. OK… I don't know what hellebore and French mercury are either. Hellebores are poisonous winter flowering plants of the buttercup family, typically having coarse divided leaves and large white, green or purple flowers. French mercury is a plant which typically flowers in the months of August and September; grows on dunghills; is a member of the castor oil plant family; and has spinach like leaves. Garlic, parsley, and leek are familiar to all. These and other medicinal plants of the Collection are indigenous to Greece and surrounding areas. The plants are abundant, readily available, and grow wild in the countryside. The treating physician simply needs to stroll through the country side and harvest the particular plant to be used that day for any particular patient.

Preparation of medicinal plants presented in the Collection are prepared by grinding, crushing, squeezing, boiling, steeping, or drying and administered singularly or in combination with other plants or substances e.g. animal fats, honeys, beer/wines, assorted minerals, especially salt and copper oxide. All modes of administration, familiar to practicing physicians today, ingestion, inhalation, injection, suppository, and topical application to the skin are used.

Pharmacological prescriptions in the Collection most typically follow a straight forward format; identification of a specific sign or symptom, followed by a recommended formulation of plant, animal, or mineral substances, followed by a recommended mode of administration. For example, a typical prescription found in the Collection will read

> "…For a child's cough: roast an egg having taken the yolk, add crushed roasted white sesame and salt grains, and give as an electuary in honey..." (400BC/1839-1862)[31].

> "…(For) promoting a quick birth: turpentine resin, honey, oil in a double amount, sweet-smelling wine, as pleasant as possible; mix these together, let it cool down, give to drink…" (400BC/1839-1862)[32].

Notice the absence of specific dosing amounts. This is typical of recipes of the Collection. Retrospective analysis of the recipes suggest this may be by design, providing novice practitioners with incomplete and insufficient information to effect a proper treatment. In order to use the Collection's recipes properly, one must complete an apprenticeship in medical training with a seasoned practitioner.

> "...Keep well in your memory drugs and their properties, both simple and compound, seeing that after all it is in the mind that also the cures of diseases; remember their modes, and their number and variety in the several cases. This in medicine is beginning, middle, and end..." (400BC/1923)[33],

Most pharmaceutical formulas in the Collection are directed to the simple management and relief of clinical signs and symptoms produced by commonly occurring disorders of the region and period. For example, chills and fevers resulting from malaria; vomiting and diarrhea resulting from dysentery; coughs and breathing impairments resulting from tuberculosis; rashes and ulcers from skin infections, infestations, or disease; and pain resulting from inflammation, infection, or trauma. A disproportionately large number of pharmaceutical formulas in the Collection are directed to the unique conditions of women.

The Hippocratic Collection and medical pharmacological formula contain within evidence an empirically driven, physically based, practical approach when providing pharmacological treatments to patients seeking care and comfort from any medical care provider. Remember the Collection is based largely upon knowledge collected from the ancient civilizations of Mesopotamia, Egypt, and Greece, and before the rule of the Roman Empire.

Theophrastus of Eresus (371 BC-287 BC) Greek natural philosopher, student of Plato and Aristotle offers his major contribution to medical pharmacology in his "Historia Plantarum" [Enquiry into Plants] (300BC/1916)[34]. This landmark, ten volume treaties provides an early organization of plants based upon plant structure, methods of reproduction, and function. Of particular relevance to the history of medical pharmacology is Book IX, which discusses the medicinal value of herbal remedies.

Theophrastus identifies approximately 70 of the 500 total plants, included in "Historia Plantarum", as having particular medicinal value. He discusses the flowering plant Colchicum, noting its medicinal value in the treatment of gout (contains the alkaloid colchicine) and is among the first to document and warn of the plant's toxicity and poisonous properties. Theophrastus documents the common use of mandrake as a narcotic to reduce pain, relieve muscle cramping, nausea, coughs, and induce sleep. He additionally warns of the toxic effects of the mandrake root and its potential to cause madness. Theophrastus additionally documents the use of the poison hemlock, reporting it can produce "…an easy and painless end…" and for which "…there is absolutely no cure…" (BK IX, xvi, 8) (300BC/1916)[34].

Recall, hemlock causes death by blocking the neuromuscular junction, similar in action to curare. Hemlock poisoning is characterized by an ascending muscular paralysis, eventually affecting the muscles of respiration, resulting in death, due to hypoxia of heart and brain.

Trivia: Greek philosopher Socrates (469 BC-399 BC) is executed by the government of Athens in 399 BC. Socrates is tried and executed as the result of his thoughtful challenges of authority and associated dogma. Specific charges are corrupting the minds of the youths of Athens and impiety (not believing in the gods of the State). He is required to drink a liquid mixture containing the known poisonous plant extract hemlock (Conium). Hemlock mixtures are used frequently during Antiquity, in the execution of individuals of higher socioeconomic/social status, convicted of committing crimes against government or society. In this case, the crime is disagreeing with established authority.

Theophrastus of Eresus's influential text, "Historia Plantarum", provides much needed guidance to practitioners beyond that provided by the Hippocratic Collections. Recall, the Collections lists plants, animal substances, and minerals along with empirically derived treatments for specific signs and symptoms. In contrast, "Historia Plantarum" offers additional information regarding the shelf life of medicinal plants "…some roots keep longer, some shorter time. Hellebore retains its usefulness for as much as thirty years…" (XIV, xiii.6-xiv.2); dosing of medicinal plants (e.g. thorn-apple) "…three twentieths of an ounce in weight is given, if the patient is to become merely sportive and to think of himself a fine fellow; twice this dose if he is to go mad outright and have delusions; thrice the dose, if he is to be permanently insane;…four times the dose is given, if the man is to be killed…" (IX,xi.5-6); as well as tolerance and diminished efficacy "…the virtues of all drugs become weaker to those who are accustomed to them, and in some cases become entirely ineffective..." (IX, xvi, 9-XVII) (300BC/1916)[34].

Aulus Celsus (25 AD-50 AD) French born, Roman encyclopedist offers his "De Mediciona Octo Libri" [Eight Books of Medicine- 45 AD]. This encyclopedia offers an extensive presentation of western medical knowledge current to the period and offers few additional insights into the historical basis of medical pharmacology. Book V is devoted exclusively to medical pharmacology and emphasizes the use of analgesics, diuretics, purgatives, and laxatives. In keeping with the organizational format of the ancient civilizations the encyclopedia lists signs and symptoms followed by recommended pharmacological treatments. Source of pharmacological active ingredients are drawn from the three traditional sources; plants, animals, and minerals. Overall, this work offers little new to pharmacology beyond summarizing well known information and demonstrating an increasing awareness of a need to document specific amounts of ingredients used singularly or in combination when preparing pharmaceuticals.

The following extract from "De Mediciona Octo Libri" is characteristic of a typical entry.

> "...A pill for pain in the chest is made from nard 4 grams, frankincense and cassia 12 grams each, myrrh and cinnamon 24 grams each, saffron 32 grams, turpentine-resin 1 gram, honey three-quarters of a liter..." (BK V, sec 25 paragraph 8) (45AD/2012)[35].

OK... for Americans and others less familiar with the metric system, a gram is equal in weight to a small, galvanized steel, wire paper clip.

Scribonius Largus (10 AD-50 AD) Sicilian pharmacologist and practicing physician offers his "Compositiones Medicamentorum" [Compounds of Medicines, circa 45 AD] (45AD/1983, 1987)[36,37]. This text lists 271 medicinal remedies formatted similarly to recipes found in the Hippocratic Collections. Specific signs or symptoms are simply followed by brief recipes identifying plants, animal substance, or minerals to be used in treatment or management. The collection is loosely grouped according to signs and symptoms e.g. fevers, headaches, coughs, gastrointestinal inflammation, hemorrhaging. There is no evidence of a rational, theory driven conceptual model guiding selections of medical ingredients, dosing, or administration. The listings are derived empirically and based upon reported effectiveness from Largus' colleagues, friends, and acquaintances. The recipes cover a broad range of conditions. Pharmacological treatments are recommended for common and usual conditions e.g. fevers (1,97), headaches (1-11), gastrointestinal inflammation (111), coughs (77), seizures (17), poisonings (165-170), and bites (213). Pharmacological treatment recommendations are also listed for trauma patients who have fallen out of trees, fallen from ladders, struck by chariots, or have had their teeth knocked out during combat (214). He provides one of the first recorded chemical treatments for the removal of tattoos (231).

Note: The numbers in parentheses above correspond to the recipe number found in "Compositiones Medicamentorum" (45AD/1983,1987)[36,37].

The following recent English translation of a recipes pertaining to the treatment of inflamed tonsils provides a representative sampling of the recipes found in "Compostinses Medicamentorum".

> " ...LXX. For Treatment of a Choking Quinsy: And the following has proven beneficial for many patients, and is certainly quite powerful and quite effective: 2 drachmas each of

costus, celery seeds, anise seeds, oil of camel grass, and cinnamon-cassia, one-half drachma of cardamom, 2 drachmas of the wild rue (two-thirds of which is the seed), one-half ounce of fissile alum, 5 medium-sized ground-up oak galls, 2 drachmas of saffron, one-half drachma of the refined residue of the oil of saffron, one-half drachma of myrrh, 4 drachmas of Cretan birthwort, 3 drachmas of cinnamon, one ounce of the ashes of a young wild swallow, and one-half drachma of spikenard. All these ingredients are to be conjoined and either pounded or otherwise produced separately each having been skimmed in Attic honey. And whenever the compound is to be used, a sufficient amount of the same honey should be added to it. The Augusta always has this compound at hand…" (45AD/1983)[38].

"Compositiones Medicamentorum" includes among its recommended pharmacological treatments, the use of bioelectricity in the treatment of pain associated with gout (162) and toothaches (11). It represents one of the early uses of bioelectricity in the treatment of pain, as an alternative or adjunct to pharmacological based pain treatments.

Scribinous Largus' "Compositiones" falls shorts when compared to the much more comprehensive works of his contemporaries e.g. Dioscorides. However, the work is instructive within the matrix of the history of medical pharmacology in providing both a glimpse of the medicinal ingredients utilized by practicing physicians of the period and the more philosophical instruction to practicing physicians, noting the responsibility of the physician to be familiar with medicinal remedies and to use the remedies as part of their routine care of patients.

Pedanius Dioscorides (40 AD-90 AD) Greek pharmacologist offers his most influential work, "De Materia Medica", circa 60 AD [Concerning Medical Substances] (60AD/1959,2000,2005)[39,40,41]. "De Materia Medica" is the precursor to all modern pharmacopeias. It serves as the gold standard of medical pharmacological knowledge for the next 1500 years. "De Materia Medica" is organized into 5 volumes and over 1000 chapters. Each chapter is devoted to a specific natural substance used for medicinal purposes. Each chapter offers a complete listing of known therapeutic indications, description of product preparation, description of major therapeutic properties, and offers dosing guidelines for each natural substance. "De Materia Medica" describes 630 plants, which is approximately twice the number of plants described in the Hippocratic Collections, and is organized in alphabetical order according to plant name. "De Materia Medica" offers over 5,300 formula prescriptions. All formulas are derived from natural substances, plants, animals, or mineral sources. Volume I describes the medicinal uses for aromatic oils, salves, and ointments. Volume II describes the medicinal use for animals, animal parts, and animal products. Volume III details the use of roots, juices, seeds, and herbs. Volume IV describes the use of narcotics and poisonous medicinal plants. Volume V describes the use for wine and metallic ores.

Pliny the Elder, aka Plinius Secundus (23 AD-79 AD) Roman natural philosopher and encyclopedist offers "Naturalis Historia" [Natural History], circa 75 AD. This encyclopedia collection is organized into 37 books and covers a broad range of subject materials, including astronomy, mathematics, anthropology, mineralogy, zoology, physiology, and botany (75AD/2012)[42]. Approximately one third of "Naturalis Historia" is devoted to materia medica.

Similar to Dioscorides' "De Materia Medica", Pliny the Elder organizes "Naturalis Hisotria" according to substances. He describes a plant, animal substance, or mineral and then offers a description of its recommended medicinal uses. More specifically, Pliny the Elder describes the opium poppy plant, provides a drawing of the plant, and then notes its juices are good for the treatment of coughs, diarrhea, and pain. This format stands in mark contrast to the format typically applied by the Ancient civilizations of Mesopotamia, Egypt, and Greece. Specifically, the Ancients describe a clinical presentation e.g. cough, diarrhea, and pain then note the juices from the opium poppy plant when ingested offer an effective treatment.

The Ancients emphasize clinical presentation of signs and symptoms then look to nature for a remedy. Pliny the Elder and Dioscorides emphasize nature i.e. the plant, animal substance, or mineral as primary and then seek to identify a disorder which can be effectively treated by it. Similar information to be sure, yet completely different ways of thinking about the information.

You, as a medical student might consider applying the same approach today. Take a body of well-established information and try to see it in an entirely different way from others. The information does not change, only the conceptualization of the information changes. The process opens new original lines of thought and can lead to new discoveries impossible when constrained by thinking similarly to all around you.

OK…back to the history of medical pharmacology.

"Naturalis Historia" is never intended to be a pharmacopeia. It is an attempt to record, as comprehensively as possible, a broad collection of knowledge known to the period. This encyclopedia offers nothing new regarding medical pharmacology content. Well established knowledge is simply reiterated e.g. the opium poppy plant has great value in the management of coughs, diarrhea, and pain; honey has great value as an antiseptic when applied topically and can when compounded with other medicinally active ingredients making them more palatable for ingestion; mineral baths offer relief to patients presenting with fever and facilitate wound healing. The strength of Pliny the Elder's "Naturalis Historia" is found not in its new content of medical pharmacological knowledge nor in its offering of a new innovative conceptual matrix, but rather in its effort to simply document as completely as possible the generally accepted medical pharmacology knowledge of the period, gathered from scholars, physicians, and lay persons alike.

Trivia: Mount Vesuvius, located in southern Italy near Naples, experiences one of its most devastating volcanic eruptions August 24, 79 AD. Pliny the Elder dies as a consequence of the eruption in his attempt to rescue volcano victims by sea (1878)[43].

Galen of Pergamum (129 AD-200 AD) Greek physician and philosopher is born and reared in the Greek academic city of Pergamum, located in northwest Turkey, a part of the Roman Empire. Pergamum is rivaled only by the City and Libraries of Alexandria, as a depository of academic knowledge and center of scholarship. Galen embraces his academic opportunities and soon establishes himself as the most prolific medical writer of Antiquity. His summaries of old knowledge, integration of old and new knowledge, willingness to challenge well established medical dogma, willingness to propose new ideas, and his shear amount of medical publications make him one of the most influential contributors to medicine ever.

Galen's contributions to medical pharmacology can be summarized as follows; he emphasizes a rational conceptual model, based upon well-reasoned thought, rather than atheoretically derived empirical observations; places emphasis upon the natural (physical) rather than supranatural (deity) explanations of body functions; emphasizes physiology and chemistry as fundamental in explaining good body health or disease; and organizes diseases, illnesses, and pharmacological ingredients into an integrated conceptual matrix which guides selection of medicinal pharmacological ingredients for medical treatment purposes.

Galen's medical pharmacology emphasizes a rational approach to acquiring new scientific information. Well-reasoned, logically derived, conceptual models are preferred over empirical models which emphasize acquiring new scientific information by way of empirical observations. Galen is outspoken in favor of the rational approach, however he recognizes the value of empirical methodologies. From a philosophical perspective, Galen is perhaps more of a centralist than he might like others to know, often arguing positions in favor and against extreme rational or empirical positions. His writings do reveal his tempered position, which emphasize a balance between reason (rational approach) and experience (empirical approach), noting a balance of the two will lead to the same scientific truths (1985)[44].

Galen's medical pharmacology is based upon a conceptual model which relies exclusively upon natural (physical) processes, governed by physics, physiology, and chemistry. Good health and disease are explained entirely as a function of physical events. An understanding of the physical processes of the body e.g. physiology and chemistry provide all of the information necessary to rationally select medicinal ingredients. Administration of the ingredients will modify fundamental physiological and biochemical processes in a predictable way. In the event of illness or disease, administration of properly selected pharmacologically active ingredients will return the body to its normal state of good physical health.

More specifically, Galen's model of normal and abnormal body function is based upon a modification of the balance doctrine, first purposed by the pre-Socratic natural philosopher Alcmaeon of Croton (circa 510 BC/1896,1952)[45,46]. Galen's slightly modified model simply states, good physical health exists in the human body when the dynamic interactions between four body humors are in balance. Diseases and illnesses result from an imbalance between these humors. The goal of treatment is to restore the dynamic balance between the four humors.

Restoring the balance between the four humors is best accomplished through changes in climate, ensuring a good diet, engaging in physical exercise, getting plenty of rest, taking relaxing medicinal mineral baths, and ingesting properly selected medications. Sound familiar? All of these recommended methods share in common an effort to facilitate the body's natural recovery from disease and illness through manipulation of body's physiological and chemical systems, based upon a predetermined conceptual model as to how the body works.

Galen offers an elaborate system which classifies pharmacological ingredients, specifically plants, animal substances, and minerals, into conceptually meaningful categories. Classification is based upon his conceptual matrix of four dynamic humors. The classification system guides selection, compounding, and dosing of appropriate pharmacological ingredients for use in medical treatments.

To understand Galen's medical pharmacology, it is necessary to have a fundamental understanding of the conceptual matrix upon which it is based. Let us briefly review the most important points here.

Galen believes the entire natural universe is made from four elements: earth, wind, fire, and water, as described by Greek philosophers Empedocles (490 BC-430 BC), Plato (423 BC-348 BC), and Aristotle (384 BC-322 BC), hundreds of years before Galen. Each element is characterized by primary and secondary qualities. There are four primary qualities: hot, cold, wet, dry. There are numerous secondary qualities e.g. density, heaviness, lightness, hardness, and brightness. Each of the four elements is characterized by two primary qualities. Specifically, earth is characterized by qualities cold and dry; wind by qualities hot and wet; fire by qualities hot and dry; and water by qualities cold and wet.

The human body, as a part of the natural universe is therefore also made from the four elements earth, wind, fire, and water and its associated pair of primary qualities. The body expresses these four primary elements as four bodily humors: black bile (earth), blood (wind), yellow bile (fire), and phlegm (water). Each bodily humor expresses the primary qualities defining each primary element. For example, the humor phlegm expresses the primary qualities of the element water, which are cold and wet and the humor yellow bile, expresses the primary qualities of fire, hot and dry.

Each of the four elements earth, wind, fire, and water originate from a primeval and eternal substance of unknown origin (1996)[47]. However, bodily humors are produced by the body from foods and as the end product of digestion. When body humors are in dynamic balance the person experiences good physical health. When body humors are not in dynamic balance a person experiences a resultant disease or illness. Within this matrix, disease and illness are conceptualized and described as a function of humors responsible for the imbalance.

For example, a bacterial pneumonia which produces excessive fluid in the lungs is considered within the conceptual matrix a disease resulting from an excessive amount of phlegm (water). Treatment is directed to restoring the healthy dynamic balance between the four humors. In this case, administration of a pharmacological ingredient which has drying properties is indicated. Drying eliminates the excess amount of phlegm (water) and returns the body to its healthy dynamic balance between body humors.

Galen classifies medicinal plants, animal substances, or minerals according to their effect on the body; heating, cooling, moistening, or drying. Each medicinal ingredient is further sub-classified according to degree, based upon the intensity of the ingredient to generate an effect; heating, cooling, moistening, or drying. Degrees are assigned on an ordinal scale from one to four. Substances of the first degree have minimal effect. Substances of the fourth degree have maximal effect. Substances of the second or third degree have intermediate effects. The system provides sufficient flexibility allowing medicinal substances to be classified according to primary effect only or combinations of primary effects. For example, poppy plant juice is classified as having cooling properties of the fourth degree, whereas as frankincense, the aromatic, milky white resin tapped from the Boswellia tree is classified as having drying properties of the first degree and heating properties of the second degree (2012)[48].

The system offers an alternative to the empirically compiled pharmacopeias, which list clinical signs and symptoms along-side of listings of recommended pharmacological ingredients to be used in treatments. Galen's degree system, for pharmacological ingredients is based upon a rational conceptual matrix as to how the body works i.e. balance of four body humors; how good health is maintained i.e. balance between four humors; the mechanisms responsible for illness and disease i.e. imbalance between the four humors; and what must be accomplished pharmacologically to restore the dynamic balance between the humors i.e. heating, cooling, moistening, or drying. Galen's degree system directs selection of pharmacological substances based upon a rational conceptual matrix, rather than empirically demonstrated associations.

Here is an example of how the system works. A patient presents with a garden variety food poisoning characterized by fever, vomiting, and diarrhea. A medical practitioner adhering to the conventional empiricist model identifies the signs and symptoms, fever, vomiting, and diarrhea then consults an empirically derived pharmacopeia, such as Book V of Aulus Celsus' "De Mediciona Octo Libri" [Eight Books of Medicine] or Pedanus Dioscorides' "De Materia Medica" [Concerning Medical Substances]. The practitioner locates the listing of signs and symptoms demonstrated and reported by the patient and then refers to the corresponding list of ingredients, which have a demonstrated history of successfully treating these particular signs and symptom.

In contrast, this same patient is recognized within Galen's system to be suffering from an excess of the humor phlegm (water). The normal physiological response of the body to is to remove the excess humor and restore balance by generating heat, producing fever and sweating and by purging the excess by way of vomiting and diarrhea. Within the Galenian model, fever, vomiting, and diarrhea are encouraged, in that they are normal body mechanisms for eliminating the excess humor. A medication selected in this particular case should facilitate the drying of the excess humor phlegm. One such selected medication might be frankincense, based upon its drying qualities. The clinical presentation and prescribed pharmacological treatment are understood within a multidimensional conceptual matrix based upon how the body is understood to work normally, what is the cause of the pathology, and properties of the pharmacological ingredients.

Galen's rational epistemological approach, tempered by recognition of strengths and weaknesses of empirical methodologies, impact the development of medical pharmacology for the next two thousand years. His original model incorporates dimensional vectors of normal body function (balance of humors), pathology (imbalance of humors), pharmacological properties of medicinal substances (hot, cold, wet, dry) and treatment (selection and administration of medicinal substances). Content knowledge generated from the model is soon regarded as dogma within the medical community and uncritically applied in clinical medical practices for the next 1500 years. Knowledge which goes unchallenged and accepted as dogma often impedes advancement of new knowledge. So too is the case here. Galen's adamant and authoritative position, he is absolutely correct absolutely and in the absence of a persuasive alternative, Galen hinders the advancement of new medical pharmacology knowledge as much as he advances it.

In summary, medical pharmacology of Antiquity is characterized by collection and consolidation of recorded medical pharmacology knowledge from the ancient civilizations of Mesopotamia, Egypt, and Greece. Records are deposited in selected cities of learning controlled by the Roman Empire. The Libraries of Alexandria are founded. The records are soon organized, studied, translated, reproduced, and modified. The Hippocratic Collections emerge from the efforts and contain over 3,100 formulated pharmaceutical recipes designed to facilitate medical treatments of illness, disease, and relieve human suffering. The Collections' recipes are simple statements which contain a clinical sign or symptom followed by a recommended combination of ingredients originating from plants, animal substances, or minerals, which have been empirically proven over time to be effective in relieving the specific clinical sign or symptom, when used in combination with a more comprehensive treatment program.

Theophrastus of Eresus, Aulus Celsus, Scribonius Largus, Pedanius Dioscorides, Pliny the Elder, and Galen of Pergamum offer influential manuscripts and texts documenting the progression of medical pharmacology from empirically derived associations (if you have a cough, take this combination of ingredients, it has helped a lot of other people who have had coughs) to rational, logically derived conceptual theoretical matrixes within which to understand the source of the pathology and to guide pharmacological treatments (your cough is the result of an imbalance in body humors; take this combination of ingredients, it will restore balance and consequently your cough will improve). Fundamental concepts in medical pharmacology are introduced. Dosing is recognized as important in generating positive treatment outcomes, eliminating toxicity, and understanding the body's response to introduction of medicinal substances. Rational, logical, theoretical models such as proposed by Galen displace empirical, experiential, atheoretical models and prove to be preferred by investigator and practicing clinicians alike, by the end of Antiquity. Illness and disease are interpreted within the matrix of natural (physical) rather than supranatural (deity) causes. Medical pharmacology is understood within the matrix of physics, chemistry, and physical laws of nature. The dogma of Galen dominates the thoughts and practices of pharmacology for the balance of Antiquity. Galenian dogma remains relatively unquestioned and unchallenged, impeding progress in medical pharmacology, for the next 1500 years.

Middle Ages (Medieval Times), 500 AD - 1400 AD.

Medical pharmacology enters a 1000 year period during which little progress is made in expanding content or process knowledge. Little new information is added to medical pharmacology beyond that already collected and summarized by the Greek and Roman encyclopedists of Antiquity. Much of what is already known is simply reiterated, slightly extended, or modified to accommodate the tremendous external influences exerted upon science and medicine by the relatively new and increasingly powerful organized religions of Christianity, Catholicism, and Islam.

A few notable advances are made and contribute to the early development of medical pharmacology as a scientific based discipline. Medical pharmacology is introduced into the medical school curriculum and required of all medical students completing a university based medical education program. Governmental regulations are implemented, requiring demonstrated competency in medical pharmacology by way of documented supervised training and examination, before a professional license is issued to practice medicine. The profession of pharmacy is founded and regulated by government, as distinct and separate from the profession of medicine.

The dominant conceptual matrix guiding medical pharmacology throughout all of the Middle Ages is the conceptual matrix offered by Galen during Antiquity. Recall, this matrix is based upon a rational epistemology, emphasizing natural rather than supranatural forces and conceptualizing pathology as the product of imbalances within the body, which can be restored through the thoughtful use of pharmacological agents.

In light of few advances in content knowledge or conceptual thought, the Middle Ages do witness a forward movement in medical pharmacology as an emerging scientific discipline. Formal training in medical pharmacology is acknowledged as necessary and essential to the competent practice of medicine. Medical pharmacology is introduced into the curriculum of the newly structured university based medical schools. Governmental regulations are imposed requiring individuals choosing to practice medicine demonstrate competency in the knowledge of medical pharmacology to medical school faculty and an independent governmental licensing board, before being permitted to practice medicine. Yes, medical licensing boards have been around for over 800 years and they expect you to know medical pharmacology, before issuing you a license to practice medicine.

The practice of compounding and dispensing medicinal remedies is parceled from the practice of medicine by governmental regulations and the profession of pharmacy is founded. The first western pharmacies are opened in the Middle East (Baghdad, 754 AD) and Europe (Trier, Germany, 1241 AD). Physicians are no longer permitted to sell medicinal remedies of their own preparation.

Geopolitical, social, economic, religious, and military factors, responsible for the recent fall of the Western Roman Empire, also slow the forward movement of medical pharmacology. Traditional city centers devoted to learning, advancement of the medical sciences, and repositories of knowledge are intentionally destroyed. Hundreds of thousands human lives are extinguished, as invading forces attempt to impose their belief systems upon others. The disturbing human behavior of taking the life of another human because the person does not agree with your own belief system is readily apparent during the Middle Ages. Most obvious examples are demonstrated by the Islamic Conquests and the Christian Crusades.

In brief, the fundamental belief and teachings of both of these newly founded, organized religions are as follows: if you do not agree with me, that my God is better than your God, then you must die; if you do not agree with me, that my way of life is better than your way of life, then you must die; if you do not agree with me, that my socio-economical-political interests are more important than yours, then you must die. So too is the case regarding scientific and medical knowledge. If your written knowledge does not agree with my beliefs, then any written record of your knowledge must be destroyed and replaced by knowledge consistent with my beliefs. Any person teaching information which is not consistent with my beliefs must die, or at the very least be controlled and prevented from disseminating the information to others. These are difficult times for those interested in the preservation of old knowledge and the pursuit of new scientific knowledge. Forward progress in medical pharmacology slows as a result.

Let us now consider briefly a few specifics.

As the Roman Empire falls so do many of the traditional city centers of learning and repositories of the written records of world knowledge. Pursuits of new knowledge and greater understanding give way to simple survival and physical preservation.

Amidst the geopolitical, social, economic, religious, and military changes, many academic scholars migrate to the Middle East. One particular and representative group of note are Greek scholars forced from the philosophical schools of Athens. In 529 AD, Emperor Justinian orders the closing of the philosophical schools. Many of the scholars relocate to the city of Jundishapur, located in southwest Persia (today Iran). Here they find academic refuge and a large hospital supportive of academic medicine. In Jundishapur, the displaced scholars soon begin the laborious task of translating Greek and Roman written records of knowledge into the languages of Persian and Syriac. Original texts, translated with relevance to medical pharmacology are the multi-authored Hippocratic Collections, Dioscorides' "De Medicina", and the numerous writings of Galen.

Translation of rescued Greek and Roman written records of science and medicine, from the original text languages into the preferred language of Persian intellectuals, Syriac, continues for the next 500 years. Many of the original records are additionally translated into Arabic. The process of translation incorporates frequent modifications of information in order to better conform to the belief systems of those translating. The process offers a mechanism of preserving medical pharmacology knowledge amassed by the Greeks and Romans and introduces the knowledge for external evaluation by individuals not directly responsible for the production of the original knowledge. The translations require tremendous amounts of effort and time. Much of the translation work is completed by the early-1000s AD. At this time many scholars return to Italy, Greece, and northern Africa, as these regions return to political and economic stability.

Little new knowledge is added, during this 500 year period of translations. Persian scholars produce several notable texts, based largely upon the translations and relating specifically to medical pharmacology. These texts will be discussed in a moment. First, we must briefly discuss an influential Greek scholar whose writings greatly influence Persian scholars.

Paulus of Aegina (625 AD-690 AD) Greek physician from the small Greek island Aegina, located approximately 17 miles from Athens and just off the Greek mainland, in a small archipelago within the Aegean Sea, has tremendous influence on the Middle East scholars. His major work, "De Medica Libri Septum" [Seven Books of Medicine], greatly influences contemporary Persian and Arabic scholars, writing on topics of medical pharmacology (circa 675AD/1847)[49]. His writings appear to be greatly influenced by the writings of Greek pharmacologist Pedanius Dioscorides, especially "De Materia Medica" [Concerning Medical Substances], and the many writings of Greek physician Galen of Pergamum. Recommended treatments offered by "De Medica Libri Septum" are based upon a balance of humors model and incorporate Galen's system of degree for selecting and compounding medicinal remedies. Descriptions are typically very brief and often fail to include dosing guidelines.

Book 7, Section III (Simples) of "De Medica Libri Septum", addresses issues of medical pharmacology. It is organized alphabetically by the primary medicinal ingredient. Each primary ingredient is followed by a brief description of the ingredient conceptualized within Galen's matrix of degrees and followed by a brief description of the ingredients primary medicinal use.

> "…Hellebore. Both kinds [black and white] are warm and dry in the third degree, are sharp, purifying, and soothing. Therefore they are effective on skin with sores; the black [hellebore] is applied to fistulas, removes their swelling in three days…" (circa 675 AD/1847p.107,1973)[49,50].

Nothing particularly new or innovative here. "De Medica Libri Septum" largely reiterates pharmacology knowledge of Antiquity and serves as a primary resource for physicians in Europe and the Middle East for the next 1,200 years.

Al-Kindi (801 AD-873 AD) non-physician and Persian scholar offers his contributions to medical pharmacology in his treatise "Libre de Gradibus" (aka "Quia Primos"). Al-Kindi extends Galen's conceptualization of degrees in an effort to better quantify properties of medicinal ingredients. The rationale to extend Galen's degree system is based upon the belief improved quantification of ingredient strength will lead to improved capabilities in compounding ingredients and consequently improved pharmacological treatments. The strength of Al-Kindi's contribution is not in the extension of Galen's degree system, which proves to be too complicated for practical use and soon abandoned, rather in its emphasis upon quantification of pharmacological ingredients and a medical pharmacology driven by a rational, conceptual matrix. Additionally, Al-Kindi extends the traditional Greek and Egyptian medical formulary to include several medicinal ingredients from India and China, thereby producing a much more internationally based formulary.

Abu Ibn al-Razi (Latinized to Rhazes) (865 AD-925 AD) Persian scholar committed to the preservation of medical knowledge offers little new in the area of medical pharmacology content knowledge. His writings reiterate that which is already known and recorded elsewhere. Razi relies heavily upon the writings of Paulus of Aegina for specific content and a guiding conceptual matrix. He accepts the balance of humors model to explain good health and disease.

His writings on medical pharmacology are presented in varying and distinctly different formats. The most recognizable of his writings, the massive 23 volume medical encyclopedia "Kitabu al Hawi fi al-tibb" [The Comprehensive Book on Medicine] offers a section on medical pharmacology, which simply list in alphabetical order, according to their Greek names botanicals, which have demonstrated medicinal effectiveness (1094 AD/1955-1971)[51]. Abu Ibn al-Razi additionally discusses the medicinal value of non-botanical substances such as copper, mercury, gold, arsenic, coral, pearl, scoria, bitumen, chalk, and clay. This comprehensive work emphasizes the value of the case study approach in generating new and evaluating old pharmacological knowledge. Much of the "Kitabu al-Hawi fi al-tibb" is simply a collection of personal observations made by Ibn al-Razi and committed to his personal notebook. After his death these observations are assembled by his students and released to the scientific and medical communities. The "Kitabu al-Hawi fi al-tibb" is translated into Latin in 1279 AD under the title "Continens Liber" and later into English as "The Virtuous Life".

Abu Ibn al-Razi additionally offers a collection of home remedies, written specifically for the non-physician, which contains several medical pharmacological treatments for common conditions e.g. colds, coughs, ear aches, stomach aches, and headaches, titled "Man la yahduruhu al-tabib" [Book for someone who does not have access to a physician] (900AD,2012)[52,53].

Here are a few examples typical of the remedies prescribed: for depression consider "…poppies or their juices (opium)…"; for a laxative "…seven drams of dried violet flowers with twenty pears, macerated and mixed well, then strain. To the filtrate, twenty drams of sugar is added for a draft…"; and for a headache with a fever " …two parts of duhn (oily extract) of rose, to be mixed with vinegar, into which a peace of linen cloth is dipped and compressed on the forehead…" (900AD/2012)[52,53]. This work reflects pharmacological knowledge the period in content and format. Additionally, the writing provides an early attempt to make arcane pharmacological knowledge available to the general public.

Abu Ibn al-Razi compiles two hospital based medical formularies for the practicing physician. The first titled "al-Adwiya al murakkaba" [Compound Drugs] offers recipes and guidance on how to compound medications from more than 300 botanical and vegetable sources, while the second serves as an abbreviated summary of the first, titled "al-Aqrabahin al-mukhtasar" [Abridged Formulary] (1966)[54].

In his manuscript "Kitab Saydalat al-tibb" [Pharmacology in Medicine] al-Razi offers his thoughts specifically on the role of medical pharmacology in the practice of medicine. He differentiates the roles of physician and pharmacologist and identifies the value of their complementary functions. He supports earlier writings of Galen, which advocates a clear division in functions between the two professions, noting the knowledge of pharmacists to be much more specialized than physicians and essential to the practice of competent medicine.

Perhaps the most valuable of al-Razi's contributions to medical pharmacology are not found in his writings reiterating specific content but rather to more general philosophical issues. Towards the end of his life he authors a much less well known manuscript titled "Shukuk ala Nazariyyat Jalinus" [Doubts about Galen]. It is here al-Razi most directly challenges the dogma of Galen and its obedient, unquestioning followers. He emphasizes the belief that good medicine requires independent thinking by its scientists and practicing physicians. To accept without independent thought, facts and reason formulated by others, is to delay progress. An interesting position in that most of al-Razi's life is devoted to reiteration of facts and reasons formulated by others. Perhaps it takes one a lifetime of participating in Normal Science to recognize true progress and advancements are made when dogma is challenged and if necessary displaced.

Ibn Sina (aka Avicenna) (980 AD-1037 AD) Persian polymath authors his comprehensive encyclopedia of medicine, "Kitab al-Qanun fi al-tibb" (1025 AD) [Canon of Medicine] (1025 AD)[55]. The encyclopedia is organized into five books. Book 2 (Simple drugs) and Book 5 (Compounded drugs) deal directly with medical pharmacology. Briefly, Book 2 discusses the nature and qualities of simple drugs, within the matrix of paired qualities e.g. hot-cold, dry-wet and the resulting effectiveness when simple ingredients of specific qualities are mixed together. Book 5 is a medical formulary of compounded remedies. Collectively the "Canon of Medicine" offers over 800 preparations, describes their properties, e.g. qualities, their mode of actions, and their indications for use. Nothing particularly new or original here.

However, in Book 2 chapter 2 a landmark contribution can be found. Ibn Sina offers seven well-reasoned guidelines to be applied whenever evaluating the effectiveness of a medication. These guidelines lay the foundation for experimental pharmacology and remain foundational to clinical trials today, over 1,200 years since first committed to paper.

The seven guidelines proposed by Ibn Sina to evaluate the efficacy of any pharmacological ingredient are originally written in Arabic. The following is a brief translational summary: 1) the drug must be pure; 2) the drug must be used on a "simple" disease; 3) the drug must be tested on at least two different types of disease; 4) the quality of the drug must correspond with the strength of the disease (see Galen's degree system); 5) the timing of observations should be measured to rule out the effects of natural healing; 6) the drug must show consistency over several trials; and 7) a drug should be tested in animals first and thereafter humans, as the effects in animals and humans may not be the same (1025 AD)[55].

Abu Ray Han al-Biruni (973 AD-1050 AD) non-physician, Persian polymath, and contemporary colleague of Ibn Sina completes "Kitab al Saydalah" (1048 AD) [The Book of Drugs] at the age of 76 years, one year before his death. This manuscript offers both an insightful discussion of professional issues and much less original listings of over 700 simple ingredients with medicinal value. The listing of simples is essentially a relisting of previous lists complied by numerous others, especially Dioscorides circa 60 AD. The listing is organized alphabetically according to ingredient and is written in Arabic. If there is unique value in Biruni's listing of simples, it is found in his inclusion of synonyms and several different language translations which accompany each entry.

Take note here of the organization of the manuscript. Notice the similarities and differences with the "Physician's Desk Reference" (PDR) widely used today.

Beyond the reiteration of simples, "Kitab al Saydalah" (1048 AD) [The Book of Drugs] offers its most useful contributions to medical pharmacology), Biruni's discussion of professional issues. (1048/2003)[56]. He recognizes the limiting value of providing scientific information only in the language which is familiar only to you and those around you. He attempts to make pharmacological knowledge more available to others by incorporating multiple languages, especially Greek, Hindi, Arabic, Persian, and Semitic, as an immediate solution, while recommending an internationally agreed standardization of terminology will provide a more permanent solution. He advocates, as have others, for the differentiation of the profession of pharmacy from the practice of clinical medicine. Recognizing both professions as essential and necessary in the treatment of illness or injury, he proposes specialize academic and practical training for pharmacist which differs from a physician.

Biruni offers a relatively succinct definition of the role of the pharmacist, which remains familiar today. In "Kitab al Saydalah" [The Book of Drugs] he defines the pharmacist "…as the professional who is specialized in the collection of all drugs, choosing the very best of each simple or compound, and in the preparation of good remedies following the most accurate methods and techniques as recommended by experts in the healing arts…" (1048AD/2003)[56]. The differentiation of professional roles of pharmacist, pharmacologist, and practicing physician establish the foundation for specialization and development of three distinct yet interdependent professions.

Trivia: The first professional pharmacy opens its doors in the Middle East in Bagdad, in 754 AD. The first professional pharmacy opens its doors in Europe, in Trier, Germany, in 1241 AD (1908)[57].

Geopolitical, social, and economic stability returns to Western Europe in 1000-1200 AD and lay the foundation for early modern European society.

The feudal system develops during the High Middle ages and provides the structure for modern European society. Recall, the feudal system is a legal-social system which structures society around the holding of land in exchange for service, typically military or labor. The system offers a hierarchal structure of social classes and details authority and legal obligations within a tiered system. The system is based upon three concepts, lords, vassals, and fiefs. In brief, a lord is the person of authority and owner of land, typically awarded to the lord by the crown for service to the crown. The vassal is a person who enters into a mutually binding legal obligation with a lord. The obligation typically includes military protection of the lord and property in exchange for certain earned privileges, for example, land ownership following a specified period of service. The land ownership secured by a vassal from a lord can then be passed to family members by way of inheritance. Fiefs are simply inheritable property or other rights granted by a lord to a vassal, which are held in fealty ("in fee") by the lord until all obligations of service are satisfied by the vassal.

The system soon restores social stability to the region and stimulates a rapidly growing economy based upon farming, commercial trade, and commerce. Return to social stability and a rapidly growing healthy economy stimulates movement back to Europe. Many of the medical, scientific, and pharmacology texts are translated from Arabic into Latin.

Of particular note are translations by Constantine the African (1020 AD-1087 AD) at the monastery of Monte Cassion, located in southern Italy near Salerno and Gerard de Sabloneta, the Italian translator from the Lombardy region of northern Italy. The Latin translations incorporate and further modify the Arabic translations which are based upon translations from the original manuscripts written in Greek. Each translation in the series modifies the text to better conform to religious belief systems dominant during the period of translations. For example, the initial Greek to Arabic translations are influenced by Islam, whereas the Arabic to Latin translations are modified by Christianity and more specifically Catholicism. Printed Latin translations are pressed in Venice and made available soon after the invention of the printing press, during the mid-1400s. So goes additional examples in the history of medicine, where economic, social, political, and religious influences modify science and medicine knowledge, whenever the knowledge is committed to a written record.

The Middle Ages witness the introduction of the university based system of education. Medical schools soon begin to associate with universities. Scuola Medica Salernitana, the medical school at Salerno, located in southern Italy is first of the schools to teach botanicals to their students. The early emphasis on teaching botanicals arise from the School's early beginning as a Benedicitne monesary in Salerno, founded in 794 AD and where the monks study botanicals and medical works of the Ancient civilizations. The Scuola Medica Salernitana distinguishes itself in 1100 AD as being the only medical school to require students to complete course work, readings, and supervised training in pharmacology. This school provides the model for medical education for all other European medical schools to follow e.g. in France, Montpellier (1181 AD) and Paris (1150 AD); in Italy, Bologna (1158 AD) and Padua (1222 AD); and in England, Oxford (1167 AD).

The Scuola Medica Salernitana is atypical and progressive. Unlike all other European medical schools of the period, it permits the admission of women. The school additonally actively encourgaes and supports a truely international based student and faculty population. To qualify for the Doctor of Medicine, a student must satisfactoraly complete a broad range curriculum of study, which includes chemistry, pharmacology, mathmatics, philosophy, and the Arts. The course of medical school study requires 10 years to complete. Emphasis is placed upon educating future physicans, in addtion to teaching them medicine. Colleges within the university at Salerno are first among all European universites to award academic degrees.

Trivia: The term "university" is derived from the Latin "universitas magistrorum et scholarium" loosely translated meaning "community of teachers and scholars".

The University based medical school model of medical education and training is firmly in place throughout Europe by the mid-1200s. Governmental regulations soon follow outlining the necessary academic and supervised clinical training requirements of all choosing to secure a professional medical license in order to practice the profession of medicine. Frederic II, King of Sicily (1194 AD-1250 AD) issues the Edict of Salerno (1241 AD), which decrees the academic and supervised clinical service training requirements for medical licensure, defines and delineates a clear separation between the professional practices of physician and pharmacist; fixes the prices of medicinal remedies sold by pharmacists; prohibits physicians from practicing pharmacy; and prohibits medical service providers from engaging in clinical medical practice or teaching of medicine without a Royal license. The Royal license is awarded after examination in the King's Court by the Masters of Salerno (1241 AD/1855)[58].

Candidate for licensure can only appear after presenting to the Court papers documenting medical training, supervision, and letters of recommendations from professors and licensed physicians with whom the candidate has studied. Acceptable medical education and training at the University requires completion of a broad curriculum, which includes the Arts. Specific requirements are listed. Students must complete three years of study "…in scientia logicali…"; five years of study in medicine; attend lectures on Hippocrates and Galen; practice under the supervision of a licensed physician for one year; provide medical advice gratis to the poor; visit patients at least twice a day; and provide medical services at night, if requested by an ill patient (1241AD/1855)[58].

By the end of the 1200s AD, additional requirements are introduced and require all physicians to complete continuing medical education training in order to keep their license. Many of the requirements decreed by the King's Court in Italy, over 800 years ago are required in modified form today throughout Europe, Canada, Australia, and the USA.

Medical pharmacology continues to refine its knowledge base through application of systematic investigations, completed primarily at university based medical schools. Increased attention is focused upon better understanding and documenting much more specifically the primary therapeutic effects of medications and their associated unwanted side effects. Medications' therapeutic and undesirable side effects are studied as functions of primary ingredients and more increasingly synergistic effects of compounding ingredients. Medicinal remedies continue to be derived from plants, animals, and minerals.

Trivia: The word "drug" is derived from the French word "drogue" during the late-1300s AD and when translated means "dried herbs" (2012)[59].

Scholasticism is coupled with the scientific method and provides the predominate epistemological model used by newly founded university based medical schools throughout Europe, until the end of the Middle Ages.

Recall, scholasticism is a method of critical thought which emphasizes reasoned dialogue and reasoned argument in establishing new knowledge. The method is heavily dependent upon rigorous conceptual analysis and extends knowledge through the process of deriving logical conclusions from premises known or assumed to be true. The scientific method on the other hand emphasizes systematic empirical observation, quantitative measurement, and rigorous experimentation.

In summary, the Middle Ages witness a period of slow advancement in content and process knowledge of medical pharmacology. Much of that which is known from Antiquity is simply reiterated and modified to better accommodate the beliefs of the new organized religions of Christianity, Catholicism, and Islam. Academic cities, along with their collections of the historical written records of knowledge are intentionally destroyed. With the fall of the Western Roman Empire, academic scholars flee to the Middle East with as much of the written record as possible. In Persia (modern-day Iran) the record is translated into Persian, Syriac, and Arabic. The scholars of the Middle East translate, evaluate, and largely reiterate medical pharmacology knowledge, recorded by Greek natural philosophers and encyclopedists of Antiquity. Separate and interdependent professional responsibilities of the medical pharmacologist, pharmacist, and physician are defined. Europe returns to a much more stable geopolitical, economical, and social environment. Universities and medical schools are founded in Europe and require demonstrated competency in medical pharmacology before graduating from medical school. Governmental regulations are established to insure all who choose to practice medicine have received didactic instruction and clinical supervision in the use of pharmacological treatments and can demonstrate competency by way of post graduate examination. Galenian dogma provides the conceptual matrix throughout the Middle Ages and hinders advancement. Scholasticism is introduced in most European universities and medical schools and offers a productive blend of rationalism and empiricism. Stabilization of Europe and introduction of university based medical education sets the stage for continued and rapid advancement in medical pharmacology during the upcoming Early Modern Period.

Early Modern, 1400 AD - 1800 AD.

Medical pharmacology matures and develops as a scientific discipline.

Herbals and botanicals continue to be the primary source of medicinal remedies. Herbals, books containing collections of plant names, their physical descriptions, and recommended use for medicinal purposes are printed and distributed throughout Europe. The Herbals no longer restricted content to local plants and include more and more plants from around the world.

Interests in the potential value of minerals and chemicals, as an alternative source of medicinal remedies to the herbals and botanicals, soon challenge the dogma of revered authorities and content knowledge in place for centuries. New models are proposed which emphasize chemistry as primary to understanding good health and explaining physical illness. The human body is conceptualized within a matrix of chemical actions, reactions, and predictably follows fundamental chemical principles.

Advances in technologies result in the invention of the printing press, intravenous injections, and navigation methods allowing for worldwide explorations by sea. The printing press permits distribution of scientific information to the masses and increasing the exchange of information between investigators. The introduction of intravenous injection arise out of academic based physiology research and offers a much more direct mode of introduction of medicinal remedies into a patient's blood circulatory system. Exploration of the world by sea brings to Europe unknown plants and medicinal remedies from populations throughout the world, especially the Americas and extends the medical pharmacology knowledge beyond geocentric Europe.

Medical schools throughout Europe now require students to complete coursework and supervised training in medical pharmacology, as part of their basic science curriculum. University research laboratories are established throughout Europe to study the chemical bases of illness, disease, and trauma and associated medicinal treatments. Advances in physiology research contribute substantially to the forward movement of medical pharmacology.

Let us consider a few specifics.

The Order of Saint Jerome (1373 AD-1833 AD) a monastic Order of the Catholic Church, founded in Spain with houses in Italy, combine beliefs and practices of organized religion with systematic investigations and recording of medicinal remedies. The Order is devoted to the study of herbals, botanicals, minerals, metals, and chemicals, in their efforts to provide the best possible care to all seeking their care. A comprehensive compilation of the Order's most effective remedies are recorded in "Libro de Secreti e Ricette" [Book of Secret Remedies] (1562)[60].

The "Book of Secrets" is written primarily in Italian, contains approximately 1,500 tested remedies, collected over a 200 year period, and organized according to the condition in need of treatment e.g. asthma, epilepsy, fevers, gout, malaria, ringworm, and syphilis. Remedies are comprised of assorted Galenic mixtures of herbs, alchemy distillates, amulets, and prayers. A modern English translation of the "Book of Secret Remedies" can be found online (1562)[60].

The value of the Order's contribution to medical pharmacology is not found in the listing of specific remedies but rather in their methodologies. The friars while embracing tradition, authority and religious dogma, suspend their faith based beliefs in favor of empirical experimentation when it comes to the evaluation of medicinal remedies. Recent analysis of the "Libro de I Secreti e Ricette" reveals, modern, twenty-first century criteria, applied in the evaluation of modern experimental therapeutics are applied equally by the friars of the Order of Saint Jerome, in Italy over 600 years ago (2002)[61].

In brief, the methods applied to evaluate each remedy are based in logic theory rather than statistical theory as conventionally applied today. Each remedy is subjected to experimental testing and evaluated against specific criteria. The criteria applied by the friars are readily recognizable by all conducting experimental therapeutics research today. Remedies are tested for reliability, to ensure the treatment result occurs consistently across different patients; linkage in time, to ensure administration of the remedy is associated with a therapeutic improvement; specificity of the remedy, to ensure a therapeutic improvement in one group of illnesses or conditions but not others; generalizability of the remedy, to ensure a therapeutic effect in observed in similar conditions; and consistency of findings, when evaluated within an experimental research design.

Herbal remedies remain the staple for medical practitioners during the 1400s. Plants continue to be boiled, steeped, ground, smoked, rubbed, inhaled, and slathered, all in an effort to effect a therapeutic relief or cure. The number and varieties of plants with medicinal properties are expanded beyond the botanicals indigenous to Europe and the Mediterranean, as the result of many sea explorations completed during the late-1400s and through the early-1600s. Explorers originating primarily from Spain, Portugal, France, and England often return to Europe, from voyages to the New Worlds of North and South America, with new plants of demonstrated medicinal value. These plants are quickly added to the European herbals. Several of these newly discovered plants and trees introduce the foundation of remedies still used today over 600 years later. For example, bark from the Cinchona tree, returned to Europe by Jesuit missionaries during the early-1600s contains the ingredient quinine, which is the ingredient still used in many parts of the world for treatment of malaria. Recall, quinine interferes with the reproduction of malaria causing protozoa and offers relief from fevers and shivers associated with malaria.

In addition to interests in the new botanicals, investigators and practitioners throughout Europe turn their focus to exploring the medicinal uses of minerals, metals, and chemicals. Much of the early work is completed by alchemists. Recall, not all alchemists are devoted exclusively to the discovery of processes to be used in the transmutation of base metals into precious metals. In particular, a sect of alchemists, Spagyrists, devote their time and energies to the discovery of medicinal remedies, based upon the application of chemical principles. Spagyrists initially investigate and develop procedures to extract medicinally therapeutic ingredients from plants utilizing fundamental chemical procedures fermentation, distillation, and chemical reactions. The resulting products are administered directly as a remedy or combined in varying formulae. Spagyrists are the precursors to the more familiar iatrogenic chemists of the 1600s whom explain conditions of health by chemical principles.

Paracelsus (1493-1531) (aka Theophrastus Phillippus Aureolus Bombastus von Hohenheim) of Switzerland is most representative of individuals of this period moving away from traditional botanicals and herbals as primary sources of medicinal remedies and replacing them with simple chemicals and minerals. He pioneers the field of iatrogenic chemistry and offers a radical, new alternative conceptual matrix to replace the long held conceptual matrixes embedded securely in medical dogma for centuries.

Trivia: Paracelsus abandons his given birth name upon completion of the baccalaureate degree in medicine from the University of Vienna at 17 years of age. The chosen name "Paracelsus" when translated means "equal to or superior to Celsus". This is in specific reference to Aulus Celsus (25 BC-50 BC), the author of the Roman medical encyclopedia "De Medicina". Oh, how a little acquired knowledge in college can instill such a sense of self-importance in such young minds. Similar self assessments can be found among some college students today.

Paracelsus, as with all who dare to challenge scientific or medical dogma, is met with much resistance from the established academic, scientific, and medical communities. His ideas, conceptualization of body organization, and approach to therapeutics shake the very core of content and process knowledge, the established scientific and medical communities hold to be true. The challenge requires attention and if possible resolution.

There is comfort, order, and ease in the passive acceptance of dogma. When dogma is challenged, it elicits intellectual discomfort. Challenges can be simply dismissed, by authorities within the profession, thereby returning a sense of order and comforting reassurance to all, or can be embraced by members of the profession. When challenges are embraced, they necessitate a reevaluation of current knowledge by members within the profession, and an open mindedness to consider alternative explanations. Sometimes it requires an admission that we had it wrong and the dogma of the past needs to be modified or displaced completely, based upon new information. In both cases, challenges to dogma will always elicit emotional responses towards the person who challenges dogma. The result can be positive or negative. What is certain is there will be a response.

Paracelsus is passionately vocal in expressing his positions on the importance of minerals and chemicals in maintaining good physical health and their value in treating disease and illness. He publically challenges and denounces the conceptual matrix proposed by Galen, which has served as the authoritative dogma for the past 1300 years, including the balance of humors model and herbal based therapeutics. He proposes instead, a model of body functioning based upon organ systems, specifying the role of each system within a conceptual matrix of body chemistry. Illness and disease are the result of impaired organ systems functioning and disruptions in normal body chemistry. Treatments are directed to restoring normal body chemistry.

More specifically, Paracelsus conceptualizes each body organ system, digestive, pulmonary, cardiovascular, renal, urinary, hepatic, neural, skeletal-muscular, as functioning much like an alchemist, separating pure from impure substances. For example, the role of the stomach is to separate nutritional substances from foods and the intestinal system functions to remove the waste materials. Illness and disease are the result of organ function failure or toxic buildup of waste materials within the system. Treatments are directed to simply restoring the normal function of the effected organ or eliminating the toxic wastes by manipulating body chemistries. Most of the chemical therapeutic interventions are dependent upon the use of minerals and metals. For example, Paracelsus recommends the use of mercury in the treatment of syphilis, the use of iron for weak anemic blood, and the internal use of antimony (a soft gray toxic metal) as an effective laxative and purge for toxic chemical build up within the body (1529,1530)[62,63].

The therapeutic use of toxic metals and chemicals, while rejected by the established medical community during the time of Paracelsus, have proven to be of value with time and can be found in use today. Consider for a moment some modern chemotherapies used in the treatment and management of cancer. How to these chemotherapies work? That is right, they chemically poison cells both healthy and cancerous. Oh how little some things have changed in medicine. Perhaps it is time for you, the new medical student to consider completely new and innovative ways in which to think about pathologies and propose conceptually new and innovative treatments.

Paracelsus devotes much of his short life to challenging medical and scientific dogma of the period. He enthusiastically encourages others to think for themselves, open their minds to new and innovative alternatives, and be willing to endure the economic and professional consequences oftentimes associated with challenging the established medical and scientific communities. As professor and department chair at the University of Basel in Switzerland, Paracelsus dramatically makes his point when, at the University, he publicly burns traditional medical textbooks and proclaims the need to move forward and no longer be constrained by the limiting conceptual models, methods, and pharmacological treatments of the past. Yes, you are right. He is immediately fired from the University.

Unable or perhaps more correctly unwilling to conform to the presses of traditional academia, Paracelsus continues his investigations into the chemical basis of good physical health and disease outside the constraining walls of the new university based European medical schools. He continues undaunted and establishes fundamental principles of medical pharmacology, many which influence thought and guide scientific investigations within the discipline for the next 500 years.

Arguably one of Paracelsus' most recognized retorts to criticism, to his anti-Galenistic use of toxic metals and chemicals in the treatment of disease, is that all medications can be considered poisons; it is only the dose amounts that determine whether medication has a therapeutic effect or a poisonous, toxic effect. Can you, as a new medical student, think of any present day medications where this applies?

Trivia: Five years before his death at 38 years of age, Paracelsus introduces the term "zink" into the professional literature for the element zinc (1526). The term is based upon the observation of sharp points, which appear on zinc crystals after smelting. The term is derived from the German word "zinke" which means pointed.

Paracelsus' challenges to medical dogma open the eyes of only a few in the established medical and scientific communities, as to the therapeutic value of minerals and medicinal chemistry as alternatives to the traditional, plant based herbals. The majority of practitioners during the mid-1500s continue to embrace the herbal approach to pharmacological treatments.

Leonhart Fuchs (1501-1566) German botanist and pharmacologist enthusiastically supports the continued use of traditional herbals in medical pharmacology. He is equally enthusiastic in his opposition to Paracelsus' ideas and suggestions to move away from herbals and consider the value of minerals and metals as potentially useful ingredients in medicinal remedies. Fuchs outlines his position in one of his first papers, titled "Errata recentiorum medicorum" [Errors of recent doctors] (1530)[64]. Here he argues against the use of noxious compounds of arcane ingredients, concocted in medieval medicine, in favor of traditional and simple plant based remedies. Twelve years later he publishes his influential herbal "De Historia Stirpium Commentarii Infignes" [Notable commentaries on the history of plants] (1542)[65]. This herbal offers detailed illustrations of medicinal plants found in Germany and other parts of Europe and contains approximately 500 plants. Fuchs is among the first Renaissance authors of herbals to recognize the great value of accurate illustrations of the living medicinal plant. In addition to assisting physicians in correctly identifying medicinal plants in the wild for collection, Fuchs recognizes the illustrations assist medical students and physicians in remembering information oftentimes forgotten when information is presented in text alone. Plants are organized in alphabetical order, followed by the recommended medicinal treatment, and accompanied by an accurate, detailed, and in later editions colored drawing of the living plant.

Fuchs describes the medicinal value of the thistle root as follows; "…a drachma in weight…" when combined with wine, offers benefit against the contagion of pestilence. When "…steeped in vinegar, is helpful against scabies, impetigo, and all blemishes of the skin difficult to cure…" (1542)[66].

Fuchs is among several university professors of the period insisting training in botany to be essential, necessary, and a part of every medical school curriculum training competent physicians. Many medical schools maintained dedicated gardens devoted to medicinal plants. Training in botany remains important in the education of medical students well into the early-1900s. Many prestigious medical schools today continue to maintain medicinal plant gardens e.g. University of California Los Angeles (UCLA) over 470 years after Fuchs emphasizes their value in the education of every medical student (2018)[67].

Valerius Cordus (1515-1544) German botanist and pharmacologist authors one of the most celebrated herbals in history. His herbal, "Dispensatorium hoc est pharmacorum conficiendorum ratio" is written in Latin and contains approximately 225 medicinal plants and minerals (1546)[68]. Soon after its initial publication, it is recognized by the government of Germany as the obligatory authoritative resource for the identification, composition, and prescription of medicinal remedies in Germany. If you practice medicine in Germany during the mid-1500s it is required by law you follow the prescription guidelines contained within this herbal.

William Turner (1508-1568) English botanist and physician adds to the growing number of herbals published during the 1500s. His herbal, "A New Herbal", like most others offers nothing particularly new or innovative (1551)[69]. The remedies are reiterations of old authoritative sources, originally described by Galen, Pliny, and Dioscorides. Illustrations appear to be copied from Leonhart Fuchs' herbal published nine years earlier. The historical value of Turner's herbal is not in its originality or new content, rather in that it is the first herbal published in English. This herbal moves information, regarding the use of botanicals for medicinal purposes, from the confines of the arcane Latin language and makes the knowledge available to all who read English.

The 1500s are the century of herbals. Plants and their medicinal value are documented by herbalists from every country in Europe and many from around the world. Worldwide sea explorations by the Spanish and Portuguese particularly into the Americas results in the discovery of new plants with demonstrated medicinal properties, many of these plants are returned to Europe. For example, bark taken from the cinchona tree, indigenous to South America, is recognized by the people of the Andes and Amazon to be an effective treatment for fevers. Jesuit missionaries bring the bark back to Europe. The bark soon becomes known simply as the "Jesuit fever bark". The active ingredient in this bark is the alkaloid quinine. It's effectiveness in treating malaria and similar fever producing disorders make it extremely valuable. The demand for the bark is so high it soon threatens the tree's survival. The bark is sold and traded at approximately the same value as gold.

Numerous herbals are published during the 1500s and medicinal remedies are dominated by plant based ingredients; however, new ideas emphasizing the use of minerals, metals, and chemistry generate excitement within medical pharmacology communities and offer an alternative to well established dogma.

Iatrochemistry with its roots in Switzerland and Flanders (northern Belgium) quickly spreads across Europe during the mid-1500s and offers an alternative to Galen based therapeutics. The idea of applying chemistry and chemical principles to the treatment of illness and disease is initially met with much resistance by the established medical communities. The powerful and influential medical faculty at the University of Paris reacts with a series of position papers, decrees, and court opinions to forbid the use of chemistry in medicine. Similar reactions are witnessed in England. However, by the 1580s, active resistance to chemistry in medicine is tempered and articles begin to appear from conservative professional societies and university based institutions, acknowledging the use and potential value of chemistry in the treatment of illness and disease.

Interests in the ideas of Paracelsus grow considerably during the late-1500s. Many of his writings are translated and offer new opportunities for reassessment and commentary by the scientific and medical communities. At the core of the interests are fundamental professional issues; the role of chemistry in medicine; reform in medical education curriculum; roles and relationships between organized religion, science, and medicine; and the role and value of ancient authority in the presence of new observations and scientific data. Two landmark publications sound the opening salvos of the confrontational debates held in the professional literature for the next one hundred years. "Idea medicinae philosophicae" [A philosophical idea in medicine] (1571)[70] argues the superior value of Paracelsus conceptual matrix and treatments to those of Galen. "Disputationes de medicina nova Paracelsi" [Discussions of the new medicine of Paracelsus] (1572-1574)[71] argues the superior value of conceptual matrix and treatments proposed by the revered ancient authorities of Aristotle and Galen. "Disputationes de medicina nova Paracelsi" injects tremendous emotion into the debate, moving beyond an objective assessment of the opposing positions and publicly damns the innovations of Paracelsus (1572-1574/2011)[71,72]. And so begins another notable and passionate debate in the history of medicine.

Internal use of metals as medicinal remedies gains increasing popularity among physicians and the general populous of Europe, during the 1600s. Perhaps the most notable is the use of antimony, a soft, gray, toxic metal (1604)[73]. The metal has a history in its use as mascara during ancient Egypt, and recommended medicinal use for treatments of assorted skin conditions, during Antiquity, as recommended by Disocorides, an emetic and diaphoretic during the Middle Ages, and an effective purge, during the early-1500s, as recommended by Paracelsus. The use of antimony is especially popular in France and England, during the 1600s and 1700s, used primarily as a purge and diaphoretic. The rationale behind the treatment is that the metal, when consumed, pulls toxic wastes from body tissues and eliminates them from the body, as the antimony moves through the digestive systems. Typically, the metal is combined and ingested with an alcohol, most typically wine.

Popularity of this treatment results in many households purchasing and regularly using a small, half pint size cup, approximately 2 inches high and 2 inches in diameter, cast in antimony. The cup is filled with wine and allowed to sit for 24 hours. The tartic acid in red wine combines with the antimony producing an effective elixir when consumed, produces therapeutic sweating, vomiting, and movement of the bowels.

"De Jure et praestantia chemicorum medicamentorum dialogus aplogeticus" [The efficacy of the medicinal chemists] (1584)[74] authored by English physician Thomas Moffett (1553-1604) offers a defense of chemistry and chemical remedies in medicine. The paper discusses fundamental strengths and weaknesses of chemical based remedies. The discussion is presented in a unique format, a discussion between two imaginary physicians. Appended to the end of the dialogue are five letters which further address issues arising from the new, chemistry based medicine. This landmark paper serves as a foundation upon which the Royal College of Physicians build their justification for inclusion of minerals, metal, and chemicals, as recognized medicinal remedies in the first edition of the heavily plant based "London Pharmacopoeia" (1618)[75].

The "London Pharmacopoeia" includes approximately 1,250 preparations, approximately equally distributed between compounded and simple remedies. The "Pharmacopoeia" creates the first standard list of medicines and their ingredients in England. It is the authoritative source for all physicians prescribing pharmacological treatments in England and its use by practicing physicians is mandated by English law.

Minerals, as medicinal remedies continue to gain attention within the medical and scientific communities during the early-1600s. The inorganic salt, magnesium sulfate or more commonly known today Epsom salt is recognized to facilitate the healing of scratches, and rashes when bathed in water and to be an effective laxative when ingested (1618)[75].

Trivia: Epsom salt is named for the town Epsom, England where the medicinal properties of the salt is first reported and recognized to have a healing effect on skin lesions of livestock bathing in the mineral waters.

Franciscus Sylvius (aka Franz de la Boe) (1614-1672) German anatomist, physiologist, and chemist establishes the first academic chemical laboratory in Europe (Leiden University, Netherlands) devoted to the study of chemical processes of life and disease processes in 1669. Sylvius conceptualizes good physical health and disease within the matrix of physical laws defined by physics and chemical actions defined by chemistry. His basic tenet guiding his research efforts is that all life and disease can be explained by understanding chemical actions. His work leads him to introduce the concept of chemical affinity, as a way to understand and explain the body's use of salts. Yes, this is the same Sylvius which describes the lateral fissure (Sylvian fissure) in the brain, separating the frontal and parietal lobes from the temporal lobes six years earlier (1663)[76].

Franciscus Sylvius, Paracelsus, and Flemish chemist Jan Baptist van Helmont (1580-1644), perhaps more than any others champion the iatrogenic chemistry movement in Europe, during the early-1500s through the mid-1600s. Their rejection of the balance of humors models and advocacy in favor of understanding the human body's normal physiology, disease conditions, and pharmacological treatments within a matrix of physical chemistry change medical pharmacology forever.

Johannes Wepfer (1620-1695) Swiss pharmacologist introduces a cautionary note to medical pharmacology with the publication of "Cicutae aquatica historia et noxae" [History and toxicology of the water hemlock] (1679)[77]. The paper offers a critical analysis of pharmacology experiments and reminds investigators and practitioners of the potential dangers and potential toxicity of pharmacological treatments. Of note, regarding the water hemlock, Wepfer reports on the death of two boys and six girls following its use in treatment, identifying and documenting hemlock's effect to interfere with normal blood coagulation. In addition to drawing attention to and detailing the often ignored toxicology of plant based remedies popular during the period, Wepfer warns of the dangers associated with the use of metals in medical treatments. He offers specific warnings against the continued use of arsenic, antimony, and mercury in medical treatments, documenting the toxicology of each metal and their destructive effect on human tissues.

Johannes Wepfer might be recognized by medical students as the person responsible for clearly implicating bleeding within the brain and blockage of main brain arteries as primary causes of stroke in his initial detailed description of four patients (1658)[78] or his works describing the vascular etiologies responsible for basal artery migraine headaches (1727)[79] or aphasias resulting from head trauma (1727)[79].

Trivia: Johannes Wepfer is friend and colleague of two investigators, also working in Schaffhausen, Switzerland, which you as a medical student might recognize from your Histology course; Johann Peyer (1653-1712) (Peyer's patch fame, 1681)[80] and Johann Brunner (1653-1727) (Brunner's gland fame, 1687)[81]. Johann Brunner is Johannes Wepfer's son in law.

Medical pharmacology matures as a new scientific discipline. The late-1700s witness the beginning of a rapid explosion of experimental and applied scientific research in Europe directed to understanding medicinal remedies within a new conceptual matrix. The new matrix is based in chemistry and is coupled with the application of the scientific method.

William Withering (1741-1799) English botanist makes specific contributions investigating the foxglove plant, exploring its potential use as a diuretic to reduce edema associated with congestive heart failure. His landmark publication "An account of the foxglove and some of its medical uses: with practical remarks on dropsy (congestive heart failure) and other diseases" specifies Digitalis purpurea as the species he recommends, when using foxglove in the treatment and management of congestive heart failure (1785)[82]. Here too he offers evidence from 163 unselected cases, from his personal caseload which demonstrate successful treatment outcomes in most and morbid toxicity in others, when foxglove is used in the medical treatment of congestive heart failure and assorted other diseases e.g. epilepsy, pulmonary consumption (tuberculosis). The book contains a collection of numerous correspondences from treating physicians, summarizing their experience with foxglove. Withering offers a synthesis of all materials, and offers specific recommendations regarding preparations, dosing amounts, warnings of potential toxicities, and specific patient constitutions predictive of favorable and unfavorable clinical treatment outcomes (1785)[82].

Erasmus Darwin (1731-1802) English physician and grandfather of famed naturalist Charles R. Darwin (1809-1882) enters the historical discussion of Digitalis, publically accusing William Withering of unprofessional behavior and poaching several of his patients. Accusations against Withering appear as Darwin attempts to claim priority for discovery in the clinical use of digitalis as an effective treatment for dropsy (congestive heart failure) and a potentially effective treatment for consumption (tuberculosis), melancholy (depression), and diabetes. Darwin formalizes his claim of priority over Withering in his address to the Royal College of Physicians in London, March 16, 1785, titled "An account of the successful use of foxglove in some dropsies and in pulmonary consumption" (1785)[83]. The paper is presented prior to the release of Withering's landmark publication on the topic titled "An account of the foxglove and some of its medical uses: with practical remarks on dropsy and other diseases" (1785)[82], released the same year.

Withering does include two identifiable cases originating from Eramus Darwin's patient case load, Mrs. H, Case IV from 1776 and Miss C, Case XII from 1777, in his collections of cases. Darwin is acknowledged in both cases as the original treating physician (1785)[82].

My reading of the original papers surrounding this particular dispute for priority and allegations of unprofessional behavior by one investigator by another leads me to the following summary conclusions. There is little evidence either man is first in recognizing the treatment value of foxglove, more specifically digitalis, as an effective treatment for congestive heart failure. The plant has been used for this purpose for hundreds of years before either man's claim of priority of discovery.

In fairness, William Withering is first to offer a systematic, scientific based study of digitalis for medical use and provides data collected over a ten year period; offers over 150 clinical cases demonstrating its effectiveness in some patients and morbid toxicities in others; offers a synthesis and summary of his investigations and his professional clinical experiences with its use; and provides written documented support of his synthesis and summary from scores of professional colleagues, reporting similar experiences in regard to treatment successes and treatment failures due to toxicity, when digitalis is used in the treatment and management of their patients. William Withering is instrumental in moving the medicinal use of digitalis from the province of folklore and anecdotal reports into the realm of systematic scientific investigation and evidence based medicine.

In equal fairness, Eramus Darwin does bring to the heightened attention of the medical and scientific communities of the late-1700s, the potential therapeutic use of digitalis, as a neglected pharmacological agent. He is not the first to do so, nor does he make any significant scientific contributions to the medical pharmacology of digitalis. If increasing an awareness of a botanical, which has been well known for hundreds of years to have potential therapeutic benefit to patients suffering specific medical conditions, then yes, Eramus Darwin, Charles Darwin's grandfather, makes that contribution.

Eramus Darwin's public claims of unprofessional and unethical behavior by William Withering appear to be fundamentally unsubstantiated, misguided, and self-promoting. When the balance of evidence is weighed, in the dispute for priority of discovery, both men go wanting. As with most discoveries throughout the history of medicine, few can be attributed to a single person and without recognition of works by others who have gone before them. So too is the case with digitalis.

Recall, digitalis achieves its therapeutic effects as both a diuretic, eliminating fluid from the body and acting directly upon the heart by inhibiting the Na+/K+/ATPase pump, which increases intracellular Ca++, thereby generating an increase in contractile force. Digitalis slows conduction through the AV node by increasing the release of acetylcholine from parasympathetic fibers onto M2 receptors in the AV-SA nodes, thereby reducing the number of electrical impulse sent from the atria to the ventricles, slowing heart rate. You remember this from your medical school physiology course, right?

John Ferriar (1761-1815) Scottish physician identifies the primary site of action of Digitalis to be the heart and recognizes the diuretic effect to be a secondary action (1799)[84]. These observations complement the works of William Withering whom details the therapeutic value and toxic side effects of digitalis 14 years earlier, yet fails to recognize its primary site of action or underlying mechanism of action. Ferriar like Withering relies upon thoughtful analysis of a series of patients he has treated over multiple years in the clinical setting. Ferriar and Withering collectively successfully answer fundamental questions essential to all medical pharmacology. Is the substance effective in treating a medical condition? What are the toxic side effects? What are the dose response relationships? What is the primary site of action? Is there a parsimonious conceptual matrix that will explain why the substance is effective in treating some conditions and not others? Can the conceptual matrix explain the physiological responses?

Johannas Reil (1759-1813) German psychiatrist calls for a scientific approach to be taken in medical pharmacology and establishes eight rules that should be followed, whenever evaluating drugs in humans. These rules lay the foundation for all experimental medical pharmacology for the next 200 years (1799,2016)[85,86]. The rules highlight the need for high integrity, knowledge, skill and skepticism of the investigator, scientific rigor, use of multiple controlled experiments, reproducibility of results, investigation of each singular drug in a compounded mixture to better understand the contribution of each simple drug, and the introduction of specialized vocabulary to facilitate the exchange of information between investigators (1799, 2016)[85,86]. Below is the English translation of rule number one.

> "…The observer must have good common sense, good understanding, judgement, know how to make observations but also have a healthy degree of skepticism. He should not allow himself to be influenced by egotism, doctrine, an attachment to his school, or any prejudice, but by the simple love of truth…" (1799/2016)[85,86].

Moving beyond empirical associations of botanicals and minerals with medical treatments, typical of pharmacology to this point in time, Reil embraces and recommends use of the scientific method and inductive reasoning. His goal is to explain the actions of drugs within the matrix of biochemical processes. Reil believes drugs affect the body and the body alters drug composition. Understanding the biochemical processes underlying these relationships is key to moving medical pharmacology forward and beyond empirical association of compounded mixtures producing effective therapeutic treatments.

Trivia: Johannas Reil is instrumental in the early development of psychiatry, emphasizing need for specialized training for all physicians choosing to provide treatment to individuals suffering disorders of mood, cognition, or thought. He coins the term "psychiatry" (1808)[87]. Johannas Reil makes numerous additional contributions in the area of neuroanatomy. He describes the insula, located deep within the lateral cerebral hemisphere fissures, which English anatomist Henry Gray renames the Island of Reil, in the first edition of Gray's Anatomy; describes the norepinephrine rich brainstem nucleus locus ceruleus (1809)[88]; identifies and names the white matter tract connecting the cortices of Wernicke's area with Broca's area, we know today as the arcuate fasciculus (1812)[89]; and many more. See the Medical Psychology or Medical Neuroscience chapters for more information on Johannas Reil.

In summary, as the 1700s come to a close in Europe, medical pharmacology as a science based-professional discipline continues to struggle with academic, professional, ethical, and medical treatment issues. The value of botanicals and herbals in medical treatment is well established and documented. The value of minerals and metals in medical treatment is established. Systematic experimental investigations are completed in efforts to establish more precisely standardized dosing guidelines, specific mechanisms of actions of pharmacological treatments are more aggressively investigated and identified, toxicology profiles of specific remedies are acknowledged and defined, professional roles and responsibilities of pharmacists, pharmacologists, and practicing physicians are more precisely defined and regulated by governmental authorities, ethical issues pertaining to the experimental use of pharmacological agents with animals and humans is debated, and most medical schools now routinely require education and supervised training in the medicinal use of pharmacological agents.

Medical pharmacology joins with academic physiology and produces scientific based advancements in understanding the effects of medications on specific tissues and organ systems. Measurement of physiological responses however remain limited, most often restricted to body temperature and pulse rate measurements. Medical pharmacology and academic pharmacology quickly recognize the demonstrated and potential benefits to each discipline working cooperatively in the common effort to understand functional biological systems. A chemistry based medical pharmacology displaces the dogma of the past. Specific active ingredients are now being identified in medicinal remedies, extracted, and refined by chemical methodologies. A more complete understanding of the how and why specific medications are effective is established and another cornerstone in the foundation of experimental and applied medical pharmacology is set into place.

Middle Modern, 1800 AD - 1900 AD.

At the beginning of the 1800s, medical pharmacology, physiology, and biology are not considered by the academic community to be exact sciences. The disciplines have yet to meet the standards satisfied by the natural sciences. Experimental based investigations and aggressive professional and academic politics, during the 1800s move medical pharmacology, physiology, and biology forward as recognized academic disciplines. In combination, these three emerging disciplines generate new knowledge, based upon fundamental principles of science, with immediate applications to the clinical treatment of medical and surgical patients.

The first half of the 1800s witness medical pharmacology moving away from the common practice of simply identifying plants and minerals and simply documenting their therapeutic value. Medical pharmacology now places emphasis upon understanding the fundamental chemical basis of ingredients in the plants responsible for the therapeutic effect. Much effort is devoted to isolating and purifying specific substances. Alkaloids are recognized during the early-1800s and attract considerable attention and much study. By the mid-1800s, attention extends to the investigation of gas based anesthesia e.g. nitrous oxide, ether, and chloroform. Pharmacology establishes scientifically sound, productive relationships with chemistry and physiology. Pharmacology founds its first academic department within the European university system and establishes itself as an independent discipline, separate from pharmacy, clinical medicine, chemistry, and physiology. Medical pharmacology continues to mature as a scientific based discipline, establishing boundaries and scope of investigations, agreed methodologies, core principles and fundamental knowledge, introduces new vocabulary, standardizes terminology, and identifies directions for future research.

The second half of the 1800s witness the founding of the discipline's first professional scientific journal devoted to experimental pharmacology. Questionable remedies are systematically eliminated from well-established pharmacopeias, based upon findings generated by experimental investigations. The late-1800s witness continued efforts to more completely establish pharmacology as a separate academic discipline, in recognition there is too much new information to be mastered by any one person or profession. The first department of pharmacology is founded within the USA university system. New knowledge is quickly translated into applied therapeutics, offering the practicing physician many new tools with which to better diagnose, treat, and manage sickness and disease. Medical pharmacology continues to mature as an independent scientific discipline.

Let us consider a few specifics.

Francois Magendie (1783-1855) French anatomist, physiologist, and pharmacologist opens the 1800s with his experimental investigations, which test his beliefs that the therapeutic and toxic effects derived from plants and minerals are derived from specific chemicals contained within the plant or mineral. Magendie believes it should be possible to isolate and extract from the plant or mineral the chemical or chemicals responsible for the medicinal effect, in their most pure forms. His beliefs are supported by experimental investigations and provide the foundation of most pharmacological studies completed during the 1800s (1809a)[90].

Francois Magendie offers additional guidance for the experimental pharmacologist emphasizing the value of the application of the scientific method, laboratory based experimentation, use of purified chemicals whenever possible, careful observation of physiological responses, and completion of experiments on animals first, followed by testing on humans. He strongly encourages the delineation of specific objectives, whenever conducting pharmacological investigations, and focused efforts directed to identifying the site of action of the drug, determining its mechanism of action, and documenting the animal's or human's physiological responses, as a function of drug dosages (1809b)[91].

The early and most influential pharmacological investigations conducted by Magendie focus upon a new class of recently identified chemical substances derived from plants, the alkaloids (1817a, 1817b,1822)[92,93,94].

Recall, alkaloids are a group of naturally occurring compounds which are typically physiologically very active and often extremely poisonous. During the 1800s, the alkaloids most often investigated by Magendie and other investigators are strychnine, atropine, caffeine, colchicine, and cocaine. Today we recognize alkaloids can be derived from sources other than plants e.g. bacteria, fungi, insects, and animals.

Pierre Pelletier (1788-1842) and Joseph Caventou (1795-1887) French chemists isolate and focus their attention on the investigation of the medically important alkaloids emetine (1817a)[92], strychnine (1818)[95], cinchonine (1820)[96], quinine (1820)[96], and caffeine (1821)[97]. Arguably, one of the most important accomplishments of the 1800s is the isolation of quinine by Pelletier and Caventou. Quinine offers an effective medical treatment for malaria. Pelletier and Caventou coin the term "quinine" and introduce the term into the medical literature and distinguish it from a similar plant alkaloid cinchonine (1820)[96]. Notice they apply the recently recommended convention of applying the suffix "ine" to naming all alkaloids derived from plants (1819)[98]. Neither Pelletier nor Caventou choose to patent their discovery of quinine, making it and its use as an effective treatment for malaria available to the world.

Perhaps you recognize the names Pelletier and Caventou from their early work in which they isolate chlorophyll, the biomolecule essential to the process used by a plant, algae, and some bacteria to capture sun light energy and transform it into chemical energy, which is then used by the plant, algae, or bacteria (photosynthesis) (1817)[99].

Friedlieb Runge (1795-1867) German chemist isolates caffeine in coffee during his search for quinine contained in coffee beans (1821)[100]. He terms the extract "kaffe base" which when translated from German into English means "the base of that which exists in coffee" (1820)[101].

One year later, Pierre Pelletier and Joseph Caventou isolate caffeine in coffee (1821)[97]. Pelletier coins the term "cafeine" (sic) derived from the French word for coffee "café" and apply the recently introduced convention of adding the suffix "ine" to all alkaline substances isolated from plants (1819,1898)[98,102]. The German term "kaffe base" and French term "café" are Anglicized into the familiar English term we now recognize as "caffeine".

Friedrich Serturner (1783-1841) German pharmacist advances pain management and moves medical pharmacology forward, isolating morphine from the opium poppy plant (Papaver somniferum). While opium has been used for thousands of years to manage pain, Serturner is first to identify, isolate, and extract the specific active chemical component which makes the opium plant so effective in managing pain. Serturner first publishes his findings on opium, at the age of 22 years (1805)[103]. This report goes largely unnoticed by the scientific and medical communities. The 1805 publication contains the following dismissive footnote by the journal's editor, renown German chemist and founder of the first pharmaceutical institute in Germany, Professor Johann Trommsdorff (1770-1837); "…Serturner's experiment may have given future research a few interesting pointers. However, the problem with opium was in no way solved…" (1805)[103]. Twelve years later, Serturner publishes his landmark paper in which he isolates pure morphine from opium, describes morphine's chemical and pharmacological properties, and reports on its physiological, cognitive, and behavioral effects when administered to animals and humans (1817)[104].

Sometimes it just takes self-confidence and persistent effort to complete the necessary work required to persuade established academic and medical communities of the value of contributions made by young investigators. I encourage you to not be easily dissuaded, if you have a fundamentally sound idea, which is not readily accepted by your professors, colleagues, or the scientific and medical communities at large. The history of medicine is filled with examples where the most innovative ideas and ideas which make the most valuable contributions are initially rejected by the established scientific and medical communities, including well respected journal editors.

Serturner in the spirit of the long practiced tradition of self experimentation and in an attempt to collect the necessary information which will lead to his influential 1817 publication, conducts a nearly catastrophic trial of morphine ingestion with himself and three friends. Much information is collected and recorded before the four are rendered unconscious. Serturner reports the outcome of his self-investigations, in part, in his 1817 paper describing the pharmacology of morphine (1817)[104]. This paper is now recognized to be a landmark paper in the history of medical pharmacology. However, at the time the paper is originally published, it is published with great reservations by the journal's editor. The published paper contains the appended dismissive editor's comment. This paper "… witnesses a lack of knowledge of science and chemistry. If there really is a substance like Mr. Serturner's morphine, then we chemists certainly have a lot to learn…" (1817)[104].

So goes another example of the continuing practice of many well established journals being resistant to publishing original papers, which challenge the accepted medical dogma of the period.

The now familiar term "morphine" is assigned by Serturner after having referred to the substance by several different terms during his 14 years of investigations 1803 to 1817. The terms include opium-saure (opium acid), meconic acid, and morphium. Serturner makes a final decision to term the substance "morphine". The term is derived from Morpheus the Greek God of sleep and dreams. Serturner incorporates the recently introduced convention of adding the suffix "ine" to all plant derived alkaloid (1819,1898)[98,102]. Morphine, an isolated extract from the opium poppy plant now offers greater control in dosing and physiological effect (primarily analgesic) when compared with use of the opium plant, as practiced for thousands of years prior to the isolation of morphine.

Serturner initially distributes morphine locally himself as an effective treatment to reduce pain. Morphine is soon manufactured and becomes commercially available from the German pharmaceutical company Merck, approximately eight years after Serturner first isolates this potent analgesic substance (1827)[105]. Serturner's discovery is recognized to be so important that in 1831 the Institute of France Academy of Sciences awards to him a monetary prize in the amount of 2,000 francs for having "…opened the way to important medical discoveries by his isolation of morphine and exposition of its character…". Millions of people have suffered much less pain as the result of Serturner's thoughtful and persistent efforts.

Attention first and second year medical students. If you have a thoughtful idea, are trying to get your first paper published and receive little encouragement from those around you remember Friedrich Serturner. You might be the one to make the next important contribution to medicine. Do not be easily discouraged. Established medical authorities and journal editors historically can be resistant to new ideas, especially if the ideas challenge prevailing medical dogma.

The discovery and study of alkaloids during the early-1800s move medical pharmacology forward as a scientific academic discipline. Alkaloids provide practicing physicians with a new class of potent medications which include now familiar substances colchicine, codeine, morphine, quinine, and atropine.

Francois Magendie is largely responsible for moving alkaloids out of the academic laboratory and into clinical medical practice. He popularizes the alkaloids as potential therapeutics and publishes a pocket size formulary for the practicing physician. The formulary deals almost entirely with the clinical use of the new alkaloids and is titled "Formulaire pour la preparation et l'emploi de plusieurs nouveaux medicamens" [Formulary for the preparation and use of several new drugs] (1822)[94]. Alkaloids remain a mainstay of medical therapeutics for the next 200 years.

Pierre Robiquet (1780-1840) French chemist adds to the rapidly growing lists of contributions made to medical pharmacology by academic chemists. Most recognized for his foundational works in identifying the building blocks of proteins, the amino acids, and first to recognize the first amino acid, asparagine (1806)[106]. Robiquet successfully identifies the second most predominant alkaloid found in opium, codeine (1832)[107]. Codeine has immediate clinical applications in the treatment of pain, coughs, and diarrhea. Today, over 185 years since it is first isolated, codeine remains by far the most widely used opiate in the world. Remember, codeine is converted by the liver into morphine, a powerful analgesic.

Trivia: The amino acid asparagine derives its name from the asparagus plant, from which it was originally extracted by Robiquet in 1806. The term "codeine" is derived from the Greek word " kodeia" meaning "head of a poppy" and is combined with the convention established in 1818 to attach the suffix "ine" to all alkaline substances isolated from plants.

Medical pharmacology of the mid-1800s continues to focus upon solutions which provide pain relief to patients. Interests in the effective painkilling analgesics popular during the first half of the 1800s is briefly supplanted by interests in gas based general anesthesia. Three gases attract the greatest amount of attention: nitrous oxide (laughing gas), ether, and chloroform. Each gas is heavily investigated as a potential anesthesia during the late-1840s, in efforts to provide surgical patients relief from pain. Controversy, rivalry, and claims for priority of discovery of these three familiar anesthesias dominate the professional literature and discussions at professional meetings throughout the mid to late-1800s (1875)[108].

Nitrous oxide is determined to be an ineffective anesthesia for most surgical procedures other than tooth extractions. Ether and chloroform prove to be effective anesthesia and gain widespread acceptance and use. Ether is the preferred in the USA while chloroform is preferred in Europe.

Nitrous oxide is first introduced into the medical literature by Joseph Priestly (1733-1804) when he isolates the gas, which he terms "nitrous air", while conducting a landmark series of experimental investigations into different kinds of airs and gases (1774-1777)[109]. Approximately 30 years later, Humphrey Davy (1728-1829) British chemist systematically investigates the gas, describes its effects, and recommends it to the medical community for use in minor surgeries (1800)[110]. The recommendation is largely ignored.

Horace Wells (1815-1848) American dentist successfully completes a series of patient studies and demonstrates its effectiveness in eliminating pain during tooth extractions (1847)[111]. Its use in dentistry quickly gains popularity in the USA, Canada, and Europe. However, nitrous oxide soon proves to be an ineffective anesthesia when used in other surgical procedures and is quickly replaced by the use of ether and chloroform.

Ether is introduced as an alternative to nitrous oxide by American dentist William Morton (1819-1868) (1846)[112]. Ether proves to be an effective anesthesia. American surgeon Henry Bigelow (1818-1890) demonstrates its effectiveness at Massachusetts General Hospital while completing the surgical removal of a tumor from a patient's neck (1846)[112]. Ether is quickly applied to a broad range of surgical procedures and proves to be extremely effective. The successful use of this anesthesia revolutionizes surgery, providing opportunity for painless surgical procedures.

William Morton quickly claims priority of discovery of ether and its application for surgical procedures. He and colleague Charles Jackson (1805-1880) immediately secure a US patent for the use of ether as an anesthesia. Morton patents ether under the name Letheon (1846)[113]. Soon it is discovered Letheon is actually ether. This creates a tremendous outcry and immediate condemnation from the medical community. Beyond the fact ether is a naturally occurring substance and therefore not patentable according to US patent laws, William Morton appears to have known Letheon to be ether, attempts to hide this fact, and attempts to profit financially from its use as an anesthesia by securing a US patent.

The legal and ethical issues produced by these events are the source of much discussion and debate within the legal and medical communities for the balance of the 1800s. Perhaps most notable is the controversy between William Morton and his mentor Charles Jackson, known simply as the Jackson and Morton controversy, addresses the issues of priority of discovery of ether, its application as an effective anesthesia in surgical procedures, and whom if anyone should benefit financially from the discoveries. In an effort to quell the dispute for priority of discovery the Institute of France Academy of Sciences offers a political compromise. Charles Jackson is awarded 2,500 francs in recognition "…for his observations and experiments on the anesthetic effects of ether…" and William Morton is awarded 2,500 francs in recognition "…for introducing it (ether) into surgical practice after the indications by Dr. Jackson…" (1863)[114]. The issues of ethical and professional behavior continue to be debated still today. As a medical student and soon to be a practicing physician, what do you think about these legal, ethical, and professional behavior issues?

Chloroform is introduced into the scientific literature during the early-1830s, independently by Eugene Souberain (1797-1859) of France (1831)[115], Justus von Liebig (1803-1873) of Germany (1832)[116], and Samuel Guthrie (1782-1848) of the USA (1832)[117]. Chloroform is thoroughly investigated by Jean-Batiste Dumas (1800-1884) generating its chemical formula ($CHCL_3$) and naming this colorless, sweet smelling, dense liquid "chloroform" (1834)[118]. It is introduced into the medical and surgical literature as an alternative anesthesia to nitrous oxide and ether by Scottish obstetrician James Simpson (1811-1870) and is initially used to eliminate pain during childbirth (1847a,1847b)[119,120]. Only a few drops are necessary to produce anesthesia. Chloroform is much less flammable than ether and offers increased safety with its use.

Although Simpson effectively demonstrates the benefit of chloroform in relieving pain during childbirth, the use of this anesthesia for this purpose is actively opposed by organized religion (1847c)[121]. In brief, the primary objection by organized religion is that God intentionally imposes pain during childbirth and man should not interfere with the intention of God (1847c)[121].

Trivia: The term "anesthesia" is coined and introduced into the medical literature by James Simpson (1847a)[119].

Rudolf Buchheim (1820-1879) German pharmacologist is first to establish pharmacology as a truly separate, scientific based discipline, recognized within a university setting. He establishes the first department of pharmacology and institute of pharmacology devoted to understanding how therapeutic drugs and poisons produce their effects. He clearly defines the professional scope and boundaries of medical pharmacology, its methodologies, and identifies its immediate and long term goals and objectives.

Simply stated Rudolf Buchheim defines pharmacology as separate and distinct from chemistry, physiology, pharmacy, or medicine. The role of pharmacology is to systematically investigate, using scientific and experimentally based methodologies, the way and extent therapeutic agents and poisons (drugs) are altered by the body (pharmacokinetics) and the way and extent these therapeutic agents and poisons (drugs) alter body functions (pharmacodynamics) (1849)[122]. He argues the necessary advantage of studying isolated substances, understanding their chemical composition, and correlating the chemistry of the drug with changes in biological tissue and organ system functions.

Buchheim further offers pharmacology a new and innovative way in which to think about and organize therapeutic substances. As an alternative to the familiar organization of material medica, he boldly proposes therapeutic substances (drugs) be classified based upon the drug's primary mode of action. The proposal, as often the case with new and innovative ideas, is met with much initial resistance and only later proves its revolutionary value. The system proves useful in organizing a rapidly expanding knowledge base generated by experimental pharmacology during the mid and late-1800s and offers medical students and practicing physicians a theoretical matrix within which to organize therapeutic agents and guide pharmacological treatments.

His vision for medical pharmacology as an academic discipline with applications for findings to be applied to the practice of medicine establishes the foundation upon which all future development in medical pharmacology will build. Arguably, no other single individual of the period effects the future direction and maturation of medical pharmacology as a scientific discipline more than Rudolf Buchheim.

Trivia: Rudolf Buchheim introduces the now familiar phrase "mode of action" into the scientific and medical literature (1843)[123]. He is an early and vocal proponent of including the study of pharmacology as necessary and essential to the education of medical students (1876)[124].

As the first half of the 1800s come to a close medical pharmacology moves away from the common practice of identifying plants and minerals and simply listing their associated medicinal value. The field moves towards a chemistry based understanding of specific active ingredients contained within plants and minerals and responsible for the therapeutic effects. Specific therapeutic agents are systematically investigated in cooperation with experimental physiologists in efforts to understand their effects upon specific biological tissues and organ systems. New physiological measurement instruments begin to quantify the physiological effects generated by introduction of specific pharmacological agents into biological systems. Alkaloids are discovered and their uses as effective analgesics are systematically investigated and introduced into clinical medicine, relieving pain for many. Anesthesias are introduced and relieve pain during surgical procedures, revolutionizing the practice of surgery. Medical pharmacology establishes itself as an independent discipline, separate from pharmacy, chemistry, physiology, and clinical medicine. Investigators from France and Germany take the lead in guiding medical pharmacology into the future. These are exciting and changing times for medical pharmacology.

The second half of the 1800s opens with continuing emphasis placed upon understanding the chemical structures of medicinal remedies and using this knowledge to guide development and synthesis of new therapeutic medicinal treatments. New technological advancements move medical pharmacology forward. The hypodermic needle syringe is introduced and offers a new delivery system to complement inhalation, intravenous infusions, suppositories, rubs, and ingestion. The modern pharmaceutical industry is founded and originates from apothecaries or chemical companies. Commercial industry becomes intimately involved in the research, development, production, and marketing of medicinal remedies. Medical pharmacology continues to develop and mature as a scientific based discipline, establishing departments of pharmacology within university and medical school settings; establishing free standing institutes devoted to the advancement of pharmacological research and new knowledge; founding its first peer review journal devoted specifically to the advancement of pharmacology as a scientific discipline; further defines itself as separate and distinct from the disciplines of chemistry, physiology, pharmacy, and clinical medicine; and refines necessary and essential educational and training requirements in pharmacology for medical students.

Alexander Wood (1817-1884) Scottish physician introduces the use of the hollow hypodermic needle and plunger syringe as a primary delivery system for subcutaneous injections of medicinal remedies (1855)[125]. The new delivery system complements existing delivery systems e.g. inhalation, intravenous injections (1667)[126], suppositories, rubs, and oral ingestion. The system is first tested in efforts to relieve localized pain. Morphine solutions are injected directly into localized sites of pain and prove to be extremely effective in relieving pain. Wood's first publication of the topic describes success in achieving relief of pain in a female suffering cervico-brachial neuralgia whom could not take opium in any other form without becoming violently ill (1855)[125].

Having successfully demonstrated the value of relieving pain via subcutaneous injection of morphine solutions, the discussion quickly turns to other issues. Does the site of injection need to be at the site of the pain? Can the injection be made elsewhere and achieve the same analgesic effect? Who should be acknowledged as most responsible for the introduction of the system to medicine? What other remedies might be administered by the subcutaneous injection method? What illnesses, diseases, or conditions might be effectively treated using the new delivery system? Each of these questions is addressed during the period of 1865 through 1870. Each question stirs passionate, heated discussions within the academic and medical communities. Medical pharmacology plays essential roles in providing experimental and clinically generated data to answer these fundamental questions and providing the necessary professional mediation between individuals within the profession who have difficulty playing well with others.

The delivery of medicinal remedies subcutaneously via a hollow needle and plunger syringe quickly becomes the next new best thing in medicine. The procedure is simple and eliminates many of the problems frequently associated with other medication delivery systems regarding absorption, distribution, metabolism, and excretion. The procedure is quickly incorporated into the treatments of a wide range of medical conditions e.g. headaches, vertigo, delirium, mania, hysteria, eclampsia, chorea, tetanus, dysentery, neuralgia, sciatica, and depression, often without sound reason. With time, experience, and systematic experimental investigations it becomes clear which conditions respond best to subcutaneous injections and why (1859,1865a,1865b,1867, 1873)[127,128,129,130,131].

Trivia: Charles Hunter (1799-1871) London surgeon coins the term "hypodermic" and introduces it into the medical literature (1859)[127]. This term replaces Alexander Wood's original term "subcutaneous" in referring to the method of injecting drugs below the skin (1858)[132].

Alexander Wood charges Charles Hunter of plagiarism and the two engage in numerous acrimonious correspondences, often published in professional medical journals (1865,1865,1865a,1865b)[133,134,135,136]. In a political effort to resolve the dispute, The Royal Medical and Chirurgical Society of London assign a special peer review committee to investigate the merits of the charges. After two years, the Committee publishes its final summary report, avoiding any official conclusions regarding the charges of plagiarism or priority for discovery. The Committee's report simply outlines clinical and experimental data to date on the pharmacokinetics and pharmacodynamics of subcutaneous injections of assorted medicinal substances compared to other delivery systems (1867)[130]. The value and pharmacology of hypodermic delivery is quickly established and the charge of plagiarism by Wood of Hunter remains unresolved.

The mid-1800s witness the founding and rapid development of the modern pharmaceutical industry. Remedies once studied in the laboratories of academia and patient bedsides are now investigated, developed, produced, marketed, and distributed by companies originating out of the apothecaries or chemical companies of Europe and the USA. Now familiar names in the pharmaceutical industry originating from apothecaries are Merck (Germany), Squibb (USA), and Eli Lilly (USA). Equally familiar named companies originating from chemical companies are Pfizer (USA), Sandoz (Switzerland), and Bayer (Germany).

Of the pharmaceutical companies originating from the apothecaries, Merck is the first to seize opportunities during the industrial revolution, now under way in Europe and the USA, to combine science with industry. Based in Germany, Merck is among the first to enter the financially lucrative business of mass production and distribution of pharmaceuticals. The Company begins its first production of massive amounts of the recently discovered alkaloids in 1827 (2012)[137]. The Company is manufacturing massive amounts of morphine from its Berlin facility by 1851 (2012)[137].

Squibb is founded by Edward Squibb (1819-1900) a US Navy physician following his service in the Mexican-American War (1846-1848). During this war he becomes so dissatisfied with the quality of medications dispensed to military physicians, he establishes a New York based laboratory and manufacturing company in 1858 and commits himself and company to development and manufacturing of high quality pharmaceuticals. Squibb plays an instrumental role in providing large amounts of medications to the Union Army, during the American Civil War (1861-1865). The Company provides a self-contained medicine chest to the Union military, containing approximately 50 medicines. Each chest contains ether and chloroform for amputations, quinine for malaria, assorted herbals for dysentery, and whisky for general medicinal purposes (2012)[138].

Eli Lilly and Company is founded in Indianapolis, Indiana during 1876 by its namesake Eli Lilly (1838-1898) for the purpose of manufacturing high quality prescription medications. Like Edward Squibb, Lilly becomes frustrated with the generally poor quality of medications dispensed during his service in the Union military during the American Civil War. The Company commits to incorporating scientific research and development into its overall business plan based on manufacturing of high quality prescription medications. Early financial success is found in the manufacturing of quinine for the treatment of malaria. Early technological advances by Eli Lilly include development of gelatin covered capsules and machinery capable of automated capsule productions (2012)[139].

Of the pharmaceutical companies originating from the commercial chemical industry, New York based Pfizer is founded in 1849. The Company enjoys early success with the release of its antihelminthic (Santonin), formulated to expel parasitic intestinal worms, a common problem in the USA during the mid-1800s. A few years later and with onset of the American Civil War, Pfizer quickly meets the needs of the Union military supplying anti-parasitic (Santonin), analgesics (morphine), anesthetics (chloroform, camphor), and antiseptics (iodine) (2012)[140].

Sandoz is founded in Basle, Switzerland during 1886 by Alfred Kern (1850-1893) and Edouard Sandoz (1853-1928) for the purpose of manufacturing commercial dyes. Within 10 years the Kern & Sandoz Company shifts its focus from commercial dyes and enters the pharmaceutical industry, manufacturing its popular antipyretic (fever reducing compound) Antipyrine. By 1899 the Company diversifies into sweeteners and begins production of saccharin (2012)[141].

Bayer is founded in Barmen, Germany by dye salesman Friedrich Bayer (1825-1880) during the summer of 1863, for the purpose of manufacture and sale of synthetic commercial dyes, primarily for the textile industry. As with other innovative dye companies of the period, Bayer establishes its own research laboratories. Bayer soon expands into pharmaceutical research, development, manufacturing, and distribution. By the end of the 1800s Bayer secures a patent and releases its anti-pyretic compound known to all physicians today, Aspirin (1899/2012)[142]. Aspirin is only available in powder form from 1899 to 1915 by prescription only. Aspirin is pressed into a tablet and made available without a prescription and over-the-counter in 1915.

Trivia: The term aspirin is derived from the German words "acetylierte Spirsaure" (acetylated salicylic acid). "A" for acetyl + "spir" from the plant genus Spiraea + "in" a common suffix appended to many medication names, originating from the Greek and Latin meaning "pertaining to". In combination, this gives us the word aspirin.

Note: Aspirin, with a capital "A" is the trade name assigned by and patented by Bayer in 1899. Once the patent expired, many begin using the generic form of Aspirin, which is denoted as aspirin, with a lower case "a".

Germany, Switzerland, and the USA establish themselves as the places of origin of the modern pharmaceutical industry. The chemistry of medicinal agents is aggressively investigated in house by the pharmaceutical companies' laboratories. Once research teams identify, extract, and purify the active therapeutic ingredients attention is refocused towards synthesizing the active ingredients and securing patents. Patents provide financial protection and great financial reward for companies successful in securing the patents. Investigations of the pharmacology of therapeutic agents moves further away from the academic scientist's laboratory and physician's patient bedside and into commercial pharmaceutical company laboratories. The way in which therapeutic remedies are identified, studied, produced, and distributed to patients suffering illness and disease changes forever.

Trivia: Before Aspirin, Bayer researchers in 1895 successfully add two acetyl groups to the naturally occurring morphine molecule and produce a new patented medication. The medication is sold over the counter as an effective cough suppressant. Adding the acetyl groups makes the substance more fat soluble, allowing for easy movement across the blood brain barrier. This new patented medication is diacetylmorphine (Heroin).

Alexander Crum Brown (1838-1922) Scottish organic chemist provides a valuable visual aide to medical pharmacology with the introduction and development of a system representing chemical compounds in diagrammatic form. He draws representations of molecules with symbols for atoms enclosed in circles and dashed line to connect atomic symbols together in a way which satisfied each atom's valence (1861,1864,1865)[143,144,145]. The diagrams provide easily interpretable representations of molecular structure and allow for quick meaningful comparisons between therapeutic compounds.

Thomas Frazer (1841-1920) English pharmacologist and Alexander Crum Brown move medical pharmacology forward emphasizing the correlation of chemical and molecular structure with therapeutic actions (1872)[146]. Understanding the chemical composition of therapeutic substances leads to synthesizing effective therapeutic substances based upon an understanding of chemical compositions and structures. Early antipyretics are among the first drugs synthesized based upon an understanding of the chemical structure of the alkaloids. Notice this rational approach stands in contrast to the empirical associations of medicinal substances and therapeutic treatments characterized by material medica, prior to the early-1800s.

Claude Bernard (1813-1878) French physiologist, perhaps most remembered for his identification of the action of curare on the neuromuscular junction (1850,1856)[147,148]; detailing the function of the pancreas and its secretions (1849)[149]; discovery of the glycogenic function of liver (1855-1856)[150]; discovery of glycogen (1857)[151]; and thoughtful analyses of fundamental biological processes of drug absorption, distribution, binding, and elimination (1858,1875)[152,153]; offers an equally important, if not greater contribution when he publishes his book titled "An Introduction to the Study of Experimental Medicine" (1865)[154]. It is here Bernard outlines the necessary scientific methodologies to be used in pharmacology to insure its development as an objective, rational, evidence based scientific discipline. It is here he recommends the use of "blinded" experimental research designs.

Trivia: Claude Bernard struggles academically as a medical student. He ranks 26 of 29 in his graduating class of 1839, from the School of Medicine at the University of Paris. After graduation he fails the necessary qualifying examination which would allow him a teaching position at the medical school. However, he makes contributions to the fields of medical pharmacology and medicine which dwarf contributions made by many academically stronger students.

Oswald Schmiedeberg (1838-1921) Russian born pharmacologist and student of Rudolf Buchheim extends Buchheim's conceptualization of the discipline of pharmacology and its role in academia and clinical medicine. Schmiedeberg makes his position clear in perhaps his most influential book "Grundriss der Arzneimittellehre" [Outline of Pharmacology] (1883)[155].

> "…The pharmacologist does not deal with therapy, the practicing clinician does. The complexity of treatment in modern medicine on one side and the scope of pharmacology on the other no longer allow anybody to represent both disciplines if he is not to become a dilettante in one of them. Without pharmacologic knowledge the physician will stumble around in the dark, whenever he employs drugs…" (1883)[155].

Oswald Schmiedeberg makes additional contributions. He and colleague Richard Koppe (unknown-) outline the effects of muscarine on cardiac tissues and recognize the effects can be antagonized by atropine, providing a rationally derived, experimentally tested antidote to muscarinic poisoning (1869)[156]. Recall, muscarinic poisoning turns on the parasympathetic nervous system and is characterized clinically by miosis (small pupils), blurred vision, increased salivation, lacrimation (tearing), excessive sweating, bronchial secretions, bronchoconstriction, abdominal cramping, and bradycardia (reduced heart rated below 60 beats per minute). Warning, be careful which wild mushrooms you eat.

Oswald Schmiedeberg with colleagues pathologists Bernard Naunyn (1839-1925) (xenobiotic metabolism pioneer) and Edwin Klebs (1831-1913) (discovers bacterium Corynebacterium diphtheriae as cause of diphtheria; bacterial genus Klebsiella is named in his honor) found the first professional scientific journal devoted to pharmacology, "Archives for Experimentelle Pathologie and Pharmakologie" [Archives for Experimental Pathology and Pharmacology] (1873)[157]. Schmiedeberg publishes numerous studies detailing the metabolism of drugs by biological tissues; discovers glucuronic acid (1879)[158], establishes in 1887 arguably the most influential institute of pharmacology in the world, the Pharmacological Institute at the University of Strasbourg located in Alsace, France and trains most pharmacology department heads of Europe and North America during the late-1800s and early-1900s.

Carl Koller (1857-1944) Bohemian (now Czech Republic) ophthalmologist introduces cocaine as an effective local anesthetic for eye surgery (1884)[159]. A few drops of a cocaine solution eliminate the involuntary reflex movements of the eye when touched and eliminates the sensation of touch. Soon, cocaine is applied in dentistry and general medical practices as a local anesthetic.

Trivia: Cocaine is contained in the original formulation of the popular carbonated cola beverage, Coca-Cola. Coca-Cola is marketed for many years as an effective treatment for headaches, fatigue, indigestion, and morphine addiction. In 1885, the inventor of Coca Cola, American pharmacist John Pemberton (1831-1888) is issued a registered trademark for Coca-Cola, by the US Patent Office, number 12,257 on May 19, 1885, as a nerve tonic (1885)[160]. Coca-Cola is initially sold as a wine (Pemberton's French Wine Coca), which contains coca extract (cocaine). With introduction of Prohibition in the State of Georgia in 1886, the pharmacist inventor of the original recipe, replaces alcohol with a non-alcoholic syrup still containing cocaine and caffeine, designed to be mixed with carbonated water. Cocaine is removed from the formula in 1906.

John Able (1857-1938) American pharmacologist and medical student of Oswald Schmiedeberg founds the first Department of Pharmacology in the United States at the University of Michigan, forty one years after the medical school opens its doors to students (1891)[161]. Two years later he moves to John Hopkins University where he founds the University's first Department of Pharmacology (1893)[162]. While at John Hopkins he completes pharmacological investigations of the recently discovered hormone epinephrine (1897,1899)[163,164]; publishes on the role of pharmacology and therapeutics in medical schools (1900)[165]; is instrumental in founding the American Society for Pharmacology and Experimental Therapeutics (ASPET) (1908)[166]; and founds the "Journal of Pharmacology and Experimental Therapeutics" (1909)[167].

Arthur Cushny (1866-1926) Scottish pharmacologist and student of Oswald Schmiedeberg, with classical training in physiology, succeeds John Able in 1893 as Chair of the Department of Pharmacology, at the University of Michigan. He authors "A textbook of pharmacology and therapeutics or the action of drugs in health and disease, for the use of students and practitioners of medicine" (1899)[168]. This is the first general textbook of pharmacology to appear in the English speaking world and is well received by the academic and medical communities. It moves pharmacology further away from the old material medica and towards a science of pharmacology based upon the modes of actions of drugs.

A review of Cushny's writings reveals he has no hesitations in rejecting medical dogma when presented in the absence of objective evidence. He is committed to establishing the new and rapidly maturing discipline of medical pharmacology, based upon a foundation of scientifically derived knowledge, and readily rejects knowledge based solely upon time honored authoritative dogma.

By the end of the 1800s medical pharmacology begins to establish itself in the Universities and medical schools of North America.

In brief summary, the 1800s witness a movement away from an empirical listing of plants and minerals along with their therapeutic effects. Movement is towards understanding the pharmacology of therapeutically active ingredients contained within the plant or mineral.

Emphasis is now placed upon understanding the chemistry of these active ingredients. Empiricism gives way to experimentalism. Alkaloids are discovered, aggressively investigated, and applied to clinical medicine. Specific and clinically important alkaloids change medicine forever e.g. quinine for malaria, morphine and codeine for pain relief. Nitrous oxide, ether, and chloroform are introduced as anesthesia. The hollow needle with a plunger syringe is introduced as an innovative way to deliver medicinal remedies. The modern, commercial, pharmaceutical industry is founded out of its origins in the apothecaries and industrial chemical industry in Europe and the USA. Pharmacology distinguishes itself as an independent, scientific based discipline, separate from pharmacy, chemistry, or medicine. The first departments of pharmacology are founded in European and American universities. Research institutes are established throughout Europe, devoted to the advancement of pharmacology research, knowledge, and training. The first scientific journal devoted specifically to pharmacology is founded and begins publication in Europe. Pharmacology and its role in medical education is debated and determined to be necessary and essential for all future physicians. Medical pharmacology is now poised for the rapid explosion of new knowledge, methodological advances, changes in conceptual matrixes, displacement of long held dogma, and maturation as a scientific discipline, as it moves purposefully into the 1900s.

Hold on. The next 100 years proves to be quite a ride for medical pharmacology.

Late Modern, 1900 AD - 2000 AD.

Medical pharmacology develops quickly during the 1900s.

The first half of the 1900s witness the founding of professional societies devoted to the advancement of pharmacology in the USA, Great Britain, and Canada. Professional scientific journals are established and devoted to the advancement of pharmacology as a science and professional discipline. Medical pharmacology struggles with its identity. Chemical receptors are conceptualized and discovered. Synaptic cell to cell signal transmission is understood within the matrix of chemical transmission and the concept of electrical sparks is displaced. Mathematical equations are introduced and become a routine component of pharmacology assisting in the calculation of fundamental pharmacokinetic functions, absorption, distribution, clearance, and elimination. The FDA is founded in the USA. Medical pharmacology soon becomes more regulated. The first prototypical injectable anticoagulant is introduced for the management of thrombosis. Hormone replacement therapy (insulin) is introduced for the management of diabetes mellitus. Antibiotics are conceptualized, aggressively investigated by academia and commercial industrial pharmaceutical companies, resulting in the introduction of synthesized antibiotics effective against numerous bacteria and formulated utilizing a rational epistemology. Sulfa based antibiotics lead the way, soon followed by cell wall inhibitors, and protein synthesis inhibitors. The first synthesized anti-cancer compounds are introduced as cytotoxic poisons, soon followed by folate inhibitors. Academia and commercial industrial pharmaceutical companies combine resources and discover cortisone to be an effective compound in the management of rheumatoid arthritis. Two classes of adrenergic receptors are conceptualized, alpha and beta, which displace pharmacology dogma and explain inhibitory and excitatory functions within the adrenergic autonomic nervous system.

The American Therapeutics Society (ATS) is founded May 1, 1900, in Washington, D.C. by 20 physicians. The Society's stated purpose is to promote the advancement of rational "...therapeutics in its broadest sense..." (1901)[169] and by "...application of any method or agency which might ameliorate, cure, a patient disease…" (1901/2012)[170]. Therapeutics are to be grounded in scientific method and empirical observation. Charlatans are to be eliminated. The ATS is among the first to question openly the potential conflict of interest, whenever accepting commercial advertisement as a means of supporting the publication of medical or scientific journals (1915)[171].

The American Society for Pharmacology and Experimental Therapeutics (ASPET) is founded by John Able and a select group of eighteen pharmacologists, meeting in John Able's laboratory, at John Hopkins University, December 28, 1908 (1908)[172]. The Society is founded for the purpose of advancing pharmacology and experimental therapeutics, as a scientific discipline within the USA. The Society quickly establishes its parent journal and begins publication of the "Journal of Pharmacology and Experimental Therapeutics" (JPET) June 1, 1909 (1909)[173].

Trivia: The term "experimental therapeutics" is a term popularized by German pharmacologist Paul Ehrlich to describe research which applies pharmacological principles to the study and treatment of disease. Recall, Ehrlich develops Salvarsan, the landmark drug for the treatment of syphilis, during the early-1900s.

The original 18 charter members of ASPET struggle to establish criteria for Society membership. Wanting to ensure the Society's focus upon experimental pharmacology and maintain its identity as an independent scientific discipline, charter members are reluctant to admit clinicians or scientists from other disciplines. Following much discussion, one requirement for membership is the individual must have published "…a meritorious investigation in pharmacology or experimental therapeutics… (and) …be actively engaged in research in these fields…". Additionally, requirements state employees of the pharmaceutical industry are explicitly and specifically to be excluded from membership "…in order to avoid every external influence, inimical to the scientific interests of pharmacology…" (1908,2007)[172,174].

John Langley (1852-1925) English physiologist with primary interests in the autonomic nervous systems, challenges pharmacology dogma that drugs have their effects on tissues by effecting endings of nerves. Langley argues it is not the nerve ending but rather a "receptive substance" on the post-synaptic neuron or target tissue which is the site of drug actions. Working with two alkaloids, pilocarpine and atropine, Langley concludes "…there is a chemical combination between drug and a constituent of the cell - the receptive substance…" which explains drug-tissue interactions; thereby introducing one of the most influential ideas in biomedical sciences of the twentieth century, the conceptual matrix of drug receptor theory (1905)[175]. As with most new and innovative ideas that challenge current dogma, Langley's proposal is met with much resistance from the scientific community. Seventy years will pass before "receptive substances" i.e. cell membrane receptor proteins, are successfully isolated during the 1970s and provide conformational evidence in support of Langley's original conceptualization.

Paul Ehrlich (1854-1915) German bacteriologist with primary interests in the relationships between bacterial toxins, antitoxins, and their potential to combat infectious diseases, introduces his formulation of a chemical receptor theory (side-chain theory). In brief, Ehrlich proposes cells have "side chains" which are capable of binding certain toxins. As "side-chains" become bound by toxins the "side-chains" are unable to fulfill their normal physiological functions. In response to binding, the cell generates additional "side-chains" which are then released into the blood-stream where they act as antibodies or antitoxins (1897)[176].

Paul Ehrlich soon generalizes his conceptual ideas of "side chains" and offers an explanation as to how drugs bind tissues and generate their therapeutic effects. Drugs contain specific chemical groups (korperklassen) which have binding capabilities specific to particular organs and tissues. Drugs are used as vehicles (lastwagen) to carry therapeutic substances to specific organs or tissue sites (1898,1902,2003)[177,178,179].

Only after John Langley's publishes his paper describing "receptive substances" and proposing a drug-cell interaction at the level of the target tissue's plasma membrane (1905)[175], does Ehrlich revises his thinking and accept the idea, drugs bind directly to target tissue cells and have their effect on tissues by way of a membrane bound "receptive substance". Ehrlich coins the term "chemoreceptor (1907)[180] to describe the membrane bound "receptive substances", first described by Langley two years earlier.

Henry Dale (1875-1968) English pharmacologist and Otto Loewi (1873-1961) German pharmacologist displace pharmacology dogma describing between cell communications and between cell signal transmissions. Prior to their seminal investigations, synapses are considered to be anatomical regions where electrical currents simply jump from one cell to another cell e.g. neuron to neuron or neuron to muscle, by electrical "sparks", as proposed and advocated by Charles Sherrington (1897,1906)[181,182]. Henry Dale and Otto Loewi demonstrate signal transmission between cells is indeed completed at the synaptic junction; however, signal transmission is not accomplished by jumping electrical "sparks", rather indirectly via a chemical intermediary (1914)[183]. Dale and Loewi share the 1936 Nobel Prize in Physiology or Medicine in recognition "…for their discoveries relating to chemical transmission of nerve impulses…" (1936)[184].

Jay McLean (1890-1957) second semester medical student at John Hopkins University discovers the injectable anticoagulant, recognized today as heparin (1916)[185]. The term "heparin" is coined by McLean's medical school professor, William Howell (1860-1945), American physiologist at John Hopkins University in 1918. The term is derived from the Greek word "hapar", meaning "liver", the organ from which Jay McLean and William Howell first isolate the anticoagulant, while studying pro-coagulate compounds. Human clinical trials are completed and an IV use heparin is marketed commercially by the Swedish pharmaceutical company Vitum AB. Heparin soon becomes the standard treatment for thrombosis and serves as the prototypical blood anticoagulant.

Recall, heparin works by binding to antithrombin, the small glycoprotein produced in the liver and which inactivates several enzymes involved in the coagulation cascade system.

Trivia: One year after Jay McLean discovers heparin, the US declares war on Germany and enters World War I. Three years after the discovery, the major league baseball team Chicago White Soxs is embroiled in scandal, during play of the 1919 World Series. Eight members of the team are banned for life from baseball, for intentionally losing games, allowing the Cincinnati Reds to win the World Series.

Additional advances are being made in medical pharmacology during the early-1920s. Most medical students are dutifully told the story of Canadian physiologists Frederick Banting and John Macleod, while working in the Department of Physiology at the University of Toronto, "discover insulin", complete the first human trials with insulin, and change the treatment of diabetes forever. The story is propagated in part by the award of the 1923 Nobel Prize in Physiology or Medicine to these two investigators "…for the discovery of insulin…" (1923)[186]. There is however another truth and one which you as future physicians are entitled. Banting nor Macleod discover insulin and are not the first to demonstrate its effective use as an antidiabetic in either animals or humans.

Nicolae Paulescu (1869-1931) Romanian physiologist successfully extracts the antidiabetic hormone, he names "pancreine", from dog and cattle pancreases and injects it into both pancreatomized and normal dogs. The venous injection of pancreine effectively lowers blood glucose in both animals (1920,1921a,1921b)[187,188,189]. Results cannot be reproduced by oral or rectal routes of administration. Paulescu injects a modified form of pancreine subcutaneously into his first human diabetic patient February 22, 1922 and additional patients three days later. The glucose lowering and antiketogenic effect of pancreine are so impressive and has such potential value in the treatment of human diabetes, he is awarded a patent for pancreine by the Romanian government six weeks later, on April 10, 1922. Nicolae Paulescu secures Romanian patent rights on "insulin" and his work is recognized by the Romanian government one month before Banting, Best, Collip, and Macleod report their first successful clinical trial with insulin at the meeting of the Association of American Physicians, in Washington D.C., May 1922.

For an extended discussion on the "discovery" and early development of insulin, see the Physiology chapter of this book.

Insulin injections provide relief to millions of patients throughout the world, suffering diabetes mellitus. Monies generated from the US and Canadian patents awarded in 1922 support research at the University of Toronto and continue today, over 95 years later. Still there is no known cure for diabetes.

Recall, diabetes mellitus is a group of metabolic disorders in which a person's blood glucose level is too high, because the body is not producing enough insulin or body cells are not responding to the insulin the body does produce. Normally, the hormone insulin is produced by the body's pancreas, regulates the uptake of glucose from blood, and moves glucose from blood into every cell of the body. Additionally, insulin functions as a signal control hormone, important in the conversion of blood glucose into its storage form in cells, glycogen. In the cases of diabetes mellitus, body cells are deprived of both of their necessary and typical primary energy sources, glucose and glycogen. Patients can reintroduce glucose control by external subcutaneous injections of the hormone insulin.

Mathematical equations are introduced and applied to pharmacokinetics. The first equations are applied to drug elimination and demonstrate elimination of alcohol from the body to be a saturatable process and follows a non-linear function curve (1924,1932)[190,191]. Something to consider the next time you have a few martinis (shaken not stirred please) or a few cold beers. Mathematical equations are applied to renal clearance of urea, five years later (1929)[192].

The United States Food and Drug Administration (FDA) is founded from the United States' Department of Agriculture Bureau of Chemistry and charged with public safety, as it relates to monitoring foods and drugs (1930)[193]. At this time, many medications being produced are combined with inferior ingredients, resulting in great variability in purity, quality, and standard of strength. Often the active ingredient is not printed on the packaging or listed in the approved United States Pharmacopoeia or National Formulary. The Agency proves to be a good idea, well-intended, and initially ineffective in accomplishing its directed objectives. The FDA will have tremendous influence in the development of medical pharmacology for the next 88 years and continues to control medical pharmacology as the official regulatory governmental agency for the development and approval of all new medications (2018)[194]

Trivia: Abraham Lincoln founded the United States Department of Agriculture (USDA) and appointed a chemist to lead the USDA's Division of Chemistry (1862), which later becomes the Bureau of Chemistry in 1901 and the FDA in 1930 (2012,2012)[195,196].

The British Pharmacological Society (BPS) is founded in 1931 by a group of 20 pharmacologists, solicited from Departments of Pharmacology and institutions conducting pharmacology research throughout all of Great Britain. The Society founding is initiated by British pharmacologists James Gunn (1882-1958), Henry Dale (1875-1968), and Walter Dixon (1871-1931). The stated purpose of the Society is "…to meet at least once a year for the reading of papers on pharmacology subjects and the discussion of questions of teaching and publications and to promote friendly relations between pharmacologist…" (2018)[197]. The Society adopts the journal of the American Society for Pharmacology and Experimental Therapeutics (ASPET), the "Journal of Pharmacology and Experimental Therapeutics" (JPET), as the Society's official journal and begins joint publication. Both the ASPET and the BPS mature quickly, establishing themselves as leaders in development of professional pharmacology. Both Society and Journal are active today and continue their professional leadership roles (2018)[198].

Trivia: Henry Dale coins terms "cholinergic" and "adrenergic" to classify neurons based upon the primary chemical used in signal transmission between neuron to neuron or neuron to target tissue, within the autonomic nervous systems (1933)[199].

Gerhard Domagk (1895-1964) German bacteriologist, working in the Bayer Laboratories in Germany, demonstrates the antibacterial properties of a brilliant orange-red industrial dye compound and ushers in a new era in medical pharmacology (1932/1986)[200]. The new compound is patented by Bayer (I.G. Farbenindustrie) and marketed as an effective bacteriostatic agent effective against Gram-positive cocci, under the trade name Prontosil Solubile. Domagk publishes his initial findings in February 1935, three years after demonstrating the compound's antibacterial properties and one month after the Bayer Company receives final approval of its German patent (1935)[201]. Hummm….

Investigators at the Pasteur Institute soon follow with publications of their own findings in November 1935, describing a simpler and less costly to manufacture compound for medical use, sulfanilamide (1935)[202]. Sulfanilamide has the additional benefit of not turning patients the reddish color of boiled lobsters, an unfortunate and permanent side effect of Prontosil. French investigators demonstrate it is necessary for the body to metabolize Prontosil into sulfanilamide, the substance responsible for the antibacterial properties, before any therapeutic antibacterial effect is evidenced (1935)[202]. Prontosil is quickly displaced by the less expensive, non-patentable sulfanilamide and ushers in a new generation of pharmaceutical treatments for bacterial infections, the sulfa drugs.

Prontosil and sulfanilamide are met with reserve and skeptical enthusiasm by the academic and medical communities. The dogma of the day identifies vaccination and immunotherapy as the accepted treatment and future direction of infectious diseases. Oh how we can at times be so confident in our knowledge and yet be so wrong. Antibiotic treatments and experimental investigations dominate medical pharmacology for the next ten years. Gerhard Domagk is awarded the 1939 Nobel Prize in Physiology or Medicine "…for the discovery of the antibacterial effects of Prontosil…" (1939)[203].

The era of synthesized antibiotics begins with the sulfa drugs and soon offers the practicing physician effective treatments against a wider range of bacterial infections and large pharmaceutical companies a huge increase in their quarterly profit margins.

Recall, sulfa drugs work by disrupting folate synthesis. Folate is necessary for production of DNA. Given bacteria must synthesize their own folate and are incapable of using external sources of folate, bacteria growth and replication is slowed, giving the patient's immune system a much better chance to destroy and remove the pathogens.

In the summer of 1938 the United States government signs into law the Food, Drug, and Cosmetic Act which greatly increases federal regulatory authority over drugs and pharmaceuticals. The Act mandates pre-market review of safety for all new drugs, prohibits false therapeutic claims in labeling, and offers the recently reorganized Food and Drug Administration (FDA) extensive powers to enforce post-market recall of ineffective drugs (1938/2018)[204]. The Act is a governmental regulatory response to the continuing problems within the United States of manufacturers providing medications with great variability in standards of strength, quality, purity of the active ingredients, and wildly unjustified and misleading marketing claims of cures for common conditions such as diabetes and tuberculosis.

The Food, Drug, and Cosmetic Act of 1938 does not require manufacturers to demonstrate the efficacy of the medication, for which it is marketed. This requirement is enacted twenty-four years later, as an amendment to the Act in 1962 (Kefauver-Harris Amendment), following the thalidomide tragedy in which thousands of babies are born deformed during 1959, after their mothers had taken thalidomide during their pregnancy, which was then marketed as a treatment for nausea. The 1962 Amendment further requires manufacturers to secure informed consent from all patients participating in clinical trials and to report all adverse drug reactions to the FDA (1962/2018)[204]. These requirements continue to be enforced today, over fifty-six years since the enactment of the Amendment.

Clinical value and commercial success of the early sulfa drugs spur competition between academic and pharmaceutical company researchers. The search for the next antibiotic is now aggressively pursued. Mechanisms of action, responsible for producing bacteriostatic and bactericidal properties are considered from a rational approach and guide much of the initial research.

Penicillin with a mechanism of action different from the sulfa drugs, disrupts essential enzymes necessary to the synthesis of the cell wall of bacteria and proves useful in the treatment of Gram positive bacteria (1940)[205].

Streptomycin disrupts protein synthesis at the level of the bacteria's ribosomes, irreversibly binding the 30S ribosomal subunit, blocking the formation of the initiation complex, which causes misreading of mRNA (1944,1945)[206,207]. Streptomycin is effective against Gram negative bacteria and the first antibiotic effective in the treatment of tuberculosis (TB). Important in that TB is a principal cause of death in USA, during the 1930s and 1940s.

Tetracyclines offer an additional protein synthesis inhibitor, irreversibly binding the 30S ribosomal subunit of bacteria, blocking the bindings of tRNA to its receptor sites on mRNA

(1948)[208]. Tetracyclines introduce the first broad spectrum antibiotics, effective against both Gran positive and Gram negative bacteria.

See the Microbiology chapter for an extended discussion of the discovery of these influential and prototypical antibiotics. Antibiotics change medicine forever.

Trivia: Benjamin Duggar (1872-1956) discovers the first of the broad spectrum tetracycline antibiotics at age 73 years. Not all major discoveries are made by young graduate students or young medical students (1948,1949)[209,210].

As a side note; recent evidence has come to light in regard to the highly visible Streptomycin controversy between Rutgers University microbiologist Selman Waksman and then Rutgers University microbiology graduate student Albert Schatz, concerning the claims of priority for the discovery and patent royalties generated from the discovery of streptomycin, the first antibiotic effective against tuberculosis (TB) (2012)[211]. Bottom line in brief, Albert Schatz's claims of priority for discovery are now confirmed beyond doubt. His snub by the Nobel Prize Committee in favor of Selman Waksman simply adds to the growing list of investigators who fail to receive due recognition for their contributions. So it goes in professional academia and science.

Anti-cancer chemotherapies introduced during the mid-1940s are representative of a shift in conceptual thought and guide pharmacology for the next seventy-five years. Rational conceptualizations, emphasizing mechanisms of actions underlying pathologies and effective pharmacological treatments, followed by rigorous experimental testing of the conceptual model, lead to rich and rapid advances in the pharmacology knowledge base.

Cancer is a broad grouping of varied diseases which share in common a disturbance in the regulation of the normal cell growth cycle. The dysregulation produces abnormal cells and abnormal biological functioning. The conceptual models guiding anti-cancer treatments during the mid-1940s are simple. Expose all cells in the body to a cytotoxic poison. The poison will kill dysregulated cancer cells and healthy cells. Rapidly dividing cells should be more effected than slowly dividing cells. Chemotherapies (poisons) should be most effective in killing cancers cells, characterized by rapid cell division. The model is tested and proves to be first among the anti-cancer treatments of the mid-1940s, demonstrating effectiveness first in treating lymphomas, using cytotoxic nitrogen mustards, chemical agents similar to the chemical warfare agent mustard gas (1946)[212].

The second major development of anti-cancer treatments, during the mid to late-1940s, is the introduction of agents which interfere with the normal synthesis of folate, a necessary biochemical ingredient (vitamin) critical for DNA metabolism. The prototypical anti-folate agent methotrexate soon proves effective in the treatment of children suffering acute lymphoblastic leukemia (ALL) by suppressing proliferation of malignant cells (1948)[213].

Advances are also beginning to be made in understanding the medical pharmacology of some autoimmune disorders. Academic pharmacology and commercial pharmaceutical companies combine resources in the mid and late-1940s, successfully identifying, isolating, and subsequently economically synthesizing the adrenal cortical steroid cortisone, and proves effective in the medical management of rheumatoid arthritis (1948)[214]. Edward Kendall (1886-1972) and Philip Hench (1896-1965) American chemists working at the Mayo Clinic, Tadeus Reichstein (1897-1996) Swiss chemist working at the University of Basel, and Merck Pharmaceuticals discover, synthesize, successfully test in humans, the adrenal cortical steroid cortisone and demonstrates its high efficacy in treating patients suffering rheumatoid arthritis (1949)[215]. Edward Kendall, Tadeus Reichstein, and Philip Hench are recognized and awarded the 1950 Nobel Prize in Physiology or Medicine "…for their discoveries relating to the hormones of the adrenal cortex, their structure and biological effects…" (1950)[216].

Raymond Ahlquist (1914-1983) American pharmacologist, working at the University of Georgia's medical school in Augusta, challenges medical pharmacology dogma. He proposes a new way to think about the mechanisms of signal transmission which occurs at the level of smooth muscles, cardiac muscles, or glands. He introduces the concept that stimulation and inhibition of these target tissues is achieved by epinephrine (adrenaline) binding different receptors located on the target tissues. He terms these new hypothetical structures alpha and beta receptors (1948,1954)[217,218]. His conceptualization and experimental data revolutionize the way in which we think about, understand, and pharmacologically manipulate the autonomic nervous systems.

Dogma of the period, based largely upon the works of Harvard Medical School based investigators Walter Cannon (1871-1945) and Arturo Rosenblueth (1900-1970), declares the excitatory and inhibitory effects observed within the adrenergic autonomic nervous system are determined by two separate neuro-hormones, one excitatory termed sympathin E and one inhibitory termed sympathin I. The neuro-hormone sympathin E produces an excitatory response and the neuro-hormone sympathin I produces an inhibitory response (1936)[219]. In effect, two different neuro-hormones have different effects, when they bind one common receptor, located on a tissue cell membrane.

Ahlquist rejects this dogma and argues against the two separate neuro-hormone model and proposes instead a single neuro-hormone model, in which a single neuro-hormone has different effects on tissues based upon different receptors located on the tissue cell membrane. In effect, one neuro-hormone can have two and opposite effects, based upon the hormone binding of different types of receptors, located on the surface of tissue cells.

Ahlquist emphatically argues there are two classes of adrenergic receptors, alpha and beta, which possess both excitatory and inhibitory functional capabilities. He offers experimental data demonstrating alpha receptors are most associated with excitatory functions of vasoconstriction and pupil dilation and the inhibitory function of intestinal relaxation. Beta receptors are most associated with the excitatory function of myocardial stimulation and the inhibitory function of vasodilatation (1948)[217].

In the same landmark paper, Ahlquist further argues the dogma of two adrenergic neuro-hormones, one excitatory one excitatory e.g. sympathin E and sympathin I is simply incorrect. The excitatory or inhibitory function is determined by the receptor not the chemical substance. He drives home his point noting the diverse effects of acetylcholine within the autonomic systems has always been ascribed to differences in the receptors and never to an excitatory or inhibitory neuro-hormone (1948)[217].

Ahlquist revolutionizes the conceptual matrix of autonomic pharmacology. The new matrix is the basis for most all therapeutic pharmacological agents introduced, effecting adrenergic autonomic system functions during the next seventy years and to present. Think about it when you are sitting in your pharmacology class or prescribing a medication to control cardiac output or lower blood pressure; injecting epinephrine (adrenaline) into your patient's IV, following a cardiac arrest to stimulate contraction of cardiac muscles; prescribing an alpha blocker to decrease peripheral vascular resistance and lower blood pressure; or prescribe an alpha agonist to increase blood pressure in your hypotensive patient.

Medical students and assistant professors take comfort; rejection is part of the academic process. Ahlquist's seminal paper challenging medical dogma, introducing alpha and beta receptors and laying the foundation upon which much of modern adrenergic pharmacology rest is immediately rejected for publication by the editors of the "Journal of Pharmacology and Experimental Therapeutics" (JPET). The paper is also submitted to the American Society for Pharmacology and Experimental Therapeutics (ASPET) for consideration of the Society's newly established John J. Abel Award in Pharmacology. The John J. Abel Award is established to recognize independence of thought by young investigators, resulting in original, outstanding research in the field of pharmacology or experimental therapeutics. Ahlquist's submission is not selected and the 1948 John J. Able Award in Pharmacology is presented to J. Garrott Allen. (1912-1992) for outstanding work in the area of irradiation injury.

In the words of Raymond Ahlquist himself, his innovative and now landmark paper in medical pharmacology, at the time it is written is "… a loser…", noting its initial rejection for publication and failure to be selected for the John J. Able Award (1978)[220]. Only with the assistance and political influence of a personal friend, noted physiologist William Hamilton (1893-1964) is the paper finally accepted for publication, five years after its original submission, and appears in the "American Journal of Physiology" (1948)[217]. Initial reaction to the paper by the established academic and medical communities is best described as overwhelmingly reserved. Another 10 years will pass before the paper's seminal contributions are widely accepted. Adrenergic pharmacology is changed forever or at least until you or someone else offers an alternative conceptual matrix.

The second half of 1900s witness the first electrical recordings of electrochemical activity occurring at the neuromuscular junction, which provides essential data in explaining the mechanisms of action of signal transmission between neurons and skeletal muscle cells; introduction of pharmaceuticals formulated specifically to alter brain chemistry, for the treatment of severe mental disorders and to enhance normal brain activity; recognition Parkinson's disease results in part from reduced dopamine activity occurring in the midbrain, which can be replenished with a pharmaceutical and typically produces significant improvement in clinical signs and symptoms; understanding of role of prostaglandins within a matrix of anti-inflammatory processes, at the cellular level; introduction of non-steroidal anti-inflammatory drugs (NSAIDs), based upon an understanding of prostaglandins; first antiviral pharmaceuticals introduced into the marketplace; discovery of G-protein second messenger systems and their role in cell signaling; understanding of the role of histamine in gastrointestinal disorders; introduction of pharmaceuticals to block specific gastrointestinal receptors offering relief for millions from gastrointestinal distress; first understanding of nitric oxide's role in cell signaling, especially in the cardiovascular system, resulting in the introduction of innovative pharmaceuticals for treatment of cardiovascular disease; investigation of serotonin's role in mood disorders, resulting in the introduction of selective serotonin reuptake inhibitors (SSRIs); introduction of brain enhancing pharmaceutical widely prescribed for students and young professional trying to get ahead in competitive academic or professional environments; and investigations into the interactions of genetic materials with pharmaceutical agents in efforts to personalize pharmaceutical treatments based upon an individual's unique genetic composition.

Bernard Katz (1911-2003) German physiologist with colleague's British neuroscientist Paul Fatt (1924-2014) and Spanish neurophysiologist Jose del Castillo (1920-2002) introduce the necessary electrophysiological technologies and conceptual matrix to explain cell to cell signaling occurring at the neuromuscular junction. Building upon the work of others, who have previously demonstrated the role of acetylcholine in neuromuscular transmission, Katz, Fatt, and del Castillo eloquently describe mechanisms of action responsible for the pre-synaptic release of acetylcholine, post-synaptic binding to receptors, and enzymatic degradation. Their innovative cellular recording technologies offer opportunities to investigate the roles of intra-cellular and extra-cellular ions before, during, and after signaling transmission (1951,1952,1954,1956)[221,222,223,224]. Their work lay the foundation for understanding normal neuromuscular synaptic transmission at the chemical level and guide the rational introduction of new pharmaceuticals designed to effect neuromuscular signaling.

Bernard Katz shares the 1970 Nobel Prize in Medicine or Physiology with Swedish pharmacologist Ulf von Euler (1905-1983) and American biochemist Julieus Axelrod (1912-2014) "… for their discoveries concerning the humoral transmitters in the nerve terminals and the mechanism for their storage, release and inactivation..." (1970)[225].

Let us briefly explore the origins of a handful of representative pharmaceuticals, introduced into the market during the 1950s, specifically warfarin (Coumadin), clorpromazine (Thorazine), monoamine oxidase inhibitors (MAOI), tricyclic antidepressants (TCA) imipramine (Tofranil), and methylphenidate (Ritalin).

Karl Link (1901-1978) American biochemist and graduate student working at the University of Wisconsin, first synthesize warfarin and secures its patent, as an effective rat poison (1947)[226]. Seven years later, warfarin (Coumadin) is approved by the FDA for use in humans as a safe and effective oral anticoagulant, effective in the treatment and management of thrombosis and embolism (1954,1956)[227,228]. Warfarin complements heparin, the prototypical IV anticoagulant discovered 38 years earlier by second semester medical student Jay McLean (1916)[185] and offers a relatively safe and effective oral anticoagulant during the mid-1950s. Warfarin (Coumadin) continues to be used today as an oral anticoagulant over 64 years after it is originally approved by the FDA. Recall, warfarin (Coumadin) achieves its therapeutic effect by blocking the formation of vitamin-K factors which are essential in the coagulation cascade and formation of blood clots.

Trivia: The name "warfarin" is derived from the foundation which funds much of the research leading to its use as an effective and safe anticoagulant in humans, the University of Wisconsin-Madison, Wisconsin Alumni Research Foundation (WARF).

Chlorpromazine (Thorazine) is introduced by the French pharmaceutical company Laboratories Rhone-Poulenc and released as a potentiator of general anesthesia for use with surgical patients (1952)[229]. The compound is soon recognized to lower body temperature during surgery (1952)[230]. This observation generates an application for treatment in patients presenting with debilitating agitation. Historically, agitated patients are oftentimes treated with exposure to cool water e.g. showers, ice packs, or cold sheet wraps in efforts to cool the body and reduce agitation. Following this logic, chlorpromazine is administered to a 24 year old, severely agitated, French, male, psychiatric inpatient at the Val de Grace military hospital, Paris, France (1952)[231]. Administration results in an immediate and calming effect.

Given its initial success in controlling agitation, chlorpromazine is soon administered to a group of 38 psychotic inpatients at Saint-Anne's Hospital in Paris and generates uniformly encouraging results (1952)[232]. This group study spurs the investigation of chlorpromazine as an effective antipsychotic pharmaceutical treatment, around the world; Italy (1952)[233], Switzerland (1953)[234], Canada (1954)[235], England (1954)[236], Germany, (1954)[237], USA (1954)[238], and Australia (1955)[239]. Clear evidence of its clinical efficacy as an antipsychotic is established by the mid-1950s, however the pharmacology of chlorpromazine, including its primary mechanism of action, blockade of brain dopamine receptors, is not understood until the early-1960s (1963)[240]. Once the pharmacology of chlorpromazine is established, new doors open for the rational development of newer antipsychotic pharmacological treatments with fewer unwanted side effects.

Monoamine oxidase inhibitors (MAOI) are a class of pharmaceuticals representative of medications introduced originally for the treatment of one disorder, which prove effective in the treatment of an entirely different disorder. The MAOIs are introduced during the early-1950s as an effective treatment for tuberculosis (TB), based upon their ability to interfere with the synthesis of the cell walls of the bacterium mycobacterium tuberculosis. This represents the rational application of a pharmaceutical based upon an a priori understanding of the compound's biological actions. However, the MAOIs are soon recognized to have additional unanticipated effects, characterized by increased sense of vitality, energy, increased appetite, weight gain, improved sleep, and euphoric mood in TB patients treated with a MAOI (1952,1953, 1957)[241,242,243]. These unanticipated side effects lead to initial experimental investigations evaluating the value of MAOI as potential agents to be used in the treatment of psychiatric disorders, specifically depression (1953,1958)[244,245].

Given the demonstrated clinical effectiveness of the MAOIs, coupled with a fundamental understanding of the pharmacology of these compounds, the monoamine models of depression are founded. These models emphasize the role of MAOI to increase brain serotonin and norepinephrine levels by interfering with the enzymatic breakdown of these two important brain neurotransmitters.

Tricyclic antidepressants (TCA) e.g. imipramine (Tofranil) are introduced during the late-1950s. TCAs represent another grouping of pharmaceuticals, originally designed and marketed for one purpose and proves unsuccessful, only later to be recognized to have therapeutic benefits for an entirely different purpose. TCAs are originally formulated, produced, and marketed by the large international Swiss pharmaceutical company J. R. Geigy AG as sedatives. The application fails and these compounds are warehoused for fifty years. In an effort to compete with Rhone-Poulenc's recently released chlorpromazine and having a similar chemical structure to the antipsychotic, clinical trials are initiated in Switzerland to evaluate their effectiveness as a sedating antipsychotic. Findings from the clinical trials reveal the compound has no value as an antipsychotic. However, the compound unexpectedly demonstrates impressive improvement in the mood of severely depressed hospitalized patients (1957,1958)[246,247].

Clinical testing in Canada, USA, and throughout Europe soon confirms the antidepressant properties of the TCA (1958,1959)[248,249]. The mechanism of action responsible for the antidepressant effects are identified several years later; reduced reuptake of norepinephrine into the presynaptic neuron, making more brain neurotransmitter available for cell to cell signaling. The TCAs provide additional confirmation to the validity of the recently proposed catecholamine-deficient hypothesis of depression, formulated in post hoc efforts to explain the anti-depressive therapeutic effect of the TCAs.

Methylphenidate (Ritalin) is first synthesized in 1944 and formulated to treat depression and chronic fatigue (1944)[250]. Eleven years later it is approved by the United States FDA for treatment of attention-deficit hyperactivity disorder (ADHD) (1955)[251]. The mechanism of action is similar to other amphetamines, increasing the release of presynaptic catecholamines norepinephrine and dopamine from brain presynaptic neurons, increasing the amount of catecholamines in the synaptic space, and altering normal brain cell to cell signaling. This pharmaceutical, like other amphetamines, increase mental alertness in most all and decreases distractibility in some. Ritalin is widely prescribed in the USA to school age children during the second half of the 1900s, in efforts by parents and physicians to enhance normal brain function, improve academic performance, and control disruptive hyperactive behaviors.

Trivia: Ritalin, the trademark name for methylphenidate, is named for the wife of the chemist who first synthesizes the compound. Her name, Marguerite Panizzon (Rita) (2008)[252].

Medical pharmacology during the 1950s is characterized by much interest in developing and releasing pharmaceuticals which can be used in the treatment and management of severe mental disorders. Few medications are available for the treatment of mental disorders before the 1950s. Pharmaceutical companies in the USA and Europe are motivated by potentially huge profit margins and physicians motivated by efforts to alleviate pain and suffering of debilitating mental disorders. Most of the pharmaceuticals released are based upon demonstrated empirical clinical efficacy with little or no understanding, by the pharmaceutical companies or prescribing physician, as to the underlying mechanisms of action producing the therapeutic effect. The mindset is very much, if it works use it; we can identify why and how it works later. Significant and rapid advances in the treatment of severe mental disorders are achieved during the 1950s. The pharmacology of the pharmaceuticals is understood much later and more slowly.

Medical treatments available to patients suffering severe mental disorders change dramatically, during the 1950s. Pharmaceuticals are introduced and displace many conventional treatments typically used to treat patients suffering severe mental disorders e.g. "sleep cures" (1900, 1922)[253,254], psychoanalysis (1921)[255], electroconvulsive shock therapies (1940)[256], and surgical trans-orbital leucotomies (1937,1944)[257,258]. Emphasis is now placed on altering brain chemistries. New technologies permit, for the first time ever, reliable measurement of small amounts of brain neurotransmitters and their metabolites e.g. spectrophotofluorimetry (1955)[259]. Focused areas of specialization begin to appear within medical pharmacology e.g. psychopharmacology and neuropharmacology. Rapid advances are being made in the identification of pharmaceuticals which demonstrate clinical benefits in the treatment and management of severe psychiatric disorders. However, understanding the pharmacology, underlying the benefits proceed much more slowly.

Julius Axelrod (1912-2004) American biochemist challenges medical pharmacology dogma during the mid-1950s and proposes a new and innovative mechanism of action to explain the removal of brain neurotransmitters released into the synaptic clef. Dogma of the period states all known brain neurotransmitters e.g. norepinephrine, epinephrine, serotonin, glutamate, acetylcholine, and GABA are removed from the synaptic cleft by enzymatic action, similar in kind to that of acetylcholine at the peripheral neuromuscular junction. Axelrod proposes an innovative alternative and offers experimental data in support. Axelrod proposes the catecholamines norepinephrine and dopamine are not removed primarily by enzymatic action, but rather by reuptake by the presynaptic neuron (1961,1966,1971)[260,261,262]. This is a big deal. It revolutionizes the way in which we think about neurotransmitter cell to cell signaling in the brain, opens new lines of investigations as to the mechanisms of action underlying brain pathologies, especially mental disorders, and offers a rational basis for the introduction of new pharmaceuticals which have primary sites of action located in the brain.

Axelrod extends his investigation to understand the mechanisms of action responsible for removing catecholamines, during peripheral sympathetic neuron to target tissues signaling and removing catecholamines when circulating throughout the body via the systemic blood supply, as endocrine cell signaling substances e.g. norepinephrine and epinephrine. Soon he provides the answer. The primary mechanisms of action for removing catecholamines is reuptake by the pre-synaptic neuron, however, there is an additional enzymatic secondary mechanism of action resulting in local degradation (1957,1958)[263,264]. Axelrod discovers and names the enzyme, now familiar to all medical students, COMT, catechol-O-methyl transferase (1959)[265]. Circulating catecholamines are ultimately removed from the system by renal excretion.

Trivia: Julieus Axelrod's application to medical school admission is rejected in 1933. He is denied promotions at the National Institutes of Health (NIH) for failure to have the required doctorate degree, although his original and innovative contributions greatly exceed others around him, whom do have the requisite professional M.D. degree.

Axelrod discovers and describes the metabolic pathway resulting in the now very recognizable analgesic effects of acetaminophen (Tylenol) (1948,1948)[266,267]. Axelrod's many additional contributions are formally recognized by the professional scientific community in 1970 with the award of the 1970 Nobel Prize in Physiology or Medicine. He shares the Prize with Bernard Katz (first to describe neuromuscular transmission (1956)[224]) and Ulf von Euler (first to discover prostaglandins (1935)[268]) "… for their discoveries concerning the humoral transmitters in the nerve terminals and the mechanism for their storage, release and inactivation…" (1970)[269]. Not too bad for someone who cannot get into medical school and is denied career promotions. Right?

Earl Sutherland (1915-1974), Theodore Rall (1928-2015) American pharmacologists, and Jacques Berthet (1926-2013) Belgian pharmacologist, working at Case Western Reserve University-School of Medicine's Department of Pharmacology, Cleveland Ohio, introduce the concept of second messengers systems, a previously unrecognized mechanism contributing to cell to cell signal transmission. To date, only surface receptors on cell membranes are recognized in signal transmission. Sutherland and Rall, while studying mechanisms of signaling between hormones and target tissues e.g. epinephrine and liver, recognize, describe, and are first to report the role of cAMP (cyclic adenosine monophosphate) as a second messenger system (1958,1958)[270,271].

Briefly, epinephrine when binding to liver tissues increases the intracellular level of cAMP which leads to conversion of inactive phosphorylase to an active enzyme, which then leads to the breakdown of stored glycogen, resulting in the release of the energy rich molecule glucose (glycogenolysis). The hormone epinephrine (first messenger) stimulates the release of intracellular cAMP (second messenger), which begins the intracellular biochemical pathway reactions which result in the final action of the tissue cells', release of glucose (1957,1958,1958,1963)[272,270,271,273]. Hormone-effector tissue signal transmissions are now understood within the matrix of second messenger cAMP systems. Earl Sutherland is awarded the 1971 Nobel Prize in Medicine or Physiology "…for his discoveries concerning the mechanisms of the action of hormones…" (1971)[274].

Arvid Carlsson (1923-2018) and Nils-Ake Hillarp (1916-1965) Swedish pharmacologists introduce and develop technologies capable of quantifying small amounts of catecholamines in biological tissues (1959)[275]. Of particular initial interests are norepinephrine and epinephrine. Carlsson and Hillarp discover central and peripheral catecholamine levels are reduced following administration of reserpine (1956,1957a,1957b)[276,277,278]. Reserpine, an alkaloid (Rauwolfia serpentine -Indian snake root) is being used during the mid-1950s as an antipsychotic and antihypertensive pharmaceutical. Its primary mechanism of action is to interfere with the neuron's ability to store norepinephrine inside of the neuron, thereby reducing the amount of neurotransmitter available for release into the synaptic clef.

Carlsson and Hillarp apply their innovative measurement technology and demonstrate different regions of the brain contain different levels of catecholamines. The basal nuclei are identified to contain particularly high levels of dopamine when compared with other brain areas. Animals administered reserpine demonstrate Parkinson's disease like signs. The Parkinsonism is reversed when the animals are administered L-dopa, a dopamine precursor compound, which crosses the blood brain barrier and elevates dopamine levels in brain (1956,1958,1959)[276,279,275]. Carlsson and colleagues soon propose L-dopa to be a potential pharmacological agent for use in the treatment of Parkinson's disease (1958)[279]. This proposal and their supporting experimental data change the treatment of Parkinson's disease forever. Their findings provide evidence in support of the recently recognized role of brain signaling substances (neurotransmitters) in regard to normal brain functioning, brain pathologies, and pharmaceutical treatments which alter brain chemistries.

Medical pharmacology redirects its focus during the 1960s away from the brain and to understanding the mechanisms of actions underlying tissue inflammation, heart disease, lung disease, and the pharmacology of rationally derived pharmaceutical treatments of these conditions.

Tissue inflammation is understood to be initiated and sustained through local chemical mediators such as prostaglandins, prostacyclins, interleukins, leukotrines, thromboxane, histamine, and bradykinin. The earlier recognition and mapping of the biochemical pathways producing these chemical mediators (1935,1962)[280,281] lead to the introduction of new non-steroidal anti-inflammatory drugs (NSAIDs) during the l960s e.g. indomethacin (1963)[282] and ibuprofen (1968)[283]. The agents are marketed as non-steroidal anti-inflammatory agents with particular efficacy in the treatment of rheumatoid arthritis and gout. The mechanisms of action of these early NSAIDs are discovered in the late-1960s (1969)[284] and open the doors for the development of more selective NSAIDs e.g. selective COX-2 inhibitors.

John Vane (1927-2004) English pharmacologist and colleagues are instrumental in identifying the mechanisms of action underlying the anti-inflammatory properties of the NSAIDs (1969)[284]. NSAIDs interfere with the synthesis of prostaglandins by interfering with the rate limiting biochemical step, mediated by the enzyme cyclooxygenase and necessary for the conversion of an omega 6 essential fatty acid (arachidonic acid) into prostaglandins (1969,1971)[284,285]. Interfering with the synthesis of the chemical mediators of inflammation e.g. prostaglandin, reduce the amount and effect of the mediator, thereby reducing inflammation in biological tissues. Adrenal steroids have long been known to reduce prostaglandin synthesis and consequently reduce inflammation; however steroids accomplish this by a mechanism of action distinctly different than the NSAIDs. Steroids depress prostaglandin synthesis by blocking the release of omega 6 essential fatty acids (arachidonic acid) from phospholipids, whereas NSAIDs interfere with the enzymatic conversion of omega 6 essential fatty acids (aracachidonic acid) into prostaglandins. John Vane shares the 1982 Nobel Prize in Physiology or Medicine with Sune Bergstrom (1916- 2004) and

Bengt Samuelsson (1934-) for "…their discoveries concerning prostaglandins and related biologically active substances…" (1982)[286].

NSAIDs are aggressively investigated, modified, and marketed by large pharmaceutical companies for the next 50 years. The early NSAIDs are soon structurally modified to be more specific, moving from nonspecific inhibitors of cycloxygenase (COX) to being able to selectively inhibit specific subtypes of cycloxygenase e.g. COX-2. Recall, COX-1 is critical for the synthesis of prostaglandins that regulate body functions such as protection of the lining of the GI tract, whereas COX-2 is critical for the synthesis of prostaglandins which serve as mediators of inflammatory cells and tissue inflammation. By 1999 NSAIDs are produced which selectively block COX-2. The popular and extremely profitable COX- 2 inhibitor celeoxib (Celebrex) with an excess of 100 million prescriptions written in the USA alone each year and generating over 3 billion dollars a year in sales, demonstrates anti-inflammatory equal to non-specific COX inhibitors e.g. aspirin, ibuprofen, while producing fewer unwanted gastrointestinal side effects (2000)[287].

Ibuprofen (Brufen, Motrin, Advil) a non-selective inhibitor of prostaglandin synthesis is formulated and patented in 1961 by the United Kingdom based company Boots Pharmaceuticals (1961)[288]. The formulation is developed as part of the Company's research efforts to formulate their own, patentable formulation of aspirin. This new NSAID is released in February 1969, under the brand name Brufen, into the UK market, requiring a physician's prescription and as an anti-inflammatory agent, useful in the treatment of rheumatoid arthritis. Five years later it is released into the USA market, under the brand name Motrin, with recommendations for use in the treatment of rheumatoid arthritis, menstrual pain (dysmenorrhea), relief of minor pains due to headaches, muscle aches, and common cold, and to assist in the temporary reduction of fevers (1974)[289]. Ibuprofen represents one of the first, non-selective (COX-1 and COX-2) inhibitor NSAIDs.

Heart disease attracts much attention during the 1960s. Two particularly notable pharmaceuticals are introduced to assist physicians with its treatment and management, Furosemide (Lasix) and Propranolol (Inderal). Recall, heart disease encompasses a large number of specific conditions and which share in common an inability of the heart to pump sufficient blood to supply body tissues. The patient complains of shortness of breath, swelling in the lower extremities, and exercise intolerance.

Furosemide (Lasix) a powerful loop diuretic is introduced first into Germany and Italy in 1963 and three years later into the USA market in 1966, as a useful pharmaceutical in the treatment of edema, congestive heart failure (CHF), and hypertension (1966)[290]. Recall, loop diuretics have their primary effect at the thick ascending loops of Henle in the kidney, where they block Na+/K+/2Cl- co-transporter systems. The effect is to reduce reabsorption of fluid and electrolytes from the kidney back into the systemic blood supply, thereby eliminating large quantities of fluid and electrolytes from the body in urine (1965)[291]. Eliminating blood volume reduces total peripheral resistance and your patient's blood pressure goes down. This pharmaceutical works great as a diuretic but can you see any potential problems? Think about the loss of electrolytes eliminated from the body in urine.

Propranolol (Inderal) is the first non-selective beta blocker introduced. It is introduced first into the UK market in 1964 and three years later into the USA market following FDA approval in 1967 (1967)[292]. This prototypical class of new pharmaceuticals proves to be effective in the treatment of heart disease. Propranolol is particularly usefulness in the management of angina (chest pains due to reduced oxygen to heart tissues), hypertension (high blood pressure), myocardial infarctions (heart attacks), arrhythmias (irregular heartbeats), and congestive heart failure (heart cannot pump enough blood to the rest of the body). Propranolol decreases cardiac output by slowing conduction from the SA through the AV node. Slowing conduction results in slowing of the heart rate. Propranolol additionally decreases the force of contraction of the cardiac ventricles, further reducing cardiac output. Propranolol is a non-selective blocker of all adrenergic receptors, beta-1, beta-2, alpha-1, and alpha-2, however its primary therapeutic effect is generated from its effect on the beta-1 receptor system.

Recall, beta blockers as a group of pharmaceuticals produce their desired therapeutic effects and oftentimes undesirable side effects by interfering with normal cell to cell signaling, mediated by the sympathetic autonomic nervous system. Norepinephrine is the primary neurotransmitter released from post-ganglionic sympathetic system neurons onto target tissues e.g. heart. Additionally, beta blockers interfere with cell to cell signaling, mediated by the neuroendocrine systems e.g. hormone epinephrine, released from the adrenal gland into the systemic blood supply, effecting alpha and beta adrenergic receptor systems, located throughout the body. Beta blockers represent a new class of pharmaceuticals, reflecting an innovative approach to the treatment and management of heart disease, distinctively different from diuretics.

James Black (1924-2010) Scottish pharmacologist working with the British pharmaceutical company Imperial Chemicals Industries builds upon the conceptual matrix proposed by American pharmacologist Raymond Ahlquist (1948)[217] and formulates propranolol (Inderal) (1962,1965, 1968)[293,294,295]. The initial formulation is soon modified due to its demonstrated carcinogenic effects in animals, however the fundamental and rational principle of blocking beta adrenergic receptors remains unchanged. Remember, while both beta-1 and beta-2 receptors are blocked, it is the beta-1 receptors located in the heart which are most responsible for the therapeutic effect.

An initial understanding of the mechanisms of action underlying propranolol and similar non-selective adrenergic receptor blockers steers James Black and Smith Kline Beecham Corporation researchers, British medicinal chemists Graham Durnat (1934-2009), John Emmett (1939-), and Robin Ganellin (1934-) to formulate a new pharmaceutical, which blocks histamine (H-2) receptors. The new pharmaceutical is cimetidine (Tagamet). Cimetidine is effective in the treatment of GI ulcers and gastroesophageal reflux disease. The formulation and development of cimetidine represents a radically different approach in the development of new pharmaceuticals. Conventionally, a new drug is formulated based upon a fortuitous discovery of a plant's ability to effect a treatment result. The active ingredient is identified, extracted, and tested in multiple compound formulations for clinical effectiveness. Often the mechanism of action responsible for producing the clinical effect is unknown. The drug is released for clinical use and only later is the mechanism of actions identified.

However with cimetidine, the process originates from a conceptual understanding of the biological mechanisms responsible for the production of acid secretion in the GI system and therefore the suspected cause of potentially life threatening gastric ulcers. The histamine molecule is identified as necessary for acid secretion in the GI system. Working within the conceptual matrix, acid is responsible for the GI irritation resulting in ulcers; then blocking the histamine receptor that mediates acid secretion should decreased acid release and gastric ulcers. By systematic testing a series of H-2 receptor antagonists (H2 blockers) the most therapeutically effective and with fewest unwanted side effects is identified and selected for marketing (1972,1978)[296,297]. This represents a revolutionary change in the way new pharmaceuticals are created. This rational method of pharmaceutical development continues to be applied by most large pharmaceutical companies today. Cimetidine becomes the first pharmaceutical to exceed 1 billion dollars in sales.

James Black shares the 1988 Nobel Prize in Physiology or Medicine with American pharmacologist Gertrude Elion (1918-1999) and American chemist George Hitchings (1905-1998) "…for their discoveries of important principals for drug treatment…" (1981)[298]. James Black is instrumental in the formulation of the H2 receptor blocker Tagamet. George Hitchings and Gertrude Elion are responsible for several additional and familiar pharmaceuticals, such as allopurinol for the management of gout and acyclovir for management of viral herpes. Perhaps it is time for a brief side note on vocabulary.

If you are like most medical students, you often believe you understand a term when in fact you really don't. What is the definition of a pharmaceutical drug? True it is a medication intended for use "…in the diagnosis, cure, mitigation, treatment, cure, or prevention of disease in man or other animals…" (2018)[299]. This is the definition of a medicinal drug. But what makes a drug a pharmaceutical drug? Pharmaceutical drugs are manufactured. Raw materials, either natural or synthesized moved through a process during which they are combined or modified or both to create a final product. All pharmaceutical drugs are drugs but not all drugs are pharmaceuticals.

Pharmaceutical drug products contain two component ingredients; active pharmacological ingredients (API) and excipients. API gives medicinal drugs their therapeutic properties. Excipients are the chemical components of medicinal drugs other than API e.g. diluents, fillers, surfactants, lubricants, disintegrants, viscosity enhancers, binders, and adhesives.

Pharmaceutical drugs are commonly classified for clinical use according to the organ system upon which they have their primary effects e.g. cardiovascular, respiratory, gastrointestinal systems. Alternatively, pharmaceutical drugs are classified according to their primary therapeutic effect e.g. analgesic (reduces pain), antipyretic (reduces fever), antibiotic (reduces bacteria). Other classification systems are based upon chemical ingredients, molecular structure, or mechanism of action e.g. propranolol hydrochloride, $C_{16}H_{21}NO_2.HCL$, beta adrenergic receptor blocker.

One system, the Anatomical Therapeutic Chemical Classification System (ATC), first introduced during the late-1960s and now regulated by the World Health Organization (WHO) combines elements of the above systems into one integrated system (2012)[300]. Therapeutic drugs are coded into groups at five levels. Level 1 defines the organ or system on which the drug principally acts, Level 2 defines therapeutic group, Level 3 defines the pharmacological subgroup, Level 4 defines chemical subgroups, and Level 5 defines the chemical substance. For example propranolol, a non-selective beta blocker is coded "C07AA, propranolol" within the ATC system. C defines the cardiovascular system, 07 defines it as a beta blocking agent, A defines it as a subtype of beta blocking agent without combination with diuretics, other vasodilators, or antihypertensive agents, the second A defines it as a non-selective beta blocker, and propranolol defines the specific chemical substance. The System provides a global standard for classifying medical substances and facilitates international exchange of information using a uniform matrix. The WHO first utilizes an early version of the ATC system to reveals marked variability in drug utilization and consumption between European countries during 1966-1967 (1968)[301].

To deal with variabilities in traditional units of measurements, a technical unit of measurement called the Defined Daily Dose (DDD) and defined as the average maintenance does per day for a drug used for its main indication in adults, is introduced and is now a part of the ATC system (ATC/DDD). The system is routinely used in drug utilizations studies worldwide and provides a standardization which facilitates the international exchange of information by using a uniform matrix.

The important point here is not the classification system itself but rather what the classification system represents within the context of the maturation of medical pharmacology as a scientific based professional discipline. Every professional discipline proceeds through a series of developmental events which define the discipline and mark its maturation. Standardization of terms to facilitate the exchange of new information is one such milestone (1962)[302].

OK…back to the history of medical pharmacology during the 1960s.

Albuterol (Ventolin) is introduced into the U.K. in 1968 and approved by the U.S. FDA for release into the U.S. market in 1981 (1981)[303]. It is an inhaled, short acting beta-2 adrenergic receptor agonist, effective in providing symptom relief to patients suffering bronchospasm associated with asthma or chronic obstructive pulmonary disease (COPD). This pharmaceutical builds upon the increased understanding of autonomic physiology and autonomic cell to cell signaling during the past thirty years and at least another two thousand year history of empirically derived treatments for asthma, which stimulate beta receptors e.g. plant based ephedrine treatments. Albuterol is released into the market without completely understanding its mechanisms of action, typical of many pharmaceutical of the period. Later the primary mechanism of action is discovered. At the cellular level it increases cAMP in the smooth muscle cells of the pulmonary air conducting system via a systems signaling system. At the functional level, it opens the conducting pathways, making it easier to breathe.

The 1970s redirect pharmacological investigations away from the NSAIDs, adrenergic and histamine blocking pharmaceuticals, popular during the 1960s, to investigations focused on understanding and subsequently manufacturing antiviral pharmaceuticals. The goal is simple; "…develop antiviral agents that are specific for the inhibition of viral multiplication without effecting normal cell division…" (1971)[304].

Acyclovir is one of the most effective and exciting prototypical selective antivirals produced during the late-1970s and based upon a rational understanding as to how viruses replicate. Acyclovir is a potent inhibitor of herpes virus replication (1977,1978)[305,306]. It is released commercially in 1982 immediately following FDA approval. Acyclovir is initially FDA approved for treatment of genital herpes (HSV2), shingles (VZV, aka HHV3), chickenpox (VZV, aka HHV3), and cold sores (HSV1) (1982)[307]. Soon Acyclovir demonstrates effectiveness against Epstein-Barr virus (1983)[308] and cytomegaloviruses (1985)[309]. The mechanism of action of acyclovir is that it acts as a specific inhibitor of herpes virus DNA polymerase (1983)[310]. More specifically, acyclovir is monophosphorylated by the herpes' enzyme thymidine kinase. This product is then di- and triphosphoylated by the host cell. The active triphosphate form of acyclovir is then incorporated into the viral DNA, causing premature DNA chain termination (2000)[311]. The virus is now unable to replicate itself. Simply an elegant system and rational pharmaceutical treatment.

The conceptual matrix upon which the development of acyclovir is based provides the foundation for many new antiviral pharmaceuticals introduced and developed during the late-1900s. Simply stated, inhibit a step in viral replication and you can control the virus. The specific manners in which pharmaceuticals interfere with the replication process varies, however the fundamental principle remains the same.

The 1980s offer a more complete understanding of second messenger systems and their roles in cell to cell signaling. G-protein mediated systems are understood within their structural organization e.g. alpha, beta, and gamma subunits, biochemical activity, and functions. Nitric oxide is understood within the matrix of paracrine signaling and influence relevant to the cardiovascular system. Selective serotonin reuptake inhibitors (SSRI) are introduced and change the pharmacological treatment of mood disorders for the next 30 years.

Martin Rodbell (1925-1998) and Alfred Gilman (1941-2015) American biochemists develop the G-protein mediated model of cell signaling. The model provides a new way to understand cell signaling (1980)[312]. No longer is cell signaling restricted to ligands binding membrane bound receptors. With the introduction and development of G-protein mediated systems, cell signaling is understood to include membrane bound receptors and a series of intracellular biochemical reactions. It is well known at this time, cell to cell signaling is accomplished by substances released from neurons (neurotransmitters) and glands (hormones) which bind to receptors on target tissue cells; however, how cells transduce the signaling substances from outside of the cell to inside of the cell and generate the effect of cell action is limited (1964,1965,1966)[313,314,315]. G-protein mediation, as a second messenger system begins to offer answers. G-protein mediated cell signaling systems explains much unexplained by membrane bound ligand-receptor models alone, offer insight into numerous pathologies which result from abnormal cell signaling e.g. diabetes, mood disorders, disorders of metabolism, and offers medical pharmacology a rational matrix within which to understand cell to cell signaling and therapeutic pharmaceuticals which modify cell signaling past, present, and future.

Martin Rodbell's contributions are built upon earlier investigation proposing G-protein mediated second messenger systems by other investigators (1969)[316]. Rodbell's conceptualization of a new second messenger system, innovative methods, and persuasive data clearly establish the role of guanosine triphosphate (GTP) in hormonal activation of adenylyl cyclase and the series of molecular events underlying G-protein mediated cell to cell signal transmission (1971a,1971b, 1971c,1974,1985)[317,318,319,320,321].

Alfred Gilman's contributions are exemplified in his recognition and description of the biochemical process responsible for G-protein mediated signal transmission, isolating the alpha, beta, and gamma subunits proposed by Martin Rodbell, subtyping G-proteins into Gs, Gi, and Gq, describing the biochemistry responsible for initiating, transducing, and terminating signal transmission of G-protein mediated systems, and developing the necessary molecular techniques which persuasively demonstrate G-proteins are necessary for hormone action (1978,1983)[322,323].

Martin Rodbell and Alfred Gilman are awarded the 1994 Nobel Prize in Physiology or Medicine "…for their discovery of G-proteins and the role of these proteins in signal transduction in cell…" (1994)[324].

Trivia: The term "G-proteins" is coined by Martin Rodbell in 1969 to describe the anticipated protein subunits, alpha, beta, and gamma, which bind intracellular guanosine diphosphate (GDP) and triphosphate (GTP), essential to the process of transducing signals across the cell.

Fred Murad (1936-), Louis Ignarro (1941-) American pharmacologists, and Robert Furchgott (1916-2009) American biochemist offer the necessary conceptual matrix and experimental data, within which to understand paracrine signaling in relaxing vascular smooth muscles. Fred Murad provides the conceptual matrix and experimental data which explains the physiological mechanism regulating smooth muscle contractions (1977a,1977b)[325,326]. Robert Furchgott is first to identify the endogenous paracrine substance responsible for regulating smooth muscle relaxation in vascular muscle and names the substance endothelium-relaxing factor (EDRF) (1980)[327]. Louis Ignarro is studying nitric oxide (NO) and recognizes it too relaxes vascular smooth muscles. Furchgott and Ignarro soon recognize the two substances EDRF and NO to be the same substance (1986,1987)[328,329]. In combination, Murad, Furchgott, and Ignarro explain the biochemical actions which underlay the clinically well-known capabilities of nitroglycerin to relax vascular smooth muscles, especially in the clinical treatment of angina. Physicians have been prescribing nitroglycerine for angina for over 100 years. Murad, Furchgott, and Ignarro now provide the answer as to how nitroglycerin accomplishes vasodilatation and its associated clinical therapeutic effects.

Recall, nitroglycerin relaxes vascular smooth muscles by conversion into nitric oxide and the associated elevation of intracellular cyclic guanosine monophosphate (cGMP) levels in the smooth muscle. The increase in cGMP leads to dephosphorization of the myosin light chains, resulting in smooth muscle relaxation (2000)[311].

Robert Furchgott, Fred Murad, and Louis Ignarro are recognized for their contributions and awarded the 1998 Nobel Prize in Physiology or Medicine "…for their discoveries concerning nitric oxide as a signaling molecule in the cardiovascular system…" (1998)[330].

The discovery and understanding of NO introduces a newly recognized biological system with immediate applications to medical pharmacology. Beyond the immediately recognizable advances in the management of cardiovascular disease, a popular pharmaceutical sildenafil (Viagra) is formulated based upon the understanding of NO and its role in relaxing vascular smooth muscle. The mechanism of action of sildenafil recall is to interfere with the enzymatic degradation of cGMP. This increases cGMP in the smooth vascular muscles producing vasodilatation. This increases blood flow to the corpus cavernosum and corpus spongiuosum (penis) in males and corpus cavernosum clitoridis in females, causing the erection.

Sildenafil (Viagra) is originally marketed by Pfizer pharmaceuticals in the U.K. for management of hypertension and angina pectoris. Phase I Clinical Testing (testing for safety in humans) demonstrate limited value in the management of angina, however it is quickly recognized to produce penile erections. Pfizer rethinks its marketing strategy and quickly decides to remarket sildenafil as a treatment for erectile dysfunction. It is patented in 1996 and within two years approved by the US FDA for treatment of erectile dysfunction. It is not long before the public recognizes sildenafil can be used to extend an erection in healthy males and joins a growing list of pharmaceuticals used for recreational purposes. Annual sales of sildenafil in the USA alone quickly peak to over 2 billion dollars a year.

Selective serotonin reuptake inhibitors (SSRIs) e.g. fluoxetine (Prozac) which is approved for the treatment of depression in December 1987 by the US FDA, represent medical pharmacology's continuing effort to develop rational pharmaceutical based treatments. Clinical trials testing during the mid-1980s demonstrate the clinical efficacy and value of these new antidepressants. Relief from suffering is provided to millions of patients. The conceptual matrix underlying the SSRIs is simple and based in the pharmacology of the 1950s. Mental disorders can and do result from disturbances in normal brain chemistries. Restore brain chemistries to normal levels and the mental disorders will resolve. Building upon the dogma of the period, a deficit monoamine model of depression, the SSRIs increase the amount of serotonin available in the synaptic cleft between brain neurons, thereby restoring the deficient amounts and returning brain chemistries to normal levels, producing the associated clinical improvements in mood and behavior (1969,1974, 1987)[331,332,333].

Models of psychopathology during the 1980s identify brain chemistries to be essential in the development, maintenance, and pharmacological treatment and typically emphasize a single or a single group of neurotransmitter systems e.g. norepinephrine, dopamine, or serotonin. The models emphasize either too much or too little neurotransmitter located in between brain neurons. Treatments are directed to blocking the neuron membrane receptor, as in the case of Thorazine; interfering with enzymatic degradation of the transmitter once inside of the synaptic clef, as in the case of the MAOIs; or blocking the presynaptic reuptake of the neurotransmitter into presynaptic neurons, as in the cases of Tofranil, Ritalin, and Prozac.

The 1990s offer investigations which further refine and detail membrane receptor pharmacology. Excitement in medical pharmacology builds during the 1990s, as the potential for manipulating genetic materials (DNA/RNA) with pharmaceuticals and offering specific, targeted pharmaceutical treatments, directed to an individual's unique DNA, captures the imaginations of investigators and clinicians alike.

Adderall (dextroamphetamine + amphetamine) is approved by the US FDA for use in the treatment and management of Attention Deficit Hyperactivity Disorder (1996)[334]. It proves extremely popular and prescribed to millions of school age children, enhancing academic performance. The mechanism of action is that of all other amphetamines, it increases the release of catecholamines from and blocks the reuptake of catecholamines dopamine and norepinephrine from pre-synaptic neurons, located in the brain, and interferes with the normal storage and enzymatic breakdown of the catecholamines inside of the neuron and in the synaptic clef. End result, it increase catecholamine levels in the brain. Pay attention. In patients with reduced catecholamine levels it helps restore a normal balance. In brains of individuals with normal brain chemistries, it transiently increases brain efficiency. Prior to the US FDA approval in 1996 for treatment of Attention Deficit Disorder, Adderall is marketed under the name of Obertol and used in the treatment and management of obesity, from the early-1960s to 1996. Adderall replaces Ritalin as the new and improved brain enhancer of the 1990s.

Donepezil (Aricept) is approved by the US FDA for the treatment and management of dementia of the Alzheimer's type (1996)[335]. It is one of the first pharmaceuticals developed out of a conceptual matrix which attempts to restore decreased levels of acetylcholine in the brains of patients suffering dementia of the Alzheimer's type. Its primary mechanism of action is to interfere with the enzymatic degradation of acetylcholine, once acetylcholine is released into the synaptic clef, between brain neurons. The rationale behind the use of this reversible acetylcholine esterase inhibitor is to increase levels of acetylcholine and return brain cell to cell signaling to normal. The model and pharmaceutical treatment are based upon the same conceptual matrix used for the past fifty years. That is, impaired brain functioning results from impaired brain chemistry, which involves a single neurotransmitter system, resulting in impaired cell to cell signaling, and which can be corrected by restoring the disordered neurotransmitter system to normal by increasing the amount of neurotransmitter in between neurons in the brain.

Aricept and other similar pharmaceuticals generate tremendous profits for the pharmaceutical companies, while attempting to meet the need for an effective pharmacological treatment of the dementias. The pharmaceutical is only partially effective and only in specific subtypes of dementia patients, suspected to be suffering Alzheimer's disease. However, its demonstrated limited effectiveness stimulates a reexamination of how we think about and treat dementia. New and innovative, alternative conceptual matrixes begin to emerge, offering welcomed and renewed hope for both patients and treating physicians.

In summary, the 1900s evidence tremendous advances in medical pharmacology as a professional scientific discipline. The first half of the 1900s witness the founding of professional societies in Europe and North America, committed to the advancement of medical pharmacology as a science based professional discipline. Scientific journals are founded and devoted to the international exchange of new knowledge in pharmacology. The chemoreceptor is discovered and its role in cell to cell signaling understood. Cell to cell signaling is recognized to be a chemical mediated process and a primary point of pharmacological treatment interventions. Heparin and insulin are discovered in university based research laboratories and quickly introduced into the practice of clinical medicine. Mathematical equations become a routine part of pharmacology. The FDA is founded and strives by way of governmental regulations to improve quality and safety of pharmaceutical drug products. Antibiotics are introduced into the market as effective treatments for bacterial infections. Germany and France take the lead, introducing sulfa drugs and the penicillins followed by North America with streptomycin and the tetracyclines. Antibiotics are understood within the matrix of their different primary sites and mechanisms of action. Chemotherapies are introduced into the treatments of cancers and are based upon rational conceptualizations of underlying pathological processes. Steroids are recognized to offer anti-inflammatory properties and prove effective in the management of rheumatoid arthritis. Alpha and beta adrenergic receptors are identified. These receptors are recognized to be key in determining whether an excitatory or inhibitory influence is effected on tissue cells. Cell to cell signaling within the autonomic nervous systems is understood.

The second half of the 1900s offers an understanding of the chemical processes of cell to cell signaling at the neuromuscular junction. Warfarin (Coumadin) is introduced as a new oral anticoagulant effective in the prevention of thrombosis and embolism. Severe mental disorders are understood within the matrix of altered brain chemistries. New pharmaceuticals are formulated to alter brain chemistries and revolutionize the medical treatments of patients suffering debilitating mental disorders. France again takes the lead with the introduction of chlorpromazine (Thorazine) for the treatment of psychosis. MAOI, TCA, and SSRIs soon follow as compounds which alter brain chemistries and prove effective in the treatment and medical management of mood disorders. Ritalin and Adderall are introduced as treatments to alter brain chemistries in children and adults suffering ADHD. Second messenger systems are introduced and understood within the matrix of biochemical processes involved in inter and intra cell signaling. Cyclic AMP is first identified as a second messenger molecule. Numerous effective pharmaceuticals are introduced into clinical medicine as the result of basic pharmacology research completed in the laboratories of universities and pharmaceutical companies. NSAID are introduced as a treatment alternative to steroids for the management of tissue inflammation. L-dopa is introduced as a treatment for Parkinson's disease. Other notable pharmaceutical examples introduced during the second half of the 1900s are Furosemide (Lasix) an effective loop diuretic for the treatment of CHF; propranolol (Inderal) the first non-selective beta blocker for treatment of heart disease; cimetidine (Tagamet) the first H2 histamine blocker for treatment of GI ulcers and gastroesophageal reflux disease; albuterol (Ventolin) the first short acting inhaled beta-2 adrenergic receptor agonist effective in providing relief from bronchospams associated with asthma; and Acyclovir one of the first effective antivirals. G-protein mediated second messenger systems are first introduced and understood within the matrix of cell signaling. Nitric oxide is understood as a relaxer of vascular smooth muscle and finally explains the mechanism of action underlying the treatment effect of nitroglycerine when used in the management of angina. Pharmaceutical companies move further away from research and development of pharmaceutical drug products with a limited treatment courses e.g. 2-3 weeks for an antibiotic and move towards development and marketing of drug products which can be used by a patient daily, over extended periods of time, and ideally the balance of the patient's life e.g. management of blood cholesterol, management of hypertension, management of heart disease, management of diabetes, management of the dementias, and yes, even management of erections for medical and recreational purposes.

Current Modern, 2000 AD - 2019 AD.

Medical pharmacology goes molecular.

Medical pharmacology engages in an explosion of research directed to understanding the molecular basis of mechanisms underlying fundamental processes in pharmacodynamics and pharmacokinetics. New and innovative conceptual matrixes are explored.

Research based discoveries exceed the capabilities of clinical medicine to integrate new discoveries into clinical practice. Practicing physicians struggle to keep abreast of new technologies and new pharmacological treatments. Practicing physicians become more dependent on pharmaceutical marketing to stay current with new information and make changes in prescribed pharmaceutical based medical treatments.

Recent advances in molecular biology and ability to quickly sequence and manipulate genetic materials open new lines of investigations and capture the imaginations of researchers, clinicians, and the general public alike. Many new and innovative treatments build upon recent advances in understanding the interrelationships among individual genetic variations and therapeutic or toxic response. Why some people with a particular pathology respond well to one pharmaceutical, while another person with the same pathology fails to respond, when given the same pharmaceutical is understood within the matrix of inter-individual variabilities in genetic materials.

Pharmacogenomics, the branch of pharmacology dealing with the influence of variabilities within genetic materials and their influence on response to medications is active and productive. New pharmaceuticals are conceptualized and developed within a rational matrix with respect to an individual genotypes. Modification of medications based upon an awareness of genotypes maximizes therapeutic effects and minimizes unwanted side effects. Today, the typical investigation focuses only on a single gene. Multiple genes and multiple gene interactions have yet to be explored.

Investigational efforts are not restricted to understanding only the genome of the patient. Efforts are committed to understanding the genome of specific pathogens. Advances in technologies have permitted the sequencing of the entire human genome and hundreds pathogens e.g. Haemophilus influenza, Helicobacter pylori, Escherichia coli, Mycobacterium tuberculosis, Chlamydia trachomatis. Modification of single base pairs within specific genes are identified and associated with specific diseases e.g. cancers, infectious disease, asthma, psychiatric disorders or specific enzymes essential to normal drug metabolism e.g. cytochrome P-450 or N-acetyltransferase (2000)[336].

The explosion of new information leaves the majority of practicing physicians stunned and overwhelmed. Clinicians want to apply new discoveries and new technologies while reporting a lack of knowledge and confidence, sufficient to integrate recent advances into clinical practice. The knowledge base upon which current and future pharmaceutical treatments are based is sufficiently unfamiliar to most clinicians few actually incorporate the advances into clinical practice (2012)[337].

Biomarkers are expanded beyond simple indicators of normal and pathological processes to now include indicators of therapeutic response to pharmaceutical treatments (2003,2007)[338,339].

Cell signaling continues to be an active area of investigation and point of pharmaceutical interventions. Conceptual models no longer are restricted to primary and second messenger signaling systems. New models introduce third and fourth messenger systems. Cell to cell and intra-cell signaling is better understood and conceptualized within the matrix of genetic variabilities and molecular biology (2010)[340].

Pharmaceutical companies redirect research investigations away from pharmaceuticals, which are used by a patient for relatively short periods of time e.g. a two to three week course of antibiotics and towards development and marketing of pharmaceuticals which are used by a patient on a daily basis for years or the balance of the patient's life e.g. cholesterol lowering agents, anticoagulants. The highest yielding commercial profits generated for large pharmaceutical companies are shifting to pharmaceuticals use by patients on a daily, long-term, multi-year schedule.

Blockbuster pharmaceuticals generate billions of dollars in sales each year, contribute to record high profits for large pharmaceutical companies. Specific conventional blockbuster drugs examples for the year 2010 are atorvastatin (Lipitor) for high cholesterol, clopindogreal (Plavix) for atherosclerosis, fluticasone and salmetrol (Advair) for asthma, etanercept (Enbrel) for rheumatoid arthritis, and valsartan (Diovan) for hypertension and congestive heart failure (2010)[341]. In 2017 pharmaceutical sells continue to rise e.g. apixaban (Eliquis) an anticoagulant generating $7.4 billion in annual sales and tadalafil (Cialis) for erectile dysfunction (frequently recreational sex) generating $1.5 billion. Specific blockbuster biologic examples for 2017 are Humira, an anti-inflammatory used for the management and treatment of rheumatoid arthritis generating global sales of $18.4 billion; rituximab (Ritxan) for non-Hodgkin's lymphoma generating global sales of $9.2 billon; Herceptin for HER2+ breast cancer global sales generating $7.4 billion; nivolumab (Opdivo) an anti-cancer treatment generating $4.9 billion, and interferon beta-1a (Avonex, Rebif) for multiple sclerosis generating global sales of $2.1 billion (2018)[342]. Pharmaceutical companies routinely realize billions of dollars in annual profits.

Biologics are revolutionizing the pharmaceutical industry. Recall, unlike conventional pharmaceutical drugs which are essentially chemicals synthesized from other chemicals, biologics are products produced from living organisms. Technological advances, during the late-1900s and early-2000s make medical use of biologics possible. Biologics can be extracted directly from living systems or produced by recombinant DNA technologies. They offer a hopeful alternative to conventional chemical based pharmaceuticals. Biologics are proving to be especially useful in the treatment of autoimmune disorders, certain cancers, diabetes, and multiple sclerosis.

Government regulations pertaining to clinical trials testing are modified to expedite the process and bring potentially medically valuable pharmaceuticals, formulated on new knowledge and technology to market more quickly and less expensively. Specifically, the US FDA introduces Phase 0 clinical trials testing. Phase 0 testing supplements the familiar FDA Phase 1, Phase 2, and Phase 3 clinical trials testing of all new pharmaceuticals (2006)[343].

Recall, FDA clinical trials Phase 1 testing requires administration of a new medication to 20-80 healthy volunteers with primary purpose to evaluate dosing parameters and identification of side effects; Phase 2 testing is completed in a larger group e.g. 100-300 people and designed to evaluate if the medication is effective in doing what it is designed to do and further evaluate safety; Phase 3 testing is completed in a much larger group e.g. 1,000-3,000 people and designed to confirm medication efficacy, monitor side effects, compare with common treatments already available on the market, and further evaluate safety; Phase 4 testing is completed after the medication is released for clinical use and evaluates post-market safety and clinical efficacy.

The new Phase 0 is completed before Phase 1 testing, completed in only a few humans (n=10), administers micro dose levels of the pharmaceutical under study, designed to assess basic pharmokinetics and pharmacodynamics in humans, and to specifically answer fundamental questions. Is the medication getting into the blood stream and having the anticipated effect on specific proteins or enzymes as postulated? No information is generated during Phase 0 regarding efficacy for treatment, dosing, side effects, or safety. Phase 0 testing is typically completed in its entirety within the course of 7 days. The rationale is to quickly determine if there is reason to continue with more expensive and time consuming traditional clinical trials testing. Recall, most pharmaceuticals which enter the traditional clinical testing phase never make it to market. Phase 0 clinical testing is designed to provide answers much earlier and less expensively in regard to making decisions to continue testing or test a different pharmaceutical. Results to date, as to how effective Phase 0 is working in accomplishing its original goals and objectives are mixed. Time will tell.

Medical schools continue to emphasize the importance of pharmacology and associated therapeutics in both the Basic Sciences and Clinical Sciences training programs. However, there is a noticeable shift occurring in the content of the medical school pharmacology courses. Most schools are embracing the new and rapid developments in molecular biology and incorporating the new knowledge base into their medical pharmacology course. A few schools are holding tight to medical dogma and continue to teach traditional medical pharmacology courses, while others experiment by eliminating the course all together, choosing to integrate medical pharmacology into a broader, less discipline based model of medical education instruction e.g. problem based learning.

Medical pharmacology is well established and recognized as a valuable scientific discipline. Advances currently being made have immediate applications to the diagnosis and treatment of patients. Pathologies and pharmaceutical treatments are understood at the molecular level. These are exciting times for medical pharmacology.

References.

[1] Dirckx, J. (1997). Stedman's concise medical dictionary for the health professional. 3rd edition. Baltimore: William and Wilkins.

[2] Online Etymology Dictionary. (2018). Pharmacology. Retrieved July 2018 from https://www.etymonline.com/word/pharmacy

[3] Gellen, M. (2010). Ancient Babylonian medicine: Theory and practice. West Sussex, United Kingdom: Wiley-Blackwell.

[4] Scurlock, J. and Anderson, B. (2005). Diagnoses in Assyrian and Babylonian medicine: Ancient sources, translations, and modern medical analyses. Chicago: University of Illinois Press.

[5] Thompson, R. (1923). Assyrian medical texts from the originals in the British Museum. London: H. Milford. Oxford University Press.

[6] Griffith, F. (1898). The Petrie papyri: Hieratic papyri from Kahun and Gurob. London: Bernard Quaritch

[7] Edwin Smith Surgical Papyrus (circa 1500 BC). [Online English translation]. Retrieved September 2011 from http://www.touregypt.net/edwinsmithsurgical.htm

[8] The Petrie Papyri: Hieratic Papyri from Kahun and Gurob (circa 1500 BC). Online English translation edited by F. Griffith. Retrieved September 2011 from http://www.archive.org/stream/hieraticpapyrifr00grifuoft#page/n7/mode/2up

[9] Ebers Papyrus (circa 1550 BC). Compendium of the whole Egyptian medicine (Georg Ebers), Columns 1-2. University of Leipzig Library, Special Collections. Leipzig, Germany.

[10] Labat, R. (1951). Traite' akkadien de diagnostics et pronostics me'dicaux. Leiden: E. J. Brill.

[11] Thompson, R. (1923). Assyrian medical texts from the originals in the British Museum. Oxford: Oxford University Press.

[12] Thompson, R. (1924). The Assyrian Herbal: A monograph on the Assyrian vegetable drugs, the subject matter of which was communicated in a paper to the Royal Society March 20, 1924. London: Luzax and Company.

[13] Thompson, R. (1949). A dictionary of Assyrian botany. A posthumous volume edited by C. J. Gadd. London: The British Academy.

[14] Kocher F. (1955). Keilschrifttexte zur assyrisch-babylonischen Drogen und Pflanzenkunde. [Cuneiform texts of Assyrian-Babylonian drug and herb lore]. Berlin: Akademie-Verlag.

[15] Kocher, F. (1963-1980). Die babylonisch-assyrische medizin in texten und untersuchungen, Bd I-VI. [The Babylonian-Assyrian texts and medical examinations] Berlin: Walter de Gruyter.

[16] Scurlock, J. and Anderson, B. (2005). Diagnoses in Assyrian and Babylonian medicine: Ancient sources, translations, and modern medical analyses. Chicago: University of Illinois Press.

[17] Levey, M. (1959). Chemistry and chemical technology in Ancient Mesopotamia. Amsterdam: Elsevier.

[18] Levey, M. (1973). Early Arabic Pharmacology: An introduction based on ancient and medieval sources. Leiden: E. J. Brill.

[19] Geller, M. (2010). Ancient Babylonian Medicine: Theory and Practice. Oxford: Wiley-Blackwell.

[20] Reisner, G. (1905). The Hearst medical papyrus, Hieratic text in 17 facsimile plates in collotype with introduction and vocabulary. Leipzig: J. C. Hinrichs.

[21] Stevens, J. (1975). Gynecology from ancient Egypt: The papyrus Kahun: A translation of the oldest treatise on gynecology that has survived from the ancient world. The Medical Journal of Australia, 2(25-26):949-952.

[22] Griffith, F. (1898(. The Petrie Papyri: Hieratic papyri from Kahun and Gurob. London: Bernard Quaritch.

[23] Joachim, H. (1890). Papyrus Ebers: Das alteste buch uber die heilkunde. [Papyrus Ebers: The oldest book on medicine]. Berlin: G. Reimer.

[24] Klein, C. (1904). The medical features of the Papyrus Ebers. Chicago: American Medical Association. Retrieved 2-20-2012 from http://www.archive.org/stream/cu31924000900849#page/n3/mode/2up

[25] Ebbell. B. (1937). The Payprus Ebers: The greatest Egyptian medical document. Copenhagen: Levin and Munksgaard. Retrieved 2-20-2012 from http://web.archive.org/web/20090312052919/http://www.macalester.edu/~cuffel/ebers.htm

[26] Hippocrates. (circa 400 BC). Hippocratic Corpus. Internet Classics. Translated by Francis Adams. Retrieved March 2012 from http://classics.mit.edu/Hippocrates/acutedis.html

[27] Adams, F. (1843). The genuine works of Hippocrates translated from the Greek by Francis Adams. London: The Sydenham Society.

[28] Jones, W. (1923). Hippocrates with an English translation by W.H.S. Jones. London: William Heinemann, Ltd.

[29] Touwaide, T. (2004). Plants and animals of Antiquity: A detective story. Paper presented at the Annual Meeting and Banquet of the Washington Academy of Sciences, Meadowlark Gardens, May 2004. Retrieved July 2018 from http://docplayer.net/27681412-Plants-and-animals-in-antiquity-a-detective-story.html

[30] Touwaide, A. (1998). Bibliographie historique de la botanique: les identificationsde plantes médicinales citées dans les traités anciens, après l'adoption du système declassification botanique de Linné (1707-1778), dans Centre Jean-Palerne. Lettre d'informations, 30 decembre 1997-janvier 1998, 2-22 et 31 juillet - septembre.

[31] Littre, E. (1839-1862). Hippocratic Collection Diseases of Women, 1.92(8.222.1-3). Paris.

[32] Littre, E. (1839-1862) Oeuvres completes d'Hippocrates, Disease of Women, 1.77; (8.170.9-172.4). Paris.

[33] Jones, W. (1923). Hippocratic Collection - Decorum VIII-X, IX; 9.238.3-6L p293. English translation by W.H.S. Jones. London: Heinemann.

[34] Theophrastus. (1916). Enquiry into plants and minor works on odours and weather signs, with an English translation by Sir Author Hort, in two volumes. The Loeb Classical Library. London: William Heinemann. Retrieved 2-28-2012 from http://www.archive.org/stream/enquiryintoplant02theouoft#page/vi/mode/2up

[35] Thayer, B. (2012). De Mediciona Octo Libri. Aulus Celsus. English translation. Retrieved 2-28-2012 from http://penelope.uchicago.edu/Thayer/E/Roman/Texts/Celsus/5*.html

[36] Largus, S. and Sconocchia, S. (1983). Scribonii Largi Compositiones. Leipzig: Teubner.

[37] Largus, S. and Helmreich, G. (1887). Scibonii Largi Compositiones. Leipzig: Teubner. Retrieved April 2012 from http://archive.org/details/scriboniilargic00helmgoog

[38] Scarborough, J. (1983). Scribonius Largus, Compositiones, 70 (2nd recipe). For quinsy and bladder stones, p7; translation from Sergio Sconocchia, ed., Scribonii Largi Compositiones. Leipzig: Teubner, p39.

[39] Gunther, R. (1959). The Greek Herbal of Dioscorides. English translation by John Goodyer 1655. New York: Hafner Publishing Company.

[40] Beck, L. (2005). Pedanius Dioscorides of Anazarbus: De material medica. Translated by Lily Y. Beck. Hildesheim: Georg Olms Verlag AG.

[41] Osbaldeston, T. (2000). Dioscorides De Materia Medica: Being an Herbal with many other medicinal materials written in Greek in the first century of the Common Era. Translation by Tess Anne Osbaldeston. Johannesburg: Ibidis Press. Retrieved April 2012 from http://www.ibidispress.scriptmania.com/box_widget.html

[42] Thayer, B. (2012). Pliny the Elder's Natural History, Books 1-35. Retrieved April 2012 from http://penelope.uchicago.edu/Thayer/E/Roman/Texts/Pliny_the_Elder/home.html

[43] Bosanquet, F. (1878). The letters of Caius Plinius Caecilius Secundus, The translation of Melmoth, revised and corrected with additional notes and a short memoir by the Rev. F.C.T. Bosanque. London: George Bell and Sons. Retrieved April 2012 from http://ancienthistory.about.com/od/pompeii/a/PlinyPompeii.htm

[44] Galen (1985). Three treatises on the nature of science. Translated by R. Walzer and M. Frede. In Hipporatis Aphorismos, I, I, K, XVIIB, p346. Indianapolis: Hacket Publishing.

[45] Wachtler, J. (1896). De Alcmaeone Crotoniata. Leipzig: Teuber.

[46] Diels, H. and Kranz, W. (1952). Die Fragmente der Vorsokratiker (in three volumes). 6th edition, Dublin and Zurich: Weidmann.

[47] Galen and DeLacy, P. (1996). On the elements according to Hippocrates. Berlin: Akademie Verlag.

[48] Kuhn, K. (2012) Claudii Galeni Opera Omnia. De simplicium medicamentorum temperamentis er facultatibus. [On the mixtures and properties of simple medications]. Volume IX. Cambridge University Press.

[49] Aegineta, P. (1847). The seven books of Paulus Aegineta. Translated from the Greek with a commentary embracing a complete view of the knowledge possessed by the Greeks, Romans, and Arabian on all subjects connected with medicine and surgery. Translated by Francis Adams in three volumes. Volume III. Printed for the Sydenham Society: London. Retrieved July 2018 from https://archive.org/stream/sevenbookspaulu01adamgoog#page/n6/search/hellebore

[50] Levey, M. (1973). Early Arabic pharmacology: An introduction based on ancient and medieval sources. Leiden: E. J. Brill.

[51] al-Razi, A. (1094). Al-Kitab al-hawi fi al-tibb [The Comprehensive Book on Medicine]. New York University, Institute for the Study of the Ancient World. MS A 17 OV1. Retrieved from http://isaw.nyu.edu/exhibitions/romance-reason/rrobjects/comprehensive-medicine-purgatives

[52] al-Razi. A. (circa 900 AD). Kitab ila man la yahduruhu al-tabib [Book for someone who does not have access to a physician]. Islamic Medical Manuscripts at the National Library of Medicine, MS. Hunt. dont. 31, item 4 and MS Marsh 137, item 2.

[53] Savage-Smith, E. (2012). A new catalogue of Arabic manuscripts in the Bodleian Library, University of Oxford: Volume 1: Medicine. Oxford: Oxford University Press.

[54] Levey, M. (1966). The Medical Formulary or Aqrabadhin of Al-Kindi. Translated with a study of its materia medica by Martin Levey. Medieval Science. Madison and Milwaukee, Wisconsin: University of Wisconsin Press.

[55] Ibn Sina, A. (1025). Kitab al-Qanun fi al-tibb [The Canon on Medicine]. MS A 53, Islamic Medical Manuscript Collection, National Library of Medicine, Bethesda, Maryland USA.

[56] Tschanz, D. (2003). A short history of Islamic Pharmacy. Journal of the International Society for the History of Islamic Medicine, 1:11-17.

[57] Ahlberg, K (1908). Den svenska farmacins historia [History of Swedish Pharamacies]. Stockholm: Wilhelm Billes Bokforlags Aktiebolag.

[58] Huillard-Breholles (1855). Hist Diplomatica Frederic II. IV. Paris.

[59] Online Etymology Dictionary. (2012). Drug. Retrieved August 2012 from http://www.etymonline.com/index.php?l=d&p=40&allowed_in_frame=0

[60] Andrea, G. (1562). Libro de I Secreti e Ricette [Book of Secret Remedies]. Original manuscript, Pryce MSE1 is located in the Department of Special Collections, Kenneth Spencer Research Library, University of Kansas, Lawrence, Kansas. English translation by Stata Norton. Retrieved 6-6-2012 from http://etext.ku.edu/view?docId=jesuatti/jesuatti.xml;brand=jesuatti;route=jesuatti

[61] Norton, S. (2002). Experimental therapeutics in the Renaissance. The Journal of Pharmacology and Experimental Therapeutics, 304(2):489-492.

[62] Paracelsus, T. (1529). Vom Holtz Guaiaco gründlicher heilung. [Guaiaco a thorough cure.] Printer Friderichen Peypus.

[63] Paracelsus, T. (1530). Von der französischen krankheit. [On the French diseae]. Printer: Drey Bucher.

[64] Fuchs, L. (1530). Errata recentiorum medicorum, LX, numero, adiectis corundum confuationibus, in studiosorum gratiam, iam primun aedita. Haganoaen aedibus Iohannis Secerii, Mense Martio.

[65] Fuchs, L. (1542). De Historia Stirpium Commentarii Infignes. Basel: Apud Ioannem Roigny.

[66] Fuchs, L. (1542). De Historia Stirpium Commentarii Infignes. Basel. Glasgow University Library Special Collection Department. Special Collection Hunterian L.1.13. English translation exert. http://special.lib.gla.ac.uk/exhibns/month/oct2002.html

[67] UCLA. (2018). Hospital's garden educates using herbal "medicine cabinet". UCLA Newsroom. Retrieved 7-27-2018 from http://newsroom.ucla.edu/stories/hospital-s-garden-educates-using-247241

[68] Cordus, V. (1546). Dispensatorium, hoc est, pharmacorum conficiendorum ratio. Nuremberg: Theobaldum Paganus.

[69] Turner, W. (1551). A new herbal. London: S. Mierdman.

[70] Severinus, P. (1571). Idea medicinae philosophicae, fundamenta continens totius doctrinae Paracelsicase, Hippocraticase et Galenica. Basile.

[71] Erastus, T. (1572-1574). Disputationes de medicina nova. Basile: P. Paracels.

[72] U.S. National Library of Medicine. (2011). The Paracelsian Debates, History of Medicine, Courtesy of the National Library of Medicine. U.S. National Library of Medicine, National Institute of Health. Bethesda Maryland. Retrieved 6-14-2012. http://www.nlm.nih.gov/exhibition/paracelsus/debates.html

[73] Valentine, B. (1604). The triumphal chariot of antimony. Translated into English by John Harding 1660. London.

[74] Moufet, T. (1584). De jure et praestantia chemicorum medicamentorum dialogus aplogeticus. Frankfort.

[75] Royal College of Physicians of London. (1618). The London Pharmacopoeia. London: Edward Griffin.

[76] Sylvius, F. (1663). Disputationum Medicarum. Amsterdam.

[77] Wepfer, J. (1679). Cicutae aquaticae historia et noxae. Commentario illustrata, Basel: J. Rodolphum Konig.

[78] Wepfer, J. (1658). Historiae apoplecticorum. Amsterdam: Jamssonio-Waesbergios.

[79] Wepfer, J., Wepfer, B., Wepfer, G. (1727). Observationes medico-practicae, de affectibus caputus ubternis and externis. Scaphusii: J. Adami Ziegleri.

[80] Peyer, J. (1681). Exercitatio anatomico-medica de glandulis intestinorum earumque usu et affectionibus. Cui subjungitur anatome ventriculi Gallinacei. Amsterdam: H. Wetstenium.

[81] Brunner, J. (1687). De glandulis in duodeno intestino detectis. Heidelberg: Bergmann.

[82] Withering, W. (1785). An account of the foxglove and some of its medical uses: With practical remarks on dropsy and other diseases. Birmingham: M. Swinney.

[83] Darwin, E. (1785). An account of the successful use of foxglove in some dropsies, and in the pulmonary consumption. Medical Transactions, College of Physicians in London, Vol 3, 255-286. London; Printed for J. Dodley, P. Elmsly, and Leigh and Sothery. http://books.google.com/books?id=I-IjAAAAcAAJ&printsec=frontcover&source=gbs_ge_summary_r&cad=0#v=onepage&q=darwin&f=false

[84] Ferriar, J. (1799). An essay on the medical properties of the digitalis purpurea, or foxglove. Manchester: Sowler and Russell.

[85] Reil, J. (1799). Beitrag zu den Prinzipien für jede künftige Pharmakologie. Röschlands Mag., 3:26–64.

[86] Gaw, A. (2016). The principles of future pharmacology: Johann Christian Reil (1759-1813) and his role in the development of clinical pharmacology. European Journal of Clinical Pharmacology, 72(1): 13-17. Supplemental material, English translation by A. Gaw (2016), Reil, J. (1799). Beitrag zu den Prinzipien fur jede künftige Pharmakologie. Röschlands Mag 3:26–64. doi:10.1007/s00228-015-1964-2

[87] Reil, J. and Hoffbauer, J. (1808). Ueber den Begriff der Medicin und ihre Verweigungen, besonders in Beziehung auf die Berichtigung der Topik der Psychiaterie. Beyträge zur Beförderung einer Kurmethode auf psychischem Wege. [Contributions to the Advancement of Psychiatric Treatment Method]. 161-279. Curtsche Buchhandlung.

[88] Reil, J. (1809). Untersuchungen uber den Bau des grossen Gehims im Menschen. Arch. Physiol., 9:136-524.

[89] Reil, J. (1812). Die vordere commissur im groben gehirn. Archiv. fur die Physiologie, 11:89-100.

[90] Magendie, F. (1809a). Examen de l'action de quelques vegetaux sur la moelle epiniere. [Examination of the action of some plants on the spinal cord]. Nouveau Bulletin Scientifique de la Société Philomatique, 1:368-405.

[91] Magendie, F. (1809b). Quelques idees générales sur les phenomenes particuliers aux corps vivants. [Some general ideas about particular phenomena in living bodies]. Bulletin des Sciences Médicales, 4:145-170.

[92] Magendie, F. and Pelletier, P. (1817a). Memoire sur l'emetine et sur les trois espèces d'ipécacuanha. Journal Générale de Médecine, de Chirurgie et de Pharmacie, 59:223-231.

[93] Magendie, F. (1817b). Recherches chimiques et physiologiques sur l'ipecacuanha. Annales de Chimie et de Physique. Paris, 4:172-185.

[94] Magendie, F. (1822). Formulaire pour la préparation et l'emploi de plusieurs nouveaux médicamentes, tels que la noix vomique, la morphine, l'acide prussique, la strychnine, la veratrine, les alcalis des quinquinas, l'iode etc. Paris: Mequignon-Marvis. English translation (1824). Formulary for the preparation and mode of employing several new remedies. Philadelphia.

[95] Pelletier, P. and Caventou, J. (1818). Note sur un nouvel alkalai. [Note on a new alkaloid]. Annales de Chimie et de Physique., 8:323-324.

[96] Pelletie, P. and Caventou, J. (1820). Suite: Des recherches chimiques sur les quinquinas. [A continuation: The chemical research on quinolones]. Annales de Chimie et de Physique., 15:337-365.

[97] Pelletier, P. (1821). Cafeine. Dictionnaire de Médecine, 4:35-36. Paris: Béchet Jeune.

[98] Meissner, C. (1819). Ueber Pflanze Alkalien: II. Ueber ein neues Pflanzae Alkali. [About alkaloid plants: A new alkaloid plant]. J. Chemie. Physik., 25:377-381.

[99] Pelletier, J. and Caventou, J. (1817). Sur la matière verte des feuilles. [On the green leaf material]. J. Pharm., 3:486-491.

[100] Runge, F. (1821). Materialien zur phytologie. p146. Berlin: G. Reimer.

[101] Runge, F. (1820). Neueste phytochemische Entdeckungen zur Begründung einer wissenschaftlichen Phytochemie [Latest phytochemical discoveries for the founding of a scientific phytochemistry]. p144–159. Berlin: G. Reimer. http://books.google.com/books?id=KLg5AAAAcAAJ&pg=P146

[102] Williams, W. (1898). New spelling in its relation to pharmacy. The druggists' circular and chemical gazette. Feb. 1898, p 32.

[103] Serturner, F. (1805). Uber die entdeckung des morphiums. [About the discovery of morphine]. Letter to the editor. Journal der Pharmacie fur Aerzte, apotheker und chemisten [Journal of pharmacy for doctors, pharmacists and chemists] Vol 13. Erfurt University Journal. Johann Trommsdorff, editor. Leipzig.

[104] Sertürner, F. (1817). Uber das morphium eine neue salzfahige grundlage, und die mekonsaure, als hampthestandtheile des opiums. [On the morphine, a new salt-viable basis, and the meconic acid, as the main constituents of opium]. Annals of Physics, New Series, 25:56-89. Leipzig: J. A. Barth.

[105] Merck, H. (1827). Pharmaceutisch-chemisches Novitaten-Cabinet: Erste lieferung, sechszehn der vorzuglichsten vegetabilischen grundlagen und deren salzfahige verbindungen. [Pharmaceutical and chemical cabinet, first delivery, sixteen of the principal vegetable bases and their saltzfahige connections].

[106] Vauquelin, L. and Robiquet, P. (1806). La découverte d'un nouveau principe vegetal dans le suc des asperges. [The discovery of a new principle in the plant juice of asparagus]. Annales de Chimie, 57:88–93.

[107] Robiquet, P. (1832). Nouvelles observations sur les principaux produits de l'opium. Annales de chimie et de physique, 51:225–267.

[108] Dunster, E. (1875). The history of anesthesia. A paper presented to the annual meeting of the Wastenaw County Medical Society, Vpslanti, Michigan, June 25. Ann Arbor: Fiske and Douglas.

[109] Priestley, J. (1974-77). Experiments and Observations on Different Kinds of Air. 3 vols. Volume I. London: W. Bowyer and J. Nichols.

[110] Davy, H. (1800). Researches, chemical, and philosophical chiefly concerning nitrous oxide or dephlogisticated nitrous air and its respiration. London: Printed for J. Johnson.

[111] Wells, H. (1847). A history of the discovery of the application of nitrous oxide gas, ether and other vapors to surgical operations. Hartford: J. Gaylord Wells.

[112] Morton, W. (1846). Demonstration performed at the operating theater of Massachusetts General Hospital, October 16, 1846.

[113] US Patent No. 4848. (1846). Issued to Charles Jackson and William Morton of Boston Massachusetts; Improvement in surgical operations, November 12, 1846.

[114] Perrier, M. and Lallemand, L. (1863). Traite d'Auaesthesie Chirurgicale. 8:668. Paris: F. Chamerot.

[115] Soubeiran, E. (1831). Recherches sur quelques combinaisons du chlore. Ann. Chim. Phys., 48:131-57.

[116] Liebig, J. (1832). Ueber die verbindungen, welche durch die einwirkung des chlors auf alkohol, aether, ölbildendes gas und essiggeist entstehen. [About the compounds formed by the action of chlorine on alcohol, ether, oil-forming gas and spirit vinegar]. Annalen der Pharmacie, 1(2):182-230.

[117] Guthrie, S. (1832). New mode of preparing a spirituous solution of chloric ether. Am. J. Sci. Arts, 21:64-5.

[118] Dumas, J. (1834). Untersuchung über die Wirkung des Chlors auf den Alkohol. [Study on the effect of chlorine on alcohol]. Annalen der Pharmacie, 107(41):650–656.

[119] Simpson, J. (1847a). Discovery of a new anesthetic agent, more efficient than sulphuric ether. London Medical Gazette, 5:906, 934-937.

[120] Simpson, J. (1847b). Discovery of a new anesthetic agent, more efficient than sulphuric ether. Lancet, November 21, 2:549-550.

[121] Simpson, J. (1847c). Answer to the religious objections advanced against the employment of anesthetic agents in midwifery and surgery. Edinburgh: Sutherland and Knox.

[122] Buchheim, R. (1849). Beitrage zur Arzneimittellehre. [Contributions to pharmacology]. Leipzig: Leopold Voss.

[123] Pereira, J. (1843). The Elements of Materia Medica and Theapeutics. 2 volumes. Philadelphia: Lea and Blanchard.

[124] Buchheim, R. (1876). Ueber die Aufgaben und die Stellung der Pharmakologie an den deutschenHochschulen. Archiv. Exp. Pathol. Pharmakol., 5:261-278.

[125] Wood, A. (1855). New method of treating neuralgia by the direct application of opiates to the painful points. Edinburgh Medical and Surgical Review, 82:265-81.

[126] Clarke, T. (1668). A letter, written to the publisher by the learned and experienced Dr. Timothy Clarke one of his Majesties physicians in ordinary, concerning some anatomical inventions and observations, particularly the origin of the injection into veins, the transfusion of bloud (sic), and the parts of generation. Phil. Trans., January 1. 3:672-682.

[127] Hunter, C. (1859). Experiments relative to the hypodermic treatment of disease. Medical Times and Gazette, 18, 234-5, 310-11, 387-8; 19:251.

[128] Hunter, C. (1865a). On the speedy relief of pain and other nervous affections by means of the hypodermic method. London: John Churchill.

[129] Hunter, C. (1865b). Hypodermic administration of certain medicines. Medical Times and Gazette, June 3: 584-587.

[130] Royal Medical and Chirurgical Society of London. (1867). Report of the Scientific Committee appointed to investigate the physiological and therapeutic effects of the hypodermic method of injection. Medico-Chirurgical Transactions, 50:561-643.

[131] Bartholow, R. (1873). Manual of hypodermic medication. Second edition, revised and enlarged. Philadelphia: J. B. Lippincott and Company.

[132] Hunter, C. (1858). On the Hypodermic Administration of Remedies in Neuralgia and Other Affections. Paper presented to the St. George's Medical Society, December 9th. Published (1860), J. E. Adlard.

[133] Wood, C. (1865). Notes, Queries and Replies. Local subcutaneous injections and the hypodermic method. Letter to the Editor of the Medical Times and Gazette. Medical Times and Gazette, July 22:107.

[134] Blandford, G. (1865). Notes, Queries, and Replies. Local Subcutaneous injections and the hypodermic method. Letter to the Editor of the Medical Times and Gazette. Medical Times and Gazette, July 22; 107.

[135] Hunter, C. (1865a). Local subcutaneous injections and the hypodermic method. Letter to the Editor. Medical Times and Gazette, July 1:22.

[136] Hunter, C. (1865b). On the speedy relief of pain and other nervous affections by means of hypodermic method. British Medical Journal, December 16:636.

[137] Merck. (2012). The history of Merck. http://www.merckgroup.com/en/company/history/history.html.

[138] Bristol-Meyer-Squibb. (2012). History. Retrieved from http://www.bms.com/ourcompany/Pages/history.aspx

[139] Eli Lilly. (2012). Heritage. Retrieved from http://www.lilly.com/about/heritage/Pages/heritage.aspx

[140] Pfizer. (2012). About Pfizer – history. Retrieved from http://www.pfizer.com/about/history/1849

[141] Sandoz. (2012). Sandoz history. Retrieved from http://www.sandoz.com/about_us/sandoz_history.shtml

[142] Bayer. (2012). History overview. Retrieved from http://www.bayer.com/en/1863-1881.aspx

[143] Brown, A. (1861). On the theory of chemical compounds. MD thesis University of Edinburgh.

[144] Brown. A. (1864). On the theory of isomeric compounds. Transactions of the Royal Society of Edinburgh, 23(3):707-719.

[145] Brown, A. (1865). On the theory of isomeric compounds. J. Chem. Soc., 18:230–245.

[146] Fraser, T. (1872). The antagonism between the actions of active substances. British Medical Journal. November 2; 2(618):485-487.

[147] Bernard, C. and Pelouze, J. (1850). Recherches sur le curare. Comptes rendus hebdomadaires de l'Académie des Sciences, Paris, 31:533-537.

[148] Benard, C. (1856). Analyse physiologique des propriétés des systèmes musculaires et nerveux au moyen de curare. Comptes rendus hebdomadaires de l'Académie des Sciences, Paris, 43:825-829.

[149] Bernard, C. (1849). Du suc pancréatique et de son rôle dans les phénomènes de la digestion. Archives générales de médecine, 19: 60-81; English translation in Medical Classics (1919), 3:581-617.

[150] Bernard, C. (1855-1856). Leçons de physiologie expérimentale appliqué à la médicine. 2 volumes. Paris: J.B. Bailliere.

[151] Benard, C. (1857). Nouvelles recherches expérimentales sur les phenomènes glycogeniques du foie. Comptes rendus de la Societe de biologie (Mémoires), Paris, 2 ser. 4:1-7; Comptes rendus hebdomadaires des seances de l'Académie des Sciences, 44:578-586, 1325-1331.

[152] Benard, C. (1857). Leçons sur les effects des substances toxiques et médicamenteuses. Paris: J. B. Bailliere et fils.

[153] Benard, C. (1875). Leçons sur les anesthésiques et sur l'asphyxie. Paris: J. B. Bailliere et fils.

[154] Bernard, C. (1865). Introduction à l'étude de la médecine expérimentale. Paris: J. B. Bailliere. English translation by Henry Copley Greene: An Introduction to the Study of Experimental Medicine, with an introduction by Lawrence J. Henderson. (1927). New York: Macmillan.

[155] Schmiedeberg, O. (1883). Grundriss der Arzneimittellehre. Leipzig: Verlag von F. C. Vogel.

[156] Schmiedeberg, O. and Koppe, R. (1869). Das Muscarin das giftige alkaloid des flugenpilzes. Leipzig: F.C.Vogel.

[157] Klebs, E., Naunyn, B., Schmiedeberg, O. (Eds). (1873). Archives of Experimental Pathology and Pharmacology, Vol 1. Leipig: F. C. Vogel.

[158] Schmiedeberg, O. and Meyer, H. (1879). Z. Physiol. Chem., 3:422.

[159] Koller, C. (1884). Uber die Verwendung des Cocaine zur Anasthesierung am auge. Weiner Medizinische Wochenschrift, 34:1276-1277. English publication (1884). On the use of cocaine for producing anesthesia on the eye. The Lancet, December 6, 124(3197):990-992.

[160] U.S. Patent Office. (1885). Alphabetic list of registrants of trademarks. Pemberton, John S. Atlanta, Ga. Nerve tonic. May 19, 12(257):423.

[161] Swain, H. (1991). One hundred years of pharmacology: Centennial 1891-1991. Prepared for the Centennial Celebration held in Ann Arbor Michigan on September 26-28, 1991 to commemorate the introduction of Pharmacology into the curricula of the American medical school. The University of Michigan, Department of Pharmacology, Ann Arbor, Michigan. Retrieved August 2012.

[162] John Hopkins University, Department of Pharmacology and Molecular Sciences, Baltimore, Maryland. Home web page, Retrieved August 2012.

[163] Able, J. and Crawford, A. (1897). On the blood-pressure-raising constituent of the suprarenal capsule. John Hopkins Hosp. Bull 8:151; Trans. Ass. American Phys., 12:461.

[164] Able, J. (1899). Ueber den blutdruckerregenden bestandtheil der nebenniere, das epinephrin. Z. physiol. [The blood pressure causing constituent of the adrenal gland, epinephrine]. Chem., 28:318.

[165] Able, J. (1900). On the teaching of pharmacology, materia medica and therapeutics in our medical schools. Philad. Med. Journal, September 6, 384-390.

[166] American Society of Pharmacology and Experimental Therapeutics. (1908). Organizational Meeting, Baltimore, Maryland. December 28, 1908. Meeting Minutes. Retrieved from ASPECT homepage August 2012. http://www.aspet.org/about/history/

[167] Able, J. (Ed.). (1909). The Journal of Pharmacology and Experimental Therapeutics. Vol 1. Baltimore: Williams and Wilkins.

[168] Cushny, A. (1899). Textbook of pharmacology and therapeutics or the action of drugs in health and disease. Philadelphia: Lea Brothers and Company.

[169] American Therapeutic Society. (1901). Constitution and By-Lays, Article II. Transactions of the American Therapeutic Society. In Transactions of the American Therapeutic Society 1900-1908 (May 1903); P. Brynberg Porter managing editor. New York: American Therapeutic Society.

[170] American Society for Clinical Pharmacology and Therapeutics (2012). ASCPT History. American Therapeutic Society Founding and Early Years 1900-1945. Retrieved from http://www.ascpt.org/AboutUs/ASCPTHistory/tabid/6634/Default.aspx

[171] Pottenger, F. (1915). President's Address, 16th Annual Meeting of the American Therapeutic Society, June 1915, San Francisco. California State Journal of Medicine, Sept., 13(9).

[172] ASPET (1908). Minutes and Records, American Society for Pharmacology and Experimental Therapeutics, Secretary, R. Hunt. Bethesda, MD.

[173] ASPET (1909). The Journal of Pharmacology and Experimental Therapeutics. 1(1):1-174. Retrieved from http://jpet.aspetjournals.org/content/1/1

[174] Parascandola, J. (2007). A brief history of ASPET on its centennial anniversary. Molecular Interventions, 7:288-302.

[175] Langley, J. (1905). On the reaction of cells and of nerve-endings to certain poisons, chiefly as regards the reaction of striated muscle to nicotine and to curare, J. Physiol., 33:374–413.

[176] Ehrlich, P. (1897). Die wertbemessung des diphtherieheilserums und deren theoretische grundlagen. Klinisches Jahrbuch., 6:299-326.

[177] Ehrlich, P. (1898). Ueber die beziehungen von chemischer constitution, verteilung und pharmakologischer Wirkung: Vortrag, gehalten im Verein für Innere Medicin am 12. December. [About the relationships of chemical constitution, distribution and pharmacological activity. Lecture presented to the Internal Medicine Association, December 12.

[178] Ehrlich, P. (1902). Ueber die Beziehungen von chemischer Constitution, Vertheilung, und pharmakologischen Wirkung. Ernst von Leyden-Festschrift, 1:645-679. Address delivered to Verein für innere Medicin, Berlin, December 12. English translation by Bolduan (1906). The relations existing between chemical constitution, distribution, and pharmacological action. Studies on Immunity, 404-442.

[179] Prull, C. (2003). Part of a scientific master plan? Paul Ehrlich and the origins of his receptor concept. Medical History, 47:332-356.

[180] Ehrlich, P. (1907). Experimental researches on specific therapy, II. Harben Lecture Series. London.

[181] Foster, M. and Sherrington, C. (1897). Textbook of Physiology. London: Macmillon.

[182] Sherrington, C. (1906). The integrative actions of the nervous system. New Haven: Yale Univ. Press.

[183] Dale, H. (1914). The action of certain esters and ethers of choline and their relation to muscarine. J. Pharmacol. Exp. Ther., 6:147-190.

[184] The Nobel Prize in Physiology or Medicine 1936. Nobelprize.org. Retrieved from http://www.nobelprize.org/nobel_prizes/medicine/laureates/1936/

[185] Maclean, J. (1916). The thromboplastic action of cephalin. Am. J. Physiology. 41:250-257.

[186] The Nobel Prize in Physiology or Medicine 1923. Nobelprize.org. Retrieved from http://www.nobelprize.org/nobel_prizes/medicine/laureates/1923/.

[187] Paulescu, N. (1920). Traite de physiologie medicale, II, Paris: Vigot Freres.

[188] Paulescu, N. (1921a). Action de l'extrait pancreatique injecte dans le sang chez un animal normal. Comptes Rendus des Seance de la Societe de Biologie et des ses filiales, 85(27):555-9.

[189] Paulescu, N. (1921b). Recherche sur le role du pancréas dans l'assimilation nutritive. Arch Intern Physiol., 17:85-103.

[190] Widnark, E. and Tandberg, J. (1924). Uber die bedingungen fur die akkumulation indifferenter narkoliken theoretische bereckerunger. J. Biochem. Z., 147:358-369.

[191] Widmark, E. (1932). Die theoretischen grundlagen und die praktische verwendbzrkeit der gerichtlichmedizinischen alkoholbestimmung. Berlin.

[192] Moller, E., NcIntosh, J., Van-Slyke, D. (1929). Studies of urea excreation. II. Relationship between urine volume and the rate ofurea excretion by normal adults. J. Clin. Invest., 6:427-434.

[193] U.S. Food and Drug Administration. (2012). About FDA. History. U.S. Department of Health and Human Services. FDA webpage http://www.fda.gov/AboutFDA/WhatWeDo/History/default.htm.

[194] United States Food and Drug Administration. (2018). Drugs. Retrieved from https://www.fda.gov/Drugs/default.htm

[195] United States Department of Agriculture. (2012). About us. Department of Agriculture Organic Act of May 15, 1862, Chapter 72, 12 Statute 387. Retrieved October 2012 from http://www.csrees.usda.gov/about/offices/legis/organic.html

[196] National Archives (2012). Records of the Food and Drug Administration (FDA). Record Group 88.2 General records of the FDA and its predecessors 1880-1942. Retrieved from http://www.archives.gov/research/guide-fed-records/groups/088.html

[197] British Pharmacological Society (2018). Our history. Retrieved from https://www.bps.ac.uk/about/who-we-are/history-of-the-society

[198] British Pharmacological Society. (2018). About BPS. Retrieved from https://www.bps.ac.uk/about/who-we-are

[199] Dale, H. (1933). Nomenclature of fibers in the autonomic system and their effects. J. Physiol., 80:10-11.

[200] Otten, H. (1986). Domagk and the development of the sulphonomides. Compound Kl 695, October, 1932. Journal of Antimicrobial Chemotherapy 17(6):689-690.

[201] Domagk, G. (1935). A contribution to the chemotherapy of bacterial infections. Deutsche medizinische Wochenschrift, February.

[202] Trefouel J., Trefouel, J., Nitti F., Bouvet, D. (1935). Activite du p-aminophenylsulfamide sur les infections streptococciques experimentales de la souris de du lapin. Comp. Rend. de Soc. Biol., Paris; 120:756-8.

[203] The Nobel Prize in Physiology or Medicine 1939. Nobelprize.org. Retrieved from http://www.nobelprize.org/nobel_prizes/medicine/laureates/1939/.

[204] U.S. Food and Drug Administration (2018). About FDA; Part III: Drugs and Foods under the 1938 Act and its Amendments. Retrieved from https://www.fda.gov/AboutFDA/History/FOrgsHistory/EvolvingPowers/ucm055118.htm

[205] Chain, E., Florey, H., Gardner, A., Heatley, N., Jennings, M., Orr-Ewing, J., Sanders, A. (1940). Penicillin as a chemotherapeutic agent. Lancet, 24:226-228.

[206] Schatz, A., Bugie, E., and Waksman, S. (1944). Streptomycin, a substance exhibiting antibiotic activity against gram-positive and gram-negative bacteria. Proc Soc. Exp. Biol. Med., 55:66-69.

[207] Schatz, A. (1945). Streptomycin, an antibiotic produced by Actinomyces griseus. Ph.D. Dissertation. Rutgers University.

[208] Duggar, B. (1948). Aureomycin: A product of the continuing search for new antibiotics. Ann. N. Y. Acad. Sci., Nov. 30, 51:177-181.

[209] Duggar, B. (1948). Aureomycin: A product of the continuing search for new antibiotics. Ann. N. Y. Acad. Sci. 51(2):177-181.

[210] Duggar, B. (1949). Aureomycin and Preparation of Same. U.S. Patent 2,482,055. Sept 13, 1949.

[211] Pringle, P. (2012). Notebook sheds light on an antibiotic contested discovery. New York Times, June 11. Experiment Eleven: Dark secrets behind the discovery of a wonder drug. Walker and Company.

[212] Goodman, L., Wintrobe, M., Dameshek, W., Goodman, M., Gilman, M., McLennan, M. (1946). Nitrogen mustard therapy: Use of Methyl-Bis (Beta-Chloroethyl) amine Hydrochloride and Tris (Beta-Chloroethyl) amine hydrochloride for Hodgkin's disease, Lymphosarcoma, Leukemia and Certain Allied and Miscellaneous Disorders. JAMA, 132(3):126-132.

[213] Farber, S. and Diamond, L. (1948). Temporary remissions in acute leukemia in children produced by folic acid antagonist, 4-aminopteroyl-glutamic acid. N. Engl. J. Med., 238, June (23):787–793.

[214] Sarett, L. (1948). A new method for the preparation of 17(α)-hydroxy-20-ketopregnanes. J. Am. Chem. Soc., 70:1454-1458.

[215] Hench, P., Kendall, E., Slocumb, C., Polley, H. (1949). The effect of a hormone of the adrenal cortex (17-hydroxy-11-dehydrocorticosterone: compound E) and the pituitary adrenocorticotropic hormone on rheumatoid arthritis. Preliminary report. Proc. Staff Meetings Mayo Clinics, 24:181-197.

[216] The Nobel Prize in Physiology or Medicine 1950". Nobelprize.org. Retrieved from http://www.nobelprize.org/nobel_prizes/medicine/laureates/1950/.

[217] Ahlquist, R. (1948). A study of the adenotrophic receptors. Am. J. Physiol. 153:586-600. http://ajplegacy.physiology.org/content/153/3/586.full.pdf+html

[218] Drill, V. (Ed.) (1954).Pharmacology in medicine. New York: McGraw-Hill Book Co.

[219] Cannon, W. and Rosenblueth, A. (1937). Autonomic neuro-effector systems. New York: Macmillan Company.

[220] Ahlquist, P. (1978). Comments on Ahlquist, P. (1948). A study of adrenotropic receptors, Amer. J. Physiology. 153:586-600, Citation Classics, November, 45. Retrieved from http://garfield.library.upenn.edu/classics1978/A1978FT95400002.pdf

[221] Fatt, P. and Katz, B. (1951). An analysis of the end-plate potential recorded with an intra-cellular electrode. J Physiol., 115:320–370.

[222] Fatt, P. and Katz, B. (1952). Spontaneous subthreshold activity at motor nerve endings. J. Physiol., 117: 109-128.

[223] Castillo, J. and Katz, B. (1954). Quantal components of the end-plate potential. J. Physiol., 124: 560–573.

[224] Castillo, J. and Katz, B. (1956). Biophysical aspects of neuromuscular transmission. Prog Biophys Biophys. Chem., 6:121-170.

[225] The Nobel Prize in Physiology or Medicine 1970. Nobelprize.org. 2 Oct 2012 http://www.nobelprize.org/nobel_prizes/medicine/laureates/1970/

[226] U.S. Patent Office. (1947). Patent 2,427,578. Warfarin. Stahmann, M., Ikawa, M., Link, K. Retrieved from http://toxnet.nlm.nih.gov/cgi-bin/sis/search/a?dbs+hsdb:@term+@DOCNO+1786

[227] U.S. Food and Drug Administration. (1954). FDA Approved Drug Products, Coumadin, Original approval date: June 8, 1954. Retrieved from http://www.accessdata.fda.gov/scripts/cder/drugsatfda/index.cfm?fuseaction=Search.DrugDetails

[228] U.S. Patent Office. (1956)/ Patent 2,765,321. Warfarin. Schroeder, C., Link, K., and Wisconsin Alumni Research Foundation. http://toxnet.nlm.nih.gov/cgi-bin/sis/search/a?dbs+hsdb:@term+@DOCNO+1786

[229] Charpentier, P., Gailliot, P., Jacob, R., Gaudechon, J., Buisson, P. (1952). Recherches sur les diméthylaminopropyl-N phénothiazines substituées. Comptes rendus de l'Academie des Sciences, 235:59–60.

[230] Laborit, H., Huguenard, P., Alluaume, R. (1952). Un nouveau stabilisateur végétatif de 4560 RP. La Presse Médicale, 60:206–8.

[231] Hamon, J., Paraire, J., Velluz, J. (1952). Remarques sur l'action du 4560 RP sur l'agitation maniaque. Annales Médico-psychologiques (Paris), 110:331–5.

[232] Delay, J. and Deniker, P. (1952b). 38 cas de psychoses traitèes par la cure prolongèe et continue de 4560 RP. CR Congr Méd Alién Neurol (France), 50:503–13.

[233] Rigotti, S. (1952). Del blocco del SN vegetativo all'ibernazione artifi ciale primi risultati di un nuevo indirizzo di terapia psichiatrica. Rassegna di Neurologia Vegetative, 9:197–210.

[234] Staehelin, J. and Kielholz, P. (1953). Largactil, ein neues vegatativen Dämpfungsmittel bei Psychischen Störungen. Schweizerische Medizinische Wochenschrift, 83:581–6.

[235] Lehmann, H. and Hanrahan, G. (1954). Chlorpromazine, new inhibiting agent for psychomotor excitement and manic states. Archives of Neurology and Psychiatry (Chicago), 71:227–37.

[236] Elkes, J. and Elkes, C. (1954). Effects of chlorpromazine on the behavior of chronically overactive psychotic patients. British Medical Journal, 2:560–76.

[237] Bente, D. and Itil, T. (1954). Zur Wirkung des Phenothiazin Körpers Megaphen auf das menschliche Hirnströmbild. Arzneimeittel Forschung, 4:418–23.

[238] Winkelman, N. (1954). Chlorpromazine in the treatment of neuropsychiatric disorders. Journal of the American Medical Association, 155:18–21.

[239] Webb, R. (1955). Largactil in psychiatry. The Medical Journal of Australia, 1:759–61.

[240] Carlsson, A. and Lindqvist, M. (1963). Effect of chlorpromazine and haloperidol on formation of 3-methoxytyramine and normetanephrine on mouse brain. Acta Pharmacologica et Toxicologica, 20:140–4.

[241] Selikoff, I.., Robitzek, E., Ornstein, G. (1952). Treatment of pulmonary tuberculosis with hydrazine derivatives of isonicotinic acid. JAMA, 150:973-80.

[242] Smith, J. (1953). The use of the isopropyl derivative of isonicotinylhydrazine (Marsilid) in the treatment of mental disease. Am. Pract., 4:519-20.

[243] Ayd, F. (1957). A preliminary report on Marsilid. Am. J. Psychiatr., 114:459.

[244] Delay, J., Laine, B., Buisson, J. (1953). Anxiety and depressive states treated with isonicotinyl hydrazide (isoniazid). Arch. Neurol. Psychiatr., 70:317-24.

[245] Loomer, H., Saunders, I., Kline, N. (1958). A clinical and pharmacodynamic evaluation of iproniazid as a psychic energizer. Psychiatr. Res. Rep. Am. Psychiatr. Assoc., 8:129-41.

[246] Kuhn, R. (1957). Uber die Behandlung depressiver Zustände mit einem Iminodibenzylderivat (G 22355). Schweiz Med Wchnschr, 87:1135-40.

[247] Kuhn, R. (1958). The treatment of depressive states with G 22355 (imipramine hydrochloride). American Journal of Psychiatry, 115:459-64.

[248] Lehmann, H., Cahn, C., De Verteuil, R. (1958). The treatment of depressive conditions with imipramine (G 22355). Can. Psychiatr. Assoc. J., 3:155-64.

[249] Ball, J. and Kiloh, L. (1959). A controlled trail of imipramine in the treatment of depressive states. Br. Med. J., 2:1052-5.

[250] Panizzon, L. (1944). La preparazione di piridil- e piperidil-arilacetonitrili e di alcuni prodotti di trasformazione (Parte Ia). Helvetica Chimica Acta, 27:1748–56.

[251] U.S. Food and Drug Administration. (1955). Drugs at FDA. Retrieved from http://www.accessdata.fda.gov/scripts/cder/drugsatfda/index.cfm?fuseaction=Search.DrugDetails

[252] Shorter, E. (2008). Before Prozac: The troubled history of mood disorders in psychiatry. New York: Oxford University Press.

[253] McLeod, N. (1900). The hormone sleep: a new departure in the treatment of acute mania. Br. Med. J., 1:134-136.

[254] Klaesi, J. (1922). Uber die therapeutische Anwendung der "Dauernarkose" mittels Somnifens bei Schizophrenen. Zeitsch Gesamte Neurol Psychiatrie. [About the therapeutic use of "prolonged anesthesia" in schizophrenics]. 74:557–592.

[255] Freud, S. (1927), The Ego and the Id. London: Hogarth.

[256] Cerletti, U. (1940). L'Elettroshock. Rivista Sperimentale di Frenatria, 1:209-310.

[257] Freeman, W. and Watts, J. (1937). Prefrontal lobotomy in the treatment of mental disorders. Southern Medical Journal, 30(1):23-31.

[258] Freeman, W. and Watts, J. (1944). Psychosurgery: An evaluation of two hundred cases over seven years. Journal of Mental Science, 90(379): 532-537.

[259] Bowman, R., Cauldield, P., Undenfriend, S. (1955). Spectrophotofluorometric assay in the visable and ultraviolet. Science, 122, (3157)32-33.

[260] Hertting, G. and Axelrod, J. (1961). The fate of tritiated-noradrenaline at the sympathetic nerve endings. Nature, 192:172-173.

[261] Glowinski, J. and Axelrod, J. (1966). Effects of drugs on the disposition of H^3-norepinephrine in the rat brain. Pharmacol Rev., 18:775-785.

[262] Axelrod, J. (1971). Noradrenaline: Fate and control of its biosynthesis. Science, 173:598-606.

[263] Axelrod, J. (1957). O-methylation of epinephrine and other catechols in vitro and in vivo. Science, 126 (3270):400–1.

[264] Axelrod, J. and Tomchick, R. (1958). Enzymatic O-methylation of epinephrine and other catechols. The Journal of Bioligcal Chemisitry, Sept., 233(3):702-5.

[265] Axelrod, J. (1959). Metbolism of epinephrine and other sympathomimetic amines. Physiology Review, 39:751-776.

[266] Axelrod J. (1948). The fate of acetanilide in man. J. Pharmacol. Exp. Ther., 94:29-38.

[267] Brodie, B. and Axelrod, J. (1948). The fate of acetanilide in man. J. Pharmacology Experimental Therapeutics, 94:429-438.

[268] von Euler, U. (1935). Uber die spezifische blutdrucksenkeride substanz des menschlichen prostataund samenblasensekreted. Journal of Molecular Medicine, 14(33):182-1183.

[269] The Nobel Prize in Physiology or Medicine 1970". Nobelprize.org. Retrieved from http://www.nobelprize.org/nobel_prizes/medicine/laureates/1970/.

[270] Rall, T. and Sutherland, E. (1958). Formation of a cyclic adenine ribonucleotide by tissue particles. J Biol Chem., 232:1065-1076.

[271] Sutherland, E. and Rall, T. (1958). Fractionation and characterization of a cyclic adenine ribonucleotide formed by tissue particles. J. Biol. Chem., 232:1077-1092.

[272] Rall, T., Earl, W., Sutherland, E., and Berthet, J. (1957). The relationship of epinephrine and glucagon to liver phosphorylase. Journal of Biological Chemistry, 224(1):463-475.

[273] Davoren, P. and Sutherland, E. (1963). The cellular location of adenyl cyclase in the pigeon erythrocyte. J. Biol. Chem., 238:3016-3023.

[274] The Nobel Prize in Physiology or Medicine 1971. Nobelprize.org. Retrieved from http://www.nobelprize.org/nobel_prizes/medicine/laureates/1971/.

[275] Carlsson, A. (1959). The occurrence, distribution, and physiological role of catecholamines in the nervous system. Pharmacol. Rev., 11:490-493.

[276] Carlsson, A, and Hillarp, N. (1956). Release of adrenalin from the adrenal medulla of rabbits treated with reserpine. Kungl Fysiogr Sallsk I Lund Forhandl., 26: 8.

[277] Carlsson, A., Lindquist, M., Magnusson, A., Waldeck, B. (1957a). 3,4-dihydroxyphenylalamine and 5-hydroxytryptophan as reserpine antagonist. Nature, 180:1200.

[278] Carlsson, A., Rosengren, E., Bertler, A., and Nilsson, J. (1957b). Effect of reserpine on the metabolism of catecholamines. In Psychotropic Drugs; Garattini, S. and Ghetti, V. editors. 363-372. Amsterdam: Elsevier.

[279] Carlsson, A, and Waldeck, B. (1958). On the presence of 3-hydroxytyramine in brain. Science 127:471.

[280] Euler, U. (1935). Kurze wissenschaftliche mitteilungen. Uberdie spezifische blutdrueksenkende substanzes menschlichen prostata-und samenglasenskretes. Klin Wochenschr., 14:1182-1183.

[281] Bergström, S., Ryhage, R., Samuelsson, B. and Sjövall, J. (1962b). The structure of prostaglandin E, F, and F_2. Acta. Chem. Scand., 16: 501-502.

[282] Hart, F. and Boardman, P. (1963). Indomethacin: A new non-steroid anti-inflammatory agent. Br. Med. J., 2(5363):965–70.

[283] Boots Pharmaceutical Company (2012). The invention of Ibuprofen. Retrieved from http://www.boots.com/en/The-history-of-Ibuprofen_1143599/.

[284] Piper, P. and Vane, J. (1969). Release of additional factors in anaphylaxis and its antagonisms by anti-inflammatory drugs. Nature, 223:29-35.

[285] Vane, J. (1971). Inhibition of prostaglandin synthesis as a mechanism of action of aspirin-like drugs. Nature, 231:232–5.

[286] Physiology or Medicine 1982 - Press Release. Nobelprize.org. 24 Sep 2012. http://www.nobelprize.org/nobel_prizes/medicine/laureates/1982/press.html

[287] Silverstein, F., Faich, G., Goldstein, J. (2000). Gastrointestinal toxicity with celecoxib vs nonsteroidal anti-inflammatory drugs for osteoarthritis and rheumatoid arthritis: the CLASS study: A randomized controlled trial. Celecoxib long-term arthritis safety study. JAMA, 284(10):1247-55.

[288] United Kingdom Patent Office London (1961). Patent number 971700, Inventors John Stewart Nicholson and Stewart Sanders Adams. Initial Application February 2, 1961; number 3999/61.

[289] US Food and Drug Administration (FDA). (2012). US Department of Health and Human Services. Retrieved from http://www.fda.gov/ohrms/dockets/ac/02/briefing/3882B2_04_Wyeth-Ibuprophen.htm

[290] U.S. Food and Drug Administration (FDA). United States Department of Health and Human Services. FDA Drug Database, Drugs@FDA, FDA approved drug products. Retrieved from http://www.accessdata.fda.gov/scripts/cder/drugsatfda/index.cfm?fuseaction=Search.DrugDetails.

[291] Suki, W., Rector, F., Seldin, D. (1965). The site of action of Furosemide and other sulfonamide diuretics in the dog. Journal of Clinical Investigation, 44(9).

[292] U.S. Food and Drug Administration. (1967). Drugs at FDA. FDA approved drug products. NDA 016419 Propranolol Hydrochloride. Retrieved from http://www.accessdata.fda.gov/scripts/cder/drugsatfda/index.cfm?fuseaction=Search.Label_ApprovalHistory#apphist

[293] Black, J. and Stephenson, J. (1962). Pharmacology of a new adrenergic beta-receptor-blocking compound (nethalide). Lancet, (2):311-4.

[294] Black, J., Duncan, W., Shanks, R. (1965). Comparison of some properties of proethalol and propranolol. British J. Pharmac. Chemotherapy, 25:577-591.

[295] Dunlop, D. and Shanks, R. (1968). Selective blockade of adrenoceptive beta receptors in the heart. Br. J. Pharmc. Chemotherapy, 32:201-218.

[296] Black, J., Duncan, W., Durrant, G., Ganelllin, C., Parsons, M. (1972). Definition and antagonism of histamine 12--receptors. Nature, 236:385-390.

[297] Brimblecombe, R., Ducan, W., Durant, G., Emmett, J., Ganellin, C., Parsons, M. (1978). Characterization and development of cimetidine as a histomine H2 receptor antagonist. Gastroenterology, 74(2 pt 2):339-347.

[298] The Nobel Prize in Physiology or Medicine 1981. Nobelprize.org. Retrieved from http://www.nobelprize.org/nobel_prizes/medicine/laureates/1988/

[299] U.S. Food and Drug Administration (FDA). (2018). Federal Food, Drug, and Cosmetic Act, Chapter 9, Section 201, Subsection 321, Definitions; 2(g)1, page 32. http://www.gpo.gov/fdsys/pkg/USCODE-2010-title21/pdf/USCODE-2010-title21-chap9-subchapII-sec321.pdf

[300] World Health Organization (WHO) (2012). Guidelines for ATC classification and DDD assignment 2012. 15th edition. WHO Collaborating Centere for Drug Statistics Methodology. Norwegian Institute of Public Health. Oslo, Norway.

[301] World Health Organization (WHO), Engel and Siderius (1968). The consumption of drugs: Report of a study 1966-1967. WHO regional Office for Europe.

[302] Kuhn, T. (1962). The Structure of Scientific Revolutions. Chicago: University of Chicago Press.

[303] U.S. Food and Drug Administration. (1981). Albuterol. New Drug Application 018473. Drugs@FDA: FDA Approved Drug Products. Retrieved from https://www.accessdata.fda.gov/scripts/cder/daf/index.cfm?event=overview.process&ApplNo=018473

[304] Schaffer, H., Vince, R, Bittner, S., Gurwara, S. (1971). Novel substrate of adenosine deaminase. Journal of Medicinal Chemistry, 14(4):367–369.

[305] Elion, G., Furman, P., Fyfe, J., de Miranda, P., Beauchamp, L., Schaeffer. H. (1977). Selectivity of action of an antiherpetic agent, 9-(2-hydroxyethoxymethyl) guanine. Proc. Natl. Acad. Sci. (USA), 74:5716-5720.

[306] Schaeffer, H., Beaucamp, L., deMiranda, P., Elion, G., Bauer, D., Collins, P. (1978). 9-(2-hydroxyeth-oxymethyl) guanine activity against viruses of the herpes group. Nature. (London). 272:583-85.

[307] U.S. Food and Drug Administration. (1982). Zovirax, NDA number 018303. Original New Drug Application approvals, October 1982. Retrieved from https://www.accessdata.fda.gov/scripts/cder/daf/index.cfm?event=reportsSearch.process&rptName=2&reportSelectMonth=10&reportSelectYear=1982&nav

[308] Pagano, J., Sixbey, J., Lin, J. (1983). Acyclovir and Epstein-Barr virus infection. Journal of Antimicrobial Chemotherapy, Sep. 12, Suppl B:113-21.

[309] Freitas, V., Smee, D., Chernow, M., Boehme R., Matthews, T. (1985). Activity of 9-(1,3-dihydroxy-2-propoxymethyl)guanine compared with that of acyclovir against human, monkey, and rodent cytomegaloviruses. Antimicrobial Agents Chemotherapy, Aug., 28(2):240-5.

[310] Gnann, J., Barton, N., Whitley, R. (1983). Acyclovir: Mechanism of action, pharmacokinetics, safety and clinical applications. Pharmacotherapy: The Journal of Human Pharmacology and Drug Therapy, Sept-Oct., 3(5):275-283.

[311] Ramachandran, A. (2000). Pharmacology recall. Baltimore: Lippincott Williams and Wilkins.

[312] Rodbell, M. (1980). The role of hormone receptors and GTP-regulatory proteins in membrane transduction. Nature, Mar. 6, 284(5751):17–22.

[313] Hechter, O. and Halkerston, I. (1964). On the action of mammalian hormones; In The Hormones, Pincus, F., Thiman, K. and Astwood, E. editors. 5: 697-825. New York: Academic Press.

[314] Robison, G., Butcher, R., Oyr, I., Morgan, H., Sutherland, E. (1965). The effect of epinephrine on adenosine 3′,5′-phosphate levels in the isolated perfused rat heart. Molecular Pharmacology, 1:168-177.

[315] Sutherland, E. and Robison, G. (1966). The role of cyclic-3',5'-AMP in responses to catecholamines and other hormones. Pharmacol. Rev., Mar; 18(1):145–161.

[316] Hardman, J. and Sutherland, E. (1969). Guanyl cyclase, an enzyme catalyzing the formation of guanosine 3′,5′-monophosphate from guanosine trihosphate. J. Biol .Chem., 244:6363-6370.

[317] Rodbell, M., Birnbaumer, L., Pohl, S., Krans, H. (1971a). The glucagon-sensitive adenyl cyclase system in plasma membranes of rat liver. V. An obligatory role of guanyl nucleotides in glucagon action. J. Biol. Chem., 246:1877-1882.

[318] Rodbell, M., Krans, H., Pohl, S., Birnbaumer, L. (1971b). The glucagon-sensitive adenyl cyclase system in plasma membranes of rat liver. III. Binding of glucagon: method of assay and specificity. J. Biol. Chem., 246:1861-1871.

[319] Rodbell, M., Krans, H., Pohl, S., Birnbaumer, L. (1971c). The glucagon-sensitive adenyl cyclase system in plasma membranes of rat liver. IV. Effects of guanyl nucleotides on binding of 125I-glucagon. J. Biol. Chem .,246:1872-1876.

[320] Robell, M., Lin, M., Salomon, Y. (1974). Evidence for interdependent action of glucagon and nucleotides on the hepatic adenylate cyclase system. The Journal of Biological Chemistry. January 10, 249(1):59-65.

[321] Rodbell, M. (1985). Programmable messengers: a new theory of hormone action. Trends Biochem. Sci., 10:461-464.

[322] Ross, E., Howlett, A., Ferguson, K., Gilman, A. (1978). Reconstitution of hormone-sensitive adenylate cyclase activity with resolved components of the enzyme. J. Biol. Chem., 253:6401-6412.

[323] Northup, J., Smigel, M., Sternweis, P., Gilman, A. (1983a). The subunits of the stimulatory regulatory component of adenylate cyclase. Resolution of the activated 45,000-dalton (alpha) subunit. J. Biol. Chem., 258:11369-11376.

[324] The Nobel Prize in Physiology or Medicine 1994. Nobelprize.org. Retrieved from http://www.nobelprize.org/nobel_prizes/medicine/laureates/1994/

[325] Katsuki, S., Arnold, W., Mittal, C., Murad, F. (1977a). Stimulation of guanylate cyclase by sodium nitroprusside, nitroglycerin and nitric oxide in various tissue preparations and comparison to the effects of sodium azide and hydroxylamine. J. Cyclic Nucl. Res., 3:23-35.

[326] Katsuki, S., Arnold, W., Mittal, C., Murad, F. (1977b). Stimulation of formation and accumulation of cyclic GMP by smooth muscle relaxing agents. Proc. of the 2nd Japanese Cyclic Nucleotide Conference, July 7- 9, 44-50.

[327] Furchgott, R. and Zawadzki, J. (1980). The obligatory role of endothelial cells in the relaxation of arterial smooth muscles by acetylcholine. Nature, 288:373-376.

[328] Ignarro, L., Byrns, R., Wood, K. (1986). Pharmacological and biochemical properties of endothelium-derived relaxing factor (EDRF): evidence that it is closely related to nitric oxide (NO) radical (abstract). Circulation, 74 (Suppl II):287.

[329] Ignarro, L., Buga, G., Wood, K., Byrns, R., Chaudhuri, G. (1987). Endothelium-derived relaxing factor produced and released from artery and vein is nitric oxide. Proc. Natl. Acad. Sci. (USA), 84:9265-9269.

[330] The Nobel Prize in Physiology or Medicine 1998. Nobelprize.org. 27 Sep 2012. http://www.nobelprize.org/nobel_prizes/medicine/laureates/1998/

[331] Lapin, J. and Oxenkrug, G. (1969). Intensification of the central serotonergic processes as a possible determinal of the thymoleptic effect. Lancet, 1:132-6.

[332] Wong, D., Horng, J., Bymaster, F., Hauser, K., Molloy, B. (1974). A selective inhibitor of serotonin uptake: Lilly 110140, 3-(ptrifluoromethylphenoxy)-N-Methyl-3-Phenylpropylamine. Life Sci., 15:471-479.

[333] Fuller, R. and Wong, D. (1987). Selective reuptake blockers in vitro and in vivo. Journal of Clinical Psychopharmacology, 7(6):36s-43s.

[334] FDA. (1996). FDA Drugs@FDA FDA Approved Drug Products, Adderall. Retrieved from https://www.accessdata.fda.gov/scripts/cder/daf/index.cfm?event=overview.process&applno=011522

[335] FDA. (1996). US Food and Drug Administration. Drugs@FDA. FDA Approved Drug Products Donepezil (Aricept) approved Nov. 25, 1996. http://www.accessdata.fda.gov/scripts/cder/drugsatfda/index.cfm?fuseaction=Search.DrugDetails

[336] Broder, S. and Venter, J. (2000). Sequencing the entire genomes of free-living organisms: The foundation of pharmacology in the new millennium. Annu. Rev. Pharmacol. Toxicol., 40:97-132.

[337] Stanek, E., Sanders, C., Taber, K., Khalid, M., Verbrugge, R., Agatep, B., Aubert, R., Epstein, R., Fruch, F. (2012). Adoption of pharmacogenomic testing by US physicians: Results of a nationwide survey. Nature, March, 91(3):450-458.

[338] Frank, R. and Hargreaves, R. (2003). Clinical biomarkers in drug discovery and development. Nature. July, vol. 2:566-580.

[339] Nutt, R., Vento, L., Ridinger, M. (2007). In vivo molecular imaging biomarkers: Clinical pharmacology's new "PET". Clinical Pharmacology and Therapeutics, 81:792-95.

[340] Jagade, J., Amrutkar, M., Katariya, D., Wankhade, A., Kale, A., Undale, V. (2010). Role of protein kinases in signal transduction and their inhibitors. Pharmacologyonline, 2:371-384.

[341] Pharma Block Busters. (2010). Pharma's top 10 blockbuster Drugs. Thursday, November 11. http://www.pharmablockbusters.info/2010/11/pharmas-top-10-blockbuster-drugs.html

[342] Stone, K. (2018). Top 10 biologic drugs in the United States. The Balance. Retrieved from https://www.thebalance.com/top-biologic-drugs-2663233

[343] U.S. Food and Drug Administration. (2006). Guidance for industry, investigators, and reviewers: Exploratory IND studies. Retrieved from http://www.fda.gov/downloads/Drugs/GuidanceComplianceRegulatoryInformation/Guidances/ucm078933.pdf

Chapter 10

Medical Pathology

Definition.

Pathology is the "…medical science and specialty practice, concerned with all aspects of disease, but with special reference to the essential nature, causes, and development of abnormal conditions, as well as the structural and functional changes that result from the disease process…" (1997)[1]. Pathology "…is a bridging discipline involving both basic science and clinical practice and is devoted to the study of the structural and functional changes in cells, tissues, and organs that underlie disease. By the use of molecular, microbiologic, immunologic, and morphologic techniques, pathology attempts to explain the whys and wherefores of the signs and symptoms manifested by patients while providing a sound foundation for rational care and therapy…" (1999)[2]. More succinctly, others define "…pathology as the objective study of disease…" (1914)[3] and a "...medical specialty concerned with the determining causes of disease and the structural and functional changes occurring in abnormal conditions…" (2012)[4].

Pathology, as taught today in most medical schools within the United States, Canada, and Europe, is organized into two broad areas of instruction, general pathology and systemic pathology. General pathology emphasizes the basic reactions of cells and tissues to disease processes. Systemic pathology emphasizes the basic reactions of organ systems to disease. Within each of these two broad categories, four dimensions of the disease process are emphasized; its causes (etiology), its mechanisms of development (pathogenesis), structural changes in cells or organs (morphological changes), and the functional consequences of these changes (clinical significance). Demonstrated competency in pathology knowledge is currently required by all medical schools and medical licensing boards throughout the world today.

Introduction.

This chapter traces the history of medical pathology from its earliest beginning, as practiced by the ancient civilizations of Mesopotamia, Egypt, and Greece to its current state today, as practiced by modern Western medicine. Emphasis is placed upon the development of medical pathology as a scientific discipline. Attention is focused upon developing an understanding and appreciation of significant events, milestone discoveries, the most influential people guiding the discipline's development throughout history, and identification of significant changes in conceptual matrixes, which have led to our current knowledge of medical pathology today.

This chapter will not review the history of all important pathologies you will cover in your medical school's pathology course. Instead, this chapter will introduce and develop the history of much broader issues of pathology. Specifically, medical pathology will be examined as a scientific discipline and specialized area of study within medicine across time. Changes in the conceptual matrix of disease, from early models emphasizing supranatural forces to recent conceptual models emphasizing changes in molecular biology are examined. Changes in technologies, ranging from early gross visual inspection, anatomical dissection, chemical assays, histological staining, tissue fixation, introduction and development of microscopes, to present day modern genetic and molecular technologies are explored in relationship to their impact upon the historical development of pathology. Changes in the primary unit of study of pathology across time from whole body, organs systems, individual tissues, cells, and genetic materials are examined and placed within a historical contextual matrix. The changes in the primary unit of study are examined. The development of pathology as a professional discipline is examined from an initial area of curiosity, through the founding of university departments of pathology, establishment of dedicated clinical pathology laboratories, the founding and development of professional scientific societies devoted to the advancement of pathology as a scientific discipline, its specialization within the practice of medicine, and its value today within the practices of modern-day medicine and surgery.

This chapter is organized chronologically for consistency with other chapters and to provide you with an opportunity to appreciate the many contributions of medical pathology as a function of time.

History.

Early Records, 3500 BC - 500 BC.

The written records of the ancient civilizations of Mesopotamia, Greece, and Egypt reveal a rich history regarding the early beginnings of medical pathology (1800BC,1550BC,1500BC,1898, 1923,2005)[5,6,7,8,9,10].

The earliest written records contain evidence of man's long standing interest in the relationships between physical health and the human body. Observations and associations are soon committed to the written record. These early records, preserved in thousands of clay tablets and assorted papyri, provide the first known attempts to establish a permanent record of the medical pathology knowledge, complementing earlier hieroglyphics drawings and the oral tradition of passing information from generation to generation.

Translations of these materials confirm ancient civilizations are aware of and do record observations of human anatomy and changes in human anatomy associated with impaired physical health, from injury and disease. Observations are made of external and internal anatomical structures, most typically noting changes in gross morphology. An empirical-inductive epistemological methodology characterizes the typical approach applied by the Ancients, whenever making or recording observations and associations. Emphasis is placed upon personal sensory experiences e.g. seeing, hearing, smelling, tasting, or touching made by the person making the observations. Individual observations are collected into a set of specific observations, from which generalized conclusions are made.

Analysis of the early records further reveal much sharing of information between ancient Mesopotamia and ancient Egypt. Both civilizations evidence an excellent knowledge of gross internal human anatomy. Egyptian papyri of the period e.g. Kahun papyrus, written circa 1800 BC, Smith papyrus, written circa 1500 BC, and Ebers papyrus, written circa 1500 BC all contain specific and detailed descriptions of associations between impaired physical health and morphological changes in anatomy. Perhaps most illustrative of these three specific papyri is the Kahun's papyrus. The papyrus provides detailed listings of clinical signs and symptoms associated with specific anatomical changes accompanying gynecological diseases and conditions.

Numerous additional examples are found in these early records, illustrating the ancient civilizations' familiarity and interests in describing relationships between changes in physical health and changes in body anatomy. Most typically entries are descriptive in kind. Descriptions are typically followed immediately by recommended treatments. Again all treatments follow the characteristic empirical-inductive model typical of this period.

For additional examples of the early records, especially revealed recently by the translation of thousands of clay tablets, documenting associations between impaired physical health, clinical signs and symptoms, changes in human body morphology, and underlying pathologies; see the Early Records sections of the Immunology and Microbiology chapters of this book.

Rapidly accumulating new information, from several modern scholars, based upon new, recent translations of the early written records from Mesopotamia, Egypt, and Greece, requires a reassessment of modern academic dogma and popular belief portraying medical knowledge of the ancient civilizations, as limited, unsophisticated, and couched in non-scientific mysticism.

The new evidence reveals these long held popular beliefs are simply no longer true. The ancient civilizations of Mesopotamia (circa 3500 BC), Egypt (circa 3200 BC), Babylonia (circa 2000 BC), and Roma (circa 750 BC) all possessed an excellent fundamental knowledge of the relationships between impaired physical health, clinical signs and symptoms, and gross morphological changes in human anatomy. The knowledge base is derived systematically from a sensory experience, empirical-inductive methodology. Fundamental relationships recorded over 2,500 years ago stand true today.

Time has come to acknowledge the new truths, set aside old truths, and embrace the recently discovered facts; the ancient civilizations of Mesopotamia, Egypt, and Greece systematically investigated relationships between changes in physical health and physical changes evidenced in the human body. They recognize the importance of the findings and committed the observed relationships to the written record. The methods used by these ancient civilizations are no more couched in mysticism than methods today. Speculations and interpretations as to the source, causes, clinical courses of disease, illness, and injury differ, however the physical findings remain the same. Medical pathology owes much to the early efforts of the ancient civilizations. Perhaps soon their contributions will be better recognized and acknowledged.

A brief word of caution here; as you move through your medical education and future practice as a physician, try to resist the temptation to attribute all that which is unfamiliar or that which you do not understand as "idiopathic" or "mystical". There is an answer; you just have to look more closely.

In brief sum, the Early Records of 3500 BC through 500 BC reveal a written record outlining the very rich beginnings of medical pathology, as a scientific discipline and its value to practicing physicians. Relationships between physical health and changes in human anatomy are observed and recognized to be sufficiently important to commit to a permanent written record. Observations rely heavily upon personal sensory experiences. An empirical-inductive epistemology is applied to the discovery of new knowledge. Much sharing of knowledge between ancient civilizations is now evident, in particular and in regard to knowledge of the relationships between changes in physical health and changes in internal and external human anatomical structures. The knowledge base and methodologies applied by the ancient civilizations, described as unsophisticated and couched in unscientific mysticism, according to relatively recent modern academic dogma, is simply incorrect. Recent modern evidence reveals the Ancients actually maintained a rather sophisticated knowledge base regarding the relationships between changes in physical health and disease. They applied a scientific methodology to the discovery of new knowledge and shared new discoveries. Time has come to displace the academic dogma of the past with new information and a more correct representation of the ancient civilizations' foundational contributions to medical pathology.

Trivia: Ancient Greece exists as a thriving civilization between 1200 BC and 300 BC. It is characterized by political, philosophical, artistic, and scientific achievements, which have tremendous influence on Western civilization. The Greek alphabet is introduced circa 750 BC, as a derivative of the earlier Phoenician alphabet. The Phoenician alphabet is a derivative of Egyptian hieroglyphics, contains 22 letters and only consonantal sounds. It is one of the earliest known alphabets and is widely used in the Mediterranean regions circa 1200 BC. The Greek alphabet introduces vowel sounds and contains 24 letters. Today, the Greek alphabet continues to be used as familiar symbols throughout all of medicine. How many letters comprise the modern English alphabet we use today? Yes, 26 letters. The word "alphabet" is compounded from the first two letters of the Greek alphabet, alpha and beta.

Antiquity, 500 BC - 500 AD.

The written records of Antiquity offer much to understanding the rich and influential beginnings of medical pathology. Arguably, no other period in the history of medical pathology has more influence in establishing the foundations upon which the discipline builds. The history of medical pathology during Antiquity can be organized into three distinct periods.

The first period, 500 BC to 50 BC, defines medical pathology. Here medical pathology establishes its foundation as a scientific discipline. Specific areas of study are identified, methods of investigation are defined and developed, specific models of disease are conceptualized, defined, and actively investigated, and medical educational programs are established to teach future physicians the content of a rapidly expanding medical pathology knowledge base.

The second period, 50 BC to 150 AD, is characterized by no real progress. No new information is contributed and much old information is destroyed. Institutions and other centers of new learning which contribute to the advancement of new knowledge and have contributed to the rapid advancement of medical pathology, during the first period are effectively disassembled and eliminated. Written records from the first period, when determined to be inconsistent with the beliefs of the many newly founded organized religions and new ruling governments, are simply destroyed. Established natural (physical) models of disease are replaced by supranatural (deity) based models of disease. In the absence of progress, old knowledge, if not destroyed is distilled and summarized at best or reinterpreted at worst to conform to the beliefs of the new ruling governments and organized religions.

The third period, 150 AD to 500 AD, also witness few advances. This period is greatly influenced by organized religion and the prolific writings by Galen and his many scribes. Nothing particularly new or innovative here. A slightly modified and extended balance of humors model dominates the conceptual matrix from which disease is understood, diagnosed, and treated. Governments and organized religions continue to ban human dissection for medical and scientific purposes. Governments and organized religions exert tremendous and repressive influences upon investigators who choose to study disease within the natural (physical) matrix. The preferred matrix from which disease is to be understood is the supranatural (deity) models, advocated by organized religions. Galen offers a modification of the balance of humors model, offering a compromise between the natural (physical) and supranatural (deity) based models of disease. His efforts are successful in appeasing influential forces, while simultaneously effectively stalling progress in medical pathology for the next 1,200 years.

Let's explore a few specifics. These are the fundamental beginnings of medical pathology.

Alcmaeon of Croton (510 BC- unknown) Greek natural philosopher founds the first medical school in Europe. The school is located in southern coastal Italy. This area is heavily populated by Greeks and is a part of several interconnected Greek settlements along the Gulf of Taranto. Recall, the Gulf of Taranto is located on the southern coast of Italy between the "heel" and the "sole" of the "boot" of Italy. It is here, at the medical school at Croton, the systematic study of anatomy and disease has many of its deepest roots. Alcmaeon assigns function to all anatomical structures and is first to propose the doctrine of balanced humors to understand normal body function and disease, noting a need for balance of humors is necessary to maintain good health. The model provides a conceptual matrix from which to understand disease. The model offers a natural (physical) cause for disease, explains clinical signs and symptoms, and offers direction for what must be done by the physician to restore good health in a patient.

Alcmaeon of Croton proposes the doctrine of balanced humors model and teaches the doctrine to medical students at his medical school at Croton, Italy, well over 100 years before Hippocrates and over 450 years before Galen, advocate the model to explain disease.

Trivia: At the approximate time Alcmaeon proposes the doctrine of humors model of disease to medical students at Croton circa 450 BC, the Acropolis and other major buildings begin construction in nearby Athens.

Hippocrates of Cos (460 BC-370 BC) Greek physician founds the medical school on Cos and emphasizes a natural (physical) rather than the supranatural (deity) basis for disease. He adopts the balance of humors model proposed by Alcmaeon of Croton, to guide diagnosis and treatment of disease, illness, and trauma. Hippocrates is an itinerate practitioner of clinical medicine and brings little new to the advancement of medical pathology. As with many individuals throughout the history of medicine, much is popularly attributed to Hippocrates with very little if any substantive historical evidence, based upon written or well documented historical records of the period.

Trivia: Cos is the second largest Greek island, located in the Aegean Sea, approximately 15 miles off the coast of Bodrum, Turkey. The island measures approximately 25 mile long and 5 miles wide.

The multi-authored Hippocratic Collection, assembled in the Libraries of Alexandria circa 300 BC, offers a clear written record describing how disease is most commonly conceptualized, evaluated, and treated during Early Antiquity, especially in and around the regions of Italy, Greece, Iran, Turkey, and Egypt. The Collection provides clear evidence, disease is indeed systematically studied during Early Antiquity and the knowledge is sufficiently important to be committed to the written record.

Reading of English translations of the Collection reveals an important distinction between the concept of disease, as conceptualized during Early Antiquity and the concept of disease, as conceptualized today 2,400 years later. Disease during Antiquity is conceptualized as a constellation of clinical signs and symptoms. Disease today is conceptualized as disordered normal biological processes which generate clinical signs and symptoms. Understand this difference and you will be better prepared to understand the matrix within which investigators and clinical practitioners think about, organized, and study disease both then and now.

The Hippocratic Collection contains organized listings of clinical signs and symptoms with clear descriptions of associated pathological processes of trauma, inflammation, infestation, and infection. Emphasis is always placed upon signs and symptoms, not the underlying process. For example, in Epidemics, Book I v, written circa 410 BC, the author describes the clinical presentation of individuals evidencing classic signs and symptoms of chronic cough, blood tinged sputum, night sweats, fever, and weigh loss. That's right; these are the typical signs and symptoms associated with infection of the lungs by the bacterium we recognize today as mycobacterium tuberculosis (TB). The author describes the condition as "…phthisis…" rather than the now more familiar term today, "tuberculosis", yet the signs and symptoms are sufficiently clear to recognize the presentation as tuberculosis (400BC,1923)[11,12]. Emphasis is on the disease "phthisis", defined by clinical signs and symptoms, rather than the disease, defined by an underlying process e.g. infection of lung tissues by the bacterium mycobacterium tuberculosis.

Pathologies contained within the Hippocratic Collection and reflective of the time period are organized and listed first by clinical signs and symptoms, followed by detailed reporting of onset, course, and resolution or lack of resolution of clinical signs and symptoms without intervention, simply observing the body's natural response. This is simply an elegant methodology. Systematically observe the relationship between clinical presentation and the human body's natural response to underlying pathologies e.g. trauma, inflammation, infestation, and infection. Do not interfere (facilitate or suppress) with the body's natural response; simply observe. Document all changes observed. Yes, most of the patients reported die from the underlying pathology and absence of effective treatment, however, the opportunity to systematically document changes in body function, as a function of pathology, independent of external interventions (treatments), and across time is impressive and informative.

Most treaties which comprise the Hippocratic Collection are reflective of the Hippocratic school of thought and its associated conceptual matrix of disease. However, many other treaties within the Collection are more reflective of the Cnidian School and its contrasting conceptual matrix of disease, emphasizing abnormal changes in organs tissues.

The Cnidian School is both an organized conceptual matrix, as well as a physical medical school. The medical school is founded circa 430 BC and offers an alternative conceptual matrix from that offered by the medical school on Cos. This school is often forgotten or even unknown to most medical students. The Cnidian medical school is physically located at the Greek settlement of

Cnidus, on the Datca peninsula, located on the southwestern coast of modern-day Turkey, and approximately 23 miles southeast of the Greek island of Cos. The school competes with the more popularly recognized medical school founded by Hippocrates on Cos, circa 430 BC. Both schools are recognized at the time to train excellent physicians and both emphasize the natural rather than supranatural causes of diseases and treatments. The schools differ substantially in their approaches and methodologies applied to understanding disease.

The Coan School (Cos) emphasizes careful observation of patient signs and symptoms, reporting onset, course, and resolution. Disease is conceptualized as a collection of signs and symptoms. Treatment interventions are minimal, allowing the body to heal itself. The assessments and treatments are patient oriented and holistic in kind. Unfortunately, while providing much valuable information on the courses of disease, most patients die.

The Cnidian School also emphasizes careful observation of patient signs and symptoms, carefully reporting onset, course, and resolution and additionally associates observations with anatomical changes observed in diseased organs. Efforts are devoted to understanding changes in patient health, as a function of anatomical changes occurring in body organs. Disease is conceptualized as both process and result. Disease is generated by pathological changes occurring in body organs. Clinical constellations of signs and symptom reflect organ pathologies. Treatments are directed to treating the diseased organ.

The Cnidian approach and method applied to understanding and treating disease stands in marked contrast to approaches and methods used at Cos. Recall, the Coan School (Cos) focuses upon understanding the patient from a holistic perspective, with attention directed to the modifying factors unique to any individual patient. Treatments are directed to maximizing conditions which will allow the body to heal itself. Treatments are individually based for each patient. The Cnidian School focuses upon understanding diseased organs and their relationships with a patient's clinical presentation. Attention is directed to identifying the underlying pathologies present within any specific organs and associating these changes with clinical signs and symptoms. Treatments are determined not from clinical signs and symptoms as at Cos, but rather by the pathologies affecting anatomical organs. Human dissection is a necessary component of the investigative method to study disease at Cnidus and an unnecessary component of the investigative methods to study disease at Cos. Both schools embrace the balance of humors doctrine and integrate this doctrine into their conceptual matrix of disease.

The medical schools at Cos and Cnidus are similar in so many ways yet maintain two very different conceptual matrixes from which to investigate and understand disease. Both models have strengths and weaknesses, both advance and obstruct progress of discovery of new knowledge, and both influence the development of medical pathology as an emerging discipline. The influence of these two schools is instrumental in laying the foundation upon which medical pathology will build for the next 2,500 years. It is here medical pathology is first embedded solidly into the foundation of medical education and becomes part of the medical school education and training of all future physicians.

The influence of both schools can be readily recognized in the treaties comprising the Hippocratic Collection. This multi-authored collection of medical treaties, written circa 400 BC represents a reasonable sampling of regional medical knowledge known at that time. Review of individual treaties readily reveals contributions by authors from both medical schools, Cos and Cnidus. Here I use the term school in both the physical sense as an institution and as the dominant conceptual matrix of thought embraced by each institution. Review reveals the marked differences between the two schools' approaches to understanding disease. For example, Epidemic, Book I, v reflects the signs and symptoms based model of disease, typical of the Coan school, whereas On Diseases of Women 1-2 is representative of the organ based model of disease, typical of the Cnidian school. Further inspection reveals marked competitiveness between schools, unchecked, and oftentimes harsh criticism of the other school's models and methods. A fundamental sense of intellectual self-righteousness is evidenced by each school when investigating and understanding human disease (173/1826/2008/2011)[13]. Oh how little things have changed in 2,500 years.

Aristotle (384 BC-322 BC) Greek natural philosopher, born in the northern Greek city of Stagira located on the Chalkidiki peninsula, lives most of his adult life in Athens, and relies upon human dissection as a primary source of knowledge. He has no problem with the dissection of the human body, given the influence of this teacher Plato (428 BC-348 BC), whom believes only the soul is sacred not the body. Aristotle proclaims all body parts have function and all function can be identified by natural observation. He further proclaims when anatomy in impaired, function is impaired. When function is impaired, anatomy is impaired (350BC,350BC)[14,15]. This concept put forth over 2,300 years ago is familiar to every medical student still today.

Herophilus of Chalcedon (335 BC-289 BC) (Chalcedon is present day Turkey) co-founds with Erasistratus of Keos, the medical school at Alexandria, Egypt, the renowned Greek city of academic learning. Human dissections are conducted on a regular basis in the medical school and Libraries of Alexandria, offering systematically collected, anatomical information from healthy and diseased human body. Herophilus is credited with completing over 600 human dissections, while in residence in Alexandria. Medical students participate in both human dissection of cadavers and vivisection of criminals. Emphasis is always placed upon understanding the relationship between anatomy and function. Herophilus is among the first to pursue pathology as a science, constantly correlating anatomical structure with disease and any associated change in normal function.

Erasistratus of Keos (304 BC-250 BC) (Keos is a small Greek island located in the Aegean Sea, southeast of the mainland of Greece) Greek, physiologist co-founds the medical school, at the port city of Alexandria, Egypt, with his more senior colleague, anatomical pathologist Herophilus of Chalcedon. Erasistratus rejects the popular balance of humors models, based upon his own observations and experimental studies completed at the medical school. In its place he proposes a modification of the doctrine of atomic structure and function model, first proposed by the pre-Socratic Greek natural philosophers Leucippus of Miletus (400 BC- unknown) and Democritus (460 BC-379 BC).

The doctrine of atomic structure and function is an innovative conceptual matrix, which directly challenges medical dogma and offers a new way in which to understand pathologies. In brief, the atomic structure model proposes the human body is composed of atoms, separated by voids of empty space. Atoms constitute the physical basis for communication between anatomical structures, not body humors. Disease results from constriction or relaxation of anatomical structure, as the result of physical changes occurring at the atomic level. Simply an elegant model of disease and one which receives very limited support from the medical and scientific communities. The model is soon overshadowed by the more popular balance of humors model.

Erasistratus is the last of the Alexandrians to report a large series of dissections of the human body. Contained within his dissection series are descriptions of the liver; one from a man who dies from abdominal dropsy (dropsy = old term for edema) and one from a man who dies from a snake bite. The liver from the man suffering abdominal dropsy is reported to be as hard as stone. The liver from the man suffering snake bite is soft and doughy in consistency (30AD/2012)[16]. Similar reports, describing changes in large organ systems are found throughout the series (1922)[17]. The findings move Erasistratus further away from conceptualizing disease within a balance of humors conceptual matrix and towards a matrix which emphasizes changes in solid organs, as primary to the disease process and can be associated with impairment in function.

Trivia: Erasistratus is a graduate of the medical school at Cnidus.

Human dissection is outlawed in Alexandria soon after the Roman invasion and destruction of the City and Libraries of Alexandria circa 47 BC. Human dissections do not reappear in this region for another 1,000 years, evidenced by the appearance of Mondino de Luzzi's manuscript "Anathomia Mondini" (1316/1474,1495,1507)[18,19,20].

As a consequence of government regulation prohibiting the use of specific medical investigational methods, in this case Roman law prohibiting human dissection, progress, development, and discovery of new knowledge in the area of medical human pathology is effectively stalled, for the next 1,000 years.

Aulus Celsus (30 BC-38 AD) Roman encyclopedist and non-physician offers his influential manuscript "De Medicina" [On Medicine] in eight volumes, circa 30 AD (30AD/2012)[21]. Arguably, this is the best surviving treaties of Alexandrian medicine known today. Of particular interests to pathology are Volumes II [Causes of disease], III [Treatment of disease], and IV [Anatomical descriptions of disease].

Volume II [Causes of disease] offers a systematic presentation of the epidemiology of disease, noting the importance of patient age, season of the year, weather conditions, and physical body characteristics as factors contributing to disease and illness. For example "…the middle period of life is the safest, for it is not disturbed by the heat of youth, nor the chill of age. Old age is more exposed to chronic diseases, youth to acute ones…"; "…winter provokes headaches, coughs, and all the affections which attack the throat, and the sides of the chest and lung…" (II,1,8); "…settled weather days are most salubrious (promote good health), rainy days better than foggy or cloudy days…the best days are those in which there is an entire absence of wind…" (II,1,3); "… the square built frame, neither thin nor fat is the fittest; for tallness as it is graceful in youth shrinks in the fullness of age; a thin frame is weak, a fat one sluggish…" (II,1,5) (30AD/2012)[21].

Volume III [Treatment of disease] offers a system of classification of disease adopted from the Greeks and organizes "…these into two species, terming some acute, other chronic…" (III,1,1) (30AD/2012)[21]. Celsus extends the classification system to four categories; acute, chronic, acute changing to chronic, and those neither chronic, acute, or acute changing to chronic. In modern terms this fourth category is labeled "not otherwise specified" NOS.

Perhaps the most recognizable observation made by Celsus pertaining to pathology and known by all medical students today is his description of the signs and symptoms associated with acute inflammation; "…Notae vero inflammationis sunt quattuor: rubor, et tumor, cum calore, et dolore…" (III,10,3 Latin edition); (redness, swelling, heat, and pain) (III,10,1 English edition) (30AD/2012)[21].

Trivia: This phrase is typically termed the four cardinal signs of inflammation. Actually, only three of these are signs, one is a symptom. That's right; redness, swelling, and heat are all signs, while pain is a symptom.

Book IV [Anatomical description of disease] reveals an excellent knowledge of internal human anatomy and the systematic study of clinical signs and symptoms associated with disease and associated changes in internal human anatomy. The first half of Book IV describes internal anatomy of gross anatomical systems e.g.

> "…from that point two passages begin: one named the windpipe, the more superficial, leads to the lung; the deeper, the gullet, to the stomach; the former takes in the breath, the latter food. Through their courses diverge, where they are joined there is a little tongue in the windpipe just below the fauces, which is raised when we breathe and when we sallow food and drink closes the windpipe. Now the actual windpipe is rigid and gristly; in the throat it is prominent, in the remaining parts it is depressed. It consists of certain little rings, arranged after the likeness of those vertebrae which are in the spine, but in such a way that whilst rough on the outer surface the inside is smooth like the gullet; descending to the praecorida it makes a junction with the lung..." (IV,1,3) 30AD/2012)[21].

The second half of Book IV offers descriptions of changes in anatomical structure associated with disease processes accompanying clinical signs and symptoms "… so far as it is necessary for a practitioner to know them…" (Book IV,2,1) (30AD/2012)[21].

Following each description, Celsus offers treatment recommendations. He organizes information according to anatomical structures, beginning with the head and systematically working down the body to the feet. The following representative entry addresses pathology of the intestines;

> "…among intestinal maladies are gripings, called by the Greeks dysenteria. The insides of the intestines ulcerate; from these blood trickles and at times is excreted with some feces which are always liquid, at time with a sort of mucus… rest must be adopted from the first, since any shaking sets up ulceration; next on an empty stomach he is to sip a cupful of wine to which has been added powdered cinquefoil root…" (IV,22,2) (30AD/2012)[21].

Note: Cinquefoil, when translated from its vulgar (common) Latin origins means five leafs and describes this herb's distinctive five serrated leaf yellow flower. The flower has the scent of honey. The roots and tannic acid present have been used as a herbal astringent to stop bleeding since the Greek natural philosopher Theophrastus (371 BC-287 BC) first names the plant and describes its medicinal properties in his manuscript "Enquiry into Plants" (300 BC/1916)[22].

An important point to reiterate here is Celsus, an encyclopedist, is summarizing medical knowledge to date. Medical pathology is very much a part of medicine at this time (circa 30 AD) and has been for at least the past 500 years. Much pathology summarized by Celsus finds its origins in the investigations and writings completed at the earliest medical schools located at Croton (southern Italy) founded circa 490 BC, Cos (Greek island) founded circa 430 BC, Cnidus (Greek settlement located in modern-dayTurkey) founded circa 430 BC, and Alexandria (Egypt) founded circa 290 BC), where relationships between disease, anatomical structure, and function are aggressively studied.

Galen of Pergamum (129 AD-200 AD) (Pergamum is present day Bergama, Turkey) adopts and modifies the Greek doctrine of balanced humors introduced by Alcmaeon of Croton 500 years earlier. The original and modified models offer rational models of disease, identify mechanisms of action responsible for the development and maintenance of disease, and guide treatment. Galen too emphasizes the natural rather than supranatural basis for disease. Echoing the observations of Greek natural philosopher Aristotle, Galen too proclaims "…a function is never impaired without the part governing the function being affected…" [On the Affected Parts] (190AD/1976)[23]. Galen is prolific in his writings yet contributes little new to the knowledge base of pathology.

Government regulations, imposed by Roman Empire law, prohibit human dissection during Galen's lifetime. Consequently, most anatomical based pathological findings reported by Galen and his many scribes are from animal vivisections and dissections. The findings are authoritatively and dogmatically generalized to humans. This process results in errors, both in normal anatomy and pathology. In combination, government regulations prohibiting human dissection, organized religion's dominant modifying influences with emphasis upon supranatural (deity based) rather than natural causes of disease, Galen's prolific writings and unwillingness to consider alternative or conflicting information, and uncritical acceptance of Galenian dogma, effectively impedes the advancement of pathology for the next 1,500 years.

As much as Galen is recognized today for of his many contributions to medicine, so too he should be recognized for impeding progress and innovative thought in medicine. Many find much comfort in uncritical acceptance of medical dogma. This statement was true during the time of Galen and true today, over 2,000 years later. Finding comfort in current medical and scientific dogma can be alluring. I encourage you, as future physicians, do not fall victim to this seductive siren.

In summary, the written record of Antiquity reveals the early foundation of medical pathology as a scientific discipline. Medical pathology identifies specific areas of investigation, methods of investigation are defined and developed, models of disease are conceptualized, defined, and actively investigated, old and new knowledge continues to be committed to the written record, knowledge continues to be shared among investigators and between surrounding civilizations, and the rapidly developing knowledge base of medical pathology becomes a required content area, for all medical students completing formal medical education programs.

Alcmaeon of Croton founds the first medical school in Europe, located in southern coastal Italy in the city of Croton. It is here, disease is systematically investigated, from a physical basis, and the first model conceptualizing disease as an imbalance of body humors is first introduced. Approximately 100 years later, the medical school on the Greek island of Cos is founded by Hippocrates and complements the more established medical school, located at the Greek settlement of Cnidus, in western Turkey.

All three schools devote considerable resources to investigating relationships between physical health and disease. All three schools make contributions to the collection of writings which will later be known as the Hippocratic Collection. The Collection is compiled in the City and Libraries at Alexandria, located on the Mediterranean coast of Egypt, located approximately 420 miles southeast of Cos and Cnidus, and approximately 100 years after Hippocrates founds the medical school on the island of Cos.

Mark differences in the conceptual matrix of disease and methods applied to study disease are soon evidenced between the schools at Croton, Cos, and Cnidus. The medical school at Croton emphasizes invasive observations and association between impaired physical health and impaired physical structure. The medical school at Cos emphasizes non-invasive observation of the body's response to disease and trauma. The medical school at Cnidus, like the medical school at Croton, emphasizes invasive observation and additionally associates impaired physical health and impaired function, specifically to abnormal changes occurring in body organs. All three schools emphasize the natural (physical) rather than the supranatural (non-physical) basis of disease and body function. All three schools embrace, in modified form, the balance of humors model of disease, first introduced by Alcmaeon of Croton circa 480 BC

Unlike the medical school faculty at Croton, Cos and Cnidus, some faculty at Alexandria challenge the dogma of the balance of humors model and offer an alternative, the doctrine of atomic structure.

Between 500 BC and 50 BC medical pathology establishes a solid foundation upon which the discipline will build for the next 3,000 years. The foundation is based upon a systematic, scientific, investigation of relationships between physical health and disease. Disease, no matter how it is conceptualized e.g. collection of clinical signs and symptoms, imbalance of body humors, abnormal changes in body organs, or physical change occurring at the atomic level, all have a physical basis and can be systematically investigated, studied and understood. Relationships between disease and physical health are stable, reproducible, and sufficiently important to be committed to the written record and shared between civilizations and generations. Familiarity with these established relationships is recognized as essential to the competent practice of clinical medicine and is established as a necessary core component of the medical education of all future physicians.

By the middle of Antiquity, circa 50 BC-150 AD, much of the knowledge established during early Antiquity is simply eliminated. The written record of pathology knowledge is destroyed whenever it is found to be inconsistent with belief systems of the new ruling governments or newly founded organized religions. Institutions of learning e.g. the Libraries of Alexandria are determined to be threats to the State and destroyed. Educational systems are too considered threats to the State, dismantled and replaced by systems consistent with the belief systems of the new ruling few. Established natural (physical) models of disease are displaced by supranatural (deity) based models. Human dissection is explicitly prohibited by new Roman law and decree from organized religions. Medical pathology experiences a period in which most all that has been established during early Antiquity by systematic, empirical, scientific investigations, is displaced by faith based belief systems of newly organized religions. In its place is substituted a new knowledge base, much more consistent with the belief systems of individuals within the new ruling governments and the leadership of organized religions. The substituted knowledge is anchored in social and theological ideologies, rather than scientific investigation.

Amidst the many changes underway during the middle of Antiquity, Roman encyclopedist Aulus Celsus offers his influential manuscript "De Medicina" [On Medicine], circa 30 AD. This series of manuscripts summarize most of the surviving knowledge from Alexandrian medicine, preserving a summary of this knowledge for future generations. His eight volume series, comprising "De Medicina" is presented without bias or prejudice. Celsus simply summarizes that which is known to be true within the broad matrix of medical knowledge for the period.

Galen modifies and extends the 500 year old doctrine of humors model of disease. He offers rational models from which to study and practice medicine, as an alternative to the empirical models of early Antiquity. In the absence of opportunity imposed by Roman law and Church decree to empirically investigate the physical (natural) relationships between changes in physical health and physical changes within the human body associated with disease and illness, Galen focuses his attention upon generation of complex rational models. The models attempt to satisfy those ascribing to a natural (physical) basis of disease, as well as those ascribing to a supranatural (deity) based model of disease. His models explain both the source of disease, guide its treatment, and explain clinical courses and outcomes. In the presence of admittedly well-reasoned models, authoritative, self-confident presentation, wide distribution, few objections from government or organized religion, and in the absence of persuasive alternatives, Galen's dogma is soon accepted and rarely challenged by the medical community, for the next 1,500 years.

Medical pathology passes through three stages of development during Antiquity. The first stage, occurs during the first half Antiquity is characterized by rapid substantial progress in establishing a new scientific based discipline committed to understanding the relationships between changes in physical health and the associated physical changes occurring within the human body.

The second stage of development, occurs during the middle of Antiquity. This second stage is characterized by intentional destruction by new governmental and organized religion leaderships of most all that has been established regarding the natural (physical) relationships between physical health and disease. Supranatural (deity) based models replace natural models (physical) models of disease.

The third stage of development, occurs during the second half of Antiquity. This stage is characterized by the writings of Galen and attempts to provide an acceptable compromise between the two extreme models of disease, the natural (physical) model from early Antiquity and the supranatural (deity) models from middle Antiquity. Unfortunately or fortunately depending upon your perspective, Galen is extremely successful, establishing medical dogma palatable to advocates of both extreme position models, consequently stifling innovative thought and significant change in medical pathology for the next 1,500 years.

Middle Ages (Medieval Times), 500 AD - 1400 AD.

The Middle Ages witness radical changes in geopolitical, social, economic, and cultural systems of Europe, the Middle East, and North Africa. The Western Roman Empire falls to invading military forces from the Middle East. Academic cities of learning, which flourished during early Antiquity e.g. Athens and the Libraries of Alexandria are destroyed by invading military forces. Rapid discovery, innovative thought, and synthesis of new and old knowledge so characteristic of Antiquity stalls. The Eastern Roman Empire soon falls to invading military forces from Western Europe. Organized religion and its belief all people in the world should follow a single chosen religion and their religion is the only one to be followed fuels the military actions of the Islamic Conquests and Christian Crusades. Pursuit of new knowledge is displaced by religious dogma and the more immediate, pressing needs to stabilize geopolitical, economic, social, and governmental systems. The once dynamic and intellectually progressive region surrounding the Mediterranean Sea struggles with newly imposed governmental and religious order. The cost of this new order is tolled, in the loss of millions of human lives and one-thousand years period of no notable advancements being made in medical pathology. Scientific investigation and thought give way to faith-based, religious beliefs, and Galenian dogma.

Well established and newly organized religions of Judaism, Christianity, Catholicism, and Islam exert their newly founded tremendous influences and impose stringent restrictions on the methods used and content studied, to understand the physical bases of disease. These organized religions uniformly reject the natural (physical) based models of disease and illness established during Antiquity. They offer an alternative, supranatural (deity) based models, to explain and understand human disease and suffering.

The supranatural deity based models of disease state diseases are produced by a supranatural deity (God) and are imposed upon individuals whom fail to conform to the teachings of an organized religion's belief system. The less conforming an individual is the more severe the disease. Relief from the disease and associated suffering is accomplished by appeasing the angered deity, through acceptance of the beliefs of the religion and conforming to its belief systems, as outlined by leaders within the particular organized religion. Each religion uniformly states, it is their particular religion and their religion only which must be followed to insure freedom from or relief from disease. Each organized religion has its own unique set of ritualistic behaviors, which when completed offer prophylactic protection against disease and provides relief when affected by disease. The supranatural models, advocated by organized religion, displace natural (physical) models of disease and systematically impede advancements in medical pathology.

Organized religions significantly influence government leaderships resulting in the imposition of governmental regulations restricting medical and scientific investigations into the natural (physical) basis of disease and illness. Human dissection, as a tool and method to understand the natural (physical) basis of disease, continues to be explicitly prohibited. Centers of learning which once generated tremendous and frequent contributions to understanding the relationships between physical health and disease are suppressed or simply eliminated.

Early during the Middle Ages and amidst the political, economic, social, and military chaos, much of the collected written knowledge of human pathology is moved from Athens and other Cities of learning to the Middle East, in efforts to preserve the written record. It is here in the Middle East many original Greek, Roman, and Egyptian papyri and tablets are translated from their languages of origin into the languages of the Middle East e.g. Persian, Syriac, and Arabic. Specific written records translated with relevance to medical pathology are the multi-authored Hippocratic Collections, Dioscorides' "De Materia Medicia", and "Galen's Corpus". Little new content or process knowledge is added during the approximate 500 year period, between 500 AD and 1000 AD. Preservation and survival, rather than innovation and discovery, best describe the first half of the Middle Ages.

As Europe and Northern Africa return to political and economic stability circa 1000 AD, marking the beginning of the second half of the Middle Ages, scholars begin to return to Italy, Greece, and Northern Africa to resume the pursuit of new knowledge. The University system of education is introduced and new medical schools are soon founded, first in southern Italy at Salerno (1100 AD) and Bologna (1158 AD) and later throughout Europe e.g. Paris (1150 AD), Oxford in England (1167 AD), Montpellier in France (1181 AD), and Padua in Italy (1222 AD).

The study of pathology quickly becomes an integral part of medical education and firmly establishes itself as a core area of instruction within the curriculum of the newly founded medical schools throughout Europe. Instruction of pathology is based almost entirely upon knowledge established before the beginning of the Middle Ages. Human dissection is reintroduced for the purpose of understanding more completely human anatomy and anatomical pathologies associated with impaired function. The medical school at Bologna requires human dissection as part of every medical student's education. The value of autopsy in aiding in the discovery of the cause of death is soon recognized and heralded by the controlling members of the university's law school (sic) faculty. Numerous human dissections are completed and add to a developing base of knowledge confirming the physical basis of disease.

The concept of disease during the Middle Ages, as taught in the new medical schools throughout Europe, is based almost exclusively upon the balance of humors models, proposed by Alcmaeon of Croton, Hippocrates, and Galen, hundreds of years earlier. Disease is the result of an imbalance in body humors. Treatments are to be directed to restoring the balance between body humors. Autopsy findings are comfortably interpreted within this conceptual matrix.

The original balance of humors models are soon expanded to incorporate belief systems of the many newly founded organized religions. The expansion accommodates both a supranatural (deity) and natural (physical) model of disease and guides treatments. In brief, this widely accepted expanded model states a supranatural force (deity) is responsible for disease and determines whom will be affected and whom will not be affected by disease. The disease is then manifest in the selected individual as an imbalance in body humors, which can be naturally (physically) observed and manipulated by treatments. Treatment is simple; appease the angered deity through completing penance, praying for forgiveness, and reassuring the deity you will live your life better conforming to the rules of the organized religion, which in doing so will satisfy the supranatural deity and good health will be returned. The ritualistic behaviors satisfy the supranatural elements of the expanded model. Restoring humors to balance, by way of bloodletting, simple and compounded medications, hot and cold baths, and similar procedures satisfy the natural (physical) elements of the expanded model. Most effective treatment strategies incorporate both supranatural and natural dimensions of the expanded model.

The expanded models, incorporating supranatural and natural dimensions offer a conceptual theoretical matrix which answers all fundamental questions regarding disease and illness. Comfort is found in knowing all the answers. Knowing the source of disease (sent from an angered deity), how it is distributed (those who fail to follow the rules of organized religions), how it is manifested and maintained (imbalance of body humors), and how it is to be treated (restore body humors to balance), eliminates the need to pursue further answers to questions which have been satisfactorily answered. No new information is needed. All important questions have been answered.

Uncritical acceptance of Galenian dogma and the faith based dogma of organized religions, do more to impede advancements in the development of medical pathology than any single or combined factors or at any other time in the history of medicine.

When you believe you know all of the answers to all of the questions, you allow yourself to be lulled by a sense of self-assurance and self-confidence. Comfortable to be certain, false confidence eliminates further investigation, eliminates continued critical analysis, and stalls progress until such time someone elects to once again challenge the dogma of the time. Don't allow yourself as a future physician to be lulled into the state of uncritical acceptance of all that which has been given to you as correct answers. Do develop and maintain your own independent assessment of all medical dogma. If dogma is left unquestioned and unchallenged, there is no advancement made in the existing current knowledge base. Do dare to challenge our current knowledge and all that we believe to be true. Think for yourself. Critically evaluate for yourself. Do not be confined by the limits of others' thoughts and analyses. Do currently accepted truths make sense to you? If not, propose and scientifically evaluate an alternative truth.

By the end of the Middle Ages and following the second devastating epidemic of the bubonic plague, which sweeps through Europe during 1347 AD through 1353 AD, university based medical schools return to the practice of human dissection and active pursuit of new knowledge, especially in the areas of anatomy and anatomical pathology. Emphasis shifts from combined supranatural/natural models of disease to primarily natural models of disease. Associations are being made between abnormal gross anatomical structure and abnormal physical health. Changes in physical structure now explain changes in physical health. The second bubonic plague epidemic in Europe is interpreted to be caused by physical rather than supranatural influences and best understood as a physical process rather than a disturbance in a spiritual, faith based process.

Recall, one of the reasons the physical (natural) models of disease, established during Antiquity are displaced by supranatural (faith based) models proposed by organized religion, during the early Middle Ages, is failure of the natural models to explain the source and cause of the plague or to guide effective treatments during the first devastating epidemic of the bubonic plague circa 542 AD. With the emphasis once again being placed on the natural processes of disease, a physical explanation for the cause of the plague, a conceptual matrix within which to guide the physical treatment of the plague, medical school curricula requiring instruction and demonstrated competency in medical pathology by all medical students completing university based medical education and training programs, medical pathology is well positioned at the end of the Middle Ages to move forward once again.

In summary, the Middle Ages witness radical changes in geopolitical, social, economic, and cultural systems of Europe, the Middle East, and North Africa. The Western Roman Empire falls to military invasions from the Middle East. The Eastern Roman Empire (Byzantine Empire) falls to military invasions from Western Europe. Organized religions exert tremendous influence upon new government leaderships and significantly restrict progress in understanding relationships between physical health and disease. Supranatural (deity) models of disease, the models favored by organized religions, displace natural (physical) models. Strict restrictions are placed upon all those who attempt to investigate opposing, natural (physical) models of disease. Human dissection is explicitly prohibited.

Academic cities, libraries, and medical schools committed to new learning are destroyed. Records of established medical knowledge are destroyed or reinterpreted to conform to religious dogma of the period. Amidst the political, economic, social, and military chaos, efforts are made by some to protect and preserve the original written record of medical pathology. Greek, Roman, and Egyptian papyri and tablets are moved from traditional cities of learning e.g. Athens and Alexandria, to the relative safety of the Middle East. Records are translated from their original languages into the languages of the Middle East. While achieving the original goal of safeguarding the original records, Middle Eastern translations further modify original content. Preservation and protection of the original Greek, Roman, and Egyptian knowledge committed to the written record rather than original innovation or discovery best describes the first 500 years of the Middle Ages.

As Europe and North Africa return to political and economic stability circa 1000 AD, scholars begin to return from the Middle East. The university system for advanced education is introduced and new medical schools are founded throughout Europe. Natural (physical) models of disease displace supranatural (deity) models as the favored model taught within the new medical schools.

Human dissection for investigational and educational purposes once again becomes part of each medical student's medical education, Medical pathology returns to the medical school curriculum and declared essential and necessary knowledge for every medical student graduating from a university based medical school. Balance of humors models are the most preferred natural model taught within the new medical schools. However, natural (physical) models are tempered and modified to accommodate the popular belief systems of organized religions. Modified rational models offer a conceptual matrix acceptable to most, provide an explanation as to the origins of disease (deity), explain how disease is expressed within the human body (imbalance of humors), and guides treatment (restore balance of humors). No additional progress is made in medical pathology until the end of the Middle Ages and the beginning of the Early Modern period circa 1400 AD.

By the end of the Middle Ages, medical pathology has returned to a conceptual matrix which emphasizes the natural (physical) rather than the supranatural (deity) based models of disease. Newly founded, university based medical schools embrace the natural (physical) models of disease and boldly investigate the relationships between physical health and physical changes in the human body. Medical pathology stumbles out of the Middle Ages into the Early Modern period and Italian Renaissance.

Early Modern, 1400 AD - 1800 AD.

Medical pathology moves forward once again.

Advances in technology and a rebirth of intellectual curiosity provide the necessary conditions to move medical pathology forward as a rapidly maturing scientific discipline. Europe embarks upon the Renaissance with its early beginnings founded in the academic and cultural cities of northern Italy. The increased availability of paper, invention of the printing press, interests in studying original ancient Greek texts of science rather than Latin translations and modifications completed during late-Antiquity and Middle Ages (Humanistic method), renewed interest in secular (worldly) rather than the supranatural phenomena, and interests in mechanical models of nature, all are applied in efforts to understand more completely the human body and changes associated with disease.

Most medical pathology practiced during the Early Modern period is best conceptualized as anatomical pathology. Human autopsies are completed, gross changes are carefully recorded, and findings are associated with patient clinical history. Results are published as series of individual cases, typical of the Italian schools or as synthesized summary of many cases, typical of the French schools. Midway through the Early Modern period, medical pathology becomes focused upon organ based systems. Organ-system based pathology parallels advances being made in organ-system based physiology of the period.

By the late-1700s investigators recognize different tissues are present in different organs and react similarly during the disease process. Systematic investigations of anatomical organ-systems based pathology soon include study of common disease processes occurring in distinctly separate and different tissues. Welcome general pathology. By the end of the Early Modern period, medical pathology moves from an emphasis on gross anatomical structures, organized into major organ systems, to examining and conceptualizing medical pathologies at the tissue level.

The dominant conceptual matrix is weighted heavily on a natural (physical) rather than a supranatural (deity) model. However, supranatural influences are not completely rejected. Often, natural (physical) changes observed in body organs and tissues continue to be understood within the matrix of Galenian dogma. Yes, there are physical changes in body organs and body tissues associated with disease, but the changes are the result of an imbalance in body humors which is initiated and maintained by a supranatural deity (God). Remember, at this time, only the earliest models proposing contagions have been proposed and not yet generally accepted by the medical or scientific communities.

Let us take a brief look at a few of the most influential people and events which guide and shape medical pathology through the Early Modern period, 1400 AD through 1800 AD.

Antonio Benivieni (1443-1502) Florentine physician offers a representative example of the Italian schools' approach to the study of the relationships between disease and associated physical changes of the human body. Working within a Galenian model of disease, emphasizing the natural (physical) basis of disease, Benivieni completes autopsies on patients presenting clinically with challenging courses or die unexpectedly. At autopsy, physical findings of these patients are recorded, detailing gross morphological changes, and are subsequently associated with the patient's clinical presentation and clinical course.

Below is an excerpt from Antonio Benivieni's now classic manuscript "De Abditis Nonnullis ac Mirandis Morborum et Sanationum Causis" [About the Hidden Causes of Disease] (1507)[24] which exemplifies the descriptive nature of medical pathology and its emphasis upon anatomical structure during the late-1400s and early-1500s.

> "…Case III… (a) woman... (with) pain in the region of the liver… consulted many physicians, but could not drive out the evil by any remedy…she departed this life…I then had her dead body cut open…There were found in the lower part of the membrane round the liver, a collection of small stones varying in shape and color. Some were round, some pointed, some square, according as position and chance had determined, and they were also marked with reddish, blue and white spots. These stones by their weight had caused the membrane to hand down in a bag a palm's length and two fingers wide. This we judged the cause of her death…." (1507)[24].

Typical of the Italian schools, this case is presented to the medical community as one of a larger collection of single case studies, compiled and published (n=111) (1507)[24]. No integrative summary of all cases is offered. Instead, the physician is to read each individual case and apply the reported observations and findings to their own individual patients, he or she may be treating. Publication of series of individual cases remains a popular format for communicating information between physicians for the next 600 years. The practice continues today.

Recognize here the importance and associated impact of the recent introduction of a new technology which makes distribution of case series readily available to a much larger readership, the printing press. The printing press, invented circa 1440 offers a flexible and affordable method to mass produce books and medical journals. Prior to the invention of the printing press, manuscripts are hand copied. Perhaps difficult to image today in a world where electronic distribution and sharing of information is immediate by way of the Internet and more specifically the World Wide Web.

As a medical student, take a moment now and think about the tremendous impact technology has had on shaping medical knowledge throughout history and how it will continue to influence medicine in the future.

OK…back to the late-1400s and early-1500s.

Jean Fernel (1497-1558) French physiologist offers a systematic, comprehensive, synthesis of medical pathological knowledge known to the period and proposes a new organizational structure. In brief, he organizes medical knowledge into three primary categories; physiology, pathology, and therapeutics. The new organizational structure is simple and conceptually elegant. Physiology concerns itself with the study of function of natural (physical) processes occurring within the human body. Pathology concerns itself with natural (physical) diseases and disease processes affecting the human body. Therapeutics concerns itself with the natural (physical) treatments and managements of patients by way of physical interventions or biologically active chemical substances.

Jean Fernel's innovative organizational structure accommodates Galenian dogma, while simultaneously offering a new conceptual matrix, within which to explain old knowledge and guide future investigations.

Fernel's conceptual model emphasize organ based systems, localization of disease, and identification of underlying biological processes producing or resulting from disease. Pathology moves from observation and description of structural anatomical changes to include examination of the underlying physical processes of disease. Synthesis and integration of anatomy with physiology is fundamental to Fernel's new pathology.

This new pathology is embraced first by the French schools and soon spreads throughout Europe as the preferred model. Fernel details his broadly influential conceptual matrix in a series of publications, first a collection of lectures "De naturali parte medicinae" [On the natural part of medicine] (1542)[25], next in two books "Medicina" (1554)[26] and "Pathologies" (1555)[27], and later published post humously, as "Universa Medicina, tribus et viginti libris absoluta" [All medicine, twenty-three books absolute] (1567)[28]. It is within these publications, the terms "physiology" and "pathology" are first introduced into the medical and scientific literature. These four publications, in their various forms provide the structure, content material, and overall conceptual matrix which guide the development of medical pathology through the next 200 years. Fernel's influence can be found in medical pathology today, now over 475 years after he first offers his conceptual matrix emphasizing physiology, pathology, and therapeutics.

Andreas Vesalius (1514-1564) Flemish anatomist and Professor of Anatomy, at the University of Paua in Italy, offers his first printing of "De humani corporis fabrica libri septem" [On the Workings of the Human Body in Seven Books] (1543)[29]. The publication offers a mechanistic view of human anatomy and is consistent with the mechanistic view of the natural world, popular at the time of publication. It is organized into seven books. Each book focuses on a functional anatomical system e.g. Book I, considers things that support the entire body, bones and ligaments; Book II, things essential for voluntary movement, muscles and ligaments; Book III, veins and arteries; Book IV, nerves; Book V, organs important for nutrition and generation; Book VI, heart and lungs; and Book VII, the brain and organs of sensation.

"De Fabrica", as Vesalius's momentous book is often referred, is a dissection manual for the human body. It does not address primarily issues of physiology, pathology, or therapeutics. It does offer instead, a detailed anatomical examination of organ systems and complete structures of the human body, which are organized loosely into functional systems. Complete and annotated English translations of the 1543 and 1555 editions of "De Fabrica" are available online by way of Northwestern University (1543/2013)[30]

The contributions to pathology offered by "De Fabrica" are many. Beyond its value as an early comprehensive human anatomy dissection manual, it articulates a return to the practices of the medical schools of Cnidia and Alexandria, circa 300 BC, when human dissection plays an essential and necessary role in advancing the knowledge of associations between impaired physical health and physical changes in human anatomy. A practice prohibited for over 1,700 years by governmental regulations and organized religion leadership decrees. "De Fabrica" challenges the dogma of Galen. It corrects many errors of normal human anatomy. "De Fabrica" offers the first mechanically printed and widely distributed manual of normal anatomy, against which changes in anatomy, as a function of disease and trauma, can be uniformly compared.

Contemporaries of Vesalius, also working as professors of anatomy in the Italian medical schools during the first half of the 1500s, rely heavily upon human dissection to make their many contributions. Perhaps as a medical student you recognize the names of Gabriele Fallopio (1523-1562) and Bartolomeo Eustachi (1500-1574). Both men rely heavily upon human dissections, in making their landmark contributions to understanding the normal anatomy and pathologies of the human reproductive system and human ear.

Accurate descriptions of human anatomy are not restricted to pathologists or anatomists. Italian Renaissance artists Leonardo da Vinci (1452-1519) and Michelangelo (1475-1564), also contemporaries of Vesalius working during the early-1500s, complete detailed anatomical human dissections and record the human form in masterful pictorial detail and exquisitely accurate sculpture.

By the mid-1500s, human dissection gains broad acceptance within the medical and scientific communities. Following one thousand years of fighting, including the Christian Crusades and Muslin Conquests, and millions of deaths in the region, resulting from organized religions leaderships repeated attempts to convince others to believe in only one God, their God, as the one and only God, and that all others are inferior, false Gods, a modicum of sensibility and stabilization returns to the region.

Complemented by a populous swell of dissatisfaction with organized religion and by extension supranatural (deity) models of disease, attention returns to the investigation of secular, natural (physical) models of disease. Soon the Roman Catholic Church reverses its longstanding objections against human dissection and sanctifies human dissection circa 1556. Additionally, London's Royal College of Physicians is given governmental and Church permission to once again dissect human cadavers, for medical and scientific purposes, as a result of recent changes brought to bear as one of many consequences of the English Reformation of organized religions e.g. Protestants breaking away from the controlling authority of the Roman Catholic Pope.

Rejuvenated by a focused return to physical models of disease, a return to acceptance of human dissection, a return to geopolitical, economical, and social stability, and a renaissance interest in new knowledge, medical pathology once again begins to make substantial progress and continues to develop as a maturing scientific discipline.

As the supranatural (deity) models of disease are displaced by natural (physical) models, there is a need to develop alternative models which not only explains the product of disease e.g. changes in gross internal anatomical structure, but also how disease is transmitted from geographical region to region or person to person. The most popular and widely accepted model of the period (mid-1500s) is the now familiar Miasma model of disease.

Miasma theory states in brief, disease results from poor environmental conditions such as foul air, contaminated water, or poor physical hygiene. These types of environmental conditions produce a noxious "air" which emanates from decomposing organic matter. It is the bad air that is responsible for disease. The model provides an explanation of transmission of disease without direct contact. Once "bad air" enters the body, an imbalance in bodily humors develops and the patient experiences the characteristic clinical signs and symptoms associated with the particular imbalance as outline by Galenian dogma. Anatomical changes result as a consequence of the imbalances in body humors. Treatments are directed to restoring balance of humors.

It is easy enough to see the reasons for the popularity of the Miasmas model of disease. It is rational, testable, and recognized by the medical community for over 1,500 years, as the preferred model within which to understand, diagnose, and treat patients suffering disease. How could it possibly be wrong?

Girolamo Fracastoro (1478-1553) Italian scholar challenges the medical dogma of the period and offers an alternative model to Miasmas theory, to explain disease. Girolamo Fracastoro offers his new theory of Contagions in "De contagion et contagiosis morbis curatione" [On contagions and the cure of contagious disease] (1546/1930)[31]. It is here Francastoro distills current knowledge on the physical causes and cures of disease and offers his conceptual matrix of Contagion theory, a forerunner of Germ theory.

In brief, Contagion theory states disease is the result of invisible, physical particles, transmitted between people, as the result of direct physical contact, indirect contact by fomites e.g. clothing, bedding, or carried through the surrounding air. The "…invisible seeds of disease…", which Fracastoro terms "semiaria", simply enter the body by contact or inhalation. The model is certainly not entirely original and can best be appreciated and understood within the matrix of medical history as an extension of Miasmas theory and as a further development and extension of earlier theories, emphasizing person to person transmission of human disease. Continuation rather than innovation best characterizes Contagion theory. As with most challenges of medical dogma, Contagion theory receives little attention from the medical community.

Understanding the cause of disease is as important as understanding the resultant changes of disease. This statement defines the future of medical pathology.

Felix Plater (1536-1614) Swiss, Professor of Medicine, and Dean of the medical school at the University of Basle (Switzerland) is perhaps most remembered for classification of psychiatric disorders (1602)[32]. He is among the first to systematically investigate mental illnesses from a scientific perspective. He is among the first pathologists to seek physiological origins to mental disorders rather than blindly accept the medical dogma of the period, mental disorders have their origins in the supranatural.

Felix Plater is first to correctly describe the underlying anatomical pathology responsible for Dupuytren contractures (1614)[33]. Plater describes this debilitating flexure of the palm and fingers 217 years before French anatomist Gullaume Dupuytren (1777-1835) describes the exact same condition and claims credit for priority of discovery (1831)[34]. Dupuytren names the condition after himself and fails to recognize Plater's earlier description. This practice, reporting conditions and pathologies previously published elsewhere by others, then publishing a case or series of cases illustrating the condition or pathology and claiming priority of discovery becomes an all too common practice, especially in Great Britain, during the 1800s. More on this practice later.

Felix Plater is first to offer autopsy evidence demonstrating sudden infant death syndrome (SIDS) is the result of an identifiable natural (physical) cause. Plater reports autopsy observations of a five month old (SIDS) infant and describes an enlarged thymus, which has compressed cervical blood vessels and trachea (1614)[35]. Plater extends his report of findings beyond a simple description of observed changes in anatomy associated with SIDS and includes an interpretation of his findings, within the conceptual matrix of a Galenian imbalance of humors model, popular during the early-1600s. Much like Felix Plater's report on the pathology underlying Dupuytren contractures, his contribution in understanding the pathology of SIDS goes largely unrecognized and unacknowledged by the medical and scientific communities, during the early-1600s.

Arnold Paltauf (1860-1893) Austrian pathologist and coroner for Vienna, (re)discovers the association and reports cases of unexplained sudden infant death syndrome (SIDS) to be characteristically associated with enlargement of the thymus and other similar lymphoid tissues (1889)[36]. Paltauf's makes his "discovery" approximately 275 years after Plater first describes the physical change in the thymus and its association with sudden infant death syndrome. Arnold Paltauf interprets his findings within the new infectious disease models, which gain considerable popularity during the late-1800s.

The same clinical syndrome (SIDS), presenting with the same observed physical changes in internal structural anatomy and interpreted within conceptual matrixes popular during each period, reflect the continuing maturation of pathology, as a maturing scientific based discipline.

Theophile Bonet (1620-1689) Swiss pathologist working within the Italian format publishes an extensive collection of 3,000 autopsies completed during the past 200 years (1679)[37]. The collection is composed of case histories and organized into four sections. Each section is organized according to gross anatomical regions of the body. Specifically, section I examines diseases of the head, section II diseases of the chest, section III diseases of the abdomen, and section IV diseases whose seat is unknown e.g. fevers and tremors. Each case is composed of an anatomical description of gross anatomical structures, notes of abnormal findings of structure, and associates autopsy pathological findings with clinical presentation before death. This publication represents the first extensive review and synthesis of autopsy findings which focus on diseased organ systems. It proves influential in its summary of known anatomical changes associated with disease.

By the late-1600s it is well established many disease states are associated with gross physical changes in normal human anatomy. Changes in anatomy are documented at autopsy and associated with patients' pre-morbid clinical presentations. Documentation remains largely descriptive in kind. Few offer new conceptual models to explain the observed physical changes. Most observed changes continue to be interpreted within the matrix of Galenian dogma and an imbalance of humors model of disease.

Herman Boerhaave (1668-1738) Dutch pathologist, working at the medical school at Leiden University, recognizes the value and growing importance for every new physician to have a fundamental command of pathology knowledge. Boerhaave insists each medical student be exposed to post-mortem examination as a routine and necessary component of the student's medical education. During each post-mortem examination, students are instructed on associations between patient clinical presentation of signs and reported symptoms and associated changes in human anatomy, as evidenced upon visual, post-mortem inspection of anatomical structures. Note the post-mortem examinations insisted upon by Boerhaave have a very different educational objective than that of anatomical dissections of a cadaver completed during the first year of medical school. Can you identify the differences in the educational objective?

Herman Boerhaave extends pathology beyond simple inspection of anatomical changes to include systematic analysis of patient excrements and fluids, for diagnostic purposes e.g. urine (1693, 1732)[38,39]. This opens new lines of investigation.

Giovanni Morgagni (1682-1771) Italian anatomist, working principally at the University of Padua and one time prosector for famed Italian anatomist Antonio Valsalva (1666-1723), offers his most influential publication "De sedibus et causis morborum per anatomen indagatis" [About the seats and causes of diseases through anatomical investigation] (1761)[40], which he publishes at 80 years of age. This influential treatise systematically describes changes in human anatomy associated with organ based disease. Structural pathological findings of 640 human autopsies are reported. The findings are associated with clinical signs and symptoms evidenced by each patient. It represents the second major treatise to focus specifically upon anatomical changes associated with human disease. Theophile Bonet's "Sepulchretum", published 82 years earlier is first to offer a comprehensive, systematically compiled series of autopsy findings focusing upon organ systems and associating autopsy findings with clinical presentation of patients (1679)[41],

To this point in time, most publications concern themselves with the identification and description of normal human anatomical structures. Theophile Bonet and Geovanni Morgagni are unique in that they are among the first and few to embrace the rich knowledge available through the study of abnormal structural anatomy. Morgagni's treatise "On the sites and causes of disease through anatomical investigation" (1761)[42] is quickly accepted by the medical and academic communities. It is soon translated from the original Latin into French (1765), English (1769)[43], and German (1771) and is used extensively throughout Europe, as the premier text for all interested in understanding the anatomical basis of human disease.

Morgagni emphasizes localization of disease to specific organ systems and considers post-mortem analysis of organs to be necessary. He conceptualizes disease within the popular doctrine of humors model and believes each disease has a final anatomical resting place. Each disease will selectively and preferentially affect a specific organ system. Structural changes within the organ are unique to the disease, much like a fingerprint and can be described. Through understanding the physical changes evidenced by an organ, one can understand disease.

Given the establishment of an anatomical substrate for human disease and clear associations with clinical signs and symptoms evidenced by the patient prior to death, the following questions are soon raised. Are the recognized anatomical changes the cause of disease or are they the result of disease? What are the biological processes which produce these changes? Can these processes be identified, described, and understood? These and similar questions guide the future direction of medical pathology.

John Hunter (1728-1793) Scottish surgeon and experimental pathologist begins to provide answers. His work exemplifies the shift in medical pathology from focus on changes in anatomy alone to include investigation of processes underlying changes in anatomy. Hunter is among the first to adamantly argue two diseases cannot exist simultaneously in the same organ. To believe otherwise "…appears to me to be founded in ignorance…" (1786)[44]. It is here Hunter test his model and investigates the possibilities of simultaneous infection by gonorrhea and syphilis.

In this same publication, Hunter first describes inflammation as both a defensive mechanism and a reparative process (1786)[44]. His thoughts and findings regarding the process of inflammation are extended in his treatise on blood, inflammation and gunshot wounds (1794)[45]. Biological processes underlying disease are now a primary focus of attention for those investigating human disease.

Matthew Baille (1761-1823) Scottish pathologist, nephew of John Hunter, moves medical pathology forward as a discipline with publication of "The morbid anatomy of some of the most important parts of the human body" (1793)[46]. This publication is first in the English language to present system based pathology in an organized textbook format and treat pathology as a separate subject, worthy in and of itself, as a new independent discipline of specialization. Ballie follows his 1793 publication six years later with an accompanying atlas of gross pathology (1799, 1803)[47,48]. Both textbook and atlas are well received by the medical community, as systematic treatments of organ based systems of pathology, yet have much less influence than Morgagni's treatise (1761)[42]. Unlike Morgagni treatise, Ballie's textbook and atlas are entirely descriptive and lack new or innovative ideas.

Mathew Baille's textbook and atlas of human pathology are formatted to provide a detailed description of gross anatomical structure, a brief clinical history of demographic information and significant signs and symptoms evidenced prior to death, and are organized according to major organ systems. They are written in the typical French School style of the period, which offers a synthesized summary of information. This stands in marked contrast to the typical Italian school format exemplified by Morgagni, in which information is presented as a series of individual cases without synthesis or summary. Which style is adopted by your medical school to present clinical pathology to you today? Which style do you as a medical student prefer? French style? Italian style? How is pathology taught in medical school today different from how pathology was taught during the 1700s?

Marie Francois Xavier Bichat (1771-1802) French anatomist moves medical pathology forward and beyond examination of gross anatomical changes associated with clinical signs and symptoms. He changes the unit of study for pathologist. Bichat introduces pathology to the study of tissues. Prior to Bichat, pathology focuses on organs and organ systems as the primary unit of study for pathologists. His methodologies e.g. cooking, drying, maceration, and exposure to chemical agents such as acids, alkaloids, and alcohol result in the separation of 21 distinct tissue types found within the human body. All of Bichat's tissues e.g. vascular, muscular, glandular can be identified and evaluated, as did Bichat, without use of a microscope. Bichat argues disease attack tissues rather than whole organ systems (1800a,1800b)[49,50]. Pathology now, at the end of the 1700s, begins to include routine assessment of body tissues, as essential to understanding associations between physical changes and disease, occurring within the human body.

Trivia: The term "tissue" is derived from the Old French word "tissu", meaning "woven material". The term is introduced into the medical literature by Marie Xavier Bichat (1800a)[49].

Much of Bichat's inspiration to analyze human body tissue is attributed to the influence of another perhaps a more recognized and familiar French physician, Philippe Pinel (1755-1826). Pinel challenges the dogma of humoral models popular during the late-1700s to explain pathology. He argues diseases must be understood within the matrix of structural lesions responsible for producing disease. Pinel reasons, given organs are composed of different elements (tissues), research need be directed to identifying the different elements of each organ and understanding how each element contributes to disease.

Pinel formalizes his conceptual matrix in his "Philosophical Nosography" (1798)[51] two years before Bichat first offers his "Traite des membranes en general de diverses membranes en particulier" [A treatise on the membranes in general and on different membranes in particular] (1800)[52]. Unlike many in academic medicine throughout history Bichat readily acknowledges Pinel's influence, "…it was reading his work that I first received this idea…" (1813)[53] referring to the study of disease at the level of individual tissues rather than organ based systems.

Pathology changes its primary unit of study across time as new technologies are introduced and conceptual matrixes are modified or replaced. Initially, a nascent medical pathology focuses the study of the entire human body. As the discipline matures the focus shifts to organ based systems. Now, in the late-1700s the unit of study shifts again to focus on investigations and analyses at the tissue level. The principle unit of study of medical pathology will shift again no less than three more times before the early-2000s.

In summary, during the Early Modern period 1400-1800, medical pathology witnesses a rebirth of intellectual curiosity and rapid advancements. Disease is conceptualized once again within the matrix of natural (physical) rather than supranatural (deity) forces. Human dissection returns to academic centers and offers new knowledge. Specific anatomical changes are identified and associated with specific diseases. Specific anatomical changes observed post-mortem are now regularly associated with patients' signs and symptoms evidenced upon clinical presentation and clinical course. Pathology's role in medicine is clarified and is identified as one of the three primary pillars of medicine, along with physiology and therapeutics. Miasma theory of disease is displaced by Contagion theory. Invention of the printing press allows for mass distribution of pathology knowledge and greatly improves communication between international investigators and clinicians.

Pathology extends beyond investigation of structural anatomy to include body fluids. Emphasis moves from description of structural changes and identified associations with clinical signs and symptoms to include investigations of the process of disease. Specific processes such as inflammation and tissue repair are aggressively investigated. Textbooks and atlases devoted specifically to pathology begin to appear. Course work in pathology and supervised human dissection experiences are now routine in European medical schools. Pathology establishes itself as valuable to the advancement of basic scientific medical knowledge and proves to be of increasing value to the practicing clinician.

Middle Modern, 1800 AD - 1900 AD.

The 1800s witness significant and rapid maturation of medical pathology as a professional discipline. Medical pathology is becoming an increasing specialized area of study and rich source of new medical and scientific knowledge. Professional societies and specialized journals devoted to the advancement of medical pathology knowledge are founded. Improved optics allow for more sophisticated use and application of the microscope. Introduction and development of Cell theory moves the principal unit of study within pathology from tissues to cells. Disease is re-conceptualized to accommodate pathologies occurring at the level of the cell. Chemistry continues to play important roles in understanding pathological changes associated with impaired physical health. Evaluations of human body fluids are now routine parts of pathological investigations. Diseases are now defined as a function of clinical signs and symptoms, as well as reliable, well documented, anatomical structural changes. Changes in normal human physiology begin to be identified, quantified, and associated with disease states and disease processes. Advancements in pathophysiology parallel rapid advances being made in normal human physiology. Technological advancements in tissue and cell staining, the fixation of biological tissue samples, and microscopy open new opportunities for discovery and sharing of new knowledge among investigators and practicing clinicians. Areas of specialization begin to develop within medical pathology and separate along lines of nationality. All substantive advances continue to be made in Europe. Medical pathology continues to mature as a professional discipline.

The early-1800s focus attention on the investigations of body fluids. Particular attention is directed to microscopic examination and chemical analyses, in efforts to better understand how body fluids change as a function of disease processes and as resultant products. Blood and urine are most studied. By the late-1830s, pathology is all about the cell. The discipline's primary unit of study shifts from organ based systems and tissues to the individual cell. Conceptualization of all biology within the matrix of the newly proposed Cell theory changes the focus of medical pathology forever. Coupled with much improved microscope optics, medical pathology makes considerable progress in the examination of disease and disease processes, at levels previously unexplored. European investigators lead the way into the new world of cellular pathology.

The mid-1800s reveal the first of many rewards resulting from recent advances in new and improved technologies, coupled with innovative thought, which challenge medical dogma. Disease and disease processes are conceptualized and studied within the matrix of Cell theory. Microscopic organisms, bacteria and parasites are identified and understood within the matrix of disease and disease process. Trichomonas vaginalis is identified in sexually transmitted disease. Blood pathologies are studied and result in the first descriptions of cellular changes underlying leukemia. Blood platelets are identified and their role in blood coagulation is first detailed. Malignant tumors are studied and understood at the microscopic level. Pathology textbooks and atlases move beyond descriptions of gross morbid anatomy to include structural changes associated with disease, at the cellular level. Pathologies are further understood within the matrix of altered normal and abnormal body physiology. New scientific and medical journals devoted specifically to pathology are founded, begin publication, and enhance the exchange of new information between investigators and among practicing physicians. These are exciting times for medical pathology.

The late-1800s are characterized by identification of such familiar pathological processes as vascular thrombosis, embolism, infarction, coagulation necrosis, and inflammation. The pathology of myocardial infarction is first described, as well as the bacterium underlying the pathology of tuberculosis (TB). Innovative cell staining techniques and new tissue fixation technologies revolutionize pathology.

Let's take a brief look at a few specific influential people, milestone discoveries, and changes in conceptual matrixes, which shape the history and future of medical pathology.

Antoine Fourcroy (1755-1809) French chemist encourages the use of body fluid chemistry, as a new way to investigate and better understand human disease (1791,1799)[54,55]. This recommendation reflects a significant change in the usual and customary methods used to investigate disease and disease processes. Most pathologists to date emphasize structural changes associated with disease and disease processes.

Johannas Reil (1759-1813) German physiologist, perhaps most recognized for his seminal contributions in the field of psychiatry, embraces the guiding words of Antoine Fourcroy. He advocates the establishment of clinical laboratories, in all medical colleges and hospitals with the charge to investigate

> "…all pathologies that can be chemically investigated…; (specifically) the different concrements in the body (calculi), urine in diabetes, dropsy (old term for edema), stone diseases (including kidney stones, gallstones), high fevers, expectorations in pulmonary consumption (old term for tuberculosis), pneumonia, diphtheria, miliary fever (acute infectious fever characterized by profuse sweating), rheumatism (old term including arthritis), intermittent fever (including malaria), and actually all discharges and their relation to the kind of the disease, its character, and course, and to the medications applied…" (1813)[56].

Clinical laboratories devoted to the collection, analysis, and study of chemical changes associated with disease and disease processes are institutionalized.

William Prout (1785-1850) British chemist establishes simple tests of urine to assist in the diagnosis of diabetes and diseases of the urinary tract (1821)[57]. He establishes relationships between chemical processes of metabolism and excretion, as measured in urine, with changes in patients' clinical status and disease state. He offers a short list of simple and readily available equipment e.g. litmus paper, test tube, specific gravity bottle, candle, stopper vials containing solutions of ammonia, potash, and nitric acid, and a watch glass (a circular, slightly concave piece of glass used in chemistry as a surface to evaporate a liquid), which can all be carried by the practicing physician in a small portable case and used to complete all diagnostic tests of urine required by the practicing physician (1825)[58]. Prout's work establishes the fundamental basis of urine analyses completed routinely in medical offices, clinics, and hospitals throughout the world today, nearly 200 years after he first introduces its value to clinical medicine.

Richard Bright (1789-1858) British pathologist offers numerous and detailed studies investigating the relationships between diseases and associated structural changes appearing in the kidneys at autopsy (1827-1831)[59]. Bright is first to report nephrogenic changes associated with edema. He establishes a clear differentiation between edema resulting from heart and kidney dysfunctions. He investigates and reports extensively on kidney diseases, especially glomerulonephritis, which is later termed Bright's disease (1877)[60]. Bright additionally is responsible for developing the first successful procedure to identify excess protein in urine (albuminuria) and applying the laboratory procedure to assist in the diagnosis of kidney disease (1827-1831,1835,1836)[61,62,63].

Richard Bright offers physicians a simple procedure to identify albuminuria. Having established an association between albuminuria and kidney disease, he encourages the use of his simple procedure. In his own words,

"…one of the most ready means of detecting albumin is the application of heat by taking a small quantity of urine in a spoon and holding it over a flame of a candle. If albumin is present, you perceive before the fluid reaches the boiling point that it becomes opaque, sometimes presenting a milky appearance at the end of the spoon, which extends inwards till it meets in the centre and then breaks into a white curd…" (1827-1831)[61].

Bright's procedure to identify albumin in urine is sensitive but not specific to kidney disease (1827-1831)[61]. Demonstrated lack of specificity in combination with prevailing medical dogma which regards illness as a general condition and not the result of localized organ dysfunction, delays acceptance and wide application of the procedure by the medical community.

Thomas Hodgkin (1798-1866) British pathologist describes the clinical presentation and post-mortem findings of seven individuals he personally examines through autopsy, two patients which he completes physical examinations while patients at Guy's Hospital in London, and seven additional cases completed elsewhere by others, in a case series report titled "On some morbid appearances of the absorbent glands and the spleen" (1832)[64]. It is here Hodgkin first reports the physical structural changes localized to the lymph nodes and spleen, which 30 years later will be named by Guy's hospital physician Samuel Wilks (1824-1911) Hodgkin's disease (1865)[65].

Trivia: Guy's Hospital is a large National Health Service teaching hospital located in central London, United Kingdom. Guy's Hospital is founded in 1721 by British publisher Thomas Guy (1644-1724). The Hospital is originally founded to treat "incurables" discharged from other hospitals. Guy's Hospital continues operation today 2019, as the major teaching hospital of the prestigious King's College London School of Medicine.

Hodgkin's disease is an older term for that which today we term Hodgkin's lymphoma. It is a cancer of the white blood cells (leukocytes) originating from the lymphoid cell line e.g. natural killer cells, B cells, and T cells. These cells are essential to the normal functioning of the human immune systems. Disturbance of the normal cell cycles of these cells compromise the body's innate and acquired capabilities to defend itself against infections.

As a medical student take time now to ensure you know the difference between leukocytes originating from the lymphoid cell line and the myeloid cell line. Now, make sure you know how these two cell lines differentially contribute to your future patients' immune systems. Can you explain these fundamental differences to a first semester medical student with confidence?

Richard Bright and Thomas Hodgkin, working in Great Britain and Robert Graves working in Ireland, continue in the tradition of the French school of clinical pathology, describing clinical presentations and associating signs and symptoms with gross changes in anatomical structure. None embrace recent advances in microscope technologies or routinely use microscopes in their study of human pathologies.

Robert Graves (1796-1853) Irish surgeon, working at Meath Hospital in Dublin, Ireland, first describes the clinical presentation of four women, which later will be known to all simply as Graves' disease (1835)[66]. This autoimmune induced disturbance of the endocrine system is well known to medical students today. Graves' description of Graves' disease does not include any reference to microscopic or visual inspection of the thyroid gland or heart. Reporting pathologies in the matrix of the traditional French school of pathology, Graves's description is restricted to clinical signs and symptoms.

Recall, Graves' disease is an autoimmune disorder in which the body produces antibodies (IgG) which selectively attack the patient's TSH receptors, located inside of the thyroid gland, binding the receptor and stimulating the chronic release of T3 and T4 into the systemic blood supply, creating a state of chronic hyperthyroidism.

Here is an excerpt from Graves' original description of the four original cases, in which he reports the now characteristic signs and symptoms of the disease which bears his name;

> "…violent and long-continued palpitations in females…so closely related by sympathy to those palpitations of the heart which are so frequent occurrence in hysterical and nervous females…beating of the heart could be heard during the paroxysm at some distance from the bed…I could hear the heart beating when my ear was distant at least four feet from her chest!... enlargement of the thyroid gland… the enlargement of the thyroid, of which I am now speaking, seems to be essentially different from goiter in not attaining a size at all equal to that observed in the latter disease… Indeed, this enlargement deserves rather the name of hypertrophy… when palpitations were violent, the gland used notably to swell and become distended…the swelling immediately begin to subside as the violence of the paroxysm of palpitation decreased…there was not the slightest evidence of any thing like inflammation of the gland… females liable to attacks of palpitations almost invariably complain of a sense of fullness, referred to the throat… inducing a sense of suffocation… (one patient evidences) some symptoms which were supposed to be hysterical…the eyeballs were apparently enlarged, so that when she slept, or tried to shut her eyes, the lids were incapable of closing. When the eyes were open, the white sclerotic could be seen, to a breath of several lines, all round the cornea… In a few months the action of the heart continuing with unceasing violence, a tumor, of a horseshoe shape, appeared on the front of the throat exactly in the situation of the thyroid gland. This was first soft, but soon attained a greater hardness, though still elastic…" (1843)[67].

Trivia: Robert Graves originally believes and investigates the origin of Graves' disease to be a pathology of the heart rather than the thyroid gland.

Robert Graves is most closely associated with the early description and discovery of the condition we recognize today as Graves' disease, however many preceded him in reporting the condition in the medical literature.

Thirty-three years before Graves offers his first publication on the condition, Italian surgeon Giuseppe Flajani (1741-1808) describes the condition in two patients. Flajani reports the first patient to evidence an obvious and palpabal "…tumor (in the front of the neck)… and… extraordinary palpitation in the region of the heart…". The second patient presents with similar signs and symptoms (1802)[68].

Twenty-five years before Graves offers his first publication on the condition, Antonio Testa (1756-1814) Italian, Professor of Medicine at the University of Bologna- School of Medicine, describes similar clinical patients, noting a coincidence of prominent eyes and disease of the heart (1810)[69].

Twenty-years before Graves offers his first publication on the condition, British physician Caleb Parry (1755-1822) describes the condition in two clinical cases. The first and most demonstrative case is a 37 year old woman who develops palpitation, tachycardia, and goiter a few months after childbirth. Parry reports "…her eyes protruded from their sockets…each systole of the heart shook the whole trunk of the body…". Parry interprets these findings to be the result of heart disease and the goiter to result from extra blood pumped from the heart and stored in the thyroid gland (1815,1825)[70, 71].

Medical students oftentimes focus on exophthalmoses (ex = prominent; opthamos = eyes; bulging eyes) as the most impressive and diagnostically important clinical sign of Graves' disease. In fact, exophthalmoses is present in only 20% of cases. In review of Robert Graves' four original patients, only one, patient number four, added at the last minute before publication and referred to Graves by friend and colleague William Stokes, actually evidence exophthalmoses (1835)[66].

Focused attention on exophthalmoses, as part of the clinical diagnostic presentation of Graves' disease patients is exacerbated by an 1840 publication, "Exophthalmos caused by hypertrophy of the cellular tissue in the orbit" (1840)[72]. In this paper, the author Karl von Basedow (1799-1854) German physician emphasizes the ocular abnormality in 3 women and 1 man. Inspection of the original published paper reveals von Basedow making only brief mention of the more common signs and symptoms and more typically associated with Graves' disease, heart palpitations and enlargement of the thyroid gland (1840)[72].

Graves' disease continues to be a relatively common presenting condition today, affecting approximately 1.2% of the general population (2017)[73]. As a future physician you are likely to be in a position to diagnose and treat this autoimmune disorder. As soon as you inform your patient of the diagnosis they will, without exception Google Graves' disease and immediately see images of patients evidencing severe exophthalmos. These images will unnecessarily frighten your patient. Do take time with your patient to inform them of the extremely low probability of exophthalmos appearing, especially given they will be receiving effective medical or surgical treatments from you.

William Stokes (1804-1878) Irish physician, colleague, and previous medical student of Robert Graves, offers additional and detailed descriptions of Graves' disease, 19 years after Graves' initial description is published. William Stokes frames Graves' disease within a matrix of cardiac theory (1854)[74].

As a medical student you might recognize William Stokes, as the physician who describes Cheyne-Stokes respirations, an abnormal pattern of breathing, characterized by progressively deeper and faster breathing followed by a brief period of apnea (1818,1854)[75,76]. This respiratory pattern cycles about once every 30 to 90 seconds and often observed in heart failure patients or any patient presenting with compromised brain stem respiratory regulation centers. The abnormal breathing pattern results from increases in blood CO_2 during the apnea phase, which is compensated by hyperventilation. If this does not make sense, take a break from reading this chapter and review your acid-base respiratory physiology.

Richard Bright, Thomas Hodgkin, and Robert Graves, three names familiar to most medical students, all make their most influential contributions during the early-1800s, without the use of the microscope. They offer case series, demonstrating associations between clinical signs and symptoms and gross organ based structural changes, Bright the kidneys, Hodgkin the lymph nodes and spleen, and Graves the heart (sic). The works of these investigators offer a fair and representative sample of the type of pathology practiced during the early-1800s. Each secures a place in the history of pathology and the minds of medical students with diseases named in recognition of their contributions.

More innovative advances are being made in France and Germany. French and German investigators embrace and apply new technologies to the study of human disease, quickly incorporating new microscope technologies and recent advances in chemical analysis of body fluids to the study of human disease.

Alfred Donne (1801-1878) French physician and microscopist is first to describe and photograph microscopic parasites found in body fluids, responsible for sexually transmitted disease e.g. Trichomonas vaginalis (1836)[77]. He is first to describe the microscopic images of fluid contained within syphilitic chancres and buboes (1836,1837)[77,78]. Four years later, while examining blood through the microscope, Donne discovers blood platelets and reports his discovery to the French Academy of Sciences (1842)[79]. Donne is an early proponent of teaching medical students how to use the microscope and its value to the practice of medicine. He incorporates projection of microscopic images into his medical school lectures and authors "Cours de microscopie complementaire des etudes medicales" [Course of microscopy complementary to medical studies, written specifically for medical students] (1844)[80]. One year later he supplements this book with an atlas, containing 86 photographed microscopic images (1845)[81]. The "Atlas" includes the first microphotographs of normal human blood cells, platelets, leukemia cells, pus, urine, sperm, mucus, sweat, saliva, human breast milk, lymph, synovial fluid, Trichomonas vaginalis, and more (1845)[81].

During the mid-1800s, the value of the microscope to the practice of medicine is questioned by the majority of physicians. Many within the medical and scientific communities actively oppose the use of the microscope. Clinicians lead the anti-microscopy movement. Beyond being the focus of many heated discussions at professional medical and scientific meetings, during the mid-1800s, the controversy all too often results in personal attacks directed against the microscopist. Alfred Donne is not immune.

Trivia: Donne is responsible for the first photographic images taken through a microscope. He presents his images on February 10, 1840 to the French Academie de Sciences (1840)[82]. Two years later he publishes an innovative manual for physicians and mothers, on the science of child care, recommending breast feeding for both nutritional value and emotional bonding between mother and child (1842)[83]. Donne recommends frequent weighing of babies, as a quantitative measure of a child's health and nutritional state (1842)[83].

Alfred Donne using the microscope, describes a disorder of white blood cell maturation, linking for the first time abnormal blood cell pathology with leukemia (1844-1845)[84]. One year later, Scottish pathologist David Craigie (1793-1866) describes the microscopic changes observed in blood cells "…large number of colorless granular, spheroidal globules varying in size…" (1845)[85]. The same year Scottish pathologist John Bennett (1812-1875) reports his detailed pathological findings of an adult patient suffering leukemia and names the condition "leucocythemia" (1845)[86]. Bennett offers the first illustration of blood cells from a leukemia patient (1852)[87]. Six weeks following Bennett's 1845 publication, 24 year old German pathologist Rudolf Virchow (1821-1902) reports his pathological findings of a patient suffering from leukemia, noting a reversal in the usual balance of white and red blood cells, "…300 red cells to one white…" (1845)[88]. Virchow follows two years later with another detailed case description, names the condition "leukemia", and too claims priority for discovery (1847)[89].

Henry Fuller (1820-1873) English physician describes a patient with enormously enlarged spleen and liver, with all blood vessels dilated and revealing pre-morbid changes in blood cells, "…in addition to natural blood corpuscles, a very large proportion of abnormal, granular, colourless globules…", characterizing the clinical physical signs and microscopic findings of the condition later termed leukemia (1846)[90]. This represents one of the first reports describing changes in blood, collected pre-mortem and viewed under the microscope from a patient suffering leukemia. Four years later Fuller is first to apply microscopic inspection blood to assist in the diagnosis of leukemia in a pre-morbid child (1850)[91].

Here begins another heated debate over claims of priority for discovery between Alfred Donne, David Craigie, John Bennett, Henry Fuller, and Rudolf Virchow (1854a,1854b,1854, 1854)[92,93,94,95]. Whom do you think makes the most rightful claim?

Claims of priority for discovery are oftentimes made without recognition of the works of those who have gone before. Few if any whom claim discovery, have not been influences by the minds and works of their predecessors. Most every new discovery is the result of the work of many and whose efforts may have been long forgotten or simply unacknowledged. So goes the nature of many ambitious individuals and throughout the history of medicine and science.

Twenty-four years will pass, from the first report of blood changes associated with leukemia, before Ernst Neumann (1834-1918) German pathologist, working at the Pathological Institute in Konigsberg (present day Kaliningrad, Russia) and Giulio Bizzozero (1846-1901) Italian pathologist, working at the University of Turin (located in Piedmont region of northwestern Italy) discover the origin of the reported abnormal blood cells to be bone marrow and determine leukemia to be a disease of bone marrow (1868,1869,1869,1870,1872)[96,97,98,99,100].

You may recall the name Giulio Bizzozero from his additional contributions e.g. discovery of the bacterium Helicobacter pylori or description of the function of platelets, during blood coagulation. You may also recall the name Ernest Neumann from his additional contributions, during the mid to late-1800s, leading to the discovery of stem cells.

Johannes Muller (1801-1858) German pathologist and physiologist is among the first to use the microscope to investigate structural changes occurring in both the healthy human body and states of disease. Initially, Muller focuses on body tissues and soon moves to analyses at the cellular level. Perhaps most remembered for his contributions in the area of sensory physiology e.g. law of specific energies; stating sensory experience perceived by a person are determined by the sensory organ-pathway systems which carries the information rather than the sensory stimulus itself (1835)[101]. His contributions in the area of histopathology are equally impressive. Muller offers one of the first detailed accounts of the microscopic observations of malignant tumors (1838)[102].

Johannes Muller embraces and inspires others to use all of the basic medical sciences e.g. chemistry, physiology, anatomy, pathology to understand the fundamental mechanisms operating within the human body in both healthy and diseased states (1833)[103]. He trains many of the most influential and recognizable investigators of the mid-1800s.

Specifically, Johannes Muller trains such notables as Theodor Schwann who develops Cell theory (1838)[104]; Julius Vogel who authors the first histopathology atlas, containing both gross and microscopic images of the same specimen (1843)[105]; Emil du Bois Reymond who discovers the action potential and pioneers electrophysiology (1848)[106]; Jakob Henle who is an early pioneer of

Contagion theory (1840)[107], authors one of the first pathology textbooks emphasizing normal organ physiology and changes as a function of disease (1846)[108], identifies the structure and functions of the loops of Henle (1862)[109]; and Herman von Helmholtz who invents the ophthalmoscope (1851)[110].

Theodor Schwann (1810-1882) German quantitative physiologist, perhaps most remembered by medical students for identifying the myelin producing cells which surrounds peripheral nervous system neurons (1839/1847)[111] later named Schwann cells. However, his contributions to medical pathology have much broader impact. Schwann plays a principal role in the development of the conceptual matrix termed Cell theory and revolutionizes the science of biology (1838,1839/1847, 1839)[104,111,112].

Cell theory states the cell is the basic unit of structure for all living things; all living things are composed of cells; and new cells are produced from preexisting cells. Cell theory is soon applied to understanding disease and disease processes. Soon Cell theory begins to displace medical dogma embraced, during the early-1800s, that disease and illness result from imbalances in vital energies, whether the vital energies are defined as four humors (Hippocrates), four temperaments (Galen), or the soul (Christian based religions). Disease begins to be understood within the matrix of structural changes occurring at the cell level and disorders of normal cellular processes. The Cell theory model is extended and modified throughout the balance of the 1800s, while the fundamental tenants of the original model remains relatively unchanged. This new conceptual matrix is supported by recent advances in technologies e.g. greatly improved microscope optics and cell staining techniques, change forever the way disease and illness are understood, studied, and treated.

Trivia: Theodor Schwann discovers and names the digestive enzyme pepsin, the enzyme which breaks down food proteins into polypeptides inside the stomach (1836)[113]. The term pepsin is derived from the Greek word "peptein", which means "to digest".

Julius Vogel (1814-1880) German pathologist publishes the first atlases of histopathology offering systematic presentations of changes at the cellular level associated with human disease (1843)[114]. Vogel follows the atlas two years later with a comprehensive text of pathology titled "Die Pathologische Anatomie des Menschlichen Korpers" [Pathological Anatomy of the Human Body] (1845,1847)[115,116]. The text contains over 100 illustrations of commonly occurring pathologies. For example, Vogel illustrates the microscopic appearances of cells taken from pulmonary tuberculosis; cancers of the breast, lungs, uterus, liver, and testis; cirrhotic liver; cells from sputum from patients suffering pneumonia and bronchitis; cells from pleura and pericardial effusions; as well as effusions associated with sexually transmitted disease.

Hermann Lebert (1813-1878) German pathologist, working primarily at the University of Paris, also publishes one of the first and influential atlas of histopathology (1845)[117]. Lebert's atlas contains illustrations of specimens, as seen with the naked eye and under the microscope. The atlas is among the first to illustrate benign tumors, cancers, infectious diseases, and inflammatory changes. Six years following publication of the "Atlas", Lebert authors an early text on cancers, with concise summaries and organ specific descriptions of benign and malignant tumors (1851)[118]. Six years later, he offers a comprehensive, two volume text covering anatomical pathology and clinical pathology (1857)[119].

Julius Vogel and Hermann Lebert, during the mid-1800s, make many of the early contributions in cellular pathology, which define cellular pathology as a productive area of scientific investigation, contributing much new basic science knowledge and offering practicing clinicians essential new knowledge to better understand, diagnose, and treat human disease.

Karl von Rokitansky (1804-1878) Austrian pathologist, Professor of Pathology with the Vienna Medical School, completes more than an estimated 40,000 autopsies. He is first to report bacteria in patients presenting with inflammation to the interior linings of the heart chambers and heart values (endocarditis) (1842)[120]. He is first to distinguishes multiple focal lesions of inflammation of the walls of the bronchiole and basal lobes of the lungs (bronchial pneumonia) and a singular, large, continuous bacterial lesion effecting a specific lobe of the lung (lobar pneumonia) (1842)[120]. Working principally as a gross pathologist he authors an influential textbook of morbid pathology, "Handbuch der athologischen anatomie" [Handbook of pathological anatomy] (1842)[120]. He is first to correctly recognize patent ductus arteriosus (PDA) as a congenital malformation (1844,1852)[120,121]. Recall, PDA results when a normal fetal blood vessel fails to close soon after birth, allowing abnormal blood flow between the descending thoracic aorta and pulmonary artery, resulting in hypoxia.

Johann Scherer (1814-1869) German clinical chemist is instrumental in demonstrating the clinical value of the analysis of blood and urine. He is first to demonstrate the chemical changes in patients' blood, accumulation of lactic acid (hyperlactatemia), under conditions of hemorrhagic and septic shock and how analysis of blood chemistry offers a reliable and effective measure of cell hypoxia (1843,1851)[122,123]. He offers many of the first clinical laboratory findings leading to a significantly improved understanding of the biological processes underlying leukemia (1851)[123]. Scherer systematically associates and details changes in body fluids, as a function of patients' clinical presentation, diagnoses, and autopsy findings (1843)[122]. Blood, urine, pus, sputum, mucus, and assorted exudates are soon subjected to routine chemical analysis. His investigations into body fluids and their changes associated with pathology, change the practice of medical pathology for the next 175 years.

Body fluids are quickly recognized to contain tremendous information regarding not only the resultant product of disease but also the process of disease. Given, body fluids are easily collected, available for repeated collection over time from the same patient, and contain much information, their collection and analysis is quickly incorporated into the evaluation, diagnosis, and management of clinical patients. Clinical laboratories are soon established in large medical institutions e.g. Wurzburg (1841), Berlin (1842), and Vienna (1844) for the purpose of analyzing body fluids. Analysis of body fluids, especially blood and urine, continue to be a routine part of most initial medical examinations conducted today, over 175 years since Johann Scherer first reports his observations of body fluids.

Trivia: Johann Scherer is first to use the term "clinical chemical laboratory" [klinisch-chemischen laboratorium]. The term first appears in the forward of this monograph [Chemical and microscopic studies in pathology] (1843)[122].

Rudolf Virchow (1821-1902) German pathologist builds upon Schwann's Cell theory and proposes a new conceptual matrix within which to study and understand disease. Rejecting medical dogma, accepting recently proposed Cell theory and its postulate the cell represents the basic unit of life; Virchow boldly proposes all human disease can and should be understood within disordered cell function. He encourages use of the microscope, an instrument many physicians of the period still believe has yet to prove its value in medicine. Virchow represents a group of forward thinking investigators who move pathology forward, focusing their attentions on the disordered cell. Rejecting the current dogma stating the fundamental unit of life to be the 21 tissues identified by Marie Bichat (1800)124 and these tissues hold the information to explain all organ based disease; Virchow aggressively pursues investigations of the disordered cell.

Trivia: Rudolf Virchow is among the first to report the changes in blood cells associated with leukemia, coins the term "leukemia", and introduces the term into the medical and scientific literature (1845,1847)[88,89].

Impatient with the speed with which submitted articles are reviewed and published and frustrated by the established German medical community's to publish several of his own papers submitted, Rudolf Virchow, in cooperation with German anatomical pathologist Benno Reinhardt (1819-1852), cofound a new scientific journal. The new journal is the "Archiv für Pathologische Anatomie und Physiologie und für Klinische Medizin" [Archives for pathological anatomy, physiology, and clinical medicine]. The new journal is devoted to the advancement of scientific knowledge in the areas of pathological anatomy, physiology, and clinical medicine (1847)125. The Journal is recognized throughout the world today, over 170 years since publishing its first issue, as a highly prestigious, highly respected, peer review, scientific journal, always open and receptive to new ideas.

In light of the many substantial contributions made by Virchow to the advancement of medical pathology, he attracts much attention during 1855 when he plagiarizes the work of Polish embryologist Robert Remak (1815-1865). In brief, Virchow claims priorities of discovery in recognition cells are the result of division of preexisting cells. The discovery is reported in the scientific and medical literature 3 years earlier by Robert Remak (1852)126. Virchow republishes Remak's work and claims it as his own. The behavior draws much attention from within the scientific community and is a hot topic of conversation at scientific and medical meetings for years to come. Medical pathology, as do most all developing professional disciplines, must wrestle with the standards and practices of individuals working within the matrix of a maturing professional discipline.

As a medical student and soon to be future practitioner of medicine, how would you deal with this event? Think about it. What are the most important issues? Should the issues be addressed? What are the risks? What are the rewards? What is the professional thing to do? What is the right thing to do? Would you get involved?

Trivia: Robert Remak is responsible for first identifying the 3 germinal cell layers, from which all mature cells in the human body will have their origins; endoderm, mesoderm, and ectoderm (1850-55)127.

Bence Jones (1813-1873) British chemical pathologist aggressively investigates and recommends the use of the examination of urine as standard procedure to assist in the diagnosis of clinical disease conditions. The urine examination is completed by way of visual inspection with the use of the light microscope and chemical analyses. He offers his first paper and describes urate crystals in the urine of patients presenting with gout (1840)128. Perhaps most remembered by medical students who have completed their pathology course work for his contributions leading to the biochemical marker associated with multiple myeloma, the Bence-Jones (B-J) protein?

Recall, the Bence-Jones protein is simply the light chain elements of the basic molecular structure of all antibodies. Remember your immunology? All antibodies maintain a similar molecular structure, composed of two heavy chains and two light chains. We name antibodies according to the slightly different structures offered by the heavy chains, IgG, IgA, IgM, IgD, and IgE. The light chains complement the heavy chains and contribute to the familiar Y structure of the antibodies (immunoglobulins, Ig). Light chains are divided into two subtypes, kappa or lambda.

Trivia: The Bence-Jones protein is designated as kappa or lambda, representing the first letter of the last names of Leonhard Korngold (1921-2010) and Rose Lipari (1929-), acknowledging their contributions in recognizing Bence-Jones protein in multiple myeloma patients (1955)[129].

Discovery of the Bence-Jones protein begins with the observations by two London primary care physicians William MacIntyre (1791-1857) and Thomas Watson (1792-1882), during 1850. Their diagnostic workups of a 45 year old male (Mr. M.), presenting with severe chest and back pains with edema, leads to collection of the patient's urine, in efforts to understand the source of the edema. When William MacIntyre initially subjects the urine to the usual and customary procedure of heating, cooling, reheating and conducts preliminary chemical analyses, he observes a peculiar reaction (1850)[130]. The reaction is discussed below.

The two physicians are sufficiently intrigued and submit independent samples of this patient's urine to colleague Bence Jones, whom is now demonstrating particular interests in the chemical analysis of urine and other body fluids for medical diagnostic purposes. The following note is attached to one of the samples submitted to Bence Jones on November 1, 1945; "…Dear Dr. Bence Jones, The tube contains urine of very high specific gravity. When boiled it becomes highly opaque. On the addition of nitric acid, it effervesces, assumes a reddish hue, and becomes quite clear; but as it cools assumes the consistence of appearance which you see. Heat reliquidfies it! What is it?…" (1847)[131].

Bence Jones systematically details the physical and chemical properties of the urine (1847, 1848)[131,132]. He recommends further investigation and association with gross structural change observed at autopsy. An autopsy is performed on Mr. M. the following year.

John Dalrymple (1803-1852) British pathologist, provides the histological and gross anatomical findings from the autopsy of patient (Mr. M.). John Dalrymple reports "...the bony structure of the ribs was cut with the greatest ease, and the bodies of the vertebrae were capable of being sliced off with the knife…" (1846)[133] . This report represents one of the first microscopic based histological analyses of a patient presenting with mollities ossium (old term for osteomalacia i.e. softening of the bones). John Dalrymple's autopsy report, in combination with clinical presentation, preliminary observations of abnormal urine by William MacIntyre and William Watson, and detailed physical and chemical urine analyses completed by Bence Jones, reveal the value of keen observations made by primary care physicians, complemented by collaborative investigations completed by pathologists, resulting in a much greater understanding of human pathologies, in this case multiple myeloma.

Recall, multiple myeloma is a cancer of the plasma cells (mature B cells). Plasma cells are responsible for producing the body's antibodies. In multiple myeloma abnormal plasma cells accumulate in bone marrow, induce pain, and interfere with production of normal blood cells. Too much calcium released from destruction of bone, coupled with impaired kidney filtration produces hypercalcemia. Too much calcium is toxic to tissues.

Trivia: The hyphen is added between his first name Bence and last name Jones, after his death and when naming the B-J protein. Identification of the B-J protein by way of urine analysis is arguably the first biochemical test for a cancer (detecting proteinuria in multiple myeloma) and preceding all others by more than 100 years.

Augustus V. Waller (1816-1870) British neurophysiologist and past medical student of Alfred Donne (1801-1878) is first to report the cellular mechanisms underlying inflammation. Augustus Waller describes the migration of white blood cells out of capillaries into surrounding tissue, as typical of the inflammatory process (1846)[134]. Waller's report is met with exceptional skepticism by the medical and scientific communities, given the medical dogma of the period is incapable of explaining how cells can possibly leave systemic blood vessels and move into surrounding tissues.

Augustus Waller is perhaps most remembered by medical students for his descriptions of the degeneration of nerve fibers, following transection of peripheral nerve fibers (Wallerian degeneration) (1850)[135].

The first half of the 1800s ends after 50 years of much progress in the advancement of medical pathology as a scientific discipline and as a medical professional specialty. New scientific journals devoted specifically to medical pathology are introduced and open the lines of communication between investigator and clinical practitioner. Introduction and development of Cell theory changes the principle unit of study in pathology from body tissues to the cell. Disease and disease states are re-conceptualized within the matrix of Cell theory. Body fluids, especially blood and urine, are aggressively investigated and offer new insights into body changes associated with human disease. Chemistry and chemical changes associated with pathological changes of disease are proposed, evaluated, identified, and incorporated into mainstream investigations. Technological advances in microscope optics allow for inspection of the body and body changes associated with disease states, unlike any time before.

Notable investigators and familiar to most medical students (or should be) Richard Bright, Thomas Hodgkin, Robert Graves, William Stokes, Theodor Schwann, Rudolf Virchow, Bence Jones, and Augustus V. Waller all make substantial contributions to the advancement of medical pathology, during the first half of the 1800s. Arguably equal, if not more important, contributions are made by less familiar others e.g. Antoine Fourcroy, Johannas Reil, William Prout, Alfred Donne, Henry Fuller, Ernst Neumann, Giulio Bizzozero, Johannes Muller, Julius Vogel, Hermann Lebert, Karl von Rokitansky, Johann Scherer, John Dalrymple, and Robert Remak.

It is not necessary to remember each investigator and their specific contribution(s). This knowledge simply provides you with an opportunity to begin to appreciate the great many whom are responsible for helping to move our knowledge in medical pathology forward and contribute to the why and how we have come to practice medicine today.

The second half of the 1800s begins with a waning of the excitement, evident during the early-1800s, to identify single chemical and microscopic diagnostic signs to correctly and reliably diagnose disease states in the clinical patient. Attention and resources are redirected, during the second half of the 1800s, away from the flurried search to identify the next single diagnostic sign to broader investigations, which systematically evaluate chemical and structural changes associated with disease and disease processes, at the cellular level. Blood and urine continue to be primary body fluids subjected to detailed study. The autopsy continues to be a primary source of information. Post-mortem findings are associated with patients' clinical presentations, most typically on a post-hoc basis and without the use of a well-reasoned theory driven conceptual matrix.

Recognition and acknowledgement of limited knowledge of normal human physiology fuels increased cooperation and exchange of information between morbid anatomists, physiologists, pathologists, and clinicians, during the second half of the 1800s. The product result is significant advancement in the knowledge base of all four disciplines and which lay the scientific foundations upon which our current understanding of disease and disease processes will build for the next 165 years.

Technological advancements contribute to the continuing progress being made in medical pathology during the second half of the 1800s. Microscope optics continue to improve. Photography, once restricted to images taken from the microscope, now is introduced into physical medicine. The punch muscle biopsy is introduced allowing for histological examination of muscle tissues at varying stages of disease processes, no longer requiring sampling only at autopsy. New stains and staining procedures are introduced to allow for improved microscopic viewing of fluids and tissues, at the cellular level. Fixation techniques are introduced, allowing for improved preservation of tissues samples and opportunities for delayed and repeated examination of specimens.

Trivia: The term photography is derived from the Greek word "photos" meaning light and "graphe" meaning drawing. Collectively, photography means drawing with light.

Let us take a brief look at a few specific influential people, milestone discoveries, and changes in conceptual matrixes, during the second half of the 1800s, which shape the history of medical pathology.

Thomas Addison (1793-1860) British pathologist exemplifies the return to the practice of the French School of pathology (sic), describing clinical presentations of patients in terms of prominent signs and symptom and then searching post-mortem, for changes in structural anatomy. Addison offers his first observations of "…a remarkable form of anemia…" describing a commonly occurring clinical presentation of signs and symptoms in patients, which upon autopsy are uniformly associated with "…a diseased condition of the supra renal glands…", (n=3) (1849)[136]. The clinical condition Addison describes and associates with structural pathology of the adrenal glands will later be recognized to be pernicious anemia.

Recall, anemia is simply a generic term applied to conditions in which your patient's blood has too few red blood cells (RBC). Reduced number of RBCs in most cases results in decreased oxygen transport to tissues. Pernicious anemia is a specific anemia, which results when your patient suffers a deficiency in vitamin B12 (cobalamin). The deficiency typically results from poor diet or an autoimmune disorder which attacks the parietal cells of the stomach, interfering with the release of intrinsic factor, which is necessary to absorb vitamin B12 from the diet into the blood system.

Addison is often credited with discovery of pernicious anemia. However, the clinical presentation and associated changes in anatomical structure are detailed elsewhere by others years before Addison's first paper on the topic appears in the British medical literature. One specific example is found in the publication by James Combe (1796-1883) Scottish pathologist. James Combe details the clinical presentation and autopsy findings of a 47 year old male presenting with anemia "…in its most idiopathic form…". The paper describes in detail the condition later to become known as "pernicious anemia". Combe's paper appears 27 years before Addison first describes the clinical presentation or autopsy findings of his patients suffering the same disorder (1822,1824)[137,138]. Which of the two names do you recognize?

James Combe, while making the original contribution, rarely receives credit. He devotes his time to the diagnosis and treatment of patients rather than engaging in the necessary politics, oftentimes required to insure credit for discovery. So goes another example of disputed claims for first discovery, politics in professional medicine, and selective bias when reporting the history of medicine.

Trivia: The term "pernicious anemia" is introduced into the medical literature by Michael Biermer (1827-1892) German internist (1872)[139]. The term "pernicious" is selected by Biermer to emphasize the insidious onset and typical fatal result of the disorder. Prior to Biermer's publication on the topic, most investigators refer to this specific anemia as simply "idiopathic anemia" (1824)[138].

Thomas Addison is perhaps most remembered for his investigations of the clinical syndrome resulting from a deficiency of secretion of adrenal-cortical hormone, from the adrenal glands, located on top of the kidneys (1849,1855)[140,141]. The clinical syndrome and associated structural pathology will be termed "Addison disease" six years later, by French internist Armand Trousseau (1801-1867), in recognition of Addison's description of the constellation of clinical signs and symptoms (1861-1862)[142]. Armand Trousseau is first to describe the structural pathology occurring in the adrenal glands and producing the clinical syndrome reported by Addison.

Today we recognize two hormones to be most affected by changes in the adrenal glands associated with Addison's disease, aldosterone and cortisol. Aldosterone is essential to maintaining normal salt and water balances in the body and crucial for maintaining normal blood pressures. Cortisol is essential to regulating (suppressing) the immune system, increasing blood sugar levels via gluconeogenesis, and regulation of the metabolism of fats, proteins, and carbohydrates.

Trivia: Thomas Addison commits suicide, June 19, 1860, jumping from his residence onto the street, fatally striking his head, following an extended period of "…melancholia, resulting from overwork of the brain…" (1860)[143].

Samuel Wilks (1824-1911) British pathologist and past medical student of Thomas Addison, embraces the value of post-mortem examination, made in combination with knowledge of the patient's clinical presentation and clinical course. He is largely responsible for conducting, collecting, organizing, synthesizing, critically evaluating, summarizing, and ultimately publishing into the medical literature, multiple series of gross autopsy findings, which reveal and demonstrate now familiar defining characteristic changes in body organ tissues. He summaries the most frequently occurring pathologies encountered in the practice of medicine during the mid to late-1800s, in his well-received text "Lectures on Pathological Anatomy" (1859)[144].

This text serves as a primary resource, for pathologists and practicing physicians, during the second half of the 1800s. "Lectures on Pathological Anatomy" is organized into the pathologies of specific organs and tissues e.g. bone, heart, arteries, skin, liver, brain, and specific "… essential disease…" conditions e.g. diabetes, apoplexy (stroke syndromes), epilepsy, chorea, delirium tremens, syphilis, mania. The organizational format is typical and representative of the period.

Three editions are offered over the course of 30 years with each updated edition occurring every 15 years (1859,1875,1891)[144,145,146].

The initial edition of "Lectures on Pathological Anatomy" reflect much of Samuel Wilks' work during which "…for the last fifteen years (I have) made a daily study of the dissection of the dead…that I have myself recorded between 2000 and 3000 inspections… and have carefully abstained from making any statement unverified by my own observation and experience…" (1859)[144]. "Lectures on Pathological Anatomy" represents one of Samuel Wilks' first attempts to reduce the variability in post-mortem findings associated with specific disease or disease processes, reported by less detail oriented investigators elsewhere.

Specific and notable contributions to medical pathology made by Samuel Wilks, often unrecognized by the medical and scientific communities, can be found in his autopsy report and description of inflammatory bowel disease (ulcerative colitis) (1859,1875)[147,148], which appears 73 years before a more recognized series of 14 patients is reported, in the landmark paper by American gastroenterologist Burrill Crohn (1884-1983), describing the same condition (1932)[149]. Today, the condition described by both men is known as Crohn's disease.

Samuel Wilks is instrumental in clarifying the underlying pathology responsible for Addison disease. Two years after Addison's death, Wilks canvasses British hospitals in search of patients diagnosed with Addison's disease. Inspection of post-mortem findings reveals errors in Addison's and others descriptions. Wilks publishes a series of 25 carefully selected cases, illustrating the principle defining characteristic anatomical changes associated with Addison disease and eliminating confounding pathologies, such as cancers of the adrenal glands (1862)[150].

Samuel Wilks is first to introduce into the medical literature the specific term "Hodgkin's disease", in reference to the pathological changes associated with this deadly malignant cancer of the lymphoid cell line, leukocytes (1856,1865)[151,152].

Samuel Wilks embraces the then popular model of reporting clinical signs and symptoms and associating the clinical presentation with gross post-mortem findings. Typically, these observations and associations are made without the guiding light of a well conceptualized theoretical matrix. Although Wilks' approach is empirical in method and post-mortem observations are made without the use of the microscope, he makes several important and oftentimes neglected observations.

Samuel Wilks contributions to medical pathology, oftentimes over looked by most medical students and practicing physicians are: being among the first if not the first to describe visceral lesions associated with syphilis appearing in addition to the more familiar skin lesion s (1863)[153]; describe the characteristic inflammation of peripheral nerves associated with chronic alcohol use (1868)[154]; offers a seminal paper on Paget's disease 7 years before James Paget (1814-1899) British pathologist offers his first paper on the same condition (1869)[155]; identifies the characteristic changes in the heart associated with bacterial endocarditis and describes the oftentimes associated systemic arterial embolisms (1870)[156]; and correctly differentiates the neuromuscular disease myasthenia gravis from the primary psychiatric disorder hysteria (1877)[157].

Trivia: James Paget originally suggest the term "osteitis deformans" for the condition, which today is known to all medical students whom have completed their Basic Science Program's pathology course, simply as Paget's disease. "…Holding, then the disease to be an inflammation of bone, I would suggest that, for brief reference, and for the present, it may be called, after its most striking character, Osteitis deformans. A better name may be given when more is known of it…" (1876, p58)[158].

James Paget acknowledges Samuel Wilks' contribution in describing the disease (Paget's disease) 7 years before Paget makes his first report of the condition. Paget includes one patient, previously reported by Wilks in 1869, in Paget's own series of 8 patients, reported in Paget's landmark paper describing Paget's disease (1876)[158]. Wilks' patient is patient #4, in Paget's series (1869, 1876)[155,158].

Guillaume Duchenne (1806-1875) French neurologist, yes, the same Duchenne as in Duchenne's muscular dystrophy, offers the first medical textbook to include photographs of patients evidencing observable physical changes associated with underlying pathologies. In the case of Duchenne's text, 16 photographs demonstrate the characteristic and unmistakable images of gross muscle atrophy of the truck and paralysis of the face (1862)[159]. The photographs are offered as an adjunct to Duchenne's textbook published one year earlier describing the use of localized electrical stimulation in the treatment of disorders of skeletal muscles (1861)[160].

Seven years later Duchenne applies the use of photography to the study of the nervous systems, offering detailed photographs of gross neuroanatomical structures and photographs taken through the microscope revealing neurohistological images of both normal and pathological neural tissues of the PNS (1864,1865)[161,162] and CNS (1868)[163]. The use of photography in medicine to demonstrate specific pathologies greatly improves the way in which medical students learn pathology and changes the format of medical pathology textbooks.

Take a moment and image trying to learn pathology or trying to read a medical pathology textbook e.g. Robbin's "Pathologic Basis of Disease", without photographic images. Aghhh!

Duchenne develops an experimental procedure for investigating movement, while initially mocked by the medical community, proves to yield tremendous amounts of new and valuable information. In brief, Duchenne applies small electrical shocks (faradic stimulation) to muscle groups and maps each muscle group's action. He demonstrates movement "…is the result of a double nervous excitation whereby muscles that exert an opposite actions (flexors and extensors) contract simultaneously, some to produce the movements and others to modulate it…" (1855)[164].

He provides a detail functional map of all major muscle groups in healthy individuals and patients suffering from assorted neuromuscular disorders and paralyses. He develops the use of electricity as a procedure with which to study normal and abnormal muscle physiology. He applies the procedure and the new knowledge generated to the clinical evaluation and treatment of patients, presenting with neuromuscular disorders and assorted paralyses. Using electrical stimulation, aka faradic stimulation, by use of two surface electrodes and a low voltage induction coil, he differentiates impaired movement resulting from CNS lesions, from peripheral nerve lesions, from lesions of the muscle itself. Duchene recognizes if a paralyzed muscle group contract upon localized faradic stimulation, then the lesion responsible for the paralysis is in the CNS. If the muscle group does not contract upon faradic stimulation, the lesion is in the peripheral nerve or muscle itself (1847)[165].

Duchenne is instrumental in developing an early "punch biopsy" procedure which allows collection of skeletal muscle tissues from clinical patients without anesthesia and for the purpose of histological inspection of the biopsied tissue using the microscope. The procedure developed by Duchenne, is a modification of a German procedure used to sample muscles for the presence of trichinosis, using the Midledorff harpoon (needle). This tissue sampling procedure allows for the microscopic inspection of pre-mortem tissues across time and at various stages of the pathological process e.g. beginning, middle, and end stages. The procedure is passionately criticized in the local media, as an unethical procedure when used with children. The procedure generates valuable new information and clarifies many early conflicting reports as to the physical changes occurring throughout the disease process of several neuromuscular disorders (1868)[166]. The procedure is the foundational base of the punch biopsy still used today.

Most medical students immediately associate the name of Duchenne with Duchenne Muscular Dystrophy (DMD), a recessive X-linked form of muscular dystrophy, resulting in a mutation of the dystrophin gene (Xp21), which codes for the protein dystrophin, a protein essential in maintaining structural integrity of muscle tissue. Recall, DMD evidences signs and symptoms during early childhood, usually before 5 years of age. Symptoms are characterized by progressive proximal muscle weakness of the legs and pelvis, eventually spreading to the arms and neck. Signs are characterized by progressive muscle mass loss, pseudo-hypertrophy of the calf muscles, difficulties engaging in most movements dependent upon skeletal muscle groups e.g. standing, walking, and climbing stairs. Muscle tissues are eventually replaced by fat and fibrotic tissues. Most effected children are wheelchair dependent by 12 years of age.

Duchenne makes his first report of this neuromuscular disorder, describing a 9 year old boy whom evidences marked hypertrophy of the calves and which Duchenne terms congenital hypertrophic paraplegia of childhood (1861)[167]. He expands and details the description seven years later, which he now terms pseudo-hypertrophic muscular dystrophy and reports the histological findings of biopsy of muscle tissues, noting the accumulation of fatty material in between muscle fibers (1868)[168]. However, like most discoveries throughout the history of medicine, Duchenne's discovery is preceded by several previous reports describing the same disorder.

Edward Meryon (1807-1880) British physician reports the same condition 10 years before Duchenne's first report of the condition (1851,1852,1864)[169,170,171]. Meryon describes the disorder as familial, affecting primarily males, demonstrates a material inheritance pattern and upon autopsy inspection reveals no observable pathology of the brain or spinal cord, and with evidence of fatty degeneration in the skeletal muscles (1852)[170]. Meryon's observations are based upon a series of nine boys from three unrelated families. Similarly, William Little (1810-1894) British physician reports the same condition, pseudo-hypertrophic muscular dystrophy in two brothers 12 and 14 years of age, eight years before Duchenne's first published report (1853)[172].

Duchenne and Meryon publically debate priority for discovery in the professional medical literature and society meetings. Edward Meryon clearly is first to describe this X- linked recessive muscular dystrophy in 1852, while Duchene published 5 extensive papers on the disorder in 1868. Duchene misrepresents the findings of Meryon, claiming Meryon studied muscular atrophy resulting from a nerve disorder rather than a muscular dystrophy. Meryon emphatically denies the assertion (1864)[173].

In perspective, Edward Meryon details the clinical presentation and histological changes of the disorder, years before Guillaume Duchenne's first report. Meryon is first to recognize the heritable nature of the disorder; first to offer a series of patients from multiple families; first to recognize the disorder appears only in boys; first to describe onset of muscle wasting and weakness begins in early childhood; first to recognize death of the patient occurs typically during early adolescence; first to recognize the disease effects muscle and not neural tissues; and first to suggest the condition be defined based upon its underlying pathological process "granular degeneration of the voluntary muscles". All of these are reported in the medical literature and society meetings years before Duchenne offers his first report on the disorder. Duchenne, however does publish many more papers on the disorder than does Meryon. Original contribution or sheer volume of published papers; whom, if either has claim for priority of discovery? You decide. Meryon muscular dystrophy or Duchenne muscular dystrophy. Oh, the politics of academic medicine.

John Down (1828-1896) British physician offers a new classification system within which to organize "… congenital mental lesions…", resulting in "…the feeble minded…idiots and imbeciles…" (1866)[174]. The proposed classification system is based upon differentiation of subgroups according to physical appearance. Characteristic physical appearances exemplified by various world ethnic groups provide the criteria for classification. For example, Down identifies physical characteristics of people originating from Ethiopia, Malaysia, Mongolia, and America. He then classifies individuals based upon physical appearance; matching their physical appearance, with the stereotyped physical appearance criteria established for each selected ethnic population. Here is an excerpt from Down's original paper (1866)[174].

"…The great Mongolian family has numerous representatives, and it is to this division, I wish, in this paper, to call special attention. A very large number of congenital idiots are typical Mongols. So marked is this, that when placed side by side, it is difficult to believe that the specimens compared are not children of the same parents. The number of idiots who arrange themselves around the Mongolian type is so great, and they present such a close resemblance to one another in mental power, that I shall describe an idiot member of this racial division, selected from the large number that have fallen under my observation.

The hair is not black, as in the real Mongol, but of a brownish colour, straight and scanty. The face is flat and broad, and destitute of prominence. The cheeks are roundish, and extended laterally. The eyes are obliquely placed, and the internal canthi more than normally distant from one another. The palpebral fissure is very narrow. The forehead is wrinkled transversely from the constant assistance which the levatores palpebrarum derive from the occipito-frontalis muscle in the opening of the eyes. The lips are large and thick with transverse fissures. The tongue is long, thick, and is much roughened. The nose is small. The skin has a slight dirty yellowish tinge, and is deficient in elasticity, giving the appearance of being too large for the body…" (1866)[174].

The classification system proposed by Down, now over 150 years ago, exemplifies reliance upon observations of patients' surface anatomy, classifications based upon shared physical signs, and an effort to bring standardized diagnostic criteria and order to a group of poorly understood underlying pathologies, effecting a nontrivial segment of the patient population.

Thomas Addison, Samuel Wilks, Guillaume Duchenne, Edward Meryon, and John Down focus their investigations upon identifying variations and changes in gross anatomical structures, then associating their gross observations with clinical signs. This approach is representative of the highly influential French School of pathology. Rudolf Virchow on the other hand champions the German School of pathology, emphasizing the study of pathology at the cellular level. Virchow rejects the proposal human disease can best be understood through the study of the 21 tissues identified by Marie Bichat (1800)[124] and boldly proposes all human disease can best be understood within the matrix of disordered cell functions.

Rudolf Virchow details his vision of a new pathology, based upon investigation of the cell and disordered cell processes, in a series of 20 lectures delivered at the Pathological Institute of Berlin, during February, March, and April 1858. The lecture series is published the same year in Germany and two years later the first English translation appears and titled "Cellular pathology as based upon physiological and pathological histology" (1858,1860)[175,176]. Pathology embraces the new directions proposed by Virchow and changes its focus of study and conceptual thought for the next 150 years.

Building upon the foundation laid by Johann Scherer and others during the mid-1800s, establishing the value of the clinical pathology laboratory, the late-1860s through early-1890s witness aggressive investigations into the normal and pathological properties of body fluids, especially human blood.

Platelets are identified and their functional role in blood coagulation is recognized. Leukocytes (white blood cells, WBC) are first identified, their functional roles within the matrix of the immune systems recognized, their physical movement from systemic blood into surrounding tissues is first reported and explained, and contribution to the formation of pus is first described and understood. Bone marrow is recognized to be the origin of red and white blood cells (erythrocytes and leukocytes). Disease of bone marrow is recognized to be unequivocally associated with leukemia. Processes and consequences of disordered blood flow are first reported and described in detail. Familiar terms such as thrombosis, embolism, and infarction are introduced into the medical literature. The microscope becomes an essential tool and provides the necessary technology to investigate pathology on the cellular level.

Julius Cohnheim (1839-1884) German pathologist revolutionizes pathology with his influential contributions regarding pus (1867)[177]. Building upon the work of others, he successfully challenges medical dogma and demonstrates movement of leukocytes (WBC) from systemic blood circulation through capillaries into surrounding tissues as part of the inflammatory process. He accomplishes this through the injection of aniline blue into the systemic blood, which is then ingested by leukocytes, and then demonstrates the presence of the aniline blue stained leukocytes in inflamed tissues by microscopic examination.

Julius Cohnheim's demonstration reflects an increasing sophistication and integration of innovative thought and methods applied by pathologists during the second half of the 1800s. It demonstrates the great value of using staining techniques applied in situ to investigate the process as well as the end result of disease. Additionally, this landmark paper reflects a conceptual shift away from an emphasis upon pathological anatomy which details morphological changes associated with disease and towards a much broader experimental physiological approach to the study of disease, which emphasizes the process of disease.

Notable additional contributions to pathology made by Julius Cohnheim are development of fresh tissue freezing techniques which are still in use today, microscopic descriptions of the neuromuscular junction (1867)[178], and insights into the process of vascular thrombosis and embolism (1872,1877)[179,180].

Franz Neumann (1834-1918) German pathologist is among the first to recognize the source of blood cells is bone marrow (1868)[181]. One year later, he details the foundational basis of hemopoiesis (1869,1870)[182,183]. Three years later, Franz Neumann applies his findings to the investigation of blood disease and unequivocally states leukemia is a disease of bone marrow (1872)[184].

Giulio Bizzozero (1846-1901) Italian pathologist and recent medical school graduate confirms microscopic observations reported by Neumann and others reporting non-nucleated red blood cells are formed from nucleated red blood cells and both RBCs and WBCs have their origins in bone marrow (1868,1869)[185,186].

Franz Neumann and Guilio Bizzozero findings are immediately rejected by the established scientific and medical communities. Their findings are at odds with conventional medical dogma. Current dogma states bone marrow is best understood as either excrement of bone (excrementum ossium) or a substance which serves as nutrition for bone. Neither accepted explanation, considers bone marrow as a source of blood cells. Contributing further to rejection of the data is dogma which states, bone is solid. Given all properly trained physicians and scientists know bone is solid, there is no way for cells to possibly travel through bone into the systemic blood circulation. Proponents and defenders of the dogma charge Neumann and Bizzozero with "…encumbering science by ill formed statements…" (1889)[187].

 So goes another example in the history of medicine of new and innovative ideas "…encumbering science by ill formed statements…". I encourage you to question that which you are taught in medical school and be willing to "encumber science" by challenging medical and scientific dogma. Thoughtful analysis and openness to new and innovative ideas will continue to move the knowledge forward, offering continued benefit to every patient you diagnose and treat in the future.

Max Schultze (1825-1874) German microscopic anatomist publishes the first accurate description of the four different types of leukocytes (WBCs) which today we know as monocytes, lymphocytes, neutrophils, and eosinophils. Additionally, in the same paper he offers the first description of platelets, noting their size to be the approximate size as the nuclei of larger cells 1865)[188]. The paper appears in a new journal founded by Schultze, "Archive fur Mikroscopische Anatomie". Schultz founds the new journal in response to his continuing frustration with editors of more established journals refusing to publish many of his papers. Beyond the fundamental contributions of distinguishing between these four WBCs, noting the granulated cells neutrophils and eosinophils are the most mobile of the four, and neutrophils are more active than eosinophils in the process of phagocytosis, is the value of the microscope as a new tool in the investigation of normal cell activities and cell mediated processes, such as the inflammatory response and phagocytosis.

Seventeen years later, Giulio Bizzozero extends the original findings of Max Schwarte, meticulously describing blood platelets and their roles and functions in the processes of adhesion, aggregation, fibrin formation, and deposition; all essential to understanding how the body normally stops bleeding (1882a)[189].

Recall from your histology course, platelets are produced in bone marrow and are small fragments of the megakaryocytes. They circulate freely throughout the blood stream, along with RBCs, WBCs, and blood plasma. When a blood vessel is damaged, the blood vessel releases cell signaling proteins which makes platelets aggregate, sticking them together, and forming a plug to fill the damaged area of the blood vessel. The typical result, bleeding stops. In disease states, when the number of platelets are low (thrombocytopenia) excessive bleeding occurs. When the number of platelets are very high (thrombocytosis) the risk of thrombosis (blood clots forming inside of a blood vessel) increases, potentially obstructing blood flow to body tissues.

Trivia: The term "platelet" is an English derivation of the Italian term used by Bizzozero "piatrine" meaning small plates (1881)[190]. The French translation of Bizzozero's paper uses the term "petite plaquettes" (1882b)[191], while the German translation is "blutplattchen" (1882a)[189].

Unknown to many medical students, Guilio Bizzozero, working at the University of Turin, is first to identify Helicobacter pylori bacterium in the gastric mucosa of the stomach fundus and duodenum (1892,1893)[192,193]. Six years later, Walery Jaworski (1849-1924) Polish gastroenterologist, working at Jagiellonian University in Krakow, identifies similar Gram negative bacterium in gastric washings from humans and is first to suggest the bacterium's role as a causal agent in human gastric disease (1899)[194].

Giulio Bizzozero and Walery Jaworski make their observations more than 86 years before the same bacterium is recognized by Barry Marshall (1951-) Australian microbiologist and Robin Warren (1937-) Australian pathologist, as the primary cause of gastritis and peptic ulcer disease in humans (1984)[195]. Barry Marshall and Robin Warren are awarded the 2005 Nobel in Physiology or Medicine, in recognition of their (re)discovery "... of the bacterium Helicobacter pylori and its role in gastritis and peptic ulcer disease..." (2005)[196].

Staining and tissue fixation procedures are greatly improved during the second half of the 1800s. Advancements in these technologies contribute significantly to extending medical pathology knowledge. The history and importance of staining and tissue fixation is discussed more fully in the Histology chapter of this text.

In brief and for perspective, staining and tissue fixation procedures become essential technologies for pathologists interested in completing investigations into disease and disease processes, at the microscopic level of analysis. Many of the now familiar stains and fixation procedures still used today are introduced and developed during the second half of the 1800s.

Six investigators and their unique contributions are briefly offered, as specific examples of staining procedures which have tremendous impact upon the development of medical pathology. You might recognize their names or stains from your medical school histology course.

Friedrich von Recklinghausen (1833-1910) German pathologist most remembered for his description of multiple neurofibromatosis (1882)[197] introduces a silver stain which allows for delineation of junctions between cells (1862)[198]. The stain also outlines connective tissue cells, revealing spaces between cells, filled with fluid, and drained by the lymphatic system.

Much more important than his brief paper describing multiple neurofibromatosis, Friedrich von Recklinghausen makes numerous and arguably more meaningful contributions to medical pathology. He systematically investigates the process of disease, rather than solely the result of disease. This reflects a significant change in direction and focus of medical pathological investigations during the late-1800s. Fredrick von Recklinghausen additionally offers a more complete understanding of the processes of thrombosis, embolism, and infarction (1883)[199]; the pathology of specific bone tumors (1889)[200]; and the pathology underlying abnormal iron deposition in body tissues (hemochromatosis) (1889)[201].

Note: Multiple neurofibromatosis is described in the medical literature by Robert Smith (1807-1873) Irish physician, 33 years before Fredrick von Recklinghausen first offers his brief paper on the condition (1849,1882)[202,197].

Heinrich Wilhelm von Waldeyer-Hartz (1836-1921) German anatomist perhaps most remembered by medical students for introducing the term "chromosome" into the medical literature (1888)[203] and popularizing the term "neuron" to describe the fundamental excitatory unit of the nervous system (1891)[204], develops the iron hematoxylin stain and applies the stain to striated muscle, revealing the striations of actin and myosin filaments (1863)[205].

Karl Weigert (1845-1904) German pathologist remembered for his many contributions describing the processes of inflammation and coagulation necrosis (1875)[206] and being first to describe the pathology of myocardial infarction (1880)[207], introduces the first stain capable of staining bacteria (1871)[208]. Eleven years later he introduces his myelin stain (1882)[209], which allows for the first time mapping of major central nervous system neuronal pathways.

Paul Ehrlich (1854-1915) German immunologist remembered for targeted therapeutic killing of organisms via chemotherapy, introduces a stain allowing for easy differentiation between the WBCs and which soon serve as the basis for diagnosing assorted diseases of blood, specifically leukemia (1878)[210].

Camillo Golgi (1843-1926) Italian pathologist recognized most immediately by medical students for his discovery of the intracellular Golgi apparatus responsible for packaging proteins (1898) and Santiago Cajal (1852-1934) Spanish pathologist remembered by most for his conceptualization and experimental investigations of the neuron doctrine, develop and refine the silver nitrate stain, allowing for visual evidence of the intricate relationship between neurons.

Hans Gram (1853-1938) Danish bacteriologist introduces his stains which allow for the differentiation of bacteria according to difference in the bacterium's cell wall (1884)[211]. His stains with little modification will prove essential in organizing bacteria e.g. Gram positive or Gram negative bacteria and guiding the selection of therapeutic interventions based upon the stain identification of bacteria for the next 135 years.

All of these stains and more are introduced during the second half of the 1800s. Staining greatly facilitates progress in the microscopic analysis of healthy and diseased cells and tissues, contributing much to the advancement of medical pathology.

Equally important are advancements in tissue preservation and fixation.

Edwin Klebs (1834-1913) German pathologist, perhaps most remembered for his identification of the bacterium Corynebacterium diphtheria as the bacterium responsible for diphtheria (1883) and Klebsiella a genus of bacteria named in recognition of his many contributions to understanding infectious diseases, introduces paraffin fixation to preserve tissues for microscopic study (1869)[212].

Ferdinand Blum (1865-1959) German physician introduces formaldehyde as a preferred fluid fixative over alcohol (1893,1894)[213,214]. Fixation and preservation advances allows for repeated examination of tissue samples and between investigators. Previously, all tissue examinations must be made within days of harvesting and before the tissues begin to naturally deteriorate.

Identification of formaldehyde as a fixative is the result of a serendipitous event recognized by Ferdinand Blum now over 125 years ago. The German based industrial chemical company, Farbwerke, formally Meister Lucius & Bruning AG purchases the license to manufacture formaldehyde. In their efforts to identify a profitable use for the compound, Ferdinand Blum is recruited to investigate formaldehyde's use as an antiseptic. Recent data out of France suggest formaldehyde might prove useful as a bactericide with applications for the treatment of wound infections. Blum investigates the use of formaldehyde in diluted solution as an antibacterial agent against Bacillus anthracis, Bacillus typhi, and Staphylococcus aureus (1893)[215]. Yes, it is an effective bactericide.

As the result of handling formaldehyde, as part of his investigations, Blum notices his fingers becoming hard, much like they do when handling alcohol. Hummm…if alcohol is used as a tissue fixative, perhaps formaldehyde might have a similar use. Indeed, not only does formaldehyde prove to be a fixative, it has properties much preferred over alcohol, in that is does not shrink or distort the tissue sample, making it a preferred fixative.

In addition to advances being made in staining and fixation techniques, medical pathologists continue identifying cell changes associated with specific diseases.

William Greenfield (1846-1919) British pathologist first reports the presence of the giant cell and identifies it to be pathognomonic of Hodgkin's disease (1878)[216]. The giant cell is rediscovered 20 years later by Carl von Sternberg (1872-1935) Austrian pathologist (1898)[217] and 24 years later by Dorothy Reed Mendenhall (1874-1964) American pathologist (1902)[218]. Most medical students today recognize the cell today simply as the Reed-Sternberg cell. The dispute and debate regarding priority of discovery and association with Hodgkin's disease continues (1972)[219].

As the 1800s begin to close, medical pathology continues to re-identify a few gross anatomical structural abnormalities underlying the clinical presentations of a few conditions, previously reported and forgotten by the medical and scientific communities.

Arthur Fallot (1850-1911) French clinician, immediately recognized by most every first year medical student and associated with the Tetralogy of Fallot (n=2) (1888)[220] exemplifies the increasingly common practice during the 1800s of investigators rediscovering a disease or condition and publishing the case(s) as if it is new information. Arthur Fallot exemplifies the traditional French School of pathology methodology, which is very much alive and well at the end of the 1800s in Europe, reporting clinical signs and symptoms, followed by post-mortem examination of the patient's body, and reporting structural abnormalities which might explain the clinical signs and symptoms. The reports are made on a purely empirical-observational and descriptive basis, often in absence of a unifying or guiding theoretical matrix.

Recall, the Tetralogy of Fallot is a collection of four congenital structural abnormalities affecting primarily the heart. The clinical presentation of babies affected is summarized simply as the Blue Baby Syndrome, reflecting the characteristic blue color of the baby's skin, as the result of impaired oxygen profusion of body tissues. In brief, the anatomical congenital abnormalities are an abnormal narrowing of the artery carrying blood from the heart to the lungs, abnormal positioning of the aorta as it leaves the heart, a hole in the septum which separates the two ventricles of the heart, and an abnormal enlargement of the walls of the right ventricle of the heart. More formally, the Tetralogy of Fallot is defined by pulmonary artery stenosis, overriding aorta, ventricular-septal deficit, and right ventricular hypertrophy. The physiological result of these four abnormalities is impaired oxygen profusion of body tissues.

The condition is dutifully remembered by every first year medical student. However, Fallot is not the first to recognize or report this constellation of congenital abnormalities or the resulting clinical presentation. The condition is first reported and published into the medical literature by Niels Stensen (1638-1686) Danish anatomist, 217 years before Fallot publishes his observations and findings (1671,1888)[221,220]. You may recognize the name Niels Stensen. He identifies and describes the duct from the parotid gland to the mouth, the "ductus stenonianus" (1662)[222]. You know this structure today as the Stensen duct.

Trivia: Arthur Fallot's medical school thesis focuses on the identification, diagnosis, treatment, prognosis, consequence, and underlying pathology of pneumothorax (1876)[223].

Trivia: Arthur Fallot never uses the term "Tetralogy of Fallot" in any of his publications, lectures, or writings. He refers to the condition as "la maladie blue" (the blue malady). The term "Tetralogy of Fallot" is introduced into the medical literature, 13 years after his death and 36 years after his 1888 publication, by Maude Abbott (1869-1940) Canadian pathologist, in acknowledgment of Fallot's description of the condition (1924)[224].

As the second half of the 1800s comes to an end, pathologists, morbid anatomists, physiologists, and practicing clinicians are working together more cooperatively, in recognition of the limited scientific knowledge regarding how the normal, healthy body works. The cooperative efforts are resulting in rapid advancements in knowledge in all four disciplines and lay the foundation for our current modern understanding of diseases and disease process. While the first half of the 1800s is all about the cell, the second half of the 1800s is all about disease process. Specific processes are investigated and understood e.g. thrombosis, embolism, infarction, atrophy, hypertrophy, coagulation necrosis.

Advances in technology during the second half of the 1800s move pathology forward. Improved optics for the microscope make it now an essential tool for every pathologist. The punch biopsy is introduced, permitting repeated examination of tissue samples, at varying stages of disease processes. New stains and staining procedures allow for greatly improved microscopic viewing of fluids and tissues at the cellular level. Stains allow for the visualization and classification of bacteria. Improved fixation techniques allow for preservation of tissue samples and opportunities for delayed and repeated examination of specimens. Photography is introduced into medicine and becomes a familiar tool in documenting physical changes throughout the disease process.

Notable investigators, familiar to most medical students (or should be), making meaningful and significant contributions during the second half of the 1800s are Thomas Addison, James Paget, Guillaume Duchenne, John Down, Rudolf Virchow, Friedrich von Recklinghausen, Camillo Golgi, Hans Gram, and Arthur Fallot. Individuals with less familiar names making arguably equally important contributions during the second half of the 1800s are Samuel Wilks, Edward

Meryon, Julius Cohnheim, Franz Neumann, Giulio Bizzozero, Max Schultze, Walery Jaworski, Heinrich Walleye, Karl Weigert, Paul Ehrlich, Ferdinand Blum, and William Greenfield.

Principle content areas investigated and preferred methodologies applied are loosely defined by nationality. Investigators working in Germany focus their investigations on the cell and identification of cell pathologies. Germany leads the way with invention and development of new technologies, while establishing innovative laboratory based techniques and procedures with immediate and valued applications for the practicing physician. Investigators working in Italy and Austria focus their investigations on body fluids. Innovative advancements are made in the chemical analysis of body fluids with applications for the practicing physician. Many of the procedures and analysis of body fluids developed during the 1800s are still used today, in the routine diagnostic practices of medicine. Investigators working in Great Britain and France embrace the traditional French School of pathology, dutifully documenting clinical signs and symptoms, then associating clinical presentation with post-mortem autopsy findings. Europe unquestionably is the leader in guiding the course of medical pathology.

American and Canadian investigators are heavily influenced by the European schools and frequently train in the established, prestigious pathology laboratories of Europe. American and Canadian investigators, especially in the universities located in the northeast and mid-west of the USA, are just beginning to make meaningful contributions, as the 1800s come to a close. A few USA universities are beginning to establish Departments of Pathology. Of particular note is the University of Philadelphia's medical school. The medical school embraces pathology from its earliest days and trains many US investigators, whom will go on to establish medical school training in pathology, at other medical schools through the USA.

Medical pathology witnesses substantial changes and advancements during the 1800s. The discipline matures as a profession and contributes meaningfully to a rapidly expanding scientific knowledge base. Human disease is more completely understood within the matrix of cause, process, and product, as the result of thoughtful challenges to medical dogma, significant advancements in technology, and the courage of a few individual researchers and clinicians to think about old problems in new and innovative ways. The 1800s are exciting times for medical pathology.

In summary, the 1800s witness the introduction and development of Cell theory. Human disease is conceptualized within the new matrix of Cell theory. The cell becomes the primary unit of study. Disease and disease states once defined solely by clinical signs and symptoms now include reliable and observable changes in biological structure and body fluid chemistries. Microscopic observations now routinely complement gross observations. Photography is introduced into medical pathology and becomes a value tool in documenting microscopic and gross physical changes accompanying disease and disease processes. Improvements in microscope technology allow for meaningful study of the microbiology underlying human disease. Specifically and by way of example, protozoan responsible for sexually transmitted disease e.g. Trichomonas vaginalis and bacterium responsible for tuberculosis (TB) e.g. Mycobaterium tuberculosis are identified. Microscopic investigations lead to the identification of structural changes in white blood cells associated with leukemia and the identification of platelets leading to understanding their essential role in blood coagulation. Fundamental processes underlying human disease states and associated pathology are identified, aggressively investigated, and detailed e.g. infarction, embolism, coagulation, necrosis, and inflammation. Common conditions e.g. myocardial infarction, are detailed beyond clinical signs and symptoms and description of resultant tissue changes, now include description of the underlying pathological processes responsible.

New cell staining and tissue fixation methods greatly facilitate the advancement of medical pathology. These improved technologies complement advances in microscope technologies allowing investigators to examine structural changes at a level of inspection previously unavailable. In addition to improved technologies to investigate structure, significant and rapid advances are concurrently being made in understanding normal human organ systems based physiology. Equipped with a better understanding of normal physiology, medical pathologists are better positioned to understand disease and disease processes affecting normal physiology. Open exchange of new knowledge between university based physiologists, medical pathologists, and practicing clinician moves all three professional disciplines rapidly forward during the 1800s. Scientific societies and journals, devoted to the scientific advancement of medical pathology, begin to appear throughout Europe and North America, offering new forums for the exchange of information between investigator and clinician. Medical pathology textbooks begin to appear in increasing numbers as new information is integrated into the existing scientific knowledge base. New medical pathology textbooks are organized into the now familiar and popular format of today; causes of disease (etiology), mechanism of development (pathogenesis), alteration of tissue (morphological changes), diagnosis, prognosis, and treatment (clinical significance). By the end of the 1800s, several university based and free standing colleges of medicine located in the USA, follow the lead of European medical schools and begin to incorporate formal didactic training and supervised experience in medical pathology into the USA medical school curriculum.

Yes, the 1800s are a period of much growth and rapid development for medical pathology.

Late Modern, 1900 AD - 2000 AD.

The 1900s witness the continuing development of medical pathology as a professional discipline. Additional professional societies and associated journals devoted to the scientific advancement of medical pathology are founded. Specialty education and training criteria are established. Formal assessment of content and process knowledge is implemented in the form of Board Specialty Examinations for physicians and scientists choosing to identify themselves as Board Certified Pathologists. Pathology is further integrated into the medical school curriculum of most all allopathic (MD) programs and medical students increasingly must demonstrate familiarity with pathology before graduating medical school or being awarded a license to independently practice medicine within the United States of America (USA) or Canada. Medical schools and universities located in the USA and Canada contribute more to pathology as a science and professional discipline than ever before and begin to rival the medical schools and universities located in Europe. The immune systems are central to most pathological investigations of the 1900s. The preferred unit of analysis moves from the cell to molecular processes within and between cells, as technological advances continue to be made throughout the 1900s. By the end of the 1900s, most all pathologies begin to be conceptualized within the matrix of potential or real contributions resulting from genetic materials.

Let's take a brief look at a few specific influential people contributing to milestone discoveries, changes in conceptual matrixes, and championing professional issues which shape the history of medical pathology during the 1900s. The names Karl Aschoff (Aschoff bodies), George Whipple (Whipple disease), Nikolai Anitschkov (cholesterol and atherosclerosis), Ernest Goodpasture (Goodpasture disease), James Ewing (Ewing sarcoma), and Albert Coons (florescent labeled antibodies and antigens), Renato Dulbecco (viruses incorporate viral DNA into DNA of cells), Stanley Robbins and Ramiz Cotran (pathology textbook), and Jack Kevorkian (euthanasia activist) are familiar to all medical students whom have completed their first medical school course in pathology. You recognize the name, you know the signs and symptoms of the disease and you know the pathological findings characteristic of each disease. Now learn something about the person most responsible and how their contributions influence the development of medical pathology.

Karl Aschoff (1866-1942) German pathologist is interested in the investigation of inflammation, both process and result. Early in his career he is particularly interested in the inflammation of the heart associated with rheumatic fever. Recall, rheumatic fever is an inflammatory disease effecting the heart, joints, skin, or central nervous system, characterized variably and most often by polyarthritis (inflammation of large joints, which is painful and migrates), carditis (inflammation of the muscles of the heart), erythema marginatium (a painless, red rash, with ragged edges), small subcutaneous nodules (painless, firm collections of collagen over bones and tendons, especially the wrist, elbow, or knee), Sydenham's chorea (abnormal, large, spontaneous movements of the arms and legs), and fever. Rheumatic fever appears most often in children, 5-15 years of age, approximately 2-4 weeks following an inadequately treated strep throat infection (Group A streptococcus bacteria). Do you remember why symptoms appear 2-4 weeks post infection? Hint: How long does the body take to produce antibodies? Rheumatic fever results from antibody cross reactivity. Your patient's antibodies generated to attack the strep infections also attack normal body tissues, which present similar identifying properties as the bacteria. See molecular mimicry in your medical pathology or immunology textbook if this is unfamiliar to you.

Karl Aschoff, initially and without the aid of the microscope, identifies 1-2 mm, fusiform shaped areas of inflammation appearing in cardiac muscle of patients presenting with rheumatic fever (1904)[225]. It is this collection of tissue bound lymphocytes and abnormal macrophages which define the pathognomonic histopathological sign of rheumatic fever. Today, we simply term these areas of inflammation Aschoff bodies.

Twenty years after his initial identification of Aschoff bodies, Karl Aschoff makes his most notable contribution. He identifies and details the cell based reticular-endothelial system of the human immune system (1922,1924)[226,227]. This contribution is oftentimes unknown or often forgotten by medical students. Building upon the earlier works of Ukrainian microbiologist Ilya Mechnikov (1845-1916) whom proposed a cell based (phagocytic) theory of immunity thirty years earlier, Aschoff challenges widely accepted medical dogma of the period. Ilya Mechnikov and Karl Aschoff argue human immunity is accomplished not by non-cell body humors and fluids e.g. blood soluble antibodies, rather it is accomplished by cell mediated processes (1892,1901,1905, 1922,1924)[228,229,230,226,227]. Karl Aschoff systematically identifies phagocytic cells within the reticular-endothelial systems, based upon their increasing order of demonstrated phagocytic activity, when presented with body antigen. The reticular-endothelial system described by Karl Aschoff is perhaps more recognizable by its current term, the mononuclear phagocytic system.

Recall, the cell based reticular-endothelial system (aka mononuclear phagocytic system, MPS) serves a primary defense against invading bacteria and viruses, assists in the removal of old and abnormal cells from the body, and complements the humoral immunity systems (i.e. antibody mediated immunity). The primary mechanism of action of the MPS is cell mediated phagocytosis, specialized cells engulfing antigen.

Equally important functions of these specialized cells is presentation of antigen to other immune cells e.g. lymphocytes. This function is essential to the production of antibodies and systematic removal of worn out red blood cells (RBCs) allowing return of hemoglobin to the body for reuse by new RBCs. The MPS cells originate from stem cells found in bone marrow. Once the cells are released from bone marrow, into the systemic blood circulation, the cells change their name to monocytes. Monocytes circulate in systemic blood until such time they migrate through blood capillaries into specific body tissues to begin their phagocytic and antigen presenting functions. Once monocytes enter body tissues, they change their name and are termed macrophages. Dependent upon the specific body tissue the macrophages occupy e.g. brain, liver, lungs, spleen, lymph nodes, the macrophage changes its name accordingly. Macrophages located in brain are termed microglia cells, in liver termed Kupffer cells, in spleen or lymph nodes termed reticular cells, and in lung termed alveolar macrophages.

The concept of cell mediated immunity is initially met by much resistance by the scientific and medical communities and only later demonstrated to be an important and essential component of the human immunological defense systems.

The professional and personal attacks against proponents of a cell mediated immune system from proponents supportive of the established dogma of a non-cellular body humor mediated immune system are brutal. Ilya Mechnikov recounts "…The polemics concerning phagocytosis might have killed or finally enfeebled me much earlier. At times (for instance, I refer to Lubarsch's attacks in 1889 and those of Pfeiffer in 1894) I was ready to rid myself of life…" (p 232) (1921)[231].

Karl Aschoff and Ilya Mechnikov are but only two investigators whom thoughtfully challenge medical and scientific dogma, necessarily respond to professional and personal criticism from the well-established medical and scientific communities, and change the future of medicine.

Trivia: Ilya Mechnikov shares the 1908 Nobel Prize in Physiology or Medicine with Paul Ehrlich "…in recognition of their work on immunity…" (1908)[232].

Much of medical pathology during the early-1900s focuses upon the scientific study of inflammation.

George Whipple (1878-1976) American pathologist, perhaps most remembered by medical students for his identification of the pathological findings of a bacterial infection which greatly impairs normal absorption of food nutrients from the intestines, Whipple's disease. Whipple disease is characterized by clinical signs and symptoms of diarrhea, weight loss, abdominal cramping, weakness, anemia, fatigue, and joint inflammation most typically occurring in middle age men. He is among the first to report the appearance of abnormal fat deposits in the walls of the small intestines and mesenteric lymphatic tissues, in the condition which he terms "intestinal lipodystrophy" and we know today simply as Whipple's disease (1907)[233].

He fails to recognize these signs to be the result of a bacterial infection and confidently attributes them to an abnormality in fat metabolism. He does speculate in his original report as to the potential contribution of the "…great number of a rod-shaped organism..." which might be causal agents and perhaps explain the observed pathological finding. Fifty-four years pass before electron microscopy technology reveal the specific bacilli and tissue macrophages underlying Whipple's disease and identifies them as the primary causal agent (1961,1961)[234,235]. The bacterium is later termed Tropheryma whippelii, originating from the Greek "trophy" meaning nourishment and "eryma" meaning barrier, given the malabsorption syndrome characteristically produced by the bacterium (1992)[236].

Less known to most medical students, George Whipple's primary research interests focus upon the investigation of anemia (1920,1925)[237,238]. He is awarded the 1934 Nobel Prize in Physiology or Medicine along with George Minot (1885-1950) and William Murphy (1892-1987) "…for their discoveries concerning liver therapy in cases of anaemia…" (1934)[239].

Trivia: Much of George Whipple's research into anemia, conducted at the newly founded University of Rochester, where he serves as Dean of the University from 1921-1954, is financed by George Eastman (1854-1932). You might recognize the name Eastman from the film and photographic equipment manufacturing company Eastman Kodak Company, founded by George Eastman in 1888 and headquartered in Rochester, New York.

Nikolai Anitschkov (1885-1964) Russian pathologist is among the first to recognize and report into the scientific literature the association between cholesterol and atherosclerosis (1884-1885, 1904,1909,1910,1913,1913)[240,241,242,243,244,245]. His initial investigations are based upon proposals by recent Nobel Prize recipient Ilya Mechnikov and Russian experimental pathologist Alexander Ignatowski (1875-1855), that an excess of protein in one's diet is potentially toxic and contributes to the acceleration of the aging process (1909)[246]. Nikolai Anischkov in his now classic experiment, feeds purified cholesterol dissolved in sunflower oil to rabbits and demonstrates the appearance of vascular pathology characteristic of the arteriosclerotic changes observed in humans (1913)[244]. So begins the century long investigations into the association of cholesterol and atherosclerosis.

Trivia: The term "atherosclerosis" is introduced into the literature by Felix Marchand (1846-1928) German pathologist (1904)[241]. The term has its origin in Greek "athero" meaning "porridge or gruel like" and "sclerosis" meaning "hardening". The term describes the accumulation of fatty substances inside artery walls, which leads to a thickening and associated loss of elasticity in the arterial vessels. This produces a chronic inflammation of the arterial wall characterized by an accumulation of macrophages in the walls of the arterial blood vessels.

Ernest Goodpasture (1886-1960) American pathologists working at Harvard University reports the rare, progressive, and usually fatal autoimmune disorder with which most medical students associate his name, Goodpasture's disease (aka anti-glomerular basement antibody disease) (1919)[247]. Recall, the condition, a type II hypersensitivity reaction, occurs when the patient's immune system antibodies attack the basement membranes of kidneys and lungs. The resulting Goodpasture's syndrome is characterized by glomerulonephritis resulting in proteinurea (protein in the urine) and ultimately kidney failure. Pulmonary signs and symptoms are typically hemoptysis (coughing up blood), anemia, and associated fatigue. Pathological findings reveal linear IgG deposits along the basement membranes in the kidneys and lungs.

Perhaps less known by most medical students is Ernest Goodpasture's later and more substantial contribution made while working at Vanderbilt University. It is here he invents the successful method for growing specific viruses and the Rickettsia bacteria, in chicken embryos (1931)[248]. The method allows for the cultured growth of the colonies necessary to complete essential works in vaccine development.

Rickettsia is a genus of Gram-negative bacteria, typically carried by ticks, fleas, and lice, and cause diseases in humans, such as Rocky Mountain spotted fever and typhus. As obligate intracellular parasites, Rickettsia cannot be grown on the usual culture mediums typically used to grow bacteria. These bacteria require host cells and within which the bacteria replicate. Investigation of viruses dominate the work of Ernest Goodpasture. Early in his career he investigates the herpes simplex (cold sores or fever blisters) virus (1923)[249]; describes intra-axonal transmission of herpes and rabies viruses (1925)[250,251]; and describes viruses producing encephalitis (1925)[252]. Five years later, in collaboration with colleague pathologist Claud Johnson (unknown-) and working at Vanderbilt University located in Nashville, Tennessee, the debate as to whether the microbial etiology of mumps is a bacterium, a spirochete, or a virus is finally resolved. Mumps, the contagious childhood disease, spread from person to person through contact with respiratory secretions, such as saliva via aerosols or fomites, resulting in the clinical signs and symptoms fever, headache, weakness, fatigue, loss of appetite, and painful swelling of the salivary glands, is the result of a filterable cytotropic virus (1935)[253].

Trivia: The term "mumps" originates from the British phrase "to mump", meaning to grin or grimace. Patients suffering the characteristic painful swelling of the parotid glands appear to be grimacing, hence the term.

The contributions of Ernest Goodpasture and other academic experimental pathologists of the early-1900s reflect the continuing maturation of medical pathology as a scientific discipline. The field witnesses a move from the systematic analysis of gross anatomical structures reflective of the contributions of Giovanni Morgagni and Matthew Baille of the mid-1700s and late-1700s, to the systematic analysis of tissues reflective of the contributions of Xavier Bichat of the late-1700s and early-1800s, to the systematic analysis of the cell and cellular pathology reflective of the contributions of Theodor Schwann and Rudolf Virchow of the mid-1800s. The contributions of Ernest Goodpasture of the early-1900s reflect movement of medical pathology into the molecular level of analysis of human disease.

James Ewing (1866-1943) American pathologist is tremendously influential in the development of medical pathology, focuses on the pathology of cancer. Early in his career, as the only Professor of Pathology at the newly founded Cornell University School of Medicine, located in New York City, he receives private endowment funding, earmarked specifically for the investigation of cancer at the medical school (Huntington Fund for Cancer Research, 1902). Soon he and his research group begin publishing numerous scientific papers addressing such issues as to the vectors of transmission, causes, diagnosis, and treatment of cancers.

Beyond his seminal contributions as an experimental pathologist e.g. transmission of tumors (1906)[254], treatment of cancer on biological principles (1912)[255], identification of the malignant bone tumor known today simply as the "Ewing sarcoma" (1920)[256], James Ewing is instrumental in founding the American Association of Cancer Research (1907)[257] and the American Cancer Society (originally termed the American Society for the Control of Cancer) (1913)[258]. He establishes active programmatic clinical research at the General Memorial Hospital for the Treatment of Cancer and Allied Diseases in 1913, which later expands and becomes known simply as the Memorial Sloan-Kettering Cancer Center, in New York City. He establishes a new scientific journal devoted specifically to the investigation of cancer, The "Journal of Cancer Research" (1916)[259]. He is an early proponent of the use of radiation as a treatment modality for the treatment of cancers (1917,1934)[260,261]. James Ewing leads the way in the USA, for cancer research during the early-1900s.

Trivia: Memorial Sloan-Kettering Cancer Center is originally founded in 1884, in New York City and committed to providing diagnostic and treatment services to patients suffering cancer and allied diseases. Originally a hospital, the New York Cancer Hospital, located on Manhattan's Upper West Side moves to its current location in 1936 on York Avenue, land donated by John D. Rockefeller, Jr.. The hospital combines with its new free standing research institute, The Sloan-Kettering Institute (SKI) (1948)[262]. Alfred Sloan (1875-1966) and Charles Kettering (1876-1958) former General Motors automobile corporate executives, provide the initial funding and financing required to establish the SKI. Today, the hospital and research institute continue to provide pioneering world class innovative research into the pathologies of cancers, compassionate treatments to all cancer patients, and offers world class training and education to professionals.

Albert Coons (1912-1978) American pathologist is first to develop technologies and methods for labeling specific antibodies with fluorescent dyes, thereby permitting the detection of antibodies, antigens, and virtually any antigenic protein in cells or tissues (1941,1942)[263,264]. The pioneering work of Albert Coons launches the clinical disciplines of diagnostic immunofluorescent microscopy for bacteriology and immunology, immunocytology, and immunohistochemistry. Medical pathology goes molecular.

Specialized training, formal examination, and demonstration of competency in content and process knowledge within medical pathology is formally introduced during the early-1990s, for physicians interested in practicing medical pathology and representing themselves as a "Board Certified" medical pathologist. Formal examination is first implemented in Scotland in 1900 and 36 years later in the USA.

Below is a copy of the specialty examination for pathology, for members of the Royal College of Physicians of Edinburgh, Scotland, choosing to identify themselves as pathologists (1900)[265]. Could you pass this exam?

Royal College of Physicians of Edinburgh

Examination for Membership
10th and 11th July 1900

Pathology

1. Describe the naked-eye and minute changes in the liver in the various forms of cirrhosis of that organ.
2. Describe the changes that take place in the brain as a consequence of thrombosis of a branch, say of the middle cerebral artery.
3. Describe the local lesion in diphtheria; give the life history of the bacillus which causes it; and mention its distribution in the body.
4. Describe the parasite of malaria; and give briefly its life history.

The American Medical Association (AMA) (1847)[266], Section of Pathology and Physiology (1901)[267], in cooperation with the American Society of Clinical Pathologist (ASCP) (1922) [268], and the newly founded American Board of Medical Specialties (ABMS) (1933)[269], work cooperatively to establish formal educational standards and examination criteria for all interested in becoming "Board Certified" in the specialty practice of pathology. As the result of these collected efforts, the

American Board of Pathology (ABP) is founded July 19, 1936 in Chicago (1936)[270]. The mission and purpose of the ABP "… as a member of the American Board of Medical Specialties, is to promote the health of the public and advance the practice and science of pathology by establishing voluntary certification standards and assessing the qualifications of those seeking to practice the specialty of pathology…" (1936)[271]. The ABP continues today setting the universally recognized standard of excellence in the evaluation and credentialing of physicians seeking recognition as "Board Certified Pathologists".

The first half of the 1900s witness increased and substantial contributions to pathology, being made from investigators located in the US and Canada. Departments of Pathology are well established in most US and Canadian universities and associated medical schools. US and Canadian based pathologists pioneer new areas of molecular investigations and rapidly incorporate new technologies into their investigations. Medical school curricula, in the US and Canada, require more classroom hours of instruction and more supervised laboratory experience in pathology than ever before. US and Canadian medical school curricula acknowledge content and process knowledge, in the area of medical pathology, as necessary and essential to the medical education of every well qualified physician. Medical pathology continues to establish itself as a valued professional, academic, scientific based discipline. Pathology is formally recognized by the American Medical Association as the practice of medicine (1943)[272] and immediately impacts the organizational structure and professional practice of clinical medicine.

Influential investigators, making substantive contributions and representative advancements during the first half of the 1900s are Karl Aschoff (cell mediated immunity), George Whipple (diet and its role in anemia), Nikolai Anischkov and Alexander Ignatowski (diet cholesterol and its role in atherosclerosis), Ernest Goodpasture (method to successfully reproduce specific viruses in laboratory), James Ewing (transmission of cancer), and Albert Coons (develops fluorescent dye technologies allowing the labeling of antibodies and antigens). Foundational work completed by these investigators continue to impact medical pathology today.

The second half of the 1900s witness the movement in medical pathology towards the molecular level of study of human pathology. Disease and disease processes are aggressively investigated at progressively increasing levels of molecular analysis. Advances in molecular technologies lowers the costs of once prohibitively expensive diagnostic procedures and offers increased availability of procedures, once completed only in the most sophisticated large academic laboratories, to be completed in the primary care physicians' office. Advances in computer technologies and internet based information exchange, allow for rapid completion of previously labor intensive procedures, and rapid dissemination of procedure results to remote locations. Medical pathology aggressively searches for relationships between human pathology and specific genetic materials. Disease and disease processes are associated with modifications in specific genes. Specific molecular changes in the DNA sequences of many disorders are identified. New conceptual matrixes emphasizing the molecular basis of pathology are proposed and tested. These are exciting times for medical pathology.

Let us take a brief look at a few specific influential people, milestone discoveries, and changes in conceptual matrixes which help shape the history of medical pathology during the second half of the 1900s.

Linus Pauling (1901-1994) American biochemist, Harvey Itano (1920-2010) American biochemist, Seymour Singer (1924-2017) American cell biologist, Ibert Wells (1921-2011)

American biochemist revolutionize the way in which human disease is conceptualized and investigated. Disease now begins to be conceptualized within the matrix of molecular biology, with particular attention focused upon disordered molecular structure and molecular processes. Familiar diseases, once defined by clinical presentation of signs and symptoms and physical changes in tissues and cells occurring at the light microscopic level, begin to be defined as a function of changes occurring at the molecular level.

For example, Sickle cell disease (SCD), once defined by its clinical signs and symptoms of shortness of breath, dizziness, headaches, coldness in the hands and feet, jaundice, pale colored mucus membranes, sudden onset of mild to severe pain, often following physical exertion, and microscopic inspection of blood, revealing abnormal shaped RBC and lower than expected blood cell counts (anemia) (1904)[273], is redefined within the emerging matrix of molecular biology by Linus Pauling, Harvey Itano, Seymour Singer, and Ibert Wells, as a disorder of abnormal protein synthesis (1949)[274]. Their now classic 1949 paper appearing in "Science", offers the first evidence human disease is caused by an abnormal protein. This finding changes the future and direction of medical pathology.

Sickle cell disease is soon understood as a point mutation of a specific gene, located at 11p15.5, coding for the beta-globin chain of hemoglobin A. This point mutation is defined by a single nucleotide substitution (A to T). The substitution changes a glutamic acid codon (GAG) to a valine codon (GTG), resulting in the abnormal protein which produces Sickle cell disease.

Trivia: The term "sickle cell anemia" is coined by medical student Verne Mason (1889-1965), while attending medical school at Johns Hopkins University (1922)[275].

Success in isolating the specific molecular abnormality responsible for Sickle cell disease triggers an avalanche of new investigations, all searching for a single gene or single molecular abnormality which will explain all other human diseases. Another 30 years will pass before the next single gene mutation is identified to be associated with a specific disease, Huntington disease (4p16.3) (1983)[276].

Jerome Lejeune (1926-1994) French geneticist investigates chromosome abnormalities, rather than gene abnormalities associated with human disease and soon recognizes children presenting with impaired intellectual abilities associated with Down's syndrome have an extra chromosome 21 (n=3) (1959)[277]. Jerome Lejeune confirms his original observation with an additional report to the French Academy of Sciences (n=9) (1959)[278]. The first association between an identified chromosomal abnormality (Trisomy 21) and impaired intellectual functioning is established. Jerome Lejeune continues his investigations and subsequently identifies additional syndromes associated with abnormal chromosomes e.g. Cri du Chat syndrome (1964)[279].

Much like the search for the next new gene associated with human disease triggered by the original sickle cell disease reports of 1949, so too is the case with chromosome anomalies. Building upon the success of identifying an abnormal number of chromosomes in the Down's syndrome patient in 1959 and improved karyotyping technologies, the search begins for additional diseases and disorders, evidencing underlying chromosomal abnormalities.

Over the course of the next two years, several syndromes are explained as the result of identifiable human chromosome abnormalities. For example, Turner syndrome results from a single X chromosome (45,X or 45,XO) (1959)[280]; Edwards syndrome results from an additional chromosome 18, Trisomy 18 (1960)[281]; Patau syndrome results from an additional chromosome 13, Trisomy 13 (1960)[282]; chronic myelogenous leukemia (CML) results form a reciprocal translocation between chromosome 9 and 22 (t(9;22) aka the Philadelphia chromosome (1960)[283].

Trivia: The currently accepted number of human chromosomes is 46 (1956)[284]. This count contains 22 pairs of autosomes and one pair of sex chromosomes (female XX or male XY). During the period 1923-1956 the accepted number of human chromosomes is 48 (1923)[285].

By the early-1960s much effort is being devoted to understanding the molecular basis of human disease.

Renato Dulbecco (1914-2012) Italian pathologist, working at the Salk Institute located in La Jolla California, discovers how tumor viruses interact with genetic material within cells. More specifically, he identifies how a virus can insert its own genes into the DNA of a cell and modify the cell's normal growth and differentiation (1963)[286,287]. This discovery opens a new line of investigation into the etiology of cancer. The prevailing scientific thought at the time of his discovery is cancer might be the end consequence of inherited genetic material. His demonstration that genetic material can be altered by a virus necessitates a reassessment of the entire conceptual matrix within which the molecular basis of cancer is investigated. Renato Dulbecco is recognized for his contributions and shares the 1975 Nobel Prize in Physiology or Medicine with American geneticist Howard Temin (1934-1994) and American immunologist David Baltimore (1938-) "...for their discoveries concerning the interaction between tumour viruses and the genetic material of the cell..." (1975)[288].

Prior to the 1975 Nobel Prize award, David Baltimore, working at Massachusetts Institute of Technology (MIT) and Howard Temin, working at the University of Wisconsin-Madison, discover the enzyme used to generate complementary DNA from an RNA template, reverse transcriptase (RTase) (1970,1970)[289,290]. Their discovery is met with much resistance from the scientific and medical communities in that it directly challenges the central dogma of molecular biology which states, DNA is transcribed into RNA, which is then translated into proteins.

The molecular basis of cancer is aggressively investigated during the 1970s and 1980s. Proto-oncogenes (normal genes which normally encode proteins that regulate cell growth and differentiation (e.g. proto-scr), oncogenes (mutated proto-oncogenes which now disrupt regulation of normal cell growth and differentiation e.g. c-src (1976,1979)[291,292] and tumor suppressor genes (genes which encode proteins that inhibit cell proliferation e.g. p53 (1979)[293,294] are identified and begin to be understood within the matrix of normal cell cycle functions and their role in the molecular basis of cancer.

Michael Bishop (1936-) and Harold Varmus (1939-) American immunologists, working at University of California San Francisco, building upon the prior works of Renato Dulbecco, David Baltimore, Howard Temin, and others are instrumental in understanding how viruses convert normal genetic material (normal genes) of normal healthy cells (proto-oncogenes) into cancer producing genetic material (cancer genes). They are recognized for their contributions with the award of the Nobel Prize in Physiology or Medicine "...for their discovery of the cellular origin of retroviral oncogenes..." (1989)[295].

New viruses producing disease are discovered and associated with specific disease syndrome. Perhaps the most recognizable virus identified during the early-1980s is the virus which causes an acquired immune deficiency syndrome (AIDS), the human immunodeficiency virus (HIV) (1983)[296].

Trivia: The virus producing AIDS, the HIV is originally named HTLV-III/LAV (human T-cell lymphotropic virus-type III/lymphadenopathy-associated virus).

Recall, acquired immunodeficiency syndrome (AIDS) is an example of a clinical syndrome generated by an infection with the human immunodeficiency virus (HIV). The HIV is a lentivirus (slowly replicating retrovirus). The retrovirus is a single stranded, positive sense, enveloped RNA virus and replicates through the process of reverse transcriptase. HIV infects the human immune system cells e.g. CD4 T-cells, macrophages, and dendritic cells. This results in a loss in cell mediated immunity and the now too familiar clinical presentation of patients to primary care physicians with AIDS.

Many of the most important advancements in medical pathology made during the period 1975-2000 are dependent upon innovative conceptualization and associated inventions of new molecular technologies. Invention and development of two procedures prove to be particularly influential in the advancement of medical pathology, production of monoclonal antibodies (MAb) and polymerase chain reaction (PCR).

George Kohler (1946-1995) German biologist and Cesar Milstein (1927-2002) Argentine biochemist introduce and develop new and innovative procedures for duplicating cells, which produce an identical antibody molecule (monoclonal antibody) (1975)[297]. The production of monoclonal antibodies provides the necessary technology to open new lines of biomedical research and offer more precise diagnosis and treatment of human disease.

Niels Jerne (1911-1994) Danish immunologist offers an innovative, integrated, conceptual matrix which addresses the specificity, development, and regulation of the immune response. His ideas and theories challenge scientific and medical dogma. In brief, he proposes the natural-selection theory regarding antibody formation; explains how cells of the immune system mature in the thymus gland; and offers a new conceptual matrix which explains how the immune response is regulated by an interactive network of antibodies and anti-antibodies. Niels Jerne challenges medical dogma and provides an innovative, testable, new conceptual matrix, within which to understand, prevent, diagnose, and treat human disease.

George Kohler, Cesar Milstein, and Niels Jerne share the 1984 Nobel Prize in Medicine or Physiology "...for theories concerning the specificity in development and control of the immune system and the discovery of the principle for production of monoclonal antibodies..." (1984)[298].

Building upon recent advances in molecular technology, human diseases are associated with identifiable changes in genetic materials and understood within the matrix of the molecular function modified by the changes in genetic material. For example, the gene responsible for the production of the protein huntingtin (4p16.3) is identified and associated with the neuro-degenerative disorder Huntington's disease (1983,1993)[299,300]. The gene responsible for the production of the protein cystic fibrosis transmembrane regulator (CFTR) (7q31.2), which regulates movement of chloride and sodium ions across epithelial membranes, such as the alveolar epithelia of the lungs, is identified and associated with cystic fibrosis (1989,1989)[301,302]. The gene responsible for the production of the protein breast cancer type 1 susceptibility protein (BCRA1) (17q21), which regulates the repair of DNA, is identified and associated with an increased risk for breast cancers (1990)[303]. The gene responsible for the production of the protein fragile X mental retardation protein (FMRP) (Xq27.3), which is essential for normal neural development is identified and associated with autism and an inherited cause of mental retardation, resulting in the fragile X syndrome (1991,1991)[304,305].

The single gene-single disease model is embraced during the early-1990s and spurs the development of a new sub-specialization within medical pathology, termed simply enough, molecular genetics. However, research soon reveals a more complex pattern of associations between human disease and genetic material. More complex models of gene-disease associations are aggressively investigated during the early-2000s. More on this later.

In the bright light of rapid advancements being made into the molecular basis of disease, a much needed, revised approach, is introduced as to how medical pathology knowledge can best be presented to medical students. The approach maximizes learning of material and increases the potential for recall of material, when placed in a clinical setting environment. By the end of the 1900s medical pathology textbooks begin to be supplemented by increased use of audiovisual materials, accessed through the World Wide Web (a partitioned space within the Internet) and companion compact discs (CDs). One medical pathology textbook requires special attention in its innovative format and that it has touched the lives of thousands and thousands of medical students, throughout the world, during the late-1900s and early-2000s is Stanley Robbins' "Pathological Basis of Disease".

Stanley Robbins (1915-2003) American pathologist, working at the Boston University College of Medicine, introduces a textbook which will change the lives of medical students and practicing physicians forever. Initially introduced and titled "Textbook of Pathology and Clinical Correlations" (1957)[306] is retitled after its third edition to "Pathological Basis of Disease" (1974)[307]. The textbook quickly becomes the gold standard against which all other medical pathology textbooks are compared. The text is unique in that it not only describes the disease within the traditional matrix of anatomical pathological changes, it offers discussion of the origin of the disease, emphasizes the mechanism of the disease process, discusses the impact of the disease process on the patient, and offers clinically relevant patho-clinical correlations in sufficient detail to make the information immediately applicable in a clinical diagnosis and treatment setting, within which most physicians practice medicine. Images and photographs are colorful and engage the student. Material is presented systematically for each organ system and contains descriptions and discussion at the gross, tissue, cell, and molecular level of analysis.

This textbook, like many innovations, is initially criticized by the established academic and medical communities as being too clinically oriented. However, medical students quickly embrace the new format and the clarity of the writing. Currently, the text is in its 11th edition (8th edition plus 3 initial editions of the text published under the title "Textbook of Pathology and Clinical Correlations") continues to make medical pathology understandable to medical students around the world today (2010)[308].

The 1900s close with the social and moral issue of euthanasia, the practice of intentionally ending a life in order to relieve pain and suffering, is planted firmly before the medical community and public at large.

Jack Kevorkian (1928-2011) American pathologist and euthanasia activist challenges the US medical community, legal system, and general public to consider one's responsibility to other human beings suffering a painful and terminal disease. The question in brief is; should a terminal patient be permitted to end their life via physician assisted suicide? Few questions elicit such emotionally charged and self-righteous answers as does this question. You as a future physician will need to make up your own mind as to where you stand on this issue.

At the end of the 1900s, the answer is clear to American pathologist and activist Jack Kevorkian; the answer is yes. At the end of the 1900s, the answer is equally clear to the USA legal system; the answer is no. Committed to his beliefs and always a champion of assisting terminal patients to end their life with dignity and physician assistance, Jack Kevorkian is arrested, tried, and convicted of second degree murder and sentenced by a USA judge to serve 10-25 years in prison for his actions. He serves eight years and released on the condition "…he not offer suicide advice to any other person…" (2007)[309].

Today, the issue of euthanasia remains unresolved in the USA. What will you do when your patient ask for your assistance, in ending their life and to end their pain and suffering, resulting from a terminal disease condition?

Several additional bioethical issues challenge the medical community as the 1900s come to a close. Who owns your patient's genetic material? Should embryonic stem cells be used in medical research? Should artificially generated genetic material be patentable? What are animal rights if any in medical research? Should physicians participate in conducting abortions? Should animals be cloned? Should humans be cloned? Medical pathology and medical pathologists continue to offer leading guidance on each issue from an informed scientific perspective.

These are exciting times for medical pathology.

Medical pathology as a discipline is alive and well at the end of the 1900s. Tremendous advancements continue to be made in the areas of molecular analysis of human disease. Genetic material is quickly being understood and information is quickly being applied to the clinical practice of medicine. New technologies permit the rapid and cost effective analysis of biological tissues and fluids, providing practicing clinicians essential information in a timely manner to guide diagnostic and treatment decisions. New scientific journals devoted to the specialty practice of medical pathology continue to be founded. Scientific and professional societies committed to the advancement of medical pathology as a scientific discipline and specialized area of medical practice thrive. Medical school curriculum continue to stay abreast of the rapid flow of new information coming from pathology, as are medical pathology residency training programs and specialty certification boards. Medical pathology is well established as a highly respected professional and scientific discipline.

Representative influential investigators making substantial contributions and representative advances during the second half of the 1900s are Linus Pauling, Harvey Itano, Seymour Singer, Ibert Wells (conceptualize basis of disease within a molecular biology matrix; human disease is caused by abnormal protein), Jerome Lejeune (chromosome abnormalities), Renato Dulbecco (DNA and cell cycle altered by virus), David Baltimore and Howard Temin (reverse transcriptase role in reproducing DNA from RNA), Michael Bishop and Harold Varmus (proto-oncogense into oncogenes), George Kohler and Cesaar Milstein (monoclonal antibodies), Niels Jerne (specificity in development and control of immune system), Stanley Robbins (textbook), and Jack Kevorkian (social-moral issue of euthanasia).

In summary, the 1900s witness continued and rapid development in medical pathology. The primary unit of study gradually shifts from the cellular level, at the beginning of the1900s to the sub-cellular molecular level by the end of the 1900s. Investigations into the process and end result of inflammation dominate much of the investigations during the early-1900s. The cell based reticular-endothelial systems (mononuclear phagocytic system) is identified and detailed. The concept of cell mediated immunity is proposed and complements the dogma of humoral models of immunity. Anemia is aggressively investigated and dietary treatments prove to be effective in its treatment. Relationships between cholesterol and atherosclerosis are established. Autoimmune disorders begin to be understood within the matrix of antibodies misinterpreting cell signaling and attack otherwise healthy tissue bound proteins. Transmission of specific viruses are understood, e.g. herpes simplex, rabies, mumps. Cancer is aggressively investigated. The American Cancer Society and Sloan-Kettering Cancer Center are founded. Specific antibodies and antigens are labeled with fluorescent dye allowing for detection of virtually any antigenic protein in cells or tissues. Medical pathology goes molecular.

Specialty examinations become the standard for excellence for individuals choosing to identify themselves as pathologists. New scientific and professional societies are founded devoted specifically to the advancement of pathology e.g. ASCP. Human disease is conceptualized within a molecular rather than cellular, tissue, or organ based matrix. Diseases are recognized to occasionally result from alterations in genetic material producing a single abnormal protein e.g. sickle cell anemia. Human chromosomes are identified and chromosome abnormalities associated with specific abnormal conditions and disease processes e.g. Down syndrome, Edwards' syndrome, chronic myelogenous leukemia. Gene abnormalities are identified for such diseases as sickle cell anemia, Huntington's disease, cystic fibrosis, breast cancer, and inherited forms of cognitive impairments e.g. fragile X syndrome. The conceptual matrix of a single gene-single disease model is embraced and aggressively explored. Viruses are recognized to insert their own DNA into the DNA of cells and modify the cells' normal growth and differentiation. Specific cancers are understood within the matrix of virus altered DNA. The enzyme reverse transcriptase, important for production of DNA from an RNA template is discovered and understood within the matrix of human disease. Proto-oncogenes, oncogenes, and tumor suppressor genes are identified and understood within the matrix of cancer. Retroviruses are identified and understood within the matrix of oncogenes. Notable technological advancements are the production of cells producing monoclonal antibodies and polymerase chain reaction procedures, allowing for rapid reproductions of segments of DNA.

Medical pathology textbook formats change, making medical pathology more digestible and offering greater clinical relevance to medical students. Medical pathology provides thoughtful leadership and guidance from within its ranks on multiple bioethical issues challenging the professional scientific and medical communities.

Current Modern, 2000 AD - 2019 AD.

Medical pathology continues to play necessary and essential roles in moving the medical knowledge base regarding human disease forward. Academic pathologists continue to contribute to understanding the process of disease as well as the end results. Clinical pathologists offer interpretations of tests and procedures completed routinely by practicing physicians around the world on a daily basis. Medical pathology remains a cornerstone in providing information essential to physicians whom choose to practice high quality medicine.

Advances in molecular technologies and information processing technologies have changed pathology forever. More information is available than ever before and must be distilled and processed. Medical pathology has gone molecular. The human genome has been sequenced and new information relevant to the competent practice of medicine in a molecular based environment is being released at unprecedented rates (2001)[310]. Pathologists are best prepared to interpret the information and assist the clinical physician in making diagnostic, treatment, and management decisions. The role of the medical pathologist is changing from diagnostic consultant to information management consultant.

The future at this time appears to be directed at understanding disease and disease processes within the matrix of molecular processes and genetic material. Diagnosis is moving towards a future of increased individualization based upon a patient's individual genetic composition, lifestyle, and demonstrated effective treatments. Diagnostic, treatment, and management decisions are increasingly based upon multifactorial computer based analyses of tremendous amounts of information which overwhelms and boggle the brightest of all human minds. The entire human genome can now be sequenced by the fastest current technology within hours. The cost has plummeted from approximately $30,000 to sequence the entire human genome only a couple of years ago to approximately $4,000 today in 2013. The cost is anticipated to drop even more within the next couple of years to approximately to $1,000 (2006,2010)[311,312]. Low cost of the sequencing of any individual's genome, coupled with the exponential understanding of what specific DNA sequences mean in regard to human disease, offer an exciting future for medical pathology and medicine in general.

Medical school curriculum are currently being revised throughout the world to accommodate the unprecedented changes occurring in the understanding of human disease and disease processes at the molecular level. Residency training programs are incorporating much more molecular pathology and genomic pathology into all its residency training programs (2010)[313]. Board certified pathologists are systematically acquiring and assimilating the new knowledge base through continuing education modules and postdoctoral fellowship training.

The future for medical pathology is certainly going to be exciting.

References.

[1] Dirckx, J. (1997). Stedman's concise medical dictionary for the health professional. 3rd edition. Baltimore: William and Wilkins.
[2] Cotran, R., Kumar, V., Collins, T. (1999). Robbins Pathological basis of disease. 6th edition. Philadelphia: W. B. Saunders Company.
[3] Morse, P. (1914). The development of pathology as a science. Detroit Medical Journal, 15(11):395-401.
[4] Pathology. (2012). In Encyclopedia Britannica. Retrieved from http://www.britannica.com/EBchecked/topic/446440/pathology
[5] The Petrie papyri: Hieratic papyri from Kahun and Gurob. (circa 1800 BC). [Online English translation]. Edited by F. Griffith. Retrieved September 2011 from http://www.archive.org/stream/hieraticpapyrifr00grifuoft#page/n7/mode/2up
[6] Ebers papyrus (circa 1550 BC). Compendium of the whole Egyptian medicine (Georg Ebers), Columns 1-2. University of Leipzig Library, Special Collections. Leipzig, Germany.
[7] Edwin Smith surgical papyrus (circa 1500 BC). [Online English translation]. Retrieved September 2011 from http://www.touregypt.net/edwinsmithsurgical.html
[8] Griffith, F. (1898). The Petrie papyri: Hieratic papyri from Kahun and Gurob. London: Bernard Quaritch.
[9] Thompson, R. (1923). Assyrian medical texts from the originals in the British Museum. London: H. Milford, Oxford University Press.

[10] Scurlock, J. and Anderson, B. (2005). Diagnoses in Assyrian and Babylonian medicine: Ancient sources, translations, and modern medical analyses. Chicago: University of Illinois Press.

[11] Hippocrates (400 BC). Hippocratic Corpus. Internet Classics. Translated by Francis Adams. Retrieved March 2012 from http://classics.mit.edu/Hippocrates/acutedis.html

[12] Jones, W. (1923). Hippocrates with an English translation by W.H.S. Jones. London: William Heinemann, Ltd.

[13] Galen, C. (173/1826/2008/2011). De methodo medendi 1.1 (Meth. Of Med. X,5,15-6,8, Kuhn, 1826); R. J. Hankinson (ed.) (2008). The Cambridge companion to Galen. Cambridge. Edited and translated by Ian Johnson and G. H. Horsley (2011). Galen: Methods of Medicine, Book 1-4. Loeb Classical Library 516.

[14] Aristotle (circa 350 BC). On the history of animals. Translated by Darcy Wentworth Thompson. Works by Aristotle from the Classics Collection at MIT. Retrieved November 2012 from http://classics.mit.edu/Aristotle/history_anim.1.i.html

[15] Aristotle (circa 350 BC). On the parts of animals. Translated by William Ogle. Works by Aristotle from the Classics Collection at MIT. Retrieved November 2012 from http://classics.mit.edu/Aristotle/parts_animals.html

[16] Celsus (circa 30) and Thayer, B. (2012). De mediciona octo libri. Aulus Celsus. English translation. Retrieved 11-15-2012 from http://penelope.uchicago.edu/Thayer/E/Roman/Texts/Celsus/5*.html.

[17] Libby, W. (1922). The history of medicine in its salient features. p52. Boston: Houghton Miffin Co.

[18] Luzzi, M. (1474). Anathomia mondini. Manuscript (1316), Printed (1474) Pavia: Petrus Maufer.

[19] Ketham, J. (1495). Fasciculus medicinae mundinus, Anatomia. Venezia: Johannes und Greorius de Greforiis.

[20] Luzzi, M. (1507). Anothomia mundini a capite usque ad pedes. Papie: Impressa per Jacob de Paucisdrapis de Burgofrancho.

[21] Celsus (circa 30) and Thayer, B. (2012). De mediciona octo libri. Aulus Celsus. English translation. Retrieved 11-15-2012 from http://penelope.uchicago.edu/Thayer/E/Roman/Texts/Celsus/5*.html

[22] Theophrastus. (300BC/1916). Enquiry into plants and minor works on odours and weather signs, with an English translation by Sir Author Hort, in two volumes. The Loeb Classical Library. London: William Heinemann. Retrieved 11-15-2012 from http://www.archive.org/stream/enquiryintoplant02theouoft#page/vi/mode/2up

[23] Galen / Siegel, R. (190AD/1976). Galen on the affected parts. Translation from the Greek text with explanatory notes. Basle: Karger.

[24] Benivieni, A. (1507). De abditis nonnullis ac mirandis morborum et sanationum causis. [About the hidden causes of disease]. Published posthumurously. Florence: Philippus Giunta. Translated by Charles Singer with a biographical appreciation by Esmond R. Long (1954). Springfield: Charles C. Thomas.

[25] Fernel, J. (1542). De naturali parte medicinae.Venetiis: Joannes Gryphius.

[26] Fernel, J. (1554). Medicina. Paris: Wechelum.

[27] Fernel, J. (1555). Pathologiae. Paris: Wechelum.

[28] Fernel, J. (1567). Universa Medicina, tribus et viginti libris absoluta [All medicine, twenty-three books absolute]. Paris: Andreas Wechelum.

[29] Vesalius, A. (1543). De corporis humani fabrica linbri septum. Basel: Johannes Oporinus.

[30] Vesalius, A., Garrison, D., & Hast, M. (1543/2013). An annotated translation of the 1543 and 1555 editions of Andreas Vesalius' De humani corporis fabrica. Northwestern University. Retrieved from http://vesalius.northwestern.edu

[31] Fracastoro, G. & Wright, W. (1546/1930).Hieronymii Fracastorii De Contagione, Libri III, Translation and notes. New York, London: G. P. Putnam's Sons.

[32] Plater, F. (1602-1608). Praxeos medicae tomi tres. [Practice of medicine volume 3]. Basel.

[33] Plater, F. (1614). Observationum in hominis affectibus plerisque, corpori and animo, functionum laesione, dolore, aliave molestia and vito incommodantibus, libri tres. [Most of the observations in the man's emotions, body, spirit, functions, injury, pain, or other discomforts and inconveniences, in three books.]. Basel: C. Waldkirch for Ludwig Konig.

[34] Dupuytren, G. (1831). De la rétraction des doigts par suite d'une affection de l'aponévrose palmaire, opération chirurgicale qui convient dans ce cas. [The retraction of the fingers as a result of a condition of the palmar aponeurosis, surgery suitable in this case]. Journal Universel et Hebdomadaire de Médecine et de Chirurgie Pratiques et des Institutions Médicales, Paris. 2(5):352-365.

[35] Plater, F. (1614). Suffocatio a struma interna abscondita, circa iugulum. [Choking from struma internal, hidden around the throat]. Observatioum in hominis affectibus plerisque corpori et animo, functionum lesione, dolore, aliave molestia er vitio incommodantinus libres tres, Part IX. Basel: Konig and Brandmulieri.

[36] Paltauf, A. (1889). Uber die beziehungen der thymus zum plotzlichen tod. [About the relationship of the thymus to sudden death]. Wiener Klinische Wochenschrift, 2:877-881.

[37] Bonet, T. (1679). Sepulchretum sive anatomica practica ex cadaveribus morbo denatis, proponens historias et observations omnium humani corporis affectuum, ipsorumque causus reconditas relevans. Quo nomine tam pathologiae genuinae, quam nosocomiae orthodoxae fundatrix, imo medicinae veteris ac novae prompturarium dici

eretur. Cum indicibus necessariis. Opus ominium medicinae et anatomiae cultorum votis hactenus expetitum summoque labore decerptum ac congestum. [Practical anatomy of corpses whom have died from disease, proposing investigations and observations of all of the human body, and their causes profound and mighty. Pathologies as well as the names and origins of drugs old and new and place to store drugs until ready for use.]. 2 volumes. Geneva: Sumptibus Leonardi Chouet.

[38] Boerhaave, H. (1693). De utilitate explorandorum in ageris excrementorum, ut signorum. [On the usefulness of examining the patient's excrements for diagnostic purposes]. (Doctoral thesis). University of Harderwijk, July 15.

[39] Boerhaave, H. (1732). Elementa chemiae [Elements of chemistry], 2 volumes. Lugduni Batavorum, Apud Isaacum Severinum. English translation, London, 1735.

[40] Morgagnus, J. (1761). De sedibus et causis morborum per anatomen indagatis, libri quinque; dissections, et animadversions, nunc primum editas complectuntur propemodum innumeras, medicis, chirugis, anatomicis profuturas. Tomus Primus duos priores continens libros. [On the seats and causes of diseases investigated by anatomy, in five books; dissection, and the observations, now issued for the first time embrace almost all physicians, surgeons, and anatomists to use. The first book contains the two previous books]. Venice: From typograhia Remondiniana.

[41] Bonet, T. (1679). Sepulchretum sive anatomia practica ex cadaveribus morbo denatis. Geneva: Leonardi Chouet.

[42] Morgagni, G. (1761). De sedibus et causis mortorum per anatomen idagatis libri quinque. Venice: Remondini.

[43] Morgagni, G. (1769). The seats and causes of diseases investigated by anatomy: in five books, containing a great variety of dissections, with remarks. To which are added very accurate and copious indexes of the principal things and names therein contained. Translated into English by B. Alexander. London: Millar and Cadell; Johnson and Payne.

[44] Hunter, J. (1786). A Treatise on the venereal disease. London: Everard Home.

[45] Hunter, J. (1794). A Treatise on the blood, inflammation and gun-shot wounds. Posthumous. London: G. Nicol.

[46] Ballie, M. (1793). The morbid anatomy of some of the most important parts of the human body. London: J. Johnson, St. Paul's Church-Yard.

[47] Ballie, M, (1799). A series of engravings with explanation which are intended to illustrate the morbid anatomy of some of the most important parts of the human body. London: W. Bulmer & Company.

[48] Ballie, M. (1808) The morbid anatomy of some of the most important parts of the body. The second American edition from the third London edition, corrected. Walpole, New Hamshire: G. W. Nichols. Retrieved from http://books.google.com/books?id=AE8SAAAAYAAJ&pg=PA1&source=gbs_toc_r&cad=4#v=onepage&q&f=false

[49] Bichat, X. (1800a). Traite des membranes en genral de diverses membranes en partilulier. [A treatise on the membranes in general and on different membranes in particular]. Paris: Brosson, Gabon, and Cie.

[50] Bichat, X. (1800b). Recherches physiologiques sur la vie et la mort. [Physiological researches on life and death]. Paris: Brosson.

[51] Pinel, P. (1798). Nosographie philosophique ou methode de l'analyse appliqué a la medicine. [Philosophical classification of diseases] Paris: J. A. Brossson.

[52] Bichat, X. (1800). Traite des membranes en general et de diverses membranes en particular. Paris: Caille et Ravier.

[53] Bichat, X. and Husson, H. (1813). A treatise on the membranes in general and on different membranes in particular. Translated into English by John Gorham Coffin. First American edition. Boston: Cummings and Hilliard.

[54] Fourcroy, A. (1791). Idees sur un nouvouveau moyen de rechercher la nature des maladies. [Ideas on how to search the new nature of diseases]. La Medecin eclairee par les sciences physique (Paris) 1:142-145.

[55] Fourcroy, A. and Vauquelin, N. (1799). Sur l'analyse des calculs urinaires humains. [On the analysis of human urinary calculi]. Ann. Chim., 32:213-222.

[56] Beneke, R. (1913). Johann Christian Reil: Gedachtnisrede bei der von der Friedrichs-Universitat veranstalteten erinnerungsfeier fur den vor 100 jahren dahingeschiedenen am 22 November , page 55 (translated from German). Halle: Max Niemeyer.

[57] Prout, W. (1821). An inquiry into the nature and treatment of gravel, calculus, and other disease of the urinary organs. London: Baldwin, Cradock, and Joy.

[58] Prout W. (1826). An inquiry into the nature and treatment of diabetes, calculus, and other affections of the urinary organs, 2nd ed. [2nd edition published in England in 1825]. Philadelphia: Towar and Hogan.

[59] Bright, R. (1827-1831). Reports of medical cases, selected with a view of illustrating the symptoms and cure of diseases by a reference to morbid anatomy. 2 volumes, London, Longmans.

[60] Wilks, S. (1877). Historical notes on Bright's disease, Addison's disease, and Hodgkin's disease. Guy's Hospital Reports. Edited by H. Howse and Frederick Taylor. Third series, vol. XXII. London: J. and A. Churchill.

[61] Bright, R. (1827-1831). Reports on medical cases selected with a view of illustrating the symptoms and cure of diseases by a reference to morbid anatomy, 1:3. London: Richard Taylor for Longman, Rees, Orme, Brown, and Green.

[62] Bright, R. (1835-1836). Cases and observations, illustrative of renal disease accompanied with the secretion of albuminous urine. London Medical Gazette, 72-74.

[63] Bright, R. (1836). Cases and observations, illustrative of renal disease accompanied with the secretion of albuminous urine. Guy's Hospital Reports, 1:338-379.

[64] Hodgkin, T. (1832). On some morbid experiences of the absorbent glands and spleen. Medical Chirurgical Transactions, 17: 68–114. Read January 20 and 24, 1832 to Royal Medical and Chirurgical Society of London. Retrieved from http://www.ncbi.nlm.nih.gov/pmc/articles/PMC2116706/

[65] Wilks S. (1865). Cases of enlargement of the lymphatic glands and spleen (or Hodgkin's disease) with remarks. Guy's Hosp Rep.11:56–67.

[66] Graves, R. (1835). Newly observed affection of the thyroid gland in females. (Clinical Lectures). London Medical and Surgical Journal (Renshaw), 7:516-517.

[67] Graves, R. (1843). Newly observed affection of the thyroid gland in females: Its connection with palpitations with fits of hysteria. In A system of clinical medicine, Lecture XL; 674-676. Dublin: Fannin and Company.

[68] Flajani, G. (1803). Sopra un tumor freddo nell'anterior parte del collo broncocele [On a cold tumor on the anterior part of the neck]. (Osservazione LXVII). In Collezione d'osservazioni e reflessioni di chirurgia. 3:270-273. Rome: Michele A Ripa Presso Lino Contedini.

[69] Testa, A. (1810). Delle malattie del cuore, loro cagioni, specie, segni e cura. [Diseases of the heart: Their causes, especially, signs and treatment.] Bologna: Giuseppe Lucchesini.

[70] Parry, C. (1815). Elements of Pathology and Therapeutics. London: Underwood.

[71] Parry, C. (1825). Enlargement of the thyroid gland in connection with enlargement or palpitations of the heart. Posthumous, in Collections from the unpublished medical writings of C. H. Parry. London, 111-129. Reprinted in Medical Classics, 1940, 5:8-30.

[72] Basedow, K. (1840). Exophthalmus durch Hypertrophie des Zellgewebes in der augenhöhle. [Exophthalmos caused by hypertrophy of the cellular tissue in the orbit]. Wochenschrift für die gesammte Heilkunde, Berlin, 6:197-204; 220-228.

[73] Pokhrel, B. & Bhusal, K. (2017). Graves' Disease. StatPearls [Internet], StatPearls Publishing, Treasue Island, Florida.

[74] Stokes, W. (1854). Increased action of the heart and of the arteries of the neck, followed by enlargement of the thyroid gland and eyeballs. In Diseases of the Heart and Aorta, p278-297. Philadelphia: Lindsay and Blakiston. Retrieved from http://archive.org/stream/diseasesheartan01stokgoog#page/n336/mode/2up

[75] Cheyne, J. (1818). A case of apoplexy in which the fleshy part of the heart was converted into fat. Dublin Hospital Reports, 2:216-223.

[76] Stokes, W. (1854). Fatty degeneration of the heart. In Diseases of the Heart and Aorta, p320–327. Dublin.

[77] Donne, A. (1836). Animalcules observes dans les matieres purulentes, et dans le produit des secretions des organs genitaux de l'homme et de la femme. [Animalculi observed in purulent fluids and secretions of genital organs from men and women]. Address to C.R. Academy of Sciences, Paris, 3:385.

[78] Donne, A. (1837). Recherches microscopiques sur la nature des mucus et la matiere des divers ecoulemens des organs genitor-urinaires, chez l'homme et chez la femme description des nouveaus animalcules decoverts dans quelques und de ces fluids. [Microscopic research on the nature of mucus and the flow of fluids of the genitourinary organs in man and women with descriptions of new animalcules discovered in some of these fluids]. Paris.

[79] Donne, A. (1842). De l'origine des globules du sang, de leur mode de formation et leur fin. C.R. Acad. Sci. (Paris), 14:366-368.

[80] Donnne, A. (1844). Cours de microscopie complementaire des etudes medicales [Course of microscopy complementary to medical studies]/ Paris: J. B. Bailliere. Retrieved from https://archive.org/details/b21470273

[81] Donne, A. (1845). Cours de microscopie complementaire des estudes medicales; anatomic microscopique et physilogie des fluides de l'economie; Atlas execute d'apres nature au microscope-daguerreotype. Paris: J.B. Bailliére

[82] Donne, A.(1840). Images photogeniques d'objects microscopiques. Comptes Rendus Acad. Science, 10:339.

[83] Donne, A. (1842). Conseils aux meres sur la maniere d'bever les enfants nouveaus nes, ou de l'education physique des enfants du premier age. Paris: J. B. Bailliere.

[84] Donne, A. (1844-5). Cours de microscopie complementaire des estudes medicales; anatomic microscopique et physilogie des fluides de l'economie; atlas execute d'apres nature au microscope-daguerreotype. Text volume published 1844 and accompanying atlas published 1845. Paris: J. B. Bailliere.

[85] Craigie, D. (1845). Case of disease and enlargement of the spleen in which death took place from the presence of purulent matter in the blood. Edinburgh Medical and Surgical Journal, 64:400-413.

[86] Bennett, J. (1845). Case 2; case of hypertrophy of the spleen and liver in which death took place from suppuration of the blood. The Edinburgh Medical and Surgical Journal, October 1, 64 413–423.

[87] Bennett, J. (1852). Leucocythemia or white cell blood. Edinburgh Medical and Surgical Journal, 72:7-82.

[88] Virchow, R. (1845). Weisses blut. In L. Froriep, R. Froriep eds. Notizen aus dem gebiete der nature und heilkunde, [White blood. In Froriep's notes from the field of science and medicine], 36:51-156. Berlin.

[89] Virchow, R. (1847). Zur pathologischen Physiologie des Blutes. II. Weisses Blut.Archives of Pathology,   Anatomy and Physiology, I:563-572.

[90] Fuller, H., Cantab, M., Cantab, L. (1846). Particulars of a case in which enormous enlargement of the spleen and liver, together with dilation of all the blood vessels of the body were found co-incident with a peculiarly altered condition of the blood. Paper presented at the Royal Medical and Chirurgical Society, Tuesday June 23, 1846. Abstract published in Lancet, 2:43-44.

[91] Fuller, H. (1850). Encephaloid tumour of the abdomen. Transactions of the Pathology Society of London, 4:224-225.

[92] Virchow, R. (1854a). Zur Geschichte der Leukamie [On the history of leukemia]. Virchow's Archives, 7:174-176.

[93] Virchow, R. (1854b). Professor Bennett uber leukamie [Professor Bennett on leukemia]. Virchow's Archives, 7:565-570.

[94] Bennett, J. (1854).Professors Kölliker and Bennett on the discovery of leucocythemia. Monthly Journal of Medical Science, 19:377-381.

[95] Kolliker, A. (1854). Professors Kölliker and Bennett on the discovery of leucocythemia. Monthly Journal of Medical Science, 2:374–377.

[96] Bizzozero, G. (1868). Sulla funzione ematopoetica del midollo delle ossa. Centralblatt Medizinische Wissenschaften, 6:885.

[97] Bizzozero, G. (1869). Sulla funzione ematopoetica del midollo delle ossa, seconda communicazione preventia. Centralblatt Medizinische Wissenschaften, 10:149-150.

[98] Neumann, E. (1869). Ueber die bedeutung des knockenmarkes fur die blutbildung. Ein beitrag zur entwicklungsgeschichte der blutkorperchen. Archives Heilkunde, 10:68-102.

[99] Neumann, E. (1870). Ein fall von leukamie mit erkrankung des knochenmarks. Archives Heilkunde II:1.

[100] Neumann, E. (1872). Ein neuer fall von leukamie mit erkrankung des knochenmarks. Archives Heilkunde, 13:502-508.

[101] Muller, J. (1835). Uber die organischen nerven der erectilen männlichen geschlechtsorgane des menschen und der saugethiere. Gelesen in der konigl Akademie der Wissenschaften zu Berlin.

[102] Muller, J. (1838). Ueber den feineren bau der krankhaften gschwülste [On the structural details of malignant tumors]. Coblenz, Germany.

[103] Muller, J. (1833). Handbuch der physiologie des menschen. [Handbook of human phyisology]. English translation by William Baly. London.

[104] Schwann T. (1838). Ueber die analogie in der structur und dem wachsthum der thiere und pflanzen. Neue Not Geb Nat Heil; Jan:33–36; Feb:25–29; Apr:21–23.

[105] Vogel J. (1841/1847). The Pathological Anatomy of the Human Body. Translated from German into English by George E. Day. Philadelphia: Lea and Blanchard.

[106] Du Bois-Reymond, E. (1848). Untersuchungen über thierische Elektricitat, Erster Band. [Studies on animal electricity. First Volume]. Berlin: Georg Reimer.

[107] Henle, F. (1840). Pathologische Untersuchungen. Berlin.

[108] Henle, F. (1846). Handbuch der rationellen pathologie. [Handbook of rational pathology]. 2 volumes in 3 parts; Braunschweig.

[109] Henle, F. (1862). Zur anatomie der niere. [On the aantomy of the kidney]. Abhandlungen der Gesellschaft der Wissenschaften zu Göttingen, 10:223-254.

[110] Helmholtz, H. (1851). Beschreibung eines Augen-Spiegels. [Description of an eye mirror]. Berlin: A Förstner'sche Verlagsbuchhandlung.

[111] Schwann, T. (1839/1847). Microscopic investigations on the accordance in the structure and growth of plants and animals. English translation by the Sydenham Society, 1847. See page 142-150. Retrieved from http://vlp.mpiwg-berlin.mpg.de/library/data/lit28715/index_html?pn=7

[112] Schwann, T. (1839). Mikroskopische untersuchungen über die uebereinstimmung in der strucktur und dem wachsthum der thiere und pflanzen. Berlin: Sander.

[113] Schwann, T. (1836). Ueber das Wesen des Verdauungsprocesses. Annals der Physik und Chemie, [About the essences of the digestive process], 38(2):358-364.

[114] Vogel, J. (1843). Icones histologiae pathologicae, Leipzig: Voss.

[115] Vogel, J. (1845). Die pathologische anatomie des menschlichen korpers. Leipzig: Berlag von Leopold-Voss.

[116] Vogel, J. (1847). The pathological anatomy of the human body. Translated from German by G. E. Day and L. M. Cantab. London: H. Bailliere. Retrieved from http://archive.org/stream/pathologicalanat00voge#page/n5/mode/2up

[117] Lebert H. (1845). Physiologie Pathologique ou Recherches Cliniques, Expérimentales et Microscopique. Paris: Bailliere.

[118] Lebert, H. (1851). Traite pratique des maladies cancéreuses et des affections curables aver le cancer. Paris: Bailliére.

[119] Lebert, H. (1857). Traite d'anatomie pathologique generale et speciale. Paris: Bailliere.

[120] Rokitawsky, K. (1842,1844,1846). Handbuch der Pathologischen Anatomie. 3 volumes. volume 1, 1843; volume 2, 1844; volume 3, 1846. Wien: Braumüller u. Seidel. Revised and illustrated edition: volume 1, 1855; volume 2, 1856; volume 3, 1861. English translation in 4 volumes, London, 1849-1854.

[121] Rokitansky, K. (1852). Ueber einige der wichtigsten krankheiten der arterien, Wien: Kaiserlich-Konigliche Hof- und Staatsdruckerei.

[122] Scherer, J. (1843). Chemische und mikroskopische untersuchungen zur pathologie angestellt an den kliniken des Julius-Hospitales zu Würzburg [Chemical and microscopic studies of pathologies employed at the clinics of the Julius Hospital in Wurzburg (Germany)]. Heidelberg: C. F. Winter.

[123] Scherer, J. (1851). Eine untersuchung des blutes bei leukämie. [Examinaiton of blood in leukemia] Verhandlungen der Physikalisch-Medicinischen Gesellschaft im Würzburg, 2:321-325.

[124] Bichat, X. (1800). Traite des membranes en general et de diverses membanes en particulier. Paris: Ricahrd, Caille et Ravier.

[125] Virchow, R. and Reinhardt, B. (1847). Archiv für pathologische anatomie und physiologie und für klinische medizin [Archives for pathological anatomy, physiology, and clinical medicine]. 1:1. Berlin: Druck und Verlag von G. Reimer.

[126] Remak, R. (1852). Ueber extracelluläre entstehung thierischer zellen und über die vermehrung derselben durch theilung. [About extracellular origin and animal cells on the same multiplication by division.]. [Müller's] Archiv. für Anatomie, Physiologie und Wissenschaftliche Medicin, Berlin, 47-57.

[127] Remak, R. (1850-55). Untersuchungen über die Entwickelung der Wirbelthiere. [Studies on the evolution of vertebrates]. 3 parts; Berlin: G. Reimer.

[128] Jones, H. B. (1840). On the presence of sulphur in cystic oxide, and an account of cystic oxide calculus. Med. Chir. Soc. Trans., 23:192-198.

[129] Korngold, L. and Lipari R. (1955). Multiple myeloma proteins II. The antigenic relationship of Bence-Jones proteins to normal gamma-globulin and cancer multiple myeloma serum proteins. Cancer, 9:262-272.

[130] Macintyre W. (1850). Cases of mollities and fragilitas ossium, accompanied with urine strongly charged with animal matter. Medical and Chirurgical Transactions of Londo., 33:211-232.

[131] Jones, H. (1847). Chemical pathology. Lancet, 2:88–92.

[132] Jones, H. (1848). On a new substance occurring in the urine of a patient with mollities ossium. Paper presented to the Royal Society of London April 22, 1847. London.

[133] Dalrymple, J. (1846). On the microscopical character of mollities ossium. Dublin Quarterly Journal of Medical Science, 2:85-95.

[134] Waller, A. (1846) Microscopical observation on the perforation of capillaries by the corpuscles of the blood and on the origin of mucus and pus globules. Philosophical Magazine (3rd Series), 29:397–405.

[135] Waller, A. (1850). Experiments on the section of the glossopharyngeal and hypoglossal nerves of the frog, and observations of the alterations produced thereby in the structure of their primitive fibres. Philosophical Transactions of the Royal Society of London, 140:423-429.

[136] Addison, T. (1849). Anaemia-disease of the suprarenal capsules. Paper presented to the South London Medical Society. March 15, 1849. London.

[137] Combe, J. (1822). History of a case of anaemia. Paper presented to the Medico-Chrugical Socoiety of Edinburgh, May 1, 1822. Retrieved from http://books.google.com/books?id=avICAAAAYAAJ&pg=PR1&lpg=PR1&dq=Transaction+of+the+Medico-Chirurgical+Society+of+Edinburgh+1824&source=bl&ots=rUVQxgoq8B&sig=7Vshh1vz22Cj3h2Qjtge4Ryz4pE&hl=en&sa=X&ei=U4kvUZWvIZSs8ATDqoH4Bw&ved=0CDAQ6AEwAQ#v=onepage&q=combe&f=false

[138] Combe, J. (1824). History of a case of anaemia. Transaction of the Medico-Chirurgical Society of Edinburgh, 1:194–204.

[139] Biermer, A. (1872). Uber eine eigentümliche form von progressiver, perniciöser anaemie. Correspondenz-Blatt für Schweizer Aerzte, Basel, 2:15-17.

[140] Addison, T. (1849). Chronics suprarenal insufficiency, usually due to tuberculosis of suprarenal capsule. London Medical Gazette, 43:517-18.

[141] Addison, T. (1855). On the constitutional and local effects of disease of the suprarenal capsule. In Collection of the published writings of the late Thomas Addison MD. (1868). London: New Sydenham Society.

[142] Trousseau, A.(1861-1862). Clinique médicale de l'Hotel-Dieu de Paris. 2 volumes, LXXXVII, Maladie d'Addison, 533-542. Paris: J. B. Bailliere.

[143] Brighton Herald Newspaper (1860). 30th June 1860 AMS 6373/9 page 3 column 7. East Sussex County. Vol. 6, no. 2 (Aug. 1860). Mr. Philip Bye, Senior Archivist of East Sussex County Council.

[144] Wilks, S. (1859). Preface. Lectures on Pathological Anatomy Delivered at Guy's Hospital during the Summer Sessions 1857–1858. London: Longman, Brown, Green, Logmans, and Roberts. Retrieved from

http://books.google.com/books?id=0iF1eCRJotIC&pg=PR7&source=gbs_selected_pages&cad=3#v=onepage&q&f=false

[145] Wilks, S. and Moxon, W. (1875). Lectures on Pathological Anatomy. 2nd ed., Philadelphia: Lindsay and Blakiston.

[146] Wilks, S. (1891). Lectures on Pathology. Edited by Marice Paul and revised by Samuel Wilks. Philadelphia: Blakiston, Son, & Co.

[147] Wilks, S. (1859). Morbid appearances in the intestine of Miss Bankes. London Medical Gazette, 2:264-265.

[148] Wilks, S. and Moxon, W. (1875). Lectures on Pathological Anatomy. 2nd ed., p.408-409. Philadelphia: Lindsay and Blakiston. Retrieved from

http://books.google.com/books?id=0iF1eCRJotIC&pg=PR7&source=gbs_selected_pages&cad=3#v=onepage&q&f=false

[149] Crohn, B., Ginsburg, L., Oppenheimer, G. (1932). Regional ileitis: A pathological and clinical entity. Journal American Medical Association, 99:1323–9.

[150] Wilks, S. (1862). On disease of the supra-renal capsules or morbus addisonnii. Guy's Hospital Reports. Series 3, vol 8. London: John Churchill, New Burlington Street. Retrieved from http://www.wehner.org/addison/wilks/p0.htm

[151] Wilks, S. (1856). Cases of lardaceous disease and some allied affections with remarks. Guy's Hospital Reports, 2:103-32.

[152] Wilks, S. (1856). Case of a peculiar enlargement of the lymphatic glands frequently associated with disease of the spleen. Guy's Hospital Reports, 2 (3):114–132 and (1865), 11:56–67.

[153] Wilks, S. (1863). On the syphilitic affections of internal organs. Guy's Hospital Reports, 3rd series, 9:1.

[154] Wilks, S. (1868). Drunkard's or alcoholic paraplegia. Medical Times and Gazette, 2:467-472.

[155] Wilks, S. (1869). A case of osteoporosis or spongy hypertrophy of the bones. Transactions of the Pathological Society of London, 20:273-7

[156] Wilkes S. (1870). Capillary embolism or arterial pyaemia. Guy's Hospital Reports, 15:29-35.

[157] Wilks, S. (1877). On cerebritis, hysteria and bulbar paralysis, as illustrative of arrest of function of the cerebrospinal centres. Guy's Hospital Reports, 22:7-55.

[158] Paget, J. (1876). On a form of chronic inflammation of bones (osteitis deformans).Medico-Chirurgical Transactions, 60:37-63 and 5 plates. Paper read to the Society November 14th, 1876.

[159] Duchenne, G. (1862). Album de photographies pathologiques complémentaire du livre Intitule d'Électrisation localisee par le docteur. Paris: Bailliére et Fils.

[160] Duchenne (de Boulogne), G. (1861). De l'electrisation localisee et de son application a la physiologie, a la pathologie et a la therapeutique. (2nd ed.). Paris: Baillière.

[161] Duchenne (de Boulogne), G. (1865). Anatomie microscopique du système nerveux. Recherche à l'aide de la photo-autographie sur pierre et sur zinc. Paris: Renouard.

[162] Duchenne (de Boulogne), G. (1864). Photo-autographie ou autographie sur métal et sur pierre de figures photo-microscopiques du système nerveux. Paris: Parent.

[163] Duchenne (de Boulogne), G. (1869). Iconographie photographique. Structure intime du système nerveux de l'homme à l'état normal et à l'état pathologique. Structure intime du bulbe a l'état normal. Premier fascicule presente a la Societe de Medecine de la Seine, le 16 Octobre 1868 et a l'Academie de Medecine de Paris.

[164] Duchenne (de Boulogne), G. (1855). De l'electrisation localisée et de son application a la physiologie, a la pathologie et a la therapeutique. (2nd edition). Paris: Baillière. English translation and edition by G.V. Poore. (1883). Selections from the clinical works of Duchenne (de Boulogne). London: The New Sydenham Society, 4-5.

[165] Duchenne (de Boulogne), G. (1847). De l'art de limiter l'excitation électrique dans les organes sans piquer ni inciser la peau, nouvelle méthode d'électrisation appelées électrisation localisée. Paris: Academie des Sciences, 4.

[166] Duchenne, G. (1868). Recherches sur la paralysie musculaire pseudo-hypertrophique, ou paralysie myosclérosique. Arch. Gen. Med., 11: 5–25, 179–209, 305–321, 421–443, 552-588.

[167] Duchenne (de Boulogne), G. (1861). De l'electrisation localisee et de son application a la physiologie, a la pathologie et à la thérapeutique. (2nd ed.). Paris: Baillière.

[168] Duchenne (de Boulogne), G. (1868). De la paralysie musculaire pseudo-hypertrophique ou paralysie myosclérotique. Arch. Gen. Med., 11:5-25, 179-209, 305-321, 421-443, 552-588.

[169] Meryon, E. (1861). On granular or fatty degeneration of the voluntary muscles. Paper presented to the Royal Medical and Chirurgical Society, December.

[170] Meryon E. (1852). On granular or fatty degeneration of the voluntary muscles. Medico-Chirurgical Transactions, 35:73-85.

[171] Meryon E. (1864). Practical and pathological researches on the various forms of paralysis. London: John Churchill and Sons.

[172] Little, W. (1843,1853). On the nature and treatment of deformities of the human frame: Being a course of lectures delivered at the Royal Orthopaedic Hospital in 1843 with numerous notes and additions to the present time. London: Longman.

[173] Meryon, E. (1864). Practical and Pathological Researches on the Various Forms of Paralysis. London: John Churchhill and Sons.

[174] Down, J. (1866). Observations on an ethnic classification of idiots. Clinical Lecture Reports, London Hospital 3: 259–262. Retrieved from http://www.neonatology.org/classics/down.html

[175] Virchow, R. (1858). Die Cellularpathologie in ihrer Begründung auf physiologische und pathologische Gewebelehre. Berlin: A. Hirschwald.

[176] Virchow, R. (1860). Cellular pathology as based upon physiological and pathological histology. Twenty lectures delivered in the Pathological Institute of Berlin, February, March, and April, 1858. English translation by Frank Chance. (2nd ed). London: John Churchill. Retrieved from http://books.google.com/books?id=nmEGHJy9uswC&printsec=frontcover&dq=pathology&hl=en&sa=X&ei=PxiQU KbPHZOk8ATNp4DwAQ&ved=0CDcQ6AEwAA

[177] Cohnhiem, J. (1867). Ueber entzündung und eiterung [By inflammation and suppuration]. Archiv für Pathologische Anatomie und Physiologie und für Klinische Medizin, 40:1-79.

[178] Cohnhiem, J. (1865). Ueber die endigung der muskelnerven, Virchows Arch. Path. Anat. Physiol., 34:194-207.

[179] Cohnhiem, J. (1872). Untersuchungen über die Embolischen Processe. Berlin: Hirschwald.

[180] Cohnheim, J. (1877). Thrombose und embolie.Vorlesungen Uber Allgemeine Pathologie. Berlin: Hirschwald.

[181] Bizzozero, G. (1868). Sulla funzione ematopoetica del midollo delle ossa. Centralblatt Medizinische Wissenschaften, 6:885.

[182] Neumann, E. (1869). Ueber die bedeutung des knockenmarkes fur die blutbildung. Ein beitrag zur entwicklungsgeschichte der blutkorperchen. Archives Heilkunde, 10:68-102.

[183] Neumann, E. (1870). Ein fall von leukamie mit erkrankung des knochenmarks.Archives Heilkunde, II, 1.

[184] Neumann, E. (1872). Ein neuer fall vonleukamie mit erkrankung des knochenmarks. Archives Heilkunde, 13:502-508.

[185] Bizzozero, G. (1868). Sulla funzione ematopetica del midollo delle ossa. Gazetta Medicia Italiana-Lombardia, 46:885.

[186] Bizzozero, G. (1869). Sulla funzione ematopoetica del midollo delle ossa, seconda communicazione preventia. centralblatt medizi-nische wissenschaften, 10:149-150.

[187] Hayem, G. (1889). Du sang et de ses alterations anatomiques. Paris: G. Masson.

[188] Schultze, M. (1865) Ein heizbarer objecttisch und seine verwendung bei untersuchungen des blutes. Archiv für Mikroscopische Anatomie, 1:1-42.

[189] Bizzozero, J. (1882a). Ueber einen neuen forrnbestandteil des blutes und dessen rolle bei der thrombose und blutgerinnung. Archiv für Pathologische Anatomie und Physiologie und für Klinische Medicin, 90:261-332.

[190] Bizzozero, G. (1881). Su di un nuovo elemento morfologico del sangue dei mammiferi e sulla sua importanza nella trombosi e nella coagulazione. Osservatore Gazetta delle Cliniche, 17:785-787.

[191] Bizzozero, G. (1882b). Sur les petites plaques du sang des mammiferes, deuxième note. Archives Italiennes de Biologie, 1:1-4.

[192] Bizzozero, G. (1892). Giornale dell'Academia di Medicinia di Torino anno LV, Seduta del 18 Marzo; 40: 205.

[193] Bizzozero, G. (1893). Ueber die schlauchförmigen drusendes magendarmkanals und die beziehungen ihres epithels zu dem oberflächenepithel der schleimhaut. Archiv Microskopische Anatomie, 42:82-152.

[194] Jaworski, W. (1899). Podrecznik chorob zołądka. [Handbook of gastric Diseases]. Wydawnictwa Dzieł Lekarskich Polskich [Polish Medical Publishing Works].

[195] Marshall, B. and Warren, J. (1984). Unidentified curved bacilli in the stomach of patients with gastritis and peptic ulceration. Lancet, 323 (8390):1311-5.

[196] The Nobel Prize in Physiology or Medicine 2005. Nobelprize.org. 5 Feb 2013.

[197] Von Recklinghausen, F. (1882). Uber die multiplen fibrome der haut und ihre beziehung zu den multiplen neuromen.Festschrift für Rudolf Virchow. Berlin: A. Hirchwald.

[198] Von Recklinghausen, F. (1862). Die lymphgefässe und ihre beziehung zum bindegewebe. Berlin, A. Hirschwald.

[199] Recklinghausen, F. (1883). Thrombose. In handbuch der allgemeinen pathologie des kreisalaufs und der ernahrung. p.117-141. Stuttgart: Ferdinand Enke.

[200] Reckinghausen, F. (1889). Demonstration von knochen mit tumor bildender ostitis deformans. [Demonstration of bone forming tumor with osteitis deformans]. Tageblatt der Naturforschenden, Versamlung, Heidelberg.

[201] Recklinghausen, F. (1889). Uber hämochromatose. Berliner klinische wochenschrift, 26:925. Tageblatt der versamlungen deutscher naturforscher und aerzte, Heidelberg, 62:324.

[202] Smith, R. (1849). A treatise on the pathology, diagnosis, and treatment of neuroma. Dublin: Hodges and Smith.

[203] Waldeyer, H. (1888). Uber karyokinese und ihre beziehungen zu den befruchtungsvorgängen. Archiv für Mikroskopische Anatomie und Entwicklungsmechanik, 32:1-122.

[204] Waldeyer, H. (1891). Ueber einige neuere forschungen im gebiete der anatomie des central nerven systems. [About some recent researches in the area of the anatomy of the central nervous system]. Deutsche Medicinische Wochenschrift, Berlin, 17:1213-1218, 1244-1246, 287-1289, 1331-1332, 1350-1356.

[205] Waldeyer, H. (1863). Untersuchungen uber den ursprung und den verlauf des achsenzylinders bei wirbellosen und wirbeltieren, sowie über dessen endverhalten in der quergestreiften muskelfaser.Zeitschrift für rationelle medicin, Leipzig and Heidelberg, 20:193-256.

[206] Weigert, K. (1875). Lehre von der coagulationsnecrose. Uber pockenähnliche gebilde in parenchymatösen organen und deren beziehung zu bakterienkolonien. Breslau.

[207] Weigert, K. (1880). Ueber die pathologische Gerinnungs-Vorgänge. Virchows Archiv für Pathologische Anatomie und Physiologie und für Klinische Medizin, 79:87-123.

[208] Weigert, K. (1871). Uber bacterien in der pockenhaut. Centralblatt für die medicinischen Wissenschaften, Berlin, 9:609-611.

[209] Weigert, K. (1882). Uber eine neue untersuchungsmethode des central nerven systems. Centralblatt für die Medicinischen Wissenschaften, Berlin, 20:753-757, 772-774.

[210] Ehrich, P. (1878). Beitrage zur theorie und praxis der histologischen farbung. [Contributions to the theory and practice of histological staining]. (Doctoral dissertation Leipzig University).

[211] Gram, H. (1884). Uber die isolierte farbung der schizomyceten in schnitt und trocken praparaten. Fortschritte der medizin, 2:185-189.

[212] Klebs, E. (1869). Die einschmelzmethode, ein beitrag zur mikroskopischen technik, Arch. Mikrosk. Anat., 5:164-166.

[213] Blum, F. (1893). Der formaldehyd als hartungsmittel. Z. Wiss. Mikrosc., 10:314.

[214] Blum, F. (1894). Notiz uber die anwendung des formaldehyds als hartungs und konservierungsmittel. Anat. Anz., 9:229.

[215] Blum, F. (1893). Der formaldehyd als antiseptic urn. Munch Med. Wochenschr., 8 Aug: 601.

[216] Greenfield, W. (1878). Specimens illustrative of the pathology of lymphadenoma and leucocythemia. Transactions of Pathological Society of London, 29:272-304.

[217] Sternberg, C. (1898). Uber eine eigenartige, unter dem bilde der pseudoleukämie verlaufende tuberkulose des lymphatischen apparates. Zeitschrift für Heilkunde, Prague, 19:21-90.

[218] Reed, D. (1902). On the pathological changes in Hodgkin's disease, with special reference to its relation to tuberculosis. Johns Hopkins Hospital Reports, Baltimore, 10:133-196.

[219] Rather, L. (1972). Who discovered the pathognomonic giant cell of Hodgkin's disease? Bulletin of the New York Academy of Medicine, 48(7):943-950.

[220] Fallot, A. (1888). Contribution a l'anatomie pathologique de la maladie bleue (cyanose cardiaque). Marseille Médical, 25:77-93, 138-158, 207-223, 341-354, 370-386, 403-420.

[221] Stensen, N. (1671). Embryo monsto affinis Parisiis dissectur. Acta Medica & Philosophica Hafniensia, 1: 202-203.

[222] Stensen, N. (1662). Observationes anatomicae, quibus varia oris, oculorum & narium vas describuntur novique salivae, lacrymarum & muci fontes deteguntur. Lugduni Batavorum (Leiden): J. Chouet.

[223] Fallot, A. (1876). Essai sur le pneumothorax. These presentee et publiquement soutenue a la Faculte de medicine de Montpellier. February 19, 1876. Montpellier: Typographie et lithographie Boehm et Fils, Imprimeurs de l'Academie des Sciences et Letters. Retrieved from http://www2.biusante.parisdescartes.fr/livanc/?p=5&cote=TMON1876x012&do=page

[224] Abbott, M. and Dawson, W. (1924). The clinical classification of congenital cardiac disease. International Clinics Series, 4(34):155.

[225] Aschoff, K. (1904). Zur Myocarditisfrage. Verhandlungen der deutschen pathologischen gesellschaft, Stuttgart, 8:46-53.

[226] Aschoff, K. (1922). Das retikulo-endotheliale system und seine beziehungen zur gallenfarbstoffbildung. [The reticulo-endothelial system and its relations with the bile pigment formation]. Münchener medizinische wochenschrift [Munich Medical Weekly], 69:1352-1356.

[227] Aschoff, K. (1924). Das reticulo-endotheliale System. Ergebnisse der Inneren Medizin, Berlin, 26:1-118.

[228] Metchnikoff, E. (1892). Lecons sur la pathologie compare de l'inflammation. Paris: G. Masson.

[229] Metchnikoff, E. (1901). L'Immunité dans les maladies infectieuses [Immunity in infectious diseases]. Paris: Masson.

[230] Metchnikoff. E. (1905). Immunity in infective diseases. Translated from the French by Francis G. Binnie. Cambridge: University Press. Retrieved from http://archive.org/stream/immunityininfec01metcgoog#page/n6/mode/2up

[231] Metchnikoff, O. (1921). Life of Ilya Mechnikov 1845-1916 by Olga Metchnikoff with a preface by Sir Ray Lankester. Boston and New York: Houghton Mifflin Company. Retrieved from http://archive.org/stream/lifeofeliemetchn00metciala#page/n7/mode/2up

[232] Metchnikoff, E. (1908). The Nobel Prize in Physiology or Medicine 1908. Nobelprize.org. 17 May 2013. Retrieved from http://www.nobelprize.org/nobel_prizes/medicine/laureates/1908/

[233] Whipple, G. (1907). A hitherto undescribed disease characterized anatomically by deposits of fat and fatty acids in the intestinal and mesenteric lymphatic tissues. Bulletin of the Johns Hopkins Hospital, Baltimore, 18:382-391.

[234] Yardley, J. and Hendrix, T. (1961). Combined electron and light microscopy in Whipple's disease: demonstration of "bacillary bodies" in the intestine. Bulletin of the Johns Hopkins Hospital, 109:80-98.

[235] Chears, W. and Ashworth, C. (1961). Electron microscopic study of the intestinal mucosa in Whipple's disease: demonstration of encapsulated bacilliform bodies in the lesion. Gastroenterology, 41:129-38.

[236] Relman, D., Schmidt, T., MacDernmott, R., Falkow, S. (1992). Identification of the uncultured bacillus of Whipple's disease. The New England Journal of Medicine, 327:293-301.

[237] Whipple, G., Hooper, C., Robscheit, F. (1920). Blood regeneration following simple anemia: I. Mixed diet Reaction. American Journal of Physiology, 53:151-166.

[238] Robscheit-Robbins, F. and Whipple, G. (1925). Blood regeneration in severe anemia. II. Favorable influence of liver, heart and skeletal muscle in diet. American Journal of Physiology, May 1, 72(3):408-418.

[239] The Nobel Prize in Physiology or Medicine 1934. Nobelprize.org. 22 May 2013. Retrieved from http://www.nobelprize.org/nobel_prizes/medicine/laureates/1934/

[240] Anitschkov, N. and Chalatov, S. (1884-1985). Uber experimentelle cholesterinsteatose und ihre bedeutung für die entstehung einiger pathologischer prozesse. [On experimental cholesterinsteatose and its importance for the development of some pathological processes]. Zentralblatt für Allgemeine Pathologie und Pathologische Anatomie, Jena, 24:1-9.

[241] Marchand, F. (1904). Ueber atherosclerosis. Verhandlungen der Kongresse fuer Innere Medizin, 21:23-59.

[242] Ignatowski, A. (1909). Ueber die wirkung der tierschen einweisse auf der aorta. Virchow's Archives of Pathological Anatomy, 198:248.

[243] Windaus A. (1910). Ueber der gehalt normaler und atheromatoser aorten an cholesterol und cholesterinester. Zeitschrift Physiol Chemie, 67:174.

[244] Anitschkow, N. and Chalatow, S. (1913). On experimental cholesterol steatosis and its significance in the origin of some pathological processes.Translated by Mary Z. Pelias. In classics in arteriosclerosis research. Arteriosclerosis, 1983, 3:178–82.

[245] Anitschkow, N. (1913). Ueber die Veranderungen der Kaninchenaorta bei experimenteller Cholesterinsteatose.Beitr. Pathol. Anat., 56:379–404.

[246] Ignatowski, A. (1909). Uber die wirkung des tierischen eiweisses auf die aorta und die paerenchymatosen organe der kaninchen. Virchows Archives of Pathological Anatomy, 198:248–270.

[247] Goodpasture, E. (1919). The significance of certain pulmonary lesions in relation to the etiology of influenza. American Journal of Medical Sciences, 158(6):863–870.

[248] Woodruff. A. and Goodpasture, E. (1931). Susceptibility of chorioallantoic membrane of chick embryos to infection with fowl-pox virus. American Journal of Pathology, 4:209-222.

[249] Teague, O. and Goodpasture, E. (1923). Experimental Herpes Zoster. The Journal of Medical Research, Dec., 44(2):185-200.7.

[250] Goodpasture, E. and Teague, O. (1923). Transmission of the virus herpes febrilis along nerves in experimentally infected rabbits. The Journal of Medical Research, Dec., 44(2):139-184.7.

[251] Goodpasture, E. (1925). A study of rabies with reference to neuronal transmission of the virus in rabbits and the structure and significance of Negri bodies. American Journal of Pathology, 1:547-584.

[252] Goodpasture, E. (1925). The pathways of infection of the central nervous system in herpetic encephalitis of rabbits contracted by contact with a comparative comment on medullary lesions in a case of human poliomyelitis. American Journal of Pathology, 1(1):29-46.

[253] Johnson, C. and Goodpasture, E. (1935). An investigation of the etiology of mumps. The Journal of Experimental Medicine, 59(1):1-19.

[254] Beebe, S. and Ewing, J. (1906). A study of the so-called infectious lymphosarcoma of dogs. The Journal of Medical Research, 15(2):209-228-5.

[255] Ewing, J. (1912). The treatment of cancer on biological principles. New York Medical Journal, 96:773.

[256] Ewing, J. (1921). Diffuse endothelioma of bone. Proceedings of the New York Pathological Society, 17-24.

[257] American Association of Cancer Research (2013). AACR: A brief history. Website retrieved 5-24-2013, http://www.aacr.org/home/about-us/centennial/aacr-history.aspx

[258] American Cancer Society. Our History: The early years. Website retrieved 5-22-2013 from http://www.cancer.org/aboutus/whoweare/our-history

[259] American Association of Cancer Research (2013). AACR: A brief history. Retrieved from http://www.aacr.org/home/about-us/centennial/aacr-history.aspx

[260] Ewing, J. (1917). Radium therapy in cancer. Journal American Medical Association, 68:1238-1247.

[261] Ewing, J. (1934). Early experiences in radiation therapy. Jameway Memorial Lectures, Paper presented to the American Radium Society, American Congress of Radiology, Chicago, Il, Sept 25-30, American Journal Roentgenology, 31:153.

[262] Memorial Sloan-Kettering Cancer Center. History and Overview. Retrieved from www.mskcc.org.

[263] Coons, A., Creech, H., Jones, R. (1941). Immunological properties of an antibody containing a fluorescent group. Proceeding Society of Experimental Biological Medicine, 47:200-202.

[264] Coons, A., Creech, H., Jones, R., Berliner, E. (1942). The demonstration of pneumococcal antigen in tissues by the use of fluorescent antibody. Journal of Immunology, 45:159-170.

[265] Royal College of Physicians of Edinburgh (2013). History. Historical Exam Papers. Specialty Examinations for Membership, Pathology, July 10th and 11th 1900. Retrieved from http://www.rcpe.ac.uk/library/exhibitions/150-years-of-membership/history/historical-exams1900.php

[266] American Medical Association. The founding of the AMA. Retrieved from http://www.ama-assn.org/ama/pub/about-ama/our-history/the-founding-of-ama.page

[267] American Medical Association. (1901). Report of General Executive Committee. Section of Pathology and Physiology. Association News. House of Delegates Proceedings, Annual Session. June 15, 1901, p.1717. Retrieved from http://ama.nmtvault.com/jsp/viewer2.jsp?doc_id=House+of+Delegates+Proceedings%2Fama_arch%2FHOD00003%2F00000019&page_name=00211717&view_width=640.0&rotation=0&query1=&collection_filter=All&collection_name=House+of+Delegates+Proceedings&zoom_factor=current

[268] American Society for Clinical Pathology. About the ASCP. Retrieved from http://www.ascp.org/About-the-ASCP

[269] American Board of Medical Specialties. ABMS history. Retrieved from http://www.abms.org/About_ABMS/ABMS_History/

[270] American Board of Pathology. Organizational History. Retrieved from http://www.abpath.org/BookletofInformation.pdf

[271] American Board of Pathology. Booklet of information 2013. Mission and Purpose. Retrieved from http://www.abpath.org/bookletofinformation.pdf

[272] American Medical Association. (1943). House of Delegates Proceedings, Annual Session 1943. p.79. Retrieved from http://ama.nmtvault.com/jsp/viewer2.jsp?doc_id=House+of+Delegates+Proceedings%2Fama_arch%2FHOD00001%2F00000036&page_name=00970079&view_width=640.0&rotation=0&query1=&collection_filter=All&collection_name=House%2Bof%2BDelegates%2BProceedings&zoom_factor=current&showThumbNails=false

[273] Herrick. J. (1904). Peculiar elongation and sickle-shaped red blood corpuscles in a case of severe anemia. Archives of Internal Medicine. 6:517-521.

[274] Pauling, L., Itano, H., Singer, S., Wells, I. (1949). Sickle cell anemia, a molecular disease. Science, Nov. 25, 110 (2865):543-548. Retrieved from http://osulibrary.oregonstate.edu/specialcollections/coll/pauling/blood/papers/1949p.15-01-large.html

[275] Mason, V. (1922). Sickle cell anemia. Journal of the American Medical Association, 79:1318-1320.

[276] Gusella, J., Wexler, N., Conneally, P., Naylor, S., Anderson, M., et al. (1983). A polymorphic DNA marker genetically linked to Huntington's disease. Nature, 306:234-338.

[277] Lejeune, J., Gautier, M., Turpin, R. (1959). Les chromosomes humains en culture de tissus. Paper presented to the Academie des Sciences, Paris (January 26). Comptes Rendus Academie des Sciences, 248:602-603.

[278] Lejeune, M., Grutier, M., Turpin, R. (1959). Estude des chromosomes somatique de nerf enfants mongoliens. Paper presented to the Academie des Sciences, Paris, March 16. Comptes Rendus Academie des Science, (16 Mars), 248:1721-1722.

[279] Lejeune, J., Lafourcade, J., Berger, R, et al. (1963). Trois cas de deletion particle du bras court d'un chromosome 5. C.R. Acad. Sci [D] Paris, 257:3098-3102.

[280] Ford, C., Jones, K., Polani, P., de Almeida, J., Briggs, J. (1959). A sex-chromosome anomaly in a case of gonadal dysgensis (Turner's syndrome). The Lancet, 273(7075):711-713.

[281] Edwards, J., Harnden, D., Cameron, A., Crosse, V., Wolff, O. (1960). A new trisomic syndrome. The Lancet, 1:787-790.

[282] Patau, K., Smith, D., Therman, E., Inhorn, S., Wagner, H. (1960). Multiple congenital anomaly caused by an extra autosome. The Lancet, 1(7128):790-793.

[283] Nowell, P. and Hungerford, D. (1960). A minute chromosome in chronic granulocytic leukemia. Science, 132 November (3438):1497.

[284] Tjio, J. and Levan, A. (1956). The chromosome number of man. Hereditas, 42:1-6.

[285] Painter, T. (1923). Studies in mammalian spermatogenesis II: The spermatogenesis of man. Journal of Experimental Zoology, 37:291–336.

[286] Dulbecco, R. (1963). Transformation of cells in vitro by viruses. Science, 15 November, 142 (3594):932-936.

[287] Dulbecco, R. (1963). Transformation of cell in vitro by viruses. Correction to Dulbecco. Science, 142 (3594): 932-936; Science, 22 November, 142(3595):1048.

[288] The Nobel Prize in Physiology or Medicine 1975. Nobelprize.org. 31 May 2013. Retrieved from http://www.nobelprize.org/nobel_prizes/medicine/laureates/1975/.

[289] Baltimore, D. (1970). RNA-dependent DNA polymerase in virions of RNA tumour viruses. Nature, 226 (5252):1209-11.

[290] Temin, H., Mizutani, S. (1970). RNA-dependent polymerase in virions of Rous sarcoma virus. Nature, 226 (5252):1211-13.

[291] Stehelin, D., Varnus, H., Bishop, J., Vogt, P. (1976). DNA related to the transforming gene(s) of avian sarcoma viruses is present in normal avian DNA. Nature, 260:170-173.

[292] Oppermann, H., Levinson, A., Varmus, H., Levintow, L., Bishop, J. (1979). Uninfected vertebrate cells contain a protein that is closely related to the product of the avian sarcoma virus transforming gene (src). Proceedings of the National Academy of Sciences USA, 76(4):1804-1808.

[293] Lane, D. and Crawford, L. (1979). T antigen is bound to a host protein in SV40-transformed cells. Nature, 278:261-3.

[294] Linzer, D. and Levine, A. (1979). Characterization of a 54K dalton cellular SV40 tumor antigen present in SV40-transformed cells and uninfected embryonal carcinoma cells. Cell, 17:43–52.

[295] Nobelprize.org. Nobelprize.org. 3 Jun 2013. Retrieved from http://www.nobelprize.org/nobel_prizes/medicine/laureates/1989/press.html

[296] Barre-Sinoussi, F., Chermann, J., Rey, F., Nugeyre, M., Chamaret, S., Gruest, J., Dauget, C., Axler-Blin, C., Vezinet-Brun, F., Rouzioux, C., Rozenbaum, W., & Montagnier, L. (1983). Isolation of a T-lymphotropic retrovirus from a patient at risk for acquired immune deficiency syndrome (AIDS). Science, 220(4599):868-71.

[297] Kohler, G. and Milstein, C. (1975). Continuous cultures of fused cells secreting antibody of predefined specificity. Nature, 256 (5517):495-497.

[298] Nobel Prize Physiology or Medicine 1984 - Press Release. Nobelprize.org. 3 Jun 2013. Retrieved from http://www.nobelprize.org/nobel_prizes/medicine/laureates/1984/press.html

[299] Gusella. J., Wexler, N., Conneally, P., Naylor, S., Anderson, M., Tanzi, R., Watkins, P., Ottina, K., Wallace, M., Sakaquchi, A., et al. (1983). A polymorphic DNA marker genetically linked to Huntington's disease. Nature, 306 (5940):234-238.

[300] The Huntington's Disease Collaborative Research Group. (1993). A novel gene containing trinucleotide repeat that is expanded and unstable on Huntington's disease chromosomes. Cell, 72(6):971-983.

[301] Kerem, B., Rommens, J., Buchanan, J., Markiewicz, D., Cox, T., Chakravarti, A., Buchwald, M., Tsui, L. (1989). Identification of the cystic fibrosis gene: Genetic analysis. Science, 8 September, 245(4922):1073-1080.

[302] Rommens, J., Iannuzzi, M., Kerem, B., Drumm, M., Melmer, G., Dean, M., Rozmahel, R., Cole, J., Kennedy, D., Hidaka, N., et al. (1989). Identification of the cystic fibrosis gene: Chromosome walking and jumping. Science, September, 245(4922):1059-1065.

[303] Hall, J., Lee, M., Newman, B., Morrow, J., Anderson, L., Huey, B., King, M. (1990). Linkage of early onset familial breast cancer to chromosome 17q21. Science, December, 250(4988):1684-1689.

[304] Oberle, I., Rousscau, F., Heitz, D., Kretz, C., Devys, D., Hanauer, A., Boue, J., Bertheas, M., Mandel, J. (1991). Instability of a 550-base pair DNA segment and abnormal methylation in fragile X syndrome. Science, 252:1097–1102.

[305] Kremer, E., Pritchard, M., Lynch, M., Yu, S., Holman, K., Baker, E., Warren, S., Schlessinger, D., Sutherland, G., Richards, R. (1991). Mapping of DNA instability at the fragile X to a trinucleotide repeat sequence (CCG). Science, 252:1711-1714.

[306] Robbins, S. (1957). Textbook of pathology with clinical applications. Philadelphia: W.B. Saunders.

[307] Robbins, S. (1974). Pathological basis of disease. Philadelphia: W.B. Saunders.

[308] Kumar, V., Abbas, A., Fausto, N., Aster, J. (2010). Robbins and Cotran pathological basis of disease. Philadelphia: Saunders Elsevier.

[309] Davey, M. (2007). Kevorkian speaks after his release from prison. The New York Times, June 4, 2007.

[310] Venter, J., Adams, M., Myers, E., Li, P. Mural, R., Sutton, G. Smith, H. Yandell, M., Evans, C., et al. (2001). Science, Feb 16; 291 (5507):1303-1351.

[311] Mardis, E. (2006). Anticipating the $1,000 genome. Genome Biology, 7:112.

[312] Davies, K. (2010). The $1000 Genome: The revolution in DNA sequencing and the new era of personalized medicine. New York: Free Press.

[313] Haspel, R., Arnaout, R., Briere, L., Kantarci, S., Marchand, K., Tonellato, P., Connolly, J., Bouguski, M., Saffitz, J. (2010). A call to action: Training pathology residents in genomics and personalized medicine. American Journal of Clinical Pathology, 133:832-834.

Index

www.ingramcontent.com/pod-product-compliance
Lightning Source LLC
Chambersburg PA
CBHW051747200326
41597CB00025B/4475